Stoelting's Anesthesia and Co-Existing Disease

SIXTH EDITION

Stoelting's Anesthesia and Co-Existing Disease

ROBERTA L. HINES, MD

Nicholas M. Greene Professor and Chairman
Department of Anesthesiology
Yale University School of Medicine
Chief of Anesthesiology
Yale-New Haven Hospital
New Haven, Connecticut

KATHERINE E. MARSCHALL, MD

Department of Anesthesiology
Yale University School of Medicine
Attending Anesthesiologist
Yale-New Haven Hospital
New Haven, Connecticut

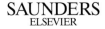

1600 John F. Kennedy Blvd.
Ste 1800
Philadelphia, PA 19103-2899

STOELTING'S ANESTHESIA AND CO-EXISTING DISEASE ISBN: 978-1-4557-0082-0
Copyright © 2012 by Saunders, an imprint of Elsevier Inc.

Notice

Knowledge and best practice in this field are constantly changing. As new research and experience broaden our understanding, changes in research methods, professional practices, or medical treatment may become necessary.

Practitioners and researchers must always rely on their own experience and knowledge in evaluating and using any information, methods, compounds, or experiments described herein. In using such information or methods, they should be mindful of their own safety and the safety of others, including parties for whom they have a professional responsibility.

With respect to any drug or pharmaceutical products identified, readers are advised to check the most current information provided (i) on procedures featured or (ii) by the manufacturer of each product to be administered to verify the recommended dose or formula, the method and duration of administration, and contraindications. It is the responsibility of practitioners, relying on their own experience and knowledge of their patients, to make diagnoses, to determine dosages and the best treatment for each individual patient, and to take all appropriate safety precautions.

To the fullest extent of the law, neither the Publisher nor the authors, contributors, or editors assume any liability for any injury and/or damage to persons or property as a matter of products liability, negligence or otherwise, or from any use or operation of any methods, products, instructions, or ideas contained in the material herein.

Previous editions copyrighted 2008, 2002, 1993, 1988, 1983.

Library of Congress Cataloging-in-Publication Data

Stoelting's anesthesia and co-existing disease. — 6th ed. / [edited by] Roberta L. Hines, Katherine E. Marschall.
   p. ; cm.
   Anesthesia and co-existing disease
   Includes bibliographical references and index.
   ISBN 978-1-4557-0082-0 (hardcover : alk. paper)
   I. Stoelting, Robert K. II. Hines, Roberta L. III. Marschall, Katherine E. IV. Title: Anesthesia and co-existing disease.
   [DNLM: 1. Anesthesia—adverse effects. 2. Anesthesia—methods. 3. Anesthetics—adverse effects. 4. Intraoperative Complications. WO 245]
   617.9'6041—dc23   2012005770

Executive Content Strategist: William Schmitt
Content Development Manager: Lucia Gunzel
Publishing Services Manager: Anne Altepeter
Senior Project Manager: Cheryl A. Abbott
Design Direction: Louis Forgione

Printed in China.

Last digit is the print number: 9   8   7   6   5   4   3   2   1

PREFACE

In 1983 the first edition of *Anesthesia and Co-Existing Disease* was published with the stated goal "to provide a concise description of the pathophysiology of disease states and their medical management that is relevant to the care of the patient in the perioperative period." The result was a very useful, basic reference text and review guide that continued through three more editions and became one of those exceptional works that is a "must have" in every anesthesiologist's personal library.

The fifth edition of *Anesthesia and Co-Existing Disease* marked a turning point in the history of the book. Drs. Robert K. Stoelting and Stephen F. Dierdorf passed the editorial "baton" to us, and we were very pleased with the response of the anesthesiology community to the publication of the fifth edition in 2008.

The continued explosion of new medical information has made another edition of this classic text necessary. In the sixth edition, all aspects of the pathophysiology and treatment of significant co-existing disease have been updated as needed. All major medical society guidelines and recommendations for the management of medical disorders that are important to the practicing anesthesiologist have been summarized. More figures and treatment algorithms have been included, and references have been made to the frontiers of medicine, that is, to those remarkable new medical and surgical treatments that will influence the practice of anesthesiology over the next several years.

We hope that our readers will continue to find this book to be "relevant to the care of the patient in the perioperative period."

Roberta L. Hines, MD
Katherine E. Marschall, MD

v

CONTRIBUTORS

Shamsuddin Akhtar, MD
Associate Professor of Anesthesiology
Director, Medical Student Education
Yale University School of Medicine
New Haven, Connecticut

Brooke E. Albright, MD
Captain, U. S. Air Force
Staff Anesthesiologist
Landstuhl Regional Medical Center
Landstuhl/Kirchberg, Germany

Sharif Al-Ruzzeh, MD, PhD
Resident in Anesthesiology
Yale-New Haven Hospital
New Haven, Connecticut

Ferne R. Braveman, MD
Professor of Anesthesiology
Vice-Chair of Clinical Affairs
Chief, Division of Obstetrics Anesthesia
Department of Anesthesiology
Yale University School of Medicine
New Haven, Connecticut

Michelle W. Diu, MD, FAAP
Assistant Professor of Anesthesiology
Yale University School of Medicine
New Haven, Connecticut

Samantha A. Franco, MD
Assistant Professor of Anesthesiology
Yale University School of Medicine
New Haven, Connecticut

Loreta Grecu, MD
Assistant Professor of Anesthesiology
Yale University School of Medicine
New Haven, Connecticut

Alá Sami Haddadin, MD, FCCP
Assistant Professor, Division of Cardiothoracic Anesthesia
    and Adult Critical Care Medicine
Medical Director, Cardiothoracic Intensive Care Unit
    Department of Anesthesiology
Yale University School of Medicine
New Haven, Connecticut

Laura L. Hammel, MD
Assistant Professor of Anesthesiology and Critical Care
University of Wisconsin Hospital and Clinics
Madison, Wisconsin

Michael Hannaman, MD
Assistant Professor, Department of Anesthesiology
University of Wisconsin School of Medicine
    and Public Health
Madison, Wisconsin

Antonio Hernandez Conte, MD, MBA
Assistant Professor of Anesthesiology
Co-Director, Perioperative Transesophageal
    Echocardiography
Cedars-Sinai Medical Center
Partner, General Anesthesia Specialists Partnership, Inc.
Los Angeles, California

Adriana Herrera, MD
Assistant Professor
Associate Program Director
Department of Anesthesiology
Yale University School of Medicine
New Haven, Connecticut

Zoltan G. Hevesi, MD, MBA
Professor of Anesthesiology and Surgery
University of Wisconsin
University of Wisconsin Hospital and Clinics
Madison, Wisconsin

Roberta L. Hines, MD
Nicholas M. Greene Professor and Chairman
Department of Anesthesiology
Yale University School of Medicine
Chief of Anesthesiology
Yale-New Haven Hospital
New Haven, Connecticut

Natalie F. Holt, MD, MPH
Assistant Professor, Department of Anesthesiology
Yale University School of Medicine
New Haven, Connecticut;
Attending Physician, West Haven Veterans Affairs
    Medical Center
West Haven, Connecticut

Viji Kurup, MD
Associate Professor, Department of Anesthesiology
Yale University School of Medicine
New Haven, Connecticut

William L. Lanier, Jr., MD
Professor of Anesthesiology
College of Medicine
Mayo Clinic
Rochester, Minnesota

Thomas J. Mancuso, MD, FAAP
Associate Professor of Anesthesia
Harvard Medical School
Senior Associate in Anesthesia
Director of Medical Education
Children's Hospital Boston
Boston, Massachusetts

Katherine E. Marschall, MD
Department of Anesthesiology
Yale University School of Medicine
Attending Anesthesiologist
Yale-New Haven Hospital
New Haven, Connecticut

Veronica A. Matei, MD
Assistant Professor of Anesthesiology
Yale University School of Medicine
New Haven, Connecticut

Raj K. Modak, MD
Assistant Professor of Cardiac and Thoracic Anesthesia
Director, Cardiac Anesthesia Fellowship Program
Department of Anesthesiology
Yale University School of Medicine
New Haven, Connecticut

Tori Myslajek, MD
Assistant Professor of Anesthesiology
Yale University School of Medicine
New Haven, Connecticut

Adriana Dana Oprea, MD
Assistant Professor of Anesthesiology
Yale University School of Medicine
New Haven, Connecticut

Jeffrey J. Pasternak, MD
Assistant Professor of Anesthesiology
College of Medicine
Mayo Clinic
Rochester, Minnesota

Wanda M. Popescu, MD
Associate Professor of Anesthesiology
Director, Thoracic Anesthesia Section
Yale University School of Medicine
New Haven, Connecticut

Ramachandran Ramani
Associate Professor of Anesthesiology
Yale University School of Medicine
New Haven, Connecticut

Robert B. Schonberger, MD, MA
Fellow, Sections of Cardiac and Thoracic Anesthesia
Department of Anesthesiology
Yale University School of Medicine
New Haven, Connecticut

Denis Snegovskikh, MD
Assistant Professor of Anesthesiology
Yale University School of Medicine
New Haven, Connecticut

Hossam Tantawy, MD
Assistant Professor of Anesthesiology
Yale University School of Medicine
New Haven, Connecticut

Russell T. Wall, III, MD
Vice-Chair and Program Director
Department of Anesthesiology
Georgetown University Hospital
Professor of Anesthesiology and Pharmacology
Senior Associate Dean
Georgetown University School of Medicine
Washington, DC

Kelley Teed Watson, MD
Clinical Assistant Professor
Yale University School of Medicine
New Haven, Connecticut;
Cardiothoracic Anesthesiologist
Department of Anesthesiology
Self Regional Healthcare
Greenwood, South Carolina

CONTENTS

Ischemic Heart Disease

SHAMSUDDIN AKHTAR ■

The prevalence of vascular disease and ischemic heart disease in the United States increases significantly with age (Figure 1-1). By some estimates 30% of patients who undergo surgery annually in the United States have ischemic heart disease. Angina pectoris, acute MI, and sudden death are often the first manifestations of ischemic heart disease, and cardiac dysrhythmias are probably the major cause of sudden death in these patients. The two most important risk factors for the development of atherosclerosis involving the coronary arteries are male gender and increasing age (Table 1-1). Additional risk factors include hypercholesterolemia, systemic hypertension, cigarette smoking, diabetes mellitus, obesity, a sedentary lifestyle, and a family history of premature development of ischemic heart disease. Psychologic factors such as type A personality and stress have also been implicated. Patients with ischemic heart disease can have chronic stable angina or acute coronary syndrome at presentation. The latter includes ST elevation myocardial infarction (STEMI) and unstable angina/non–ST elevation myocardial infarction (UA/NSTEMI).

STABLE MYOCARDIAL ISCHEMIA (ANGINA PECTORIS)

The coronary artery circulation normally supplies sufficient blood flow to meet the demands of the myocardium in response to widely varying workloads. An imbalance between coronary blood flow (supply) and myocardial oxygen consumption (demand) can precipitate ischemia, which frequently manifests as angina pectoris. Stable angina typically develops in the setting of partial occlusion or significant

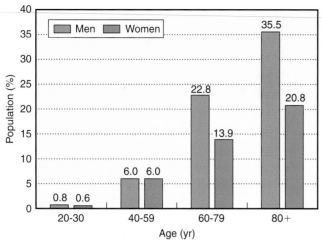

FIGURE 1-1 Prevalence of coronary heart disease by age and gender in the United States (2005 to 2008). *(Data from the National Center for Health Statistics and National Heart, Lung, and Blood Institute.)*

TABLE 1-1   Risk factors for development of ischemic heart disease

Male gender
Increasing age
Hypercholesterolemia
Hypertension
Cigarette smoking
Diabetes mellitus
Obesity
Sedentary lifestyle
Genetic factors/family history

TABLE 1-2   Common causes of acute chest pain

System	Condition
Cardiac	Angina
	Rest or unstable angina
	Acute myocardial infarction
	Pericarditis
Vascular	Aortic dissection
	Pulmonary embolism
	Pulmonary hypertension
Pulmonary	Pleuritis and/or pneumonia
	Tracheobronchitis
	Spontaneous pneumothorax
Gastrointestinal	Esophageal reflux
	Peptic ulcer
	Gallbladder disease
	Pancreatitis
Musculoskeletal	Costochondritis
	Cervical disc disease
	Trauma or strain
Infectious	Herpes zoster
Psychologic	Panic disorder

(>70%) chronic narrowing of a segment of coronary artery. When the imbalance becomes extreme, congestive heart failure, electrical instability with cardiac dysrhythmias, and MI may result. Angina pectoris reflects intracardiac release of adenosine, bradykinin, and other substances during ischemia. These substances stimulate cardiac nociceptive and mechanosensitive receptors, whose afferent neurons converge with the upper five thoracic sympathetic ganglia and somatic nerve fibers in the spinal cord, and ultimately produce thalamic and cortical stimulation that results in the typical chest pain of angina pectoris. These substances also slow atrioventricular nodal conduction and decrease cardiac contractility, which improves the balance between myocardial oxygen demand and supply. Atherosclerosis is the most common cause of impaired coronary blood flow resulting in angina pectoris.

Diagnosis

Angina pectoris is typically described as retrosternal chest discomfort, pain, pressure, or heaviness. The chest discomfort often radiates to the neck, left shoulder, left arm, or jaw and occasionally to the back or down both arms. Angina may also be perceived as epigastric discomfort resembling indigestion. Some patients describe angina as shortness of breath, mistaking a sense of chest constriction as dyspnea. The need to take a deep breath, rather than to breathe rapidly, often identifies shortness of breath as an anginal equivalent. Angina pectoris usually lasts several minutes and is crescendo-decrescendo in nature. A sharp pain that lasts only a few seconds or a dull ache that lasts for hours is rarely caused by myocardial ischemia. Physical exertion, emotional tension, and cold weather may induce angina. Rest and/or nitroglycerin relieve it. *Chronic stable angina* refers to chest pain or discomfort that does not change appreciably in frequency or severity over 2 months or longer. *Unstable angina,* by contrast, is defined as angina at rest, angina of new onset, or an increase in the severity or frequency of previously stable angina without an increase in levels of cardiac biomarkers. Sharp retrosternal pain exacerbated by deep breathing, coughing, or change in body position suggests pericarditis. There are many causes of noncardiac chest pain (Table 1-2). Noncardiac chest pain is often exacerbated by chest wall movement and is associated with tenderness over the involved area, which is often a costochondral junction. Esophageal spasm can produce severe substernal pressure that may be confused with angina pectoris and may also be relieved by administration of nitroglycerin.

ELECTROCARDIOGRAPHY

During myocardial ischemia, the *standard 12-lead electrocardiogram* (ECG) demonstrates ST-segment depression (characteristic of subendocardial ischemia) that coincides in time with anginal chest pain. This may be accompanied by transient symmetrical T-wave inversion. Patients with chronically inverted T waves resulting from previous MI may manifest a return of the T waves to the normal upright position (*pseudonormalization* of the T wave) during myocardial ischemia. These ECG changes are seen in 50% of patients. *Variant angina,* that is, angina that results from *coronary vasospasm* rather than *occlusive coronary artery disease,* is diagnosed by ST elevation during an episode of angina pectoris.

Exercise ECG is useful for detecting signs of myocardial ischemia and establishing their relationship to chest pain. The test also provides information about exercise capacity. The appearance of a new murmur of mitral regurgitation or a decrease in blood pressure during exercise adds to the diagnostic value of the test. Exercise testing is not always feasible, either because of the inability of a patient to exercise or the presence of conditions that interfere with interpretation of the exercise ECG (paced rhythm, left ventricular hypertrophy, digitalis administration, or preexcitation syndrome). Contraindications to exercise stress testing include severe aortic stenosis, severe hypertension, acute myocarditis, uncontrolled heart failure, and infective endocarditis.

The exercise ECG is most likely to indicate myocardial ischemia when there is at least 1 mm of horizontal or down-sloping ST-segment depression during or within 4 minutes after exercise. The greater the degree of ST-segment depression, the greater is the likelihood of significant coronary artery disease. When the ST-segment abnormality is associated with angina pectoris and occurs during the early stages of exercise and persists for several minutes after exercise, significant coronary artery disease is very likely. Exercise ECG is less accurate but more cost effective than imaging tests for detecting ischemic heart disease. A negative stress test result does not exclude the presence of coronary artery disease, but it makes the likelihood of three-vessel or left main coronary disease extremely low. Exercise ECG is less sensitive and specific in detecting ischemic heart disease than nuclear cardiology techniques (Table 1-3).

NUCLEAR CARDIOLOGY TECHNIQUES

Nuclear stress imaging is useful for assessing coronary perfusion. It has greater sensitivity than exercise testing for detection of ischemic heart disease. It can define vascular regions in which stress-induced coronary blood flow is limited and can estimate left ventricular systolic size and function. Tracers such as thallium and technetium can be detected over the myocardium by single-photon emission computed tomography (SPECT) techniques. A significant coronary obstructive lesion causes less blood flow and thus less tracer activity. Exercise perfusion imaging with simultaneous ECG testing is superior to exercise ECG alone (see Table 1-3). Exercise increases the difference in tracer activity between normal and underperfused regions, because coronary blood flow increases markedly with exercise except in those regions distal to a coronary artery obstruction. Imaging is carried out in two phases: the first is immediately after cessation of exercise to detect regional ischemia, and the second is 4 hours later to detect reversible ischemia. Areas of persistently absent uptake signify an old MI. The size of the perfusion abnormality is the most important indicator of the significance of the coronary artery disease detected.

TABLE 1-3 ■ Sensitivity and specificity of stress testing*		
Modality	**Sensitivity**	**Specificity**[†]
Exercise electrocardiography	0.68	0.77
Exercise SPECT	0.88	0.72
Adenosine SPECT	0.90	0.82
Exercise echocardiography	0.85	0.81
Dobutamine echocardiography	0.81	0.79

Data from Gibbons RJ, Abrams J, Chatterjee K, et al. ACC/AHA 2002 guideline update for the management of patients with chronic stable angina: a report of the American College of Cardiology/American Heart Association Task Force on Practice Guidelines. Circulation. 2003;107: 149–158. (Committee to Update the 1999 Guidelines for the Management of Patients with Chronic Stable Angina).
SPECT, Single-photon emission computed tomography.
*Without correction for referral bias.
[†]Weighted average pooled across individual trials.

Many patients who are at increased risk of coronary events cannot exercise because of peripheral vascular or musculoskeletal disease, deconditioning, dyspnea on exertion due to pulmonary disease, or prior stroke. Noninvasive imaging tests for the detection of ischemic heart disease are usually recommended when exercise ECG is not possible or interpretation of ST-segment changes would be difficult. Administration of atropine, infusion of dobutamine, or institution of artificial cardiac pacing produces a rapid heart rate to create cardiac stress. Alternatively, cardiac stress can be produced by administering a coronary vasodilator such as adenosine or dipyridamole. These drugs dilate normal coronary arteries but evoke minimal or no change in the diameter of atherosclerotic coronary arteries. After cardiac stress is induced by these interventions, radionuclide tracer scanning is performed to assess myocardial perfusion.

ECHOCARDIOGRAPHY

Echocardiographic wall motion analysis can be performed immediately after stressing the heart either pharmacologically or with exercise. New ventricular wall motion abnormalities induced by stress correspond to sites of myocardial ischemia, thereby localizing obstructive coronary lesions. In contrast, exercise ECG can indicate only the *presence* of ischemic heart disease and does not reliably predict the *location* of the obstructive coronary lesion. One can also visualize global wall motion under baseline conditions and under cardiac stress. Valvular function can be assessed as well. Limitations imposed by poor visualization have been improved by newer contrast-assisted technologies that have improved the accuracy of stress echocardiography.

STRESS CARDIAC MAGNETIC RESONANCE IMAGING

Pharmacologic stress imaging with cardiac magnetic resonance imaging compares favorably with other methods and is being used clinically in some centers, especially when other modalities cannot be used effectively.

ELECTRON BEAM COMPUTED TOMOGRAPHY

Calcium deposition occurs in atherosclerotic vessels. Coronary artery calcification can be detected by electron beam computed tomography. Although the sensitivity of electron beam computed tomography is high, it is not a very specific test and yields many false-positive results. Its routine use is not recommended.

CORONARY ANGIOGRAPHY

Coronary angiography provides the best information about the condition of the coronary arteries. It is indicated in patients with known or possible angina pectoris who have survived sudden cardiac death, those who continue to have angina pectoris despite maximal medical therapy, and those who are being considered for coronary revascularization, as well as for the definitive diagnosis of coronary disease for occupational reasons (e.g., in airline pilots). Coronary angiography is also useful for establishing the diagnosis of nonatherosclerotic coronary artery disease such as coronary artery spasm, Kawasaki's disease, radiation-induced vasculopathy, and primary coronary artery dissection. Among patients with chronic stable angina 25% will have significant single-, double-, or triple-vessel coronary artery disease, 5% to 10% will have left main coronary artery disease, and 15% will have no flow-limiting obstructions.

The important prognostic determinants in patients with coronary artery disease are the anatomic extent of the atherosclerotic disease, the state of left ventricular function (ejection fraction), and the stability of the coronary plaque. Left main coronary artery disease is the most dangerous anatomic lesion and is associated with an unfavorable prognosis when managed with medical therapy alone. Greater than 50% stenosis of the left main coronary artery is associated with a mortality rate of 15% per year.

Unfortunately, coronary angiography cannot predict which plaques are most likely to rupture and initiate acute coronary syndromes. *Vulnerable plaques,* that is, those most likely to rupture and form an occlusive thrombus, have a thin fibrous cap and a large lipid core containing a large number of macrophages. The presence of vulnerable plaque predicts a greater risk of MI regardless of the degree of coronary artery stenosis. Indeed, acute MI most often results from rupture of a plaque that had produced less than 50% stenosis of a coronary artery. Currently, there is no satisfactory test to measure the stability of plaques.

Treatment

Comprehensive management of ischemic heart disease has five aspects: (1) identification and treatment of diseases that can precipitate or worsen ischemia, (2) reduction of risk factors for coronary artery disease, (3) lifestyle modification, (4) pharmacologic management of angina, and (5) revascularization by coronary artery bypass grafting (CABG) or percutaneous coronary intervention (PCI) with or without placement of intracoronary stents. The goal of treatment of patients with chronic stale angina is to achieve complete or almost complete elimination of anginal chest pain and a return to normal activities with minimal side effects.

TREATMENT OF ASSOCIATED DISEASES

Conditions that increase oxygen demand or decrease oxygen delivery may contribute to an exacerbation of previously stable angina or worsen existing angina. These conditions include fever, infection, anemia, tachycardia, thyrotoxicosis, heart failure, and cocaine use. Treatment of these conditions is critical to the management of stable ischemic heart disease.

REDUCTION OF RISK FACTORS AND LIFESTYLE MODIFICATION

The progression of atherosclerosis may be slowed by cessation of smoking; maintenance of an ideal body weight by consumption of a low-fat, low-cholesterol diet; regular aerobic exercise; and treatment of hypertension. Lowering the low-density lipoprotein (LDL) cholesterol level by diet and/or drugs such as statins is associated with a substantial decrease in the risk of death due to cardiac events. Drug treatment is appropriate when the LDL cholesterol level exceeds 130 mg/dL. The goal of treatment is a decrease in LDL to less than 100 mg/dL. Patients with ischemic heart disease may benefit from even lower LDL levels (<70 mg/dL), which can be achieved by a combination of diet and statin therapy. Hypertension increases the risk of coronary events as a result of direct vascular injury, left ventricular hypertrophy, and increased myocardial oxygen demand. Lowering the blood pressure from hypertensive levels to normal levels decreases the risk of MI, congestive heart failure, and stroke. In combination with lifestyle modifications, β-blockers, and calcium channel blockers are especially useful in managing hypertension in patients with angina pectoris. If left ventricular dysfunction accompanies hypertension, an angiotensin-converting enzyme (ACE) inhibitor or an angiotensin receptor blocker (ARB) is recommended.

MEDICAL TREATMENT OF MYOCARDIAL ISCHEMIA

Antiplatelet drugs, nitrates, β-blockers, calcium channel blockers, and ACE inhibitors are used in the medical treatment of angina pectoris.

Three classes of *antiplatelet drugs* are widely used in the management of ischemic heart disease: aspirin, thienopyridines (clopidogrel and prasugrel), and platelet glycoprotein IIb/IIIa inhibitors (eptifibatide, tirofiban, and abciximab). A fourth class of antiplatelet drug, which affects platelet cyclic adenosine monophosphate (dipyridamole), is not widely used. A new class of short-acting, reversible platelet inhibitors (cangrelor and ticagrelor) is currently under development.

Aspirin inhibits the enzyme cyclooxygenase-1 (COX-1); this results in inhibition of thromboxane A_2, which plays an important role in platelet aggregation. This inhibition of COX-1 is irreversible, lasts for the duration of platelet life span (around 7 days), and can be produced by low dosages of aspirin. Low-dose aspirin therapy (75 to 325 mg/day) decreases the risk of cardiac events in patients with stable or unstable angina pectoris and is recommended for all patients with ischemic heart disease. Clopidogrel inhibits the adenosine diphosphate (ADP) receptor P2Y₁₂ and inhibits platelet aggregation in response to ADP release from activated platelets (Figure 1-2). Clopidogrel-induced inhibition of ADP receptors is irreversible and also lasts for the duration of the platelet's life span. Seven days after cessation of this drug 80% of platelets will have recovered normal aggregation function. Clopidogrel is a prodrug that is metabolized into an active compound in the liver. Due to genetic differences in the enzymes that metabolize clopidogrel to the active drug, significant variability in its activity has been observed. By some estimates, 10% to 20% of patients taking aspirin and clopidogrel demonstrate *hypo*responsiveness (resistance) or *hyper*responsiveness. Furthermore, some drugs, such as proton pump inhibitors, can affect the enzyme that metabolizes clopidogrel to its active compound and thereby can reduce the effectiveness of clopidogrel. Clopidogrel can be used in patients who have a contraindication to or are intolerant of aspirin. Prasugrel also inhibits the ADP P2Y₁₂ receptor irreversibly. However, the pharmacokinetics of prasugrel are more predictable. It is rapidly absorbed,

has a faster onset of action, and demonstrates less interindividual variability in platelet responses compared with clopidogrel. It also is more potent than clopidogrel, and a higher risk of bleeding has been associated with its use. Platelet glycoprotein IIb/IIIa receptor antagonists (abciximab, eptifibatide, tirofiban) inhibit platelet adhesion, activation, and aggregation. Short-term administration of antiplatelet drugs is particularly useful after placement of an intracoronary stent.

Organic *nitrates* decrease the frequency, duration, and severity of angina pectoris and increase the amount of exercise required to produce ST-segment depression. The antianginal effects of nitrates are greater when used in combination with β-blockers or calcium channel blockers. Nitrates dilate coronary arteries and collateral blood vessels and thereby improve coronary blood flow. Nitrates also decrease peripheral vascular resistance, which reduces left ventricular afterload and myocardial oxygen consumption. The venodilating effect of nitrates decreases venous return and hence left ventricular preload and myocardial oxygen consumption. They also have potential antithrombotic effects. Nitrates are contraindicated in the presence of hypertrophic cardiomyopathy or

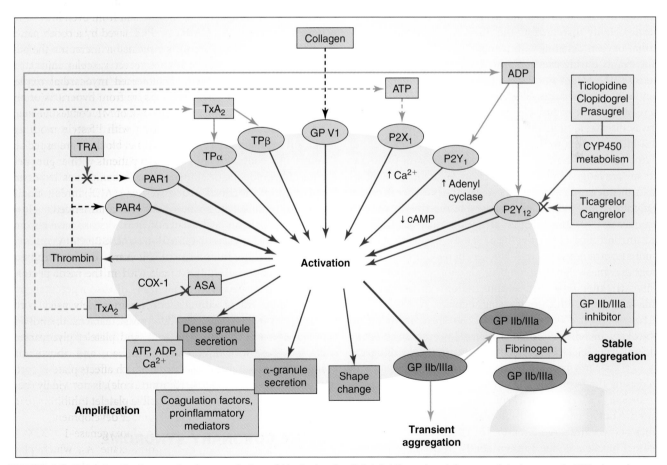

FIGURE 1-2 Platelet activation mechanisms and sites of blockade of antiplatelet therapies. ↑, Increased; ↓, decreased; *ADP,* adenosine diphosphate; *ASA,* acetylsalicylic acid; *ATP,* adenosine triphosphate; *cAMP,* cyclic adenosine monophosphate; *COX-1,* cyclooxygenase-1; *CYP450,* cytochrome P450; *GP,* glycoprotein; *GPVI,* [glycoprotein VI]; *P2X₁, P2Y₁,* purinergic receptors; *PAR,* protease-activated receptor; *TP,* thromboxane receptor; *TRA,* [thrombin recepter agonist]; *TxA₂,* thromboxane A₂. *(From Cannon CP, Braunwald E. Unstable angina and non-ST elevation myocardial infarction. In: Bonow RO, Mann DL, Zipes DP, et al, eds.* Braunwald's Heart Disease. *Philadelphia, PA: Saunders; 2012.)*

severe aortic stenosis and should not be used within 24 hours of sildenafil, tadalafil, or vardenafil because this combination may produce severe hypotension. Administration of sublingual nitroglycerin by tablet or spray produces prompt relief of angina pectoris. The most common side effect of nitrate treatment is headache. Hypotension may occur after nitrate administration in hypovolemic patients. For long-term therapy, long-acting nitrate preparations (isosorbide, nitroglycerin ointment or patches) are equally effective. The therapeutic value of organic nitrates is compromised by the development of tolerance. To avoid nitrate tolerance, a daily 8- to 12-hour interval free of nitrate exposure is recommended.

β-Blockers are the principal drug treatment for patients with stable angina pectoris. They have antiischemic, antihypertensive, and antidysrhythmic properties. Long-term administration of β-blockers decreases the risk of death and myocardial reinfarction in patients who have had an MI, presumably by decreasing myocardial oxygen demand. This benefit is present even in patients in whom β-blockers were traditionally thought to be contraindicated, such as those with congestive heart failure, pulmonary disease, or advanced age. Drug-induced blockade of β_1-adrenergic receptors (atenolol, metoprolol, acebutolol, bisoprolol) results in heart rate slowing and decreased myocardial contractility that are greater during activity than at rest. The result is a decrease in myocardial oxygen demand with a subsequent decrease in ischemic events during exertion. The decrease in heart rate also increases the length of diastole and thereby coronary perfusion time. β_2-Adrenergic blockers (propranolol, nadolol) can increase the risk of bronchospasm in patients with reactive airway disease. Despite differences between β_1 and β_2 effects, all β-blockers seem to be equally effective in the treatment of angina pectoris. The most common side effects of β-blocker therapy are fatigue and insomnia. Heart failure may be intensified. β-Blockers are contraindicated in the presence of severe bradycardia, sick sinus syndrome, severe reactive airway disease, second- or third-degree atrioventricular heart block, and uncontrolled congestive heart failure. Diabetes mellitus is not a contraindication to β-blocker therapy, although these drugs may mask signs of hypoglycemia. Abrupt withdrawal of β-blockers after prolonged administration can worsen ischemia in patients with chronic stable angina.

Long-acting calcium channel blockers are comparable to β-blockers in relieving anginal pain. However, *short-acting* calcium channel blockers such as verapamil and diltiazem are not. Calcium channel blockers are uniquely effective in decreasing the frequency and severity of angina pectoris due to coronary artery spasm (*Prinzmetal's* or *variant angina*). They are not as effective as β-blockers in decreasing the incidence of myocardial reinfarction. The effectiveness of calcium channel blockers is due to their ability to decrease vascular smooth muscle tone, dilate coronary arteries, decrease myocardial contractility and oxygen consumption, and decrease systemic blood pressure. Many calcium channel blockers such as amlodipine, nicardipine, isradipine, felodipine, and long-acting nifedipine are potent vasodilators and are useful in treating both hypertension and angina. Common side effects of calcium channel blocker therapy are hypotension, peripheral edema, and headache. Calcium channel blockers are contraindicated in patients with severe congestive heart failure or severe aortic stenosis. They must be used cautiously if given in combination with β-blockers, because both classes of drugs have significant depressant effects on heart rate and myocardial contractility.

Excessive angiotensin II plays a significant role in the pathophysiology of cardiac disorders. It can lead to development of myocardial hypertrophy, interstitial myocardial fibrosis, increased coronary vasoconstriction, and endothelial dysfunction. Angiotensin II also promotes inflammatory responses and atheroma formation. *ACE inhibitors* are important not only in the treatment of heart failure but also in the treatment of hypertension and in cardiovascular protection. ACE inhibitors are recommended for patients with coronary artery disease, especially those with hypertension, left ventricular dysfunction, or diabetes. Angiotensin receptor blockers offer similar benefits. Contraindications to ACE inhibitor use include documented intolerance or allergy, hyperkalemia, bilateral renal artery stenosis, and renal failure.

REVASCULARIZATION

Revascularization by CABG or PCI with or without placement of intracoronary stents is indicated when optimal medical therapy fails to control angina pectoris. Revascularization is also indicated for specific anatomic lesions—in particular, left main coronary artery stenosis of more than 50% or the presence of a 70% or greater stenosis in an epicardial coronary artery. Revascularization is also indicated in patients with significant coronary artery disease with evidence of impaired left ventricular contractility (ejection fraction of <40%). The presence of hypokinetic or akinetic areas in the left ventricle connotes a poor prognosis. Extensive myocardial fibrosis from a prior MI is unlikely to be improved by revascularization. However, some patients with ischemic heart disease have chronically impaired myocardial function (*hibernating myocardium*) that demonstrates improvement in contractility following surgical revascularization. In patients with stable angina pectoris and one- or two-vessel coronary artery disease, a percutaneous intervention with or without stent placement, or surgical coronary artery bypass may be used for revascularization. CABG is preferred over PCI in patients with significant left main artery disease, those with three-vessel coronary artery obstruction, and patients with diabetes who have two- or three-vessel coronary artery disease. Operative mortality rates for CABG surgery currently range from 1.5% to 2%.

ACUTE CORONARY SYNDROME

Acute coronary syndrome represents a hypercoagulable state. Focal disruption of an atheromatous plaque triggers the coagulation cascade with subsequent generation of thrombin and partial or complete occlusion of the coronary artery by a thrombus. Imbalance of myocardial oxygen supply and demand leads to ischemic chest pain. Patients who have isch-emic chest pain can be categorized based on the findings of a 12-lead ECG. Patients with ST elevation at presentation are considered to have STEMI. Patients who have ST-segment depression or nonspecific changes on the ECG can be catego-rized based on the levels of cardiac-specific troponins or myo-cardial creatine kinase (CK-MB). Elevation of cardiac-specific biomarker levels in this situation indicates NSTEMI. If levels of cardiac-specific biomarkers are normal, then unstable angina is present (Figure 1-3). STEMI and UA/NSTEMI are treated differently and have different prognoses. Many more patients have UA/NSTEMI than have STEMI at presentation. The dif-ferent kinds of MI often occur in different clinical situations.

ST Elevation Myocardial Infarction

Mortality rates from STEMI have declined steadily because of early therapeutic interventions such as angioplasty, throm-bolysis and aspirin, heparin, and statin therapy. However, the mortality rate of acute MI remains significant. The short-term mortality rate of patients with STEMI who receive aggressive reperfusion therapy is about 6.5%. Data from the general med-ical community show a mortality rate of 15% to 20% (these patients have not received reperfusion therapy). Advanced age consistently emerges as one of the principal determinants of early mortality in patients with STEMI. Coronary angiog-raphy has documented that nearly all STEMIs are caused by thrombotic occlusion of a coronary artery.

The long-term prognosis after an acute MI is determined principally by the severity of residual left ventricular dysfunc-tion, the presence and degree of residual ischemia, and the presence of malignant ventricular dysrhythmias. Most deaths that occur during the first year after hospital discharge take place within the first 3 months. Ventricular function can be substantially improved during the first few weeks after an acute MI, particularly in patients in whom early reperfusion was achieved. Therefore, measurement of ventricular function 2 to 3 months after an MI is a more accurate predictor of long-term prognosis than measurement of ventricular function during the acute phase of the infarction.

PATHOPHYSIOLOGY

Atherosclerosis is being increasingly recognized as an inflam-matory disease. The presence of inflammatory cells in athero-sclerotic plaques suggests that inflammation is important in the cascade of events leading to plaque rupture. Indeed, serum markers of inflammation, such as C-reactive protein and fibrinogen, are increased in those at greatest risk of developing coronary artery disease.

STEMI occurs when coronary blood flow decreases abruptly. This decrease in blood flow is attributable to acute thrombus formation at a site when an atherosclerotic plaque fissures, ruptures, or ulcerates. This creates a local environment that favors thrombogenesis. Typically, vulnerable plaques— that is, those with rich lipid cores and thin fibrous caps—are most prone to rupture. A platelet monolayer forms at the site

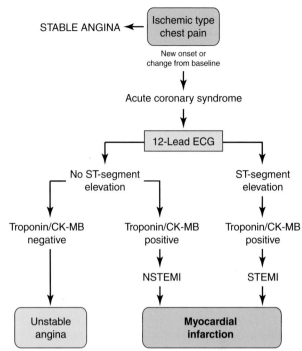

FIGURE 1-3 Terminology of acute coronary syndrome. *CK-MB, Creatine kinase, myocardial-bound isoenzyme; ECG, electrocardio-gram; NSTEMI, non–ST elevation myocardial infarction; STEMI, ST elevation myocardial infarction. (Adapted from Alpert JS, Thygesen K, Antman E, et al. Myocardial infarction redefined—a consensus document of the Joint European Society of Cardiology/American College of Cardiology Committee for the redefinition of myocardial infarction. J Am Coll Cardiol. 2000;36:959-969.)*

of ruptured plaque, and various chemical mediators such as collagen, ADP, epinephrine, and serotonin stimulate platelet aggregation. The potent vasoconstrictor thromboxane A_2 is released, which further compromises coronary blood flow. Glycoprotein IIb/IIIa receptors on the platelets are activated, which enhances the ability of platelets to interact with adhe-sive proteins and other platelets and causes growth and stabili-zation of the thrombus. Further activation of coagulation leads to strengthening of the clot by fibrin deposition. This makes the clot more resistant to thrombolysis. It is rather paradoxical that plaques that rupture and lead to acute coronary occlusion are rarely of a size that causes significant coronary obstruc-tion. By contrast, flow-restrictive plaques that produce angina pectoris and stimulate development of collateral circulation are less likely to rupture. Rarely, STEMI develops as a result of acute coronary spasm or coronary artery embolism.

DIAGNOSIS

With recent advances in the techniques for detecting MI, the criteria for diagnosing an acute, evolving, or recent MI have been revised (Table 1-4). Diagnosis of acute MI requires the typical rise and subsequent fall in plasma levels of biochemical markers of myocardial necrosis in combination with at least one of the following: (1) ischemic symptoms, (2) develop-ment of pathologic Q waves on the ECG, (3) ECG changes

TABLE 1-4 ■ Revised definition of myocardial infarction

CRITERIA FOR ACUTE, EVOLVING, OR RECENT MYOCARDIAL INFARCTION

Either of the following criteria satisfies the diagnosis for acute, evolving, or recent myocardial infarction:
1. Typical rise and/or fall of biochemical markers of myocardial necrosis with at least one of the following:
   a. Ischemic symptoms
   b. Development of pathologic Q waves on the electrocardiogram (ECG)
   c. ECG changes indicative of ischemia (ST-segment elevation or depression)
   d. Imaging evidence of new loss of viable myocardium or new regional wall motion abnormality
2. Pathologic findings of an acute myocardial infarction

CRITERIA FOR HEALING OR HEALED MYOCARDIAL INFARCTION

Either of the following criteria satisfies the diagnosis for healing or healed myocardial infarction:
1. Development of new pathologic Q waves on serial ECGs. The patient may or may not remember previous symptoms. Levels of biochemical markers of myocardial necrosis may have normalized, depending on the length of time that has passed since the infarction developed.
2. Pathologic findings of a healed or healing infarction.

Adapted from Thygesen K, Alpert JS, White HD, et al. Universal definition of myocardial infarction. *Circulation*. 2007;116:2634-2653.

TABLE 1-5 ■ Biomarkers for evaluation of patients with ST elevation myocardial infarction

Biomarker	Range of time to initial elevation	Mean time to peak elevation*	Time to return to normal
FREQUENTLY USED IN CLINICAL PRACTICE			
CK-MB[†]	3-12 hr	24 hr	48-72 hr
Troponin I[‡]	3-12 hr	24 hr	5-10 day
Troponin T	3-12 hr	12 hr–2 days	5-14 day
INFREQUENTLY USED IN CLINICAL PRACTICE			
Myoglobin	1-4 hr	6-7 hr	24 hr
CK-MB tissue isoform	2-6 hr	18 hr	Unknown
CK-MM tissue isoform	1-6 hr	12 hr	38 hr

Modified from Antman EM, Anbe DT, Armstrong PW, et al. ACC/AHA guidelines for the management of patients with ST-elevation myocardial infarction. A report of the American College of Cardiology/American Heart Association Task Force on Practice Guidelines (Committee to Revise the 1999 Guidelines for the Management of Patients with Acute Myocardial Infarction). *Circulation*. 2004;110:e82-e292.
*Nonreperfused patients.
[†]Increased sensitivity can be achieved by sampling every 6 or 8 hr.
[‡]Multiple assays available for clinical use; the clinician should be familiar with the cutoff value used in his or her institution.

indicative of ischemia (ST-segment elevation or depression), and (4) imaging evidence of a new loss of viable myocardium or new regional wall motion abnormality.

Almost two thirds of patients describe new-onset angina pectoris or a change in their anginal pattern during the 30 days preceding an acute MI. The pain is often more severe than the previous angina pectoris and does not resolve with rest. Other potential causes of severe chest pain (pulmonary embolism, aortic dissection, spontaneous pneumothorax, pericarditis, cholecystitis) should be considered (see Table 1-2). About a quarter of patients, especially the elderly and those with diabetes, have no or only mild pain at the time of MI.

On physical examination, patients typically appear anxious, pale, and diaphoretic. Sinus tachycardia is usually present. Hypotension caused by left or right ventricular dysfunction or cardiac dysrhythmias may be present. Rales signal congestive heart failure due to left ventricular dysfunction. A cardiac murmur may indicate ischemic mitral regurgitation.

Laboratory Studies

Troponin is a cardiac-specific protein and biochemical marker for acute MI. An increase in the circulating concentration of troponin occurs early after myocardial injury. Levels of cardiac troponins (troponin T or I) increase within 3 hours after myocardial injury and remain elevated for 7 to 10 days (Table 1-5). Elevated troponin levels and the ECG are powerful predictors of adverse cardiac events in patients with anginal pain. Troponin is more specific than CK-MB for determining myocardial injury. The currently accepted definition of MI

recommends assessing the magnitude of the infarction by measuring how much the cardiac biomarker level is elevated above the normal reference range (Figure 1-4).

Imaging Studies

Patients with typical ECG evidence of acute MI do not require evaluation with echocardiography. However, echocardiography is useful in patients with left bundle branch block or an abnormal ECG in whom the diagnosis of acute MI is uncertain and in patients with suspected aortic dissection. Echocardiography will demonstrate regional wall motion abnormalities in most patients with acute MI. The time required to perform myocardial perfusion imaging and the inability to differentiate between new and old MI limits the utility of radionuclide imaging in the early diagnosis of acute MI.

TREATMENT

Early treatment of acute MI reduces morbidity and mortality. Initial steps include evaluating hemodynamic stability, obtaining a 12-lead ECG, and administering oxygen to all patients suspected of having acute MI. Pain relief, usually provided by intravenous morphine and/or sublingual nitroglycerin, is necessary to reduce catecholamine release and the resultant increase in myocardial oxygen requirements. Aspirin (or clopidogrel for those intolerant of aspirin) is administered to decrease further thrombus formation. Prasugrel can be used as an alternative to clopidogrel. Platelet glycoprotein IIb/IIIa inhibitors can be used if urgent surgical intervention is likely. β-Blockers relieve ischemic chest pain, infarct size, and

FIGURE 1-4 Rate and extent of rise of cardiac troponin and myocardial creatine kinase (CK-MB) levels after a typical acute myocardial infarction (AMI). Cardiac microinfarctions can raise the troponin levels without increasing the CK-MB levels. *(From Antman EM. ST-segment myocardial infarction: pathology, pathophysiology, and clinical features. In: Bonow RO, Mann DL, Zipes DP, et al, eds. Braunwald's Heart Disease. Philadelphia, PA: Saunders; 2012:Figure 54-14.)*

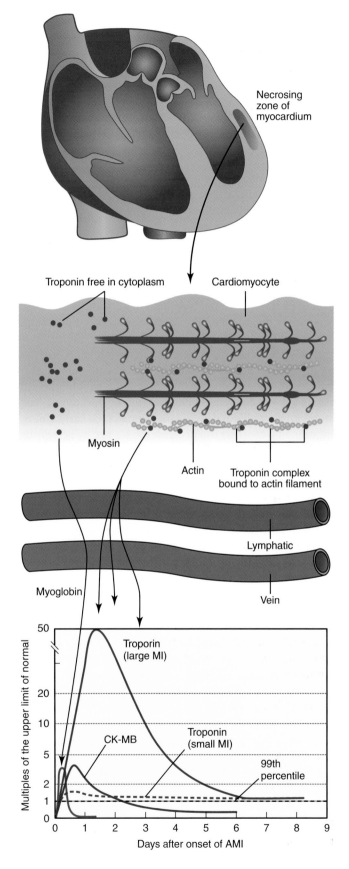

life-threatening dysrhythmias. β-Blockers are administered to patients in *hemodynamically stable condition* who are *not* in heart failure, in a low cardiac output state, or at risk of cardiogenic shock. β-Blockers are *not* given to those with heart block. The primary goal in management of STEMI is to reestablish blood flow in the obstructed coronary artery as soon as possible. This can be achieved by reperfusion therapy or coronary angioplasty with or without placement of an intracoronary stent. The time to reperfusion therapy strongly influences the outcome of an acute STEMI.

Reperfusion Therapy

Thrombolytic therapy with streptokinase, tissue plasminogen activator, reteplase, or tenecteplase should be initiated within 30 to 60 minutes of hospital arrival, and within 12 hours of symptom onset. Thrombolytic therapy restores normal antegrade blood flow in the occluded coronary artery. Dissolution of the clot by thrombolytic therapy becomes much more difficult if therapy is delayed. The most feared complication of thrombolytic therapy is intracranial hemorrhage. This is most likely in elderly patients (>75 years of age) and in those with uncontrolled hypertension. Patients who have gastrointestinal bleeding or have recently undergone surgery are also at increased risk of bleeding complications.

Percutaneous Coronary Intervention

PCI may be preferable to thrombolytic therapy for restoring flow to an occluded coronary artery if appropriate resources are available. Ideally, angioplasty should be performed within 90 minutes of arrival at the health care facility and within 12 hours of symptom onset. It is the modality of choice in patients with a contraindication to thrombolytic therapy and those with severe heart failure and/or pulmonary edema. About 5% of patients who undergo immediate PCI require emergency cardiac surgery because of failed angioplasty or because the coronary artery anatomy precludes an intervention. The combined use of intracoronary stents and antiplatelet drugs (aspirin, clopidogrel or prasugrel, and a platelet glycoprotein IIb/IIIa inhibitor) during emergency PCI provides the maximum chance of achieving normal antegrade coronary blood flow, and this therapy decreases the need for a subsequent revascularization procedure.

Coronary Artery Bypass Graft Surgery

CABG can restore blood flow in an occluded coronary artery, but reperfusion can be achieved faster with thrombolytic therapy or coronary angioplasty. Emergency CABG is usually reserved for patients in whom angiography reveals coronary anatomy that precludes PCI, patients with a failed angioplasty, and those with evidence of infarction-related ventricular septal rupture or mitral regurgitation. Patients with ST-segment elevation who develop cardiogenic shock, left bundle branch block, or a posterior wall MI within 36 hours of an acute STEMI are also candidates for early revascularization. Mortality from CABG is significant during the first 3 to 7 days after an acute MI.

Adjunctive Medical Therapy

Intravenous heparin therapy is commonly administered for 48 hours after thrombolytic therapy to decrease the risk of thrombus regeneration. A disadvantage of unfractionated heparin is the variability in the dose response due to its binding with plasma proteins other than antithrombin. Low-molecular-weight heparin provides a more predictable pharmacologic effect, a long plasma half-life, and a more practical means of administration (subcutaneous), without the need to monitor the activated partial thromboplastin time. Thus, low-molecular-weight heparin is an excellent alternative to unfractionated heparin. Direct thrombin inhibitors such as bivalirudin can be used in patients with a history of heparin-induced thrombocytopenia. Administration of β-blockers is associated with a significant decrease in early (in-hospital) and long-term mortality and myocardial reinfarction. Early administration of β-blockers can decrease infarct size by decreasing heart rate, blood pressure, and myocardial contractility. In the absence of specific contraindications, it is recommended that patients receive β-blockers as early as possible after an acute MI. β-Blocker therapy should be continued indefinitely.

All patients with a large anterior wall MI, clinical evidence of left ventricular failure, an ejection fraction of less than 40%, or diabetes should be treated with ACE inhibitors, or an angiotensin II receptor blocker if they are intolerant of ACE inhibitors.

In the absence of ventricular dysrhythmias, prophylactic administration of lidocaine or other antidysrhythmic drugs is not recommended. Calcium channel blockers should not be administered routinely but should be reserved for patients with persistent myocardial ischemia despite optimal use of aspirin, β-blockers, nitrates, and heparin. Glycemic control is part of the standard care of diabetic patients with an acute MI. Routine administration of magnesium is not recommended, but magnesium therapy is indicated in patients with torsade de pointes ventricular tachycardia. Statins have strong immune-modulating effects and should be started as soon as possible after MI, especially in patients receiving long-term statin therapy.

Unstable Angina/Non–ST Elevation Myocardial Infarction

UA/NSTEMI results from a reduction in myocardial oxygen supply. Typically, five pathophysiologic processes may contribute to the development of UA/NSTEMI: (1) rupture or erosion of a coronary plaque that leads to nonocclusive thrombosis; (2) dynamic obstruction due to vasoconstriction (Prinzmetal's variant angina, cold, cocaine use); (3) worsening coronary luminal narrowing due to progressive atherosclerosis, in-stent restenosis, or narrowing of coronary artery bypass grafts; (4) inflammation (vasculitis); (5) myocardial ischemia due to increased oxygen demand (sepsis, fever, tachycardia, anemia). Most culprit arteries have less than 50% stenosis. Embolization of platelets and clot fragments into the coronary microvasculature leads to microcirculatory ischemia and infarction that can result in elevation of cardiac biomarker levels without elevation of the ST segments on a 12-lead ECG.

DIAGNOSIS

UA/NSTEMI has three principal presentations: angina at rest (usually lasting more than 20 minutes unless interrupted by antianginal medication), chronic angina pectoris that becomes more frequent and more easily provoked, and new-onset angina that is severe, prolonged, or disabling. UA/NSTEMI can also present with hemodynamic instability or congestive heart failure. Signs of congestive heart failure (S_3 gallop, jugular venous distention, rales, peripheral edema) or ischemia-induced papillary muscle dysfunction causing acute mitral regurgitation may be evident. Fifty percent of patients with UA/NSTEMI have significant ECG abnormalities, including transient ST-segment elevation, ST depression, and T-wave inversion. Significant ST-segment depression in two or more contiguous leads and/or deep symmetrical T-wave inversion, especially in the setting of chest pain, is highly consistent with a diagnosis of myocardial ischemia and UA/NSTEMI. Elevated levels of cardiac biomarkers establish the diagnosis of acute MI. Approximately two thirds of patients who would have been classified as having unstable angina have now been found to show evidence of myocardial necrosis based on sensitive cardiac enzymes assays and should be classified as having NSTEMI.

TREATMENT

Management of UA/NSTEMI is directed at decreasing myocardial oxygen demand and limiting thrombus formation by inhibiting platelet activation and aggregation. Bed rest, supplemental oxygen, analgesia, and β-blocker therapy are indicated. Calcium channel blockers can also be used. Sublingual or intravenous nitroglycerin may improve myocardial oxygen supply. Aspirin, clopidogrel, or prasugrel and 48 hours of heparin therapy are strongly recommended to decrease further thrombus formation. Glycoprotein IIb/IIIa agents may be used as an alternative or in addition to other antiplatelet drugs in certain clinical situations. Thrombolytic therapy is *not indicated* in UA/NSTEMI and has been shown to *increase* mortality. Older age (>65 years), positive finding for cardiac biomarkers, rales, hypotension, tachycardia, and decreased left ventricular function (ejection fraction of <40%) are associated with increased mortality. Patients at high risk include the elderly, those with ischemic symptoms in the preceding 48 hours, those with prolonged chest pain (>20 minutes), those with heart failure or hemodynamic instability, those with sustained ventricular dysrhythmias, those who had a PCI within the past 6 months or had prior CABG surgery, those with elevated troponin levels, and those with angina at low-level activity. These patients are considered for early invasive evaluation, which includes coronary angiography and revascularization by PCI or CABG, if needed. Patients with mild to moderate renal insufficiency (creatinine clearance of >30 mL/min) may also benefit from early invasive treatment. Patients at lower risk are treated medically and undergo stress testing at a later time. Coronary angiography is often considered for patients who demonstrate significant ischemia on stress testing.

COMPLICATIONS OF ACUTE MYOCARDIAL INFARCTION

Cardiac Dysrhythmias

Cardiac dysrhythmias, especially ventricular dysrhythmias, are a common cause of death during the early period following acute MI.

Ventricular fibrillation occurs in 3% to 5% of patients with acute MI, usually during the first 4 hours after the event. Rapid defibrillation with 200 to 300 J of energy is necessary when ventricular fibrillation occurs. Prophylactic lidocaine is not necessary if electrical defibrillation can be promptly accomplished. Amiodarone is regarded as one of the most effective antidysrhythmic drugs for control of ventricular tachydysrhythmias, especially after MI. Administration of β-blockers may decrease the early occurrence of ventricular fibrillation. Hypokalemia is a risk factor for ventricular fibrillation. Ventricular fibrillation is often fatal when it occurs in patients with co-existing hypotension and/or congestive heart failure.

Ventricular tachycardia is common in acute MI. Short periods of nonsustained ventricular tachycardia do not appear to predispose a patient to sustained ventricular tachycardia or ventricular fibrillation. Sustained or hemodynamically significant ventricular tachycardia *must* be treated promptly with electrical cardioversion. Asymptomatic ventricular tachycardia can be treated with intravenous lidocaine or amiodarone. Implantation of a cardioverter-defibrillator may be indicated in patients who experience recurrent ventricular tachycardia or ventricular fibrillation despite adequate revascularization.

Atrial fibrillation and *atrial flutter* are the most common atrial dysrhythmias seen with acute MI. They occur in about 20% of patients. Precipitating factors include hypoxia, acidosis, heart failure, pericarditis, and sinus node ischemia. Atrial fibrillation may also result from atrial ischemia or from an acute increase in left atrial pressure as a result of left ventricular dysfunction. The incidence of atrial fibrillation is decreased in patients who receive thrombolytic therapy. When atrial fibrillation is hemodynamically significant, cardioversion is necessary. If atrial fibrillation is well tolerated, β-blockers or calcium channel blockers are indicated to control the ventricular response.

Sinus bradycardia is common after acute MI, particularly in patients with inferior wall MI. This may reflect increased parasympathetic nervous system activity or acute ischemia of the sinus node or atrioventricular node. Treatment with atropine and/or a temporary cardiac pacemaker is needed only when there is hemodynamic compromise from the bradycardia. *Second- or third-degree atrioventricular heart block* occurs in about 20% of patients with inferior wall MI. Complete heart block requires temporary cardiac pacing.

Pericarditis

Acute pericarditis is a common complication that occurs 1 to 4 days after MI in 10% to 15% of patients. It may cause chest pain that can be confused with continuing or recurrent angina. However, in contrast to the pain of myocardial ischemia, the pain of pericarditis is pleuritic, gets worse with inspiration or lying down, and may be relieved by changes in posture. A pericardial friction rub can be heard but is often transient and positional. Diffuse ST-segment and T-wave changes may be present on the ECG. In the absence of a significant pericardial effusion, treatment of pericarditis is aimed at relieving the chest pain. Aspirin or indomethacin is recommended initially. Corticosteroids can relieve symptoms dramatically but are usually reserved for refractory cases, and it is recommended that steroid therapy be deferred for at least 4 weeks after an acute MI. *Dressler's syndrome* (*post–MI syndrome*) is a delayed form of pericarditis developing several weeks to months after an acute MI. It is thought to be immune mediated.

Mitral Regurgitation

Mitral regurgitation due to ischemic injury to the papillary muscles and/or the ventricular muscle to which the papillary muscles attach can occur after acute MI. Severe mitral regurgitation is rare and usually results from partial or complete rupture of a papillary muscle. Severe mitral regurgitation is 10 times more likely to occur after an inferior wall MI than after an anterior wall MI. Severe acute mitral regurgitation typically results in pulmonary edema and cardiogenic shock. Total papillary muscle rupture usually leads to death within 24 hours. Prompt surgical repair is required. Treatments that decrease left ventricular afterload and improve coronary perfusion, such as an intraaortic balloon pump or intravenous nitroprusside, can decrease the regurgitant volume and increase forward flow and cardiac output until surgery can be accomplished.

Ventricular Septal Rupture

Ventricular septal rupture is more likely after anterior wall rather than inferior wall MI. The characteristic holosystolic murmur of ventricular septal rupture may be difficult to distinguish from the murmur of severe mitral regurgitation. The diagnosis can be made by echocardiography. As soon as the diagnosis of ventricular septal rupture is made, intraaortic balloon counterpulsation should be initiated. Emergency surgical repair is necessary when the ventricular defect is associated with hemodynamic compromise. The mortality rate associated with surgical repair of a post-MI ventricular septal defect is about 20%. It is better to wait at least a week before surgical repair is undertaken in patients in hemodynamically stable condition. If the defect is left untreated, mortality approaches 90%.

Congestive Heart Failure and Cardiogenic Shock

Acute MI is often complicated by some degree of left ventricular dysfunction. The term *cardiogenic shock* is restricted to an advanced form of acute heart failure in which the cardiac output is insufficient to maintain adequate perfusion of the brain, kidneys, and other vital organs. Hypotension and oliguria persist after relief of anginal pain, abatement of excess sympathetic nervous system activity, correction of hypovolemia, and treatment of dysrhythmias. Systolic blood pressure is low, and there may be associated pulmonary edema and arterial hypoxemia. Cardiogenic shock is usually a manifestation of infarction of more than 40% of the left ventricular myocardium. In the setting of an acute MI, the mortality of cardiogenic shock exceeds 50%.

Important in the management of cardiogenic shock is the diagnosis and prompt treatment of potentially reversible mechanical complications of MI. These include (1) rupture of the left ventricular free wall, septum, or papillary muscles; (2) cardiac tamponade; and (3) acute, severe mitral regurgitation. Echocardiography is extremely helpful in diagnosing and quantifying these pathologic conditions. Treatment of cardiogenic shock is dependent on blood pressure and peripheral perfusion. Norepinephrine, vasopressin, dopamine, or dobutamine may be administered in an attempt to improve blood pressure and cardiac output. If the blood pressure is adequate, nitroglycerin can be used to decrease left ventricular preload and afterload. Concomitant pulmonary edema may require the use of morphine, diuretics, and mechanical ventilation. Restoration of some coronary blood flow to the zone around the infarction by thrombolytic therapy, PCI, or surgical revascularization may be indicated. Circulatory assist devices can help sustain viable myocardium and support cardiac output until revascularization can be performed. Left ventricular assist devices improve cardiac output much more than intraaortic balloon counterpulsation, but intraaortic balloon pumps are much more widely available. The intraaortic balloon pump is programmed to the ECG so that it deflates just before systole and inflates during diastole. Inflation of the balloon during diastole increases diastolic blood pressure and thus improves coronary blood flow and myocardial oxygen delivery. Deflation of the balloon just before systole augments left ventricular ejection and decreases left ventricular afterload. Infusion of a combination of inotropic and vasodilator drugs may serve as a pharmacologic alternative to mechanical counterpulsation.

Myocardial Rupture

Myocardial rupture usually causes acute cardiac tamponade. This typically occurs within the first week after an MI and presents with sudden hemodynamic collapse or sudden death. In an extremely small percentage of cases, it is possible to have time for medical stabilization and emergency surgery.

Right Ventricular Infarction

Right ventricular infarction occurs in about one third of patients with acute inferior wall MI. Isolated right ventricular infarction is very unusual. The right ventricle has a more favorable oxygen supply/demand ratio than the left ventricle because of its smaller muscle mass and its improved oxygen delivery, which results from delivery of coronary blood flow during both systole and diastole. The clinical triad of hypotension, increased jugular venous pressure, and clear lung fields in a patient with an inferior wall MI is virtually pathognomonic for right ventricular infarction. *Kussmaul's sign* (distention of the jugular vein on inspiration) is often seen. Right ventricular dilation, right ventricular asynergy, and abnormal interventricular septal motion can be seen on echocardiography.

Recognition of right ventricular infarction is important, because certain pharmacologic treatments for left ventricular failure may worsen right ventricular failure. In particular, administration of vasodilators and diuretics is very undesirable. Initial therapy for right ventricular failure consists of intravenous fluids. If hypotension persists, then inotropic support, with or without intraaortic balloon counterpulsation, may be necessary. Cardiogenic shock, although uncommon, is the most serious complication of right ventricular infarction. Improvement in right ventricular function generally occurs over time, which suggests reversal of "ischemic stunning" of the right ventricular myocardium. About one third of patients with right ventricular infarction develop atrial fibrillation. Heart block may occur in as many as 50% of these patients. Both of these situations may produce severe hemodynamic compromise. Third-degree atrioventricular heart block should be treated promptly with temporary atrioventricular sequential pacing, in recognition of the value of atrioventricular synchrony in maintaining ventricular filling in the ischemic, and therefore noncompliant, right ventricle.

Stroke

Infarction of the anterior wall and apex of the left ventricle results in thrombus formation there in as many as one third of patients. The risk of systemic embolization and the possibility of an *ischemic stroke* are very significant in these patients. Echocardiography is used to detect a left ventricular thrombus. The presence of such a thrombus is an indication for immediate anticoagulation with heparin followed by 6 months of anticoagulation with warfarin.

Thrombolytic therapy is associated with *hemorrhagic stroke* in 0.3% to 1% of patients. The stroke is usually evident within the first 24 hours after treatment and is associated with a high mortality rate.

PERIOPERATIVE IMPLICATIONS OF PERCUTANEOUS CORONARY INTERVENTION

Percutaneous coronary angioplasty (PTCA) was introduced as an alternative to CABG to mechanically open stenosed coronary arteries. It was effective, but restenosis of the angioplasty site occurred in 15% to 60% of patients. To solve the problem of abrupt coronary closure after angioplasty, bare metal stents were introduced. However, coronary restenosis due to neointimal hyperplasia was observed in 10% to 30% of patients with bare metal stents. Stents coated with drugs (*drug-eluting stents*) were then introduced to reduce neointimal hyperplasia and subsequent stenosis. Today, at least three polymer-based drug-eluting stents are available: (1) the Cypher sirolimus-eluting stent, (2) the Taxus paclitaxel-eluting stent, and (3) the Endeavor zotarolimus-eluting stent. The drugs in these stents prevent cell division and hence reduce neointimal hyperplasia. The two principal issues related to PCI with stent placement are thrombosis and an increased risk of bleeding due to dual antiplatelet therapy.

Percutaneous Coronary Intervention and Thrombosis

Mechanically opening a blood vessel by angiography causes vessel injury, especially destruction of the endothelium. This makes the area prone to thrombosis. It takes about 2 to 3 weeks for the vessel to reendothelialize after balloon angioplasty. After bare metal stent placement, reendothelialization can take up to 12 weeks, and a drug-eluting stent may not be completely endothelialized even after 1 year. Thus, thrombosis after angioplasty and stent placement is a major concern.

Stent thrombosis is categorized by the time interval between its occurrence and the PCI: *acute* (within 24 hours), *subacute* (between 2 and 30 days), *late* (between 30 days and a year), and *very late* (after a year). Early stent thrombosis is usually mechanical in origin and due to coronary artery dissection or underexpansion of the stent. In contrast, late stent thrombosis is typically related to stent malposition, abnormal reendothelialization, or hypersensitivity. Platelets play an important role in the pathophysiology of stent thrombosis, and use of antiplatelet drugs is critical in these patients until the stent becomes less prone to thrombosis. Platelets can be activated by many triggers, and there is significant redundancy and crosstalk between these pathways. Thus, multiple pathways must be blocked to achieve clinically effective platelet inhibition.

The discontinuation of antiplatelet therapy increases the risk of stent thrombosis. Dual antiplatelet therapy (aspirin with clopidogrel) is better in preventing stent thrombosis compared with aspirin alone. Clopidogrel discontinuation is the most significant independent predictor of stent thrombosis, with the probability of an event increased by more than

14 times after discontinuation. Patients with drug-eluting stents who stopped clopidogrel during the first month after PCI were 10 times more likely to have a fatal outcome during the next 11 months. Current recommendations for dual antiplatelet therapy are the following: it is needed for at least 2 weeks after balloon angioplasty without stenting, for at least 6 weeks after bare metal stent placement, and for at least 1 year after drug-eluting stent placement.

Other factors can predispose a patient to stent thrombosis, and these may be important in the perioperative period. Patients at risk for stent thrombosis include those with acute coronary syndrome, low ejection fraction, diabetes, renal impairment, advanced age, prior brachytherapy, and cancer. Factors related to coronary anatomy (length of the stents, placement of multiple stents, bifurcated lesions) may also predispose patients to stent thrombosis. Elective surgery and emergency surgery both increase the risk of stent thrombosis because of the prothrombotic state during the perioperative period.

Surgery and Risk of Stent Thrombosis

SURGERY AND BARE METAL STENTS

The frequency of major adverse cardiovascular events (death, MI, stent thrombosis, or the need for repeat revascularization) used to be 10.5% when noncardiac surgery was performed within 4 weeks of PCI. It decreased to 3.8% when surgery was performed between 31 and 90 days after PCI and to 2.8% when performed more than 90 days after PCI. The risk of death, MI, stent thrombosis, and urgent revascularization is increased by 5% to 30% if surgery is performed within 6 weeks of bare metal stent placement.

SURGERY AND DRUG-ELUTING STENTS

In the nonsurgical population, the chance of late stent thrombosis is higher after placement of a drug-eluting stent than after placement of a bare metal stent. This is attributed to the delayed endothelialization seen with drug-eluting stents. The incidence of major adverse cardiac events is quite significant if dual antiplatelet therapy is discontinued and noncardiac surgery is performed within 1 year of drug-eluting stent placement.

The risk of adverse events is higher in patients who undergo emergency surgery. In patients with bare metal stents, emergency surgery increases the adverse event rate threefold over elective surgery. For patients with drug-eluting stents, data indicate a 3.5-fold increase in adverse events.

Risk of Bleeding with Antiplatelet Agents

It is predictable that patients who are taking antiplatelet drugs will have a higher chance of bleeding, which can be of major concern in the perioperative period. The risk of spontaneous bleeding increases in patients who are receiving antiplatelet agents. It has been shown that continuing aspirin therapy increases the risk of bleeding by a factor of 1.5, but the severity of adverse events is not increased. The risk of bleeding in patients undergoing noncardiac surgery who are taking clopidogrel has not been extensively studied. The addition of clopidogrel to aspirin increases the relative risk of bleeding by 50%. So far no increase in mortality has been noted except for intracranial surgery.

Bleeding versus Stent Thrombosis in the Perioperative Period

Discontinuing antiplatelet therapy causes a significant increase in coronary, cerebrovascular, and peripheral vascular events. However, in the perioperative patient, the risk of bleeding has to be weighed against the risk of thrombosis. In many situations the risk of coronary thrombosis is high and the consequence of thrombosis could be catastrophic; on the other hand, although the risk of bleeding is increased, bleeding could be manageable and does not contribute to significant morbidity and mortality. In such cases it may be prudent to continue antiplatelet therapy. However, some individuals are more prone to bleeding or need to undergo procedures in which bleeding can have severe consequences. These include neurosurgery, spinal cord decompression, aortic aneurysm surgery, and prostatectomy, among others. In such cases the risk of bleeding may outweigh the risk of thrombosis, so antiplatelet therapy should be stopped before these operations (at least 5 to 7 days before surgery for clopidogrel) and resumed as soon as feasible postoperatively. Some patients come for surgery receiving antiplatelet therapy for secondary prevention of cardiovascular events. These patients have no stents, so the risk of bleeding will outweigh the risk of cardiovascular events. Antiplatelet drugs can be temporarily withheld for high-risk surgery.

Management of Patients with Stents

Five factors should be considered when caring for a patient with a coronary stent: (1) timing of the operation after PCI, also called the *PCI-to-surgery interval;* (2) continuation of dual antiplatelet therapy; (3) perioperative monitoring strategies; (4) anesthetic technique; and (5) immediate availability of an interventional cardiologist.

PCI-TO-SURGERY INTERVAL

The risk of stent thrombosis is significant in the first month after stent placement and progressively decreases as the time from PCI to surgery increases. The longer one waits after stent placement the better it is. For patients with bare metal stents, waiting *at least 6 weeks* (preferably 90 days) before elective surgery is recommended. In patients with drug-eluting stents waiting *at least 1 year* before elective noncardiac surgery is recommended (Table 1-6).

CONTINUATION OF DUAL ANTIPLATELET THERAPY

Dual antiplatelet therapy should be continued for at least 6 weeks in patients with bare metal stents and 1 year in patients with drug-eluting stents. If dual antiplatelet therapy needs to be stopped, at least aspirin therapy should be continued. Aspirin should be stopped before elective surgery only

TABLE 1-6 ■ Recommended time intervals to wait for elective noncardiac surgery after coronary revascularization

Procedure	Time to wait for elective surgery
Angioplasty without stenting	2-4 wk
Bare metal stent placement	At least 6 wk; 12 wk preferable
Coronary artery bypass grafting	At least 6 wk; 12 wk preferable
Drug-eluting stent placement	At least 12 mo

when absolutely indicated. Although less than 6 weeks after bare metal stent placement and less than 1 year after drug-eluting stent placement is considered a highly vulnerable period for stent thrombosis, stent thrombosis can happen at any time. Intraoperative and postoperative monitoring should be based on the risk of surgery, overall patient condition, and the interval between PCI and surgery. Patients who are in the vulnerable period should be monitored very closely, especially if antiplatelet therapy was discontinued for the surgery. In a bleeding patient, platelets can be administered to counteract the effects of antiplatelet drugs, but the effectiveness of the platelet infusions will depend on the timing of the last dose of clopidogrel. Platelet transfusions can be administered as soon as 4 hours after discontinuation of clopidogrel, but they will be most effective 24 hours after the last dose of clopidogrel.

PERIOPERATIVE MONITORING STRATEGIES

Practitioners should have a high index of suspicion for cardiac events and concentrate on monitoring for myocardial ischemia and infarction. Intraoperative continuous ECG monitoring with ST analysis is very helpful in monitoring for myocardial ischemia. Any angina in a patient with a stent should prompt evaluation to rule out acute MI, and an urgent cardiology evaluation should be sought.

ANESTHETIC TECHNIQUE

Use of neuraxial anesthetic techniques in patients who are receiving dual antiplatelet therapy is controversial. However, both the American Society of Regional Anesthesia and the European Society of Anaesthesiologists have adopted a conservative approach in this matter. Use of neuraxial blockade is not encouraged in patients who are receiving dual antiplatelet therapy. The risk of developing a spinal hematoma exists not only at the time of placement of the catheter, but also at the time of its removal. Recommended waiting times before placement or removal of an epidural catheter and administration of antiplatelet agents are given in Table 1-7.

IMMEDIATE AVAILABILITY OF AN INTERVENTIONAL CARDIOLOGIST

Although many MIs in the perioperative period are silent, any angina in a patient with a stent should prompt evaluation to rule out acute MI, and an urgent cardiology evaluation should

TABLE 1-7 ■ Recommended time intervals for withholding antiplatelet therapy before and after neuraxial puncture or catheter removal

Drug	Time *before* puncture/ catheter manipulation or removal	Time *after* puncture/ catheter manipulation or removal
Clopidogrel	7 days	After catheter removal
Ticlopidine	10 days	After catheter removal
Prasugrel	7-10 days	6 hr after catheter removal
Ticagrelor	5 days	6 hr after catheter removal

Data from recommendations of the European Society of Anaesthesiology.

be sought. There should ideally be immediate access to interventional cardiology services. Once the diagnosis of acute MI or acute stent thrombosis is made or considered, triage to interventional cardiology within 90 minutes is strongly recommended. Mortality increases substantially if reperfusion is delayed. Ambulatory surgical facilities, endoscopy suites, and other non–hospital-based operating locations without these resources on site should develop a relationship with interventional cardiologists that can facilitate rapid transfer if needed.

PERIOPERATIVE MYOCARDIAL INFARCTION

The incidence of perioperative cardiac injury is a cumulative result of the patient's preoperative medical condition, the specific surgical procedure, the expertise of the surgeon, the diagnostic criteria used to define MI, and the overall medical care at a particular institution. The risk of perioperative death due to cardiac causes is less than 1% in patients who do not have ischemic heart disease. The incidence of perioperative MI in patients who undergo elective high-risk vascular surgery is between 5% and 15%. The risk is even higher for emergency surgery. Patients who undergo *urgent* hip surgery have an incidence of perioperative MI of 5% to 7%, whereas fewer than 3% of patients who undergo *elective* total hip or knee arthroplasty have a perioperative MI. Perioperative MIs are associated with a 20% mortality.

Pathophysiology

Ischemia occurs early in the postoperative period and is associated with development of a perioperative MI. Contemporary studies indicate that most perioperative MIs occur in the first 24 to 48 hours after surgery. Many postoperative MIs are NSTEMIs and can be diagnosed by release of cardiac biomarkers and/or ECG changes. These MIs are usually preceded by tachycardia and ST depression and are often silent. Patients

with more severe coronary artery disease are at greater risk. These observations support the hypothesis that perioperative myocardial injury develops as a consequence of increased myocardial oxygen demand (increased blood pressure and heart rate) in the context of underlying compromised myocardial oxygen supply.

Another hypothesis suggests that perioperative MI is the result of sudden development of a thrombotic process associated with vulnerable plaque rupture. This hypothesis is based on postoperative autopsy studies and angiographic evidence of thrombi in coronary arteries that are not critically stenosed. Endothelial injury at the site of a plaque rupture triggers the cascade of platelet aggregation and release of mediators. Aggregation of platelets and activation of other inflammatory and noninflammatory mediators potentiates thrombus formation and leads to dynamic vasoconstriction distal to the thrombus. The combined effects of dynamic and physical blood vessel narrowing cause ischemia and/or infarction. In the postoperative period, changes in blood viscosity, catecholamine concentrations, cortisol levels, endogenous tissue plasminogen activator concentrations, and plasminogen activator inhibitor levels create a prothrombotic state. Changes in heart rate and blood pressure as a result of the stress response can increase the propensity for a plaque to fissure and develop endothelial damage. In combination, these factors can precipitate thrombus formation in an atherosclerotic coronary artery and lead to the development of an STEMI. Thus, two different pathophysiologic mechanisms can be responsible for perioperative MI. One could be related to acute coronary thrombosis, and the other could be the consequence of increased myocardial oxygen demand in the setting of compromised myocardial oxygen supply. These processes are not mutually exclusive. However, one process or the other usually predominates in a particular patient (Figure 1-5).

Diagnosis

In the perioperative period, ischemic episodes often are not associated with chest pain. In addition, many postoperative ECGs are nondiagnostic. Nonspecific ECG changes, new-onset dysrhythmias, and noncardiac hemodynamic instability can further obscure the clinical picture of acute coronary syndrome in the perioperative period. Therefore, the diagnosis of perioperative MI may be quite difficult.

An acute increase in troponin levels should be considered to indicate MI in the perioperative setting. An increase in cardiac troponin level is a marker of myocardial injury, and there is a good correlation between the duration of myocardial ischemia and the increase in the level of cardiac-specific troponin. There is also a significant association between increased troponin levels and short- and long-term morbidity and mortality in surgical patients. This association exists for cardiac death, MI, myocardial ischemia, congestive heart failure, cardiac dysrhythmias, and stroke. Even relatively minor cardiovascular complications such as uncontrolled hypertension, palpitations, increased fatigue, and shortness of breath

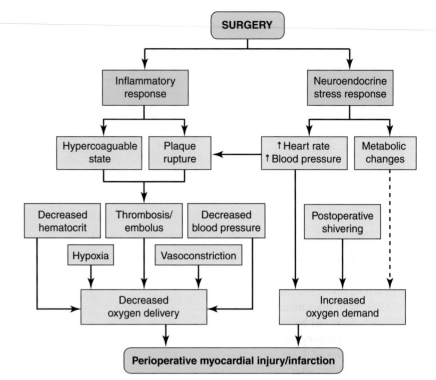

FIGURE 1-5 Factors that can contribute to perioperative myocardial infarction. ↑, Increased.

are correlated with increased levels of cardiac-specific troponins. An increase in troponin level postoperatively, even in the absence of clear cardiovascular signs and symptoms, is an important finding that requires careful attention and referral to a cardiologist for further evaluation and management.

PREOPERATIVE ASSESSMENT OF PATIENTS WITH KNOWN OR SUSPECTED ISCHEMIC HEART DISEASE

History

The preoperative history taking is meant to elicit the severity, progression, and functional limitations imposed by ischemic heart disease. It should focus on determining the presence of major, intermediate, and minor clinical risk factors in a particular patient (Table 1-8). Myocardial ischemia, left ventricular dysfunction, and cardiac dysrhythmias are usually responsible for the signs and symptoms of ischemic heart disease. Symptoms such as angina and dyspnea may be absent at rest, which emphasizes the importance of evaluating the patient's response to various physical activities such as walking or climbing stairs. Limited exercise tolerance in the absence of significant lung disease is good evidence of decreased cardiac reserve. If a patient can climb two to three flights of stairs without symptoms, it is likely that cardiac reserve is adequate. Dyspnea after the onset of angina pectoris suggests the presence of acute left ventricular dysfunction caused by myocardial ischemia. In some patients myocardial ischemia does not evoke chest pain or discomfort. This *silent* myocardial ischemia usually occurs at a heart rate and blood pressure substantially lower than that present during exercise-induced ischemia. It is estimated

TABLE 1-8   Clinical predictors of increased perioperative cardiovascular risk

MAJOR

Unstable coronary syndromes
Acute or recent MI with evidence of important ischemic risk based on clinical symptoms or noninvasive study
Unstable or severe angina
Decompensated heart failure
Significant dysrhythmias
High-grade atrioventricular block
Symptomatic ventricular dysrhythmias in the presence of underlying heart disease
Supraventricular dysrhythmias with uncontrolled ventricular rate
Severe valvular heart disease

INTERMEDIATE

Mild angina pectoris
Previous MI based on history or Q waves on ECG
Compensated or previous heart failure
Diabetes mellitus (particularly insulin dependent)
Renal insufficiency

MINOR

Advanced age (>70 years)
Abnormal ECG (left ventricular hypertrophy, left bundle branch block, ST-T abnormalities)
Rhythm other than sinus
Low functional capacity
History of stroke
Uncontrolled systemic hypertension

Adapted from Fleisher LA, Beckman JA, Brown KA, et al. ACC/AHA 2006 guideline update on perioperative cardiovascular evaluation for noncardiac surgery: focused update on perioperative beta-blocker therapy: a report of the American College of Cardiology/American Heart Association Task Force on Practice Guidelines. *Circulation.* 2006;113:2662-2674, with permission. *ECG,* Electrocardiogram; *MI,* myocardial infarction.

that nearly three quarters of ischemic episodes in patients with symptomatic ischemic heart disease are not associated with angina pectoris and 10% to 15% of acute MIs are silent. It is important to recognize the presence of incipient congestive heart failure preoperatively, because the added stresses of anesthesia, surgery, fluid replacement, and postoperative pain may result in overt congestive heart failure.

A history of MI is an important piece of information. It is common practice to delay elective surgery for some time (at least 30 days) following MI. Retrospective studies of large groups of adult patients have suggested that the incidence of myocardial reinfarction during the perioperative period is influenced by the time elapsed since the previous MI. Acute MI (1 to 7 days previously), recent MI (8 to 30 days previously), and unstable angina are associated with the highest risk of perioperative myocardial ischemia, MI, and cardiac death.

It is important to determine whether a patient has undergone cardiac revascularization with PCI and stent placement or CABG. Stent placement (drug-eluting or bare metal stent) is routinely followed by postprocedure antiplatelet therapy to prevent acute coronary thrombosis and maintain the long-term patency of the vessel. It is prudent to delay elective noncardiac surgery for 6 weeks after PCI with bare metal stent placement and as long as 12 months with drug-eluting stent placement. Ideally, elective noncardiac surgery should be delayed for 6 weeks after coronary bypass surgery (see Table 1-6).

The presence of aortic stenosis is associated with a two- to three-fold increase in the risk of perioperative cardiac morbidity and mortality. Patients with critical aortic stenosis have the highest risk of cardiac decompensation after noncardiac surgery. Mitral valve disease is associated with less risk of perioperative complications. The presence of prosthetic valves should be noted, since patients with these valves will require perioperative endocarditis prophylaxis and adjustment of their anticoagulation regimens.

The history taking should also elicit information relevant to co-existing noncardiac disease. For example, patients with ischemic heart disease are likely to have peripheral vascular disease. A history of syncope may reflect cerebrovascular disease, a seizure disorder, or cardiac dysrhythmias. Cough is often pulmonary rather than cardiac in origin. It may be difficult to differentiate dyspnea caused by cardiac dysfunction from that caused by chronic lung disease, although patients with ischemic heart disease more often complain of orthopnea and paroxysmal nocturnal dyspnea. Chronic obstructive pulmonary disease is likely in patients with a long history of cigarette smoking. Diabetes mellitus often co-exists with ischemic heart disease. Renal insufficiency (creatinine level of >2.0 mg/dL) increases the risk of perioperative cardiac events.

Medical treatment for ischemic heart disease is designed to decrease myocardial oxygen requirements, improve coronary blood flow, stabilize plaque, prevent thrombosis, and remodel the injured myocardium. These goals are achieved by the use of β-blockers, nitrates, calcium entry blockers, statins, antiplatelet drugs, and ACE inhibitors. Effective β-blockade is suggested by a resting heart rate of 50 to 60 beats per minute.

Routine physical activity is expected to increase the heart rate by 10% to 20%. There is no evidence that β-blockers enhance the negative inotropic effects of volatile anesthetics. β-Blocker therapy should be continued throughout the perioperative period. Atropine or glycopyrrolate can be used to treat excessive bradycardia caused by β-blockers during the perioperative period. Isoproterenol is the specific pharmacologic antagonist for excessive β-blocker activity. The postoperative period is a time when inadvertent withdrawal of β-blocker therapy may occur and result in rebound hypertension and tachycardia.

Significant hypotension has been observed in patients receiving long-term treatment with ACE inhibitors who undergo general anesthesia. Many recommend withholding ACE inhibitors for 24 hours before surgery involving significant fluid shifts or blood loss. Hypotension attributable to ACE inhibitors is usually responsive to fluids or sympathomimetic drugs. If hypotension is refractory to these measures, treatment with vasopressin or one of its analogues may be required.

Antiplatelet drugs are an essential component in the pharmacotherapy of acute coronary syndrome and long-term management of ischemic heart disease. The use of dual antiplatelet therapy precludes neuraxial anesthesia and increases the risk of perioperative bleeding, which may require platelet transfusion in certain clinical situations.

Physical Examination

The physical examination of patients with ischemic heart disease often yields normal findings. Nevertheless, signs of right and left ventricular dysfunction must be sought. A carotid bruit may indicate cerebrovascular disease. Orthostatic hypotension may reflect attenuated autonomic nervous system activity because of treatment with antihypertensive drugs. Jugular venous distention and peripheral edema are signs of right ventricular dysfunction. Auscultation of the chest may reveal evidence of left ventricular dysfunction such as an S_3 gallop or rales.

Specialized Preoperative Testing

Specialized preoperative cardiac testing includes ECG, echocardiography, radionuclide ventriculography, thallium scintigraphy, high-speed CT, MRI, and positron emission tomography scanning. Such testing is reserved for patients in whom the results are critical for guiding therapy during the perioperative period.

EXERCISE ELECTROCARDIOGRAPHY

Preoperative evaluation that includes tests that stimulate an increase in heart rate is appealing, because perioperative increases in myocardial oxygen consumption and the development of myocardial ischemia are often accompanied by tachycardia. Preoperative stress testing and/or the exercise tolerance of a patient can indicate the risk of perioperative myocardial ischemia. Preoperative exercise stress testing is not usually indicated in patients with stable coronary artery disease and acceptable exercise tolerance.

ECHOCARDIOGRAPHY

Preoperative transthoracic or transesophageal echocardiography is useful for diagnosing left ventricular dysfunction and assessing valvular heart disease. Results of resting echocardiography do not contribute appreciably to the information provided by routine clinical and ECG data in predicting adverse outcomes. Echocardiographic wall motion analysis during infusion of dipyridamole or dobutamine or atropine (pharmacologic stress testing) is a good technique for evaluating ischemic heart disease, particularly in patients with no history of MI. Dobutamine stress echocardiography provides comparable, if not better, results than myocardial perfusion scintigraphy and provides additional information about valvular function.

THALLIUM SCINTIGRAPHY

Physical limitations, such as claudication or joint disease, may impair the ability of a patient to exercise. This limits the usefulness of exercise stress testing. Dipyridamole-thallium testing mimics the coronary vasodilator response associated with exercise. Like stress echocardiography, it is a useful test in patients with limited exercise capacity. Defects or "cold spots" on the nuclear scan denote areas of myocardial ischemia or infarction. The cost effectiveness of thallium scintigraphy is best when this test is restricted to patients who cannot exercise and whose risk of perioperative cardiac complications cannot be estimated based on other clinical factors.

RADIONUCLIDE VENTRICULOGRAPHY

Radionuclide ventriculography quantitates left and right ventricular systolic and diastolic function. The ejection fraction determined by radionuclide ventriculography does not provide information that can be used to predict the risk of perioperative myocardial ischemia, but an ejection fraction of less than 50% may predict an increased risk of postoperative congestive heart failure.

COMPUTED TOMOGRAPHY AND MAGNETIC RESONANCE IMAGING

High-speed CT can visualize coronary artery calcification. Intravenous administration of radiographic contrast media enhances the clarity of the images. MRI provides even greater image clarity and can delineate the proximal portions of the coronary arterial circulation. However, CT and MRI are more expensive and less mobile than other modalities of cardiac evaluation.

POSITRON EMISSION TOMOGRAPHY

Positron emission tomography is a highly sophisticated technique that demonstrates regional myocardial blood flow and metabolism. It can be used to delineate the extent of coronary artery disease and myocardial viability.

MANAGEMENT OF ANESTHESIA IN PATIENTS WITH KNOWN OR SUSPECTED ISCHEMIC HEART DISEASE UNDERGOING NONCARDIAC SURGERY

The preoperative management of patients with ischemic heart disease or risk factors for ischemic heart disease is geared toward the following goals: (1) determining the extent of ischemic heart disease and any previous interventions (CABG, PCI), (2) assessing the severity and stability of the disease, and (3) reviewing medical therapy and noting any drugs that can increase the risk of surgical bleeding or contraindicate use of a particular anesthetic technique. The first two goals are important in risk stratification.

Risk Stratification

For patients in stable condition undergoing elective major noncardiac surgery, six independent predictors of major cardiac complications have been identified and included in the Lee Revised Cardiac Risk Index (Table 1-9). These six predictors are high-risk surgery, history of ischemic heart disease, history of congestive heart failure, history of cerebrovascular disease, preoperative insulin-dependent diabetes mellitus, and preoperative serum creatinine level higher than 2.0 mg/dL. The higher the number of risk factors present, the greater the probability of perioperative cardiac complications such as cardiac death, cardiac arrest or ventricular fibrillation, complete heart block, acute MI, and pulmonary edema (Figure 1-6). These risk factors have been incorporated into the American

---

TABLE 1-9 ■ Cardiac risk factors in patients undergoing elective major noncardiac surgery

1. High-risk surgery
   Abdominal aortic aneurysm
   Peripheral vascular operation
   Thoracotomy
   Major abdominal operation
2. Ischemic heart disease
   History of myocardial infarction
   History of a positive finding on exercise testing
   Current complaints of angina pectoris
   Use of nitrate therapy
   Presence of Q waves on electrocardiogram
3. Congestive heart failure
   History of congestive heart failure
   History of pulmonary edema
   History of paroxysmal nocturnal dyspnea
   Physical examination showing rales or S_3 gallop
   Chest radiograph showing pulmonary vascular redistribution
4. Cerebrovascular disease
   History of stroke
   History of transient ischemic attack
5. Insulin-dependent diabetes mellitus
6. Preoperative serum creatinine concentration >2 mg/dL

Adapted from Lee TH, Marcantonio ER, Mangione CM, et al. Derivation and prospective validation of a simple index for prediction of cardiac risk of major noncardiac surgery. *Circulation.* 1999;100:1043-1049, with permission.

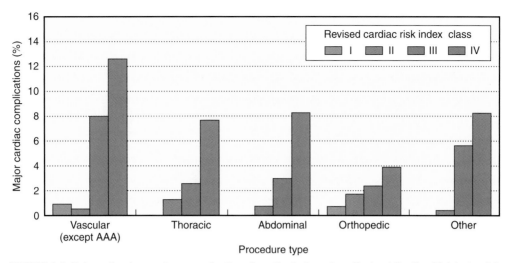

FIGURE 1-6 Rates of major cardiac complications in patients in various Revised Cardiac Risk Index risk classes according to the type of surgery performed. Note that, by definition, patients undergoing abdominal aortic aneurysm (AAA), thoracic, and abdominal procedures are excluded from risk class I because these operations are all considered high-risk surgery. In all subsets, there was a statistically significant trend toward greater risk with higher risk class. *(Adapted from Lee TH, Marcantonio ER, Mangione CM, et al. Derivation and prospective validation of a simple index for prediction of cardiac risk of major noncardiac surgery. Circulation. 1999;100:1043-1049.)*

College of Cardiology/American Heart Association (ACC/AHA) guidelines for perioperative cardiovascular evaluation for noncardiac surgery. The principal theme of the guidelines is that preoperative intervention is rarely necessary simply to lower the risk of surgery. *An intervention is indicated or not indicated irrespective of the need for surgery.* Preoperative testing should be performed only if it the result is likely to influence perioperative management. Although no prospective, randomized study has been conducted to prove the efficacy of these guidelines, they offer a paradigm that has been widely adopted by clinicians.

The ACC/AHA guidelines provide a multistep algorithm for determining the need for preoperative cardiac evaluation. The first step assesses the urgency of the surgery. The need for emergency surgery takes precedence over the need for additional workup (Figure 1-7). Subsequent steps of the ACC/AHA guidelines integrate risk stratification according to clinical risk factors, functional capacity, and surgery-specific risk factors. Clinical risk factors identified from the history, physical examination, and review of the ECG are grouped into three categories: (1) Major clinical risk factors (unstable coronary syndrome, decompensated heart failure, significant dysrhythmias, severe valvular heart disease) may require delay of elective surgery and cardiologic evaluation. Intensive preoperative management is necessary if surgery is urgent or emergent. (2) Moderate clinical risk factors (stable angina pectoris, previous MI identified by history or pathologic Q waves, compensated or previous heart failure, insulin-dependent diabetes mellitus, renal insufficiency) are well-validated markers of an enhanced risk of perioperative cardiac complications. (3) Minor clinical risk factors (hypertension, left bundle branch block, nonspecific ST-T wave changes, history of stroke) are recognized

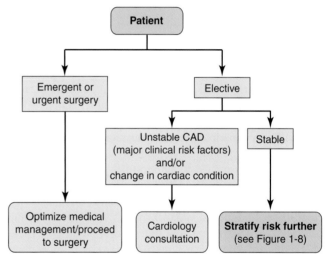

FIGURE 1-7 Algorithm for preoperative assessment of patients with ischemic heart disease. Patients requiring urgent or emergent surgery are identified before proceeding to the operating room with medical management. In patients scheduled for elective surgery, the presence of major clinical risk factors or a change in medical condition may prompt further evaluation before surgery. *CAD,* Coronary artery disease.

markers of coronary artery disease that have not been proven to independently increase perioperative cardiac risk.

Functional capacity or exercise tolerance can be expressed in metabolic equivalent of the task (MET) units. The O_2 consumption ($\dot{V}O_2$) of a 70-kg, 40-year-old man in a resting state is 3.5 mL/kg/min or 1 MET. Perioperative cardiac risk is increased in patients with poor functional capacity, that is, those who are unable to meet a 4-MET demand during normal daily activities. These individuals may be able to perform

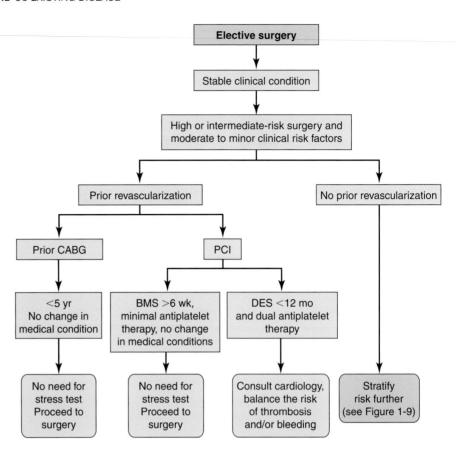

FIGURE 1-8 Algorithm for preoperative assessment of patients with ischemic heart disease scheduled for elective intermediate-to high-risk surgery who are in stable clinical condition with moderate clinical risk factors. Determine whether previous coronary intervention was performed and assess the stability of the cardiac condition. If no change in cardiac condition has occurred, proceed with surgery with medical management. For patients with intracoronary stents, determine the date of insertion and location of the stent(s), the kind of stent(s), and the status of current antiplatelet therapy. Patients receiving antiplatelet therapy may require consultation with the cardiologist and the surgeon. *BMS,* Bare metal stent; *CABG,* coronary artery bypass graft; *DES,* drug-eluting stent; *PCI,* percutaneous coronary intervention.

some activities, such as baking, slow ballroom dancing, golfing (riding in a cart), or walking at a speed of approximately 2 to 3 mph, but are unable to perform more strenuous activity without developing chest pain or significant shortness of breath. The ability to participate in activities requiring more than 4 METs indicates good functional capacity.

The surgery-specific risk of noncardiac surgical procedures is graded as high, intermediate, or low. High-risk surgery includes emergency major surgery, aortic and other major vascular surgery, peripheral vascular surgery, and prolonged surgery associated with large fluid shifts and/or blood loss. These operations are reported to carry a cardiac risk of more than 5%. Intermediate-risk surgery includes endovascular aortic surgery, carotid endarterectomy, head and neck surgery, intraperitoneal and intrathoracic surgery, orthopedic surgery, and prostate surgery. Such operations are reported to be associated with a cardiac risk of less than 5%. Low-risk procedures such as endoscopic surgery, superficial surgery, cataract surgery, breast surgery, and ambulatory surgery are reported to carry a less than 1% risk of perioperative cardiac events.

According to the most recent ACC/AHA guidelines, a select subgroup of patients should be considered for further cardiac evaluation preoperatively. Patients who have major clinical risk factors require cardiology consultation, workup, and optimization of care before elective surgery. If a patient previously underwent a revascularization procedure (CABG or PCI) and there has been no change in the patient's clinical status, the patient can proceed to surgery (Figure 1-8). It

is recommended that patients who are scheduled to undergo elective high-risk surgery and have low exercise tolerance and three or more moderate clinical risk factors be sent for further cardiologic workup (Figure 1-9). Patients scheduled for intermediate-risk surgery with low exercise tolerance and three or more moderate clinical risk factors or those with low functional capacity and one or two clinical risk factors may be considered for further evaluation *if it will affect perioperative management.* Patients scheduled for elective low-risk surgery or those with minor clinical risk factors can proceed to surgery without further workup. Many patients who need further preoperative evaluation may not be candidates for exercise stress testing but can be referred for pharmacologic stress testing. Nuclear imaging can better detect myocardium at risk.

Preoperative coronary angiography is most suitable in a patient with a positive stress test result that suggests significant myocardium at risk. The aim of the angiographic study would be to identify significant coronary artery disease, that is, left main or severe multivessel coronary artery disease. Further management in such a patient would be dictated by the patient's clinical condition, the overall risk of an intervention, and available resources.

Management after Risk Stratification

The fundamental reason for risk stratification is to identify patients at increased risk so as to manage them with pharmacologic and other perioperative interventions that can lessen

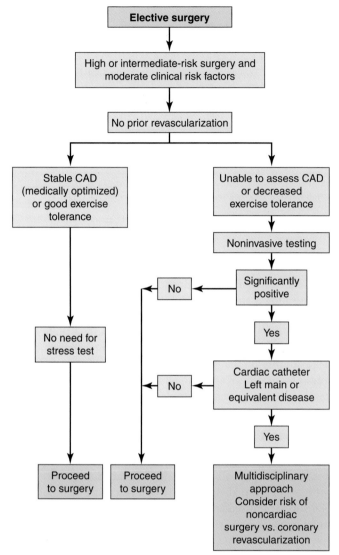

FIGURE 1-9 Algorithm for preoperative assessment of patients scheduled for intermediate- to high-risk surgery who have moderate clinical risk factors and poor exercise tolerance (or exercise tolerance cannot be established). Consider noninvasive stress testing to determine whether significant myocardium is at risk. If significant myocardium is at risk, consider coronary angiography. For patients with one or two clinical risk factors, consider noninvasive stress testing only if it will affect patient management; otherwise proceed to surgery with medical management. *CAD,* Coronary artery disease.

the risk and severity of perioperative cardiac events. Three therapeutic options are available before elective noncardiac surgery: (1) revascularization by surgery, (2) revascularization by PCI, and (3) optimal medical management.

In nonoperative settings, treatment strategies such as PCI (with or without stenting), CABG surgery, and medical therapy have proven efficacious in improving long-term morbidity and mortality. Patients with significant ischemic heart disease who come for noncardiac surgery are likely to be candidates for one or more of these therapies regardless of their need for surgery. Optimal medical management can improve perioperative outcomes. Coronary intervention should be guided by the patient's cardiac condition and by the potential consequences of delaying surgery for recovery from the revascularization.

CORONARY ARTERY BYPASS GRAFTING

For CABG surgery to be beneficial before noncardiac surgery, the institutional risk of that particular noncardiac operation should be greater than the combined risk of coronary catheterization and coronary revascularization, plus the generally reported risk of that noncardiac operation. The indications for preoperative surgical coronary revascularization are the same as those in the nonoperative setting.

PERCUTANEOUS CORONARY INTERVENTION

It was thought that PCI before elective noncardiac surgery could improve perioperative outcomes. However, PCI, which is now often accompanied by stenting and dual antiplatelet therapy, poses its own unique set of problems that need to be considered in patients who are scheduled to undergo elective noncardiac surgery. There is no value in preoperative coronary intervention in a patient with stable ischemic heart disease.

PHARMACOLOGIC MANAGEMENT

The reason to formulate a risk stratification index is so that individuals at high risk will be identified and treated to reduce their risk of perioperative cardiac complications. In view of the serious limitations of current PCIs and lack of utility of CABG and PCI in patients with stable coronary artery disease, very few patients with stable coronary artery disease will undergo revascularization before surgery. Most patients with stable coronary artery disease and/or risk factors for coronary artery disease will be managed pharmacologically, as will patients with significant ischemic heart disease who come for emergent or urgent surgery.

Several pharmacologic agents have been used to reduce perioperative myocardial injury. These are drugs that have demonstrated pharmacologic efficacy in the management of coronary ischemia in the nonsurgical setting. Nitroglycerin may be helpful in the management of active perioperative ischemia. However, prophylactic use of nitroglycerin has not been shown to be efficacious in reducing perioperative morbidity and mortality.

Perioperative use of β-blockers has been shown to be efficacious in reducing perioperative cardiac morbidity and mortality in high-risk patients undergoing vascular surgery. However, recent trials have not shown efficacy of high-dose, *acutely administered,* perioperative β-blockers in reducing overall mortality in patients undergoing noncardiac surgery, but they did show better perioperative *cardiac* outcomes with β-blocker use. However a higher mortality and stroke rate has been noted with β-blocker use. Currently the only class I recommendation (action that should be taken) for perioperative administration of β-blockers is to continue their use in patients who are already receiving β-blockers.

TABLE 1-10 ■ Recommendations for perioperative β-blocker use

	Already receiving β-blockers	Major clinical risk factors or signs of ischemia on preoperative stress testing	Multiple moderate clinical risk factors	Single moderate clinical risk factor
Vascular surgery	++	+	+	±
High- or intermediate-risk surgery	++	+	±	±
Low-risk surgery	*	*	*	*

Adapted from Fleisher LA, Beckman JA, Brown KA, et al. 2009 ACCF/AHA focused update on perioperative beta blockade incorporated into the ACC/AHA 2007 Guidelines on Perioperative Cardiovascular Evaluation and Care for Noncardiac Surgery: a report of the American College of Cardiology Foundation/American Heart Association Task Force on Practice Guidelines. *Circulation*. 2009;120(21):e169-e276.

++, Class I recommendation—β-blockers should be used; +, class IIa recommendation—β-blockers should probably be used; ±, class IIb recommendation—β-blockers may be used.

*Insufficient data available.

Patients undergoing vascular surgery who have multiple risk factors or are found to have reversible ischemia on preoperative testing may benefit from perioperative administration of β-blockers. Although there are some differences between the European and the AHA guidelines, both agree that if β-blockers are used for prophylactic purposes in the perioperative period, they should be initiated at least a week before elective surgery, and *acute* administration of high-dose β-blockers in high-risk populations is not recommended (Table 1-10). Questions regarding the choice of β-blocker and the target heart rate are still unresolved. For ease of dosing and consistency of effect, longer-acting β-blockers such as atenolol or bisoprolol may be more efficacious in the perioperative period.

Patients with vascular disease should receive statin therapy for secondary prevention regardless of the need for noncardiac surgery. Clinical trials have demonstrated a beneficial effect of perioperative statin use. European guidelines recommend starting therapy 1 to 4 weeks before high-risk surgery. Discontinuation of statins in the perioperative period may cause a rebound effect that may be harmful. Thus, it is recommended that statins be continued perioperatively.

α_2-Agonists, by virtue of their central action, have analgesic, sedative, and sympatholytic effects. Perioperative use of α_2-agonists may be considered in patients who cannot tolerate β-blockers.

Controlling hyperglycemia in patients undergoing cardiac surgery and in patients in intensive care units has been associated with improved outcomes. The recent discoveries regarding the nonmetabolic effects of insulin and the harmful effects of hyperglycemia make it prudent to actively manage hyperglycemia with insulin. This is especially important in patients who are at high risk of cardiac injury. The goal is to keep the perioperative glucose level below 180 mg/dL. Because several pathophysiologic mechanisms can trigger a perioperative MI, it seems reasonable to think that multimodal therapy with β-blockers or α_2-agonists, statins, and insulin may be more beneficial than treatment with any single drug (Figure 1-10).

Preoperative anxiety reduction can be achieved by both conversational and pharmacologic means. Patients are more likely to arrive in the operating room in a relaxed state if there has been a preoperative visit during which the anesthetic to be used was explained in detail and all questions and concerns were addressed. The goal of drug-induced sedation and anxiolysis is maximum sedation and/or amnesia without significant circulatory or ventilatory depression.

Intraoperative Management

The basic challenges during induction and maintenance of anesthesia in patients with ischemic heart disease are (1) to prevent myocardial ischemia by optimizing myocardial oxygen supply and reducing myocardial oxygen demand, (2) to monitor for ischemia, and (3) to treat ischemia if it develops. Intraoperative events associated with persistent tachycardia, systolic hypertension, sympathetic nervous system stimulation, arterial hypoxemia, or hypotension can adversely affect the patient with ischemic heart disease (Table 1-11). Perioperative myocardial injury is closely associated with heart rate in vascular surgery patients. A rapid heart rate increases myocardial oxygen requirements and decreases diastolic time for coronary blood flow and therefore oxygen delivery. The increased oxygen requirements produced by hypertension are offset to some degree by improved coronary perfusion. Hyperventilation must be avoided, because hypocapnia may cause coronary artery vasoconstriction. Maintenance of the balance between myocardial oxygen supply and demand is more important than which specific anesthetic technique or drugs are selected to produce anesthesia and muscle relaxation. Although isoflurane may decrease coronary vascular resistance, predisposing to coronary steal syndrome, there is no evidence that this drug increases the incidence of intraoperative myocardial ischemia.

It is important to avoid persistent and excessive changes in heart rate and blood pressure. A common recommendation is to keep the heart rate and blood pressure within 20% of the normal awake value for that patient. However, many episodes

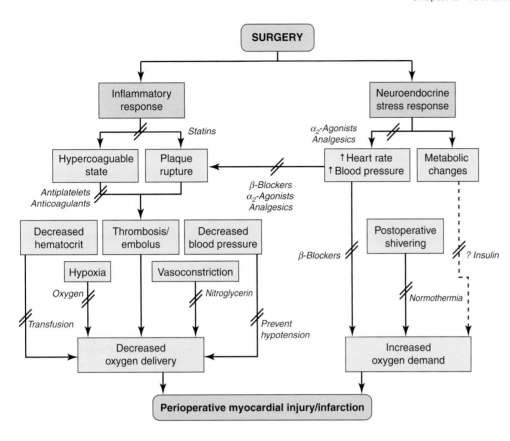

FIGURE 1-10 Interventions that can modulate triggers of perioperative myocardial injury. ↑, Increased; ↓, decreased.

TABLE 1-11 ▪ Intraoperative events that influence the balance between myocardial oxygen delivery and myocardial oxygen requirements

DECREASED OXYGEN DELIVERY

Decreased coronary blood flow
Tachycardia
Hypotension
Hypocapnia (coronary artery vasoconstriction)
Coronary artery spasm
Decreased oxygen content
Anemia
Arterial hypoxemia
Shift of the oxyhemoglobin dissociation curve to the left

INCREASED OXYGEN REQUIREMENTS

Sympathetic nervous system stimulation
Tachycardia
Hypertension
Increased myocardial contractility
Increased afterload
Increased preload

---

of intraoperative myocardial ischemia occur in the absence of hemodynamic changes. These episodes of myocardial ischemia may be due to regional decreases in myocardial perfusion and oxygenation. It is unlikely that this form of ischemia can be prevented by the anesthesiologist.

INDUCTION OF ANESTHESIA

Induction of anesthesia in patients with ischemic heart disease can be accomplished with an intravenous induction drug. Ketamine is not a likely choice, because the associated increase in heart rate and blood pressure transiently increases myocardial oxygen requirements. Tracheal intubation is facilitated by administration of succinylcholine or a nondepolarizing muscle relaxant.

Myocardial ischemia may accompany the sympathetic stimulation that results from direct laryngoscopy and endotracheal intubation. Keeping the duration of direct laryngoscopy short (≤15 seconds) is useful in minimizing the magnitude and duration of the circulatory changes associated with tracheal intubation. If the duration of direct laryngoscopy is not likely to be brief or if hypertension already exists, it is reasonable to consider administering drugs to minimize the sympathetic response. Laryngotracheal lidocaine, intravenous lidocaine, esmolol, fentanyl, and dexmedetomidine have all been shown to be useful for blunting the increase in heart rate evoked by tracheal intubation.

MAINTENANCE OF ANESTHESIA

In patients with normal left ventricular function, tachycardia and hypertension are likely to develop in response to intense stimulation, such as during direct laryngoscopy or painful surgical stimulation. Achieving controlled myocardial depression using a volatile anesthetic may be useful in such patients to minimize the increase in sympathetic nervous system activity.

Overall, volatile anesthetics may be beneficial in patients with ischemic heart disease because they decrease myocardial oxygen requirements and precondition the myocardium to tolerate ischemic events, or they may be detrimental because they lead to a decrease in blood pressure and an associated reduction in coronary perfusion pressure. The AHA guidelines state that it can be beneficial to use volatile anesthetic agents during noncardiac surgery for the maintenance of general anesthesia in patients in hemodynamically stable condition at risk for myocardial ischemia.

The use of nitrous oxide in patients with a history of coronary artery disease has been questioned since the early 1990s when animal and human studies showed an increase in pulmonary vascular resistance, diastolic dysfunction, and subsequent myocardial ischemia with its use. A large multicenter study is currently underway to better define the harmful effects of nitrous oxide.

Patients with severely impaired left ventricular function may not tolerate anesthesia-induced myocardial depression. Opioids may be selected as the principal anesthetic in these patients. The addition of nitrous oxide, a benzodiazepine, or a low-dose volatile anesthetic may be needed, because amnesia cannot be ensured with an opioid anesthetic. However, the addition of nitrous oxide or a volatile anesthetic may be associated with myocardial depression.

Regional anesthesia is an acceptable technique in patients with ischemic heart disease. However, the decrease in blood pressure associated with epidural or spinal anesthesia must be controlled. Prompt treatment of hypotension that exceeds 20% of the preblock blood pressure is necessary. Potential benefits of use of a regional anesthetic include excellent pain control, a decreased incidence of deep venous thrombosis in some patients, and the opportunity to continue the block into the postoperative period. However, the incidence of perioperative cardiac morbidity and mortality does not appear to be significantly different for general and regional anesthesia.

Hemodynamic goals of intraoperative therapy with β-blockers are unclear, and potential interactions with anesthetics that cause myocardial depression and vasodilation must be considered. It seems prudent to maintain the intraoperative heart rate at less than 80 beats per minute.

The choice of a nondepolarizing muscle relaxant in patients with ischemic heart disease is influenced by the impact these drugs can have on the balance between myocardial oxygen delivery and myocardial oxygen requirements. Muscle relaxants with minimal or no effect on heart rate and systemic blood pressure (vecuronium, rocuronium, cisatracurium) are attractive choices for patients with ischemic heart disease. The histamine release and resulting decrease in blood pressure caused by atracurium make it less desirable. Myocardial ischemia has been described in patients with ischemic heart disease given pancuronium, presumably because of the modest increase in heart rate and blood pressure produced by this drug. However, the circulatory changes produced by pancuronium may be useful in offsetting the negative inotropic and chronotropic effects of some anesthetic drugs.

Reversal of neuromuscular blockade with an anticholinesterase-anticholinergic drug combination can be safely accomplished in patients with ischemic heart disease. Glycopyrrolate, which has much less chronotropic effect than atropine, is preferred in these patients.

MONITORING

Type of perioperative monitoring is influenced by the complexity of the operative procedure and the severity of the ischemic heart disease. The most important goal in selecting monitoring methods for patients with ischemic heart disease is to select those that allow *early* detection of myocardial ischemia. Most myocardial ischemia occurs in the absence of hemodynamic alterations, so one should be cautious in endorsing routine use of expensive or complex monitors to detect myocardial ischemia.

The simplest, most cost-effective method for detecting perioperative myocardial ischemia is electrocardiography. The diagnosis of myocardial ischemia focuses on changes in the ST segment, characterized as elevation or depression of at least 1 mm and T-wave inversions. However, other factors such as alterations in electrolytes can also produce such changes. The degree of ST-segment depression parallels the severity of myocardial ischemia. Because visual detection of ST-segment changes is unreliable, computerized ST-segment analysis has been incorporated into ECG monitors. Traditionally, monitoring of *two* leads (leads II and V_5) has been the standard, but it appears that monitoring *three* leads (leads II, V_4, and V_5, or else V_3, V_4, and V_5) improves the ability to detect ischemia. There is a correlation between the lead of the ECG that detects myocardial ischemia and the anatomic distribution of the diseased coronary artery (Table 1-12). For example, the V_5 lead (fifth intercostal space in the anterior axillary line) reflects myocardial ischemia in the portion of the left ventricle supplied by the left anterior descending

TABLE 1-12 ■ Relationship of electrocardiogram (ECG) leads to areas of myocardial ischemia

ECG lead	Coronary artery responsible for ischemia	Area of myocardium that may be involved
II, III, aVF	Right coronary artery	Right atrium Right ventricle Sinoatrial node Inferior aspect of left ventricle Atrioventricular node
I, aVL	Circumflex coronary artery	Lateral aspect of left ventricle
V_3-V_5	Left anterior descending coronary artery	Anterolateral aspect of left ventricle

coronary artery (Figure 1-11). Lead II is more likely to detect myocardial ischemia occurring in the distribution of the right coronary artery. Lead II is also very useful for analysis of cardiac rhythm disturbances.

Events other than myocardial ischemia that can cause ST-segment abnormalities include cardiac dysrhythmias, cardiac conduction disturbances, digitalis therapy, electrolyte abnormalities, and hypothermia. However, in patients with known or suspected coronary artery disease, it is reasonable to assume that intraoperative ST-segment changes represent myocardial ischemia. The occurrence and duration of intraoperative ST-segment changes in high-risk patients are linked to an increased incidence of perioperative MI and adverse cardiac events. Interestingly, the overall incidence of myocardial ischemia is *lower* in the *intraoperative* period than that in the preoperative or postoperative period.

Intraoperative myocardial ischemia can manifest as an acute increase in pulmonary artery occlusion pressure due to changes in left ventricular compliance and left ventricular systolic performance. If myocardial ischemia is global or involves the papillary muscle, V waves may appear in the pulmonary artery occlusion pressure tracing. Nonischemic causes of increased pulmonary artery occlusion pressure include an acute increase in ventricular afterload, an increase in pulmonary venous resistance, and mitral regurgitation due to

nonischemic mechanisms. If only small regions of left ventricular myocardium become ischemic, overall ventricular compliance and pulmonary artery occlusion pressure will remain unchanged, so the *pulmonary artery catheter* is a relatively *insensitive* method of monitoring for myocardial ischemia. In addition, pulmonary artery occlusion pressure is measured only intermittently, and the pulmonary artery diastolic pressure is even less sensitive than the pulmonary artery occlusion pressure in detecting a change in left ventricular compliance. Pulmonary artery catheter measurements are more useful as a guide in the treatment of myocardial dysfunction. They can be used to guide fluid replacement, to measure cardiac output, and to calculate systemic vascular resistance and thereby evaluate the effectiveness of vasopressor, vasodilator, or inotropic therapy.

Indications for placing a pulmonary artery catheter are influenced by the information likely to be derived from it. Use of a pulmonary artery catheter has not been shown to be associated with improved cardiac outcomes. Nevertheless, the value and safety of pulmonary artery catheterization in selected patients are widely accepted. Central venous pressure and pulmonary artery occlusion pressure are correlated in patients with ischemic heart disease when the ejection fraction is more than 50%. However, if the ejection fraction is less than 50%, there is no longer a predictable correlation.

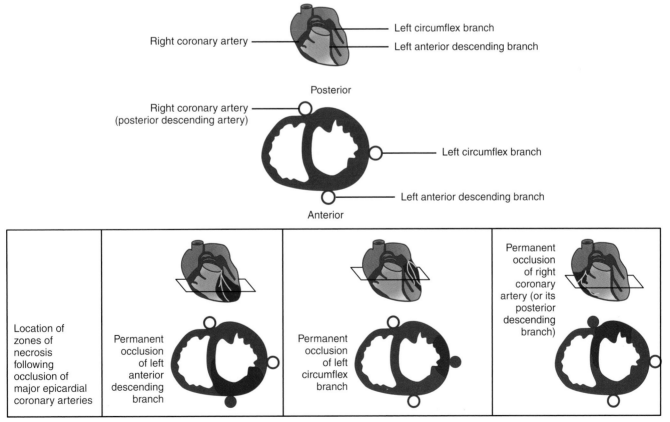

FIGURE 1-11 Correlation of sites of coronary occlusion and zones of necrosis. *(From Antman EM. ST-segment myocardial infarction: pathology, pathophysiology, and clinical features. In: Bonow RO, Mann DL, Zipes DP, et al, eds. Braunwald's Heart Disease. Philadelphia, PA: Saunders; 2012:Figure 54-4.)*

The development of new regional ventricular wall motion abnormalities is the accepted standard for the intraoperative diagnosis of myocardial ischemia. These regional wall motion abnormalities occur before ECG changes are seen. However, segmental wall motion abnormalities may also occur in response to events other than myocardial ischemia. The limitations of *transesophageal echocardiography* include its cost, the need for extensive training in interpreting the images, and the fact that the transducer cannot be inserted until after induction of anesthesia, so there is a critical period during which myocardial ischemia may develop in the absence of this monitoring.

INTRAOPERATIVE MANAGEMENT OF MYOCARDIAL ISCHEMIA

Treatment of myocardial ischemia should be instituted when there are 1-mm ST-segment changes on the ECG. Prompt pharmacologic treatment of changes in heart rate and/or blood pressure is indicated. Nitroglycerin is an appropriate choice when myocardial ischemia is associated with a normal or modestly elevated blood pressure. In this situation, the nitroglycerin-induced coronary vasodilation and decrease in preload facilitate improved subendocardial blood flow, but the nitroglycerin-induced decrease in afterload does not decrease systemic blood pressure to the point that coronary perfusion pressure is jeopardized. A persistent increase in heart rate in the setting of normal or high blood pressure can also be treated by administration of a β-blocker such as esmolol.

Hypotension is treated with sympathomimetic drugs to restore coronary perfusion pressure. In addition to administration of vasoconstrictor drugs, fluid infusion can be useful to help restore blood pressure. Regardless of the treatment, prompt restoration of blood pressure is necessary to maintain pressure-dependent flow through narrowed coronary arteries. In an unstable hemodynamic situation, circulatory support with inotropes or an intraaortic balloon pump may be necessary. It may also be necessary to plan for early postoperative cardiac catheterization.

Postoperative Management

Although significant advances have been made in researching and refining preoperative evaluation and risk management strategies, evidence-based strategies that can be adopted in the postoperative period to improve outcome have not yet been developed.

The goals of postoperative management are the same as those for intraoperative management: prevent ischemia, monitor for myocardial injury, and treat myocardial ischemia or infarction. Any situation that leads to prolonged and significant hemodynamic perturbations can stress the heart. Intraoperative hypothermia may predispose to shivering on awakening, leading to abrupt and dramatic increases in myocardial oxygen requirements. Pain, hypoxemia, hypercarbia, sepsis, and hemorrhage also lead to increased myocardial oxygen demand. The resulting oxygen supply/demand imbalance in patients with ischemic heart disease can precipitate myocardial ischemia, infarction, or death. Although most adverse cardiac events occur within the first 48 hours postoperatively, delayed cardiac events can occur within the first 30 days and can be the result of secondary stresses. It is imperative that patients taking β-blockers continue to receive these drugs throughout the perioperative period.

Prevention of hypovolemia and hypotension is necessary postoperatively, and not only an adequate intravascular volume but also an adequate hemoglobin concentration must be maintained. Oxygen content and oxygen delivery depend significantly on the concentration of hemoglobin in blood. The degree of anemia that can be safely tolerated in patients with ischemic heart disease remains to be defined.

The timing of ventilatory weaning and tracheal extubation is another aspect of care that requires careful consideration. Early extubation is possible and desirable in many patients as long as they fulfill the criteria for extubation. However, patients with ischemic heart disease can become ischemic during emergence from anesthesia and/or weaning from mechanical ventilation. Any increase in heart rate and/or blood pressure must be managed diligently. Pharmacologic therapy with a β-blocker or a combined α- and β-blocker, such as labetalol, can be very helpful.

Continuous ECG monitoring is useful for detecting postoperative myocardial ischemia, which is often silent. Postoperative myocardial ischemia predicts adverse in-hospital and long-term cardiac events. It should be identified, evaluated, and managed, preferably in consultation with a cardiologist.

CARDIAC TRANSPLANTATION

Cardiac transplantation is most often performed in patients with end-stage heart failure due to an idiopathic or ischemic cardiomyopathy. Preoperatively, the ejection fraction is often less than 20%. Irreversible pulmonary hypertension is a contraindication to cardiac transplantation, and most centers do not consider candidates older than 65 years of age for this procedure. Active infection and recent pulmonary thromboembolism with pulmonary infarction are additional contraindications to heart transplantation.

Management of Anesthesia

Patients may come for cardiac transplantation with inotropic, vasodilator, or mechanical circulatory support. Most patients coming for cardiac transplantation will not be in a fasting state and should be considered as having a full stomach. They should be in hemodynamically stable condition before induction of anesthesia. Etomidate is preferred as an induction agent because it has little effect on hemodynamics. An opioid technique is often chosen for maintenance of anesthesia. Volatile anesthetics may produce undesirable degrees of myocardial depression and peripheral vasodilation. Nitrous oxide is rarely used because significant pulmonary hypertension is often present. In addition, there is concern about air embolism because large blood vessels are opened during the surgical procedure. Nondepolarizing neuromuscular blocking drugs that do not cause histamine release are usually selected. The ability of pancuronium to increase heart rate and systemic blood pressure modestly may be desirable in some patients. Many patients undergoing cardiac transplantation have coagulation disturbances due to passive congestion of the liver as a result of chronic congestive heart failure.

The operative technique includes cardiopulmonary bypass and anastomosis of the aorta, pulmonary artery, and left and right atria. Immunosuppressive drugs are usually begun during the preoperative period. Intravascular catheters must be placed using strict aseptic technique. It is necessary to withdraw the central venous or pulmonary artery catheter into the superior vena cava when the native heart is removed. The catheter is then repositioned into the donor heart. These catheters are often inserted into the central circulation via the left internal jugular vein so that the right internal jugular vein is available as an access site when needed to perform endomyocardial biopsies during the postoperative period. Transesophageal echocardiography is used to monitor cardiac function intraoperatively.

After cessation of cardiopulmonary bypass, an inotropic drug may be needed briefly to maintain myocardial contractility and heart rate. Therapy to lower pulmonary vascular resistance may also be necessary and includes administration of a pulmonary vasodilator such as isoproterenol, a prostaglandin, nitric oxide, or a phosphodiesterase inhibitor. The denervated transplanted heart initially assumes an intrinsic heart rate of about 110 beats per minute, which reflects the absence of normal vagal tone. Stroke volume responds to an increase in preload by the Frank-Starling mechanism. These patients tolerate hypovolemia poorly. The transplanted heart does respond to direct-acting catecholamines, but drugs that act by indirect mechanisms, such as ephedrine, have a less intense effect. Vasopressin may be needed to treat severe hypotension unresponsive to catecholamines. The heart rate does not change in response to administration of anticholinergic or anticholinesterase drugs. About one quarter of patients develop bradycardia after transplantation that requires insertion of a permanent cardiac pacemaker.

Postoperative Complications

Cardiac transplant patients may require β-adrenergic stimulants for 3 to 4 days after transplantation. Early postoperative morbidity related to heart transplantation surgery usually involves sepsis and/or rejection. The most common early cause of death is opportunistic infection as a result of immunosuppressive therapy. Transvenous right ventricular endomyocardial biopsies are performed to provide early warning of asymptomatic allograft rejection. Congestive heart failure and development of dysrhythmias are late signs of rejection. Cyclosporine treatment can be associated with drug-induced hypertension that is often resistant to antihypertensive therapy. Nephrotoxicity is another complication of cyclosporine

and tacrolimus therapy. Long-term corticosteroid use may result in skeletal demineralization and glucose intolerance.

Late complications of cardiac transplantation include development of coronary artery disease in the allograft and an increased incidence of cancer. *Diffuse obliterative coronary arteriopathy* affects cardiac transplant recipients over time, and the ischemic sequelae of this form of coronary artery disease are the principal limitations to long-term survival. The arterial disease is restricted to the allograft and is present in about one half of cardiac transplant recipients after 5 years. The accelerated appearance of this coronary artery disease likely reflects a chronic rejection process in the vascular endothelium. This process is not unique to cardiac allografts and is thought to be analogous to the chronic immunologically mediated changes seen in other organ allografts (chronic rejection of the kidney, bronchiolitis obliterans in the lungs, vanishing bile duct syndrome in the liver). The clinical sequelae of this obliterative coronary artery disease include myocardial ischemia, left ventricular dysfunction, cardiac dysrhythmias, and sudden death. The prognosis for transplant recipients with angiographically established coronary artery disease is poor.

Any medical regimen involving long-term immunosuppression is associated with an increased incidence of cancer, especially lymphoproliferative and cutaneous cancers. Malignancy is responsible for a significant portion of the mortality of heart transplant patients. Most posttransplantation lymphoproliferative disease is related to infection with the Epstein-Barr virus.

Anesthetic Considerations in Heart Transplant Recipients

Heart transplant patients present unique anesthetic challenges because of the hemodynamic function of the transplanted denervated heart, the side effects of immunosuppressive therapy, the risk of infection, the potential for drug interactions given the complex drug regimens, and the potential for allograft rejection.

Allograft rejection results in progressive deterioration of cardiac function. The presence and degree of rejection should be noted preoperatively. The presence of infection must also be noted preoperatively, because infection is a significant cause of morbidity and mortality in these patients. Invasive monitoring requires the use of strict aseptic technique. When hepatic and renal function are normal, there is no contraindication to the use of any anesthetic drug.

The transplanted heart has no sympathetic, parasympathetic, or sensory innervation, and the loss of vagal tone results in a higher than normal resting heart rate. Two P waves are detectable on the ECG after heart transplantation. The native sinus node remains intact if a cuff of atrium is left in place to permit surgical anastomosis to the grafted heart. Because the native P wave cannot traverse the suture line, it has no influence on the chronotropic activity of the heart. Carotid sinus massage and Valsalva's maneuver have no effect on heart rate. There is no sympathetic response to direct laryngoscopy and tracheal intubation, and the denervated heart has a blunted heart rate response to light anesthesia or intense pain. The transplanted heart is unable to increase its heart rate immediately in response to hypovolemia or hypotension but responds instead with an increase in stroke volume via the Frank-Starling mechanism. The needed increase in cardiac output is dependent on venous return until the heart rate increases after several minutes in response to the effect of circulating catecholamines. Because α- and β-adrenergic receptors are intact on the transplanted heart, it will eventually respond to circulating catecholamines.

Cardiac dysrhythmias may occur in heart transplant patients, perhaps reflecting a lack of vagal innervation and/or increased levels of circulating catecholamines. At rest, the heart rate reflects the intrinsic rate of depolarization of the donor sinoatrial node in the absence of any vagal tone. First-degree atrioventricular block (an increased PR interval) is common after cardiac transplantation. Some patients may require a cardiac pacemaker for treatment of bradydysrhythmias. A surgical transplantation technique that preserves the anatomic integrity of the right atrium by using anastomoses at the level of the superior and inferior vena cava rather than at the mid-atrial level results in better preservation of sinoatrial node and tricuspid valve function. Afferent denervation renders the cardiac transplant patient incapable of experiencing angina pectoris in response to myocardial ischemia.

RESPONSE TO DRUGS

Catecholamine responses are different in the transplanted heart because the intact sympathetic nerves required for normal uptake and metabolism of catecholamines are absent. The density of α and β receptors in the transplanted heart is unchanged, however, and responses to direct-acting sympathomimetic drugs are intact. Epinephrine, isoproterenol, and dobutamine have similar effects in normal and denervated hearts. Indirect-acting sympathomimetics such as ephedrine have a blunted effect in denervated hearts.

Vagolytic drugs such as atropine do not increase the heart rate. Pancuronium does not increase the heart rate, and neostigmine and other anticholinesterases do not slow the heart rate of denervated hearts.

PREOPERATIVE EVALUATION

At presentation heart transplant recipients may have ongoing rejection manifesting as myocardial dysfunction, accelerated coronary atherosclerosis, or dysrhythmias. All preoperative drug therapy must be continued, and proper functioning of a cardiac pacemaker must be confirmed. Cyclosporine-induced hypertension may require treatment with calcium channel–blocking drugs or ACE inhibitors. Cyclosporine-induced nephrotoxicity may present as an increased creatinine concentration. In such cases anesthetic drugs excreted mainly by renal clearance mechanisms should be avoided. Proper hydration is important and should be confirmed preoperatively, because heart transplant patients are preload dependent.

MANAGEMENT OF ANESTHESIA

Experience suggests that heart transplant recipients undergoing noncardiac surgery have monitoring and anesthetic requirements similar to those of other patients undergoing the same surgery. Intravascular volume must be maintained intraoperatively, because these patients are preload dependent and the denervated heart is unable to respond to sudden shifts in blood volume with an increase in heart rate. Invasive hemodynamic monitoring may be considered if the planned procedure is associated with large fluid shifts. Transesophageal echocardiography is an alternative to invasive hemodynamic monitoring in these patients. General anesthesia is usually selected because there may be an impaired response to the hypotension associated with spinal or epidural anesthesia. Anesthetic management includes avoidance of significant vasodilation and acute reductions in preload. Although volatile anesthetics may produce myocardial depression, they are usually well tolerated in heart transplant patients who do not have significant heart failure. Despite reports of cyclosporine-induced enhanced neuromuscular blockade, it does not appear that these patients require different dosing of muscle relaxants than normal patients. Careful attention must be paid to appropriate aseptic technique because of the increased susceptibility to infection.

KEY POINTS

- The exercise ECG is most likely to indicate myocardial ischemia when there is at least 1 mm of horizontal or down-sloping ST-segment depression during or within 4 minutes after exercise. The greater the degree of ST-segment depression, the greater the likelihood of significant coronary disease. When the ST-segment abnormality is associated with angina pectoris and occurs during the early stages of exercise and persists for several minutes after exercise, significant coronary artery disease is very likely.

- Noninvasive imaging tests for the detection of ischemic heart disease are used when exercise ECG is not possible or interpretation of ST-segment changes would be difficult. Administration of atropine, infusion of dobutamine, institution of cardiac pacing, or administration of a coronary vasodilator such as adenosine or dipyridamole creates cardiac stress. After stress is induced, either echocardiography to assess myocardial function or radionuclide imaging to assess myocardial perfusion is performed.

- β-Blockers are the principal drug treatment for patients with angina pectoris. Long-term administration of β-blockers decreases the risk of death and myocardial reinfarction in patients who have had an MI, presumably by decreasing myocardial oxygen demand. This benefit is present even in patients in whom β-blockers were traditionally thought to be contraindicated, such as those with congestive heart failure, pulmonary disease, or advanced age.

- Patients with acute coronary syndrome can be categorized based on a 12-lead ECG. Patients with ST elevation at presentation are considered to have STEMI. Patients who have

ST-segment depression or nonspecific ECG changes can be classified based on the level of cardiac-specific troponins or CK-MB. Elevation of cardiac-specific biomarkers indicates NSTEMI. If levels of cardiac-specific biomarkers are normal, then unstable angina is present.

■ STEMI occurs when coronary blood flow decreases abruptly. This decrease in blood flow is attributable to acute thrombus formation at a site where an atherosclerotic plaque fissures, ruptures, or ulcerates, which creates a local environment that favors thrombogenesis. Typically, vulnerable plaques—that is, those with rich lipid cores and thin fibrous caps—are most prone to rupture. Plaques that rupture are rarely of a size that causes significant coronary obstruction. By contrast, flow-restrictive plaques that produce angina pectoris and stimulate development of collateral circulation are less likely to rupture.

■ The primary goal in the management of STEMI is reestablishment of blood flow in the obstructed coronary artery as soon as possible. This can be achieved by reperfusion therapy or coronary angioplasty with or without placement of an intracoronary stent. Thrombolytic therapy is associated with hemorrhagic stroke in 0.3% to 1% of patients.

■ Administration of β-blockers after an acute MI is associated with a significant decrease in early (in-hospital) and long-term mortality and myocardial reinfarction. Early administration of β-blockers can decrease infarct size by decreasing heart rate, blood pressure, and myocardial contractility. In the absence of specific contraindications, it is recommended that all patients receive intravenous β-blockers as soon as possible after acute MI.

■ NSTEMI and unstable angina result from a reduction in myocardial oxygen supply. Rupture or erosion of an atherosclerotic coronary plaque leads to thrombosis, inflammation, and vasoconstriction. Embolization of platelets and clot fragments into the coronary microvasculature leads to microcirculatory ischemia and infarction and results in elevation of cardiac biomarker levels.

■ Infarction of the anterior wall and/or apex of the left ventricle can result in intracardiac thrombus formation in as many as one third of patients. Echocardiography can be used to detect this thrombus. The presence of a left ventricular thrombus is an indication for immediate anticoagulation with heparin followed by 6 months of anticoagulation with warfarin.

■ Most postoperative MIs are NSTEMIs and can be diagnosed by ECG changes and/or release of cardiac biomarkers. Two different pathophysiologic mechanisms may be responsible for perioperative MI. One is related to acute coronary thrombosis, and the other is the consequence of increased myocardial oxygen demand in the setting of compromised myocardial oxygen supply.

■ Acute MI (1 to 7 days previously), recent MI (8 to 30 days previously), and unstable angina are associated with the highest risk of perioperative myocardial ischemia, MI, and cardiac death.

■ Coronary artery stent placement (drug-eluting or bare metal stent) is routinely followed by dual antiplatelet therapy to prevent acute coronary thrombosis and maintain long-term patency of the vessel. Elective noncardiac surgery should be delayed for 6 weeks after a PCI with bare metal stent placement and for at least 12 months after a PCI with drug-eluting stent placement to allow endothelialization of the stent and completion of dual antiplatelet therapy.

■ The simplest, most cost-effective method for detecting perioperative myocardial ischemia is ECG. The diagnosis of myocardial ischemia focuses on changes in the ST segment characterized as elevation or depression of at least 1 mm. The degree of ST-segment depression parallels the severity of myocardial ischemia. T-wave inversion can also be associated with myocardial ischemia. Events other than myocardial ischemia that can cause ST-segment abnormalities include cardiac dysrhythmias, cardiac conduction disturbances, digitalis therapy, electrolyte abnormalities, and hypothermia.

■ The transplanted heart has no sympathetic, parasympathetic, or sensory innervation, and the loss of vagal tone results in a higher than normal resting heart rate. Carotid sinus massage and Valsalva's maneuver have no effect on heart rate. There is no sympathetic response to direct laryngoscopy and tracheal intubation, and the denervated heart has a blunted heart rate response to light anesthesia or intense pain. The transplanted heart is unable to increase its heart rate immediately in response to hypovolemia or hypotension. It responds instead with an increase in stroke volume via the Frank-Starling mechanism. The needed increase in cardiac output is then dependent on venous return. After several minutes, the heart rate increases in response to the effect of circulating catecholamines. Because α- and β-adrenergic receptors are intact on the transplanted heart, it eventually responds to circulating catecholamines.

■ One of the late complications of cardiac transplantation is the development of coronary artery disease in the allograft. Diffuse obliterative coronary arteriopathy affects cardiac transplant recipients over time, and the ischemic sequelae of this form of coronary disease are the principal limitations to long-term survival. The arterial disease is restricted to the allograft and is present in about one half of cardiac transplant recipients after 5 years. The accelerated appearance of this coronary artery disease likely reflects a chronic rejection process in the vascular endothelium.

RESOURCES

Anderson JL, Adams CD, Antman EM, et al. 2011 ACCF/AHA focused update incorporated into the ACC/AHA 2007 Guidelines for the Management of Patients with Unstable Angina/Non–ST-Elevation Myocardial Infarction: a report of the American College of Cardiology Foundation/ American Heart Association Task Force on Practice Guidelines. *Circulation*. 2011;123(18):e426-e579.

Antman EM. ST-segment myocardial infarction: pathology, pathophysiology, and clinical features. In: Bonow RO, Mann DL, Zipes DP, et al. eds. *Braunwald's Heart Disease*. Philadelphia, PA: Saunders; 2012.

Barash P, Akhtar S. Coronary stents: factors contributing to perioperative major adverse cardiovascular events. *Br J Anaesth*. 2010;105(suppl 1):i3-i15.

Cannon CP, Braunwald E. Unstable angina and non–ST elevation myocardial infarction. In: Bonow RO, Mann DL, Zipes DP, et al. eds. *Braunwald's Heart Disease*. Philadelphia, PA: Saunders; 2012.

Fleisher LA, Beckman JA, Brown KA, et al. 2009 ACCF/AHA focused update on perioperative beta blockade incorporated into the ACC/AHA 2007 Guidelines on Perioperative Cardiovascular Evaluation and Care for Noncardiac Surgery: a report of the American College of Cardiology Foundation/American Heart Association Task Force on Practice Guidelines. *Circulation*. 2009;120(21):e169-e276.

Gibbons RJ, Abrams J, Chatterjee K, et al. ACC/AHA 2002 guideline update for the management of patients with chronic stable angina—summary article: a report of the American College of Cardiology/American Heart Association Task Force on Practice Guidelines (Committee on the Management of Patients with Chronic Stable Angina). *J Am Coll Cardiol*. 2003;41:159-168.

Kushner FG, Hand M, Smith Jr SC, et al. 2009 focused updates: ACC/AHA guidelines for the management of patients with ST-elevation myocardial infarction (updating the 2004 guideline and 2007 focused update) and ACC/AHA/SCAI guidelines on percutaneous coronary intervention (updating the 2005 guideline and 2007 focused update): a report of the American College of Cardiology Foundation/American Heart Association Task Force on Practice Guidelines. *Circulation*. 2009;120(22):2271-2306.

Opie L, Poole-Wilson P. Beta-blocking agents. In: Opie L, Gersh BJ, eds. *Drugs for the Heart*. Philadelphia, PA: Saunders; 2009.

Poldermans D, Bax JJ, Boersma E, et al. Guidelines for pre-operative cardiac risk assessment and perioperative cardiac management in non-cardiac surgery: the Task Force for Preoperative Cardiac Risk Assessment and Perioperative Cardiac Management in Non-cardiac Surgery of the European Society of Cardiology (ESC) and endorsed by the European Society of Anaesthesiology (ESA). *Eur Heart J*. 2009;30(22):2769-2812.

Thygesen K, Alpert JS, White HD, et al. Universal definition of myocardial infarction. *Circulation*. 2007;116:2634-2653.

Valvular Heart Disease

ADRIANA HERRERA ∎

The prevalence of valvular heart disease in the United States is currently around 2.5% and is expected to increase significantly with the aging of the population. This form of heart disease continues to be an important cause of perioperative morbidity and mortality. In the past 25 years there have been major advances in understanding the natural history of valvular heart disease and in improving cardiac function in patients with valvular disorders. The development of better noninvasive methods of monitoring ventricular function, improved prosthetic heart valves, and better techniques for valve reconstruction as well as the formulation of guidelines for selecting the proper timing for surgical intervention have resulted in better outcomes in these patients.

Valvular heart disease places a hemodynamic burden on the left and/or right ventricle that is initially tolerated as a result of various compensations of the cardiovascular system. However, hemodynamic overload eventually leads to cardiac muscle dysfunction, congestive heart failure (CHF), or even sudden death. Management of patients with valvular heart disease during the perioperative period requires an understanding of the hemodynamic alterations that accompany valvular dysfunction. The most frequently encountered cardiac valve lesions produce pressure overload (mitral stenosis, aortic stenosis) or volume overload (mitral regurgitation, aortic regurgitation) on the left atrium or left ventricle. Anesthetic management during the perioperative period is based on the likely effects of drug-induced changes in cardiac rhythm and rate, preload, afterload, myocardial contractility, systemic blood pressure, systemic vascular resistance, and pulmonary vascular resistance relative to the pathophysiology of the specific valvular lesion.

PREOPERATIVE EVALUATION

Preoperative evaluation of patients with valvular heart disease includes assessment of (1) the severity of the cardiac disease, (2) the degree of impaired myocardial contractility, and (3) the presence of associated major organ system disease. Recognition of compensatory mechanisms for maintaining cardiac

TABLE 2-1   New York Heart Association functional classification of patients with heart disease

Class	Description
I	Asymptomatic
II	Symptoms with ordinary activity but comfortable at rest
III	Symptoms with minimal activity but comfortable at rest
IV	Symptoms at rest

output such as increased sympathetic nervous system activity and cardiac hypertrophy as well as consideration of current drug therapy are important. The presence of a prosthetic heart valve introduces special considerations in the preoperative evaluation, especially if noncardiac surgery is planned.

History and Physical Examination

Questions designed to define exercise tolerance are necessary to evaluate cardiac reserve in the presence of valvular heart disease and to provide a functional classification according to the criteria established by the New York Heart Association (Table 2-1). When myocardial contractility is impaired, patients complain of dyspnea, orthopnea, and easy fatigability. A compensatory increase in sympathetic nervous system activity may manifest as anxiety, diaphoresis, and resting tachycardia. CHF is a frequent companion of chronic valvular heart disease, and its presence is detected by noting basilar chest rales, jugular venous distention, and a third heart sound. Typically, elective surgery is deferred until CHF can be treated and myocardial contractility optimized.

Disease of a cardiac valve rarely occurs without an accompanying murmur, reflecting turbulent blood flow across the valve. The character, location, intensity, and direction of radiation of a heart murmur provide clues to the location and severity of the valvular lesion. During systole, the aortic and pulmonic valves are open, and the mitral and tricuspid valves are closed. Therefore, a heart murmur that occurs during systole is due to stenosis of the aortic or pulmonic valves or incompetence of the mitral or tricuspid valves. During diastole, the aortic and pulmonic valves are closed, and the mitral and tricuspid valves are open. Therefore, a diastolic heart murmur is due to stenosis of the mitral or tricuspid valves or incompetence of the aortic or pulmonic valves.

Cardiac dysrhythmias are seen with all types of valvular heart disease. Atrial fibrillation is common, especially with mitral valve disease associated with left atrial enlargement. Atrial fibrillation may be paroxysmal or chronic.

Angina pectoris may occur in patients with valvular heart disease even in the absence of coronary artery disease. It usually reflects increased myocardial oxygen demand due to ventricular hypertrophy. The demands of this thickened muscle mass may exceed the ability of even normal coronary arteries to deliver adequate amounts of oxygen. Valvular heart disease and ischemic

heart disease frequently co-exist. Fifty percent of patients with aortic stenosis who are older than 50 years of age have associated ischemic heart disease. The presence of coronary artery disease in patients with mitral or aortic valve disease worsens the long-term prognosis, and mitral regurgitation due to ischemic heart disease is associated with an increased mortality.

Drug Therapy

Modern drug therapy for valvular heart disease may include β-blockers, calcium channel blockers, and digitalis for heart rate control; angiotensin-converting enzyme inhibitors and vasodilators to control blood pressure and afterload; and diuretics, inotropes, and vasodilators as needed to control heart failure. Antidysrhythmic therapy may also be necessary. Certain cardiac lesions such as aortic and mitral stenosis require a slow heart rate to prolong the duration of diastole and improve left ventricular filling and coronary blood flow. The regurgitant valvular lesions such as aortic and mitral regurgitation require afterload reduction and a somewhat faster heart rate to shorten the time for regurgitation. Atrial fibrillation requires a controlled ventricular response so that activation of the sympathetic nervous system, as during tracheal intubation or in response to surgical stimulation, does not cause sufficient tachycardia to significantly decrease diastolic filling time and stroke volume.

Laboratory Data

The electrocardiogram (ECG) often exhibits characteristic changes due to valvular heart disease. Broad and notched P waves (P mitrale) suggest the presence of left atrial enlargement typical of mitral valve disease. Left and right ventricular hypertrophy can be diagnosed by the presence of left or right axis deviation and high voltage. Other common ECG findings include dysrhythmias, conduction abnormalities, and evidence of active ischemia or previous myocardial infarction.

The size and shape of the heart and great vessels and pulmonary vascular markings can be evaluated by chest radiography. On a posteroanterior chest radiograph cardiomegaly can be established if the heart size exceeds 50% of the internal width of the thoracic cage. Abnormalities of the pulmonary artery, left atrium, and left ventricle can be noted along the left heart border, and right atrial and right ventricular enlargement along the right heart border. Enlargement of the left atrium can result in elevation of the left mainstem bronchus. Valvular calcifications may be identified. Vascular markings in the peripheral lung fields are sparse in the presence of significant pulmonary hypertension.

Echocardiography with color flow Doppler imaging is essential for noninvasive evaluation of valvular heart disease (Table 2-2). It is particularly useful in evaluating the significance of cardiac murmurs such as systolic ejection murmurs when aortic stenosis is suspected and in detecting the presence of mitral stenosis. It permits determination of cardiac anatomy and function, presence of hypertrophy, cavity dimensions, valve area, transvalvular pressure gradients, and the magnitude of valvular regurgitation.

TABLE 2-2 ■ **Utility of echocardiography in evaluation of valvular heart disease**

Determine significance of cardiac murmurs
Identify hemodynamic abnormalities associated with physical findings
Determine transvalvular pressure gradient
Determine valve area
Determine ventricular ejection fraction
Diagnose valvular regurgitation
Evaluate prosthetic valve function

TABLE 2-3 ■ **Complications associated with prosthetic heart valves**

Valve thrombosis
Systemic embolization
Structural failure
Hemolysis
Paravalvular leak
Endocarditis

Cardiac catheterization can provide information about the presence and severity of valvular stenosis and/or regurgitation, coronary artery disease, and intracardiac shunting and can help resolve discrepancies between clinical and echocardiographic findings. Transvalvular pressure gradients determined at the time of cardiac catheterization indicate the severity of the valvular heart disease. Mitral and aortic stenosis are considered to be severe when transvalvular pressure gradients are more than 10 mm Hg and 50 mm Hg, respectively. However, when CHF accompanies aortic stenosis, transvalvular pressure gradients may be smaller because of the inability of the dysfunctional left ventricular muscle to generate a large gradient. In patients with mitral stenosis or mitral regurgitation, measurement of pulmonary artery pressure and right ventricular filling pressure may provide evidence of pulmonary hypertension and right ventricular failure.

Presence of Prosthetic Heart Valves

Prosthetic heart valves may be mechanical or bioprosthetic. Mechanical valves are composed primarily of metal or carbon alloys and are classified according to their structure, such as caged-ball, single tilting-disk, or bileaflet tilting-disk valves. Bioprostheses may be heterografts, composed of porcine or bovine tissues mounted on metal supports, or homografts, which are preserved human aortic valves.

Prosthetic valves differ from one another with regard to durability, thrombogenicity, and hemodynamic profile. Mechanical valves are very durable, lasting at least 20 to 30 years, whereas bioprosthetic valves last about 10 to 15 years. Mechanical valves are highly thrombogenic and require long-term anticoagulation. Because bioprosthetic valves have a low thrombogenic potential, long-term anticoagulation often is not necessary. Mechanical valves are preferred in patients who are young, have a life expectancy of more than 10 to 15 years, or require long-term anticoagulation therapy for another reason, such as atrial fibrillation. Bioprosthetic valves are preferred in elderly patients and in those who cannot tolerate anticoagulation.

ASSESSMENT OF PROSTHETIC HEART VALVE FUNCTION

Prosthetic heart valve dysfunction is suggested by a change in the intensity or quality of prosthetic valve clicks, the appearance of a new murmur, or a change in the characteristics of an existing murmur. *Transthoracic echocardiography* can be used to assess sewing ring stability and leaflet motion of bioprosthetic valves, but mechanical valves may be difficult to evaluate with this method because of echo reverberations from the metal. *Transesophageal echocardiography* may provide higher-resolution images, especially of a prosthetic valve in the mitral position. Magnetic resonance imaging can be used if prosthetic valve regurgitation or a paravalvular leak is suspected but not adequately visualized by echocardiography. Cardiac catheterization permits measurement of transvalvular pressure gradients and effective valve area of bioprosthetic valves.

COMPLICATIONS ASSOCIATED WITH PROSTHETIC HEART VALVES

Prosthetic heart valves can be associated with significant complications whose presence should be considered during the preoperative evaluation (Table 2-3). Because of the risk of thromboembolism, patients with mechanical prosthetic heart valves require long-term anticoagulant therapy. Subclinical intravascular hemolysis, evidenced by an increased serum lactate dehydrogenase concentration, decreased serum haptoglobin concentration, and reticulocytosis, is noted in many patients with normally functioning mechanical heart valves. The incidence of pigmented gallstones is increased in patients with prosthetic heart valves, presumably as a result of chronic low-grade intravascular hemolysis. Severe hemolytic anemia is uncommon, and its presence usually indicates valvular dysfunction or endocarditis. Antibiotic prophylaxis is necessary to decrease the perioperative risk of infective endocarditis.

MANAGEMENT OF ANTICOAGULATION IN PATIENTS WITH PROSTHETIC HEART VALVES

Patients may need to discontinue anticoagulation before surgery. However, this temporary discontinuation of anticoagulant therapy puts patients with mechanical heart valves or atrial fibrillation at risk of arterial or venous thromboembolism due to a rebound hypercoagulable state and to the prothrombotic effects of surgery. The risk of thromboembolism is estimated to be about 5% to 8%. Anticoagulation may be continued in patients with prosthetic heart valves who are scheduled for minor surgery in which blood loss is expected to be minimal. When major surgery is planned, however, warfarin is typically discontinued 3 to 5 days preoperatively. Intravenous unfractionated heparin or subcutaneous low-molecular-weight heparin is administered after discontinuation of warfarin and continued until the day before or the day of surgery. The heparin can be restarted postoperatively when the risk of bleeding has lessened and can be continued until effective anticoagulation is again achieved with oral therapy. When possible, elective surgery should be avoided in the first month after an acute episode of arterial or venous thromboembolism.

Anticoagulant therapy is particularly important in parturients with prosthetic heart valves, because the incidence of arterial embolization is greatly increased during pregnancy. However, warfarin administration during the first trimester can be associated with fetal defects and fetal death. Therefore, warfarin is discontinued during pregnancy and subcutaneous standard or low-molecular-weight heparin is administered until delivery. Low-dose aspirin therapy is safe for the mother and fetus and can be used in conjunction with the heparin therapy.

Prevention of Bacterial Endocarditis

The American Heart Association (AHA) has made recommendations for prevention of infective endocarditis for the past half-century. The most recent Guidelines for the Prevention of Infective Endocarditis (2007) represent a radical departure from prior recommendations and dramatically reduce the indications for antibiotic prophylaxis. These guidelines are based on the best available evidence regarding this medical problem. Current scientific data suggest that infective endocarditis is more likely to result from frequent exposure to bacteremia associated with daily activities than from bacteremia associated with dental, gastrointestinal, or genitourinary tract procedures. For example, maintenance of good oral health and oral hygiene reduces bacteremia associated with normal daily activities (chewing, teeth brushing, flossing, use of toothpicks, etc.) and is more important than prophylactic antibiotics in reducing the risk of endocarditis. Endocarditis prophylaxis may prevent an exceedingly small number of cases of endocarditis, if any, in at-risk patients. It also appears that the risk of antibiotic-associated adverse events exceeds the benefits of endocarditis prophylaxis overall and that the common use of antibiotic prophylaxis promotes the emergence of antibiotic-resistant organisms.

Experts feel that infective endocarditis prophylaxis should be administered not to individuals with a high cumulative lifetime risk of contracting endocarditis but rather to individuals *at highest risk of adverse outcomes if they develop endocarditis*. It appears that only a very small group of patients with heart disease are likely to have the most severe forms and complications of endocarditis. The conditions associated with this high risk are listed in Table 2-4. The new AHA guidelines target endocarditis prophylaxis *only to patients with these conditions*. The recommendations regarding which antibiotic to use for endocarditis prophylaxis are not dissimilar from previous recommendations.

In summary, the major changes in the updated AHA guidelines for infective endocarditis prophylaxis are these: (1) Antibiotic prophylaxis for infective endocarditis is recommended

TABLE 2-4   Cardiac conditions associated with the highest risk of adverse outcomes from endocarditis for which prophylaxis for dental procedures is reasonable
1. Prosthetic cardiac valve or prosthetic material used for cardiac valve repair
2. Previous infective endocarditis
3. Congenital heart disease Unrepaired cyanotic congenital heart disease, including palliative shunts and conduits Completely repaired congenital heart defect with prosthetic material or device, whether placed by surgery or by catheter intervention, during the first 6 months after the procedure* Repaired congenital heart disease with residual defects at the site or adjacent to the site of a prosthetic patch or prosthetic device (which inhibit endothelialization)
4. Cardiac transplantation recipients who develop cardiac valvulopathy

From Wilson W, Taubert KA, Gewitz M, et al. Prevention of infective endocarditis: guidelines from the American Heart Association. *Circulation.* 2007;116:1736-1754, with permission.
Except for the conditions listed above, antibiotic prophylaxis is no longer recommended for any other form of congenital heart disease.
*Prophylaxis is reasonable because endothelialization of prosthetic material occurs within 6 months after the procedure.

only under a very few conditions. (2) Antibiotic prophylaxis *is* recommended for dental procedures that involve manipulation of gingival tissues or the periapical regions of the teeth, or perforation of the oral mucosa. (3) Antibiotic prophylaxis *is* recommended for invasive procedures, that is, those that involve incision or biopsy of the respiratory tract or infected skin, skin structures, or musculoskeletal tissue. (4) Antibiotic prophylaxis *is not* recommended for genitourinary or gastrointestinal tract procedures.

MITRAL STENOSIS

The most common cause of mitral stenosis is rheumatic heart disease. The incidence of rheumatic fever in developed countries is very low, but the disease continues to be common in developing countries. Mitral stenosis primarily affects females. Diffuse thickening of the mitral leaflets and subvalvular apparatus, commissural fusion, and calcification of the annulus and leaflets are typically present. This process occurs slowly, and many patients do not become symptomatic for 20 to 30 years after the initial episode of rheumatic fever. Over time, the mitral valve becomes stenotic, and CHF, pulmonary hypertension, and right ventricular failure may develop.

Much less common causes of mitral stenosis include carcinoid syndrome, left atrial myxoma, severe mitral annular calcification, endocarditis, cor triatriatum, rheumatoid arthritis, systemic lupus erythematosus, congenital mitral stenosis, and iatrogenic mitral stenosis after mitral valve repair. Patients with mitral stenosis typically exhibit dyspnea on exertion, orthopnea, and paroxysmal nocturnal dyspnea as a result of high left atrial pressure. Left ventricular contractility is usually normal. Rheumatic heart disease presents as isolated mitral stenosis in about 40% of patients. If aortic and/or mitral regurgitation accompany mitral stenosis, there is often evidence of left ventricular dysfunction.

Pathophysiology

The normal mitral valve orifice area is 4 to 6 cm². Mitral stenosis is characterized by mechanical obstruction to left ventricular diastolic filling secondary to a progressive decrease in the size of the mitral valve orifice. This valvular obstruction produces an increase in left atrial volume and pressure. With mild mitral stenosis, left ventricular filling and stroke volume are maintained at rest by an increase in left atrial pressure. However, stroke volume will decrease during stress-induced tachycardia or when effective atrial contraction is lost, as with atrial fibrillation. Symptoms usually develop when mitral valve area is less than 1.5 cm². As the disease progresses the pulmonary venous pressure is increased in association with the increase in left atrial pressure. The result is transudation of fluid into the pulmonary interstitial space, decreased pulmonary compliance, and increased work of breathing, which leads to progressive dyspnea on exertion. Overt pulmonary edema is likely when the pulmonary venous pressure exceeds plasma oncotic pressure. If the increase in left atrial pressure is gradual, there is an increase in lymphatic drainage from the lungs and thickening of the capillary basement membrane that enables patients to tolerate an increased pulmonary venous pressure without development of pulmonary edema. Over time changes in the pulmonary vasculature result in pulmonary hypertension, and eventually right-sided heart failure may occur. Left ventricular function is usually preserved. Episodes of pulmonary edema typically occur with atrial fibrillation, sepsis, pain, and pregnancy.

Diagnosis

Echocardiography is used to assess the anatomy of the mitral valve, including the degree of leaflet thickening, calcification, changes in mobility, and extent of involvement of the subvalvular apparatus. The severity of mitral stenosis is assessed by calculation of mitral valve area and measurement of the transvalvular pressure gradient. Echocardiography also allows evaluation of cardiac chamber dimensions, pulmonary hypertension, left and right ventricular function, and other valvular disease, and examination of the left atrial appendage for the presence or absence of thrombus.

Patients with mitral stenosis usually become symptomatic when the size of the mitral valve orifice has decreased at least 50%. When the mitral valve area is less than 1 cm², a mean atrial pressure of about 25 mm Hg is necessary to maintain adequate left ventricular filling and resting cardiac output. Pulmonary hypertension is likely if the left atrial pressure is above 25 mm Hg over the long term. When the mitral transvalvular pressure gradient is higher than 10 mm Hg (normal value is <5 mm Hg), it is likely that mitral stenosis is severe.

When mitral stenosis is severe, any additional stress such as fever or sepsis may precipitate pulmonary edema.

Clinically, mitral stenosis is recognized by the characteristic opening snap that occurs early in diastole and by a rumbling diastolic heart murmur best heard at the apex or in the left axilla. Vibrations set in motion by the opening of the mobile but stenosed valve cause the opening snap. Calcification of the valve and greatly reduced leaflet mobility result in disappearance of the opening snap. Left atrial enlargement is often visible on chest radiographs as straightening of the left heart border and elevation of the left mainstem bronchus. The "double density" of an enlarged left atrium, mitral calcification, and evidence of pulmonary edema or pulmonary vascular congestion may also be seen. Broad notched P waves on the ECG suggest left atrial enlargement. Atrial fibrillation is present in about one third of patients with severe mitral stenosis.

Stasis of blood in the distended left atrium predisposes patients with mitral stenosis to a higher risk of *systemic* thromboembolism. *Venous* thrombosis is also more likely because of the decreased physical activity of these patients.

Treatment

When symptoms of mild mitral stenosis develop, diuretics can decrease the left atrial pressure and relieve symptoms. If atrial fibrillation occurs, heart rate control may be achieved with digoxin, β-blockers, calcium channel blockers, or a combination of these medications. Control of the heart rate is critical because tachycardia impairs left ventricular filling and increases left atrial pressure. Anticoagulation is required in patients with mitral stenosis and atrial fibrillation, because the risk of embolic stroke in such patients is about 7% to 15% per year. Warfarin is administered to a target international normalized ratio (INR) of 2.5 to 3.0. Surgical correction of mitral stenosis is indicated when symptoms worsen and pulmonary hypertension develops.

Mitral stenosis can sometimes be corrected by percutaneous balloon valvotomy. If heavy valvular calcification or valve deformity is present, surgical commissurotomy, valve reconstruction, or valve replacement is performed. In patients with concomitant severe tricuspid regurgitation (due to pulmonary hypertension), tricuspid valvuloplasty or ring annuloplasty can be performed together with the mitral valve surgery.

Management of Anesthesia

Management of anesthesia for noncardiac surgery in patients with mitral stenosis includes prevention and treatment of events that can decrease cardiac output or produce pulmonary edema (Table 2-5). The development of atrial fibrillation with a rapid ventricular response significantly decreases cardiac output and can produce pulmonary edema. Treatment consists of cardioversion or intravenous administration of amiodarone, β-blockers, calcium channel blockers, or digoxin. Excessive perioperative fluid administration, placement in Trendelenburg's position, or

TABLE 2-5	Intraoperative events that have a significant impact on mitral stenosis

Sinus tachycardia or a rapid ventricular response during atrial fibrillation

Marked increase in central blood volume, as associated with overtransfusion or head-down positioning

Drug-induced decrease in systemic vascular resistance

Hypoxemia and hypercarbia that may exacerbate pulmonary hypertension and evoke right ventricular failure

autotransfusion via uterine contraction increases central blood volume and can precipitate CHF. In patients with severe mitral stenosis, a sudden decrease in systemic vascular resistance may not be tolerated, because the normal response to hypotension—that is, a reflex increase in heart rate—itself decreases cardiac output. If necessary, systemic blood pressure and systemic vascular resistance can be maintained with vasoconstrictor drugs such as phenylephrine. Use of vasopressin may also be considered since it has minimal effect on pulmonary artery pressure. Pulmonary hypertension and right ventricular failure may be precipitated by numerous factors, including hypercarbia, hypoxemia, lung hyperinflation, and an increase in lung water. Right ventricular failure may require support with inotropic and pulmonary vasodilating drugs.

PREOPERATIVE MEDICATION

Preoperative medication can be used to decrease anxiety and its associated tachycardia, but it must be appreciated that patients with mitral stenosis may be more susceptible than normal patients to the ventilatory-depressant effects of these drugs. Preoperative administration of anticholinergics is not recommended, because the resultant tachycardia will be poorly tolerated.

Drugs used for heart rate control should be continued until the time of surgery. Diuretic-induced hypokalemia can be detected and treated preoperatively. Orthostatic hypotension may be evidence of diuretic-induced hypovolemia. It may be acceptable to continue anticoagulant therapy for minor surgery, but major surgery associated with significant blood loss requires discontinuation of anticoagulation.

Neuroaxial anesthesia is an acceptable technique in the absence of anticoagulation. Other regional techniques such as peripheral nerve blocks may also be used safely. The American Society of Regional Anesthesia and Pain Medicine (ASRA) evidence-based guidelines on regional anesthesia in the patient receiving anticoagulation or thrombolytic therapy (third edition) should be followed as needed. Use of neuroaxial anesthesia requires measures to avoid hypotension, maintain adequate preload, and avoid tachycardia. Compared with spinal anesthesia, epidural anesthesia may allow better control of the level of sympathectomy and reduction in blood pressure.

INDUCTION OF ANESTHESIA

Induction of general anesthesia can be achieved using any intravenous induction drug with the exception of ketamine, which should be avoided because of its propensity to increase the heart rate. Tracheal intubation and muscle relaxation should be accomplished by administration of neuromuscular blockers that do not induce either tachycardia or hypotension from histamine release. Short-acting β-blockers may be necessary to treat episodes of tachycardia during induction. Cardioversion to treat new-onset atrial fibrillation with hemodynamic instability may be needed.

MAINTENANCE OF ANESTHESIA

Maintenance of anesthesia is best accomplished using drugs with minimal effects on heart rate, myocardial contractility, and systemic and pulmonary vascular resistance. Often a nitrous/narcotic anesthetic or a balanced anesthetic that includes a low concentration of a volatile anesthetic can achieve this goal. Nitrous oxide can evoke some pulmonary vasoconstriction and increase pulmonary vascular resistance if pulmonary hypertension is present.

Pharmacologic reversal of the effects of nondepolarizing muscle relaxants should be accomplished slowly to help ameliorate any drug-induced tachycardia caused by the anticholinergic drug in the mixture. Light anesthesia and/or surgical stimulation can result in sympathetic stimulation producing tachycardia and systemic and pulmonary hypertension. Pulmonary vasodilator therapy may be necessary if pulmonary hypertension is severe. Intraoperative fluid replacement must be carefully titrated, because these patients are very susceptible to volume overload and development of pulmonary edema.

MONITORING

Use of invasive monitoring depends on the complexity of the operative procedure and the magnitude of physiologic impairment caused by the mitral stenosis. Monitoring of asymptomatic patients without evidence of pulmonary congestion need be no different from monitoring of patients without valvular heart disease. On the other hand, transesophageal echocardiography can be useful in patients with symptomatic mitral stenosis undergoing major surgery, especially if significant blood loss is expected. Continuous monitoring of intraarterial pressure, pulmonary artery pressure, and left atrial pressure (pulmonary artery occlusion pressure) should be considered. Such monitoring helps confirm the adequacy of cardiac function, intravascular fluid volume, ventilation, and oxygenation. Patients with significant pulmonary hypertension are at greater risk of pulmonary artery rupture from manipulation of a pulmonary artery catheter, so measurement of pulmonary artery occlusion pressure should be done infrequently and very carefully.

POSTOPERATIVE MANAGEMENT

In patients with mitral stenosis, the risk of pulmonary edema and right heart failure continues into the postoperative period, so cardiovascular monitoring should continue as well. Pain and hypoventilation with subsequent respiratory acidosis and hypoxemia may be responsible for increasing heart rate and pulmonary vascular resistance. Decreased pulmonary compliance and increased work of breathing may necessitate a period of mechanical ventilation, particularly after major thoracic or abdominal surgery. Relief of postoperative pain with neuro-axial opioids can be very useful in selected patients. Anticoagulation therapy should be restarted as soon as the risk of perioperative bleeding has diminished.

MITRAL REGURGITATION

Mitral regurgitation due to rheumatic fever is usually associated with some degree of mitral stenosis. Isolated mitral regurgitation can be associated with ischemic heart disease or result from papillary muscle dysfunction, mitral annular dilation, or rupture of chordae tendineae. Other causes of mitral regurgitation include endocarditis, mitral valve prolapse, trauma, congenital heart disease (such as an endocardial cushion defect), left ventricular hypertrophy, cardiomyopathy, myxomatous degeneration, systemic lupus erythematosus, rheumatoid arthritis, ankylosing spondylitis, and carcinoid syndrome.

Pathophysiology

The basic hemodynamic derangement in mitral regurgitation is a decrease in forward left ventricular stroke volume and cardiac output. A portion of every stroke volume is regurgitated through the incompetent mitral valve back into the left atrium, which results in left atrial volume overload and pulmonary congestion. Patients with a regurgitant fraction of more than 0.6 are considered to have severe mitral regurgitation. The fraction of left ventricular stroke volume that regurgitates into the left atrium depends on (1) the size of the mitral valve orifice; (2) heart rate, which determines the duration of ventricular ejection; and (3) pressure gradients across the mitral valve. Such gradients are related to left ventricle compliance and impedance to left ventricular ejection into the aorta. Pharmacologic interventions that increase or decrease systemic vascular resistance have a major impact on the regurgitant fraction in patients with mitral regurgitation.

Patients with isolated mitral regurgitation are less dependent on properly timed left atrial contraction for left ventricular filling than are patients with co-existing mitral or aortic stenosis. Patients with rheumatic fever–induced mitral regurgitation are most likely to exhibit marked left atrial enlargement and atrial fibrillation. Myocardial ischemia as a result of mitral regurgitation is uncommon, because the increased left ventricular wall tension is quickly dissipated as the stroke volume is rapidly ejected into the aorta and left atrium. When mitral regurgitation develops gradually, the volume overload produced by mitral regurgitation transforms the left ventricle into a larger, more compliant chamber that is able to deliver a larger stroke volume. This occurs through a dissolution of collagen weave, remodeling of the extracellular matrix, rearrangement of myocardial fibers, and addition of new sarcomeres with the development of ventricular hypertrophy. Development of ventricular hypertrophy and increased compliance of the left atrium permit the accommodation of the regurgitant volume without a major increase in left atrial pressure. This allows patients to maintain cardiac output and remain free of pulmonary congestion, and to be asymptomatic for many years. The combination of mitral regurgitation and mitral stenosis results in volume and pressure overload of the left atrium and a markedly increased left atrial pressure. Atrial fibrillation, pulmonary edema, and pulmonary hypertension develop much earlier in these patients than in those with isolated mitral regurgitation.

Because there has been no time for development of left atrial or left ventricular compensation, *acute* mitral regurgitation presents as pulmonary edema and/or cardiogenic shock.

Diagnosis

Mitral regurgitation is recognized clinically by the presence of a holosystolic apical murmur with radiation to the axilla. Cardiomegaly can also be detected on physical examination. Severe mitral regurgitation can produce left atrial and left ventricular hypertrophy detectable on ECG and chest radiograph. Echocardiography confirms the presence, severity, and often the cause of the mitral regurgitation. Left atrial size and pressure, left ventricular wall thickness, cavitary dimensions, ventricular function, and pulmonary artery pressure can be measured. In addition, the left atrial appendage can be evaluated for the presence of thrombus. Many methods exist to determine the severity of mitral regurgitation. These include color flow and pulsed wave Doppler echocardiographic examination of the mitral valve with calculation of regurgitant volume and regurgitant fraction and measurement of the area of the regurgitant jet. The presence of a V wave in a pulmonary artery occlusion pressure waveform reflects regurgitant flow through the mitral valve, and the size of this V wave correlates with the magnitude of the mitral regurgitation.

If the severity of mitral regurgitation is in doubt or mitral valve surgery is planned, cardiac catheterization, including coronary angiography, is necessary.

Treatment

Unlike stenotic valve lesions, regurgitant cardiac valve lesions often progress insidiously, causing left ventricular damage and remodeling before symptoms have developed. Early surgery may be warranted to prevent left ventricular muscle dysfunction from becoming severe or irreversible. Survival may be prolonged if surgery is performed before the ejection fraction is less than 60% or before the left ventricle is unable to contract to an end-systolic dimension of 45 mm (normal <40 mm). Patients with an ejection fraction of less than 30% or a left ventricular end-systolic dimension of more than 55 mm do not experience improvement with mitral valve surgery. *Symptomatic* patients should undergo mitral valve surgery even if the ejection fraction is normal. Mitral valve repair, if possible, is preferred to mitral valve replacement because it restores valve competence, maintains the functional aspects of the mitral valve apparatus, and avoids insertion of a prosthesis. The mitral valve apparatus is very important in supporting left ventricular function. The

TABLE 2-6   Anesthetic considerations in patients with mitral regurgitation

Prevent bradycardia
Prevent increases in systemic vascular resistance
Minimize drug-induced myocardial depression
Monitor the magnitude of regurgitant flow with a pulmonary artery catheter (size of the V wave) and/or echocardiography

absence of the subvalvular apparatus causes distortion of left ventricular contractile geometry and impairment of left ventricular ejection. In patients in whom the valve and its apparatus cannot be preserved, valve replacement is done, but there is a postoperative decline in left ventricular ejection fraction.

Although vasodilators are useful in the medical management of acute mitral regurgitation, there is no apparent benefit to long-term use of these drugs in *asymptomatic* patients with chronic mitral regurgitation. For *symptomatic* patients, angiotensin-converting enzyme inhibitors or β-blockers (particularly carvedilol) and biventricular pacing have all been shown to decrease functional mitral regurgitation and improve symptoms and exercise tolerance.

Management of Anesthesia

Management of anesthesia for noncardiac surgery in patients with mitral regurgitation includes prevention and treatment of events that may further decrease cardiac output (Table 2-6). The goal is to improve forward left ventricular stroke volume and decrease the regurgitant fraction. Maintenance of a normal to slightly increased heart rate is recommended. Bradycardia may result in severe left ventricular volume overload. Increases in systemic vascular resistance can also cause decompensation of the left ventricle. Afterload reduction with a vasodilator drug such as nitroprusside with or without an inotropic drug will improve left ventricular function. In most patients, cardiac output can be maintained or improved with modest increases in heart rate and modest decreases in systemic vascular resistance. The decrease in systemic vascular resistance caused by regional anesthesia may be beneficial in some patients. Preoperative sedation and anticholinergics are usually well tolerated.

INDUCTION OF ANESTHESIA

Induction of anesthesia can be achieved with an intravenous induction drug. Dosing should be adjusted to prevent an increase in systemic vascular resistance or a decrease in heart rate, because both of these hemodynamic changes reduce cardiac output. Selection of a muscle relaxant should follow the same principles. Pancuronium produces a modest increase in heart rate, which can contribute to maintenance of forward left ventricular stroke volume.

MAINTENANCE OF ANESTHESIA

Volatile anesthetics can be administered to attenuate the undesirable increases in systemic blood pressure and systemic vascular resistance that can accompany surgical stimulation.

The increase in heart rate and decrease in systemic vascular resistance plus the minimal negative inotropic effects associated with isoflurane, desflurane, and sevoflurane make them all acceptable choices for maintenance of anesthesia. When myocardial function is severely compromised, use of an opioid-based anesthetic is another option because of the minimal myocardial depression that opioids produce. However, potent narcotics can produce significant bradycardia, and this would be very deleterious in the presence of severe mitral regurgitation. Mechanical ventilation should be adjusted to maintain near-normal values on acid-base and respiratory parameters. The pattern of ventilation must provide sufficient time between breaths for adequate venous return. Maintenance of intravascular fluid volume is very important for maintaining left ventricular volume and cardiac output. Neuraxial techniques will result in afterload reduction, decreasing the regurgitant volume. Other regional techniques are also considered safe for these patients. ASRA guidelines for regional anesthesia in patients receiving anticoagulation therapy should be followed.

MONITORING

Anesthesia for surgery in patients with asymptomatic mitral regurgitation does not require invasive monitoring. However, in the presence of severe mitral regurgitation, the use of invasive monitoring is helpful for detecting the adequacy of cardiac output and the hemodynamic response to anesthetic and vasodilating drugs and for facilitating intravenous fluid replacement. Mitral regurgitation produces a V wave on the pulmonary artery occlusion pressure waveform. Changes in V wave amplitude can assist in estimating the magnitude and direction of changes in the degree of mitral regurgitation. However, pulmonary artery occlusion pressure may be a poor measure of left ventricular end-diastolic volume in patients with *chronic* mitral regurgitation. With *acute* mitral regurgitation, the left atrium is less compliant, and pulmonary artery occlusion pressure does correlate with left atrial and left ventricular end-diastolic pressure. Transesophageal echocardiography is another useful technique for monitoring mitral valve and left ventricular function during major surgery.

MITRAL VALVE PROLAPSE

Mitral valve prolapse (MVP) is defined as the prolapse of one or both mitral leaflets into the left atrium during systole with or without mitral regurgitation. It is associated with the auscultatory findings of a midsystolic click and a late systolic murmur. MVP is the most common form of valvular heart disease, affecting 1% to 2.5% of the U.S. population. It is more common in young women. MVP can be associated with Marfan's syndrome, rheumatic carditis, myocarditis, thyrotoxicosis, and systemic lupus erythematosus. Although it is usually a benign condition, MVP can have devastating complications such as cerebral embolic events, infective endocarditis, severe mitral regurgitation requiring surgery, dysrhythmias, and sudden death. Patients with MVP and abnormal mitral valve morphology appear to be the subset of patients at risk for these complications.

Diagnosis

The definitive diagnosis of MVP is based on echocardiographic findings. It has been defined as valve prolapse of 2 mm or more above the mitral annulus. MVP can occur with or without leaflet thickening and with or without mitral regurgitation. Patients with redundant and thickened leaflets have a primary (anatomic) form of MVP. This form of MVP typically occurs in patients with connective tissue diseases or in elderly men. Patients with mild bowing and normal-appearing leaflets have a normal variant (functional) form of MVP, and their risk of adverse events is probably no different from that of the general population.

Patients with MVP may experience anxiety, orthostatic symptoms, palpitations, dyspnea, fatigue and atypical chest pain. Cardiac dysrhythmias, both supraventricular and ventricular, may occur and respond well to β-blocker therapy. Cardiac conduction abnormalities are not uncommon.

Management of Anesthesia

Management of anesthesia for noncardiac surgery in patients with MVP follows the same principles outlined earlier for patients with mitral regurgitation. Management is influenced primarily by the degree of mitral regurgitation. Interestingly, the degree of MVP can be affected by left ventricular dimensions and is more dynamic than mitral valvular disease. A larger ventricle will often have less prolapse (and regurgitation) than a smaller ventricle. So events that affect how much the left ventricle fills or empties with each cardiac cycle will affect the amount of mitral regurgitation. Perioperative events that enhance left ventricular *emptying* include (1) increased sympathetic activity that increases myocardial contractility, (2) decreased systemic vascular resistance, and (3) assumption of the upright posture. Hypovolemia reduces left ventricular *filling*. Events that *decrease* left ventricular emptying and *increase* left ventricular volume may *decrease* the degree of MVP. These include hypertension or vasoconstriction, drug-induced myocardial depression, and volume resuscitation.

PREOPERATIVE EVALUATION

In the absence of symptoms, the finding of a systolic click and murmur does not warrant a preoperative cardiologic consultation.

Preoperative evaluation of patients with a diagnosis of MVP should focus on distinguishing patients with purely functional disease from those with significant mitral regurgitation. Functional MVP is most often present in women younger than 45 years of age. Some patients may be taking β-blockers to control dysrhythmias, and these drugs should be continued throughout the perioperative period. Patients with a history of transient neurologic events who are in sinus rhythm with no

atrial thrombi are likely to be taking daily aspirin therapy (81 to 325 mg/day), whereas patients with atrial fibrillation and/or left atrial thrombis and/or previous stroke are likely to be taking warfarin. Although the ECG frequently shows premature ventricular contractions, repolarization abnormalities, and QT interval prolongation, there is no evidence that these findings predict or are associated with adverse intraoperative events.

Older men with an anatomic form of MVP can have symptoms of mild to moderate CHF, including exercise intolerance, orthopnea, and dyspnea on exertion. These patients may be taking diuretics and angiotensin-converting enzyme inhibitors. Physical examination often reveals a midsystolic to holosystolic murmur, an S_3 gallop, and signs of pulmonary congestion.

SELECTION OF ANESTHETIC TECHNIQUE

Most patients with MVP have normal left ventricular function and tolerate all forms of general and regional anesthesia. Volatile anesthetic–induced myocardial depression can be useful for offsetting the vasodilation that could decrease left ventricular volume and increase mitral prolapse and/or regurgitation. There is no contraindication to the use of regional anesthesia in patients with MVP. The decrease in systemic vascular resistance should be anticipated, and administration of fluids should offset any changes in left ventricular volume that could affect the degree of prolapse and regurgitation.

INDUCTION OF ANESTHESIA

When an intravenous induction drug is selected, the need to avoid a significant or prolonged decrease in systemic vascular resistance must be considered. Etomidate causes minimal myocardial depression and minimal alterations in sympathetic nervous system activity, so it is an attractive choice for induction of anesthesia in the presence of hemodynamically significant MVP. Ketamine, because of its ability to stimulate the sympathetic nervous system and enhance left ventricular emptying, may cause an increase in prolapse and regurgitation.

MAINTENANCE OF ANESTHESIA

Maintenance of anesthesia must minimize sympathetic nervous system activation resulting from painful intraoperative stimuli. Volatile anesthetics combined with nitrous oxide and/or opioids are useful for attenuating sympathetic nervous system activity, but their doses must be titrated to minimize a significant decrease in systemic vascular resistance.

Patients with hemodynamically significant MVP may not tolerate the dose-dependent myocardial depression of volatile anesthetics. However, low concentrations (about 0.5 minimum alveolar concentration) of isoflurane, desflurane, and sevoflurane can decrease the regurgitant fraction. In patients with severe mitral regurgitation, vasodilators such as nitroprusside or nitroglycerin may be carefully titrated to maximize forward left ventricular flow and decrease left ventricular end-diastolic volume and left atrial pressure. There are no clinical data to support the use of one muscle relaxant over another in the presence of isolated MVP, but drug-induced hemodynamic alterations such as vagolysis or histamine release deserve consideration when selecting a specific drug.

Unexpected ventricular dysrhythmias can occur during anesthesia, especially during operations performed with the patient in the head-up or sitting position. Presumably, in these positions, there is an increase in left ventricular emptying and accentuation of valve prolapse. Lidocaine and β-blockers can treat these dysrhythmias.

Maintenance of proper fluid balance blunts the decrease in venous return caused by positive pressure ventilation. Proper fluid balance also helps prevent an increase in the degree of prolapse. If vasopressors are needed, an α-agonist such as phenylephrine is acceptable. Use of an anesthetic technique that includes controlled hypotension would be unwise, because the change in systemic vascular resistance would enhance the degree of MVP.

MONITORING

Routine monitoring is all that is necessary in the majority of patients with MVP. An intraarterial catheter and pulmonary artery catheter or transesophageal echocardiography are needed only in patients with significant mitral regurgitation and left ventricular dysfunction.

AORTIC STENOSIS

Aortic stenosis is a common valvular lesion in the United States, and its incidence is increasing as the U.S. population grows older. Two factors are associated with development of aortic stenosis. The first is degeneration and calcification of the aortic leaflets and subsequent stenosis. This is a process of aging. The second factor is the presence of a bicuspid rather that a tricuspid aortic valve. Aortic stenosis develops earlier in life (30 to 50 years of age) in individuals with a *bicuspid* aortic valve than in those with a *tricuspid* aortic valve (60 to 80 years of age). Other causes include rheumatic heart disease and infective endocarditis. Aortic stenosis is associated with risk factors similar to those of ischemic heart disease, such as systemic hypertension and hypercholesterolemia.

Pathophysiology

Obstruction to ejection of blood into the aorta caused by a decrease in the aortic valve area necessitates an increase in left ventricular pressure to maintain stroke volume. The normal aortic valve area is 2.5 to 3.5 cm^2. Transvalvular pressure gradients higher than 50 mm Hg and an aortic valve area of less than 0.8 cm^2 are characteristic of *severe* aortic stenosis. Aortic stenosis is almost always associated with some degree of aortic regurgitation.

Angina pectoris may occur in patients with aortic stenosis despite the absence of coronary disease. This is due to an increase in myocardial oxygen requirements because of concentric left ventricular hypertrophy and the increase in myocardial work necessary to offset the afterload produced by the stenotic valve. In addition, myocardial oxygen delivery

is decreased because of the compression of subendocardial blood vessels by the increased left ventricular pressure.

Since the initial study by Goldman and colleagues in 1977 showing that patients with aortic stenosis had an increased risk of perioperative cardiac complications, many studies have demonstrated that patients with aortic stenosis have an increased risk of perioperative mortality and of nonfatal myocardial infarction regardless of the presence or absence of risk factors for coronary artery disease. The perioperative risk attributable to aortic stenosis is independent of the risk attributable to coronary artery disease.

The origin of syncope in patients with aortic stenosis is controversial but may reflect an exercise-induced decrease in systemic vascular resistance that remains uncompensated because cardiac output is limited by the stenotic valve. CHF can be due to systolic and/or diastolic dysfunction (Figure 2-1).

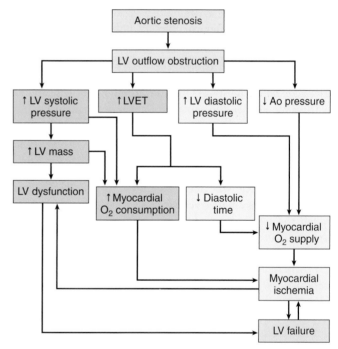

FIGURE 2-1 Pathophysiology of aortic stenosis. Left ventricular (LV) outflow obstruction results in an increased LV systolic pressure, increased LV ejection time (LVET), increased LV diastolic pressure, and decreased aortic (Ao) pressure. Increased LV systolic pressure with LV volume overload increases LV mass, which may lead to LV dysfunction and failure. Increased LV systolic pressure, LV mass, and LVET increase myocardial O_2 consumption. Increased LVET results in a decrease of diastolic time (myocardial perfusion time). Increased LV diastolic pressure and decreased Ao diastolic pressure decrease coronary perfusion pressure. Decreased diastolic time and coronary perfusion pressure decrease myocardial O_2 supply. Increased myocardial O_2 consumption and decreased myocardial O_2 supply produce myocardial ischemia, which causes LV function to deteriorate further. ↑, Increased; ↓, decreased. *(From Boudoulas H, Gravanis MB. Valvular heart disease. In: Gravanis MB, ed. Cardiovascular Disorders: Pathogenesis and Pathophysiology. St Louis, MO: Mosby; 1993:64.)*

Diagnosis

The classic clinical symptoms of *critical* aortic stenosis are angina pectoris, syncope, and dyspnea on exertion, a manifestation of CHF. The onset of these symptoms has been shown to correlate with an average time to death of 5, 3, and 2 years, respectively. About 75% of symptomatic patients will die within 3 years if they do not have a valve replacement. On physical examination, auscultation reveals a characteristic systolic murmur heard best in the aortic area. This murmur may radiate to the neck and mimic a carotid bruit. Because patients with aortic stenosis frequently have concomitant carotid artery disease, this finding deserves special attention. Because many patients with aortic stenosis are asymptomatic, it is important to listen for the systolic murmur of aortic stenosis in older patients scheduled for surgery. Chest radiography may show a prominent ascending aorta due to poststenotic aortic dilation. The ECG may demonstrate left ventricular hypertrophy.

Echocardiography with Doppler examination of the aortic valve provides a more accurate assessment of the severity of aortic stenosis than does clinical evaluation, and patients can be followed echocardiographically to assess the progression of their disease. Findings include identification of a trileaflet versus a bileaflet aortic valve, thickening and calcification of the aortic valve, decreased mobility of the aortic valve leaflets, left ventricular hypertrophy, and left ventricular systolic or diastolic dysfunction. Aortic valve area and transvalvular pressure gradients can be measured. Cardiac catheterization (and coronary angiography) may be necessary when the severity of aortic stenosis cannot be determined by echocardiography.

Exercise stress testing may be an additional strategy to evaluate asymptomatic patients with moderate to severe aortic stenosis to identify those with poor exercise tolerance and/or an abnormal blood pressure response to exercise. Patients with exercise-induced symptoms might benefit from aortic valve replacement.

Treatment

In asymptomatic patients with aortic stenosis, it appears to be safe to continue medical management and to delay valve replacement surgery until symptoms develop. However, there is a small risk of sudden death or rapid progression of symptoms and then sudden death. Mortality approaches 75% within 3 years after development of critical aortic stenosis unless the aortic valve is replaced. Even though most patients with aortic stenosis are elderly, the risks of valve replacement surgery are acceptable unless there are also serious comorbid diseases that can worsen outcome. Aortic valve replacement relieves the symptoms of aortic stenosis dramatically, and the ejection fraction usually increases. Coronary revascularization is often done at the time of aortic valve replacement in patients with both aortic stenosis and coronary artery disease.

Percutaneous aortic balloon valvotomy has been shown to be beneficial in adolescents and young adults with congenital or rheumatic aortic stenosis. However, adults with acquired aortic stenosis experience only temporary relief of symptoms with this procedure. Balloon valvotomy may occasionally be useful for palliation of aortic stenosis in patients who are not candidates for aortic valve replacement.

Management of Anesthesia

Patients with aortic stenosis coming for noncardiac surgery are at high risk of major perioperative cardiac complications, and the risk of these complications increases with the complexity of the surgery. Hence, it is important to ascertain the severity of the aortic stenosis preoperatively. Management of anesthesia in patients with aortic stenosis includes the prevention of hypotension and any hemodynamic change that will decrease cardiac output (Table 2-7).

Normal sinus rhythm must be maintained, because the left ventricle is dependent on a properly timed atrial contraction to produce an optimal left ventricular end-diastolic volume. Loss of atrial contraction, as during junctional rhythm or atrial fibrillation, may produce a dramatic decrease in stroke volume and blood pressure. The heart rate is important because it determines the time available for ventricular filling, for ejection of the stroke volume, and for coronary perfusion. A sustained increase in heart rate decreases the time for left ventricular filling and ejection and reduces cardiac output. A decrease in heart rate can cause overdistention of the left ventricle. Hypotension reduces coronary blood flow and results in myocardial ischemia and further deterioration in left ventricular function and cardiac output. Aggressive treatment of hypotension is mandatory to prevent cardiogenic shock and/or cardiac arrest. Cardiopulmonary resuscitation is *not* effective in patients with aortic stenosis because it is difficult, if not impossible, to create an adequate stroke volume across a stenotic aortic valve with cardiac compression.

INDUCTION OF ANESTHESIA

General anesthesia is often selected in preference to epidural or spinal anesthesia because the sympathetic blockade produced by regional anesthesia can lead to significant hypotension.

Induction of anesthesia can be accomplished with an intravenous induction drug that does not decrease systemic vascular resistance. An opioid induction agent may be useful if left ventricular function is compromised. Other good choices

TABLE 2-7 ■ Anesthetic considerations in patients with aortic stenosis

Maintain normal sinus rhythm
Avoid bradycardia or tachycardia
Avoid hypotension
Optimize intravascular fluid volume to maintain venous return and left ventricular filling

include benzodiazepines and etomidate. Ketamine may induce tachycardia and should be avoided.

MAINTENANCE OF ANESTHESIA

Maintenance of anesthesia can be accomplished with a combination of nitrous oxide and volatile anesthetic and opioids or with opioids alone. The primary goal is to maintain systemic vascular resistance and cardiac output. Drugs that depress sinus node automaticity can produce junctional rhythm and loss of properly timed atrial contraction, which can cause a significant reduction in cardiac output. If left ventricular function is impaired, it is prudent to avoid any drugs that can cause additional depression of myocardial contractility. A decrease in systemic vascular resistance is also very undesirable. Maintenance of anesthesia with nitrous oxide plus opioids or with opioids alone in high doses is recommended for patients with marked left ventricular dysfunction. Neuromuscular blocking drugs with minimal hemodynamic effects are best. Intravascular fluid volume should be maintained at normal levels, since these patients are preload dependent.

Hypotension should be treated aggressively with α-agonists such as phenylephrine that do not cause tachycardia and therefore maintain diastolic filling time. The onset of junctional rhythm or bradycardia requires prompt treatment with glycopyrrolate, atropine, or ephedrine. Persistent tachycardia can be treated with β-blockers such as esmolol. Supraventricular tachycardia should be promptly terminated by cardioversion. Lidocaine, amiodarone, and a defibrillator should be immediately available, since these patients have a propensity to develop ventricular dysrhythmias.

MONITORING

Intraoperative monitoring of patients with aortic stenosis must include ECG leads that reliably detect cardiac rhythm and left ventricular myocardial ischemia. The complexity of the surgery and the severity of the aortic stenosis influence the decision to use an intraarterial catheter, a central venous catheter, a pulmonary artery catheter, or transesophageal echocardiography. Such monitoring techniques help to determine whether intraoperative hypotension is due to hypovolemia or heart failure. Pulmonary artery occlusion pressure may overestimate left ventricular end-diastolic volume because of the decreased compliance of the hypertrophied left ventricle.

AORTIC REGURGITATION

Aortic regurgitation results from failure of aortic leaflet coaptation caused by disease of the aortic leaflets or of the aortic root. Common causes of leaflet abnormalities are infective endocarditis, rheumatic fever, bicuspid aortic valve, and the use of anorexigenic drugs. Abnormalities of the aortic root causing aortic regurgitation include idiopathic aortic root dilation, hypertension-induced aortoannular ectasia, aortic dissection, syphilitic aortitis, Marfan's syndrome, Ehlers-Danlos syndrome, rheumatoid arthritis, ankylosing spondylitis, and psoriatic arthritis. Acute aortic regurgitation is usually the result of endocarditis or aortic dissection.

Pathophysiology

The basic hemodynamic derangement in aortic regurgitation is a decrease in cardiac output because of regurgitation of a part of the ejected stroke volume from the aorta back into the left ventricle during diastole. This results in a combined pressure and volume overload on the left ventricle. The magnitude of the regurgitant volume depends on (1) the time available for the regurgitant flow to occur, which is determined by the heart rate; and (2) the pressure gradient across the aortic valve, which is dependent on the systemic vascular resistance. The magnitude of aortic regurgitation is decreased by tachycardia and peripheral vasodilation. With aortic regurgitation, the entire stroke volume is ejected into the aorta. Because the pulse pressure is proportional to the stroke volume and aortic elastance, the increased stroke volume increases systolic pressure, and systolic hypertension increases afterload. The left ventricle compensates by developing hypertrophy and enlarging to accommodate the volume overload. Because of the increased oxygen requirements necessitated by left ventricular hypertrophy and the decrease in aortic diastolic pressure, which reduces coronary blood flow, angina pectoris may occur in the absence of coronary artery disease.

The left ventricle can usually tolerate the chronic volume overload. However, if left ventricular failure occurs, left ventricular end-diastolic volume increases dramatically and pulmonary edema develops. A helpful indicator of left ventricular function in the presence of aortic regurgitation is the echocardiographically determined end-systolic volume and ejection fraction, both of which remain normal until left ventricular function becomes impaired. Indeed, surgery is recommended before the ejection fraction decreases to less than 55% and left ventricular end-systolic volume increases to more than 55 mL.

Compared to patients with chronic aortic regurgitation, patients with acute aortic regurgitation experience severe volume overload in a ventricle that has not had time to compensate. This typically results in coronary ischemia, rapid deterioration in left ventricular function, and heart failure (Figure 2-2).

Diagnosis

Aortic regurgitation is recognized clinically by its characteristic diastolic murmur, heard best along the right sternal border, and peripheral signs of a hyperdynamic circulation, including a widened pulse pressure, decreased diastolic blood pressure, and bounding pulses. In addition to the typical murmur of aortic regurgitation, there may be a low-pitched diastolic rumble (Austin-Flint murmur) that results from fluttering of the mitral valve caused by the regurgitant jet. As with mitral regurgitation, symptoms of aortic regurgitation may not appear until left ventricular dysfunction is present. Symptoms at this stage are manifestations of left ventricular failure (dyspnea, orthopnea, fatigue) and coronary ischemia.

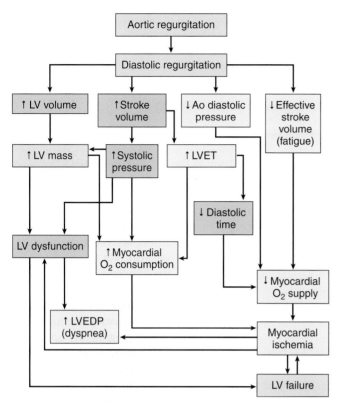

FIGURE 2-2 Pathophysiology of aortic regurgitation. Aortic regurgitation results in an increased left ventricular (LV) volume, increased stroke volume, increased aortic (Ao) systolic pressure, and decreased effective stroke volume. Increased LV volume results in an increased LV mass, which may lead to LV dysfunction and failure. Increased LV stroke volume increases systolic pressure and prolongs LV ejection time (LVET). Increased LV systolic pressure results in a decrease in diastolic time. Decreased diastolic time (myocardial perfusion time), diastolic aortic pressure, and effective stroke volume reduce myocardial O_2 supply. Increased myocardial O_2 consumption and decreased myocardial O_2 supply produce myocardial ischemia, which causes further deterioration in LV function. ↑, Increased; ↓, decreased; *LVEDP,* left ventricular end-diastolic pressure. *(From Boudoulas H, Gravanis MB: Valvular heart disease. In: Gravanis MB, ed. Cardiovascular Disorders: Pathogenesis and Pathophysiology. St Louis, MO: Mosby; 1993:64.)*

With chronic aortic regurgitation, evidence of left ventricular enlargement and left ventricular hypertrophy may be seen on the chest radiograph and ECG. Echocardiography will reveal any anatomic abnormalities of the aortic valve, including leaflet perforation or prolapse, and will identify any abnormalities in the aortic root and aortic annulus. Left ventricular size, volume, and ejection fraction can be measured, and Doppler examination can be used to identify the presence and severity of aortic regurgitation. Many methods exist to quantify aortic regurgitation. These include regurgitant jet width as a percentage of overall left ventricular outflow tract width, pressure half-time, and diastolic flow reversal in the descending aorta. Cardiac catheterization and cardiac magnetic resonance imaging may be useful for grading aortic regurgitation if echocardiography is insufficient.

TABLE 2-8 ■ Anesthetic considerations in patients with aortic regurgitation
Avoid bradycardia
Avoid increases in systemic vascular resistance
Minimize myocardial depression

Treatment

Surgical replacement of a diseased aortic valve is recommended before the onset of permanent left ventricular dysfunction, even if patients are asymptomatic. The operative mortality for isolated aortic valve replacement is approximately 4%. It is higher if there is concomitant aortic root replacement or coronary artery bypass grafting or if there are substantial comorbidities. The mortality rate of *asymptomatic* patients with normal left ventricular size and function is less than 0.2% per year. In contrast, *symptomatic* patients have a mortality rate greater than 10% per year. In acute aortic regurgitation, immediate surgical intervention is necessary, because the acute volume overload results in heart failure. Alternatives to aortic valve replacement with a prosthetic valve include a pulmonic valve autograft (Ross procedure) and aortic valve reconstruction.

Medical treatment of aortic regurgitation is designed to decrease systolic hypertension and left ventricular wall stress and improve left ventricular function. Intravenous infusion of a vasodilator such as nitroprusside and an inotropic drug such as dobutamine may be useful for improving left ventricular stroke volume and reducing regurgitant volume. Long-term therapy with nifedipine or hydralazine can be beneficial and may delay the need for surgery in asymptomatic patients with good left ventricular function.

Management of Anesthesia

Management of anesthesia for noncardiac surgery in patients with aortic regurgitation is designed to maintain forward left ventricular stroke volume (Table 2-8). The heart rate must be kept above 80 beats per minute because bradycardia, by increasing the duration of diastole and thereby the time for regurgitation, produces acute left ventricular volume overload. An abrupt increase in systemic vascular resistance can also precipitate left ventricular failure. The compensations for aortic regurgitation may be tenuous, and anesthetic-induced myocardial depression may upset this delicate balance. If left ventricular failure occurs, it is treated with a vasodilator to reduce afterload and an inotrope to increase contractility. Overall, modest increases in heart rate and modest decreases in systemic vascular resistance are reasonable hemodynamic goals during anesthesia. General anesthesia is the usual choice for patients with aortic regurgitation.

INDUCTION OF ANESTHESIA
Induction of anesthesia in the presence of aortic regurgitation can be achieved with an inhaled anesthetic or an intravenous induction drug. Ideally the induction drug should not decrease the heart rate or increase systemic vascular resistance.

In the absence of severe left ventricular dysfunction, maintenance of anesthesia is often provided with nitrous oxide plus a volatile anesthetic and/or opioid. The increase in heart rate, decrease in systemic vascular resistance, and minimal myocardial depression associated with isoflurane, desflurane, and sevoflurane make these drugs excellent choices in patients with aortic regurgitation. In patients with severe left ventricular dysfunction, high-dose opioid anesthesia may be preferred. Bradycardia and myocardial depression from concomitant use of nitrous oxide or a benzodiazepine are risks of the high-dose narcotic technique. Neuromuscular blockers with minimal or no effect on blood pressure and heart rate are typically used, although the modest increase in heart rate associated with pancuronium administration could be helpful in patients with aortic regurgitation.

Mechanical ventilation should be adjusted to maintain normal oxygenation and carbon dioxide elimination and provide adequate time for venous return. Intravascular fluid volume should be maintained at normal levels to provide for adequate preload. Bradycardia and junctional rhythm require prompt treatment with intravenous atropine.

Surgery in patients with asymptomatic aortic regurgitation may not require invasive monitoring. Standard monitors should be adequate to detect rhythm disturbances or myocardial ischemia. In the presence of severe aortic regurgitation, monitoring with a pulmonary artery catheter or transesophageal echocardiography is helpful for detecting myocardial depression, for facilitating intravascular volume replacement, and for measuring the response to administration of a vasodilating drug.

TRICUSPID REGURGITATION

Tricuspid regurgitation is usually *functional,* caused by tricuspid annular dilation secondary to right ventricle enlargement or pulmonary hypertension. Other causes include infective endocarditis (typically associated with intravenous drug abuse and unsterile injection), carcinoid syndrome, rheumatic heart disease, tricuspid valve prolapse, and Ebstein's anomaly. Tricuspid valve disease is often associated with mitral or aortic valve disease. Mild tricuspid regurgitation can be a normal finding at any age and is very commonly seen in highly trained athletes.

Pathophysiology

The basic hemodynamic consequence of tricuspid regurgitation is right atrial volume overload. The high compliance of the right atrium and vena cava result in only a minimal increase in right atrial pressure even in the presence of a large regurgitant volume. Even surgical removal of the tricuspid valve can be well tolerated. Signs of tricuspid regurgitation include jugular venous distention, hepatomegaly, ascites, and peripheral edema. The treatment of functional tricuspid regurgitation is aimed at the cause of the lesion, that is, at improving lung function, relieving left-sided heart failure, or reducing pulmonary hypertension. Surgical intervention for isolated tricuspid valve disease is rarely done but would be considered if other cardiac surgery is planned. A tricuspid annuloplasty or valvuloplasty may be performed. Tricuspid valve replacement is rarely performed.

Management of Anesthesia

Management of anesthesia in patients with tricuspid regurgitation includes maintenance of intravascular fluid volume and central venous pressure in the high-normal range to facilitate adequate right ventricular preload and left ventricular filling. Positive pressure ventilation and vasodilating drugs may be particularly deleterious if they significantly reduce venous return. Events known to increase pulmonary artery pressure, such as hypoxemia and hypercarbia, must also be avoided.

A specific anesthetic drug combination or technique cannot be recommended for management of patients with tricuspid regurgitation. Agents that produce some pulmonary vasodilation and those that maintain venous return are best. Nitrous oxide can be a weak pulmonary artery vasoconstrictor and could increase the degree of tricuspid regurgitation, so it is best avoided. Intraoperative monitoring should include measurement of right atrial pressure to guide intravenous fluid replacement and to detect changes in the amount of tricuspid regurgitation in response to administration of anesthetic drugs. With high right atrial pressures, the possibility of right-to-left intracardiac shunting through a patent foramen ovale must be considered. Taking meticulous care to avoid infusion of air through intravenous fluid systems can reduce the risk of a systemic air embolism.

TRICUSPID STENOSIS

Tricuspid stenosis is rare in the adult population. The most common cause in adults is rheumatic heart disease with co-existing tricuspid regurgitation and often mitral or aortic valve disease. Carcinoid syndrome and endomyocardial fibrosis are even rarer causes of tricuspid stenosis. Tricuspid stenosis increases right atrial pressure and increases the pressure gradient between the right atrium and right ventricle. Right atrial dimensions are increased, but the right ventricular dimensions are determined by the degree of volume overload from concomitant tricuspid regurgitation. Evaluation by echocardiography and color flow Doppler imaging helps estimate the severity of the stenosis.

PULMONIC VALVE REGURGITATION

Pulmonic valve regurgitation results from pulmonary hypertension with annular dilatation of the pulmonic valve. Other causes include connective tissue diseases, carcinoid syndrome, infective endocarditis, and rheumatic heart disease. Pulmonary regurgitation is rarely symptomatic.

PULMONIC STENOSIS

Pulmonic stenosis is usually congenital (either as part of a complex congenital cardiac lesion or as an isolated congenital defect) and detected and corrected in childhood. An acquired form can be due to rheumatic fever, carcinoid syndrome, infective endocarditis, or previous surgery or other interventions. Significant obstruction can cause syncope, angina, right ventricular hypertrophy, and right ventricular failure. Surgical valvotomy can be used to relieve the obstruction. Echocardiography is essential for evaluation and management.

NEW FRONTIERS IN THE TREATMENT OF VALVULAR HEART DISEASE

Aortic valve replacement in patients with critical aortic stenosis can be lifesaving. Aortic valve replacement has traditionally been accomplished via open heart surgery and the use of cardiopulmonary bypass. Patients who are deemed to be at very high risk or even inoperable because of age and multiple comorbid conditions have been treated medically or by balloon aortic valvotomy. This treatment might provide short-term relief of symptoms but does not alter the natural history of severe aortic stenosis. The need for alternative treatment options for this population of patients with valvular heart disease is now being addressed. During the last decade several different procedures have been developed to treat valvular heart disease without open heart surgery and cardiopulmonary bypass.

Transcatheter aortic valve implantation (TAVI) is a procedure that can be performed percutaneously via the femoral artery (retrograde and less invasive) or via puncture of the apex of the left ventricle (antegrade and more invasive) (Figure 2-3). An article by Leon and colleagues with a link to a video animation of this procedure is listed in the Resources section at the end of the chapter. The approach is chosen with consideration of iliac artery size; the presence of aortic or iliac disease, pathologic changes in the left ventricular apex, or pericardial disease; and any history of left thoracotomy or mediastinal or chest radiation. General anesthesia may be used for the transfemoral approach and is essential for the transapical approach. Transesophageal echocardiography is used initially to determine the aortic valve pathologic features, annulus size, and left ventricular function, and to detect the presence of mitral regurgitation and aortic atheromas. After implantation of the valve, echocardiography is used to assess prosthesis position; to determine the degree of aortic regurgitation, if any; and to detect the presence of perivalvular leaks, aortic dissection, mitral regurgitation, left ventricular dysfunction, or new regional wall motion abnormalities. Further research is needed to develop less traumatic devices with features providing cerebral protection to reduce the frequency of neurologic complications, which is currently rather high.

Compared with medical therapy or balloon valvotomy, transcatheter aortic valve implantation is associated with a lower 30-day and 1-year mortality from all causes, a greater improvement in cardiac symptoms, and a reduced need for repeat hospitalizations for cardiac reasons. Major complications of transcutaneous aortic valve replacement include

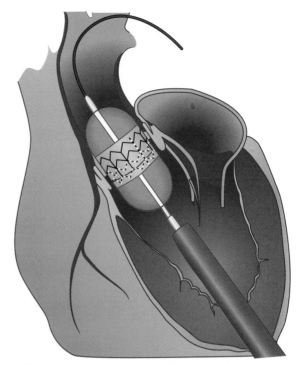

FIGURE 2-3 Schematic illustration of transapical aortic valve implantation. The prosthesis is being dilated at the annular level within the native aortic valve cusps. Transapical sheath insert is secured with a purse-string suture. *(From Walther T, Falk V, Borger MA, et al. Minimally invasive transapical beating heart aortic valve implantation—proof of concept.* Eur J Cardiothorac Surg. *2007;31:9-15.)*

stroke, cognitive dysfunction, aortic dissection, bleeding, femoral or iliac artery injury, and perivalvular leaks.

Percutaneous balloon valvotomy has been used for quite some time to correct mitral stenosis. For mitral regurgitation, however, the recommendation in symptomatic patients and those with evidence of left ventricular dysfunction is mitral valve repair (ring annuloplasty) or mitral valve replacement via open heart surgery and cardiopulmonary bypass. Medical management only improves symptoms; it does not affect the progression of the disease. Clinical trials of devices that can perform percutaneous repair of the mitral valve are underway.

Transcatheter pulmonic valve placement has been used in selected patients with pulmonary insufficiency and right ventricular outflow tract problems. Successful percutaneous placement of this valve is associated with a reduction in right ventricular outflow tract obstruction, improved right ventricular pressure and/or volume unloading, and improved overall right ventricular function, biventricular function, and functional capacity. The procedure has been performed under general anesthesia with minimal hemodynamic instability. Transesophageal echocardiography has been found helpful during this procedure.

Additional randomized clinical trials are needed to compare all of these new treatments for valvular heart disease with traditional methodologies and to measure the long-term outcomes in terms of both longevity and quality of life.

KEY POINTS

- The most frequently encountered cardiac valve lesions produce pressure overload (mitral stenosis, aortic stenosis) or volume overload (mitral regurgitation, aortic regurgitation) on the left atrium or left ventricle.

- Angina pectoris may occur in patients with valvular heart disease even in the absence of coronary artery disease. It usually reflects increased myocardial oxygen demand due to ventricular hypertrophy. The demands of this thickened muscle mass may exceed the ability of even normal coronary arteries to deliver adequate amounts of oxygen.

- Certain cardiac lesions such as aortic and mitral stenosis require a slow heart rate to prolong the duration of diastole and improve left ventricular filling and coronary blood flow. The regurgitant valvular lesions such as aortic and mitral regurgitation require afterload reduction and somewhat faster heart rate to shorten the time for regurgitation.

- Prosthetic valves differ from one another with regard to durability, thrombogenicity, and hemodynamic profile. Mechanical valves are very durable, lasting at least 20 to 30 years, whereas bioprosthetic valves last about 10 to 15 years. Mechanical valves are highly thrombogenic and require long-term anticoagulation. Because bioprosthetic valves have a low thrombogenic potential, long-term anticoagulation is not necessary.

- In 2007, major changes were made in the AHA Guidelines for Prevention of Infective Endocarditis. Antibiotic prophylaxis is now recommended *only for those patients who are at highest risk of adverse outcomes if they were to develop infective endocarditis.*

- Management of anesthesia for noncardiac surgery in patients with mitral stenosis includes prevention and treatment of events that can decrease cardiac output or produce pulmonary edema. The development of atrial fibrillation with a rapid ventricular response significantly decreases cardiac output and can produce pulmonary edema. Excessive perioperative fluid administration, placement in Trendelenburg's position, or autotransfusion via uterine contraction increases central blood volume and can precipitate CHF. A sudden decrease in systemic vascular resistance may not be tolerated because the normal response to hypotension—that is, a reflex increase in heart rate—itself decreases cardiac output.

- The basic hemodynamic derangement in mitral regurgitation is a decrease in forward left ventricular stroke volume and cardiac output. A portion of every stroke volume is regurgitated through the incompetent mitral valve back into the left atrium, which results in left atrial volume overload and pulmonary congestion. Patients with a regurgitant fraction of more than 0.6 have severe mitral regurgitation. Pharmacologic interventions that increase or decrease systemic vascular resistance have a major impact on the regurgitant fraction in patients with mitral regurgitation.

- MVP is defined as the prolapse of one or both mitral leaflets into the left atrium during systole with or without mitral regurgitation; it is associated with the auscultatory findings of a midsystolic click and a late systolic murmur. MVP is the most common form of valvular heart disease, affecting 1% to 2.5% of the U.S. population. It is usually a benign condition.

- Management of anesthesia in patients with aortic stenosis includes the prevention of hypotension and any hemodynamic change that will decrease cardiac output. Normal sinus rhythm must be maintained, because the left ventricle is dependent on a properly timed atrial contraction to produce an optimal left ventricular end-diastolic volume. Loss of atrial contraction may produce a dramatic decrease in stroke volume and blood pressure. The heart rate is important because it determines the time available for ventricular filling, for ejection of the stroke volume, and for coronary perfusion. A sustained increase in heart rate decreases the time for left ventricular filling and ejection and reduces cardiac output. Hypotension reduces coronary blood flow and results in myocardial ischemia and further deterioration in left ventricular function and cardiac output. Aggressive treatment of hypotension is mandatory to prevent cardiogenic shock and/or cardiac arrest.

- The basic hemodynamic derangement in aortic regurgitation is a decrease in cardiac output because of regurgitation of a part of the ejected stroke volume from the aorta back into the left ventricle during diastole. This results in a combined pressure and volume overload on the left ventricle. The magnitude of the regurgitant volume depends on (1) the time available for the regurgitant flow to occur, which is determined by the heart rate; and (2) the pressure gradient across the aortic valve, which is dependent on systemic vascular resistance. The magnitude of aortic regurgitation is decreased by tachycardia and peripheral vasodilation.

RESOURCES

Billings FT, Kodali SK, Shanewise JS. Transcatheter aortic valve implantation: anesthetic considerations. *Anesth Analg.* 2009;108:1453-1462.

Bonow RO, Carabello BA, Kanu C, et al. ACC/AHA 2006 guidelines for the management of patients with valvular heart disease: a report of the American College of Cardiology/American Heart Association Task Force on Practice Guidelines (writing committee to revise the 1998 guidelines for the management of patients with valvular heart disease): developed in collaboration with the Society of Cardiovascular Anesthesiologists: endorsed by the Society for Cardiovascular Angiography and Interventions and the Society of Thoracic Surgeons. *Circulation.* 2006;114:e84-e231.

Feldman T, Foster E, Glower DG, et al. Percutaneous repair or surgery for mitral regurgitation. *N Engl J Med.* 2011;364:1395-1406.

Kertai MD, Bountioukos M, Boersma E, et al. Aortic stenosis: an underestimated risk factor for perioperative complications in patients undergoing noncardiac surgery. *Am J Med.* 2004;116:8-13.

Leon MB, Smith CR, Mack M, et al. Transcatheter aortic-valve implantation for aortic stenosis in patients who cannot undergo surgery. *N Engl J Med.* 2010;363:1597-1607. A link to an animation of the transcatheter aortic valve implantation (TAVI) procedure is available on the *New England Journal of Medicine* web page containing this article http://www.nejm.org/doi/full/10.1056/NEJMoa1008232.

McElhinney DB, Hellenbrand WE, Zahn EM, et al. Short- and medium-term outcomes after transcatheter pulmonary valve placement in the expanded multicenter US Melody valve trial. *Circulation.* 2010;122:507-516.

Perrino AC, Reeves ST. *A Practical Approach to Transesophageal Echocardiography.* 2nd ed. Philadelphia, PA: Lippincott Williams & Wilkins; 2007.

Walther T, Volkman F, Borger MA, et al. Minimally-invasive transapical heart aortic valve implantation—proof of concept. *Eur J Cardiothorac Surg.* 2007;31:9-15.

Wilson W, Taubert KA, Gewitz M, et al. Prevention of infective endocarditis: guidelines from the American Heart Association. *Circulation.* 2007;116:1736-1754.

Wong MCG, Clark DJ, Horrigan HE, et al. Advances in percutaneous treatment of adult valvular heart disease. *Intern Med J.* 2009;39:465-474.

CHAPTER 3

Congenital Heart Disease

SAMANTHA A. FRANCO ■
ROBERTA L. HINES ■

Congenital anomalies of the heart and cardiovascular system occur in 7 to 10 per 1000 live births (0.7% to 1.0%). Congenital heart disease is the most common form of congenital disease and accounts for approximately 30% of all congenital diseases that occur. With the decline in rheumatic heart disease, congenital heart disease has become the principal cause of heart disease, with 10% to 15% of affected children having associated congenital anomalies of the skeletal, genitourinary, or gastrointestinal system. Nine congenital heart lesions comprise more than 80% of congenital heart disease, with a wide range of more unusual and complex lesions accounting for the remainder (Table 3-1). The population of adults with congenital heart disease, surgically corrected or uncorrected, is estimated to exceed 1 million persons in the United States. As the success rate of cardiac surgery increases, more patients with complex cardiac defects will survive into adulthood and undergo noncardiac surgery and cardiac catheterization.

Transthoracic and transesophageal echocardiography has facilitated early, accurate diagnosis of congenital heart disease, assessment of the intraoperative and postoperative course, and evaluation of the ventricular function response to anesthetics in these patients. Fetal cardiac ultrasonography has permitted prenatal diagnosis of congenital heart defects, allowing subsequent perinatal management. Imaging modalities such as cardiac magnetic resonance imaging and three-dimensional echocardiography have increased the understanding of complex cardiac malformations and allow visualization of blood flow and vascular structures. Cardiac catheterization and selective angiocardiography are the most definitive diagnostic procedures available for use in patients with congenital heart disease. Advances in molecular biology have provided new understanding of the genetic basis of congenital heart disease. Chromosomal abnormalities are associated with an estimated 10% of congenital cardiovascular lesions. Two thirds of these lesions occur in patients with trisomy 21; the other one third is found in patients with karyotypic abnormalities, such as trisomy 13 and trisomy 18, and in patients with Turner's syndrome. The remaining 90% of congenital cardiovascular lesions are postulated to be multifactorial in origin and to occur as a result of interactions of several genes with or without the influence of external factors (rubella, ethanol abuse, lithium use, maternal diabetes mellitus). A widely used acronym, *CATCH-22* (cardiac defects, abnormal facies, thymic hypoplasia, cleft palate, hypocalcemia), describes a congenital

TABLE 3-1 ■ Classification and incidence of congenital heart disease	
Disease	**Incidence (%)**
ACYANOTIC DEFECTS	
Ventricular septal defect	35
Atrial septal defect	9
Patent ductus arteriosus	8
Pulmonary stenosis	8
Aortic stenosis	6
Coarctation of the aorta	6
Atrioventricular septal defect	3
CYANOTIC DEFECTS	
Tetralogy of Fallot	5
Transposition of the great vessels	4

TABLE 3-2 ■ Signs and symptoms of congenital heart disease
INFANTS
Tachypnea
Failure to gain weight
Heart rate >200 beats per minute
Heart murmur
Congestive heart failure
Cyanosis
CHILDREN
Dyspnea
Slow physical development
Decreased exercise tolerance
Heart murmur
Congestive heart failure
Cyanosis
Clubbing of digits
Squatting
Hypertension

TABLE 3-3 ■ Common problems associated with congenital heart disease
Infective endocarditis
Cardiac dysrhythmias
Complete heart block
Hypertension (systemic or pulmonary)
Erythrocytosis
Thromboembolism
Coagulopathy
Brain abscess
Increased plasma uric acid concentration
Sudden death

TABLE 3-4 ■ Congenital heart defects resulting in a left-to-right intracardiac shunt or its equivalent
Secundum atrial septal defect
Primum atrial septal defect (endocardial cushion defect)
Ventricular septal defect
Aorticopulmonary fenestration

heart disease syndrome attributed to defects in chromosome 22. An increased incidence of congenital heart disease in the offspring of affected adult patients suggests a role for single-gene defects in isolated congenital heart disease.

Signs and symptoms of congenital heart disease in infants and children often include dyspnea, slow physical development, and the presence of a cardiac murmur (Table 3-2). The diagnosis of congenital heart disease is apparent during the first week of life in approximately 50% of affected neonates and before 5 years of age in virtually all remaining patients. Echocardiography is the initial diagnostic step if congenital heart disease is suspected. Certain complications are likely to accompany congenital heart disease (Table 3-3). For example, infective endocarditis is a risk associated with most congenital cardiac anomalies, and guidelines for antibiotic prophylaxis have been developed (see later). Cardiac dysrhythmias are not usually a prominent feature of congenital heart disease.

ACYANOTIC CONGENITAL HEART DISEASE

Acyanotic congenital heart disease is characterized by a left-to-right intracardiac shunt (Table 3-4). The ultimate result of this intracardiac shunt, regardless of its location, is increased pulmonary blood flow with pulmonary hypertension, right ventricular hypertrophy, and eventually congestive heart failure. The younger the patient at the time of correction, the greater the likelihood that pulmonary vascular resistance will normalize. In older patients, if pulmonary vascular resistance is one third or less of the systemic vascular resistance, corrective surgery is likely to prevent or, in some cases, even cause slight regression of pulmonary vascular disease. The onset and severity of clinical symptoms vary with the site and magnitude of the vascular shunt.

Atrial Septal Defect

Atrial septal defect (ASD) accounts for about one third of the congenital heart disease detected in adults, with a frequency in females of two to three times that observed in males. Anatomically, an ASD may take the form of ostium secundum in the region of the fossa ovalis (often located near the center of the interatrial septum and varying from a single opening to a fenestrated septum) (Figure 3-1), ostium primum (endocardial cushion defect characterized by a large opening in the interatrial septum), or sinus venosus located in the upper atrial septum. Secundum ASDs account for 75% of all ASDs. Coronary sinus ASDs, associated with persistent left-sided superior vena cava, occur but are rare. Additional cardiac abnormalities may occur with each type of defect and include mitral valve prolapse (ostium secundum) and mitral

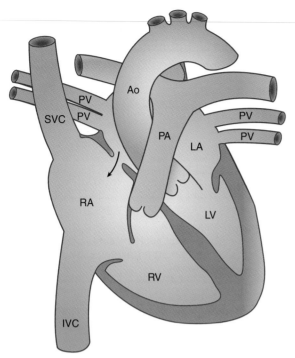

FIGURE 3-1 Secundum atrial septal defect located in the center of the interatrial septum. Blood flow is along a pressure gradient from the left atrium (LA) to the right atrium (RA). The resulting left-to-right intracardiac shunt is associated with increased blood flow through the pulmonary artery (PA). A decrease in systemic vascular resistance or an increase in pulmonary vascular resistance decreases the pressure gradient across the defect, which leads to a decrease in the magnitude of the shunt. *Ao,* Aorta; *IVC,* inferior vena cava; *LV,* left ventricle; *PV,* pulmonary vein; *RV,* right ventricle; *SVC,* superior vena cava.

regurgitation resulting from a cleft in the anterior mitral valve leaflet (ostium primum). Most ASDs occur as a result of spontaneous genetic mutations.

The physiologic consequences of ASDs are the same regardless of the anatomic location and reflect the shunting of blood from one atrium to the other; the direction and magnitude of the shunt are determined by the size of the defect and the relative compliance of the ventricles. A small defect (<0.5 cm in diameter) is associated with a small shunt and no hemodynamic sequelae. When the diameter of the ASD approaches 2 cm, it is likely that left atrial blood is being shunted to the right atrium (the right ventricle is more compliant than the left ventricle), which results in increased pulmonary blood flow. A systolic ejection murmur audible in the second left intercostal space may be mistaken for an innocent flow murmur in a child who has otherwise been well. As the volume of pulmonary blood flow increases with time, pulmonary valve closure is delayed, and the second heart sound is typically widely split and fixed. A pediatric cardiologist should evaluate a child with a loud systolic murmur and wide splitting of the second heart sound. A heart murmur is usually detected at age 6 to 8 weeks. The electrocardiogram (ECG) may reflect right axis deviation and incomplete right bundle branch block. Atrial fibrillation

and supraventricular tachycardia may accompany an ASD that remains uncorrected into adulthood. The chest radiograph is likely to reveal prominent pulmonary arteries and mild to moderate cardiomegaly. Transesophageal echocardiography and color flow Doppler echocardiography are both useful for detecting and determining the location of ASDs.

SIGNS AND SYMPTOMS

Because they initially produce no symptoms or striking findings on physical examination, ASDs may remain undetected for years. A small defect with minimal right-to-left shunting (ratio of pulmonary flow to systemic flow is <1.5) usually causes no symptoms and therefore does not require closure. When pulmonary blood flow is 1.5 times the systemic blood flow, the ASD should be closed either percutaneously via cardiac catheterization or surgically with open sternotomy and cardiopulmonary bypass to prevent right ventricular dysfunction and irreversible pulmonary hypertension. Symptoms resulting from large ASDs include dyspnea on exertion, supraventricular dysrhythmias, right heart failure, paradoxical embolism, and recurrent pulmonary infections. Abdominal viscera may become congested because of increased right-sided pressures and circulating volume. Prophylaxis against infective endocarditis is not recommended for patients with ASDs unless a concomitant valvular abnormality (mitral valve prolapse or mitral valve cleft) is present.

MANAGEMENT OF ANESTHESIA

An ASD associated with a left-to-right intracardiac shunt has only minor implications for the management of anesthesia. For example, as long as the systemic blood flow remains normal, the pharmacokinetics of inhaled drugs are not significantly altered despite the increased pulmonary blood flow. Conversely, increased pulmonary blood flow can dilute drugs injected intravenously. It is unlikely, however, that this potential dilution will alter the clinical response to these drugs because the pulmonary circulation time is brief.

Any change in systemic or pulmonary vascular resistance during the perioperative period will have important implications for the patient with an ASD. For example, drugs or events that produce prolonged increases in systemic vascular resistance should be avoided, because this change favors an increase in the magnitude of the left-to-right shunt at the atrial level. This is particularly true for a primum ASD associated with mitral regurgitation. Use of high fractional concentrations of inspired oxygen will decrease pulmonary vascular resistance and increase pulmonary blood flow and left-to-right shunt. Conversely, decreases in systemic vascular resistance, as produced by volatile anesthetics or increases in pulmonary vascular resistance due to positive pressure ventilation of the lungs, tend to decrease the magnitude of the left-to-right shunt.

Another consideration in the management of anesthesia in the presence of ASDs is the need to provide prophylactic antibiotics to protect against infective endocarditis when a cardiac valvular abnormality is present. In addition, meticulously avoiding the entrance of air into the circulation, as can occur through tubing used to deliver intravenous solutions, is imperative. Transient supraventricular dysrhythmias and atrioventricular conduction defects are common during the early postoperative period after surgical repair of an ASD, which may warrant a temporary use of a pacemaker and/or pharmacologic management.

Ventricular Septal Defect

Ventricular septal defect (VSD) is the most common congenital cardiac abnormality in infants and children (Figure 3-2), occurring in 50% of all children with congenital heart disease and in 20% as an isolated lesion. In the adult population, VSDs are the most common congenital heart defect excluding a bicuspid aortic valve. A large number of VSDs close spontaneously by the time a child reaches 2 years of age. Anatomically, approximately 70% of these defects are located in the membranous portion of the intraventricular septum; 20% in the muscular portion of the septum; 5% just below the aortic valve, causing aortic regurgitation; and 5% near the junction of the mitral and tricuspid valves (atrioventricular canal defect).

Echocardiography with Doppler flow ultrasonography confirms the presence and location of the VSD, and color flow mapping provides information about the magnitude and direction of the intracardiac shunt. Cardiac catheterization and angiography confirm the presence and location of the VSD and determine the magnitude of the intracardiac shunting and the pulmonary vascular resistance.

SIGNS AND SYMPTOMS

The physiologic significance of a VSD depends on the size of the defect, the pressure in the right and left ventricular chambers, and the relative resistance in the systemic and pulmonary circulations. If the defect is small, there is minimal functional disturbance because pulmonary blood flow is only modestly increased. If the defect is large, the ventricular systolic pressures equalize, and the relative vascular resistances of these two circulations determine the magnitude of systemic and pulmonary blood flow. Initially, systemic vascular resistance exceeds pulmonary vascular resistance, and left-to-right intracardiac shunting predominates, with corresponding pulmonary artery, left atrial, and left ventricular volume overload. Over time, the pulmonary vascular resistance increases, and the magnitude of the left-to-right intracardiac shunting decreases; eventually, the shunt may become right to left with the development of arterial hypoxemia (cyanosis).

The murmur of a moderate to large VSD is holosystolic and is loudest at the lower left sternal border. The ECG and chest radiographic findings remain normal in the presence of a small VSD. When the VSD is large, there is evidence of left atrial and ventricular enlargement on the ECG. If pulmonary hypertension develops, the QRS axis shifts to the right, and signs of right atrial and ventricular enlargement are noted on the ECG. The chest radiograph may then exhibit chamber enlargement to varying degrees, depending on the volume of the shunt, and increased pulmonary vascularity.

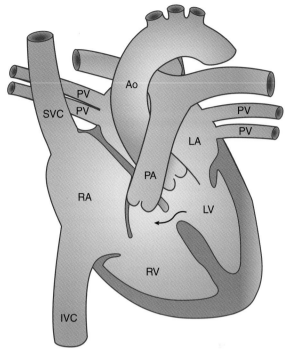

FIGURE 3-2 Ventricular septal defect located just below the muscular ridge that separates the body of the right ventricle (RV) from the pulmonary artery (PA) outflow tract. Blood flow is along a pressure gradient from the left ventricle (LV) to the RV. The resulting left-to-right intracardiac shunt is associated with pulmonary blood flow that exceeds the stroke volume of the LV. A decrease in systemic vascular resistance decreases the pressure gradient across the defect and reduces the magnitude of the shunt. *Ao,* Aorta; *IVC,* inferior vena cava; *LA,* left atrium; *PV,* pulmonary vein; *RA,* right atrium; *SVC,* superior vena cava.

The natural history of a VSD depends on the size of the defect and the pulmonary vascular resistance. Adults with small defects and normal pulmonary arterial pressures are generally asymptomatic, and pulmonary hypertension is unlikely to develop. These patients are at risk of developing infective endocarditis even though they may not meet the criteria for surgical correction of the VSD. In the absence of surgical correction, a large VSD eventually leads to left ventricular failure or pulmonary hypertension with associated right ventricular failure. Surgical closure of the defect is recommended in these patients if the magnitude of the pulmonary hypertension is not prohibitive. Once the pulmonary/systemic vascular resistance ratio exceeds 0.7, the risk of surgical closure becomes prohibitive.

MANAGEMENT OF ANESTHESIA

Antibiotic prophylaxis to protect against infective endocarditis is indicated when noncardiac surgery is planned in patients with unrepaired VSDs. The pharmacokinetics of inhaled and injected drugs is not significantly altered by a VSD. As with an ASD, acute and persistent increases in systemic vascular resistance or decreases in pulmonary vascular resistance are undesirable, because these changes can accentuate the magnitude of the left-to-right intracardiac shunt at the ventricular level. In this regard, volatile anesthetics (which decrease systemic vascular resistance) and positive pressure ventilation (which increases pulmonary vascular resistance) are well tolerated. However, there may be increased delivery of depressant drugs to the heart if coronary blood flow is increased to supply the hypertrophied ventricles. Conceivably, the technique of increasing the inspired concentrations of volatile anesthetics to achieve rapid induction of anesthesia, as is often done in children without cardiac defects, could result in excessive depression of the heart before central nervous system depression is achieved in children with VSD.

Right ventricular infundibular hypertrophy may be present in patients with VSDs. Normally, this is a beneficial change because it increases the resistance to right ventricular ejection, which leads to a decrease in the magnitude of the left-to-right intracardiac shunt. Nevertheless, perioperative events that exaggerate this obstruction to right ventricular outflow, such as increased myocardial contractility or hypovolemia, must be minimized. Therefore, these patients are often anesthetized with volatile anesthetics. In addition, the use of halothane, isoflurane, and sevoflurane, with a fractional concentration of inspired oxygen of 1.0, did not change echocardiographically derived pulmonary/systemic blood flow ratios in 30 biventricular patients with left-to-right shunts. In addition, intravascular fluid volume should be maintained by prompt replacement with crystalloid or colloid (depending on the clinical scenario).

Anesthesia for placement of a pulmonary artery band to reduce overcirculation and pulmonary blood flow is often achieved with drugs that provide minimal cardiac depression. If bradycardia or systemic hypotension develops during surgery, it may be necessary to remove the pulmonary artery band promptly. Continuous monitoring of the systemic blood pressure using an intraarterial catheter is helpful. Use of positive end-expiratory pressure may be beneficial in the presence of congestive heart failure but should be discontinued when the pulmonary artery band is in place. The high mortality rate associated with pulmonary artery banding has led to attempted complete surgical correction at an early age. Third-degree atrioventricular heart block may follow surgical closure if the cardiac conduction system is near the VSD. Premature ventricular beats may reflect the electrical instability of the ventricle due to surgical ventriculotomy. The risk of ventricular tachycardia is low, however, if postoperative ventricular filling pressures are normal.

Patent Ductus Arteriosus

A patent ductus arteriosus (PDA) is present when the ductus arteriosus (which arises just distal to the left subclavian artery and connects the descending aorta to the left pulmonary artery) fails to close spontaneously shortly after birth (Figure 3-3). In the fetus, the ductus arteriosus permits pulmonary arterial blood to bypass the deflated lungs and enter the descending aorta for oxygenation in the placenta. In full-term newborns, the ductus arteriosus closes within 24 to 48

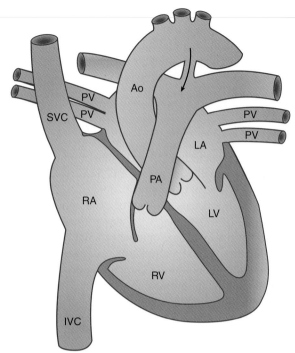

FIGURE 3-3 Patent ductus arteriosus connecting the arch of the aorta (Ao) with the pulmonary artery (PA). Blood flow is from the high-pressure Ao into the PA. The resulting Ao-to-PA shunt (left-to-right shunt) leads to increased pulmonary blood flow. A decrease in systemic vascular resistance or an increase in pulmonary vascular resistance decreases the magnitude of the shunt through the ductus arteriosus. *IVC,* Inferior vena cava; *LA,* left atrium; *LV,* left ventricle; *PV,* pulmonary vein; *RA,* right atrium; *RV,* right ventricle; *SVC,* superior vena cava.

hours after delivery, but in preterm newborns, the ductus arteriosus frequently fails to close. When the ductus arteriosus fails to close spontaneously after birth, the result is continuous flow of blood from the aorta to the pulmonary artery. The pulmonary/systemic blood flow ratio depends on the pressure gradient from the aorta to the pulmonary artery, the pulmonary/systemic vascular resistance ratio, and the diameter and length of the ductus arteriosus. The PDA can usually be visualized by echocardiography, with Doppler studies confirming the continuous flow into the pulmonary circulation. Cardiac catheterization and angiography make it possible to quantify the magnitude of the shunting and the pulmonary vascular resistance and to visualize the PDA.

SIGNS AND SYMPTOMS

Most patients with a PDA are asymptomatic and have only modest left-to-right shunts. This cardiac defect is often detected during a routine physical examination, at which time the characteristic continuous systolic and diastolic murmur is best heard at the left infraclavicular area or left upper sternal border. If the left-to-right shunt is large, there may be evidence of left ventricular hypertrophy on the ECG and chest radiograph. If pulmonary hypertension develops, right ventricular hypertrophy is apparent. The potential adverse effects of an untreated PDA include ventricular hypertrophy with congestive heart failure, pulmonary vascular disease including Eisenmenger's syndrome with shunt flow reversal, poor physical growth, infective endocarditis, aneurysmal dilatation of the ductus, and ductal calcification. Surgical ligation of a PDA is associated with low mortality and is unlikely to require cardiopulmonary bypass. Without surgical closure, most patients remain asymptomatic until adolescence, when pulmonary hypertension and congestive heart failure may occur. Once severe pulmonary hypertension develops, surgical or percutaneous closure is contraindicated.

TREATMENT

It is estimated that 70% of preterm infants delivered before 28 weeks of gestation require medical or surgical closure of a PDA. Surgical ligation of a PDA can be performed in neonatal intensive care units with low morbidity and mortality rates. Nevertheless, the risks of surgical closure are significant and include intracranial hemorrhage, infections, and recurrent laryngeal nerve paralysis, especially in infants born at less than 28 weeks of gestation. Inhibition of prostaglandin synthesis with nonselective cyclooxygenase-1 or cyclooxygenase-2 inhibitors appears to be an effective medical alternative to surgery for closure of a PDA in neonates. Indomethacin, a nonselective cyclooxygenase inhibitor used for this purpose, has reduced the need for surgery by 60% and is the first line of therapy for PDA. Adverse side effects of indomethacin include decreased mesenteric, renal, and cerebral blood flow; hence, a single standard indomethacin regime is not the ideal for every premature infant. Ibuprofen is a nonselective cyclooxygenase inhibitor that can be used effectively to treat PDA and has less effect on organ blood flow than indomethacin.

MANAGEMENT OF ANESTHESIA

Antibiotic prophylaxis for protection against infective endocarditis is recommended for patients with PDAs who are scheduled for noncardiac surgery. When surgical closure of the PDA is planned through a left thoracotomy, appropriate preparations must be made in anticipation of the possibility of large blood loss should control of the PDA be lost during attempted ligation. The decrease in systemic vascular resistance produced by volatile anesthetics may improve systemic blood flow by decreasing the magnitude of the left-to-right shunt. Likewise, positive pressure ventilation of the patient's lungs is well tolerated, as pulmonary vascular resistance, thereby decreasing the pressure gradient across the PDA. Conversely, increases in systemic vascular resistance or decreases in pulmonary vascular resistance should be avoided, because these changes will increase the magnitude of the left-to-right shunt.

Ligation of the PDA is often associated with significant systemic hypertension during the postoperative period. This hypertension can be managed with continuous infusion of vasodilating drugs such as nitroprusside. Long-acting antihypertensive drugs can be gradually substituted for nitroprusside if systemic hypertension persists.

Death occurs in fewer than 1% of patients undergoing surgical closure. Injuries to the recurrent laryngeal nerve (hoarseness), the left phrenic nerve (paralysis of the left hemidiaphragm), or the thoracic duct (chylothorax) are among the complications. Recanalization (reopening) of the ductus is possible, although rare, occurring after ligation alone and without division.

Aorticopulmonary Fenestration

Aorticopulmonary fenestration is characterized by a communication between the left side of the ascending aorta and the right wall of the main pulmonary artery, just anterior to the origin of the right pulmonary artery. This communication is due to failure of the aorticopulmonary septum to fuse and completely separate the aorta from the pulmonary artery. Clinical and hemodynamic manifestations of an aorticopulmonary communication are similar to those of a large PDA. The diagnosis is facilitated by echocardiography and angiocardiography. Treatment is surgical and requires the use of cardiopulmonary bypass. Management of anesthesia follows the same principles as described for patients with PDAs.

Aortic Stenosis

Bicuspid aortic valves occur in 2% to 3% of the U.S. population, and an estimated 20% of these patients have other cardiovascular abnormalities, such as PDA or coarctation of the aorta (see Chapter 2). The deformed bicuspid aortic valve is not stenotic at birth, but with time, thickening and calcification of the leaflets occur (usually not apparent before 15 years of age) with resulting immobility. Transthoracic echocardiography with Doppler flow studies permits accurate assessment of the severity of the aortic stenosis and of left ventricular function. Cardiac catheterization is performed to determine whether concomitant coronary artery disease is present.

SIGNS AND SYMPTOMS

Aortic stenosis is associated with a systolic murmur that is audible over the aortic area (second right intercostal space) and often radiates into the neck. Most patients with congenital aortic stenosis are asymptomatic until adulthood. Infants with severe aortic stenosis, however, may have congestive heart failure. Findings in patients with supravalvular aortic stenosis (SVAS) may include a characteristic appearance in which the facial bones are prominent, the forehead is rounded, and the upper lip is pursed. Patients with congenital SVAS may also have associated peripheral pulmonary artery stenoses in conjunction with Williams-Beuren syndrome, characterized by distinctive personality and behavioral traits, elfin facies, and transient neonatal hypercalcemia. Strabismus, inguinal hernia, dental abnormalities, and moderate mental retardation are commonly present. The nonsyndromic form of SVAS is much less common. Of note, in congenital SVAS, myocardial ischemia has been implicated in the majority of cases of sudden death in conjunction with anesthesia or sedation. Identifying these patients remains problematic, but cardiac magnetic resonance imaging with echocardiography has proved useful in addition to the gold standard of cardiac catheterization. In congenital aortic stenosis the ECG typically reveals left ventricular hypertrophy. Depression of the ST segment on the ECG is likely during exercise, particularly if the pressure gradient across the aortic valve is more than 50 mm Hg. Chest radiographs show left ventricular hypertrophy with or without poststenotic dilation of the aorta. Angina pectoris in the absence of coronary artery disease reflects the inability of coronary blood flow to meet increased myocardial oxygen requirements of the hypertrophied left ventricle. Syncope can occur when the pressure gradient across the aortic valve exceeds 50 mm Hg. In the presence of aortic stenosis, the myocardium must generate an intraventricular pressure that is two to three times normal, whereas pressure in the aorta remains within a physiologic range. The resulting concentric myocardial hypertrophy leads to increased myocardial oxygen requirements. Furthermore, the high velocity of blood flow through the stenotic area predisposes to the development of infective endocarditis and is associated with poststenotic dilation of the aorta. In adults with symptomatic aortic stenosis (syncope, angina pectoris, congestive heart failure), the indicated treatment is surgical valve replacement.

MANAGEMENT OF ANESTHESIA

Anesthetic management requires careful attention to maintaining an age-appropriate heart rate, sinus rhythm, preload, contractility, and systemic vascular resistance, and avoiding increases in pulmonary vascular resistance. Drugs with vagolytic activity (atropine) and sympathomimetic activity (pancuronium) should be avoided, and the dose of atropine or glycopyrrolate given with a reversal agent should be carefully chosen so as to avoid significant tachycardia. Supraventricular tachycardia, dysrhythmias, and hypotension should be treated aggressively.

Pulmonic Stenosis

Pulmonic stenosis producing obstruction to right ventricular outflow is valvular in 90% of patients; in the remainder, it is supravalvular or subvalvular. Supravalvular pulmonic stenosis often co-exists with other congenital cardiac abnormalities (ASD, VSD, PDA, tetralogy of Fallot). It is a common feature of Williams's syndrome, which is characterized by infantile hypercalcemia and mental retardation. Subvalvular pulmonic stenosis usually occurs in association with a VSD. Valvular pulmonic stenosis is typically an isolated abnormality, but it may occur in association with a VSD. Severe pulmonic stenosis is characterized by transvalvular pressure gradients of more than 80 mm Hg or right ventricular systolic pressures of more than 100 mm Hg. Echocardiography and Doppler flow studies can determine the site of the obstruction and the severity of the stenosis. Treatment of pulmonic stenosis is with percutaneous balloon valvuloplasty.

SIGNS AND SYMPTOMS

In asymptomatic patients, pulmonic stenosis is detected by the presence of a loud systolic ejection murmur, best heard at the second left intercostal space. The intensity and duration of the cardiac murmur parallel the severity of the pulmonic stenosis. Dyspnea may occur on exertion, and eventually right ventricular failure with peripheral edema and ascites develops. If the foramen ovale is patent, right-to-left intracardiac shunting of blood may occur, causing cyanosis and clubbing.

MANAGEMENT OF ANESTHESIA

Management of anesthesia is designed to avoid increases in right ventricular oxygen requirements. Therefore, excessive increases in heart rate and myocardial contractility are undesirable. The impact of changes in pulmonary vascular resistance is minimized by the presence of fixed obstruction of the pulmonic valve. As a result, increases in pulmonary vascular resistance due to positive pressure ventilation of the lungs are unlikely to produce significant increases in right ventricular afterload and oxygen requirements. These patients are extremely difficult to resuscitate if cardiac arrest occurs because external cardiac compression is not highly effective in forcing blood across a stenotic pulmonic valve. Therefore, decreases in systemic blood pressure should be promptly treated with sympathomimetic drugs. Likewise, cardiac dysrhythmias or increases in heart rate that become hemodynamically significant should be rapidly corrected.

Coarctation of the Aorta

Coarctation of the aorta typically consists of a discrete, diaphragm-like ridge extending into the aortic lumen and is described by its relationship to the ductus arteriosus (preductal, juxtaductal, postductal). A postductal coarctation extends just distal to the left subclavian artery at the site of the aortic ductal attachment (ligamentum arteriosum) and is most likely to manifest in young adults. Less commonly, the coarctation is immediately proximal to the left subclavian artery (preductal); this situation is most likely to present in infants. Coarctation of the aorta is more common in males and may occur in conjunction with a bicuspid aortic valve, PDA, mitral stenosis or regurgitation, aneurysms of the circle of Willis, and gonadal dysgenesis (Turner's syndrome).

SIGNS AND SYMPTOMS

Since most adults with coarctation of the aorta are asymptomatic, the problem usually is diagnosed during a routine physical examination when systemic hypertension is detected in the arms in association with diminished or absent femoral arterial pulses. Characteristically, systolic blood pressure is higher in the arms than in the legs, but the diastolic pressure is similar, which results in widened pulse pressure in the arms. The femoral arterial pulses are weak and delayed. Systemic hypertension presumably reflects ejection of the left ventricular stroke volume into the fixed resistance created by the narrowed aorta. A harsh systolic ejection murmur is present along the left sternal border and in the back, particularly over the area of the coarctation. In the presence of preductal coarctation of the aorta, there is no difference in the systemic blood pressures in the arms and legs since extensive collateral arterial circulation to the distal body through the internal thoracic, intercostal, scapular, and subclavian arteries is present. In such cases, a systolic murmur may be heard in the back, reflecting this collateral blood flow.

The ECG shows signs of left ventricular hypertrophy. On the chest radiograph, increased collateral flow through the intercostal arteries causes symmetrical notching of the posterior third of the third through eighth ribs. Notching is not seen in the anterior ribs because the anterior intercostal arteries are not located in costal grooves. The coarctation may be visible as an indentation of the aorta with prestenotic or poststenotic dilation of the aorta, producing the "reversed E," or "3," sign. The coarctation may be visualized with echocardiography, and Doppler examination makes it possible to estimate the transcoarctation pressure gradient. Computed tomography, magnetic resonance imaging, and contrast aortography provide precise anatomic information regarding the location and length of the coarctation and the degree of collateral circulation.

When clinical symptoms of a previously unrecognized coarctation of the aorta manifest, they usually include headache, dizziness, epistaxis, and palpitations. Occasionally, diminished blood flow to the legs causes claudication. Women with coarctation of the aorta are at increased risk of aortic dissection during pregnancy. Complications of coarctation of the aorta include systemic hypertension, left ventricular failure, aortic dissection, premature ischemic heart disease presumably related to chronic hypertension, infective endocarditis, and cerebrovascular accidents caused by rupture of intracerebral aneurysms. Patients with known coarctation of the aorta should be given prophylactic antibiotics in accordance with the recommended guidelines.

TREATMENT

Surgical resection of the coarctation of the aorta should be considered for patients with a transcoarctation pressure gradient of more than 30 mm Hg. Although balloon dilation is a therapeutic alternative, the procedure is associated with a higher incidence of subsequent aortic aneurysm and recurrent coarctation than is surgical resection.

MANAGEMENT OF ANESTHESIA

Management of anesthesia for surgical resection of coarctation of the aorta must consider (1) the adequacy of perfusion to the lower portion of the body during cross-clamping of the aorta, (2) the propensity for systemic hypertension during cross-clamping of the aorta, and (3) the risk of neurologic sequelae due to ischemia of the spinal cord. Blood flow to the anterior spinal artery is augmented by radicular branches of the intercostal arteries and may be compromised during cross-clamping of the aorta for surgical resection of coarctation of the aorta. Paraplegia after surgical resection of coarctation of the aorta is a rare complication. Continuous monitoring of systemic blood pressure above and below the coarctation is achieved by placing

a catheter in the right radial artery and in a femoral artery. By monitoring these pressures simultaneously, it is possible to evaluate the adequacy of the collateral circulation during periods of aortic cross-clamping. Mean arterial pressures in the lower extremities should be at least 40 mm Hg to ensure adequate blood flow to the kidneys and spinal cord. If the systemic blood pressure cannot be maintained above this level, it may be necessary to use partial circulatory bypass. Somatosensory evoked potentials are useful for monitoring spinal cord function and the adequacy of its blood flow during cross-clamping of the aorta. Nevertheless, case reports of paraplegia despite normal somatosensory evoked potentials suggest that monitoring posterior (sensory) cord function does not ensure adequate blood flow to the anterior (motor) portion of the spinal cord. Excessive increases in systolic blood pressure during cross-clamping of the aorta may adversely increase the work of the heart and make surgical repair more difficult. In this situation, the use of volatile anesthetics is helpful for maintaining normal systemic blood pressures. If systemic hypertension persists, continuous intravenous infusions of nitroprusside should be considered. The disadvantages of lowering the systemic blood pressure to normal levels are excessively decreased perfusion pressure in the lower part of the body and inadequate blood flow to the kidneys and spinal cord.

POSTOPERATIVE MANAGEMENT

Immediately postoperative complications include paradoxical hypertension, possible sequelae of a bicuspid aortic valve (infective endocarditis and aortic regurgitation), and paraplegia. Baroreceptor reflexes, activation of the renin-angiotensin-aldosterone system, and excessive release of catecholamines have been implicated as possible causes of immediately postoperative systemic hypertension. Regardless of the cause, intravenous administration of nitroprusside with or without esmolol effectively controls the systemic blood pressure during the early postoperative period. Longer-acting antihypertensive drugs may be needed if hypertension persists. If a thoracic epidural catheter has been placed, local anesthetics or clonidine may be effective adjuvants to control blood pressure. Paraplegia manifesting during the immediately postoperative period is assumed to reflect ischemic damage to the spinal cord during the aortic cross-clamping required for surgical resection of the coarctation. Left recurrent laryngeal nerve injury, manifesting as stridor or hoarseness, or left phrenic nerve injury may prolong the need for airway and respiratory support. Abdominal pain may occur during the postoperative period and is presumably due to sudden increases in blood flow to the gastrointestinal tract, which leads to increased vasoactivity. Early feeding is not recommended because of the concerns about postcoarctation mesenteric arteritis.

The incidence of persistent or recurrent systemic hypertension and the survival rate are influenced by the patient's age at the time of surgery. Most of the patients who undergo surgery during childhood are normotensive 5 years later, whereas those who undergo surgery after 40 years of age often manifest persistent systemic hypertension.

TABLE 3-5	Congenital heart defects resulting in a right-to-left intracardiac shunt

Tetralogy of Fallot
Eisenmenger's syndrome
Ebstein's anomaly (malformation of the tricuspid valve)
Tricuspid atresia
Foramen ovale

CYANOTIC CONGENITAL HEART DISEASE

Cyanotic congenital heart disease is characterized by a right-to-left intracardiac shunt (Table 3-5) with associated decreases in pulmonary blood flow and the development of arterial hypoxemia. The magnitude of shunting determines the severity of arterial hypoxemia. Erythrocytosis secondary to chronic arterial hypoxemia results in a risk of thromboembolism, especially when the hematocrit exceeds 70%. Patients with secondary erythrocytosis may exhibit coagulation defects, most likely due to deficiencies of vitamin K–dependent clotting factors in the liver and defective platelet aggregation. Development of a brain abscess is a major risk in patients with cyanotic congenital heart disease. The onset of a brain abscess often mimics a stroke. Survival in the presence of a right-to-left intracardiac shunt requires a communication between the systemic and pulmonary circulations. Tetralogy of Fallot is the prototype of these defects and is included in the "5 Ts," or common cyanotic congenital heart defects (tetralogy of Fallot, transposition of the great arteries, tricuspid atresia, total anomalous pulmonary venous connection, and truncus arteriosus). Most children with cyanotic congenital heart disease do not survive to adulthood without surgical intervention. Principles for the management of anesthesia are the same for all the cyanotic congenital cardiac defects.

Tetralogy of Fallot

Tetralogy of Fallot, the most common cyanotic congenital heart defect, accounting for about 10% of all congenital heart disease cases, is characterized by a large single VSD, an aorta that overrides the right and left ventricles, obstruction to right ventricular outflow (subvalvular, valvular, supravalvular, pulmonary arterial branches), and right ventricular hypertrophy (Figure 3-4). Several abnormalities may occur in association with tetralogy of Fallot, including right aortic arch in 25% of cases, ASD (pentalogy of Fallot) in 15% of patients, and coronary arterial anomalies. Right ventricular hypertrophy occurs because the VSD permits continuous exposure of the right ventricle to the high pressures present in the left ventricle. Right-to-left intracardiac shunting occurs because of increased resistance to flow in the right ventricular outflow tract, the severity of which determines the magnitude of the shunt. Because the resistance to flow across the right ventricular outflow tract is relatively fixed, changes in systemic vascular resistance (drug induced) may affect the magnitude of the shunt. Decreases in systemic vascular resistance increase

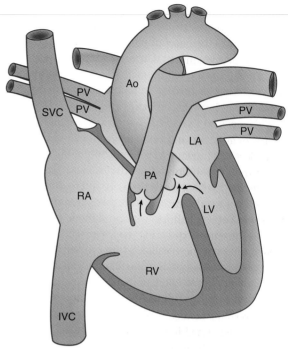

FIGURE 3-4 Anatomic cardiac defects associated with tetralogy of Fallot. Defects include (1) ventricular septal defect, (2) aorta (Ao) overriding the pulmonary artery (PA) outflow tract, (3) obstruction to blood flow through a narrowed PA or stenotic pulmonic valve, and (4) right ventricular hypertrophy. Obstruction to PA outflow results in a pressure gradient that favors blood flow across the ventricular septal defect from the right ventricle (RV) to the left ventricle (LV). The resulting right-to-left intracardiac shunt combined with obstruction to ejection of the stroke volume from the RV leads to marked decreases in pulmonary blood flow and the development of arterial hypoxemia. Any event that increases pulmonary vascular resistance or decreases systemic vascular resistance increases the magnitude of the shunt and accentuates arterial hypoxemia. *IVC*, Inferior vena cava; *LA*, left atrium; *PV*, pulmonary vein; *RA*, right atrium; *SVC*, superior vena cava.

right-to-left intracardiac shunting and accentuate arterial hypoxemia, whereas increases in systemic vascular resistance (squatting) decrease left-to-right intracardiac shunting with resultant increases in pulmonary blood flow.

DIAGNOSIS

Echocardiography is used to establish the diagnosis, assess for the presence of associated abnormalities, and determine the level and severity of the obstruction to right ventricular outflow, the size of the main pulmonary artery and its branches, and the number and location of the VSDs. Right-to-left shunting through the VSD is visualized by color Doppler imaging, and the severity of the right ventricular outflow tract obstruction can be determined by spectral Doppler measurement. Cardiac catheterization further confirms the diagnosis and permits confirmation of anatomic and hemodynamic data, including the location and magnitude of the right-to-left shunt, the level and severity of the right ventricular outflow obstruction, the anatomic features of the right ventricular outflow obstruction, the anatomic features of the right ventricular outflow tract and the main pulmonary artery and its branches, and the origin and course of the coronary arteries. Magnetic resonance imaging can also provide much of this information.

SIGNS AND SYMPTOMS

Typically the infant with tetralogy of Fallot may be pink (not cyanotic) as a neonate and develops cyanosis between 2 and 6 months of age. The most common auscultatory finding is a systolic ejection murmur heard along the left sternal border resulting from blood flow across the stenotic pulmonic valve or right ventricular outflow tract. In contrast to pulmonic stenosis with an intact ventricular septum, the murmur of tetralogy of Fallot becomes shorter and less intense with increasing severity of pulmonic stenosis. During a hypercyanotic spell, the murmur disappears or becomes very soft. A holosystolic murmur of VSD may be heard in the left lower sternal border in some children. Congestive heart failure rarely develops, because the large VSD permits equilibration of intraventricular pressures and cardiac workload. Chest radiographs show evidence of decreased lung vascularity, and the heart is boot shaped with an upturned right ventricular apex and a concave main pulmonary arterial segment. The ECG is characterized by changes indicative of right axis deviation and right ventricular hypertrophy. Arterial oxygen desaturation is present even when the patient breathes 100% oxygen (PaO_2 is usually <50 mm Hg), indicating central cyanosis. Compensatory erythropoiesis is proportional to the magnitude of the arterial hypoxemia. The $PaCO_2$ and arterial pH are usually normal. Squatting is a common feature of children with tetralogy of Fallot. It is speculated that squatting increases the systemic vascular resistance by kinking the large arteries in the inguinal area. The resulting increase in systemic vascular resistance tends to decrease the magnitude of the right-to-left intracardiac shunt, which leads to increased pulmonary blood flow and subsequent improvement in arterial oxygenation.

Hypercyanotic Attacks

Hypercyanotic attacks are characterized by sudden spells of arterial hypoxemia associated with worsening cyanosis, increasing rate and depth of respirations (hyperpnea), and, in some instances, loss of consciousness, seizures, cerebrovascular accidents, and even death. These attacks can occur without obvious provocation but are often associated with crying, defecation, feeding, or exercise. Their mechanism is not known, but the most likely explanation is a sudden decrease in pulmonary blood flow due to spasm of the infundibular cardiac muscle or decreased systemic vascular resistance. They can occur any time between 1 month and 12 years of age, but the peak incidence is at 2 to 3 months.

Treatment of hypercyanotic attacks is influenced by the cause of the pulmonary outflow obstruction. When symptoms reflect a dynamic infundibular obstruction (spasm), appropriate treatment is administration of β-adrenergic antagonists such as esmolol or propranolol. Indeed, long-term oral propranolol therapy is indicated in patients who have recurrent hypercyanotic attacks caused by spasm of the outflow tract muscle. If the cause is decreased systemic vascular resistance, treatment is intravenous administration of fluids and/or phenylephrine. Emergently, the infant may be placed in the knee-chest position. Sympathomimetic drugs that display β-agonist properties are not selected because they may accentuate the spasm of the infundibular cardiac muscle. Recurrent hypercyanotic attacks indicate the need for surgical correction of the abnormalities associated with tetralogy of Fallot.

These attacks do not occur in adolescents or adults. Adults with tetralogy of Fallot manifest dyspnea and limited exercise tolerance. They may also have complications of chronic cyanosis, including erythrocytosis, hyperviscosity, abnormalities of hemostasis, cerebral abscess or stroke, and infective endocarditis.

Cerebrovascular Accident

Cerebrovascular accidents are common in children with severe tetralogy of Fallot. Cerebrovascular thrombosis or severe arterial hypoxemia may be the explanation for these adverse responses. Dehydration and polycythemia may contribute to thrombosis. Hemoglobin concentrations exceeding 20 g/dL are common in these patients.

Cerebral Abscess

A cerebral abscess is suggested by the abrupt onset of headache, fever, and lethargy followed by persistent emesis and the appearance of seizure activity. The most likely cause is arterial seeding into areas of previous cerebral infarction.

Infective Endocarditis

Infective endocarditis is a constant danger in patients with tetralogy of Fallot and is associated with a high mortality rate. Antibiotics should be administered to protect against this serious possibility whenever dental or surgical procedures are planned in these patients in keeping with standard guidelines.

TREATMENT

Treatment of tetralogy of Fallot is complete surgical correction when patients are extremely young (closure of the VSD with a Dacron patch and relief of right ventricular outflow obstruction by placement of a synthetic graft). Infants with pulmonary atresia undergo Rastelli's procedures. Without surgery, mortality exceeds 50% by 3 years of age. Pulmonic regurgitation caused by an incompetent pulmonic valve usually results from surgical correction of the cardiac defects characteristic of tetralogy of Fallot but poses no major hazard unless the distal pulmonary arteries are hypoplastic, in which case volume overload of the right ventricle secondary to regurgitant blood flow may result. Platelet dysfunction and hypofibrinogenemia are common in these patients and may contribute to postoperative bleeding problems. Right-to-left intracardiac shunting often develops through the foramen ovale during the postoperative period. Shunting through the foramen ovale acts as a safety valve if the right ventricle is unable to function with the same efficiency as the left ventricle.

In the past, infants underwent one of three palliative procedures to increase pulmonary blood flow. All three palliative procedures involved anastomosis of a systemic artery to a pulmonary artery in an effort to increase pulmonary blood flow and improve arterial oxygenation. These palliative procedures are Waterston's operation (side-to-side anastomosis of the ascending aorta and the right pulmonary artery), Potts's operation (side-to-side anastomosis of the descending aorta to the left pulmonary artery), and the Blalock-Taussig operation (end-to-side anastomosis of the subclavian artery to the pulmonary artery). Often, however, these procedures are associated with long-term complications such as pulmonary hypertension, left ventricular volume overload, and distortion of the pulmonary arterial branches. Nevertheless, if the patient does not meet the criteria for correction at the time, these preliminary measures may be undertaken. Balloon pulmonary valvuloplasty has been employed in some patients with tetralogy of Fallot to augment pulmonary blood flow and to allow for growth and development of the pulmonary arterial system and left ventricle so that a total surgical corrective procedure can be performed at a later time with a greater chance of success.

MANAGEMENT OF ANESTHESIA

Management of anesthesia in patients with tetralogy of Fallot requires a thorough understanding of those events and drugs that can alter the magnitude of the right-to-left intracardiac shunt. For example, when shunt magnitude is acutely increased, there are associated decreases in pulmonary blood flow and Pao_2. Furthermore, the magnitude of the right-to-left shunt may alter the pharmacokinetics of both inhaled and injected drugs.

The magnitude of a right-to-left intracardiac shunt can be increased by (1) decreased systemic vascular resistance, (2) increased pulmonary vascular resistance, and (3) increased myocardial contractility, which accentuates infundibular obstruction to ejection of blood by the right ventricle. In many respects, resistance to ejection of blood into the pulmonary artery outflow tract is relatively fixed, and hence the magnitude of the shunt is inversely proportional to the systemic vascular resistance. Pharmacologically induced responses that decrease systemic vascular resistance (response to volatile anesthetics, histamine release, ganglionic blockade, α-adrenergic blockade) increase the magnitude of the right-to-left shunt and accentuate arterial hypoxemia. Pulmonary blood flow can be decreased by increases in pulmonary vascular resistance that accompany such intraoperative ventilatory maneuvers as intermittent positive airway pressure or positive end-expiratory pressure. Furthermore, the loss of negative intrapleural pressure on opening the chest increases pulmonary vascular resistance and the magnitude of the shunt. Nevertheless, the advantages of controlled ventilation of the lungs during operations usually offset this potential hazard. Indeed, arterial oxygenation does not predictably deteriorate in patients with tetralogy of Fallot, either with the institution of positive pressure ventilation of the lungs or after opening of the chest.

Preoperative Preparation

Preoperatively, it is important to avoid dehydration by maintaining oral feedings in extremely young patients or by providing intravenous fluids before the patient's arrival in the operating room. Crying associated with intramuscular administration of drugs used for preoperative medication can lead to hypercyanotic attacks. Treatment with β-adrenergic antagonists should be continued until the induction of anesthesia in patients receiving these drugs for prophylaxis against hypercyanotic attacks.

Induction of Anesthesia

Induction of anesthesia in patients with tetralogy of Fallot is often accomplished with ketamine (3 to 4 mg/kg IM or 1 to 2 mg/kg IV). The onset of anesthesia after ketamine injection may be associated with improved arterial oxygenation; this presumably reflects increased pulmonary blood flow resulting from ketamine-induced increases in systemic vascular resistance, which can lead to a decrease in the magnitude of the right-to-left intracardiac shunt. Ketamine has also been alleged to increase pulmonary vascular resistance, which would be undesirable in patients with a right-to-left shunt. The efficacious response to ketamine of patients with tetralogy of Fallot, however, suggests that this concern is not clinically significant. Tracheal intubation is facilitated by administration of muscle relaxants. It should be remembered that the onset of action of drugs administered intravenously may be more rapid in the presence of right-to-left shunts because the dilutional effect in the lungs is decreased. For this reason, it may be prudent to decrease the rate of intravenous injection of depressant drugs in these patients.

Induction of anesthesia with a volatile anesthetic such as sevoflurane is acceptable but must be accomplished with caution and careful monitoring of systemic oxygenation. Although decreased pulmonary blood flow speeds the achievement of anesthetic concentrations, the hazard of decreased systemic blood pressure plus decreased systemic vascular resistance is great. Indeed, hypercyanotic attacks can occur during administration of low concentrations of volatile anesthetics. Halothane is the preferred inhalational anesthetic because it decreases contractility and maintains systemic vascular resistance.

Maintenance of Anesthesia

Maintenance of anesthesia is often achieved with nitrous oxide combined with ketamine. The advantage of this combination is preservation of the systemic vascular resistance. Nitrous oxide may also increase pulmonary vascular resistance, but this potentially adverse effect is more than offset by its beneficial effects on systemic vascular resistance (no change or modest increase). The principal disadvantage of using nitrous oxide is the associated decrease in the inspired oxygen concentration. Theoretically, increased inspired oxygen concentrations could decrease pulmonary vascular resistance, leading to increased pulmonary blood flow and improved Pao_2. Therefore, it seems prudent to limit the inspired concentration of nitrous oxide to 50%. The use of an opioid or benzodiazepine may also be considered during maintenance of anesthesia, but the dose and rate of administration must be adjusted to minimize decreased systemic blood pressure and systemic vascular resistance.

Intraoperative skeletal muscle paralysis may be provided with pancuronium in view of its ability to maintain systemic blood pressure and systemic vascular resistance. An increase in heart rate associated with pancuronium is helpful for maintaining left ventricular cardiac output. Careful consideration should be given to selecting alternative nondepolarizing neuromuscular blocking drugs, because some drugs administered rapidly in high dose may evoke histamine release with associated decreases in systemic vascular resistance and systemic blood pressure.

Ventilation of the patient's lungs should be controlled, but it must be appreciated that excessive positive airway pressure may adversely increase the resistance to blood flow through the lungs. Intravascular fluid volume must be maintained with intravenous fluid administration, because acute hypovolemia may increase the magnitude of the right-to-left intracardiac shunt. In view of the predictable erythrocytosis, it is probably not necessary to consider blood replacement until approximately 20% of the patient's blood volume has been lost. It is crucial that meticulous care be taken to avoid infusion of air through the tubing used to deliver intravenous solutions because it could lead to systemic air embolization. α-Adrenergic agonist drugs such as phenylephrine must be available to treat undesirable decreases in systemic blood pressure caused by decreased systemic vascular resistance.

PATIENT CHARACTERISTICS FOLLOWING SURGICAL REPAIR OF TETRALOGY OF FALLOT

Although patients with surgically repaired tetralogy of Fallot are usually asymptomatic, their survival is often shortened because of sudden death, presumably from cardiac causes. Ventricular cardiac dysrhythmias are common in patients following surgical correction of tetralogy of Fallot. Patients with surgically repaired tetralogy of Fallot often develop atrial fibrillation or flutter. Right bundle branch block is frequent, whereas third-degree atrioventricular heart block is uncommon. Pulmonic regurgitation may develop as a consequence of surgical repair of the right ventricular outflow tract and may eventually lead to right ventricular hypertrophy and dysfunction. An aneurysm may form at the site where the right ventricular outflow tract was repaired.

Eisenmenger's Syndrome

Patients in whom a left-to-right intracardiac shunt is reversed, as a result of increased pulmonary vascular resistance, to a level that equals or exceeds the systemic vascular resistance are said to have Eisenmenger's syndrome. It is presumed that exposure of the pulmonary vasculature to increased blood flow and pressure, as may accompany a VSD or ASD, results in pulmonary obstructive disease. As obliteration of the pulmonary vascular bed progresses, the pulmonary vascular resistance increases until it equals or exceeds systemic vascular resistance and the intracardiac shunt is reversed. Shunt reversal occurs in approximately 50% of patients with an untreated VSD and approximately 10% of patients with an untreated ASD. The murmur associated with these cardiac defects disappears when Eisenmenger's syndrome develops.

SIGNS AND SYMPTOMS

Cyanosis and decreased exercise tolerance occur as right-to-left intracardiac shunting develops. Palpitations are common and are most often due to the onset of atrial fibrillation or atrial flutter. Arterial hypoxemia stimulates erythrocytosis, which leads to increased blood viscosity and associated visual disturbances, headache, dizziness, and paresthesias. Hemoptysis may occur as a result of pulmonary infarction or rupture of dilated pulmonary arteries, arterioles, or aorticopulmonary collateral vessels. Abnormal coagulation and thrombosis often accompany arterial hypoxemia and erythrocytosis. The possibility of a cerebrovascular accident or brain abscess is increased. Syncope most likely reflects inadequate cardiac output. Sudden death is a risk in patients with Eisenmenger's syndrome. The ECG shows right ventricular hypertrophy.

TREATMENT

No treatment has proved effective in producing sustained decreases in pulmonary vascular resistance, although intravenous epoprostenol may be beneficial. Phlebotomy with isovolemic replacement should be undertaken in patients with moderate or severe symptoms of hyperviscosity. Pregnancy is discouraged in women with Eisenmenger's syndrome. Lung transplantation with repair of the cardiac defect or combined heart–lung transplantation is an option for selected patients with this syndrome. The presence of irreversibly increased pulmonary vascular resistance contraindicates surgical correction of the congenital heart defect that was responsible for the original left-to-right intracardiac shunt.

MANAGEMENT OF ANESTHESIA

Management of anesthesia in patients with Eisenmenger's syndrome undergoing noncardiac surgery is based on maintenance of preoperative levels of systemic vascular resistance and recognition that increases in right-to-left intracardiac shunting are likely if sudden vasodilation occurs. These patients pose a challenge to anesthesiologists because of their inability to adapt to sudden changes in hemodynamics because their pulmonary vascular bed is fixed. Since many agents used for induction and maintenance of general anesthesia depress myocardial function and reduce systemic vascular resistance, the choice should be limited to those that cause the least hemodynamic disturbance, such as ketamine or opioids with etomidate. Continuous intravenous infusions of norepinephrine have been reported to maintain systemic vascular resistance during the perioperative period. Minimization of blood loss leading to hypovolemia and prevention of iatrogenic paradoxical embolization are important considerations. It may be useful to perform prophylactic phlebotomy with isovolemic replacement in patients with hematocrits higher than 65%. Preoperative administration of antiplatelet drugs is not encouraged, because intraoperative blood loss may be associated with the impaired coagulation that accompanies chronic arterial hypoxemia and erythrocytosis. Opioids have been administered safely for preoperative and postoperative analgesia.

Laparoscopic procedures may pose an increased risk to these patients because insufflation of the peritoneal cavity with carbon dioxide may cause increases in $Paco_2$ that result in acidosis, hypotension, and cardiac dysrhythmias. Efforts to maintain normocapnia may be accompanied by increases in airway pressures and pulmonary vascular resistance, especially as the intraabdominal pressure increases. These events may be further exaggerated by placing the patient in the head-down position. Early tracheal extubation of these patients is preferable because of the deleterious effects of positive pressure ventilation.

Despite the potential for undesirable decreases in systemic blood pressure and systemic vascular resistance, the successful management of anesthesia using epidural anesthesia has been described in patients undergoing tubal ligation and cesarean section. If epidural anesthesia is selected, it seems prudent not to add epinephrine to the local anesthetic solution injected into the epidural space. This recommendation is based on the observation that peripheral β-agonist effects produced by the epinephrine absorbed from the epidural space into the systemic circulation can exaggerate decreases in systemic blood pressure and systemic vascular resistance associated with epidural anesthesia. Slowly titrated local anesthetics combined with epidural opioids may avoid the abrupt decline in systemic vascular resistance and provide adequate analgesia depending upon the surgical procedure.

Ebstein's Anomaly

Ebstein's anomaly is an abnormality of the tricuspid valve in which the posterior and septal valve leaflets are malformed or displaced downward into the right ventricle and may adhere to the myocardium. The anterior tricuspid leaflet is abnormally large and sail-like, and may have multiple fenestrations. As a result, the right ventricle has a small distal effective portion and an atrialized proximal portion. The tricuspid valve is usually regurgitant but may also be stenotic. Most patients with Ebstein's anomaly have an interatrial communication (ASD, patent foramen ovale) through which there may be right-to-left shunting of blood and associated pulmonary atresia or VSDs. Ebstein's anomaly is a rare condition, accounting for fewer than 1% of all congenital heart anomalies.

The severity of the hemodynamic derangements in patients with Ebstein's anomaly depends on the degree of displacement and the functional status of the tricuspid valve leaflets.

As a result, the clinical presentation of Ebstein's anomaly varies from congestive heart failure in neonates to the absence of symptoms in adults in whom the anomaly is discovered incidentally. Neonates often manifest cyanosis and congestive heart failure that worsens after the ductus arteriosus closes and thereby decreases pulmonary blood flow. Most neonates with symptomatic Ebstein's anomaly will not survive without surgical intervention in infancy. Older children with Ebstein's anomaly may be diagnosed because of an incidental murmur, whereas adolescents and adults are likely to come to attention because of supraventricular dysrhythmias that lead to congestive heart failure, worsening cyanosis, and occasionally syncope. Patients with Ebstein's anomaly and an interatrial communication are at risk of paradoxical embolization, brain abscess, congestive heart failure, and sudden death.

The severity of cyanosis depends on the magnitude of the right-to-left shunt. A systolic murmur caused by tricuspid regurgitation is usually present at the left lower sternal border. Hepatomegaly resulting from passive hepatic congestion due to increased right atrial pressures may be present. The ECG is characterized by tall and broad P waves (resembling right bundle branch block), and first-degree atrioventricular heart block is common. Paroxysmal supraventricular and ventricular tachydysrhythmias may occur, and as many as 20% of patients with Ebstein's anomaly have ventricular preexcitation by way of accessory electrical pathways between the atrium and ventricle (Wolff-Parkinson-White syndrome). In patients with severe disease (marked right-to-left shunting and minimally functional right ventricle), marked cardiomegaly is present that is largely due to right atrial enlargement.

Echocardiography is used to assess right atrial dilation, the distortion of the tricuspid valve leaflets, and the severity of the tricuspid regurgitation or stenosis. The presence and magnitude of interatrial shunting can be determined by color Doppler imaging studies. Enlargement of the right atrium may be so massive that the apical portions of the lungs are compressed, which results in restrictive pulmonary disease. Chest radiographs in symptomatic infants with Ebstein's anomaly often will demonstrate significant enlargement of the right atrium and cardiomegaly, which creates the appearance of a globe-shaped, "wall-to-wall" heart that fills the chest cavity.

The hazards of pregnancy in parturient women with Ebstein's anomaly include deterioration in right ventricular function due to increased blood volume and cardiac output, increased right-to-left shunting and arterial hypoxemia if an ASD is present, and cardiac dysrhythmias. Pregnancy-induced hypertension may result in the development of congestive heart failure in these women.

Treatment of Ebstein's anomaly is based on the prevention of associated complications, including antibiotic prophylaxis against infective endocarditis and administration of diuretics and digoxin for management of congestive heart failure. Patients with supraventricular dysrhythmias are treated pharmacologically or with catheter ablation if an accessory pathway is present. In severely ill neonates with Ebstein's anomaly, an arterial shunt from the systemic circulation to the pulmonary circulation is created to increase pulmonary blood flow and thus decrease cyanosis. Further staged procedures to create a univentricular heart (Glenn's shunt and Fontan's procedure) may also be considered in these cases. Repair or replacement of the tricuspid valve in conjunction with closure of the interatrial communication is recommended for older patients who have severe symptoms despite medical therapy. Complications of surgery to correct Ebstein's anomaly include third-degree atrioventricular heart block, persistence of supraventricular dysrhythmias, residual tricuspid regurgitation after valve repair, and prosthetic valve dysfunction when the tricuspid valve is replaced.

MANAGEMENT OF ANESTHESIA

Hazards during anesthesia in patients with Ebstein's anomaly include accentuation of arterial hypoxemia due to increases in the magnitude of the right-to-left intracardiac shunt and the development of supraventricular tachydysrhythmias. The hemodynamic consequences in Ebstein's anomaly are determined by the functional status of the tricuspid valve, the size of the ASD or patent foramen ovale, impairment of right and/or left ventricular function, and the presence of Wolff-Parkinson-White syndrome. Also, since tachyarrhythmic sudden death is a threat regardless of the severity of Ebstein's anomaly, electrophysiologic evaluation is often warranted and radiofrequency ablation may be performed to avoid recurrent arrhythmia and instability in the perioperative period. A defibrillator and antidysrhythmics should be immediately available before the induction of anesthesia to potentially terminate any possible arrhythmias. Light premedication also assists in reducing the incidence of anxiety-induced tachycardia. Increased right atrial pressures may indicate the presence of right ventricular failure. In the presence of a probe-patent foramen ovale (present in approximately 30% of patients), an increase in right atrial pressure above the pressure in the left atrium can lead to a right-to-left intracardiac shunt through the foramen ovale. Unexplained arterial hypoxemia or paradoxical air embolism during the perioperative period may be due to shunting of blood or air through a previously closed foramen ovale. The anesthetic plan must also focus on the maintenance of right ventricular function and avoidance of an increase in pulmonary vascular resistance, hence curtailing hypoxemia, hypercarbia, and acidemia. Agents that lower pulmonary vascular resistance, such as nitrates and nitric oxide, may be beneficial in patients with severe pulmonary hypertension. The delayed onset of pharmacologic effects after intravenous administration of drugs during anesthesia most likely reflects pooling and dilution in an enlarged right atrium. The pooled blood also acts as a depot, releasing administered medication subsequently; this may have profound hemodynamic effects, so that care in dosing and patience in induction of anesthesia are required. Epidural analgesia with slow titration of local anesthetic has been used safely for labor and delivery.

Tricuspid Atresia

Tricuspid atresia is defined as congenital absence or agenesis of the morphologic tricuspid valve and is characterized by arterial hypoxemia, a small right ventricle, a large left ventricle, and marked decreases in pulmonary blood flow. Poorly oxygenated blood from the right atrium passes through an ASD into the left atrium, mixes with oxygenated blood, and then enters the left ventricle, from which it is ejected into the systemic circulation. Pulmonary blood flow is via a VSD, PDA, or bronchial vessels. The relative position of the great vessels is quite variable and has been the basis for classification of this anomaly: type I is characterized by normally related great arteries; type II shows dextro-transposition of the great arteries; type III has transposition of the great arteries other than dextro-transposition (such as double-outlet right or left ventricle, levo-malposition of the great arteries); and type IV is distinguished by truncus arteriosus. Patients with transposition may have associated pulmonary outflow tract obstruction, either subvalvular or valvular, whereas patients with normally related great arteries often have obstruction at the VSD level. Hence, within each type there may be one or more subgroups: (1) cases with pulmonary atresia, (2) cases with pulmonary stenosis or hypoplasia, and (3) cases with normal pulmonary arteries and no stenosis.

SIGNS AND SYMPTOMS

Approximately one half of patients with tricuspid atresia have symptoms on the first day of life, and 80% exhibit symptoms by the end of the first month of life. The magnitude of the pulmonary blood flow determines the type and timing of the clinical presentation. In infants (and children) with decreased pulmonary blood flow, the physical examination reveals central cyanosis, clubbing (in older children), tachypnea or hyperpnea, normal pulses, a prominent *a* wave in the jugular venous pulse (if there is interatrial obstruction), no hepatic enlargement, and no clinical signs of congestive heart failure. A holosystolic murmur suggestive of VSD may be heard in the left lower sternal border or continuous PDA murmur. In those with increased pulmonary blood flow, examination reveals tachypnea, tachycardia, decreased femoral pulses (if associated with coarctation of the aorta), minimal cyanosis, hepatomegaly, prominent *a* waves, VSD and/or PDA murmurs, and clinical signs of congestive heart failure. In addition, difficulty feeding, failure to thrive, diaphoresis, and recurrent respiratory tract infections may also be seen in these patients. Chest radiographic findings depend on the total pulmonary blood flow and provide no consistent pattern diagnostic of tricuspid atresia. The ECG in an infant with cyanotic tricuspid atresia shows signs of right atrial enlargement, left axis deviation, and left ventricular hypertrophy. Left axis deviation is seen in 80% of patients with type I anatomy (normally related great vessels) and in fewer than 50% of patients with type II (transposition) anatomy. Echocardiography shows the atretic tricuspid valve with the enlarged right atrium, left atrium, and left ventricle, and Doppler flow studies identify obstruction across the VSD and the right ventricular outflow tract and estimate pulmonary artery pressures. Cardiac catheterization and angiography are useful if issues are not clarified by the noninvasive studies.

TREATMENT

Since these patients often come to attention as neonates, they are frequently managed based on the degree of pulmonary blood flow and associated symptoms. The cyanotic neonate or neonate with decreased but ductal-dependent pulmonary blood flow may require prostaglandin to maintain patency and receive a Blalock-Taussig type of shunt until reaching an acceptable age or stage of development for more definitive treatment. Patients with symptomatic pulmonary congestion may initially be managed medically with diuretics, and once in stable condition, they may undergo temporizing treatment via pulmonary artery banding, then staged correction via Glenn's shunt placement and finally Fontan's operation. Ultimately, either of two types of Fontan's procedure is used to treat tricuspid atresia. One is the classical internal conduit with anastomosis of the right atrial appendage to the right pulmonary artery to bypass the right ventricle and provide a direct atriopulmonary communication. The other is the extracardiac Fontan's procedure, which also diverts inferior vena caval flow into the pulmonary arteries. This operation is also used to treat pulmonary artery atresia.

MANAGEMENT OF ANESTHESIA

Management of anesthesia in patients undergoing Fontan's procedures has been successfully achieved with opioids or volatile anesthetics. Immediately after cardiopulmonary bypass and continuing into the early postoperative period, it is important to maintain increased right atrial pressures (16 to 20 mm Hg) to facilitate pulmonary blood flow. An increase in pulmonary vascular resistance resulting from acidosis, hypercarbia, hypothermia, peak airway pressures higher than 15 cm H_2O, or reactions to the tracheal tube may cause right-sided heart failure. Early tracheal extubation and spontaneous ventilation are desirable. Positive inotropic drugs (dopamine) with or without vasodilators (nitroprusside) are often required to optimize cardiac output and maintain low pulmonary vascular resistance. Pleural effusions, ascites, and edema of the lower extremities are not uncommon postoperatively and usually resolve within a few weeks. Right atrial pressure that is equal to the pulmonary artery pressure remains elevated after this operation, averaging 15 mm Hg.

Although absence of a contractile right ventricle is compatible with long-term survival, the adaptability of the circulatory system is restricted. This decreased capacity of a single ventricle to respond to an increased workload may have a significant impact on the management of these patients during another operation. In this regard, subsequent management of anesthesia in patients who have undergone Fontan's procedures is facilitated by monitoring the central venous pressure (which equals the pulmonary artery pressure in

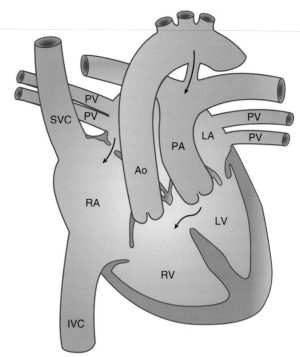

FIGURE 3-5 Transposition of the great arteries. The right ventricle (RV) and left ventricle (LV) are not connected in series. Instead, the two ventricles function as parallel and independent circulations, with the aorta (Ao) arising from the RV and the pulmonary artery (PA) arising from the LV. Survival is not possible unless mixing of blood between the two circulations occurs through an atrial septal defect, ventricular septal defect, or patent ductus. *IVC,* Inferior vena cava; *LA,* left atrium; *PV,* pulmonary vein; *RA,* right atrium; *SVC,* superior vena cava.

these patients) to assess the intravascular fluid volume and to detect sudden impairment of left ventricular function and increased pulmonary vascular resistance. The value of monitoring the central venous pressure reflects the absence of a contractile right ventricle and the impaired ability of a single ventricle to adapt to acute increases in afterload, which may necessitate prompt administration of positive inotropic drugs. Insertion of a thermodilution pulmonary artery catheter in patients after Fontan's procedure may be technically difficult because of the unusual anatomy. No information is available regarding the accuracy of thermodilution cardiac output measurements in such patients. Peak and mean airway pressure must be maintained, because this will increase pulmonary vascular resistance and may decrease carbon dioxide significantly.

Transposition of the Great Arteries

Transposition of the great arteries constitutes 5% of all congenital heart disease and 10% of all neonatal cyanotic congenital heart disease. Transposition of the great arteries results from failure of the truncus arteriosus to spiral, so that the aorta arises from the anterior portion of the right ventricle and the pulmonary artery arises from the left ventricle (Figure 3-5).

There is complete separation of the pulmonary and systemic circulations such that systemic venous blood traverses the right atrium, right ventricle, aorta, and systemic circulation; and pulmonary venous blood traverses the left atrium, left ventricle, pulmonary artery, and lungs. Thus, the circulation is parallel instead of normal in-series circulation. Survival is possible only if there is communication between the two circulations in the form of a VSD, ASD, or PDA.

SIGNS AND SYMPTOMS

Clinical symptoms depend on the type. Infants in group I, who have transposition of the great arteries with intact ventricular septum, usually exhibit cyanosis in the first week of life (sometimes within hours to days of life) or may otherwise be asymptomatic; they will, with time, become tachypneic and develop respiratory distress. The right ventricular impulse will be increased, and either no murmur or a grade I-II/VI nonspecific systolic ejection murmur may be auscultated. Infants in group II, who have transposition of the great arteries with VSD, show symptoms of congestive heart failure (tachypnea, tachycardia, sweating, and poor feeding) between 4 to 8 weeks with relatively minimal cyanosis. Congestive heart failure reflects left ventricular failure resulting from volume overload created by the left-to-right intracardiac shunt necessary for survival. A grade III-IV/VI holosystolic murmur at the left lower sternal border and mid-diastolic flow rumble (murmur) at the apex may be present. Infants in group III have transposition of the great arteries with VSD and pulmonary stenosis, and presentation varies based on the severity of the stenosis. If the pulmonary stenosis is severe, the presentation may present similar to that of patients with tetralogy of Fallot. With moderate pulmonary stenosis, the presentation is late with longer survival, and those with mild stenosis may exhibit signs of congestive heart failure similar to group II patients. The ECG is likely to demonstrate right axis deviation and right ventricular hypertrophy because the right ventricle is the systemic ventricle. Classically, the cardiac silhouette on the chest radiograph is described as being "egg shaped with a narrow stalk." Echocardiography is generally helpful in diagnosis and assessment.

TREATMENT

The immediate management of transposition of the great arteries involves creating intracardiac mixing or increasing the degree of mixing. This goal is accomplished with infusions of prostaglandin E$_1$ to maintain patency of the ductus arteriosus and/or balloon atrial septostomy (Rashkind's procedure). Administration of oxygen may decrease pulmonary vascular resistance and increase pulmonary blood flow. Diuretics and digoxin are administered to treat congestive heart failure.

Two surgical switch procedures have been used to treat complete transition of the great arteries. The surgical procedure first used, known as *Mustard's* or *Senning's operation,* generally involved resection of the atrial septum and its replacement with a baffle to direct the systemic venous blood into the left ventricle and the pulmonary venous blood across the tricuspid valve into the right ventricle. This operation has been replaced by the arterial switch operation in which the pulmonary artery and ascending aorta are transected above the semilunar valves and reanastomosed with the right and left ventricles; the coronary arteries are then reimplanted so that the aorta is connected to the left ventricle and the pulmonary artery is connected to the right ventricle. The arterial switch operation has some advantages over the venous switch procedure in that arrhythmias are less frequent and the left ventricle rather than the right ventricle serves as a pump to the systemic circuit.

MANAGEMENT OF ANESTHESIA

Management of anesthesia in the presence of transposition of the great arteries must take into account the separation of the pulmonary and systemic circulations. Drugs administered intravenously are distributed with minimal dilution to organs such as the heart and brain. Therefore, doses and rates of injection of intravenously administered drugs may have to be decreased. Conversely, the onset of anesthesia produced by inhaled drugs is delayed because only small amounts of the inhaled drug reach the systemic circulation. In the final analysis, induction and maintenance of anesthesia are often accomplished with ketamine combined with muscle relaxants to facilitate tracheal intubation. Ketamine can be supplemented with opioids or benzodiazepines for maintenance of anesthesia. Nitrous oxide has limited application in these patients, because it is important to administer oxygen at high inspired concentrations. The potential cardiac-depressant effects of volatile anesthetics detract from the use of these drugs. Selection of muscle relaxants is influenced by the desire to avoid histamine-induced changes in systemic blood pressure. The ability of pancuronium to increase the heart rate and systemic blood pressure modestly may be useful.

Dehydration must be avoided during the perioperative period. These patients may have hematocrits in excess of 70%, which may contribute to the high incidence of cerebral venous thrombosis. This finding suggests that oral fluids should not be withheld from these patients for prolonged periods. An intravenous infusion should be initiated during the preoperative period. Atrial dysrhythmias and conduction disturbances may occur postoperatively.

Mixing of Blood between the Pulmonary and Systemic Circulations

Rare congenital heart defects that result in mixing of blood from the pulmonary and systemic circulations manifest as cyanosis and arterial hypoxemia of varying severity depending on the magnitude of the pulmonary blood flow. As a result of the mixing of blood from both circulations, pulmonary arterial blood has a higher oxygen saturation than that of systemic venous blood, and systemic arterial blood has a lower oxygen saturation than that of pulmonary venous blood.

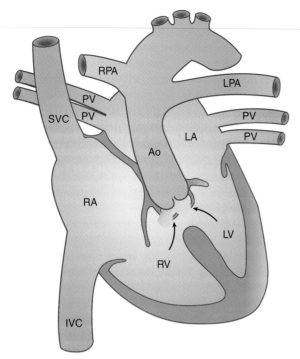

FIGURE 3-6 Truncus arteriosus in which the pulmonary artery and aorta (Ao) arise from a single trunk that overrides the left ventricle (LV) and right ventricle (RV). This trunk receives blood from both ventricles by virtue of a ventricular septal defect. *IVC,* Inferior vena cava; *LA,* left atrium; *LPA,* left pulmonary artery; *PV,* pulmonary vein; *RA,* right atrium; *RPA,* right pulmonary artery; *SVC,* superior vena cava.

Truncus Arteriosus

Truncus arteriosus refers to the congenital cardiac defect in which a single arterial trunk serves as the origin of the aorta and pulmonary artery (Figure 3-6). This single arterial trunk overrides both ventricles, which are connected through a VSD. Mortality is high, with a median survival of approximately 5 to 6 weeks.

SIGNS AND SYMPTOMS

The spectrum of severity is based on the origin of the pulmonary arteries from the truncal artery. A main pulmonary artery may arise from the truncal artery (type I truncus arteriosus), the branch pulmonary arteries may arise separately but in close proximity (type II), or the branch pulmonary arteries may arise widely separate from the lateral aspects of the truncal artery (type III). Truncus arteriosus results in unrestrictive left-to-right shunting of blood and pulmonary overcirculation. Presenting signs and symptoms of truncus arteriosus include cyanosis and arterial hypoxemia, failure to thrive, and congestive heart failure early in life. Peripheral pulses may be accentuated owing to the rapid diastolic runoff of blood into the pulmonary circulation. Auscultation of the chest and evaluation of the ECG do not give predictable information and are not diagnostic. Chest radiography reveals cardiomegaly and increased vascularity of the lung fields. The diagnosis is confirmed by angiocardiography performed during cardiac catheterization.

TREATMENT

Surgical treatment of truncus arteriosus includes banding of the right and left pulmonary arteries if pulmonary blood flow is excessive. In addition, an associated VSD can be closed so only left ventricular output enters the truncus arteriosus. When this is done, a Dacron conduit with a valve is also placed between the right ventricle and pulmonary artery.

MANAGEMENT OF ANESTHESIA

Management of anesthesia in the presence of truncus arteriosus is influenced by the magnitude of the pulmonary blood flow. When pulmonary blood flow is increased, the use of positive end-expiratory pressure is beneficial and may serve to decrease the symptoms of congestive heart failure. Increased pulmonary blood flow may be associated with evidence of myocardial ischemia on the ECG. When myocardial ischemia that occurs intraoperatively does not respond to intravenous administration of phenylephrine or fluids, or the use of positive end-expiratory pressure, consideration may be given to temporary banding of the pulmonary artery to increase systemic and coronary blood flow. Patients with decreased pulmonary blood flow and arterial hypoxemia should be managed in the same way as patients with tetralogy of Fallot.

Partial Anomalous Pulmonary Venous Return

Partial anomalous pulmonary venous return is characterized by the presence of left or right pulmonary veins that empty into the right side of the circulation rather than the left atrium. In approximately one half of cases, the aberrant pulmonary veins drain into the superior vena cava. This abnormality results in left-to-right shunting of blood at the atrial level as well as right ventricular and right atrial dilatation. In the remaining cases, pulmonary veins enter the right atrium, inferior vena cava, azygos vein, or coronary sinus. Partial anomalous pulmonary venous return may be more common than appreciated, as suggested by the presence of this anomaly in approximately 0.5% of routine autopsy cases.

The onset and severity of symptoms produced by this abnormality depend on the amount of pulmonary blood flow routed through the right side of the heart. Fatigue and exertional dyspnea are the most frequent initial manifestations, usually appearing during early adulthood. Cyanosis and congestive heart failure are likely if more than 50% of the pulmonary venous flow enters the right side of the circulation. With prolonged right atrial dilatation, right ventricular dysfunction and atrial arrhythmias can occur.

Angiography is the most useful technique for confirming the diagnosis of partial anomalous pulmonary venous return. Cardiac catheterization usually demonstrates normal intracardiac pressures and increased oxygen saturations of blood in the right side of the heart. Treatment is by surgical repair.

Total Anomalous Pulmonary Venous Return

Total anomalous pulmonary venous return (total anomalous pulmonary venous connection, or TAPVC) is characterized by drainage of all four pulmonary veins into the systemic venous system. The most common presentation of this defect—supracardiac TAPVC—accounting for approximately one half of cases, is drainage of the four pulmonary veins into the left innominate vein in association with a left-sided superior vena cava. Oxygenated blood reaches the left atrium by way of an ASD. PDA is present in approximately one third of patients. Intracardiac TAPVC is present when the pulmonary venous return enters a common confluence that then empties into the coronary sinus. Coronary venous return, pulmonary venous return, and systemic venous return empty into the right atrium. The left atrium receives mixed systemic and pulmonary venous return via an ASD. Infracardiac TAPVC is present when the pulmonary venous confluence drains inferiorly to the ductus venosus, which empties into the inferior vena cava and connects to the liver's portal vein system. The right atrium receives mixed systemic and pulmonary venous return, whereas the left atrium is supplied by the right atrium via an ASD.

SIGNS AND SYMPTOMS

TAPVC presents clinically as congestive heart failure in 50% of patients by 1 month of age and in 90% by 1 year. Those with obstructed pulmonary venous return are severely cyanotic, developing respiratory distress, tachypnea, grunting, and retractions of the rib cage muscles, whereas those with unobstructed flow may initially be asymptomatic with mild cyanosis. Murmur indicative of an ASD is also present. The ECG demonstrates signs of right atrial and right ventricular enlargement. The chest radiograph may show evidence of cardiomegaly and pulmonary edema. Echocardiography can demonstrate enlargement of the right atrium and right ventricle and assess the size and flow across the ASD. It is definitively diagnosed by angiocardiography. Cardiac catheterization can also detect whether there is pulmonary venous obstruction and whether the ASD is restrictive. Mortality is approximately 80% by 1 year of age unless the TAPVC is surgically corrected using cardiopulmonary bypass and aortic cross-clamping.

MANAGEMENT OF ANESTHESIA AND TREATMENT

Management of anesthesia in the presence of TAPVC may include application of positive end-expiratory pressure to the airways in an attempt to decrease excessive pulmonary blood flow. Patients who have pulmonary edema should undergo positive pressure ventilation through an endotracheal tube before cardiac catheterization. Operative manipulation of the right atrium, which is tolerated by healthy patients, may result in obstruction to flow into the right atrium in these patients, manifesting as sudden decreases in systemic blood pressure and the onset of bradycardia. Intravenous transfusions may be hazardous, because any increase in right atrial pressure is transmitted directly to the pulmonary veins, which can lead to pulmonary edema. Surgical repair takes advantage of the fact that in virtually all types of TAPVC, the pulmonary veins return to a common confluence behind the left atrium. The common pulmonary vein confluence is connected by the surgeon to the back of the left atrium, which results in normal connection of pulmonary veins to the left atrial chamber. The ASD is then closed. Postoperatively, atrioventricular conduction disturbances, atrial tachydysrhythmias, and sinus bradycardia are sometimes encountered. Elevated pulmonary vascular resistance with decreased cardiac output and pulmonary hypertension may develop, requiring hyperventilation, increased sedation, and administration of inhaled nitric oxide. Extracorporeal membrane oxygenation support is sometimes required in the early postoperative period.

Hypoplastic Left Heart Syndrome

Hypoplastic left heart syndrome is characterized by left ventricular hypoplasia, mitral valve hypoplasia, aortic valve atresia, and hypoplasia of the ascending aorta. Extracardiac congenital anomalies do not usually accompany this syndrome. There is complete mixing of pulmonary venous and systemic venous blood in a single ventricle, which is connected in parallel to both the pulmonary and systemic circulations. Systemic blood flow is dependent on a PDA. In addition to ductal patency, infant survival depends on a balance between systemic vascular resistance and pulmonary vascular resistance, because both circulations are supplied from a single ventricle in a parallel fashion. An abrupt decrease in pulmonary vascular resistance after delivery results in increased pulmonary blood flow at the expense of systemic blood flow (pulmonary steal phenomenon). When this occurs, coronary and systemic blood flow is inadequate, which leads to metabolic acidosis, high-output cardiac failure, and ventricular fibrillation, despite increasingly high Pao_2 values (Figure 3-7). Alternatively, any postnatal event that leads to increased pulmonary vascular resistance can decrease the pulmonary blood flow so severely that arterial hypoxemia worsens, leading to progressive metabolic acidosis and circulatory collapse (see Figure 3-7). Because rapid changes in pulmonary vascular resistance occur during the postnatal period, the necessary fine balance between pulmonary vascular resistance and systemic vascular resistance is unstable and difficult to maintain.

SIGNS AND SYMPTOMS

The common presentation of newborns with hypoplastic left heart syndrome at birth is cardiovascular collapse and shock. The peripheral pulses are weak, without a major difference between the brachial and femoral pulses. There is usually a mild to moderate degree of cyanosis, but no differential cyanosis. The chest radiograph shows cardiomegaly and plethoric lung fields. The ECG documents right ventricular hypertrophy and reduced left ventricular forces. If the diagnosis is suspected, infusion of prostaglandin normally maintains patency of the ductus arteriosus and prevents further cardiovascular compromise, progressive acidosis, and death.

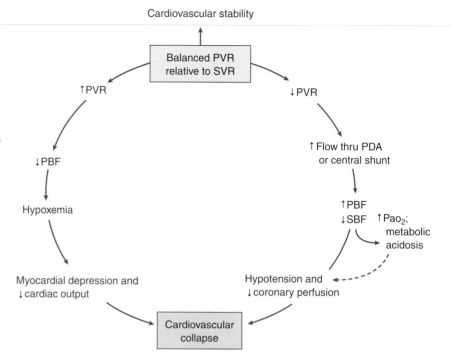

FIGURE 3-7 Cardiovascular stability in the presence of hypoplastic left heart syndrome requires a balance between pulmonary vascular resistance (PVR) and systemic vascular resistance (SVR). An abrupt decrease in PVR after delivery can result in excessive pulmonary blood flow (PBF) relative to systemic blood flow (SBF) with cardiovascular collapse despite the absence of arterial hypoxemia. Conversely, postnatal changes that increase PVR can lead to cardiovascular collapse in the presence of arterial hypoxemia. *PDA,* Patent ductus arteriosus. *(From Hansen DD, Hickey PR. Anesthesia for hypoplastic left heart syndrome: use of high-dose fentanyl in 30 neonates. Anesth Analg. 1986;65:127-132, with permission.)*

TREATMENT

Administration of cardiac inotropes and sodium bicarbonate may be necessary. Ultimately, treatment of hypoplastic left heart syndrome is surgical, beginning with a palliative procedure that eliminates the need for continued patency of the ductus arteriosus.

Stage I, or the initial palliative procedure, consists of reconstructing the ascending aorta using the proximal pulmonary artery (Figure 3-8). A systemic-to-pulmonary shunt to provide pulmonary blood flow is placed between the reconstructed aorta and the distal pulmonary artery (Blalock-Taussig shunt). Typically, infants are placed on cardiopulmonary bypass to permit induction of whole-body hypothermia; reconstruction of the aorta is then accomplished during 40 to 60 minutes of circulatory arrest. The central shunt is placed after reinstitution of cardiopulmonary bypass and during rewarming. The completed palliative procedure leaves the single right ventricle connected in parallel to the systemic circulation and pulmonary circulation. This classic Norwood procedure places a nonvalved tube from the right ventricle to the left pulmonary artery (Sano's modification), and later to the right pulmonary artery. Controversy continues as to the advantages and disadvantages of either approach. At present there is no significant difference in 1-year survival after any of these procedures. At about 4 to 6 months of age, children who underwent stage I palliation experience severe cyanosis because of the very limited pulmonary blood flow. It is then common practice to proceed to surgical creation of a bidirectional cavopulmonary (Glenn) shunt with interruption of the original Blalock-Taussig shunt or the conduit from the right ventricle to the pulmonary artery. At around 2 to 5 years of age, children with hypoplastic left heart syndrome who have undergone stage

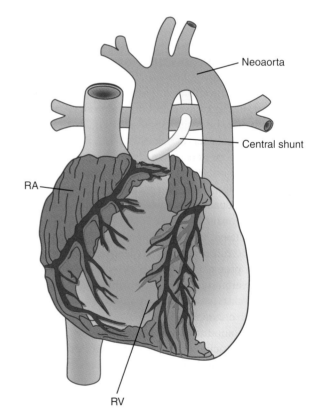

FIGURE 3-8 Anatomy after the first-stage palliative procedure for hypoplastic left heart syndrome during the neonatal period. The ascending aorta has been reconstructed from the proximal pulmonary artery to form a neoaorta. *RA,* Right atrium; *RV,* right ventricle. *(From Hansen DD, Hickey PR. Anesthesia for hypoplastic left heart syndrome: use of high-dose fentanyl in 30 neonates. Anesth Analg. 1986;65:127-132, with permission.)*

I and II surgery will become increasingly fatigued and short of breath with cyanosis after mild to moderate activity. The stage is now set for correction with Fontan's procedure when pulmonary vascular resistance has decreased to adult levels (see the section on tricuspid atresia). Execution of Fontan's procedure plus elimination of the systemic-to-pulmonary shunt separates the two circulations and facilitates development of normal arterial oxygen saturation.

MANAGEMENT OF ANESTHESIA

Umbilical artery and intravenous catheters are usually placed before infants with uncorrected hypoplastic left heart syndrome arrive in the operating room. After monitoring is instituted, induction of anesthesia is often accomplished with fentanyl (50 to 75 mcg/kg IV) administered simultaneously with pancuronium.

These infants are vulnerable to the development of ventricular fibrillation resulting from inadequate coronary blood flow before the palliative procedure. The danger of ventricular fibrillation and borderline cardiac status argues against the use of volatile anesthetics in these infants. A high PaO_2 implies excessive pulmonary blood flow at the expense of the systemic circulation. Indeed, if the initial PaO_2 is more than 100 mm Hg, maneuvers to increase pulmonary vascular resistance and decrease pulmonary blood flow are instituted. For example, a decrease in the volume of ventilation leads to increases in $PaCO_2$ and decreases in the arterial pH, which results in increased pulmonary vascular resistance and decreased pulmonary blood flow. If the PaO_2 remains unacceptably high, institution of positive end-expiratory pressure leads to increased lung volumes and further increases in pulmonary vascular resistance. In extreme cases, temporary occlusion of one pulmonary artery serves to decrease the PaO_2.

Dopamine or isoproterenol is administered when necessary for inotropic support at the conclusion of cardiopulmonary bypass. The selection of specific inotropic drugs is influenced by pulmonary vascular resistance. The most frequent problem after cardiopulmonary bypass is too little pulmonary blood flow with associated arterial hypoxemia (PaO_2 of <20 mm Hg). Methods to improve the PaO_2 include hyperventilation of the lungs to produce a low $PaCO_2$ (20 to 25 mm Hg) and to increase the arterial pH, plus infusion of isoproterenol to decrease pulmonary vascular resistance. A PaO_2 higher than 50 mm Hg after cardiopulmonary bypass may indicate inadequate systemic blood flow and the likely occurrence of progressive metabolic acidosis unless steps are taken to decrease pulmonary blood flow. In the setting of refractory cardiovascular and hemodynamic instability, there may be an indication for ECMO, but debate continues as to the selection of patients for this therapy.

MECHANICAL OBSTRUCTION OF THE TRACHEA

The trachea can be obstructed by circulatory anomalies that produce a vascular ring or by dilation of the pulmonary artery secondary to absence of the pulmonic valve. These lesions must be considered when evaluating a child with unexplained stridor or other evidence of upper airway obstruction. The possibility of an undiagnosed vascular ring should be considered in the differential diagnosis of airway obstruction that follows placement of a nasogastric tube or an esophageal stethoscope.

Double Aortic Arch

Double aortic arch results in a vascular ring that can produce pressure on the trachea and esophagus. Compression resulting from this pressure can be manifested as inspiratory stridor, difficulty mobilizing secretions, and dysphagia. Patients with this cardiac defect usually prefer to lie with the neck extended because flexion of the neck often accentuates compression of the trachea.

Surgical transection of the smaller aortic arch is the treatment of choice for symptomatic patients. During surgery, the tracheal tube should be placed beyond the area of tracheal compression if this can be safely accomplished without producing endobronchial intubation. It must be appreciated that esophageal stethoscopes or nasogastric tubes can cause occlusion of the trachea if the tracheal tube remains above the level of vascular compression. Clinical improvement after surgical transection is often prompt. In addition to hemodynamic factors, weaning from mechanical ventilation should take into account the risk of tracheomalacia caused by prolonged compression of the trachea, which can jeopardize the patency of the trachea.

Aberrant Left Pulmonary Artery

Tracheal or bronchial obstruction can occur when the left pulmonary artery is absent and the arterial supply to the left lung is derived from a branch of the right pulmonary artery passing between the trachea and esophagus. This anatomic arrangement has been referred to as *vascular sling* because a complete ring is not present. The sling can cause obstruction of the right main bronchus, the distal trachea, or rarely the left main bronchus.

Clinical manifestations of an aberrant left pulmonary artery include stridor, wheezing, and occasionally arterial hypoxemia. Unlike with a true vascular ring, esophageal obstructions are rare, and the stridor produced by this defect is usually present during exhalation rather than inspiration. Chest radiographs may demonstrate an abnormal separation between the esophagus and the trachea. Hyperinflation or atelectasis of either lung may be present. Angiography is the most accurate approach for confirming the diagnosis.

Surgical division of the aberrant left pulmonary artery at its origin and redirection of its course anterior to the trachea, with anastomosis to the main pulmonary artery, is the treatment of choice. During the first months of life, surgical correction with deep hypothermia without cardiopulmonary bypass may be considered. Theoretically, continuous positive airway pressure or positive end-expiratory pressure should relieve the airway obstruction and associated stridor in these cases.

Absent Pulmonic Valve

Absence of the pulmonic valve results in dilation of the pulmonary artery, which can result in compression of the trachea and left main bronchus. This lesion may occur as an isolated defect or in conjunction with tetralogy of Fallot. Symptoms include signs of tracheal obstruction and occasionally the development of arterial hypoxemia and congestive heart failure. Any increase in pulmonary vascular resistance, as may occur with arterial hypoxemia or hypercarbia, accentuates airway obstruction. Tracheal intubation and maintenance of 4 to 6 mm Hg of continuous positive airway pressure can be used to keep the trachea distended, which reduces the magnitude of airway obstruction. Definitive treatment consists of inserting a tubular graft with an artificial pulmonic valve.

THE ADULT PATIENT WITH CONGENITAL HEART DISEASE UNDERGOING NONCARDIAC SURGERY

Because of improvements in medical and surgical care, increasing numbers of children with congenital heart disease are living into adulthood. In the United States alone there are more adult patients with congenital heart disease than pediatric patients with these disorders, and the number of surviving citizens is estimated to be between 1 million and 2.9 million. The prevalence of severe congenital heart disease in adult patients increased by 85% from 1985 to 2000, significantly outpacing that in the pediatric population. Although survival into adulthood has improved for patients with congenital heart disease, attributable to more profound knowledge of the multisystem effects of congenital heart disease as well as better surgical and percutaneous techniques, the fact that the median age of the congenital heart disease population in 2002 was 40 years and that of the severe congenital heart disease population was 29 years indicates that survival is not normal in this cohort. The majority of the mortality and morbidity in these patients can be attributed to chronic difficulties, namely, cardiovascular causes such as chronic heart failure. In two large cohorts, hospitalization rates were 50%, twice that of the general population. Long-term cardiac complications include pulmonary hypertension, ventricular dysfunction, dysrhythmias and conduction defects, residual shunts, valvular lesions (regurgitation and stenosis), hypertension, and aneurysms. A significant number of these patients require additional cardiac surgeries to address residual lesions, such as atrioventricular valve regurgitation, pulmonary valve regurgitation, outflow tract obstruction, or arrhythmias. Noncardiac sequelae include developmental abnormalities, central nervous system abnormalities such as seizure disorders from prior thromboembolic or cerebrovascular events, secondary erythrocytosis, cholelithiasis,

nephrolithiasis, hearing or visual loss, and restrictive and obstructive lung disease. Debate continues as to whether these patients are best served in children's hospitals, since the procedures are often performed by pediatric cardiac surgeons, or in adult centers, where there is familiarity with some of the comorbidities in adults not seen as often in children, such as atherosclerotic coronary disease, peripheral vascular disease, deep venous thrombosis, and emphysema. In either case, adult patients with congenital heart disease should be treated optimally by clinicians with expertise in the physiology of congenital heart disease and its manifestations in the mature individual. Therefore, knowledge of and experience with the physiology of adult congenital heart disease and its challenges is paramount for the anesthesiologist during the perioperative period.

Management of Anesthesia

PREOPERATIVE EVALUATION

Adult congenital heart disease patients can be viewed on a continuum in which some patients have defects that have not been corrected, some have received palliative repairs (e.g., partial or total cavopulmonary shunts), and others have undergone complete correction. In nearly all cases, congenital heart disease in adults should be viewed as a systemic condition with associated multiorgan dysfunction. Perioperative risk is substantially increased in adults with congenital heart disease, particularly those with poor functional status, pulmonary hypertension, congestive heart failure, and cyanosis. In addition to obtaining the basic preoperative information, the anesthesiologist should be familiar with the patient's specific anatomy and physiology as determined by echocardiographic and cardiac catheterization results. The most common lesions seen in adult patients with congenital heart disease are (1) conotruncal abnormalities after repair (of tetralogy of Fallot, truncus arteriosus, double-outlet right ventricle), (2) coarctation of the aorta after repair, (3) transposition of the great arteries after an atrial or arterial switch procedure, (4) complex single ventricles after Fontan's procedure, (5) pulmonary valve stenosis, (6) congenital aortic valve stenosis, (7) atrioventricular canal defects (complete and partial) after repair, (8) secundum ASDs, (9) congenitally corrected transposition of the great arteries, and (10) sinus venosus ASDs with partial anomalous pulmonary venous return.

With each lesion, there are unique manifestations require a meticulous perioperative plan. *Premedication* is advantageous in those adult congenital heart disease patients with anxiety because of multiple prior procedures or developmental delay (trisomy 21) but must be undertaken cautiously, because hypercapnia and hypoventilation can increase pulmonary vascular resistance and be deleterious to patients with pulmonary hypertension or systemic-to-pulmonary shunts. *Endocarditis prophylaxis* is also an important perioperative factor for these patients, and new guidelines from the American Heart Association (AHA) are discussed in the last section.

Dysrhythmias are common in adults with congenital heart disease; for example, supraventricular dysrhythmias occur in 20% to 45% of patients who have undergone previous atrial surgery (late ASD closure, Mustard's or Fontan's procedure) or who have atrial dilatation. The most common form of tachyarrhythmia observed is intraatrial reentrant tachycardia originating from the right atrium, which can be resistant to pharmacologic treatment and lead to rapid hemodynamic deterioration. Ventricular dysrhythmias may be seen in adult congenital heart disease patients who have significantly depressed right or left ventricular function. Some patients may require permanent pacemakers or an intracardiac defibrillator.

Pulmonary hypertension poses another risk factor to adults with congenital heart disease. It can be due to pulmonary venous hypertension secondary to elevated ventricular end-diastolic pressure, elevated pulmonary venous atrial pressure, or pulmonary vein stenosis. Although some patients may have decreased oxygen saturation resulting from residual shunt or poor lung function, the main cause of pulmonary hypertension in adults with congenital heart disease is the presence of chronic large and nonrestrictive shunts. The increased blood flow and near systemic pressure to the pulmonary vasculature can lead to irreversible vascular changes and elevated pulmonary vascular resistance. Eisenmenger's syndrome, for instance, is pulmonary hypertension resulting from chronic left-to-right shunting. Predictors of mortality in these patients include poor functional status, younger age at presentation or development of symptoms, syncope, supraventricular dysrhythmias, elevated right atrial pressures, low oxygen saturation (<85%), renal insufficiency, severe right ventricular dysfunction, and trisomy 21.

Heart failure, namely, right-sided and left-sided failure, is a common complication of both corrected and uncorrected congenital heart disease. Abnormal cardiac autonomic nervous system regulation and altered hemodynamics contribute to the development of heart failure in these patients. Approaches for the management of left ventricular failure are well documented, and such management should be optimized in the perioperative period. Unlike for left ventricular failure, there are no evidence-based guidelines for the management of heart failure in patients with a systemic right ventricle (congenitally corrected transposition of the great arteries and single ventricles).

Coagulation and bleeding abnormalities may also be apparent in adults with congenital heart disease. Cyanotic patients often have low levels of circulating vitamin K–dependent clotting factors, factor V, and von Willebrand factor, which leads to an elevated international normalized ratio and a prolonged activated partial thromboplastin time. However, because of decreased flow and increased blood viscosity, they do not have an elevated bleeding time. The increased bleeding risk does not counteract the risk of thrombosis due to secondary erythrocytosis, which develops as a compensatory response to chronic hypoxia and from overproduction of erythropoietin. As a result, the increased whole-blood viscosity with increased red cell mass and decreased plasma volume leads to reduced flow-through in the small arterioles and capillaries. In the perioperative setting, preoperative fasting might exacerbate symptoms of hyperviscosity and increase the risk of cerebrovascular thrombosis; hence, adequate hydration with intravenous fluids is paramount in these fasting patients, and in some cases, preoperative phlebotomy might be advisable when hematocrit levels exceed 65%. Coagulation status must also be assessed and potentially corrected in patients undergoing moderate or major surgery.

INTRAOPERATIVE MANAGEMENT

The intraoperative anesthetic strategy depends on the complexity of the congenital heart disease, prior surgery, the patient's functional status, and the type of operation being performed. In addition to direct examination, standard monitoring with pulse oximetry, ECG, arterial blood pressure measurement, capnography, and temperature measurement should be used in all patients, with careful consideration of the underlying anatomy and physiology. For example, in those patients with hypoplastic left heart syndrome who have undergone three stages of repair (Blalock-Taussig shunt, Glenn's shunt, and Fontan's procedure), placement of a central venous catheter, as well as interpretation of its readings obtained, may be complicated. In patients with Fontan circulation, for example, central venous pressure reflects mean pulmonary artery pressure. In patients with an intraatrial baffle (e.g., Mustard's or Senning's procedure), pulmonary artery catheter placement may be difficult or impossible. Intraarterial monitoring may be essential in adult congenital heart disease patients, especially those with Eisenmenger's syndrome, intracardiac shunts, or systemic-to-pulmonary shunts, who are sensitive to sudden changes in preload and systemic and pulmonary vascular resistance. However, vascular access may be challenging because of the presence of scar tissue from prior vessel catheterization. Finally, transesophageal echocardiography may be useful to monitor intravascular volume status and ventricular function.

Unless the patient is having a primary or staged cardiac repair, there are no evidence-based recommendations to guide the anesthetic management of the adult congenital heart disease patient undergoing surgery. However, intraoperative management should promote tissue oxygen delivery by preventing arterial desaturation, maintaining a balance between pulmonary and systemic flows, and optimizing hematocrit. Most intravenous agents depress myocardial contractility and decrease systemic vascular resistance, which could have a deleterious effect on tissue oxygen delivery during induction of anesthesia. The use of ketamine has been shown to be beneficial in children with congenital heart disease and pulmonary hypertension undergoing sevoflurane anesthesia because it maintains ventricular performance and systemic vascular resistance without increasing pulmonary vascular resistance, but it has been associated with an increase in pulmonary vascular resistance in adults without congenital heart disease. Overall choice of anesthetic agent should be guided by the patient's underlying physiology and current presentation, and by the goal of balancing systemic and pulmonary blood flow. *Intracardiac and systemic-to-pulmonary shunts* can provide challenges to case management. For example, in patients with cyanotic heart disease, ventilation with high airway pressures can increase pulmonary vascular resistance, compromise venous return, and exacerbate right-to-left shunt physiology. Placement in Trendelenburg's position can increase central venous (superior vena cava) pressure and cause cerebral hypoperfusion in a patient with a Glenn shunt or Fontan circulation. In those adult patients with large ASDs, inadequate anesthesia and sympathetic nervous system stimulation might increase systemic vascular resistance, exacerbate left-to-right shunting, and reduce cardiac output. Adult congenital heart disease patients with *univentricular* physiology and anatomy, and pulmonary hypertension, such as those with Eisenmenger's syndrome, can be the most challenging in terms of intraoperative anesthetic management. As another example, adults with congenital heart disease who have undergone Fontan's procedure generally have passive, nonpulsatile flow from both the inferior and superior vena cava to the pulmonary artery; hence, any factor that increases pulmonary vascular resistance will decrease pulmonary blood flow and lead to arterial desaturation. Prevention and treatment of pulmonary hypertensive crisis includes hyperventilation (with 1.0 fractional inspired oxygen concentration), correction of acidosis, avoidance of sympathetic nervous system stimulation, maintenance of normothermia, minimization of intrathoracic pressure, and use of inotropic support. Inhaled nitric oxide may be useful for sudden increases in pulmonary vascular resistance in high-risk patients. Regional anesthesia may be an alternative for certain procedures, but a caveat to the use of spinal and epidural anesthesia is the decrease in systemic vascular resistance in patients with unrestrictive intracardiac shunts. The anesthesiologist must also be prepared for an increased intraoperative bleeding risk, such as in patients with Fontan circulation with associated liver dysfunction, as well as potential thrombosis in patients with secondary erythrocytosis.

POSTOPERATIVE MANAGEMENT

Adults with congenital heart disease should be stratified to the appropriate postoperative environment based on the severity of disease, type of procedure, and perioperative course through consultation among the anesthesiologist, the surgeon, and, optimally, the patient's congenital heart disease cardiology specialist. The major postoperative risks are the same as those in the preoperative and intraoperative settings, such as bleeding, thrombosis, worsening pulmonary hypertension, and dysrhythmias. Patients who have severe congenital heart disease and/or have undergone high-risk surgery should be managed in an intensive care unit experienced in caring for adults with congenital heart disease. To date there are no evidence-based guidelines for perioperative management of adults with congenital heart disease; hence, clinical trials are warranted to improve the anesthetic care of these unique yet challenging patients.

INFECTIVE ENDOCARDITIS ANTIBIOTIC PROPHYLAXIS IN PATIENTS WITH REPAIRED AND UNREPAIRED CONGENITAL HEART DISEASE

Of particular interest to adults with congenital heart disease are the modified recommendations for infective endocarditis prophylaxis. Current recommendations have resulted in a more restrictive use of such prophylaxis. The AHA has recently published updated guidelines for the prevention of infective endocarditis. After reviewing the literature for the past 40 years, its expert panel found that very few cases of endocarditis could have been prevented by antibiotic prophylaxis. The guidelines now emphasize the use of infective endocarditis prophylaxis in patients at high risk, particularly those with prosthetic cardiac materials. These include patients with prosthetic valves or prosthetic material used for valve repair, palliative shunts, and conduits; completely repaired congenital heart disease with prosthetic material or a device placed during surgery or by catheter intervention during the first 6 months after the procedure; and repaired congenital heart disease with residual defects at or adjacent to the site of a prosthetic patch or prosthetic device (which inhibit endothelialization). In addition, infective endocarditis prophylaxis is recommended for those with previous infective endocarditis, unrepaired congenital heart disease, or cyanotic congenital heart disease, and for cardiac transplantation recipients who develop cardiac valvulopathy. Except for patients with the aforementioned conditions, antibiotic prophylaxis is no longer recommended for patients with congenital heart disease. In addition, the committee concluded that for patients with these underlying cardiac conditions at highest risk for adverse outcomes from infective endocarditis, prophylaxis is reasonable for all dental procedures involving manipulation of the gingival tissue, the periapical region of teeth, or perforation of the oral mucosa. Prophylaxis is not recommended based solely on an increased lifetime risk of acquiring infective endocarditis. The committee also does not recommend administering antibiotics solely to prevent infective endocarditis in patients undergoing genitourinary or gastrointestinal tract operations. These new guidelines have been designed to clearly define appropriate indications for infective endocarditis prophylaxis and to provide more uniform recommendations.

KEY POINTS

- Congenital heart disease is the most common form of congenital disease and accounts for approximately 30% of all congenital diseases that occur.
- Ventricular septal defects (VSDs) remain the most commonly encountered congenital cardiac abnormality in infants and children.
- Transthoracic and transesophageal echocardiography facilitates early and accurate diagnosis of congenital heart disease.

- Advances in molecular biology have provided new insights into the genetic basis of congenital heart disease.
- In patients with acyanotic or cyanotic congenital heart disease, an understanding of the relationship between systemic and pulmonary vascular resistance is essential to determine appropriate anesthetic management. For example, in patients with cyanotic heart disease, ventilation with high airway pressures can increase pulmonary vascular resistance, compromise venous return, and exacerbate right-to-left shunt physiology. Placement in Trendelenburg's position can increase central venous (superior vena cava) pressure and cause cerebral hypoperfusion in a patient who has a Glenn shunt or has undergone Fontan's procedure. In those patients with large ASDs, inadequate anesthesia and sympathetic nervous system stimulation might increase systemic vascular resistance, exacerbate left-to-right shunting, and reduce cardiac output.
- New modalities for decreasing pulmonary vascular resistance have had a significant impact on the treatment of patients with intracardiac and systemic-to-pulmonary shunts, whether in acyanotic or cyanotic congenital heart disease. Management of pulmonary vascular resistance and hence prevention of pulmonary hypertension is essential for better hemodynamic stability in the intraoperative and postoperative environment as well as for improved long-term outcomes. Prevention and treatment of pulmonary hypertensive crisis in congenital heart disease patients includes hyperventilation (with 1.0 fractional inspired oxygen concentration), correction of acidosis, avoidance of sympathetic nervous system stimulation, maintenance of normothermia, minimization of intrathoracic pressure, and use of inotropic support. Inhaled nitric oxide may be useful for sudden increases in pulmonary vascular resistance in patients at high risk.
- As innovation and expertise continue to improve survival, the growing adult patient population with repaired congenital heart defects provides a unique challenge to the anesthesiologist. Familiarity and experience with congenital heart disease anatomy and physiology in adults, in addition to a profound understanding of perioperative complications such as bleeding and thrombosis risk, pulmonary hypertension, heart failure, and dysrhythmias, are essential for effective anesthetic management.
- The American Heart Association published updated new guidelines for infective endocarditis prophylaxis in patients with repaired and unrepaired congenital heart defects. The guidelines now emphasize the use of antibiotic prophylaxis in patients at high risk, particularly those with prosthetic cardiac materials (as discussed), a history of infective endocarditis, unrepaired congenital heart defects, or cyanotic congenital heart disease as well as cardiac transplant recipients who develop cardiac valvulopathy. The committee concluded that for patients with these underlying cardiac conditions who are at highest risk for adverse outcomes from infective endocarditis, prophylaxis is reasonable for all dental procedures involving manipulation of the gingival tissue, the periapical region of teeth, or perforation of the oral mucosa but is not recommended solely to prevent infective endocarditis in patients undergoing genitourinary or gastrointestinal tract operations.

RESOURCES

Alsenaidi K, Gurofsky R, Karamlou T, et al. Management and outcomes of double aortic arch in 81 patients. *Pediatrics*. 2006;118(5):1336-1341.

Ammash NM, Connolly HM, Abel MD, et al. Noncardiac surgery in Eisenmenger syndrome. *J Am Coll Cardiol*. 1999;33:222-227.

Anand KJS, Hickey PR. Halothane-morphine compared with high-dose sufentanil for anesthesia and postoperative analgesia in neonatal cardiac surgery. *N Engl J Med*. 1992;326:1-9.

Andropoulos DB, Stayer SA, Skjonsby BS, et al. Anesthetic and perioperative outcome of teenagers and adults with congenital heart disease. *J Cardiothorac Vasc Anesth*. 2002:731-736.

Baum VC, Perloff JK. Anesthetic implications of adults with congenital heart disease. *Anesth Analg*. 1993;76:1342-1358.

Brickner ME, Hillis LD, Lange RA. Congenital heart disease in adults. *N Engl J Med*. 2000;342:256-263.

Burch TM, McGowan FX, Kussman BD, et al. Congenital supravalvular aortic stenosis and sudden death associated with anesthesia: what's the mystery? *Anesth Analg*. 2008;107:1848-1854.

Cannesson M, Earing MG, Collange V, et al. Anesthesia for noncardiac surgery in adults with congenital heart disease. *Anesthesiology*. 2009;111(2):432-440.

Clyman RI. Ibuprofen and patent ductus arteriosus. *N Engl J Med*. 2000;343:728-730.

Diaz LK, Andropoulos DB. New developments in pediatric cardiac anesthesia. *Anesthesiol Clin North Am*. 2005;23:655-676.

Greeley WJ, Stanley TE, Ungerleider RM, et al. Intraoperative hypoxemic spells in tetralogy of Fallot, an echocardiographic analysis of diagnosis and treatment. *Anesth Analg*. 1989;68:815-819.

Groves ER, Groves JB. Epidural analgesia for labour in a patient with Ebstein's anomaly. *Can J Anaesth*. 1995;42:77-79.

Hansen DD, Hickey PR. Anesthesia for hypoplastic left heart syndrome: use of high-dose fentanyl in 30 neonates. *Anesth Analg*. 1986;65:127-132.

Hosking MP, Beynen F. Repair of coarctation of the aorta in a child after a modified Fontan's operation: anesthetic implications and management. *Anesthesiology*. 1989;71:312-315.

Khairy P, Poirier N, Mercier LA. Univentricular heart. *Circulation*. 2007; 115:800-812.

Landzberg MJ, Murphy Jr DJ, Davidson Jr WR, et al. Task force 4: organization of delivery systems for adults with congenital heart disease. *J Am Coll Cardiol*. 2001;37:1187-1193.

Larson CP. Anesthesia in neonatal cardiac surgery. *N Engl J Med*. 1992;327:124.

Minette MS, Sahn DJ. Ventricular septal defects. *Circulation*. 2006; 114:2190-2197.

Mullen MP. Adult congenital heart disease. *Sci Am Med*. 2000:1-10.

Perloff JK, Warnes CA. Challenges posed by adults with repaired congenital heart disease. *Circulation*. 2001;103:2637-2643.

Sinha PK, Kumar B, Varma PK. Anesthetic management for surgical repair of Ebstein's anomaly along with coexistent Wolff-Parkinson-White syndrome in a patient with severe mitral stenosis. *Ann Card Anaesth*. 2010;13(2):154-158.

Spinnato JA, Kraynack BJ, Cooper MW. Eisenmenger's syndrome in pregnancy: epidural anesthesia for elective cesarean section. *N Engl J Med*. 1981;304:1215-1216.

Stumper O. Hypoplastic left heart syndrome. *Heart*. 2010;96(3):231-236.

Triedman JK. Arrhythmias in adults with congenital heart disease. *Heart*. 2002;87:383-389.

Van Overmeire B, Smets K, Lecoutere D, et al. A comparison of ibuprofen and indomethacin for closure of patent ductus arteriosus. *N Engl J Med*. 2000;343:674-681.

Warnes CA, Liberthson R, Danielson GK, et al. Task force 1: the changing profile of congenital heart disease in adult life. *J Am Coll Cardiol.* 2001;37:1170-1175.

Weiss BM, Zemp L, Seifert B, et al. Outcome of pulmonary vascular disease in pregnancy: a systematic overview from 1978 through 1996. *J Am Coll Cardiol.* 1998;31:1650-1659.

Wilson W, Taubert KA, Gewitz M, et al. Prevention of infective endocarditis: guidelines from the American Heart Association: a guideline from the American Heart Association Rheumatic Fever, Endocarditis, and Kawasaki Disease Committee, Council on Cardiovascular Disease in the Young, and the Council on Clinical Cardiology, Council on Cardiovascular Surgery and Anesthesia, and the Quality of Care and Outcomes Research Interdisciplinary Working Group. *Circulation.* 2007;116:1736-1754.

Wong RS, Baum VC, Sangivan S. Truncus arteriosus: recognition and therapy of intraoperative cardiac ischemia. *Anesthesiology.* 1991;74:378-380.

Abnormalities of Cardiac Conduction and Cardiac Rhythm

KELLEY TEED WATSON ∎

ANATOMY OF INTRINSIC CARDIAC PACEMAKERS AND THE CONDUCTION SYSTEM

The conduction system of the heart is composed of a set of very specialized cells that initiate and conduct electrical signals through the heart with precise coordination and great speed. As an electrical impulse moves along the conduction system, a wave of depolarization is propagated throughout the heart, causing progressive contraction of cardiac muscle cells (Figure 4-1).

The sinoatrial (SA) node is the primary site for impulse initiation. Impulses initiated in the SA node are rapidly conducted across the right and left atria, causing them to contract. The electrical impulse then travels between the fibrous atrioventricular (AV) rings, where it slows down briefly at the AV node. The impulse then continues down the interventricular septum, branching into right and left portions and ending in an even smaller branching network of fibers called the *His-Purkinje system*.

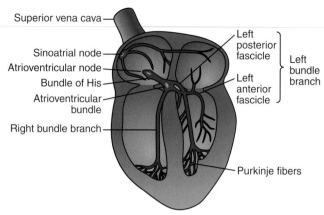

FIGURE 4-1 Anatomy of the conduction system for transmission of cardiac electrical impulses.

The SA node is located at the junction of the superior vena cava and the right atrium, and is richly innervated by sympathetic and parasympathetic nerve endings. In 60% of individuals, the arterial blood supply to the SA node comes from the right coronary artery; in the remaining 40%, the blood supply is from the left circumflex coronary artery.

The AV rings are the tough fibrous frames that support the delicate tissue of the tricuspid and mitral valves. These rings essentially insulate the conduction tissue of the AV node, thus allowing conduction through the normal pathway while preventing aberrant electrical conduction between the atria and ventricles. In addition, the AV node has a long refractory period to prevent overstimulation of the ventricles in the event of abnormally rapid atrial impulses.

The AV node is located in the septal wall of the right atrium, anterior to the coronary sinus and above the insertion of the septal leaflet of the tricuspid valve. It is also innervated by both parasympathetic and sympathetic nerves. The blood supply to the AV node comes from the right coronary artery in 85% to 90% of the population and from the left circumflex coronary artery in the remaining 10% to 15%. The AV node slows the conduction velocity of the electrical impulse, which allows time for atrial contraction, the so-called atrial kick, to contribute an additional 20% to filling of the ventricles in late diastole. After a brief slowing of the electrical impulse at the AV node, the impulse continues down the conduction tract along the bundle of His.

The bundle of His quickly divides into two branches, right and the left bundles, within the interventricular septum. The right bundle branch (RBB) is a relatively thin bundle of fibers that courses down the right ventricle and then branches near the right ventricular apex. Because of this late branching, the RBB is more vulnerable to interruption than the left bundle branch (LBB), which branches early and widely.

The LBB divides into two fascicles: the left anterior superior fascicle and the left posterior inferior fascicle. The left and right bundles both receive blood supply from branches of the left anterior descending coronary artery. Infarction in the territory of the left anterior descending coronary artery can often affect the left anterior superior fascicle and the RBB, but rarely the left posterior inferior fascicle, because that portion receives additional blood supply from the posterior descending coronary artery. This is why disruption of the more robust LBB in the form of a left bundle branch block (LBBB) usually indicates more extensive cardiac disease or damage than a right bundle branch block (RBBB). The distal branches of the right and left bundles interlace into a network of Purkinje fibers.

ELECTROPHYSIOLOGY OF THE CONDUCTION SYSTEM

On a cellular level, impulses are conducted through the heart by a process of progressive depolarization. In the resting state, the inside of a cardiac cell is negative relative to the outside. Cardiac muscle cells have a resting membrane potential of −80 to −90 mV. The resting gradient is maintained by membrane-bound sodium–potassium–adenosine triphosphatase (Na^+,K^+-ATPase) that concentrates potassium intracellularly and extrudes sodium extracellularly. The membrane potential increases when the sodium and calcium channels open in response to shifts in the charge on neighboring cell membranes. At the point at which the membrane potential reaches +20 mV, an action potential (or depolarization) occurs. After depolarization, cells are refractory to subsequent action potentials for a period of time corresponding to phase 4 of the depolarization potential (Figure 4-2).

Electrocardiography

The essential monitor for diagnosis of cardiac conduction abnormalities and rhythm disturbances is the electrocardiogram (ECG). An ECG is a tracing made by a machine that uses electrodes on the skin to amplify the movement of electrical potentials through the heart. The direction of the electrical signal relative to a ground electrode determines the direction of the deflection seen on the ECG. Positive signals are represented by deflections above the isoelectric line and negative signals are represented as deflections below the isoelectric line.

The type and configuration of the deflections determine the type of rhythm. The normal ECG tracing, called *sinus rhythm*, is made up of three parts: the P wave (atrial depolarization), the QRS complex (ventricular depolarization), and the T wave (ventricular repolarization). The time between atrial depolarization and the initiation of ventricular depolarization is the PR interval. The normal reference range for the PR interval is 0.12 to 0.20 seconds. The QRS complex corresponds to the wave of depolarization as it emerges from the AV node and moves downward to depolarize the right and left ventricles. The QRS is normally 0.05 to 0.10 seconds in duration. Abnormal intraventricular conduction is suggested by a QRS complex that exceeds 0.12 seconds. The segment between the end of the S wave (end of ventricular depolarization) and the beginning of the T wave is the ST segment.

The ST segment represents the time between ventricular depolarization and the start of ventricular repolarization. It is normally isoelectric but can be elevated to 1 mm in the

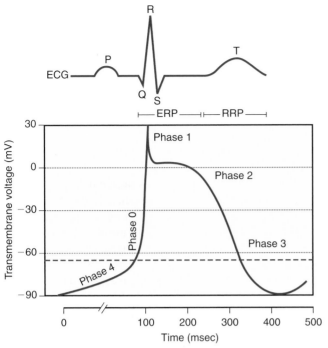

FIGURE 4-2 Transmembrane action potential occurring in an automatic cardiac cell and the relationship of this action potential to events depicted on the electrocardiogram (ECG). Phase 4 is characterized by spontaneous depolarization from the resting membrane potential (−90 mV) until the threshold potential (*broken line*) is reached. Depolarization (phase 0) occurs when the threshold potential is reached and corresponds to the QRS complex on the ECG. Phases 1 through 3 represent repolarization, with phase 3 corresponding to the T wave on the ECG. The effective refractory period (ERP) is the time during which cardiac impulses cannot be conducted, regardless of the intensity of the stimulus. During the relative refractory period (RRP), a strong stimulus can initiate an action potential. The action potential developed in a contractile cardiac cell differs from that occurring in an automatic cardiac cell in that phase 4 is not characterized by spontaneous depolarization.

absence of any cardiac abnormality. However, it is *never* normal for the ST segment to be depressed. The T-wave deflection should be in the same direction as the QRS complex and should not exceed 5 mm in amplitude in standard leads or 10 mm in precordial leads. Normal values for the QT interval should be corrected for the heart rate (QTc) because the QT interval varies inversely with heart rate. A normal QTc is less than 0.47 seconds. As a general rule, the QT interval is less than one half of the preceding R-R interval.

CARDIAC DYSRHYTHMIAS

Cardiac rhythms that show abnormalities in rate, interval length, or conduction path are referred to as *dysrhythmias*. Dysrhythmias are usually classified according to heart rate and the site of the abnormality. The clinical significance of these abnormalities for the anesthesiologist depends on the effect they have on vital signs and the potential for deterioration into life-threatening

rhythms. In healthy adults, a wide variation in heart rate can be tolerated, because normal compensatory mechanisms serve to maintain cardiac output and blood pressure. In patients with cardiac disease, however, dysrhythmias and conduction disturbances can overwhelm normal compensatory processes and result in hemodynamic instability, cardiac and other end-organ ischemia, congestive heart failure, and even death.

MECHANISMS OF TACHYDYSRHYTHMIAS

A cardiac rhythm higher than 100 beats per minute is considered a tachydysrhythmia. Tachydysrhythmias can result from three mechanisms: (1) increased automaticity in normal conduction tissue or in an ectopic focus, (2) reentry of electrical potentials through abnormal pathways, and (3) triggering of abnormal cardiac potentials due to afterdepolarizations.

Automaticity

The fastest pacemaker in the heart is normally the SA node. The SA node spontaneously discharges at a rate of 60 to 100 beats per minute. Other pacemakers can be accelerated and overdrive the SA node as a result of disease states or iatrogenic influences such as mechanical or drug stimulation. A sustained rhythm resulting from accelerated firing of a pacemaker other than the SA node is called an *ectopic rhythm*. Clinically, dysrhythmias resulting from an ectopic focus often have a gradual onset and termination. Cardiac dysrhythmias caused by enhanced automaticity result from repetitive firing of a focus other than the sinus node.

Abnormal automaticity is not confined to secondary pacemakers within the conduction system. Almost any cell in the heart may exhibit automaticity under certain circumstances. The automaticity of cardiac tissue changes when the slope of phase 4 depolarization shifts or the resting membrane potential changes. Sympathetic stimulation causes an increase in heart rate by increasing the slope of phase 4 of the action potential and by decreasing the resting membrane potential. Conversely, parasympathetic stimulation results in a decrease in the slope of phase 4 depolarization and an increase in resting membrane potential to slow the heart rate.

Reentry Pathways

Reentry pathways account for most premature beats and tachydysrhythmias. Reentry or triggered dysrhythmias require two pathways over which cardiac impulses can be conducted at different velocities (Figure 4-3). Extra pathways called *accessory tracts* can exist around the AV node and can conduct impulses bypassing the AV node and normal infranodal conduction tract. These accessory tracts are usually remnants of tissue left from the embryologic formation of the heart.

Normally, passage through the AV node is the slowest portion of the conduction system. In a reentry circuit, there is anterograde (forward) conduction over the slower normal conduction pathway and retrograde (backward) conduction over a

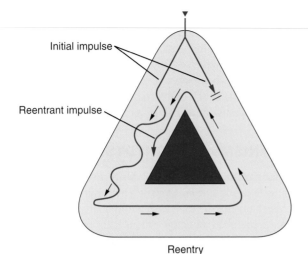

FIGURE 4-3 Essential requirement for initiation of reentry excitation is a unilateral block that prevents uniform anterograde propagation of the initial cardiac impulse. Under appropriate conditions, this same cardiac impulse can traverse the area of blockade in a retrograde direction and become a reentrant cardiac impulse. *(Adapted from Akhtar M. Management of ventricular tachyarrhythmias. JAMA. 1982;247:671-674.)*

TABLE 4-1   ■   Perioperative causes of sinus tachycardia
PHYSIOLOGIC INCREASE IN SYMPATHETIC TONE
Pain
Anxiety or fear
Light anesthesia
Hypovolemia or anemia
Arterial hypoxemia
Hypotension
Hypoglycemia
Fever or infection
PATHOLOGIC INCREASE IN SYMPATHETIC TONE
Myocardial ischemia or infarction
Congestive heart failure
Pulmonary embolus
Hyperthyroidism
Pericarditis
Pericardial tamponade
Malignant hyperthermia
Ethanol withdrawal
DRUG-INDUCED INCREASE IN HEART RATE
Atropine or glycopyrrolate
Sympathomimetic drugs
Caffeine
Nicotine
Cocaine or amphetamines

faster accessory pathway. Pharmacologic or physiologic events may alter the balance between conduction velocities and refractory periods of the dual pathways, resulting in the initiation or termination of reentrant dysrhythmias. Reentrant dysrhythmias tend to be paroxysmal with abrupt onset and termination.

Triggering by Afterdepolarizations

Afterdepolarizations are oscillations in membrane potential that occur during or after repolarization. Normally, these membrane oscillations dissipate. However, under special circumstances they can trigger a complete depolarization. Once triggered, the process may continue and result in a self-sustaining dysrhythmia. Triggered dysrhythmias associated with *early* afterdepolarizations are enhanced by slow heart rates and are treated by accelerating the heart rate with positive chronotropic drugs or pacing. Conversely, triggered dysrhythmias associated with *delayed* afterdepolarizations are enhanced by fast heart rates and can be suppressed with drugs that lower the heart rate.

SUPRAVENTRICULAR DYSRHYTHMIAS

Sinus Dysrhythmia

Occasionally an ECG will show a sinus rhythm that appears irregular. This normal variant is called *sinus dysrhythmia*. The variation in heart rate is in response to intrathoracic pressure changes during inspiration and expiration known as the *Bainbridge reflex*. Inspiration accelerates the heart rate and expiration slows it down. It is a normal variant and carries no risk of deterioration into a more dangerous rhythm. Sinus

dysrhythmia is common in children and young people but tends to decrease with age.

Sinus Tachycardia

SIGNS, SYMPTOMS, AND DIAGNOSIS

Sinus tachycardia occurs at a heart rate of 100 to 160 beats per minute. The ECG during sinus tachycardia shows a normal P wave before every QRS complex. The PR interval is normal unless a co-existing conduction block exists. Typically, it is a nonparoxysmal increase in heart rate that speeds up and slows down gradually. Sinus tachycardia is caused by acceleration of SA node discharge secondary to sympathetic stimulation.

Sinus tachycardia without manifestations of hemodynamic instability is not life-threatening. It can occur as part of the normal physiologic response to stimuli such as fear or pain or as a pharmacologic response to medications or substances such as atropine or caffeine. Since it does increase myocardial oxygen demand, it can contribute to myocardial ischemia and congestive heart failure in susceptible patients. Sinus tachycardia can also occur as a compensatory mechanism in the setting of significant heart disease such as congestive heart failure or myocardial infarction (Table 4-1). In these circumstances, the increased heart rate is usually a physiologic effort to increase cardiac output. Sinus tachycardia is the most common supraventricular dysrhythmia associated with acute myocardial infarction, occurring in 30% to 40% of these patients.

PERIOPERATIVE MANAGEMENT

Treatment of sinus tachycardia is directed toward correcting any underlying causes of increased sympathetic stimulation. Sinus tachycardia in patients with ischemic heart disease, diastolic dysfunction, or congestive heart failure can lead to significant clinical deterioration because of the increased oxygen demand, increased wall stress, and inability to increase myocardial perfusion in many of these patients. Many causes of sinus tachycardia such as hypovolemia are clinically obvious, but some of the most serious causes, such as infection, hypoxia, myocardial ischemia, and congestive heart failure, may be less apparent. If a specific cause of sinus tachycardia can be determined, it should be treated.

Avoidance of vagolytic drugs, such as pancuronium, can aid in management of sinus tachycardia intraoperatively. Although sinus tachycardia is generally well tolerated in young healthy patients, supplemental oxygen should be administered to increase oxygen supply in response to the increased oxygen demand. If a patient is not hypovolemic, intravenous administration of a β-blocker may be employed to lower the heart rate and decrease myocardial oxygen demand.

Caution must be exercised in the use of β-blockers in patients susceptible to bronchospasm. β-Blocker–mediated decreases in heart rate can cause an abrupt and dangerous decrease in blood pressure in patients with impaired cardiac function. Such patients may be unable to increase their stroke volume to compensate for the reduction in heart rate.

Premature Atrial Beats

SIGNS, SYMPTOMS, AND DIAGNOSIS

Premature atrial contractions (PACs) arise from ectopic foci in the atria. PACs are recognized on the ECG by the presence of early, abnormally shaped P waves. The PR interval is variable. Most often the duration and configuration of the corresponding QRS complex is normal, because activation of the ventricles occurs through the normal conduction pathway. Aberrant conduction of atrial impulses can occur, resulting in a QRS complex that is widened and may mimic that associated with a premature ventricular contraction (PVC). PACs, unlike PVCs, are *not* followed by a compensatory pause. The occurrence of PACs is *not* a risk factor for progression to a life-threatening dysrhythmia.

Typical symptoms of PACs include an awareness of a "fluttering" or a "heavy" heart beat. Precipitating factors include excessive caffeine, emotional stress, alcohol, nicotine, recreational drugs, and hyperthyroidism. PACs are common in patients of all ages with and without heart disease. They often occur at rest and become less frequent with exercise. They are more common in patients with chronic lung disease, ischemic heart disease, and digitalis toxicity. PACs are the second most common dysrhythmia associated with acute myocardial infarction.

PERIOPERATIVE MANAGEMENT

Avoidance of precipitating drugs or toxins can reduce the incidence of PACs. Underlying predisposing conditions should be treated. PACs are usually hemodynamically insignificant and do not require acute therapy unless they are associated with initiation of a tachydysrhythmia. In this situation treatment is directed at controlling or converting the tachydysrhythmia.

Anesthetic management of the patient with PACs should include avoidance of excessive sympathetic stimulation and drugs that might induce PACs. Pharmacologic treatment is required only if the PACs trigger secondary dysrhythmias. PACs can usually be suppressed with calcium channel blockers or β-blockers. The secondary dysrhythmias triggered by PACs are treated with drugs or maneuvers that improve heart rate control and/or convert the dysrhythmia to sinus rhythm.

Supraventricular Tachycardia

SIGNS, SYMPTOMS, AND DIAGNOSIS

Supraventricular tachycardia (SVT) is a tachydysrhythmia (average heart rate of 160 to 180 beats per minute) initiated and sustained by tissue at or above the AV node. Unlike sinus tachycardia, SVT is usually paroxysmal and may begin and end very abruptly. AV nodal reentrant tachycardia (AVNRT) is the most common type of SVT and accounts for 50% of diagnosed SVTs. AVNRT is most commonly due to a reentry circuit in which there is anterograde conduction over the slower AV nodal pathway and retrograde conduction over a faster accessory pathway. Other mechanisms for SVT include enhanced automaticity of secondary pacemaker cells and triggered impulse initiation by afterdepolarizations. Atrial fibrillation and atrial flutter are SVTs, but their electrophysiology and treatment are distinctly different from those of other forms of SVT, so they are discussed separately.

Common symptoms during an episode of SVT include light-headedness, dizziness, fatigue, chest discomfort, and dyspnea. Fifteen percent of patients with SVT experience overt syncope. SVT occurs most often in the absence of structural heart disease in younger individuals and occurs three times more often in women than in men. Polyuria can be associated with SVT or any atrial tachycardia that causes AV dyssynchrony. The polyuria is caused by increased secretion of atrial natriuretic peptide. This happens because atrial pressures increase from contraction of the atria against closed AV valves and atrial stretch receptors are activated.

PERIOPERATIVE MANAGEMENT

If the patient is in hemodynamically stable condition, the initial treatment of SVT can consist of vagal maneuvers such as carotid sinus massage or Valsalva's maneuver. Termination by a vagal maneuver suggests reentry as the causative mechanism. If conservative treatment is not effective, pharmacologic treatment directed at blocking AV nodal conduction is indicated. Clinical factors guide the choice of drug treatment, but adenosine, calcium channel blockers, and β-blockers are commonly used to terminate SVT (Figure 4-4).

Adenosine has a unique advantage over other intravenous drugs used to treat SVT because it has a very rapid onset (15 to 30 seconds) and very brief duration of action (10 seconds). Most AVNRT episodes can be terminated by a single dose

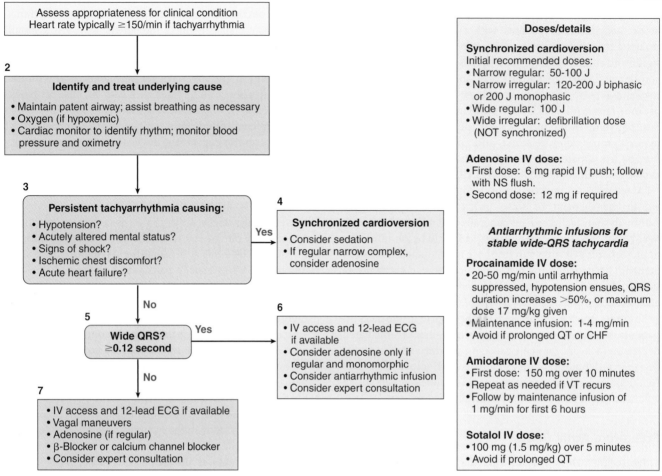

FIGURE 4-4 Algorithm for treatment of adult tachycardia (with pulse). *CHF,* Congestive heart failure; *ECG,* electrocardiogram; *IV,* intravenous; *NS,* normal saline; *VT,* ventricular tachycardia. *(From Neumar RW, Otto CW, Link MS, et al. Part 8: adult advanced cardiovascular life support: 2010 American Heart Association Guidelines for Cardiopulmonary Resuscitation and Emergency Cardiovascular Care. Circulation. 2010;122:S751.)*

of adenosine. Multifocal atrial tachycardia, atrial flutter, and atrial fibrillation do not respond to adenosine. Heart transplant recipients require a reduction in dosage because of denervation hypersensitivity. Conversely, patients taking theophylline may require higher dosages of adenosine to produce a therapeutic effect because of competition with adenosine for receptor sites.

Intravenous administration of calcium channel–blocking drugs such as verapamil and diltiazem is also useful for terminating SVT. These drugs offer the advantage of a longer duration of action than adenosine. However, side effects, including peripheral vasodilation and negative inotropy, can contribute to an undesirable degree of hypotension. Intravenous β-blockers can also be used to control or convert SVT. Intravenous digoxin is not clinically useful in acute control of SVT because digoxin has a delayed peak effect and a narrow therapeutic window. Electrical cardioversion is indicated for SVT unresponsive to drug therapy or SVT associated with hemodynamic instability. Long-term medical treatment of patients with repeated episodes of SVT includes calcium

channel blockers, digoxin, and/or β-blockers. Radiofrequency catheter ablation may also be used to treat patients with recurrent or recalcitrant AVNRT.

Anesthetic management for a patient with SVT should focus on avoiding factors known to produce ectopy, such as increased sympathetic tone, electrolyte imbalances, and acid-base disturbances. Because SVT is usually paroxysmal, monitoring of vital signs to detect any progression to hemodynamic instability and verbal reassurance (if the patient is awake) is usually all that is needed until an episode of SVT terminates. One should evaluate and treat any potential aggravating factors and anticipate the need for antidysrhythmics and/or cardioversion.

Multifocal Atrial Tachycardia

SIGNS, SYMPTOMS, AND DIAGNOSIS

Multifocal atrial tachycardia (MAT) is an irregular rhythm that electrophysiologically reflects the presence of multiple ectopic

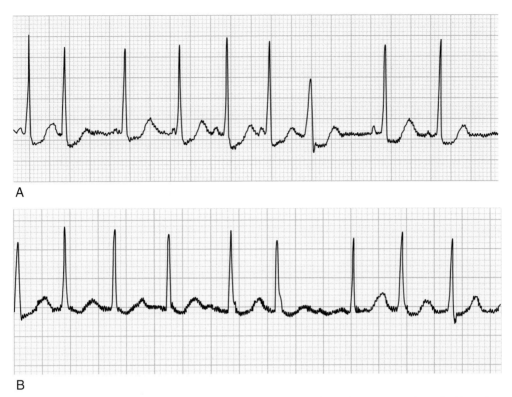

FIGURE 4-5 Comparison of the electrocardiogram appearance of multifocal atrial tachycardia (**A**) and atrial fibrillation (**B**). Both rhythms are irregular. However, note several distinct P-wave morphologies and varying PR intervals with multifocal atrial tachycardia. There are no distinct P waves with atrial fibrillation.

atrial pacemakers. The ECG shows P waves with three or more different morphologies, and the PR intervals vary. This rhythm is frequently confused with atrial fibrillation, but unlike atrial fibrillation, the rate is not excessively rapid (Figure 4-5). The atrial rhythm is usually between 100 and 180 beats per minute.

MAT is most commonly seen in patients experiencing an acute exacerbation of chronic lung disease. It can also be associated with methylxanthine toxicity (theophylline and caffeine), congestive heart failure, sepsis, and metabolic or electrolyte abnormalities.

PERIOPERATIVE MANAGEMENT

MAT usually responds to treatment of the underlying pulmonary decompensation with bronchodilators and supplemental oxygen. An improvement in arterial oxygenation tends to decrease the activity of the ectopic foci that cause MAT. Pharmacologic treatment of MAT has limited success and is considered secondary.

Magnesium sulfate 2 g IV over 1 hour followed by 1 to 2 g IV per hour by infusion has shown some success in decreasing atrial ectopy and converting MAT to sinus rhythm. Verapamil 5 to 10 mg IV over 5 to 10 minutes slows the ventricular rate and will convert to sinus rhythm in some patients. Likewise, β-blockers such as esmolol or metoprolol can decrease the ventricular rate but at the risk of worsening the situation by provoking bronchospasm in susceptible patients. Theophylline use can exacerbate this condition. Cardioversion has *no effect* on the multiple sites of ectopy that produce this dysrhythmia.

In summary, patients with MAT who must undergo urgent surgery benefit from optimization of their pulmonary function and arterial oxygenation. Avoidance of medications or procedures that could worsen the pulmonary status and avoidance of hypoxemia are the mainstays of anesthetic management.

Atrial Flutter

SIGNS, SYMPTOMS, AND DIAGNOSIS

Atrial flutter is characterized by an organized atrial rhythm with an atrial rate of 250 to 350 beats per minute with varying degrees of AV block. The rapid P waves create a sawtooth appearance on ECG and are called *flutter waves*. The flutter waves are particularly noticeable in leads II, III, aVF, and V_1. The flutter waves are not separated by an isoelectric baseline. The ventricular rate may be regular or irregular depending on the rate of conduction. Most commonly, patients have 2:1 AV conduction so, for example, an atrial rate of 300 beats per minute with 2:1 conduction results in a ventricular rate of 150 beats per minute. Characteristically, the ventricular rate is about 150 beats per minute. Atrial flutter frequently occurs in association with other dysrhythmias such as atrial fibrillation or atrial tachycardia. Reciprocating deterioration of atrial flutter into atrial fibrillation and then reversion of atrial fibrillation into atrial flutter is common.

Atrial flutter is usually associated with structural heart disease. It occurs in approximately 30% of patients with atrial fibrillation and may be associated with more intense symptoms than atrial fibrillation because of the more rapid ventricular response. About 60% of patients experience atrial flutter in association with an acute exacerbation of a chronic condition such as pulmonary disease, acute myocardial infarction, ethanol intoxication, or thyrotoxicosis, or after cardiothoracic surgery. In many instances treatment of the underlying disease process restores sinus rhythm.

If atrial flutter is hemodynamically significant, the treatment is cardioversion. Often less than 50 J (monophasic) is adequate to convert the rhythm to sinus. In a patient in hemodynamically stable condition, overdrive pacing using transesophageal or atrial electrodes can be used for conversion to sinus rhythm. Patients with atrial flutter lasting longer than 48 hours should receive anticoagulant therapy and should be evaluated by transesophageal echocardiography for the presence of an atrial thrombus before any attempt at cardioversion is made.

Pharmacologic control of the ventricular response and conversion to sinus rhythm can be challenging in patients with atrial flutter. Ventricular rate control should be the initial goal of therapy. This is done to prevent deterioration in AV conduction from 2:1 to 1:1, which represents a doubling of the heart rate. Such an increase in heart rate can cause severe hemodynamic instability. If there is 1:1 conduction with a ventricular rate of 300 beats per minute or faster, reentry is the most likely mechanism and procainamide administration should be considered. More commonly, intravenous drug therapy for ventricular rate control includes amiodarone, diltiazem, and verapamil. All of these drugs are helpful in controlling the ventricular rate, but none of these agents is likely to convert atrial flutter to sinus rhythm.

PERIOPERATIVE MANAGEMENT

If atrial flutter occurs before induction of anesthesia, surgery should be postponed if possible until control of the dysrhythmia has been achieved. Management of atrial flutter occurring during anesthesia or surgery depends on the hemodynamic stability of the patient. If the atrial flutter is hemodynamically significant, treatment requires cardioversion. Synchronized cardioversion starting at 50 J (monophasic) is indicated. Pharmacologic control of the ventricular response with intravenous amiodarone, diltiazem, or verapamil may be attempted if vital signs are stable. The choice of pharmacologic agent depends on the co-existing medical conditions of the patient.

Atrial Fibrillation

SIGNS, SYMPTOMS, AND DIAGNOSIS

Atrial fibrillation occurs when multiple areas of the atria continuously depolarize and contract in a disorganized manner. There is no coordinated depolarization or contraction, only a quivering of the atrial walls. The dysrhythmia is characterized on the ECG by chaotic atrial activity with no discernible P waves (see Figure 4-5). Atrial fibrillation may be triggered by other atrial tachycardias and commonly occurs in association with atrial flutter. Rapid, disordered atrial activation and irregular electrical input to the AV node result in sporadic AV nodal conduction and irregularly irregular ventricular contraction. Ventricular response rates as high as 180 beats per minute can occur in patients with normal AV node function. Extremely rapid ventricular responses in excess of 180 beats per minute can be seen in patients with accessory AV nodal bypass tracts. In this situation, the QRS complex is often wide, and the ECG can resemble ventricular tachycardia or ventricular fibrillation.

Atrial fibrillation can be a sustained or an episodic dysrhythmia. Predisposing conditions include rheumatic heart disease (especially mitral valve disease), hypertension, hyperthyroidism, ischemic heart disease, chronic obstructive pulmonary disease, alcohol intake (holiday heart syndrome), pericarditis, pulmonary embolus, and atrial septal defect. In some instances, treating the underlying disorder eliminates the atrial fibrillation. Increased left atrial size and mass are positive predictors for atrial fibrillation. Atrial fibrillation may be identified on physical examination or ECG in a patient with no associated symptoms. However, most patients are symptomatic. Symptoms may be vague, such as generalized weakness and fatigue, or prominent, such as palpitations, angina pectoris, shortness of breath, orthopnea, and hypotension.

PERIOPERATIVE MANAGEMENT

Atrial fibrillation is the most common sustained cardiac dysrhythmia in the general population, affecting 2.2 million people in the United States. The incidence of atrial fibrillation increases with age: it is present in 1% of individuals younger than 60 years of age, increases to 5% in those 70 to 75 years, and exceeds 10% in those older than 80 years. The most common underlying cardiovascular diseases associated with atrial fibrillation are systemic hypertension and ischemic heart disease. Valvular heart disease, congestive heart failure, and diabetes mellitus are independent risk factors for the development of atrial fibrillation. Long-term atrial fibrillation increases an individual's risk of heart failure.

Loss of coordinated atrial contraction promotes stasis of blood within the left atrium and can lead to the formation of atrial thrombi. Atrial thrombi and the potential for thromboembolic stroke are the most serious clinical dangers of atrial fibrillation. Patients with atrial thrombus are usually treated with anticoagulants. The prophylactic regimen chosen for each patient is determined by risk stratification for thromboembolism based on age and concomitant heart disease. In the acute setting, intravenous heparin is most commonly administered. For long-term anticoagulation therapy, warfarin is most often used. Warfarin is a vitamin K antagonist, with a narrow therapeutic window that necessitates frequent monitoring of clinical effect (international normalized ratio). It also interacts with numerous foods and medications. An alternative to warfarin emerged in 2010 with U.S. Food and Drug Administration (FDA) approval of the first new oral anticoagulant to become available in 50 years. Dabigatran (Pradaxa) is now available for the prevention of stroke and systemic embolization in patients with atrial fibrillation. Dabigatran is a thrombin inhibitor with a half-life of 12 to 17 hours. There is no specific antidote for dabigatran effects. However, transfusion of fresh frozen plasma or packed red blood cells and surgical intervention to control bleeding are supportive therapies recommended for severe hemorrhage associated with dabigatran therapy.

A large proportion of patients with new-onset atrial fibrillation experience spontaneous conversion to sinus rhythm within 24 to 48 hours. Therapy goals for new-onset atrial fibrillation include ventricular rate control and electrical or pharmacologic cardioversion. Control of ventricular response is typically achieved with drugs that slow AV nodal conduction. The most commonly used drugs for this purpose are β-blockers, calcium channel blockers, and digoxin. β-Blockers are useful in the prevention of recurrent atrial fibrillation, provide good heart rate control, and reduce symptoms during subsequent episodes of atrial fibrillation. Potential side effects of β-blocker therapy are hypotension and bronchospasm. Calcium channel–blocking drugs such as diltiazem and verapamil can rapidly reduce the ventricular rate during atrial fibrillation. These drugs have negative inotropic effects and must be used with caution in patients prone to heart failure. Digoxin can be useful to control ventricular rate but is not effective for conversion of atrial fibrillation to sinus rhythm. In the acute setting of rapid atrial fibrillation, the usefulness of digoxin is limited due to the fact that its peak therapeutic effects are delayed by several hours. Side effects associated with digitalis therapy are dose related and most commonly include AV block and ventricular ectopy.

Pharmacologic cardioversion is most effective if initiated within 7 days of the onset of atrial fibrillation. Several drugs are efficacious in converting atrial fibrillation to sinus rhythm, including amiodarone, propafenone, ibutilide, and sotalol. The preferred drug for patients with significant heart disease, including ischemic heart disease, left ventricular hypertrophy, left ventricular dysfunction, and heart failure, is amiodarone. The efficacy of intravenous amiodarone in producing chemical cardioversion ranges from 34% to 69% for a bolus dose and 55% to 95% when the bolus is followed by a continuous drug infusion. Amiodarone also suppresses atrial ectopy and recurrence of atrial fibrillation and improves the success rate of electrical cardioversion. Adverse effects of short-term amiodarone administration include bradycardia, hypotension, and phlebitis at the site of administration. Potential long-term side effects include visual disturbances, thyroid dysfunction, pulmonary toxicity, and skin discoloration. Electrical cardioversion is the most effective method for converting atrial fibrillation to normal sinus rhythm and is indicated in patients with co-existing symptoms of heart failure, angina pectoris, or hemodynamic instability.

If new-onset atrial fibrillation occurs before induction of anesthesia, surgery should be postponed if possible until ventricular rate control or conversion to sinus rhythm has been achieved. Intraoperative management of atrial fibrillation depends on the hemodynamic stability of the patient. If the atrial fibrillation is hemodynamically significant, the treatment is cardioversion. Synchronized cardioversion at 100 to 200 J (biphasic) is indicated. If vital signs are stable, the primary goal should be rate control with a β-blocker or calcium channel blocker if there are no clinical contraindications. The drug of choice for rate control in a patient with a known or suspected electrical accessory pathway and preexcitation is procainamide or amiodarone. Pharmacologic conversion to sinus rhythm with intravenous amiodarone may be attempted if vital signs allow.

Atrial fibrillation is the most common postoperative tachydysrhythmia and frequently occurs early in the postoperative period (first 2 to 4 days), especially in elderly patients following cardiothoracic surgery. Patients with chronic atrial fibrillation should continue to receive their antidysrhythmic drugs perioperatively with close attention to serum magnesium and potassium levels, particularly if the patient is taking digoxin. Careful coordination with the primary care team is needed to manage the transition on and off of intravenous and oral anticoagulation.

VENTRICULAR DYSRHYTHMIAS

Ventricular Ectopy (Premature Ventricular Beats)

SIGNS, SYMPTOMS, AND DIAGNOSIS

Ventricular premature beats arise from single (unifocal) or multiple (multifocal) foci located below the AV node. Characteristic ECG findings include a premature and wide QRS complex, no preceding P wave, ST segment and T-wave deflection opposite to the QRS deflection, and a compensatory pause before the next sinus beat. PVCs can be benign and self-limiting or progressive and detrimental. The vulnerable period of the ECG complex (corresponding to the relative refractory period of the cardiac action potential) occurs at approximately the middle third of the T wave. PVCs that occur during this time may initiate repetitive beats that can deteriorate into a sustained rhythm such as ventricular tachycardia or ventricular fibrillation. This clinical situation is known as the *R-on-T phenomenon*.

Ventricular ectopy can occur as short episodes with spontaneous termination or as a sustained period of bigeminy or trigeminy. The occurrence of more than three consecutive PVCs is considered ventricular tachycardia. The most common symptoms associated with ventricular ectopy are palpitations, near syncope, and syncope. The volume of blood ejected during a PVC is smaller than that ejected during a sinus beat because of lack of the atrial contribution to ventricular filling during diastole (loss of "atrial kick"). There is a compensatory pause after a PVC before the P wave of the next sinus beat. The stroke volume of the sinus beat following the compensatory pause is larger than normal.

PERIOPERATIVE MANAGEMENT

Typically, benign ventricular premature beats occur at rest and disappear with exercise. An increased frequency of PVCs with exercise may be an indication of underlying heart disease. The prognostic significance of ventricular ectopy depends on the presence and severity of co-existing structural heart disease. The incidence of PVCs in a healthy population ranges from 0.5% in those younger than 20 years to 2.2% in those older than 50 years. In the absence of structural heart disease, asymptomatic ventricular ectopy is benign with no demonstrable risk of sudden death even in the presence of ventricular tachycardia.

The occurrence of six or more PVCs per minute and repetitive or multifocal forms of ventricular ectopy, even if asymptomatic, indicate an increased risk of developing a life-threatening ventricular tachydysrhythmia. The most common pathologic conditions associated with this type of dysrhythmia are arterial hypoxemia, myocardial ischemia or infarction, valvular heart disease, cardiomyopathy, QT interval prolongation, digitalis toxicity, and electrolyte abnormalities, especially hypokalemia and hypomagnesemia. Excessive caffeine, alcohol, and cocaine use can also cause PVCs (Table 4-2).

Ventricular premature beats should be treated when they are frequent, are polymorphic, occur in runs of three or more, or exhibit the R-on-T phenomenon, because these characteristics are associated with an increased incidence of progression to ventricular tachycardia and ventricular fibrillation. Primary steps in the treatment of ventricular premature beats include elimination or correction of the underlying cause, discontinuation of prodysrhythmic drugs or drugs that prolong the QT interval, and elimination of any iatrogenic mechanical irritation of the heart such as from intracardiac catheters. A defibrillator should be immediately available in case clinical deterioration into a life-threatening dysrhythmia occurs.

With the exception of β-blockers, currently available antidysrhythmic drugs have not been shown in randomized clinical trials to be effective in the primary long-term management of ventricular dysrhythmias. Many antidysrhythmic drugs have prodysrhythmic effects and/or prolong the QT interval. In fact, prolongation of depolarization (QT interval) can precipitate and increase the propensity for dysrhythmias. Amiodarone, lidocaine, and other antidysrhythmics are not indicated unless PVCs progress to ventricular tachycardia or are frequent enough to cause hemodynamic instability. Drug therapy is not effective in suppression of ventricular dysrhythmias caused by mechanical irritation of the heart.

During administration of an anesthetic, if a patient exhibits six or more PVCs per minute and repetitive or multifocal forms of ventricular ectopy, there is an increased risk of development of a life-threatening dysrhythmia. The immediate availability of a defibrillator should be confirmed. The differential diagnosis of possible causes of PVCs includes acidosis, electrolyte imbalance, use of prodysrhythmic drugs, and mechanical irritation such as from cardiac surgery or intracardiac or intrathoracic catheters. Treatment should be aimed at elimination of as many of these causative factors as possible. Amiodarone, lidocaine, and other antidysrhythmics are indicated only if the PVCs progress to ventricular tachycardia or are frequent enough to cause hemodynamic instability.

TABLE 4-2	Conditions and factors associated with the development of ventricular premature beats

Normal heart
Arterial hypoxemia
Myocardial ischemia
Myocardial infarction
Myocarditis
Sympathetic nervous system activation
Hypokalemia
Hypomagnesemia
Digitalis toxicity
Caffeine
Cocaine
Alcohol
Mechanical irritation (central venous or pulmonary artery catheter)

β-Blockers are the most successful drugs in suppressing ventricular ectopy.

Ventricular Tachycardia

SIGNS, SYMPTOMS, AND DIAGNOSIS

Ventricular dysrhythmias occur in 70% to 80% of persons older than age 60 and are often asymptomatic. The prognosis depends on the presence or absence of structural heart disease. In the perioperative environment, mechanical ventilation, drug therapy, insertion of central catheters, and other interventions can be iatrogenic causes of ventricular dysrhythmias. The risk of sudden death in patients with structurally normal hearts experiencing ventricular dysrhythmias is low. However, treatment with a β-blocker or calcium channel blocker can suppress the dysrhythmia and alleviate symptoms. Catheter ablation or implantation of a cardioverter or defibrillator are options for treatment of drug-refractory ventricular tachycardia.

Ventricular tachycardia (also called *monomorphic ventricular tachycardia*) is present when three or more consecutive ventricular premature beats occur at a heart rate of more than 120 beats per minute (usually 150 to 200 beats per minute). Ventricular tachycardia can occur as a nonsustained, paroxysmal rhythm or as a sustained rhythm. The rhythm is regular with wide QRS complexes and no discernible P waves (Figure 4-6). SVT can sometimes be difficult to distinguish from ventricular tachycardia, especially if there is aberrant conduction or if the patient has an RBBB or LBBB. Ventricular tachycardia is common after an acute myocardial infarction and in the presence of inflammatory or infectious diseases of the heart. Digitalis toxicity may also appear as ventricular tachycardia.

Torsade de pointes (TdP; also called *polymorphic ventricular tachycardia*) is a distinct form of ventricular tachycardia initiated by a ventricular premature beat in the setting of abnormal ventricular repolarization (prolongation of the QT interval). Drugs that prolong repolarization, such as phenothiazines,

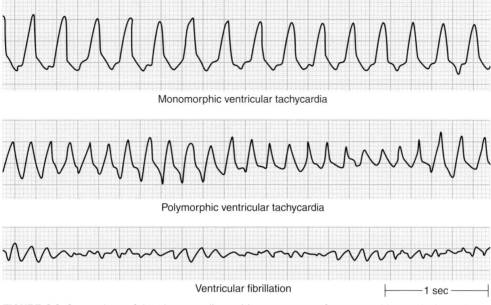

Monomorphic ventricular tachycardia

Polymorphic ventricular tachycardia

Ventricular fibrillation ├────── 1 sec ──────┤

FIGURE 4-6 Comparison of the electrocardiographic appearance of monomorphic ventricular tachycardia, polymorphic ventricular tachycardia (torsade de pointes), and ventricular fibrillation.

tricyclic antidepressants, certain antiemetics, and most antidysrhythmics, predispose to development of TdP.

PERIOPERATIVE MANAGEMENT

On occasion, it may be impossible to differentiate monomorphic ventricular tachycardia from SVT based on clinical symptoms, vital signs, or ECG findings. Patients with symptomatic or unstable monomorphic ventricular tachycardia or SVT should undergo cardioversion immediately. Cardioversion can begin at an output of 100 J (monophasic) and increase in increments of 50 to 100 J as necessary. If vital signs are stable but the ventricular tachycardia is persistent or recurrent after cardioversion, then administration of amiodarone 150 mg over 10 minutes is recommended. This may be repeated as needed to a maximum total dose of 2.2 g in 24 hours. Recommended alternative drugs include procainamide, sotalol, and lidocaine. Pulseless ventricular tachycardia or polymorphic ventricular tachycardia under any circumstances requires initiation of cardiopulmonary resuscitation (CPR) and immediate defibrillation using 360 J (monophasic).

The occurrence of paroxysmal nonsustained ventricular tachycardia during anesthesia should prompt an investigation into potential causes. A plan to improve reversible factors should be implemented. At any point, episodic ventricular tachycardia can progress to stable ventricular tachycardia or deteriorate into unstable ventricular tachycardia, pulseless ventricular tachycardia, or ventricular fibrillation. The occurrence of sustained ventricular tachycardia with or without a pulse demands immediate action. In addition to electrical therapy and drug treatment, endotracheal intubation and evaluation and correction of acid-base and electrolyte disturbances should be undertaken as clinically appropriate.

Ventricular Fibrillation

SIGNS, SYMPTOMS, AND DIAGNOSIS

Ventricular fibrillation is the most common cause of sudden cardiac death. Most victims have underlying ischemic heart disease. In patients with acute coronary ischemia, those receiving β-blockers, angiotensin-converting enzyme inhibitors, and statins have ventricular tachycardia or ventricular fibrillation less often than those not receiving these drugs. Ventricular tachycardia often precedes the onset of ventricular fibrillation. The gold standard for long-term treatment of recurrent episodic ventricular tachycardia or fibrillation is implantation of a permanent automatic pacemaker-cardioverter-defibrillator with adjuvant drug therapy as a second-line treatment.

Ventricular fibrillation is a rapid, grossly irregular ventricular rhythm with marked variability in QRS cycle length, morphology, and amplitude (see Figure 4-6). This rhythm is incompatible with life because there is no associated stroke volume or cardiac output. A pulse or blood pressure *never* accompanies ventricular fibrillation. If a patient with presumed ventricular fibrillation is awake or responsive, the ECG must be reevaluated before treatment decisions are made.

PERIOPERATIVE MANAGEMENT

Ventricular fibrillation during anesthesia is a critical event. CPR must be initiated immediately. Electrical defibrillation is the only effective method to convert ventricular fibrillation to a rhythm capable of generating a cardiac output. Defibrillation involves delivery of an electrical current through the heart to depolarize all myocardial cells at once. Ideally, a single pacemaker focus will then restore myocardial synchrony. This treatment should be instituted as soon as possible, because cardiac output, coronary blood flow, and cerebral blood flow are extremely low during ventricular fibrillation, even with ideally performed external cardiac compressions. The single most important factor affecting survival in patients experiencing ventricular fibrillation is time to defibrillation. Survival is best if defibrillation occurs within 3 to 5 minutes of cardiac arrest.

When ventricular fibrillation is refractory to electrical treatment, administration of epinephrine 1 mg IV or vasopressin 40 units IV may improve the response to electrical defibrillation. Adjunctive therapy with amiodarone, lidocaine, or, in the case of TdP, magnesium may be indicated. Standardized advanced cardiac life support (ACLS) algorithms (Figure 4-7) should be followed for electrical, pharmacologic, and adjunctive therapy.

In any pulseless arrest, contributing factors should be sought and treated. The differential diagnosis includes hypoxia, hypovolemia, acidosis, hypokalemia, hyperkalemia, hypoglycemia, hypothermia, drug or environmental toxins, cardiac tamponade, tension pneumothorax, coronary ischemia, pulmonary embolus, and hemorrhage.

VENTRICULAR PREEXCITATION SYNDROMES

The normal conduction system of the heart from atria to ventricles is a single conduction pathway through the AV node and His-Purkinje system. Some patients have alternate (accessory) conduction pathways that function as electrically active muscle bridges bypassing the normal conduction pathway and creating a potential avenue for reentrant tachycardias. These accessory pathways are congenital and most likely represent remnants of fetal AV muscular connections left by incomplete development of the annulus fibrosus.

Wolff-Parkinson-White Syndrome

SIGNS, SYMPTOMS, AND DIAGNOSIS

Since Wolff-Parkinson-White (WPW) syndrome was first described in 1930, the understanding of WPW syndrome and reentrant tachycardias has improved enormously. WPW syndrome occurs in 1% of the general population. It is more common in patients with Ebstein's malformation of the tricuspid valve, hypertrophic cardiomyopathy, and transposition of the great vessels. There is a bimodal age distribution in initial symptoms, with the first peak in early childhood, then a second in young adulthood. Paroxysmal palpitations with or without dizziness, syncope, dyspnea, or angina pectoris are common during the tachydysrhythmias associated with this syndrome. The initial manifestation of WPW syndrome occurs during pregnancy in some women. Other patients have the first manifestation of WPW syndrome during the perioperative period. The incidence of sudden cardiac death in patients with WPW syndrome is 0.15% to 0.39% per patient-year, but it is very unusual for sudden death to be the initial manifestation of WPW syndrome.

PERIOPERATIVE MANAGEMENT

The diagnosis of WPW syndrome is reserved for conditions characterized by both preexcitation and tachydysrhythmia. Ventricular preexcitation causes an earlier than normal deflection of the QRS complex called a *delta wave*. Delta waves can mimic the Q waves of a myocardial infarction.

AVNRT is the most common tachydysrhythmia seen in patients with WPW syndrome. It accounts for 95% of the dysrhythmias seen with this syndrome. This tachydysrhythmia is usually triggered by a PAC. AVNRT is classified as either orthodromic (narrow QRS complex) or antidromic (wide QRS complex). *Orthodromic* AVNRT is much more common (90% of 95% of cases) and has a narrow QRS complex because the cardiac impulse is conducted from the atrium through the normal AV node–His-Purkinje system. These impulses return from the ventricle to the atrium using the accessory pathway. Treatment of orthodromic AVNRT in conscious patients in stable condition should begin with vagal maneuvers such as carotid sinus massage or Valsalva's maneuver. If vagal maneuvers are unsuccessful, adenosine, verapamil, β-blockers, or amiodarone may be used as clinically appropriate.

In the less common *antidromic* form of AVNRT, the cardiac impulse is conducted from the atrium to the ventricle through the accessory pathway and returns from the ventricles to the atria via the normal AV node. The wide QRS complex seen in antidromic AVNRT makes it difficult to distinguish this dysrhythmia from ventricular tachycardia on ECG. Treatment of antidromic AVNRT is intended to block conduction of the cardiac impulse along the accessory pathway. Drugs that slow AV nodal conduction, such as adenosine, calcium channel blockers, β-blockers, lidocaine, and digoxin, may *increase* conduction along the accessory pathway and are *contraindicated*. Facilitation of conduction over the accessory pathway may produce a marked increase in ventricular rate. Treatment of antidromic AVNRT in patients with stable vital signs includes intravenous administration of procainamide 10 mg/kg IV infused at a rate not to exceed 50 mg/min. Procainamide slows conduction of cardiac impulses along the accessory pathway and may slow the ventricular response rate and terminate the wide-complex tachydysrhythmia. Electrical cardioversion is indicated if the ventricular response cannot be controlled by drug therapy.

Atrial fibrillation and atrial flutter are uncommon in WPW syndrome but are potentially lethal because they can result in very rapid ventricular response rates and deteriorate into ventricular fibrillation. The mechanism responsible is anterograde conduction from the atria to the ventricles through the accessory pathway. There is no mechanism along the accessory pathway to slow the conduction speed. The result is extremely rapid ventricular rates that often degenerate into ventricular fibrillation and death. Atrial fibrillation in the setting of WPW syndrome can be treated with intravenous procainamide. Verapamil and digoxin are *contraindicated* in this situation because they may actually accelerate conduction through the accessory pathway, making the situation worse. Electrical cardioversion is preferred in the presence of hemodynamic

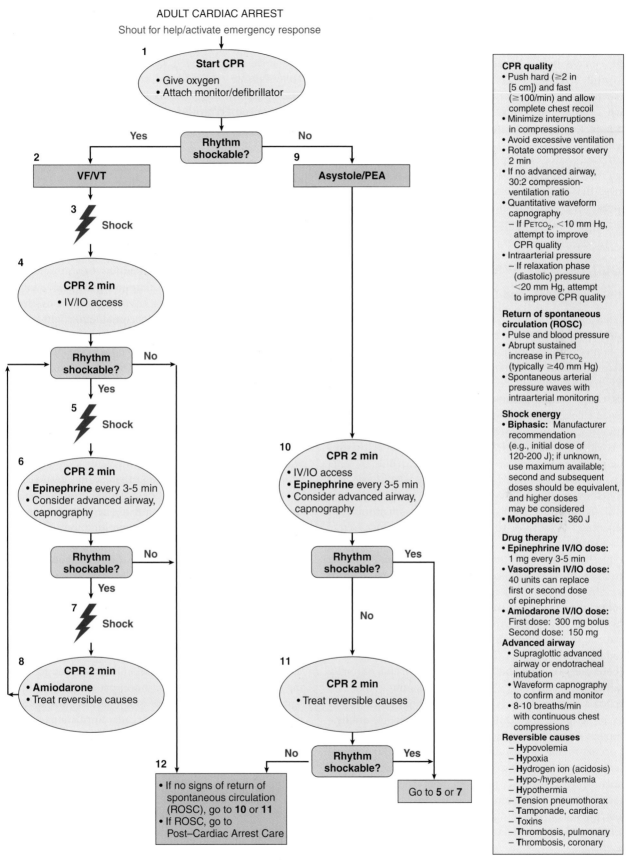

FIGURE 4-7 Algorithm for treatment of adult cardiac arrest. *CPR,* Cardiopulmonary resuscitation; *ET,* endotracheal; *IV/IO,* intravenous/intraosseous; *PEA,* pulseless electrical activity; *P*ETCO2, extrapolated end-tidal carbon dioxide pressure; *VF,* ventricular fibrillation; *VT,* ventricular tachycardia. *(From Neumar RW, Otto CW, Link MS, et al. Part 8: adult advanced cardiovascular life support: 2010 American Heart Association Guidelines for Cardiopulmonary Resuscitation and Emergency Cardiovascular Care. Circulation. 2010;122:S736.)*

instability. Long-term management of tachydysrhythmias in patients with WPW syndrome usually involves radiofrequency catheter ablation of the accessory pathway. The procedure is curative in 95% of patients and has a low complication rate. Antidysrhythmic drugs may be used as adjuvant therapy.

Patients with known WPW syndrome coming for surgery should continue to receive their antidysrhythmic medications. The goal during management of anesthesia is to avoid any event (e.g., increased sympathetic nervous system activity due to pain, anxiety, or hypovolemia) or drug (digoxin, verapamil) that could enhance anterograde conduction of cardiac impulses through an accessory pathway. Appropriate antidysrhythmic drugs and equipment for electrical cardioversion-defibrillation must be immediately available.

PROLONGED QT SYNDROME

Signs, Symptoms, and Diagnosis

By definition, a patient with long QT syndrome (LQTS) has a prolongation of the QTc exceeding 460 milliseconds. The prolongation of repolarization in LQTS results in a dispersion of refractory periods throughout the myocardium. This abnormality in repolarization allows afterdepolarizations to trigger PVCs. Under certain circumstances, the triggered PVCs initiate a ventricular reentry rhythm manifesting as polymorphic ventricular tachycardia, also known as *torsade de pointes* (TdP). TdP is electrocardiographically characterized by a "twisting of the peaks" or rotation around the ECG baseline. In other words, there is a constantly changing cycle length, axis, and morphology of the QRS complexes around the isoelectric baseline during TdP (see Figure 4-6). This dysrhythmia may be repetitive, episodic, or sustained and may degenerate into ventricular fibrillation.

Typically, women have longer QT intervals than men. This difference is more pronounced at slower heart rates. The incidence of congenital and acquired prolonged QT syndromes is higher in women. Not surprisingly, the incidence of TdP is also higher in women. The strongest predictor of the risk of syncope or sudden death in patients with congenital prolonged QT syndrome is a QTc exceeding 500 milliseconds.

There are two types of LQTS: congenital and acquired. Acquired iatrogenic LQTS is far more common than the inherited forms of LQTS. Acquired LQTS may be caused by many prescription medications such as antibiotics, antidysrhythmics, antidepressants, and antiemetics. Data suggest that TdP occurs in 1% to 10% of patients receiving QT-prolonging antidysrhythmic drugs. However, the incidence of TdP is much lower in patients receiving noncardiovascular QT-prolonging drugs. LQTS can be associated with hypokalemia, hypomagnesemia, severe malnutrition, hypertrophic cardiomyopathy, and intracranial catastrophes such as subarachnoid hemorrhage.

There are several genetic syndromes that manifest a long QT interval. The two most common are the Romano-Ward and Timothy syndromes. These are inherited as autosomal dominant disorders and usually present as syncope in late childhood. Manifestations can occur as early as the first year of life or as late as the sixth decade. A rarer autosomal recessive form of prolonged QT syndrome, called *Jervell and Lange-Nielsen syndrome,* is associated with congenital deafness. Syncope is the hallmark symptom of the inherited forms of prolonged QT syndrome. These syncopal events are commonly associated with stress, emotion, exercise, or other situations that lead to increased sympathetic stimulation.

Perioperative Management

Treatment of LQTS includes correction of electrolyte abnormalities, particularly those of magnesium or potassium. Any drugs associated with QT prolongation should be discontinued. Cardiac pacing is a treatment option in LQTS, because TdP is often preceded by bradycardia. Programming a pacemaker to pace at a higher backup rate than usual can prevent the bradycardia that precedes TdP and abort the dysrhythmia. Pacing is usually employed in combination with β-blocker therapy. Studies have shown a considerable reduction in cardiac events and mortality in congenital LQTS patients treated with β-blocker therapy (from 50% to <5% over a 10-year period). In recent years, implantable cardioverter-defibrillators (ICDs) with pacing capability have emerged as the lifesaving therapy for patients with recurrent symptoms and recalcitrant TdP despite ventricular suppression therapy with β-blockers.

A preoperative ECG to rule out LQTS is useful in a patient with a history of unexplained syncope or a family history of sudden death. The choice of anesthetic drugs deserves special attention in the case of LQTS, since many common anesthetic drugs cause some prolongation of the QTc. Isoflurane and sevoflurane have been shown to prolong the QTc in otherwise healthy children and adults. Currently, however, there is insufficient information to favor one volatile anesthetic over another. Droperidol and other antiemetic drugs also increase the QT interval. Events known to prolong the QT interval should be avoided, such as abrupt increases in sympathetic stimulation associated with preoperative anxiety and noxious stimulation intraoperatively, acute hypokalemia due to iatrogenic hyperventilation, and administration of drugs known to prolong the QTc. Consideration may be given to establishing β-blockade before induction in patients believed to be at particular risk. A defibrillator should be available, because the likelihood of perioperative ventricular fibrillation is increased.

MECHANISMS OF BRADYDYSRHYTHMIAS

Sinus Bradycardia

SIGNS, SYMPTOMS, AND DIAGNOSIS

Bradycardia is defined as a heart rate of less than 60 beats per minute (Table 4-3). Trained athletes often exhibit resting bradycardia, as may normal individuals during sleep. However, an inability to increase the heart rate adequately during exercise, bradycardia associated with symptoms (such as syncope,

TABLE 4-3   Perioperative causes of sinus bradycardia

Vagal stimulation
    Oculocardiac reflex: traction on eye muscles
    Celiac plexus stimulation: traction on the mesentery
    Laryngoscopy
    Abdominal insufflation
    Nausea
    Pain
    Electroconvulsive therapy
Drugs
    β-Blockers
    Calcium channel blockers
    Opioids (fentanyl, sufentanil)
Succinylcholine
Hypothermia
Hypothyroidism
Athletic heart syndrome
Sinoatrial nodal disease or ischemia

dizziness, and chest pain), or a heart rate of less than 40 beats per minute in the absence of physical conditioning or sleep is considered abnormal. Bradydysrhythmias are most commonly caused by SA node dysfunction or dysfunction in the conduction system below the SA node.

Dysfunction of the SA node, also referred to as *sick sinus syndrome,* is a common cause of bradycardia. Sick sinus syndrome with symptomatic bradycardia is the most common reason for insertion of a permanent cardiac pacemaker. The prevalence of sinus node dysfunction may be as high as 1 in 600 patients older than 65 years of age. Many patients with sick sinus syndrome are asymptomatic; others experience syncope or palpitations. Episodes of SVT may punctuate periods of bradycardia, which accounts for another common name for sinus node dysfunction: *tachycardia-bradycardia (tachy-brady) syndrome.* In patients with ischemic heart disease, periods of bradycardia may contribute to the development of congestive heart failure, whereas periods of tachycardia can contribute to the development of hypertension and angina pectoris. The rate of progression to second- or third-degree AV heart block in patients with sick sinus syndrome is approximately 1% to 5% per year.

The ECG during sinus bradycardia demonstrates a regular rhythm with a normal-appearing P wave before each QRS complex and a heart rate of 60 beats per minute or less. The SA node usually fires between 60 and 100 times per minute and overdrives other potential pacemakers in the heart. However, if the SA node does not fire, other slower pacemaker cells may take over primary pacemaker function. There is normally a pause in electrical activity before a secondary slower pacemaker begins to fire. Each group of potential pacemaker cells has an intrinsic rate. Cells near the AV node, so called *junctional pacemakers,* fire at 40 to 60 beats per minute. Ventricular cells below the AV node can act as an ectopic pacemaker but fire at a very slow rate in the range of 30 to 45 beats per minute.

PERIOPERATIVE MANAGEMENT

In asymptomatic patients with sinus bradycardia, no treatment is required. However, these patients should be monitored for worsening bradycardia or hemodynamic deterioration. In mildly symptomatic patients, any potential contributing factors such as excess vagal tone or drugs should be eliminated. In severely symptomatic patients—that is, those with chest pain or syncope—immediate transcutaneous or transvenous pacing is indicated. Atropine 0.5 mg IV every 3 to 5 minutes (to a maximum of 3 mg) may be given to increase heart rate but should not delay initiation of pacing. It should be noted that small doses of atropine (<0.5 mg IV) can cause a further *slowing* of the heart rate. In the event that cardiac pacing is delayed or pacing capabilities are limited, an epinephrine or dopamine infusion may be titrated to response while cardiac pacing is awaited. If atropine is ineffective, glucagon may be useful if the bradycardia is due to β-blocker or calcium channel blocker overdose. Glucagon stimulates glucagon-specific receptors on the myocardium that increase cyclic adenosine monophosphate (cAMP) levels and increase myocardial contractility, heart rate, and AV conduction. Suggested dosing of glucagon is 50 to 70 mcg/kg (3 to 5 mg in a 70-kg patient) every 3 to 5 minutes until clinical response is achieved or a total dose of 10 mg is reached. To maintain clinical effect, this should be followed with a continuous infusion at 2 to 10 mg/hr.

Bradycardia during neuraxial blockade can occur in patients of any age and any American Society of Anesthesiologists (ASA) physical status class, whether or not they are sedated. The incidence of profound bradycardia and cardiac arrest during neuraxial anesthesia is approximately 1.5 per 10,000 cases. By contrast, cardiac arrest during general anesthesia occurs at a rate of 5.5 per 10,000 cases. Bradycardia or asystole may develop suddenly (within seconds or minutes) in a patient with a previously normal or even increased heart rate, or the heart rate slowing may be progressive. Bradycardia can occur at any time during neuraxial blockade but most often occurs approximately an hour after anesthetic administration. The risk of bradycardia and asystole may persist into the postoperative period even after the sensory and motor blockade has diminished. Oxygen saturation is usually normal before the onset of bradycardia. Approximately half of patients who experience arrest during neuraxial anesthesia complain of shortness of breath, nausea, restlessness, light-headedness, or tingling of the fingers and manifest deterioration in mental status before arrest.

The exact mechanism responsible for bradycardia and asystole during spinal and epidural anesthesia is not known. One proposed mechanism is termed the *Bezold-Jarisch response.* This is a paradoxical reflex-induced bradycardia resulting from decreased venous return and activation of vagal reflex arcs mediated by baroreceptors and stretch receptors. Another possible mechanism is the unopposed parasympathetic nervous system activity that results from the anesthetic-induced sympathectomy. Blockade of cardiac accelerator fibers originating from thoracic sympathetic ganglia (T1 to T4) may alter the balance of autonomic nervous system input to the heart and lead to relatively unopposed parasympathetic influences on the SA node and AV node, which slows the heart rate.

Bradydysrhythmias associated with spinal or epidural anesthesia should be treated aggressively. Bradycardia can occur despite prophylactic therapy with atropine and/or intravenous fluids. Recalcitrant bradycardia necessitates transcutaneous or transvenous pacing. Secondary factors such as hypovolemia, opioid administration, sedation, hypercarbia, concurrent medical illnesses, and long-term use of medications that slow the heart rate can contribute to the development of bradycardia. In the clinical setting of severe bradycardia, preparation should be made for management of asystole, which is treated with CPR. Pharmacologic management should follow ACLS protocols and include treatment with atropine, epinephrine, and/or vasopressin as appropriate (Figure 4-8).

Junctional Rhythm

SIGNS, SYMPTOMS, AND DIAGNOSIS

Junctional or nodal rhythm is due to the activity of a cardiac pacemaker in the tissues surrounding the AV node. Junctional pacemakers usually have an intrinsic rate of 40 to 60 beats per minute. The impulse initiated by a junctional pacemaker travels to the ventricles along the normal conduction pathway but can also be conducted retrograde into the atria. The site of the junctional pacemaker determines whether the P wave precedes the QRS complex (with a shortened PR interval), follows the QRS complex, or is buried within the QRS complex and is not visible. The diagnosis of junctional rhythm may be an incidental finding on ECG. Junctional rhythm can be suspected if on physical examination the jugular venous pulsation shows cannon *a* waves.

If the junctional rhythm has an accelerated rate, it is called a *junctional tachycardia* or *accelerated nodal (junctional)*

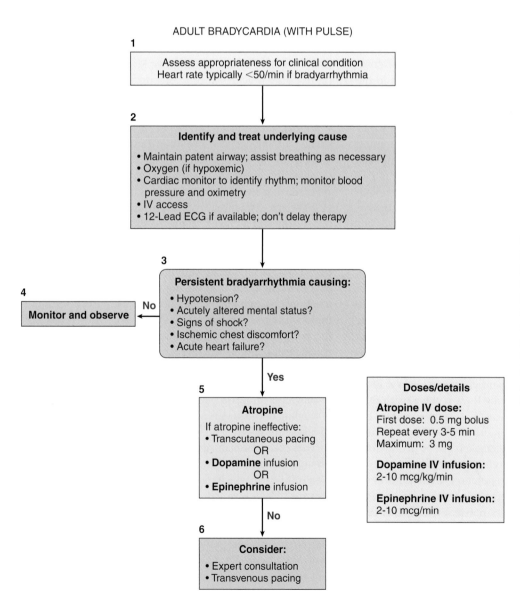

FIGURE 4-8 Algorithm for treatment of adult bradycardia (with pulse). *ECG*, Electrocardiogram; *IV*, intravenous. *(From Neumar RW, Otto CW, Link MS, et al. Part 8: adult advanced cardiovascular life support: 2010 American Heart Association Guidelines for Cardiopulmonary Resuscitation and Emergency Cardiovascular Care. Circulation. 2010;122:S749.)*

rhythm. Junctional tachycardia is a narrow-complex tachycardia at a rate usually lower than 120 beats per minute. Junctional rhythms can cause AV dyssynchrony, loss of atrial kick, and in some circumstances rapid ventricular rates. This can result in symptoms such as fatigue, generalized weakness, angina pectoris, impaired cardiac output, congestive heart failure, pulmonary edema, and hypotension.

PERIOPERATIVE MANAGEMENT

Junctional rhythm can occur in association with many different disorders. It is often an escape rhythm because of depressed sinus node function, SA block, or delayed conduction in the AV node. Junctional tachycardia can result from increased automaticity of junctional tissues in the setting of digitalis toxicity or cardiac ischemia. Junctional rhythm that occurs in association with myocarditis, myocardial ischemia, or digitalis toxicity should be managed by treating the underlying disorder. Junctional rhythms are not uncommon during general anesthesia using halogenated anesthetic vapors and, in this setting, require no treatment. Even in the setting of acute myocardial infarction, junctional rhythms are usually considered benign and require no treatment. However, in certain patients the loss of AV synchrony during a junctional rhythm will result in myocardial ischemia, heart failure, or hypotension. Atropine at a dose of 0.5 mg can be used to accelerate the heart rate if a slow junctional rhythm becomes hemodynamically significant.

CONDUCTION DISTURBANCES

Conduction disturbances are usually classified by the site and degree of blockade. An intact cardiac conduction system normally ensures conduction of each sinus impulse from the atria to the ventricles. Abnormalities of the conduction system can disrupt this process and lead to heart block. Assessing the site of the conduction abnormality and the risk of progression to complete heart block are core issues in treating a patient with heart block.

A variety of acute and chronic conditions can cause or contribute to heart block. These include acute myocardial infarction (especially in the distribution of the right coronary artery), digitalis toxicity, excessive β-blockade or calcium channel blockade, myocarditis, rheumatic fever, mononucleosis, Lyme disease, and infiltrative diseases such as sarcoidosis and amyloidosis.

First-Degree Atrioventricular Heart Block

SIGNS, SYMPTOMS, AND DIAGNOSIS

First-degree AV block is defined as a PR interval of longer than 0.2 seconds. Each P wave is conducted and has a corresponding QRS complex of normal duration. There is a delay in the passage of the cardiac impulse through the AV node. First-degree AV block is often a result of minor degenerative changes in the cardiac conduction system that accompany normal aging. Other causes include myocardial ischemia (involving the blood supply

to the AV node), inferior wall myocardial infarction, drugs affecting AV node conduction (digitalis and amiodarone), and processes that enhance parasympathetic nervous system activity and vagal tone. First-degree AV block can be found in patients with and without structural heart disease. Patients with first-degree AV block are usually asymptomatic and appear to have no significant increase in mortality compared with matched controls. The Framingham Heart Study followed long-term outcomes of individuals with first-degree heart block, and the results suggested an increased risk of atrial fibrillation in this population.

PERIOPERATIVE MANAGEMENT

Anesthetic management of the patient with first-degree heart block should be aimed at avoiding any clinical situation or drug that increases vagal tone or slows AV conduction. Atropine administration can speed conduction of cardiac impulses through the AV node. However, in patients with significant heart disease, the increase in heart rate produced by atropine may contribute to myocardial ischemia. In patients with risk factors such as coronary ischemia and systemic infection, these clinical conditions should be treated and medically optimized before surgery. Digoxin levels should be checked before surgery, and serum potassium should be maintained at normal levels in patients receiving digoxin.

Second-Degree Atrioventricular Heart Block

SIGNS, SYMPTOMS, AND DIAGNOSIS

Second-degree AV block can be suspected when a P wave is present without a corresponding QRS complex. Second-degree AV heart block can be categorized as Mobitz type I (Wenckebach) block or Mobitz type II block. Mobitz type I block shows progressive prolongation of the PR interval until a beat is entirely blocked (dropped beat) followed by a repeat of this sequence. In contrast, Mobitz type II block is characterized by sudden and complete interruption of conduction (dropped QRS) without PR prolongation. Mobitz type II block is usually associated with permanent damage to the conduction system and may progress to third-degree block, especially in the setting of acute myocardial infarction.

Mobitz type I (Wenckebach) block demonstrates progressive prolongation of the PR interval until a beat is dropped. This type of block is often transient and *asymptomatic*. It is thought to occur because each successive depolarization produces a prolongation of the refractory period of the AV node. This process continues until an atrial impulse reaches the AV node during its absolute refractory period and conduction of that impulse is blocked completely. A pause allows the AV node to recover and then the process resumes. The prognosis for Mobitz type I block is good, since reliable secondary pacemakers in the AV node usually take over pacing duties and maintain adequate cardiac output. Mobitz type I block does not require treatment unless the decreased ventricular rate results in signs of hypoperfusion. Symptomatic patients may be treated with atropine as needed. If atropine is unsuccessful, pacing may be indicated. Mobitz type I block can be a result of myocardial ischemia or infarction, myocardial fibrosis or calcification, or infiltrative or inflammatory diseases of the myocardium, or can occur after cardiothoracic surgery. It can also be associated with the use of certain drugs such as calcium channel blockers, β-blockers, digoxin, and sympatholytic drugs.

Mobitz type II block is a complete interruption in the conduction of a cardiac impulse, usually at a point below the AV node in the bundle of His or in a bundle branch. Mobitz type II block is usually *symptomatic,* with palpitations and near syncope being common complaints. Mobitz type II block has a less favorable prognosis because there is a substantial risk of progression to third-degree AV block. Reliable secondary pacemakers are not present in Mobitz type II block or in third-degree heart block, because these disorders are associated with serious disease involving the infranodal conduction system.

PERIOPERATIVE MANAGEMENT

Therapeutic decisions for patients with second-degree heart block depend on the ventricular response and the symptoms of the patient. The heart rate in Mobitz type I block is usually good and rarely does it progress to third-degree heart block. In the presence of an acceptable ventricular rate and an adequate cardiac output, no treatment is needed.

Mobitz type II block has a high rate of progression to third-degree heart block and can manifest as a slow escape rhythm insufficient to sustain an acceptable cardiac output. Placement of a cardiac pacemaker is necessary under these circumstances. Treatment for Mobitz type II block includes transcutaneous or transvenous cardiac pacing. Atropine is unlikely to improve bradycardia caused by Mobitz type II block.

Bundle Branch Blocks

Conduction disturbances at various levels of the His-Purkinje system are called *bundle branch blocks* or *intraventricular conduction defects.* Bundle branch blocks can be chronic or intermittent. Intraventricular conduction disturbances are usually associated with significant structural heart disease, especially dilated cardiomyopathies. They are a marker of poor prognosis, both in terms of heart failure and increased mortality.

RIGHT BUNDLE BRANCH BLOCK

Signs, Symptoms, and Diagnosis

RBBB is present in approximately 1% of hospitalized adult patients. It does not always imply cardiac disease and is often of no clinical significance. In patients without structural heart disease, RBBB is more common than LBBB. However, RBBB can be associated with structural heart disease such as atrial septal defect, valvular heart disease, and ischemic heart disease. The intraventricular conduction delay resulting from RBBB is seldom symptomatic and rarely progresses to advanced AV block.

RBBB is due to a disruption of the cardiac impulse as it travels over the RBB. It is recognized on the ECG by a widened QRS complex (>0.1 second in duration) and an rSR′ configuration in leads V_1 and V_2. There is also a deep S wave in leads I and V_6. *Bifascicular heart block* is present when RBBB exists in combination with block of either the left anterior or left posterior fascicle of the LBB. RBBB in association with left anterior hemiblock is more common than RBBB with left posterior hemiblock. This is because anatomically the posterior fascicle usually has a dual blood supply, whereas the anterior fascicle does not. Indications of RBBB with left anterior hemiblock are present on approximately 1% of all adult ECGs. The combination of RBBB and left posterior hemiblock is infrequent, and each year approximately 1% to 2% of patients with this form of block show progression to third-degree heart block.

Perioperative Management

Acute treatment of RBBB or RBBB with left anterior hemiblock consists of observation and elimination of drugs or clinical factors known to contribute to conduction disturbances. Pacing capability should be available in the event of progression to complete heart block.

A theoretical concern in patients with bifascicular heart block is that perioperative events (changes in blood pressure, arterial oxygenation, serum electrolyte concentrations) might compromise impulse conduction in the remaining fascicle and lead to third-degree heart block. There is no evidence, however, that surgery performed with general or regional anesthesia predisposes patients with preexisting bifascicular heart block to the development of third-degree heart block. Prophylactic placement of a cardiac pacemaker is *not* necessary.

LEFT BUNDLE BRANCH BLOCK

Signs, Symptoms, and Diagnosis

LBBB is recognized on the ECG as a QRS complex of longer than 0.12 seconds in duration and the absence of Q waves in leads I and V_6. Abnormal conduction of impulses through the fascicles of the LBB can be characterized as unifascicular—that is, a hemiblock—or as complete. Block of the left anterior fascicle is the most common hemiblock. Left posterior hemiblock is uncommon because the posterior fascicle of the LBB is larger and better perfused than the anterior fascicle. Although hemiblock is a form of intraventricular heart block, the duration of the QRS complex is normal or only minimally prolonged when a hemiblock is present.

LBBB, in contrast to RBBB, has more ominous clinical implications. LBBB is often associated with ischemic heart disease, hypertension, and valvular heart disease. Patients with isolated LBBB rarely show progression to advanced AV block. The appearance of LBBB has been observed during anesthesia, particularly during hypertensive or tachycardic episodes, and may be a sign of myocardial ischemia. It is very difficult to diagnose a myocardial infarction by ECG in the presence of LBBB, because ST-segment and T-wave changes (repolarization abnormalities) are already present as part of the bundle branch block pattern. An SVT can be mistaken for ventricular tachycardia in a patient with LBBB because the QRS complexes are characteristically wide.

Perioperative Management

LBBB is often a marker of serious heart disease, such as hypertension, coronary artery disease, aortic valve disease, or cardiomyopathy. Treatment of these contributing disorders can decrease the incidence of LBBB in susceptible patients. Isolated LBBB is often asymptomatic, and some patients have LBBB only after a critical heart rate is reached.

The presence of LBBB has special implications if insertion of a pulmonary artery catheter is planned. Third-degree heart block can occur if the central catheter induces RBBB in a patient with preexisting LBBB. RBBB (usually transient) occurs during insertion of a pulmonary artery catheter in approximately 2% to 5% of patients.

Third-Degree Atrioventricular Heart Block

SIGNS, SYMPTOMS, AND DIAGNOSIS

Third-degree heart block, also known as *complete heart block,* is the complete interruption of AV conduction. There is no conduction of cardiac impulses from the atria to the ventricles. Continued activity of the ventricles is due to impulses from an ectopic pacemaker distal to the site of the conduction block. If the conduction block is near the AV node, the heart rate is usually 45 to 55 beats per minute and the QRS complex is narrow. When the conduction block is below the AV node (infranodal), the heart rate is usually 30 to 40 beats per minute and the QRS complex is wide.

In patients with isolated chronic RBBB, the progression to complete AV block is rare. Patients with bifascicular block (RBBB and left anterior or posterior fascicular block) or complete LBBB have a 6% incidence of progression to complete heart block. In the setting of acute myocardial infarction, the development of new bifascicular block plus first-degree AV block is associated with a very high risk (40%) of progression to complete heart block. Approximately 8% of patients with acute inferior wall myocardial infarction develop complete heart block. It is usually transient, although it may last for several days. These patients should undergo temporary cardiac pacing. ECG evidence of alternating bundle branch blocks, even if asymptomatic, is a sign of advanced conduction system disease and an indication for permanent pacing.

The onset of third-degree AV block may be signaled by an episode of vertigo or syncope. Other symptoms include weakness and dyspnea. A syncopal episode caused by third-degree heart block is called a *Stokes-Adams attack.* Congestive heart failure can occur from the decreased cardiac output and bradycardia that accompanies third-degree AV block.

The most common cause of third-degree AV block in adults is fibrotic degeneration of the distal cardiac conduction system associated with aging (Lenègre's disease). Degenerative and calcific changes in more proximal conduction tissue adjacent to the mitral valve annulus can also interrupt cardiac conduction (Lev's disease).

PERIOPERATIVE MANAGEMENT

Caution must be exercised when administering antidysrhythmic drugs to patients with third-degree AV block before pacemaker placement, because the drugs may suppress the ectopic ventricular pacemaker that is responsible for maintaining the heart rate. Treatment of third-degree AV block during anesthesia consists of transcutaneous or transvenous cardiac pacing. If the block persists, placement of a permanent cardiac pacemaker is indicated. Preoperative placement of a transvenous pacemaker or the availability of transcutaneous cardiac pacing is necessary before an anesthetic is administered for insertion of a permanent cardiac pacemaker. Isoproterenol may be needed to maintain an acceptable heart rate and act as a "chemical pacemaker" until a permanent pacemaker is implanted and functional.

TREATMENT OF CARDIAC DYSRHYTHMIAS

Antidysrhythmic Drugs

Antidysrhythmic drugs are administered when correction of identifiable precipitating events is not sufficient to suppress dysrhythmias. These drugs act by altering various electrophysiologic characteristics of myocardial cells. The majority of antidysrhythmia drugs work by one of three mechanisms: (1) suppressing automaticity in pacemaker cells by decreasing the slope of phase 4 depolarization, (2) prolonging the effective refractory period to eliminate reentry circuits, or (3) facilitating impulse conduction along normal conduction pathways to prevent conduction over a reentrant pathway. ECG changes, such as an increased PR interval or a prolonged QRS duration, are relatively common side effects of antidysrhythmic drug therapy.

Abnormal physiologic parameters should be corrected before initiating antidysrhythmic drug therapy or inserting a cardiac pacemaker. Establishment of physiologic acid-base values, normalization of serum electrolyte concentrations, and stabilization of autonomic nervous system activity are important and maximize the possibility of reestablishing normal sinus rhythm.

ADENOSINE

Adenosine is formed by serial dephosphorylation of adenosine triphosphate. It is an α-agonist and the drug of choice for pharmacologic termination of hemodynamically stable AVNRT. Sixty percent of patients respond at a dose of 6 mg, and an additional 32% of patients respond at a dose of 12 mg. Its therapeutic effect is short, lasting approximately 10 seconds. This extremely short half-life results from rapid active transport of the drug into red blood cells and endothelial cells, where it is metabolized. To be effective, adenosine should be injected rapidly and flushed quickly through the intravenous tubing with saline.

Common side effects of adenosine include facial flushing, dyspnea, and chest pressure. Generally, these effects are transient, lasting less than 60 seconds. Less common side effects include nausea, light-headedness, headache, sweating, palpitations, hypotension, and blurred vision.

Several drugs influence the clinical effectiveness of adenosine. Caffeine and theophylline antagonize the actions of adenosine. On the other hand, dipyridamole pretreatment increases the potency of adenosine. Carbamazepine also potentiates the action of adenosine. Patients with a heart transplant require only one third to one fifth the usual dose of adenosine because the transplanted heart is denervated. Administration of adenosine is contraindicated in patients with sick sinus syndrome and second- or third-degree heart block unless the patient has a functioning cardiac pacemaker.

ATROPINE

Atropine sulfate is a vagolytic drug that is a competitive antagonist at muscarinic cholinergic receptor sites. It is used to increase heart rate and blood pressure. Potential adverse side effects of atropine administration include tachycardia, sedation (especially in the elderly), urinary retention, and increased intraocular pressure in patients with closed-angle glaucoma. There is no evidence that atropine is detrimental to the treatment of asystolic arrest or pulseless electrical activity. However, evidence does not support any clinical benefit from atropine use in these situations. Therefore, it has been removed from ACLS recommendations for pharmacologic treatment of asystole and pulseless electrical activity.

Atropine is recommended in the treatment of symptomatic bradycardia as a temporizing measure while awaiting initiation of transcutaneous or transvenous pacing. The recommended dose is 0.5 mg IV every 3 to 5 minutes as needed to a maximum total dose of 3 mg. Doses of less than 0.5 mg in adults can worsen bradycardia. Heart rate effects appear within seconds of administration and last 15 to 30 minutes. Atropine is not effective in patients who have undergone cardiac transplantation.

AMIODARONE

Amiodarone is an antidysrhythmic structurally similar to thyroxine and procainamide. It acts on sodium, potassium, and calcium channels to produce α- and β-blocking effects that result in prolongation of the refractory period in myocardial cells. Amiodarone is useful in controlling ventricular rate in patients with atrial fibrillation. It is also indicated for treatment of ventricular fibrillation and pulseless ventricular tachycardia unresponsive to defibrillation, CPR, and vasopressors. In this situation, amiodarone improves the likelihood of successful defibrillation. Amiodarone is metabolized in the liver and slows the metabolism and increases the blood levels of other drugs metabolized by the liver, such as warfarin, digoxin, diltiazem, quinidine, procainamide, disopyramide, mexiletine, and propafenone. The dose recommended for cardiac arrest unresponsive to CPR, defibrillation, and vasopressor therapy is an initial dose of 300 mg IV. It can be followed by a second dose of 150 mg IV.

β-ADRENERGIC BLOCKERS

β-Blockers ameliorate the effects of circulating catecholamines and decrease heart rate and blood pressure. These cardioprotective effects are particularly important in patients with acute coronary syndromes. β-Blockers are indicated in patients with preserved left ventricular function who require ventricular rate control in atrial fibrillation, atrial flutter, and narrow-complex tachycardias originating at or above the AV node.

Side effects of β-blockade include bradycardia, AV conduction delays, and hypotension. Contraindications to β-blocker therapy include second- or third-degree heart block, hypotension, severe congestive heart failure, and reactive airway disease. β-Blockers should not be used in the treatment of atrial fibrillation or atrial flutter associated with WPW syndrome, since they may contribute to clinical deterioration in this situation by decreasing conduction through the AV node and speeding conduction through the accessory bypass tract.

CALCIUM CHANNEL BLOCKERS

Verapamil and diltiazem are calcium channel blockers. Verapamil inhibits the influx of extracellular calcium across myocardial and vascular smooth muscle cell membranes. It inhibits vascular smooth muscle contraction and causes marked vasodilation in coronary and other peripheral vascular beds.. Verapamil slows conduction and increases refractoriness of the AV node and is useful in controlling ventricular rate in patients with atrial tachydysrhythmias and in terminating reentrant dysrhythmias.

Verapamil is indicated for the treatment of narrow-complex tachycardia (SVT) in patients in whom vagal maneuvers and adenosine therapy have failed. It is also indicated for ventricular rate control with atrial flutter or atrial fibrillation. It is contraindicated in patients with an accessory bypass tract, such as those with WPW syndrome, since it can accelerate conduction through the accessory tract and thereby increase the ventricular rate to dangerously high levels. Calcium channel blockers have negative inotropic properties and should be avoided in patients with left ventricular dysfunction.

Verapamil can prolong the PR interval and is not effective in treating tachycardias originating below the AV node. The initial dose of verapamil is typically 2.5 to 5 mg IV over 2 minutes. This can be repeated if needed to a maximum total dose of 0.15 mg/kg. Hemodynamic effects peak in 5 minutes and persist for 20 to 30 minutes. If calcium channel blockers are administered to patients already receiving β-blockers, additive effects can result in iatrogenic second- or third-degree heart block.

Diltiazem has a similar mechanism of action and similar clinical indications as verapamil. However, diltiazem has less negative inotropic effect and causes less peripheral vasodilation than verapamil. The degree of AV node inhibition is similar for both drugs. The recommended dose for diltiazem is 0.25 mg/kg IV over 2 minutes. This can be repeated if needed. Successful dysrhythmia treatment can be followed by a maintenance infusion at 5 to 15 mg/hr.

DIGOXIN

Digoxin is a cardiac glycoside that was approved by the FDA in 1952 and has been used since that time for the treatment of congestive heart failure and atrial fibrillation. Digoxin inhibits the myocardial cell membrane Na^+,K^+-ATPase pump. Useful pharmacologic effects of digoxin include positive inotropy, slowing of conduction through the AV node, and lengthening of the refractory period of the AV node.

The inotropic effects of digoxin are due to an increase in intracellular calcium that allows for greater activation of contractile proteins. In addition to having positive inotropic effects, digoxin also increases phase 4 depolarization and shortens the action potential. This decreases conduction velocity through the AV node and prolongs the AV nodal refractory period.

Digoxin is effective in controlling the ventricular rate in atrial fibrillation, although it does not convert atrial fibrillation to sinus rhythm. Onset of therapeutic effects after intravenous administration of digoxin occurs in 5 to 30 minutes, with the peak effect at 2 to 6 hours after injection. Digoxin has a low therapeutic/toxic ratio (therapeutic index), especially in the presence of hypokalemia.

High serum digoxin levels can cause a variety of symptoms and signs, including life-threatening dysrhythmias. Coexisting disease states that can contribute to digoxin toxicity include hypothyroidism, hypokalemia, and renal dysfunction. A digoxin-specific antibody is available for treatment of severe digitalis toxicity.

DOPAMINE

Dopamine is a catecholamine precursor to norepinephrine and epinephrine present in nerve terminals and the adrenal medulla. It has direct dose-related effects on α, β, and dopaminergic receptors. At low doses (3 to 5 mcg/kg/min), dopamine increases renal, mesenteric, coronary, and cerebral blood flow through the activation of dopaminergic receptors. At moderate doses (5 to 7 mcg/kg/min), β effects predominate, producing increased heart rate, contractility, and cardiac output with a decrease in systemic vascular resistance. At high doses (>10 mcg/kg/min), α receptor stimulation causes peripheral vasoconstriction and a reduction in renal blood flow.

Dopamine is a second-line drug for the treatment of symptomatic bradycardia unresponsive to atropine. Like atropine, it should be considered a temporizing measure while awaiting initiation of transcutaneous or transvenous pacing. The dose recommended in this situation is 2 to 10 mcg/kg/min titrated to heart rate response. Caution must be exercised if infusion is through a peripheral intravenous line, because skin necrosis can result from extravasation at the injection site.

EPINEPHRINE

Epinephrine is a catecholamine produced by the adrenal medulla. Epinephrine is a potent mast cell stabilizer and bronchodilator and is useful in the treatment of severe bronchospasm and anaphylactic reactions. It is also a potent vasopressor that is useful during CPR. Its clinical effects vary with dosage. Increased contractility and heart rate occur at all dosages, but the effect on systemic vascular resistance is dose dependant. At low dosages (10 to 150 mcg/kg/min) the systemic vascular resistance may decrease or stay the same, but at high dosages (>150 mcg/kg/min) the systemic vascular resistance increases. The α effects of epinephrine can be beneficial during CPR to increase coronary and cerebral perfusion.

Epinephrine is indicated in the treatment of cardiac arrest because of its α-adrenergic vasoconstrictor properties. Studies have shown a higher likelihood of return to spontaneous circulation in patients treated with epinephrine than in those not given epinephrine during cardiac arrest from sustained ventricular fibrillation, pulseless electrical activity, or asystole.

The suggested dose is 1 mg IV every 3 to 5 minutes during adult cardiac arrest. Occasionally, larger doses may be needed to treat cardiac arrest resulting from β-blocker or calcium channel blocker overdose. Epinephrine should be given through central venous catheters if at all possible, because extravasation from a peripheral intravenous line can cause tissue necrosis.

In addition to the intravenous route, epinephrine can be administered by the intratracheal route. The dose for intratracheal use is 2 to 2.5 mg diluted in 5 to 10 mL of sterile water (which provides better drug absorption than saline). Other drugs that may be given intratracheally include lidocaine, atropine, naloxone, and vasopressin.

Epinephrine is a second-line drug in the treatment of symptomatic bradycardia unresponsive to atropine. The recommended dosage is an infusion of 2 to 10 mcg/min titrated to heart rate response. Like atropine, it should be considered a temporizing measure while awaiting initiation of transcutaneous or transvenous pacing.

ISOPROTERENOL

Isoproterenol is a potent bronchodilator and sympathomimetic structurally similar to epinephrine. Functionally, it has potent β_1- and β_2-agonist actions but lacks any α-adrenergic properties. The actions of isoproterenol are mediated intracellularly by cAMP. Stimulation of β_1 receptors produces positive inotropic and chronotropic effects. Characteristically isoproterenol administration causes the systolic blood pressure to increase and the diastolic blood pressure to decrease. This is attributed to drug-induced peripheral vasodilation. This vasodilatory effect does increase coronary blood flow, but the increased oxygen demand resulting from a higher heart rate outweighs the potential benefit of any increase in myocardial blood flow. Isoproterenol increases myocardial excitability and automaticity, which potentially favors dysrhythmias.

Isoproterenol is a second-line drug in the treatment of symptomatic bradycardia unresponsive to atropine. The recommended dosage is 2 to 10 mcg/min by continuous infusion titrated to heart rate effect. Because of its direct action on β receptors, isoproterenol is useful to treat symptomatic bradycardia in heart transplant recipients. An initial intravenous dosage of 1 mcg/min is titrated slowly upward until the desired effect is achieved.

LIDOCAINE

Lidocaine is a unique drug with many useful applications in the field of anesthesiology. Lidocaine is an amide local anesthetic commonly employed in regional anesthetic nerve blockade. However, the same sodium channel–blocking effects that make it a good local anesthetic make it a useful antidysrhythmic drug when administered intravenously. Lidocaine may be used in the treatment of cardiac arrest associated with ventricular fibrillation or pulseless ventricular tachycardia if amiodarone is not available. The recommended dose is 1.0 to 1.5 mg/kg IV. If ventricular fibrillation or pulseless ventricular tachycardia persists, half this dose can be repeated at 5- to 10-minute intervals to a maximum total dose of 3 mg/kg. Therapeutic doses of lidocaine have minimal negative inotropic effects.

Lidocaine is rapidly redistributed out of the plasma and myocardium, so multiple loading doses may be needed to achieve therapeutic blood levels. Clinical duration of action is 15 to 30 minutes after a loading dose. To sustain therapeutic effect, lidocaine must be administered by continuous infusion (1 to 4 mg/min). When administered in combination with other antidysrhythmic drugs, lidocaine can cause some myocardial depression or sinus node dysfunction.

During lidocaine therapy, monitoring of mental status is desirable, because the first signs of toxicity are usually central nervous system symptoms such as tinnitus, drowsiness, dysarthria, or confusion. At higher blood levels, signs of central nervous system depression such as sedation and respiratory depression predominate and may be accompanied by seizures. Lidocaine undergoes extensive first-pass hepatic metabolism, so clinical conditions that result in decreased hepatic blood flow, such as general anesthesia, congestive heart failure, liver disease, and advanced age, can result in higher than normal blood levels. Certain drugs such as cimetidine can also cause an increase in the plasma concentration of lidocaine.

MAGNESIUM

Magnesium functions in the body as a cofactor in the control of sodium and potassium transport. With regard to its antidysrhythmic properties, there are a few observational studies supporting the use of magnesium in the termination of TdP ventricular tachycardia associated with QT prolongation. However, there is no evidence that magnesium is effective in treating ventricular tachycardia associated with a normal QT interval. In ventricular fibrillation or pulseless ventricular tachycardia associated with TdP, magnesium can be given in a dose of 1 to 2 g over 5 minutes. If a pulse is present with the torsade, then the same dose can be administered, but more slowly.

PROCAINAMIDE

Procainamide is an antidysrhythmic drug that slows conduction, decreases automaticity, and increases the refractoriness of myocardial cells. It can be used in patients with preserved ventricular function to treat the following conditions: ventricular tachycardia with a pulse, atrial flutter or fibrillation, atrial fibrillation in WPW syndrome, and SVT resistant to adenosine and vagal maneuvers.

Procainamide can be administered at a rate of 50 mg/min IV until the dysrhythmia is suppressed, significant

hypotension occurs, or the QRS complex is prolonged by 50%. The duration of action after a bolus dose is 2 to 4 hours. Procainamide must be used with caution in patients with QT prolongation and in combination with other drugs that prolong the QT interval. To maintain therapeutic effect, procainamide can be given as a maintenance infusion at a rate of 1 to 4 mg/min. Dosage should be reduced in renal failure.

SOTALOL

Sotalol is a nonselective β-blocker. It prolongs the duration of the action potential and increases the refractoriness of cardiac cells. Sotalol can be used in the treatment of ventricular tachycardia and atrial fibrillation or atrial flutter in patients with WPW syndrome. The dose is 1.5 mg/kg IV over 5 minutes. Potential side effects include bradycardia, hypotension, and QT prolongation.

VASOPRESSIN

Vasopressin is a potent peripheral vasoconstrictor that works independently of α- or β-adrenergic mechanisms. It is an endogenous antidiuretic hormone that in high concentrations produces direct peripheral vasoconstriction by activating smooth muscle vasopressin (V_1) receptors. Currently, epinephrine and vasopressin are recommended interchangeably to treat cardiac arrest. If vasopressin is chosen, the dose is 40 units IV. Vasopressin may replace the first or second dose of epinephrine in the treatment of cardiac arrest. Vasopressin therapy may be useful in maintaining systemic vascular resistance in patients who have severe sepsis or acidosis or have undergone cardiopulmonary bypass when other drug treatments have failed.

TWENTY-PERCENT LIPID EMULSION

Infusion of lipid emulsion has been shown to increase the survival of rats and mice following bupivacaine overdose. The first reported case of its use in an adult human to successfully treat a bupivacaine-related cardiac arrest was in 2006. Since then, with accumulation of more data and experience, "lipid rescue" had become a widely accepted treatment. More study and experience are needed to standardize optimal dosing. However, the suggested initial dose is 1 mL/kg over 1 minute while chest compressions and related ACLS maneuvers are continued. The dose can be repeated every 3 to 5 minutes to a maximum of 3 mL/kg. After conversion to sinus rhythm, a maintenance infusion of 0.25 mL/kg/min is suggested until hemodynamic recovery occurs. This therapy has been used successfully in resuscitation of patients experiencing cardiac arrest resulting from local anesthetics other than bupivacaine.

Transcutaneous Pacing

The first external pacemaker was developed in the early 1950s by Boston cardiologist Paul M. Zoll. Although it represented a huge technologic advance for modern science, the device was impractical for long-term use because of the high current required, the skin irritation caused by the delivery pads, and significant patient discomfort during pacing. These limitations of transcutaneous pacing are still valid for the current generation of transcutaneous pacers.

If transcutaneous pacing is needed, the chest and back electrodes should be placed over areas of lower skeletal muscle mass, and low-density constant-current impulses should be delivered. This improves the likelihood of effective cardiac stimulation and minimizes painful skeletal muscle or cutaneous stimulation. Despite its drawbacks, transcutaneous pacing is an effective temporizing measure to treat bradydysrhythmias until a transvenous pacemaker can be placed or a more permanent mode of cardiac pacing can be implemented.

Electrical Cardioversion

Electrical *cardioversion* is the delivery of an electrical discharge synchronized to the R wave of the ECG. The purpose of cardioversion is to recoordinate the electrical pathways of the heart by delivering a single dominant burst of electricity on the R wave of the ECG. The electrical discharge or "shock" is transmitted through two chest electrodes configured as hand-held paddles or adhesive pads on the chest in the anterior and apical positions or in the anterior and posterior positions. The shock is coordinated with the R wave on the ECG so that the stimulus is not delivered during the relative refractory period of the ventricle—that is, during the T wave—to prevent the R-on-T phenomenon and its associated ventricular tachycardia or ventricular fibrillation.

Synchronized cardioversion is used to treat acute unstable supraventricular tachycardias (such as SVT, atrial flutter, and atrial fibrillation) and to convert chronic stable rate-controlled atrial flutter or atrial fibrillation to sinus rhythm. Cardioversion can also be used to treat monomorphic ventricular tachycardia with a pulse present. Of note, digitalis-induced dysrhythmias are refractory to cardioversion, and attempts at cardioversion in this situation could trigger more serious ventricular dysrhythmias. Digitalis-induced dysrhythmias should be treated by correction of acid-base status and electrolyte abnormalities, and administration of digitalis-binding antibody if needed.

In patients with atrial fibrillation, cardioversion carries the risk of systemic embolization. Therefore, it is recommended that elective cardioversion be preceded by anticoagulation if the dysrhythmia has been present for longer than 48 hours. Before elective cardioversion, patients fast for at least 6 hours and electrolyte imbalances are corrected. Normally, elective cardioversion is performed under intravenous sedation-amnesia or very brief general anesthesia with standard monitoring. Propofol and short-acting benzodiazepines are commonly used for this procedure. Antidysrhythmic drugs, advanced airway equipment, and emergency cardiac pacing–defibrillation devices should be immediately available, because ventricular ectopy or bradycardia can occur after cardioversion.

Defibrillation

In contrast to cardioversion, electrical *defibrillation* is used to correct dysrhythmias when it is not possible or reasonable to synchronize the electrical current to the ECG because there is no R wave (no defined QRS complexes) or the patient is pulseless. The position of the paddles or pads is the same as for cardioversion. Defibrillation-cardioversion electrodes should not be placed directly over pacemakers or ICD pulse generators. Delivery of a high current near a pacemaker or ICD can cause the device to malfunction and can block and/or divert the current path and result in suboptimal current delivery to the myocardium. In addition, all permanently implanted cardiac devices should be evaluated after defibrillation or cardioversion to ensure proper function.

Maximizing the success of defibrillation involves decreasing thoracic impedance, positioning the electrodes properly, and selecting proper electrode size. When transthoracic impedance is too high, an energy shock will not achieve defibrillation. Defibrillation electrodes come in several sizes, and as a rule of thumb, it is best to use the largest pads available that can fit on the chest and not overlap. To reduce impedance, conductive gels should always be used with defibrillation paddles. Self-adhesive defibrillation pads have an integrated conductive surface that reduces impedance. In some patients, electrode contact with the skin can be suboptimal and leave gaps or air pockets between the defibrillator paddles and the skin. The air interface increases impedance and can be very dangerous, because the electrical charge can ignite in an oxygen-rich environment. Routine use of self-adhesive defibrillation pads or gel pads with paddles and attention to elimination of air pockets at the interface can minimize the risk of current arcing and fire. At times, particularly in an excessively hairy patient, the pad area may need to be shaved to achieve good electrode contact. In addition to the impedance caused by the chest wall (the skin and fat overlying the bone), the electrical current encounters some increase in impedance from air spaces within the lung tissue in the current path. The defibrillator current is therefore ideally delivered when the lungs are deflated, that is, during exhalation.

Modern defibrillators are classified according to the type of waveform delivered and may be monophasic or biphasic. The first-generation defibrillators were monophasic. Most modern defibrillators are biphasic devices. Neither type of defibrillator has been shown to be more successful in terminating pulseless rhythms or improving survival. A current dose of 360 J is indicated for transthoracic defibrillation using a monophasic defibrillator. Biphasic defibrillators deliver lower currents (120 to 200 J) than monophasic devices. The optimal energy dose delivered by a biphasic defibrillator is not standardized; the manufacturer of each device has dose suggestions specific to its equipment. In the absence of a recommended dose, 200 J should be used. The single most important factor determining survival after cardiac arrest due to ventricular fibrillation is the time between arrest and the first defibrillation attempt. In witnessed cardiac arrest due to ventricular fibrillation, patients who undergo defibrillation within the first 3 minutes have a survival rate of 74%.

Radiofrequency Catheter Ablation

In radiofrequency catheter ablation, an intracardiac electrode catheter inserted percutaneously under local anesthesia through a large vein (femoral, subclavian, internal jugular, or cephalic) is used to produce small, well-demarcated areas of thermal injury that destroy the myocardial tissue responsible for initiation or maintenance of dysrhythmias. Cardiac dysrhythmias amenable to radiofrequency catheter ablation include reentrant supraventricular dysrhythmias and some ventricular dysrhythmias. Radiofrequency catheter ablation is usually considered after pharmacologic therapy has failed or has not been tolerated by the patient. The procedure is usually performed under conscious sedation with routine monitoring.

Permanently Implanted Cardiac Pacemakers

The first successful human cardiac pacemaker implantation in the United States was performed in Buffalo, New York, by Dr. William Chardack in 1960. Permanent cardiac pacing was originally designed for the management of Stokes-Adams (syncopal) attacks in patients with complete heart block. Currently, the most common indication for permanent pacemaker insertion is sinus node dysfunction (sick sinus syndrome). Cardiac pacing is the only long-term treatment for symptomatic bradycardia regardless of cause.

In the past decade, there have been great advances in the durability, reliability, and complexity of cardiac implanted electronic devices (CIEDs). However, the basic components of an artificial cardiac pacemaker have not changed in over 50 years. These devices are made up of a pulse generator capable of producing electrical impulses, one or more sensing and pacing electrodes located in the right atrium and right ventricle, and a battery power source. Electrical impulses originating in the pulse generator are transmitted through specialized leads to excite endocardial cells and produce a propagating wave of depolarization in the myocardium. The pulse generator is powered by a small lithium-iodide battery. The lithium-iodide batteries used in pulse generators can last up to 10 years, but battery depletion requires surgical replacement of the entire pulse generator. The pulse generator for endocardial leads is usually implanted in a subcutaneous pocket below the clavicle. The generator for epicardial leads is often implanted in the abdominal wall.

All implanted cardiac devices are designed to detect and respond to low-amplitude electrical signals. Extraneous signals produced by external electrical or magnetic fields can influence the function of CIEDs and are known as *electromagnetic interference* (EMI). Even with vast improvements in EMI shielding of CIEDs, the potential for microwaves, electrocautery, or magnetic resonance imaging to produce inhibition of ventricular pacing is still clinically relevant. There are no known CIED concerns involving exposure to plain radiography, ultrasonography, fluoroscopy, or mammography. Many artificial cardiac pacemakers are designed to convert to an asynchronous mode rather than be completely inhibited when an external electrical field is encountered.

The endocardial leads can be unipolar or bipolar. In a unipolar pacing system there is one electrode that is an active lead. Current flows from the negative pole (active lead) to stimulate the heart, then returns to the positive pole (the casing of the pulse generator). The current returns to the positive pole by traveling through myocardium to complete the circuit. This separation between the positive and negative poles leads to the unipolar system's susceptibility to EMI (Figure 4-9). In a bipolar lead system, there are two separate electrodes (positive and negative) in the same chamber in very close proximity to each other, so the distance the current travels to complete the circuit is very small, and hence there is very little chance that extraneous signals will intrude into or affect the lead circuit.

EMI can be any strong external electrical or magnetic force in close proximity to a CIED. EMI signals enter device circuits primarily through the leads. Unipolar systems are more prone to EMI because there is a larger separation between the positive and negative poles. Other factors influencing the susceptibility of a device to EMI include field strength, patient body mass, and the proximity and orientation of the device to the EMI field. Potential effects of EMI depend on the pacing mode and the lead involved, but range from cessation of pacing to inappropriate triggering of pacemaker activity. Improved shielding of pacemakers and use of mostly bipolar lead systems has eliminated many problems related to EMI.

PACING MODES

A five-letter generic code is used to describe the various characteristics of cardiac pacemakers. The first letter denotes the cardiac chamber(s) being paced (*A*, atrium; *V*, ventricle; *D*, dual chamber). The second letter denotes the cardiac chamber(s) in which electrical activity is being sensed or detected (*O*, none; *A*, atrium; *V*, ventricle; *D*, dual). The third letter indicates the

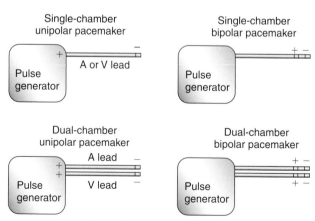

FIGURE 4-9 Unipolar and bipolar lead systems. *A,* Atrial; *V,* ventricular. (*From Stone ME, Apinis A. Current perioperative management of the patient with a cardiac rhythm management device. Semin Cardiothorac Vasc Anesth. 2009;13:32.*)

response to sensed signals (*O,* none; *I,* inhibition; *T,* triggering; *D,* dual—inhibition and triggering). The fourth letter, *R,* denotes activation of rate response features, and the fifth position denotes the chamber(s) in which multisite pacing is delivered. The most common pacing modes are AAI, VVI, and DDD.

Asynchronous Pacing

Asynchronous pacing is the simplest form of pacing. It can be AOO, VOO, or DOO. In this mode, the lead(s) fire at a fixed rate regardless of the patient's underlying rhythm. This pacing mode can be used safely in patients with no intrinsic ventricular activity because there is no risk of the R-on-T phenomenon. Asynchronous pacing may compete with a patient's intrinsic rhythm, and the continuous pacing activity decreases battery life and necessitates more frequent battery and pulse generator replacement.

Single-Chamber Pacing

The choice of pacing mode depends on the primary indication for the artificial pacemaker. Single-chamber pacemakers can be atrial or ventricular. If the patient has SA node disease and no evidence of disease in the AV node or bundle of His, an atrial pacemaker (AAI) can be placed. Use of atrial pacing modes requires a functioning AV node, and then AAI pacing can maintain AV synchrony. However, it has been estimated that approximately 8% of patient with SA node dysfunction will progress to AV node dysfunction within 3 years.

Individuals experiencing episodes of symptomatic bradycardia caused by SA node or AV node disease may benefit from placement of a single-chamber ventricular (VVI) pacemaker. This mode of pacing senses the native R wave, and if it is present, pacemaker discharge is inhibited (Figure 4-10). It is often used in patients with complete heart block with chronic atrial flutter or fibrillation, and in patients with long ventricular pauses. A factor to consider in the patient with a single-chamber ventricular pacemaker is the potential for pacemaker syndrome.

Pacemaker syndrome is a constellation of symptoms caused by the loss of AV synchrony. Symptoms include syncope, weakness, lethargy, cough, orthopnea, paroxysmal nocturnal dyspnea, hypotension, and pulmonary edema. DDD pacing minimizes the incidence of pacemaker syndrome and can be used to alleviate symptoms of pacemaker syndrome by restoring AV synchrony.

Dual-Chamber Pacing

Technical advances in cardiac pacing have included the creation of dual-chamber devices, rate-response algorithms, and implantable cardioverter-defibrillators with pacing capability. These advances have expanded the indications for cardiac pacing beyond symptomatic bradycardia to include neurogenic syncope, hypertrophic obstructive cardiomyopathy, and cardiac resynchronization therapy for congestive heart failure.

Disease of the AV node or His bundle, or ongoing drug treatment to slow AV nodal conduction, requires a dual-chamber (DDD or DDI) system. Disorders such as neurocardiogenic syncope (resulting from carotid sinus hypersensitivity), vasovagal syncope, and hypertrophic cardiomyopathy can also be successfully treated with dual-chamber pacemakers.

Dual-chamber pacing is also known as *physiologic pacing* because it maintains AV synchrony. This improves cardiac output by maintaining the contribution of atrial systole to ventricular filling. AV synchrony also maintains appropriate valve closure timing, which reduces the risk of significant mitral and/or tricuspid insufficiency. Several studies suggest that patients receiving dual-chamber pacing have a decreased risk of atrial fibrillation and heart failure.

Cardiac resynchronization therapy using biatrial or biventricular pacing is being employed in patients with electromechanical asynchrony and intraventricular conduction block. The criteria for cardiac resynchronization therapy include the presence of drug-refractory heart failure (symptoms at rest or with minimal exertion), left ventricular ejection fraction of less than 35%, left ventricular dilation, and prolongation of the QRS complex to more than 130 milliseconds.

DDD Pacing. Dual-chamber pacemakers have two leads, one placed in the right atrium and one located in the right ventricle. DDD pacing is based on electrical feedback from the leads in the atrium and ventricle. If a native atrial signal is sensed, the atrial pacemaker output is inhibited, and if no intrinsic atrial signal is sensed, the pacemaker output is triggered. Likewise, if intrinsic ventricular activity is sensed at the end of a programmable AV interval, the intrinsic ventricular activity inhibits pacemaker output. If intrinsic ventricular activity is not sensed, the pacemaker triggers a spike (Figure 4-11). The DDD pacing mode permits the pacemaker to respond to increases in sinus node discharge rate, such as during exercise.

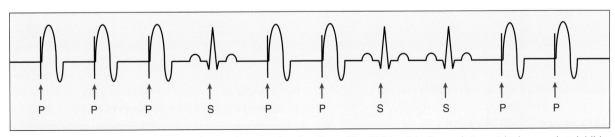

FIGURE 4-10 Electrocardiographic evidence of pacemaker function with a VVI (ventricular pacing, ventricular sensing, inhibition) pacemaker. *P,* Paced beat; *S,* sensed beat. *(From Allen M. Pacemakers and implantable cardioverter defibrillators. Anaesthesia. 2006;61:885.)*

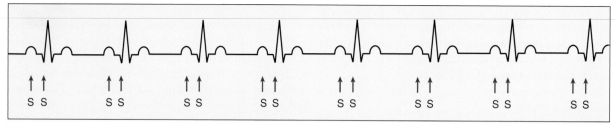

A

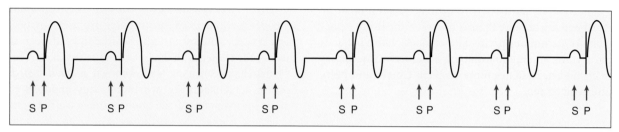

B

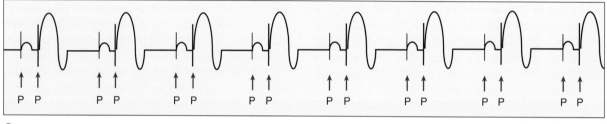

C

FIGURE 4-11 Electrocardiographic evidence of pacemaker function with a DDD (dual pacing, dual sensing, inhibition and triggering) pacemaker. **A,** Patient has intrinsic atrial and ventricular activity that is sensed by the pacemaker. **B,** Patient has intrinsic activity that is not conducted to the ventricle, so the pacemaker senses the atrial activity and paces the ventricle. **C,** Patient has no atrial or ventricular activity sensed by the pacemaker, so the pacemaker paces both the atrium and the ventricle. *P,* Paced beat; *S,* sensed beat. *(Allen M. Pacemakers and implantable cardioverter defibrillators. Anaesthesia. 2006;61:886.)*

Programming the dual-chamber leads to have an adjustable AV interval provides an important benefit in maintaining AV synchrony over a wide range of heart rates. Loss of AV synchrony has many deleterious effects, including reducing cardiac output by 20% to 30% or more, increasing atrial pressure resulting from contraction of the atria against closed mitral and tricuspid valves, and activation of baroreceptors that may induce reflex peripheral vasodilation.

DDI Pacing. In the DDI pacing mode, there is sensing in both the atrium and ventricle, but the only response to a sensed event is inhibition (inhibited pacing of the atrium and ventricle). DDI pacing is useful when there are frequent atrial tachydysrhythmias that might be inappropriately tracked by a DDD pacemaker and result in rapid ventricular rates.

RATE-ADAPTIVE PACEMAKERS

Patients with sinus node disease, AV node disease, or lower conduction system disease whose heart rates do not respond to increases in metabolic demands should be considered candidates

for rate-adaptive pacing systems. In the late 1990s pacemaker technology expanded to include the capability of matching the pacing rate to activity levels. This is called *rate-adaptive pacing* and is considered for patients who do not have an appropriate heart rate response to exercise *(chronotropic incompetence)*. This syndrome can be caused by drug treatment with negative chronotropic drugs such as β-blockers or calcium channel blockers or by pathologic processes such as sick sinus syndrome.

Normally, AV synchrony contributes more to cardiac output at rest and at low levels of exercise, whereas rate adaptation (i.e., a higher heart rate) is more important at higher levels of exercise. Sensors within rate-adaptive pacemakers detect changes in movement (using a piezoelectric crystal) or minute ventilation (by transthoracic impedance) as physical or physiologic signs of exercise. In response, the device makes rate adjustments to mimic the response of a normal sinus node.

ANESTHESIA FOR CARDIAC PACEMAKER INSERTION

Most pacemakers are inserted under conscious sedation in the cardiac catheterization laboratory or under monitored anesthesia care in the operating room. Routine anesthetic monitoring is employed. A functioning cardiac pacemaker should be in place or transcutaneous cardiac pacing available before administration of anesthetic drugs. Drugs such as atropine and isoproterenol should be available should a decrease in heart rate compromise hemodynamics before the new pacemaker is functional.

The incidence of complications related to pacemaker insertion is approximately 5%. An artificial cardiac pacemaker can be inserted intravenously using endocardial leads or via a subcostal incision or median sternotomy (after cardiac surgery) using epicardial or myocardial leads. Early complications are often associated with the venous access and/or surgical access necessary to place the leads. Perioperative complications include pneumothorax, hemothorax, and air embolism. Pneumothoraces are often small and asymptomatic. However, tension pneumothorax should always be considered if hypotension or pulseless electrical activity develops during or immediately after pacemaker placement. Hemothorax can result from trauma to the great vessels or other vascular structures. Arterial cannulation must be immediately recognized and treated with manual compression or arterial repair. Arterial damage can be minimized by placing a small guidewire under fluoroscopic guidance before placing the much larger introducer sheath. Variable amounts of air can be introduced into the low-pressure venous system during the procedure. Small amounts are generally well tolerated, but larger air embolism can result in respiratory distress, oxygen desaturation, hypotension, and cardiac arrest.

Permanently Implanted Cardioverter-Defibrillators

IMPLANTED CARDIOVERTER-DEFIBRILLATORS AND CARDIAC RESYNCHRONIZATION THERAPY

The ICD system consists of a pulse generator and leads for dysrhythmia detection and current delivery. In addition to internal defibrillation, an ICD can deliver antitachycardia or antibradycardia pacing and synchronized cardioversion. Detailed diagnostic data concerning intracardiac electrograms and event markers are stored in the memory of the device and can be retrieved for analysis. The pulse generator is a small computer powered by a lithium battery that is sealed within a titanium case. The transvenous leads consist of pacing and sensing electrodes and one or two defibrillation coils. The defibrillation circuit is completed by the titanium case of the pulse generator, which acts as a defibrillation electrode. The pulse generator is usually implanted into a subcutaneous pocket. The position of the pulse generator is important because the position affects the defibrillation wave front. The left pectoral region is the ideal location for the pulse generator. Right-sided implantation can result in a significantly higher defibrillation threshold. ICDs employ electrical defibrillation as the sole method for treatment of ventricular fibrillation.

The ICD uses a specialized lead in the right ventricle that senses ventricular depolarization. It amplifies, filters, and rectifies the signal and then compares it with the programmed sensing thresholds and the R-R interval algorithms. If the device detects ventricular fibrillation, the capacitor charges, a secondary algorithm is fulfilled by signal analysis to confirm the rhythm, and then the shock is delivered. This secondary confirmatory process prevents inappropriate shocks in response to self-terminating events or spurious signals. The process takes approximately 10 to 15 seconds from dysrhythmia detection to shock delivery. During this time, the patient may experience presyncope or syncope.

A defibrillator coding system exists similar to the one used for pacemakers. The first letter is the chamber shocked (*O*, none; *A*, atrium; *V*, ventricle; *D*, dual). The second letter indicates the *antitachycardia* pacing chamber (*O*, none; *A*, atrium; *V*, ventricle; *D*, dual). The third position indicates the tachycardia detection mechanism (*E*, electrogram; *H*, hemodynamic). The fourth position denotes the *antibradycardia* pacing chamber (*O*, none; *A*, atrium; *V*, ventricle; *D*, dual).

Implantable ICDs were approved by the FDA in 1985. Currently there are over 1.5 million Americans living with a pacemaker and over 500,000 living with an ICD. The indications for the implantation of an ICD have changed dramatically over the past few years. An increase in ICD implantation occurred after clinical trials showed a survival benefit for ICDs placement compared with antidysrhythmic drug therapy in survivors of cardiac arrest not caused by transient or reversible factors such as acute myocardial infarction, use of prodysrhythmic drugs, or electrolyte disturbances.

Another turning point in the use of ICDs came when multiple clinical trials showed that using cardiac resynchronization therapy decreased heart failure events and mortality in appropriately selected patients. The goal of cardiac resynchronization therapy, also called *biventricular pacing,* is to use multisite pacing to improve electromechanical synchrony. In the pathophysiology of congestive heart failure, ventricular electrical dyssynchrony progresses to mechanical dyssynchrony as the left ventricular contraction becomes increasingly inefficient. This can be further worsened by a prolongation of AV conduction, which leads to AV dyssynchrony and a decrease in the atrial contribution to left ventricular filling.

Cardiac resynchronization therapy uses three pacing leads: right atrial, right ventricular, and a coronary sinus lead (or an additional atrial or ventricular lead depending on the sites of dysfunction). By adjusting the timing of each lead, AV synchrony is optimized. Cardiac resynchronization therapy is now a mainstay of treatment in patients who have left ventricular dysfunction (ejection fraction of ≤35%), QRS prolongation (≥120 milliseconds), and moderate to severe heart failure symptoms (New York Heart Association functional class III or IV) while receiving optimal medical therapy. Cardiac resynchronization therapy with or without a defibrillator component has been shown to reduce hospitalizations and all-cause mortality in these patients.

Approximately half of patients receiving an ICD will have an adverse event related to the device within the first year after implantation. Lead-related problems such as failure to sense or pace, inappropriate therapy, and dislodgment remain the most common problems. One of the most devastating complications is infection associated with the ICD components. The estimated infection rate is approximately 0.6%, which is similar to the infection rate associated with pacemaker implantation. Device-related infection requires explantation of the entire ICD system.

ANESTHESIA FOR INSERTION OF IMPLANTABLE CARDIOVERTER-DEFIBRILLATORS

Preparation for the care of a patient for ICD placement is the same as that for pacemaker insertion. Some of these procedures are done under general anesthesia because of the increased risks associated with repeated defibrillation during threshold testing. The nature and severity of the patient's co-existing medical conditions dictate the extent of monitoring and the necessary clinical preparations.

SURGERY IN PATIENTS WITH CARDIAC IMPLANTABLE ELECTRONIC DEVICES

The presence of any type of CIED—whether an artificial cardiac pacemaker or ICD—for any indication—whether pacing, cardioversion, defibrillation, or resynchronization—in a patient scheduled for surgery unrelated to the device introduces special considerations for preoperative evaluation and subsequent management of anesthesia to ensure patient safety and preservation of proper device placement and function. These CIED recommendations apply to all forms of anesthetic care, from conscious sedation and monitored anesthesia care to regional and general anesthesia.

Potential adverse outcomes associated with perioperative CIED-related issues include hypotension, tachydysrhythmias or bradydysrythmias, myocardial damage, myocardial ischemia or infarction, device malfunction, delay or cancellation of surgery, readmission to a health care facility for management of device malfunction, extended hospital stay, increased patient and hospital costs, and avoidable increased consumption of hospital resources.

Preoperative Evaluation

A patient with a preexisting CIED coming for surgery has at least one of three underlying cardiac problems: sustained or intermittent bradydysrhythmia, tachydysrhythmia, or heart failure. Regardless of the indication for the device, any patient with a CIED requiring anesthetic care must undergo a detailed systematic preoperative evaluation. Although treatment decisions are made based on the clinical scenario, the preoperative evaluation of a patient with a CIED should include determination of the type of device present, identification of the clinical indication for the device, appraisal of the patient's degree of dependence on the device (for patients requiring pacing for bradycardia), and assessment of device function.

In determining whether the patient has a CIED, patient history and physical examination, medical records, chest radiographs, and ECGs or a rhythm strip can often aid in confirming the presence of a device and establishing the type of device, clinical indication, and in some instances the patient's

level of dependence. Strong evidence indicating that a patient is CIED dependent includes a history of bradycardia symptoms, a history of AV node ablation, and little or no spontaneous ventricular activity on ECG, that is, the majority of beats are paced on ECG. A preoperative history of presyncope, or syncope in a patient with a pacemaker could reflect pacemaker dysfunction. The rate of discharge of an atrial or ventricular *asynchronous* (fixed-rate) cardiac pacemaker (usually 70 to 72 beats per minute) is a useful indicator of pulse generator function. A 10% decrease in heart rate from the initial heart rate setting may reflect battery depletion. An irregular heart rate could indicate competition of the pulse generator with the patient's intrinsic heart rate or failure of the pulse generator to sense R waves.

The best way to determine CIED function preoperatively is CIED interrogation by a qualified consultant. However, in the event that this is not possible, clinical evidence such as pacing spikes present on the ECG that successfully create paced beats may suffice. The ECG is not a diagnostic aid if the intrinsic heart rate is greater than the preset pacemaker rate. In such cases, proper function of a ventricular synchronous or sequential artificial cardiac pacemaker is best confirmed by electronic evaluation. Beyond the routine indications for antibradycardia pacing or antitachycardia defibrillation, many pacemaker-defibrillators are implanted for resynchronization therapy to treat heart failure. This has made management decisions increasingly complex, so early involvement of a qualified consultant is desirable. Ideally, perioperative assessment and planning for the patient with a CIED should be coordinated with a cardiologist and the pacemaker representative for that specific device.

Management of Anesthesia

It is estimated that in the population of patients with CIEDs 50% have coronary artery disease, 20% have hypertension, and 10% have diabetes. Achieving good clinical outcomes in CIED patients requires evaluation and optimal treatment of co-existing diseases in addition to management of the issues directly involving the CIED. There are several major areas of concern that must be addressed regarding the CIED to ensure safety during the administration of anesthesia. Is EMI likely to occur during the surgery? Does the CIED need to be reprogrammed? Are temporary pacing equipment and a defibrillator immediately available?

In addition to patient-specific issues concerning CIEDs, adverse outcomes related to the functionality of the device are also important to consider. These include the potential for damage to the pulse generator or leads (circuitry), damage to the tissue around the device (burns, thermal changes effecting impedance), failure of the device to pace or defibrillate, inappropriate pacing or defibrillation, and inadvertent electrical reset to backup pacing modes.

The most common CIED-related problem encountered in the perioperative period is interference with device function resulting from EMI. The most common effects of EMI are inhibition of pacing and resetting of the device to asynchronous pacing. EMI can cause more serious problems, however, such as inappropriate defibrillation or complete device failure.

Three procedures that have been reported to have some association with EMI-induced dysfunction in CIEDs are electrocautery, radiofrequency ablation, and MRI. Choice of anesthetic technique is not thought to influence CIED function directly, but physiologic changes (acid-base, electrolytes) and hemodynamic shifts (heart rate, heart rhythm, hypertension, coronary ischemia) can induce changes in CIED function and adversely affect patient outcomes.

Most literature suggests reprogramming the CIED to an asynchronous mode before surgery if the patient is *pacemaker dependent*. However, there are no controlled studies examining the clinical effect of reprogramming a pacemaker to asynchronous mode under these circumstances. Any inadvertent exposure to a source of electric current or magnetic field can cause damage to the pulse generator, the leads, or the tissue surrounding any part of the device. Improved shielding of cardiac pacemakers has reduced the problems associated with EMI from electrocautery, but the use of monopolar electrocautery remains the principal concern intraoperatively in patients with CIEDs. There are reports suggesting that CIED reprogramming may be beneficial if electrocautery will be used, but this point is controversial.

Use of "coagulation" settings in monopolar electrocautery causes more EMI problems than use of "cutting" settings. It is beneficial to keep the electrocautery current as low as possible and to apply electrocautery in short bursts, especially if current is being applied in close proximity to the pulse generator. The recommendation is to avoid using cautery in the area of the pulse generator and leads if that is possible. The cautery device generating the EMI field need not actually *touch* the patient to adversely effect the CIED. Use of bipolar electrocautery or the ultrasonic Harmonic scalpel is associated with lower rates of EMI effects on the pulse generator and leads. The current return pad (grounding pad) should be placed so that the current path does not cross the chest or CIED system. The grounding electrode for electrocautery should be as far as possible from the pulse generator to minimize detection of the cautery current by the pulse generator.

Application of a magnet to a pacemaker often results in asynchronous pacemaker function at a fixed rate. Although asynchronous pacing can maintain a reliable heart rate in pacemaker-dependent patients, for some patients the asynchronous rate may be excessive and contribute to hypertension, coronary ischemia, or congestive heart failure. Asynchronous pacing carries the risk of producing the R-on-T phenomenon. If a magnet is used, it must remain in place to maintain the asynchronous mode of pacing. Removal of the magnet results in reversion to the baseline device program. The magnet-induced rate varies by manufacturer and can be altered by programming.

Application of a magnet to a cardioverter-defibrillator rarely alters the antibradycardia pacing capabilities, but most often

TABLE 4-4	Factors that can alter the depolarization threshold of cardiac pacemakers
Factors increasing the threshold	**Factors decreasing the threshold**
Hyperkalemia	Hypokalemia
Acidosis or alkalosis	Increased catecholamine levels
Antidysrhythmic medication (e.g., quinidine, procainamide, lidocaine, propafenone)	Sympathomimetic drugs
Hypoxia	Anticholinergics
Hypoglycemia	Glucocorticoids
Local anesthetics (lidocaine)	Stress or anxiety
Myocardial ischemia	Hyperthyroidism
Myocardial infarction (scar tissue)	Hypermetabolic states
Acute inflammation around lead tip during first month after implantation	
Hypothermia	

suspends antitachycardia therapy (defibrillation). It is difficult to accurately assess the effect of a magnet on a cardioverter-defibrillator CIED without electronic interrogation. Some ICDs have no magnet response; others can be permanently disabled by magnet exposure. Recommendations for patients with ICDs who undergo a procedure with a high risk of EMI include suspending the antitachycardia functions—that is, turning off the defibrillator—and electronically adjusting the pacing modes as appropriate in pacemaker-dependent individuals.

The choice of drugs for anesthesia is not altered by the presence of a properly functioning CIED, nor is there any evidence that anesthetic drugs alter the stimulation threshold of CIEDs. Nevertheless, it is prudent to avoid events such as hyperventilation that can acutely change the serum potassium concentration (Table 4-4). Conceivably, succinylcholine could increase the stimulation threshold because of the associated acute increase in serum potassium concentration. Succinylcholine could also inhibit a normally functioning cardiac pacemaker by causing contraction of skeletal muscle groups (myopotentials) that the pulse generator could interpret as intrinsic R waves. Clinical experience suggests that succinylcholine is usually a safe drug to use in patients with artificial cardiac pacemakers and that, if myopotential inhibition does occur, it is generally transient.

Monitoring of the patient with a CIED should always follow the ASA standards and should include continuous ECG monitoring and continuous monitoring of a peripheral pulse. This can be done with a pulse oximeter, manual palpation of a pulse, auscultation of heart sounds, or intraarterial catheterization. Verification of the presence of a pulse is necessary to confirm continued cardiac activity in the event of disruption of the ECG signal by EMI.

No special laboratory testing or radiographs are needed for CIED patients unless otherwise clinically indicated. At times a chest radiograph can be useful to evaluate the location and external condition of pacemaker electrodes. If the patient is known to have a biventricular pacemaker, a chest radiograph to confirm the position of the coronary sinus lead is helpful when insertion of a central line or pulmonary artery catheter is planned. There have been reports of coronary sinus and endocardial lead dislodgement in association with these procedures. The danger of lead dislodgment is minimal a month or longer after lead implantation. Epicardial leads are not at risk in this situation. The presence of a *temporary* transvenous cardiac pacemaker creates a situation in which there is a direct connection between an external electrical source and the endocardium. This could introduce the risk of ventricular fibrillation resulting from microshock. There are case reports of inappropriately high pacing rates in CIEDs containing active minute ventilation sensors for rate-adaptive pacing caused by EMI from a cardiac monitor. The consensus is that all rate-adaptive modes should be turned off preoperatively.

MRI scanning of patients with CIEDs is controversial and is generally regarded as contraindicated. However, 50% to 75% of patients with cardiac devices will likely need to undergo MRI at some point in their lifetimes, so this is becoming an important concern. There is insufficient evidence at present to standardize management of the patient with a CIED needing MRI scanning. If MRI must be performed, care should be coordinated among the ordering physician, radiologist, and pacemaker specialist or cardiologist.

Management of EMI associated with radiofrequency ablation includes keeping the radiofrequency current path, which runs from the electrode tip to the current return pad, as far away from the pulse generator as possible. Some suggest keeping the ablation electrode at least 5 cm away from the pacer leads.

Recommendations for patients undergoing lithotripsy include keeping the focus of the lithotripsy beam away from the pulse generator. It has been suggested that there may be some benefit to disabling atrial pacing if the lithotripsy system triggers on the R wave, but there is no clinical evidence to support this practice at this time.

There is insufficient evidence to standardize care for CIED patients needing radiation therapy. The recommendation currently is to keep the device out of the radiation field. In some patients this will require pulse generator relocation. Most manufacturers recommend verification of appropriate pulse generator function at the completion of radiation therapy. Potential CIED problems from radiation therapy include pacemaker failure and "runaway" pacemaker. Runaway pacemaker is the sudden rapid and erratic pacing that can occur in the event of multiple internal component malfunctions. Most modern pacemakers limit the upper rate of pacing to 210 beats per minute.

No clinical studies have reported EMI or permanent CIED malfunction in association with electroconvulsive therapy, but care should be coordinated with a cardiologist. The device should be interrogated and the antitachycardia functions suspended. Because electroconvulsive therapy can be associated with considerable swings in blood pressure and heart rate, a backup external defibrillator and temporary pacing capability should be immediately available. The myopotentials produced during seizures may inhibit pacemaker activity. In pacemaker-dependent patients, programming to asynchronous mode is recommended.

Other potential sources of EMI during anesthetic care include current from peripheral nerve stimulators or evoked potential monitors, large tidal volumes, shivering, and medication-induced muscle fasciculations.

If emergency defibrillation is necessary in a patient with a CIED (permanent cardiac pacemaker or ICD that is turned off), an effort should be made to keep the defibrillation current away from the pulse generator and lead system. This can be facilitated by placing the electrode pads in an anterior–posterior position. It is suggested that, if the situation allows, before performing defibrillation or cardioversion in a patient with an ICD in a magnet-disabled treatment mode, all sources of EMI be eliminated and the magnet be removed to reactivate the antitachycardia capabilities of the device. The patient can then be observed for appropriate CIED function. The primary goal is care of the patient, of course, with care of the CIED being secondary, but in most circumstances the two are not mutually exclusive. An acute increase in pacing threshold and loss of capture may follow external defibrillation. If this occurs, transcutaneous cardiac pacing or temporary transvenous pacing may be required.

Postoperative management of the patient with a CIED consists of interrogating the device and restoring appropriate baseline settings, including antitachycardia therapy in patients with ICDs. This should be done as soon as possible after the procedure, either in the postanesthesia care unit or the intensive care unit. There have been no reports of permanently reprogrammed CIEDs attributed to EMI. Nevertheless, cardiac rate and rhythm should be monitored throughout the immediately postoperative period, including during transport from the anesthetizing location to the recovery area. Backup cardioversion–defibrillation and pacing equipment should be immediately available. Postoperative CIED checks may not be needed if surgery did not include use of EMI-generating devices, no electronic preoperative device reprogramming was done, no blood transfusions were administered, and no intraoperative problems were identified that related to CIED function.

KEY POINTS

- Cardiac dysrhythmias are classified according to heart rate and the site of origin of the abnormality. Conduction disturbances are classified by site and degree of blockade. The clinical significance of these abnormalities depends on their effect on vital signs (hemodynamic instability, cardiac and end-organ ischemia, congestive heart failure) and/or their potential for deterioration into life-threatening rhythms.

■ Tachydysrhythmias can result from three mechanisms: (1) increased automaticity in normal conduction tissue or in an ectopic focus, (2) reentry of electrical potentials through abnormal pathways, and (3) triggering of abnormal cardiac potentials due to afterdepolarizations.

■ Atrial fibrillation is the most common sustained cardiac dysrhythmia in the general population (0.4% to 1% incidence), affecting 2.2 million people in the United States. Rapid, disordered atrial activation and irregular electrical input to the AV node results in sporadic AV nodal conduction and irregular ventricular contraction. Ventricular response rates as high as 180 beats per minute can occur in patients with normal AV node function.

■ Bradycardia during neuraxial blockade can occur in patients of any age, any ASA physical status class, and any degree of sedation. The incidence of profound bradycardia and cardiac arrest during neuraxial anesthesia is approximately 1.5 per 10,000 cases. By contrast, cardiac arrest during general anesthesia occurs at a rate of 5.5 per 10,000 cases.

■ Ventricular fibrillation is a rapid, grossly irregular ventricular rhythm with marked variability in QRS cycle length, morphology, and amplitude. This rhythm is incompatible with life because there is no associated stroke volume or cardiac output. A pulse or blood pressure *never* accompanies ventricular fibrillation. Electrical defibrillation is the only effective method to convert ventricular fibrillation to a rhythm capable of generating a cardiac output.

■ Antidysrhythmic drugs work by one of three mechanisms: (1) suppressing automaticity in cardiac pacemaker cells by decreasing the slope of phase 4 depolarization, (2) prolonging the effective refractory period to eliminate reentry circuits, and (3) facilitating impulse conduction along the normal conduction pathway to prevent conduction over a reentrant pathway. ECG changes, such as a prolonged PR interval or a prolonged QRS duration, are relatively common side effects of antidysrhythmic drug therapy.

■ Mobitz type I (Wenckebach) block is distinguished by progressive prolongation of the PR interval until a beat is dropped. A pause allows the AV node to recover and then the process resumes. In contrast, Mobitz type II block is characterized by sudden and complete interruption of conduction without PR prolongation. Mobitz type II block is usually associated with permanent damage to the conduction system and may progress to third-degree block.

■ Third-degree heart block (complete heart block) is characterized by complete absence of conduction of cardiac impulses from the atria to the ventricles. Continued activity of the ventricles is related to impulse generation from an ectopic focus distal to the site of block. If the conduction block is near the AV node, the heart rate is usually 45 to 55 beats per minute and the QRS complex has a normal width. If the conduction block is below the AV node (infranodal), the heart rate is usually 30 to 40 beats per minute and the QRS complex is wide.

■ The ICD system consists of a pulse generator and leads for dysrhythmia detection and current delivery. In addition to internal defibrillation, an ICD can deliver antitachycardia or antibradycardia pacing and synchronized cardioversion.

■ All CIEDs are designed to detect and respond to low-amplitude electrical signals. Extraneous signals produced by external electrical or magnetic fields can influence the function of CIEDs. Strong electromagnetic fields, such as occur in electrocautery, MRI, and radiofrequency ablation, pose the highest risk of interference with CIED function.

RESOURCES

Allen M. Pacemakers and implantable cardioverter defibrillators. *Anaesthesia.* 2006;61:883-890.

Apfelbaum JL, Belott P, Cajon E, et al. Practice advisory for the perioperative management of patients with cardiac implantable electronic devices: pacemakers and implantable cardioverter-defibrillators. *Anesthesiology.* 2011;114:247-261.

Blomstrom-Lundqvist C, Scheinman MM, Aliot EM, et al. ACC/AHA/ESC guidelines for the management of patients with supraventricular arrhythmias—executive summary. A report of the American College of Cardiology/American Heart Association Task Force on Practice Guidelines and the European Society of Cardiology Committee for Practice Guidelines. Developed in collaboration with NASPE-Heart Rhythm Society. *J Am Coll Cardiol.* 2003;42:1493-1531.

Crossley GH, Poole JE, Rozner MA, et al. The Heart Rhythm Society (HRS)/American Society of Anesthesiologists (ASA) expert consensus statement on the perioperative management of patients with implantable defibrillators, pacemakers and arrhythmia monitors: facilities and patient management. *Heart Rhythm.* 2011;8(7):1114-1154.

Fuster A, Ryden LE, Cannom DS, et al. ACC/AHA/ESC 2006 guidelines for the management of patients with atrial fibrillation: a report of the American College of Cardiology/American Heart Association Task Force on Practice Guidelines and the European Society of Cardiology Committee for Practice Guidelines. Developed in collaboration with the European Heart Rhythm Association and the Heart Rhythm Society. *Circulation.* 2006;114:e257-e354.

Kopp SL, Horlocker TT, Warner ME, et al. Cardiac arrest during neuraxial anesthesia: frequency and predisposing factors associated with survival. *Anesth Analg.* 2005;100:855-865.

Neumar RW, Otto CW, Link MS, et al. Part 8: adult advanced cardiovascular life support: 2010 American Heart Association Guidelines for Cardiopulmonary Resuscitation and Emergency Cardiovascular Care. *Circulation.* 2010;122:S729-S767.

Rosenblatt MA, Abel M, Fischer GW, et al. Successful use of a 20% lipid emulsion to resuscitate a patient after a presumed bupivacaine-related cardiac arrest. *Anesthesiology.* 2006;105:217-218.

Stone ME, Apinis A. Current perioperative management of the patient with a cardiac rhythm management device. *Semin Cardiothorac Vasc Anesth.* 2009;13:31-43.

Wann LS, Curtis AB, Ellenbogen KA, et al. 2011 ACCF/AHA/HRS focused update on the management of patients with atrial fibrillation (update on dabigatran): a report of the American College of Cardiology/American Heart Association Task Force on Practice Guidelines. *Circulation.* 2011;123:144-150.

Zipes DP, Camm AJ, Borggrefe M, et al. ACC/AHA/ESC 2006 guidelines for management of patients with ventricular arrhythmias and the prevention of sudden cardiac death: a report of the American College of Cardiology/American Heart Association Task Force and the European Society of Cardiology Committee for Practice Guidelines. *Circulation.* 2006;114:e385-e484.

Systemic and Pulmonary Arterial Hypertension

VERONICA A. MATEI ■
ALÁ SAMI HADDADIN ■

SYSTEMIC HYPERTENSION

An adult is considered to have hypertension when the systemic blood pressure measures 140/90 mm Hg or higher on at least two occasions a minimum of 1 to 2 weeks apart (Table 5-1). Prehypertension is defined as the presence of a systolic blood pressure of 120 to 139 mm Hg or a diastolic blood pressure of 80 to 89 mm Hg.

These definitions are based on the Seventh Report of the Joint National Committee on Prevention, Detection, Evaluation, and Treatment of High Blood Pressure (JNC 7). An updated report (JNC 8) is under development. Based on the JNC 7 definitions, systemic hypertension is the most common circulatory derangement in the United States, affecting about 30% of adults. The incidence of systemic hypertension increases progressively with age and is higher in the African American population (Figure 5-1). Hypertension is a significant risk factor for the development of ischemic heart disease (Figure 5-2) and a major cause of congestive heart failure (Figure 5-3), cerebrovascular accident (stroke), arterial aneurysm, and end-stage renal disease. It is estimated that fewer than one third of people with hypertension in the United States are aware of their condition and are adequately treated.

Isolated systolic hypertension is increasingly being recognized as a significant independent risk factor for cardiovascular disease in all decades of life. Control of systolic blood pressure is being encouraged, particularly in elderly patient populations in which isolated systolic hypertension is prevalent.

The pulse pressure—that is, the difference between the systolic blood pressure and diastolic blood pressure—is emerging as a new marker of the degree of vascular stiffness. Increased pulse pressure is a cardiovascular risk factor, and some studies have linked an increased pulse pressure with intraoperative hemodynamic instability and adverse postoperative outcomes.

Pathophysiology

Systemic hypertension is characterized as *essential* or *primary hypertension* when a cause for the increased blood pressure cannot be identified. It is termed *secondary hypertension* when an identifiable cause is present.

ESSENTIAL HYPERTENSION

Essential hypertension, which accounts for more than 95% of all cases of hypertension, is characterized by a familial incidence and inherited biochemical abnormalities. Pathophysiologic factors implicated in the genesis of essential hypertension include increased sympathetic nervous system activity in response to stress, overproduction of sodium-retaining hormones and vasoconstrictors, high sodium intake, inadequate dietary intake of potassium and calcium, increased renin secretion, deficiencies of endogenous vasodilators such as prostaglandins and nitric oxide (NO), and the presence of medical diseases such as diabetes mellitus

TABLE 5-1 ■ Classification of systemic blood pressure in adults		
Category	Systolic blood pressure (mm Hg)	Diastolic blood pressure (mm Hg)
Normal	<120	<80
Prehypertension	120-139	80-89
Stage 1 hypertension	140-159	90-99
Stage 2 hypertension	≥160	≥100

Data from Chobanian AV, Bakris GL, Black HR, et al; Joint National Committee on Prevention, Detection, Evaluation, and Treatment of High Blood Pressure; National Heart, Lung, and Blood Institute; National High Blood Pressure Education Program Coordinating Committee. Seventh report of the Joint National Committee on Prevention, Detection, Evaluation and Treatment of High Blood Pressure. *Hypertension*. 2003;42:1206-1252.

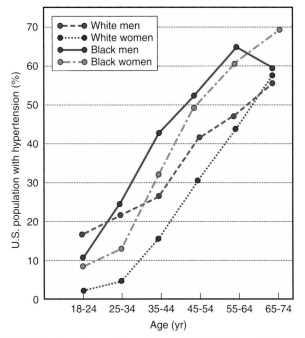

FIGURE 5-1 Prevalence of hypertension (>160/90 mm Hg) in the adult population in the United States. *(Data from Tjoa HI, Kaplan NM. Treatment of hypertension in the elderly. JAMA. 1990;264:1015-1018.)*

and obesity. The final common pathway in the pathophysiology of essential hypertension is salt and water retention. Hypertension, insulin resistance, dyslipidemia, and obesity often occur concomitantly, and an estimated 40% of patients with hypertension also have hypercholesterolemia. Alcohol and tobacco use are associated with an increased incidence of essential hypertension. Obstructive sleep apnea, which is present in a substantial proportion of the adult population, causes temporary increases in blood pressure in association with hypoxemia, arousal, and activation of the sympathetic nervous system. There is evidence that obstructive sleep apnea leads to sustained hypertension independent of known confounding factors such as obesity. Indeed, an

estimated 30% of hypertensive patients manifest obstructive sleep apnea.

A history of ischemic heart disease, angina pectoris, left ventricular hypertrophy, congestive heart failure, cerebrovascular disease, stroke, peripheral vascular disease, or renal insufficiency suggests end-organ disease resulting from chronic, poorly controlled essential hypertension. Laboratory evaluation is intended to document target organ damage and includes blood urea nitrogen and serum creatinine assays to quantify renal function. Hypokalemia in the presence of essential hypertension suggests primary hyperaldosteronism. Fasting blood glucose concentration should be evaluated, because half of hypertensive patients exhibit glucose intolerance. An electrocardiogram is useful for detecting evidence of ischemic heart disease or left ventricular hypertrophy.

SECONDARY HYPERTENSION

Secondary hypertension has a demonstrable cause but accounts for fewer than 5% of all cases of systemic hypertension. Renal artery stenosis leading to renovascular hypertension is the most common cause of secondary hypertension. This and other common causes of secondary hypertension with their notable signs and symptoms are listed in Table 5-2. A more comprehensive list of causes of secondary hypertension is provided in Table 5-3.

Treatment of Essential Hypertension

The standard goal of therapy for essential hypertension is to decrease systemic blood pressure to less than 140/90 mm Hg. In the presence of concurrent diabetes mellitus or renal disease, current guidelines (JNC 7) recommend lowering the blood pressure to less than 130/80 mm Hg, but this is somewhat controversial.

Decreasing blood pressure by lifestyle modification and pharmacologic therapy is intended to decrease morbidity and mortality. Treatment resulting in normalization of blood pressure has been particularly successful in decreasing the incidence of stroke. Decreasing blood pressure also decreases the morbidity and mortality associated with ischemic heart disease (Figure 5-4). It slows or prevents progression to a more severe stage of hypertension and decreases the risk of congestive heart failure and renal failure. The benefits of antihypertensive drug therapy appear to be greater in elderly patients than in younger patients.

Patients with concomitant risk factors (hypercholesterolemia, diabetes mellitus, tobacco use, family history of hypertension, age >60 years) and evidence of target organ damage (angina pectoris, prior myocardial infarction, left ventricular hypertrophy, cerebrovascular disease, nephropathy, retinopathy, peripheral vascular disease) are most likely to benefit from pharmacologic antihypertensive therapy. Patients who do not manifest clinical evidence of cardiovascular disease or target organ damage may benefit from a trial of lifestyle modification and subsequent reevaluation before initiation of pharmacologic therapy.

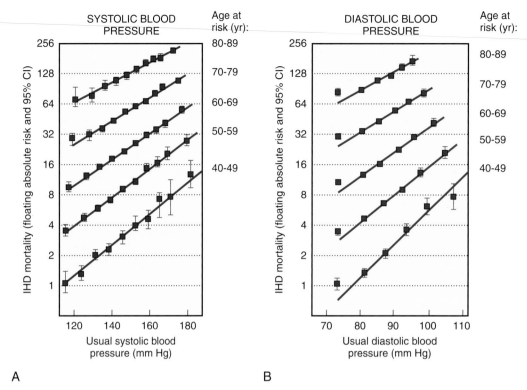

FIGURE 5-2 Ischemic heart disease *(IHD)* mortality rate in each decade of age versus usual blood pressure at the start of that decade. Mortality rates are termed *floating* because multiplication by a constant appropriate for a particular population would allow prediction of the absolute rate in that population. *CI,* Confidence interval. *(Data from Lewington S, Clarke R, Qizilbash N, et al. Age-specific relevance of usual blood pressure to vascular mortality: a meta-analysis of individual data for one million adults in 61 prospective studies.* Lancet. *2002;360:1903-1913.)*

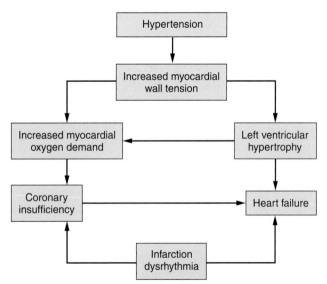

FIGURE 5-3 Chronically increased systemic blood pressure initiate a series of pathophysiologic changes that may culminate in congestive heart failure.

LIFESTYLE MODIFICATION

Lifestyle modifications of proven value in lowering blood pressure include weight reduction or prevention of weight gain, moderation of alcohol intake, increase in physical activity, adherence to recommendations for dietary calcium and potassium intake, and moderation in dietary salt intake. Smoking cessation is critical, because smoking is an independent risk factor for cardiovascular disease.

Weight loss may be the most efficacious of all nonpharmacologic interventions in the treatment of hypertension. A 10-kg weight loss decreases the systolic and diastolic blood pressure by an average of 6.0 mm Hg and 4.6 mm Hg, respectively. Weight loss also enhances the efficacy of antihypertensive drug therapy. Alcohol consumption is associated with an increase in blood pressure, and excessive use of alcohol may cause resistance to antihypertensive drugs. However, moderate alcohol ingestion has been shown to decrease overall cardiovascular risk in the general population. At least 30 minutes of moderate-intensity physical activity, such as brisk walking or bicycling, can lower blood pressure in both normotensive and hypertensive individuals.

There is an inverse relationship between dietary potassium and calcium intake and blood pressure in the general population. Dietary salt restriction (such as the Dietary Approaches to Stop Hypertension [DASH] eating plan) is associated with small but consistent decreases in systemic blood pressure (Figure 5-5). It is possible that sodium restriction is most beneficial in lowering blood pressure in a subset of patients with low renin activity, such as the elderly and African Americans.

TABLE 5-2 ▪ **Common causes of secondary hypertension**

Causes	Clinical findings	Laboratory evaluation
Renovascular disease	Epigastric or abdominal bruit Severe hypertension in young patient	MRA Aortography Duplex ultrasonography CT angiography
Hyperaldosteronism	Fatigue Weakness Headache Paresthesia Nocturnal polyuria and polydipsia	Urinary potassium Serum potassium Plasma renin Plasma aldosterone
Aortic coarctation	Elevated blood pressure in upper limbs relative to lower limbs Weak femoral pulses Systolic bruit	Aortography Echocardiography MRI or CT
Pheochromocytoma	Episodic headache, palpitations, and diaphoresis Paroxysmal hypertension	Plasma metanephrines Urinary catecholamines Spot urine metanephrines Adrenal CT/MRI scan
Cushing's syndrome	Truncal obesity Proximal muscle weakness Purple striae Moon facies Hirsutism	Dexamethasone suppression test Urinary cortisol Adrenal CT scan Glucose tolerance test
Renal parenchymal disease	Nocturia Edema	Urinary glucose, protein, and casts Serum creatinine Renal ultrasonography Renal biopsy
Pregnancy-induced hypertension	Peripheral and pulmonary edema Headache Seizures Right upper quadrant pain	Urinary protein Uric acid Cardiac output Platelet count

CT, Computed tomography; *MRA,* magnetic resonance angiography; *MRI,* magnetic resonance imaging.

TABLE 5-3 ▪ **Other causes of secondary hypertension**

SYSTOLIC AND DIASTOLIC HYPERTENSION

Renal disorders
  Renal transplantation
  Renin-secreting tumors
Endocrine disorders
  Acromegaly
  Hyperparathyroidism
Obstructive sleep apnea
Postoperative hypertension
Neurologic disorders
  Increased intracranial pressure
  Spinal cord injury
  Guillain-Barré syndrome
  Dysautonomia
Drugs
  Glucocorticoids
  Mineralocorticoids
  Cyclosporine
  Sympathomimetics
  Tyramine and monoamine oxidase inhibitors
  Nasal decongestants
Sudden withdrawal from antihypertensive drug therapy (central acting and β-adrenergic antagonists)

ISOLATED SYSTOLIC HYPERTENSION

Aging with associated aortic rigidity
Increased cardiac output
  Thyrotoxicosis
  Anemia
  Aortic regurgitation
Decreased peripheral vascular resistance
  Arteriovenous shunts
  Paget's disease

Sodium restriction can minimize diuretic-induced hypokalemia and may enhance the control of blood pressure with diuretic therapy. Additional benefits of salt restriction include protection from osteoporosis and fractures through a decrease in urinary calcium excretion and favorable effects on left ventricular remodeling. Salt substitutes in which sodium is replaced with potassium are useful for hypertensive patients who do not have renal dysfunction.

PHARMACOLOGIC THERAPY

Initiation of drug therapy should occur in tandem with lifestyle modification. After drug therapy is started, patients are seen every 1 to 4 weeks to titrate the antihypertensive drug dose and then every 3 to 4 months once the desired degree of blood pressure control has been achieved. Use of long-acting drugs is preferable, because patient adherence and consistency of blood pressure control are superior with once-daily dosing. As reported by JNC 7, thiazide diuretics are recommended as initial therapy for uncomplicated hypertension (Figure 5-6). Thiazide diuretics can also increase the efficacy of multidrug regimens. Hypertensive patient may have other medical conditions that present *compelling* indications for antihypertensive therapy with drugs of a particular class (Table 5-4). For example, hypertension in patients with heart failure is typically treated with an angiotensin-converting enzyme (ACE) inhibitor or an angiotensin receptor antagonist (ARB). These compelling indications were identified based on the results of several outcome studies. If monotherapy is unsuccessful, a second drug, usually of a different class, is added. A large variety of antihypertensive drugs are available, and many of these drugs present unique and potentially significant advantages and side effects (Table 5-5).

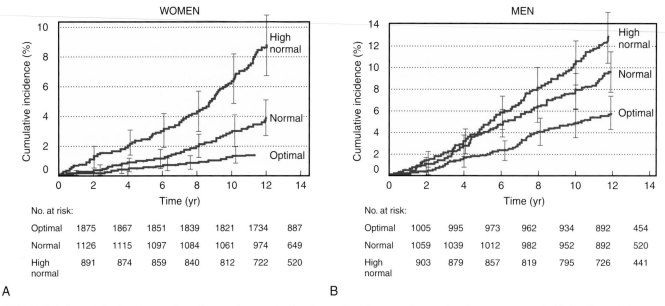

FIGURE 5-4 Cumulative incidence of cardiovascular events (death resulting from cardiovascular disease, myocardial infarction, stroke, or congestive heart failure) in women (**A**) and men (**B**) without hypertension according to blood pressure category at the baseline examination. Optimal blood pressure, <120/80 mm Hg; normal blood pressure, <130/85 mm Hg; high-normal blood pressure, <140/90 mm Hg. *(Adapted from Vasan RS, Larson MG, Leip EP, et al. Impact of high-normal blood pressure on the risk of cardiovascular disease. N Engl J Med. 2001;345:1291-1297.)*

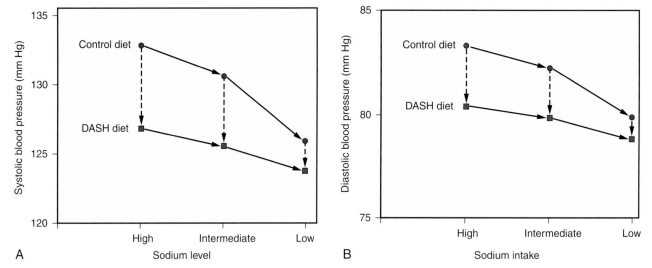

FIGURE 5-5 Effect on systolic blood pressure (**A**) and diastolic blood pressure (**B**) of reduced sodium intake and adherence to the Dietary Approaches to Stop Hypertension (DASH) diet. *(Data from Sacks FM, Svetkey LP, Vollmer WM, et al: Effects on blood pressure of reduced dietary sodium and the Dietary Approaches to Stop Hypertension [DASH] diet. N Engl J Med. 2001;344:3-10.)*

Recent trials have documented the benefits of antihypertensive therapy in very elderly patients—that is, those older than 80 years—in reducing cardiovascular risk and mortality. Such therapy may also benefit cognitive function. As a result of these data, new guidelines have been issued for the treatment of hypertension in octogenarians.

Treatment of Secondary Hypertension

Treatment of secondary hypertension is often surgical. Pharmacologic therapy is reserved for patients in whom surgery is not possible. Certain disease entities, such as pheochromocytoma, may require a combined pharmacologic and surgical approach for optimal outcome.

SURGICAL THERAPY

Surgery is used to treat identifiable causes of secondary hypertension such as renovascular hypertension, hyperaldosteronism, Cushing's disease, and pheochromocytoma. Surgery includes correction of renal artery stenosis via angioplasty or direct repair for renovascular hypertension, and adrenalectomy for adrenal adenoma or pheochromocytoma.

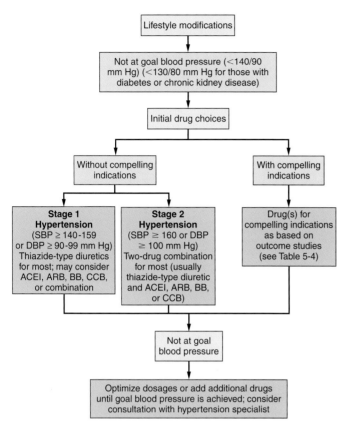

FIGURE 5-6 Algorithm for treatment of hypertension. *ACEI,* Angiotensin-converting enzyme inhibitor; *ARB,* angiotensin receptor blocker; *BB,* β-blocker; *CCB,* calcium channel blocker; *DBP,* diastolic blood pressure; *SBP,* systolic blood pressure. *(Data from Chobanian AV, Bakris GL, Black HR, et al. Joint National Committee on Prevention, Detection, Evaluation, and Treatment of High Blood Pressure; National Heart, Lung, and Blood Institute; National High Blood Pressure Education Program Coordinating Committee. Seventh report of the Joint National Committee on Prevention, Detection, Evaluation, and Treatment of High Blood Pressure. Hypertension. 2003;42:1206-1252.)*

PHARMACOLOGIC THERAPY

For patients in whom renal artery repair is not possible, blood pressure control may be accomplished with ACE inhibitors alone or in combination with diuretics. Renal function and serum potassium concentration must be carefully monitored when ACE inhibitor therapy is initiated in these patients. Primary hyperaldosteronism in women can be treated with an aldosterone antagonist such as spironolactone. Amiloride is used to treat hyperaldosteronism in men, because spironolactone may cause gynecomastia.

Hypertensive Crises

DEFINITION

Hypertensive crises typically present with a blood pressure of more than 180/120 mm Hg and can be categorized as either a hypertensive urgency or a hypertensive emergency, based on the presence or absence of impending or progressive target organ damage. Patients with chronic systemic hypertension can tolerate a higher systemic blood pressure than previously normotensive individuals and are more likely to experience urgencies rather than emergencies.

HYPERTENSIVE EMERGENCY

Patients with evidence of acute or ongoing target organ damage (encephalopathy, intracerebral hemorrhage, acute left ventricular failure with pulmonary edema, unstable angina,

dissecting aortic aneurysm, acute myocardial infarction, eclampsia, microangiopathic hemolytic anemia, or renal insufficiency) require prompt pharmacologic intervention to lower the systemic blood pressure. Encephalopathy rarely develops in patients with chronic hypertension until the diastolic blood pressure exceeds 150 mm Hg. However, parturient woman with pregnancy-induced hypertension may develop signs of encephalopathy with a diastolic blood pressure of less than 100 mm Hg. Even in the absence of symptoms, a parturient with a diastolic blood pressure higher than 109 mm Hg is considered to have a hypertensive emergency and requires immediate treatment. The goal of treatment in hypertensive emergencies is to decrease the diastolic blood pressure promptly but gradually. A precipitous decrease in blood pressure to normotensive levels could provoke coronary or cerebral ischemia. Typically, mean arterial pressure is reduced by about 20% within the first hour of treatment and then more gradually over the next 2 to 6 hours to a target blood pressure of about 160/110 mm Hg if tolerated as indicated by the absence of symptomatic hypoperfusion of target organs.

HYPERTENSIVE URGENCY

Hypertensive urgencies are situations in which the blood pressure is severely elevated, but the patient is not exhibiting evidence of target organ damage. These patients can have headache, epistaxis, or anxiety at presentation. Selected

TABLE 5-4 ■ Compelling indications for specific classes of antihypertensive drugs

Comorbid condition	Class of antihypertensive drugs
Previous myocardial infarction	ACE inhibitor Aldosterone antagonist β-Blocker
Heart failure	ACE inhibitor Aldosterone antagonist ARB β-Blocker Diuretic
High risk of coronary artery disease	ACE inhibitor β-Blocker Calcium channel blocker Diuretic
Diabetes	ACE inhibitor ARB β-Blocker Calcium channel blocker Diuretic
Chronic kidney disease	ACE inhibitor ARB
Recurrent stroke prevention	ACE inhibitor Diuretic

ACE, Angiotensin-converting enzyme; ARB, angiotensin receptor blocker.

TABLE 5-5 ■ Commonly used antihypertensive drugs

Class	Subclass	Generic name	Trade name
Diuretics	Thiazides	Chlorothiazide Hydrochlorothiazide Indapamide Metolazone	Diuril HydroDiuril, Microzide Lozol Zaroxolyn, Mykrox
	Loop	Bumetanide Furosemide Torsemide	Bumex Lasix Demadex
	Potassium sparing	Amiloride Spironolactone Triamterene	Midamor Aldactone Dyrenium
Adrenergic antagonists	β-Blockers	Atenolol Bisoprolol Metoprolol Nadolol Propranolol Timolol	Tenormin Zebeta Lopressor Corgard Inderal Blocadren
	α_1-Blockers	Doxazosin Prazosin Terazosin	Cardura Minipress Hytrin
	Combined α- and β-blockers	Carvedilol Labetalol	Coreg Normodyne, Trandate
	Centrally acting	Clonidine Methyldopa	Catapres Aldomet
Vasodilators		Hydralazine	Apresoline
Angiotensin-converting enzyme inhibitors		Benazepril Captopril Enalapril Fosinopril Lisinopril Moexipril Quinapril Ramipril Trandolapril	Lotensin Capoten Vasotec Monopril Prinivil, Zestril Univasc Accupril Altace Mavik
Angiotensin receptor blockers		Candesartan Eprosartan Irbesartan Losartan Olmesartan Telmisartan Valsartan	Atacand Teveten Avapro Cozaar Benicar Micardis Diovan
Calcium channel blockers	Dihydropyridine	Amlodipine Felodipine Isradipine Nicardipine Nifedipine Nisoldipine Clevidipine	Norvasc Plendil DynaCirc Cardene Adalat, Procardia Sular Cleviprex
	Nondihydropyridine	Diltiazem Verapamil	Cardizem, Dilacor, Tiazac Calan, Isoptin SR, Covera

patients may benefit from oral antihypertensive therapy, because nonadherence to the medication regimen or unavailability of prescribed medications is often the reason behind the hypertensive urgency.

PHARMACOLOGIC THERAPY

The initial choice of drug for treatment of a hypertensive emergency is based on an analysis of all of the patient's medical conditions and the symptoms and signs at presentation (Table 5-6). Placement of an intraarterial catheter to continuously monitor systemic blood pressure is recommended during treatment with potent vasoactive drugs. The goal is to decrease the blood pressure by no more than 20% to 25% initially so that target organ hypoperfusion is prevented. For most types of hypertensive emergencies, sodium nitroprusside 0.5 to 10.0 mcg/kg/min IV is a drug of choice. The immediate onset and short duration of action allow effective minute-by-minute titration of blood pressure, but sodium nitroprusside use can be complicated by lactic acidosis and cyanide toxicity. Nicardipine infusion is another option and may improve both cardiac and cerebral ischemia. The dopamine (D_1 receptor–specific) agonist fenoldopam increases renal blood flow and inhibits sodium reabsorption, which makes it an excellent drug in patients with renal insufficiency. Esmolol infusion can be effective alone or in combination with other drugs. Labetalol, an α- and β-blocker, can also be very effective in the acute treatment of malignant hypertension.

TABLE 5-6 ■ Treatment of hypertensive emergencies

Cause/manifestation	Primary agents	Cautions	Comments
Encephalopathy and intracranial hypertension	Nitroprusside, labetalol, fenoldopam, nicardipine	Cerebral ischemia may result from lower blood pressure due to altered autoregulation Risk of cyanide toxicity with nitroprusside Nitroprusside increases intracranial pressure	Lower blood pressure may lessen bleeding in intracerebral hemorrhage Elevated blood pressure often resolves spontaneously
Myocardial ischemia	Nitroglycerin	Avoid β-blockers in acute congestive heart failure	Include morphine and oxygen therapy
Acute pulmonary edema	Nitroglycerin, nitroprusside, fenoldopam	Avoid β-blockers in acute congestive heart failure	Include morphine, loop diuretic, and oxygen therapy
Aortic dissection	Trimethaphan, esmolol, vasodilators	Vasodilators may cause reflex tachycardia and increase pulsatile force of left ventricular contraction	Goal is lessening of pulsatile force of left ventricular contraction
Renal insufficiency	Fenoldopam, nicardipine	Tachyphylaxis occurs with fenoldopam	May require emergent hemodialysis Avoid ACE inhibitors and ARBs
Preeclampsia and eclampsia	Methyldopa, hydralazine Magnesium sulfate Labetalol, nicardipine	Lupuslike syndrome with hydralazine Risk of flash pulmonary edema Calcium channel blockers may reduce uterine blood flow and inhibit labor	Definitive therapy is delivery ACE inhibitors and ARBs are contraindicated during pregnancy due to teratogenicity
Pheochromocytoma	Phentolamine, phenoxybenzamine, propranolol	Unopposed α-adrenergic stimulation following β-blockade worsens hypertension	
Cocaine intoxication	Nitroglycerin, nitroprusside, phentolamine	Unopposed α-adrenergic stimulation following β-blockade worsens hypertension	

ACE, Angiotensin-converting enzyme; ARB, angiotensin receptor blocker.

Clevidipine (Cleviprex), a third-generation dihydropyridine calcium channel blocker with ultrashort duration of action and selective arteriolar vasodilating properties has recently been approved by the Food and Drug Administration. The pharmacokinetics and pharmacodynamics of clevidipine are favorable for use of this drug in clinical situations in which tight blood pressure control is essential.

Management of Anesthesia in Patients with Essential Hypertension

Despite earlier suggestions that antihypertensive medications be discontinued preoperatively, it is now accepted that most drugs that effectively control systemic blood pressure should be continued throughout the perioperative period to ensure optimum blood pressure control. A summary of the anesthetic management of patients with hypertension is presented in Table 5-7.

PREOPERATIVE EVALUATION

Preoperative evaluation of patients with essential hypertension should determine the adequacy of blood pressure control, and the drug therapy that has rendered the patient normotensive should be continued throughout the perioperative period.

It seems reasonable to adhere to the concept that hypertensive patients should be made normotensive before elective

TABLE 5-7 ■ Management of anesthesia for hypertensive patients

PREOPERATIVE EVALUATION

Determine adequacy of blood pressure control
Review pharmacology of drugs being administered to control blood pressure
Evaluate for evidence of end-organ damage
Continue drugs used for control of blood pressure

INDUCTION AND MAINTENANCE OF ANESTHESIA

Anticipate exaggerated blood pressure response to anesthetic drugs
Limit duration of direct laryngoscopy
Administer a balanced anesthetic to blunt hypertensive responses
Consider placement of invasive hemodynamic monitors
Monitor for myocardial ischemia

POSTOPERATIVE MANAGEMENT

Anticipate periods of systemic hypertension
Maintain monitoring of end-organ function

surgery. The incidence of hypotension and evidence of myocardial ischemia during maintenance of anesthesia is increased in patients who are hypertensive before induction of anesthesia. It is not clear if hypertension per se has a significant impact on surgical risk. Chronic hypertension is a cardiovascular,

TABLE 5-8   Risk of general anesthesia and elective surgery in hypertensive patients

Preoperative systemic blood pressure status	Incidence of perioperative hypertensive episodes (%)	Incidence of postoperative cardiac complications (%)
Normotensive	8*	11
Treated and rendered normotensive	27	24
Treated but remain hypertensive	25	7
Untreated and hypertensive	20	12

Data from Goldman L, Caldera DL. Risk of general anesthesia and elective operation in the hypertensive patient. *Anesthesiology*. 1979;50:285-292.
*P < .05 compared with other groups in the same column.

cerebrovascular, and renal risk factor, and this, in turn, may increase surgical risk.

The magnitude of blood pressure changes during anesthesia is greater in hypertensive than in normotensive patients. Intraoperative *hypotension* may be particularly problematic. Co-existing hypertension may increase the incidence of postoperative myocardial reinfarction in patients with a history of myocardial infarction as well as the incidence of neurologic complications in patients undergoing carotid endarterectomy. However, intraoperative *hypertension* commonly occurs in patients with a history of hypertension, whether or not the blood pressure is controlled preoperatively (Table 5-8). There is no evidence that the incidence of postoperative complications is increased in hypertensive patients with a diastolic blood pressure as high as 110 mm Hg who undergo elective surgery.

There are no universally accepted guidelines for postponement of elective surgery in patients in whom blood pressure control is less than optimal. A diastolic blood pressure of 100 to 115 mm Hg is most often used as a criterion for postponement of elective surgery. In hypertensive patients with signs of target organ damage, postponement of an elective procedure is justified if that end-organ damage can be improved or if further evaluation of that damage could alter the anesthetic plan. Of course, the urgency of the surgery has to be taken into account when evaluating a hypertensive surgical patient and optimizing the patient's condition.

It is not uncommon for the blood pressure on admission to the hospital to be increased (white coat syndrome), reflecting patient anxiety. Subsequently measured blood pressures are often lower. Interestingly, the subset of patients who manifest anxiety-related hypertension are likely to have exaggerated pressor responses to direct laryngoscopy and are more likely than others to develop perioperative myocardial ischemia or to require antihypertensive therapy during the perioperative period.

End-organ damage (angina pectoris, left ventricular hypertrophy, congestive heart failure, cerebrovascular disease, stroke, peripheral vascular disease, renal insufficiency) should be evaluated preoperatively. Patients with essential hypertension should be presumed to have ischemic heart disease until proven otherwise. Renal insufficiency secondary to chronic hypertension is a marker of a widespread hypertensive disease process.

It is useful to review the pharmacology and potential side effects of the drugs being used for antihypertensive therapy. Many of these drugs interfere with autonomic nervous system function. Preoperatively, this may appear as orthostatic hypotension. During anesthesia, exaggerated decreases in blood pressure seen with blood loss, positive pressure ventilation, or changes in body position reflect impaired vascular compensation because of these autonomic-inhibitory effects. Administration of vasopressors, such as phenylephrine and ephedrine, results in predictable and appropriate blood pressure responses in these patients.

Another compelling reason to continue antihypertensive therapy throughout the perioperative period is to avoid the risk of rebound hypertension should certain drugs, especially β-adrenergic antagonists and clonidine, be abruptly discontinued. Antihypertensive agents that act independently of the autonomic nervous system, such as ACE inhibitors, are not associated with rebound hypertension.

Bradycardia may be a manifestation of a selective alteration in sympathetic nervous system activity. There is no evidence, however, that heart rate responses to surgical stimulation or surgical blood loss are absent in patients treated with antihypertensive drugs. Decreased anesthetic requirements parallel the sedative effects produced by clonidine. Hypokalemia (<3.5 mEq/L) despite potassium supplementation is a common preoperative finding in patients being treated with diuretics. However, this drug-induced hypokalemia does not appear to increase the incidence of cardiac dysrhythmias in the perioperative period. Hyperkalemia can be seen in patients being treated with ACE inhibitors or ARBs who are also receiving potassium supplementation or have renal dysfunction.

Angiotensin-Converting Enzyme Inhibitors

There is a risk of hemodynamic instability and hypotension during anesthesia in patients receiving ACE inhibitors. Three systems exist to maintain normal blood pressure. After blunting of autonomic responses by induction of general anesthesia and blunting of the renin-angiotensin-aldosterone system by an ACE inhibitor, the only system remaining to support blood pressure is the vasopressin system, and so blood pressure is likely to be volume dependent (Figure 5-7). ACE inhibitors may also decrease cardiac output by attenuating the venoconstrictor effect of angiotensin on capacitance vessels. This will result in a decrease in venous return. Maintenance of intravascular fluid volume is crucial during surgery in patients undergoing long-term treatment with these drugs. Surgical procedures involving major fluid shifts have been associated

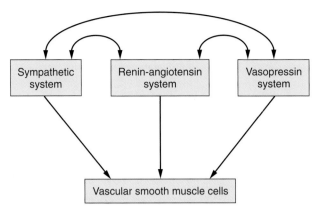

FIGURE 5-7 Vasopressor systems in blood pressure regulation. Three different vasopressor systems are involved in blood pressure regulation. Each acts on the same target—the vascular smooth muscle cell—by inducing an increase in free cytosolic calcium followed by cell contraction. Each system is related to the others and may act as a compensatory mechanism. *(Data from Colson P, Ryckwaert F, Coriat P. Renin angiotensin system antagonists and anesthesia.* Anesth Analg. *1999;89:1143-1155.)*

with hypotension in patients being treated with ACE inhibitors. This hypotension has been responsive to fluid infusion and administration of sympathomimetic drugs. Hypotension resistant to such measures may require administration of vasopressin or a vasopressin analogue. Careful titration of anesthetic drugs may prevent or limit the hypotension attributable to ACE inhibitors. It may be prudent to discontinue ACE inhibitors 24 to 48 hours preoperatively in patients at high risk of intraoperative hypovolemia and hypotension. The major disadvantage of drug discontinuation is a potential loss of blood pressure control.

Angiotensin Receptor Blockers

ARBs effectively treat hypertension by preventing angiotensin II from binding to its receptor. As with ACE inhibitors, blockade of the renin-angiotensin-aldosterone system by ARBs increases the potential for hypotension during anesthesia. Hypotension requiring vasoconstrictor treatment occurs more often after induction of anesthesia in patients continuing ARB treatment than in those in whom treatment was discontinued on the day before surgery. In addition, the hypotensive episodes experienced by patients treated with ARBs may be refractory to management with conventional vasoconstrictors such as ephedrine and phenylephrine, which necessitates the use of vasopressin or one of its analogues. For these reasons, it is recommended that ARBs be discontinued the day before surgery.

INDUCTION OF ANESTHESIA

Induction of anesthesia with rapidly acting intravenous drugs may produce significant hypotension due to peripheral vasodilation in the presence of a decreased intravascular fluid volume, as is likely in the presence of diastolic hypertension. Hypotension during induction is more pronounced in patients

continuing ACE inhibitor or ARB therapy up until the time of surgery.

Direct laryngoscopy and tracheal intubation can produce significant hypertension in patients with essential hypertension, even if these patients had been rendered normotensive preoperatively. Evidence of myocardial ischemia is likely to occur in association with the hypertension and tachycardia that can accompany laryngoscopy and intubation. Intravenous induction drugs do not predictably suppress the circulatory responses evoked by tracheal intubation. Patients at high risk for developing myocardial ischemia may benefit from maneuvers that suppress tracheal reflexes and blunt the autonomic responses to tracheal manipulation, such as deep inhalation anesthesia or injection of an opioid, lidocaine, β-blocker or vasodilator before laryngoscopy. In addition, the duration of laryngoscopy is important in limiting the pressor response to this painful stimulus. Ensuring that direct laryngoscopy does not exceed 15 seconds in duration helps minimize blood pressure changes.

MAINTENANCE OF ANESTHESIA

The hemodynamic goal for hypertensive patients during maintenance of anesthesia is to minimize wide fluctuations in blood pressure. Management of intraoperative blood pressure lability is as important as preoperative control of blood pressure in these patients.

Regional anesthesia can be used in hypertensive patients. However, a high sensory level of anesthesia with its associated sympathetic denervation can unmask unsuspected hypovolemia.

Intraoperative Hypertension

The most likely intraoperative blood pressure change is hypertension produced by noxious stimulation, that is, light anesthesia. Indeed, the incidence of perioperative hypertensive episodes is increased in patients diagnosed with essential hypertension, even if the blood pressure was controlled preoperatively. Volatile anesthetics are useful in attenuating sympathetic nervous system activity responsible for these pressor responses. Volatile anesthetics produce a dose-dependent decrease in blood pressure, which reflects a decrease in systemic vascular resistance and/or myocardial depression. There is no evidence that one volatile anesthetic drug is preferable to another for control of intraoperative hypertension.

A nitrous oxide–opioid technique can be used for maintenance of anesthesia, although it is likely that a volatile agent will be needed at times to control hypertension, especially during periods of abrupt change in surgical stimulation. Antihypertensive medication administered by bolus or by continuous infusion is an alternative to the use of a volatile anesthetic for blood pressure control intraoperatively. No specific neuromuscular blocker has been shown to be best for patients with hypertension. Pancuronium can modestly increase blood pressure, but there is no evidence that this pressor response is exaggerated in the presence of essential hypertension.

Intraoperative Hypotension

Hypotension during maintenance of anesthesia may be treated by decreasing the depth of anesthesia and/or by increasing intravascular volume. Administration of sympathomimetic drugs such as ephedrine or phenylephrine may be necessary to restore vital organ perfusion pressures until the underlying cause of hypotension can be ascertained and corrected. Despite the suppressant effect of many antihypertensive drugs on the autonomic nervous system, extensive clinical experience has confirmed that the response to sympathomimetic drugs is both appropriate and predictable. Intraoperative hypotension in patients being treated with ACE inhibitors or ARBs is responsive to administration of intravenous fluids, sympathomimetic drugs, and/or vasopressin. Cardiac rhythm disturbances that result in loss of sequential atrioventricular contraction, such as junctional rhythm and atrial fibrillation, can also create hypotension and must be treated promptly.

Monitoring

Monitoring in patients with essential hypertension is influenced by the complexity of the surgery. ECG is particularly useful for identifying the occurrence of myocardial ischemia during periods of intense painful stimulation such as laryngoscopy and tracheal intubation. Invasive monitoring with an intraarterial catheter and a central venous or pulmonary artery catheter may be useful if extensive surgery is planned and there is evidence of left ventricular dysfunction or other significant end-organ damage. Transesophageal echocardiography is an excellent technique for monitoring left ventricular function and adequacy of intravascular volume replacement, but it requires specific equipment and specially trained personnel, and it may not be universally available.

POSTOPERATIVE MANAGEMENT

Postoperative hypertension is common in patients with essential hypertension. This hypertension requires prompt assessment and treatment to decrease the risk of myocardial ischemia, cardiac dysrhythmias, congestive heart failure, stroke, and excessive bleeding. Hypertension that persists despite adequate treatment of postoperative pain may necessitate administration of an intravenous antihypertensive medication. Gradually, conversion can be made to the patient's usual regimen of oral antihypertensive medication.

PULMONARY ARTERIAL HYPERTENSION

This section deals with idiopathic pulmonary arterial hypertension. See Chapters 2, 6, and 9 for discussion of pulmonary hypertension associated with heart or lung disease. Pulmonary arterial hypertension (PAH) used to be considered a very rare disease, but it is now noted more commonly. PAH may have an incidence of 2.4 cases per million people per year and a prevalence of 15 cases per million people (about 6 cases per million people for idiopathic PAH).

TABLE 5-9   Calculation of pulmonary vascular resistance

$\dfrac{(\overline{PAP} - PAOP) \times 80}{CO}$	PVR is expressed in dynes/sec/cm^{-5}, with normal PVR = 50-150 dynes/sec/cm^{-5}
$\dfrac{(\overline{PAP} - PAOP)}{CO}$	PVR is expressed in Wood units (mm Hg/L/min), with normal PVR = 1 Wood unit

CO, Cardiac output (L/min); PAOP, pulmonary artery occlusion pressure (mm Hg); $\overline{PAP}$, mean pulmonary artery pressure (mm Hg); PVR, pulmonary vascular resistance.

Idiopathic PAH is a devastating clinical condition, with a median period of survival after diagnosis of 2.8 years. Most patients succumb to progressive right ventricular (RV) failure. Patients with idiopathic PAH are at risk of perioperative RV failure, hypoxemia, and coronary ischemia. Their risk may be as high as 28% for respiratory failure, 12% for cardiac dysrhythmias, 11% for congestive heart failure, and 7% for overall perioperative mortality for noncardiac surgery.

Definition, Nomenclature, and Classification

PAH is defined hemodynamically as a mean pulmonary artery pressure of more than 25 mm Hg at rest with a pulmonary capillary wedge pressure, left atrial pressure, or left ventricular end-diastolic pressure of 15 mm Hg or less, and a pulmonary vascular resistance (PVR) of more than 3 Wood units (Table 5-9). The definition of exercise-related PAH is awaiting better scientific support.

The 2008 Fourth World Symposium on Pulmonary Arterial Hypertension produced a document updating the classification of pulmonary hypertension (Table 5-10). In the current classification, the use of the terms *primary* and *secondary pulmonary hypertension* are avoided, and the term *idiopathic PAH* (IPAH) is preferred. IPAH refers to sporadic cases of PAH with no familial context and no identifiable risk factor. In the new classification the term *heritable PAH* replaces the term *familial PAH*. Most patients with heritable PAH have mutations in bone morphogenetic protein receptor type 2 (BMPR2).

Clinical Presentation and Evaluation

PAH often presents with vague symptoms, including breathlessness, weakness, fatigue, and abdominal distention. Syncope and angina pectoris are indicative of severe limitations in cardiac output and possible myocardial ischemia. Chest pain likely reflects reduced coronary blood flow to a markedly hypertrophied right ventricle. As the cardiac output becomes fixed and eventually falls, patients may have episodes of syncope or nearsyncope. On physical examination, the patient may exhibit a parasternal lift, murmurs of pulmonic insufficiency and/or tricuspid regurgitation, a pronounced pulmonic component of S$_2$, an S$_3$ gallop, jugular venous distention with a large *a* wave in the jugular venous pulsation, peripheral edema, hepatomegaly, and

TABLE 5-10 ■ Updated clinical classification of pulmonary hypertension

1. PULMONARY ARTERIAL HYPERTENSION (PAH)

Idiopathic PAH
Heritable
  BMPR2
  ALK1, endoglin (with or without hereditary hemorrhagic
    telangiectasia)
  Unknown
Drug and toxin induced
Associated with
  Connective tissue diseases
  HIV infection
  Portal hypertension
  Congenital heart disease
  Schistosomiasis
  Chronic hemolytic anemia
Persistent pulmonary hypertension of the newborn
Pulmonary venoocclusive disease (PVOD) and/or pulmonary
  capillary hemangiomatosis (PCH)

2. PULMONARY HYPERTENSION OWING TO LEFT HEART DISEASE

Systolic dysfunction
Diastolic dysfunction
Valvular disease

3. PULMONARY HYPERTENSION OWING TO LUNG DISEASES AND/OR HYPOXIA

Chronic obstructive pulmonary disease
Interstitial lung disease
Other pulmonary diseases with mixed restrictive
  and obstructive pattern
Sleep-disordered breathing
Alveolar hypoventilation disorders
Chronic exposure to high altitude
Developmental abnormalities

4. CHRONIC THROMBOEMBOLIC PULMONARY HYPERTENSION (CTEPH)

5. PULMONARY HYPERTENSION WITH UNCLEAR MULTIFACTORIAL MECHANISMS

Hematologic disorders: myeloproliferative disorders,
  splenectomy
Systemic disorders: sarcoidosis, pulmonary Langerhans cell
  histiocytosis, lymphangioleiomyomatosis, neurofibromatosis,
  vasculitis
Metabolic disorders: glycogen storage disease, Gaucher's
  disease, thyroid disorders
Other: tumoral obstruction, fibrosing mediastinitis, chronic
  renal failure on hemodialysis

Reprinted with permission from Simonneau G, Robbins IM, Berghetti M, et al. Updated clinical classification of pulmonary hypertension. *J Am Coll Cardiol*. 2009;54:S43-S54.
ALK1, Activin receptor–like kinase type 1; *BMPR2*, bone morphogenetic protein receptor type 2; *HIV*, human immunodeficiency virus.

TABLE 5-11 ■ Clinical findings in pulmonary hypertension

Diagnostic modality	Key findings
Chest radiograph	Prominent pulmonary arteries
	Right atrial and right ventricular enlargement
	Parenchymal lung disease
Electrocardiography	P pulmonale
	Right axis deviation
	Right ventricular strain or hypertrophy
	Complete or incomplete right bundle branch block
Two-dimensional echocardiography	Right atrial enlargement
	Right ventricular hypertrophy, dilation, or volume overload
	Tricuspid regurgitation
	Elevated estimated pulmonary artery pressures
	Congenital heart disease
Pulmonary function tests	Obstructive or restrictive pattern
	Low diffusing capacity
$\dot{V}/\dot{Q}$ scan	Ventilation/perfusion mismatching
Pulmonary angiography	Vascular filling defects
Chest CT scan	Main pulmonary artery size of >30 mm
	Vascular filling defects
	Mosaic perfusion defects
Abdominal ultrasonography or CT scan	Cirrhosis
	Portal hypertension
Blood tests	Antinuclear antibody positive
	Rheumatoid factor positive
	Platelet dysfunction
	HIV positive
Sleep study	High respiratory disturbance index

Reprinted with permission from Dincer HE, Presberg KW. Current management of pulmonary hypertension. *Clin Pulm Med*. 2004;11:40-53. *CT*, Computed tomography; *HIV*, human immunodeficiency virus; $\dot{V}/\dot{Q}$, ventilation/perfusion.

ascites. Uncommonly, the left recurrent laryngeal nerve can become paralyzed because of compression by a dilated pulmonary artery (Ortner's syndrome). The laboratory evaluation and diagnostic studies used in the workup of pulmonary hypertension of any cause are listed in Table 5-11. A 6-minute walk test can be performed to assess functional status and noninvasively follow the progress of therapy. Right-sided heart catheterization provides a definitive means to determine disease severity and to ascertain which patients can respond to vasodilator therapy. A potent vasodilator such as prostacyclin, NO, adenosine, or prostaglandin E$_1$ is administered. The result of the vasodilator test is considered positive, that is, the patient shows a response, if PVR and mean pulmonary arterial pressure both decrease acutely by 20% or more. Only about one fourth of patients show a favorable response to the vasodilator test.

Physiology and Pathophysiology

The normal pulmonary circulation can accommodate flow rates ranging from 6 to 25 L/min with minimal changes in pulmonary artery pressure. PAH develops as a result of pulmonary

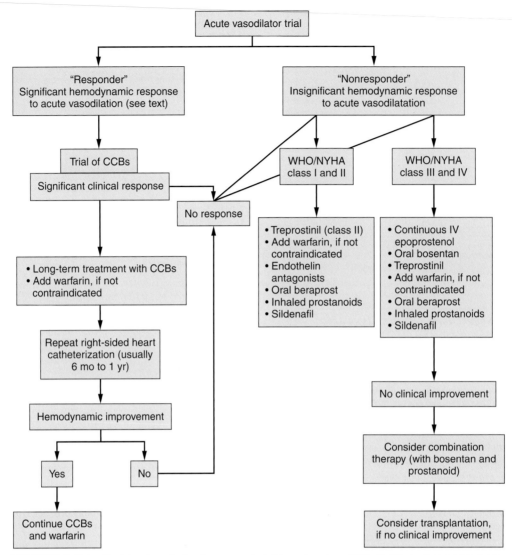

FIGURE 5-8 Outpatient treatment of pulmonary arterial hypertension. *CCBs,* Calcium channel blockers; *IV,* intravenous; *NYHA,* New York Heart Association; *WHO,* World Health Organization. *(Data from Dincer HE, Presberg KW. Current management of pulmonary hypertension.* Clin Pulm Med. *2004;11:40-53.)*

vasoconstriction, vascular wall remodeling, and thrombosis in situ. Vasoconstrictor–vasodilator response imbalance and proliferation–apoptosis imbalance play an important role in the development of PAH and are the basis for current treatment strategies.

RV wall stress increases in response to the increase in afterload produced by pulmonary hypertension. RV stroke volume and thus the volume available for left ventricular filling is reduced, which leads to a reduction in cardiac output and *systemic hypotension.* RV dilation in response to increased wall stress results in annular dilation of right-sided heart valves, producing tricuspid regurgitation and/or pulmonic insufficiency. The right ventricle usually receives coronary blood flow during both systole and diastole. However, RV myocardial perfusion can be dramatically limited as RV wall stress increases and RV systolic pressure approaches systemic systolic blood pressure.

Patients with PAH are at risk of hypoxemia because of three mechanisms: (1) as right-sided pressures increase, right-to-left shunting can occur through a patent foramen ovale; (2) in the presence of a relatively fixed cardiac output, the increased oxygen extraction associated with exertion produces hypoxemia; and (3) ventilation/perfusion mismatch can result in perfusion of poorly ventilated alveoli. If hypoxic pulmonary vasoconstriction occurs, overall pulmonary hypertension will be worsened.

Treatment of Pulmonary Hypertension

A sample treatment algorithm is presented in Figure 5-8.

OXYGEN, ANTICOAGULATION, AND DIURETICS

Oxygen therapy can be helpful in reducing hypoxic pulmonary vasoconstriction. In patients with pulmonary hypertension, oxygen therapy improves survival and reduces progression of pulmonary hypertension. Anticoagulation may be recommended because of the increased risk of thrombosis and thromboembolism resulting from sluggish pulmonary blood flow, dilation of the right side of the heart, venous stasis, and limitations in physical activity imposed by this disease. Diuretics can be used to decrease preload in patients with right-sided heart failure, especially when hepatic congestion, ascites, and severe peripheral edema are present. A sodium-restricted diet is recommended, particularly in patients with RV failure. Routine influenza immunizations are also recommended.

CALCIUM CHANNEL BLOCKERS

The first class of drugs to provide dramatic long-term benefit in patients with PAH was calcium channel blockers. Calcium channel blockers are administered to patients who exhibit a positive response to a vasodilator trial in the cardiac catheterization laboratory. Nifedipine, diltiazem, and amlodipine are the most commonly used calcium channel blockers for this purpose and have been shown to improve 5-year survival.

PHOSPHODIESTERASE INHIBITORS

Phosphodiesterase inhibitors produce pulmonary vasodilation and improve cardiac output. Sildenafil (Viagra) administration has been associated with improved exercise capacity and reduction in RV mass, although long-term mortality benefits have not yet been proven. Tadalafil (Adcirca), a long-acting phosphodiesterase 5 inhibitor, is similarly well tolerated.

Phosphodiesterase inhibitors inhibit the hydrolysis of cyclic guanosine monophosphate (cGMP), reducing intracellular calcium concentration and producing smooth muscle relaxation. They are effective when given alone and can augment the efficacy of inhaled NO.

INHALED NITRIC OXIDE

Inhaled NO in concentrations of 20 to 40 ppm can be used to treat PAH. When inhaled, NO diffuses into vascular smooth muscle, where it activates guanylate cyclase; this increases intracellular cGMP, which reduces the intracellular calcium concentration and results in smooth muscle relaxation. After diffusing into the intravascular space, NO binds to hemoglobin-forming nitrosyl methemoglobin, which is rapidly metabolized to methemoglobin and excreted by the kidneys. All NO is rendered inactive in the pulmonary circulation, which eliminates systemic effects. Because it is administered via inhalation, NO is preferentially distributed to well-ventilated alveoli, causing vasodilation in these areas. This improves ventilation/perfusion matching and improves oxygenation. NO has been shown to increase oxygenation and lower pulmonary arterial pressure in acute respiratory distress syndrome and in other conditions associated with severe pulmonary hypertension, but it has not been shown to reduce mortality in these situations. Problems associated with NO administration include rebound pulmonary hypertension, platelet inhibition, methemoglobinemia, formation of toxic nitrate metabolites, and the complex technical requirements for its application.

PROSTACYCLINS

Prostacyclins are systemic and pulmonary vasodilators that also have antiplatelet activity. The prostacyclins reduce PVR and improve cardiac output and exercise tolerance. However, complications such as worsened intrapulmonary shunting, rebound pulmonary hypertension, systemic hypotension, infection, and bronchospasm can occur. Prostacyclins can be administered by continuous infusion in the short term and by a pump attached to a permanent indwelling central venous catheter for the long term, by inhalation, and by intermittent subcutaneous injection. All prostacyclins produce a significant improvement in cardiopulmonary hemodynamics, at least in the short term, but have not yet provided evidence of sustained improvement or a decrease in mortality. Currently used prostacyclins include epoprostenol (Flolan), treprostinil (Remodulin), and iloprost (Ventavis).

ENDOTHELIN RECEPTOR ANTAGONISTS

Endothelin interacts with two receptors: endothelin A receptors and endothelin B receptors. The endothelin A receptors cause pulmonary vasoconstriction and smooth muscle proliferation, whereas the endothelin B receptors produce vasodilation via enhanced endothelin clearance and increased production of NO and prostacyclin. Endothelin receptor antagonists have been shown to lower pulmonary artery pressure and PVR; to improve RV function, exercise tolerance, quality of life; and to reduce mortality. The only endothelin receptor antagonist currently available for general use in the United States is bosentan (Tracleer). Selective endothelin receptor A antagonists are under development.

SURGICAL TREATMENT

RV assist devices can be used in severe pulmonary hypertension and right-sided heart failure. Balloon atrial septostomy is an investigational procedure that creates an atrial septal defect and allows right-to-left shunting of blood to decompress the right side of the heart at the expense of an expected and generally well-tolerated decrease in arterial oxygen saturation. This has been shown to improve exercise tolerance. Currently, this procedure is reserved for treatment of terminal right-sided heart failure and as a bridge to cardiac transplantation. The benefits of extracorporeal membrane oxygenation are well established in children, but this modality has not found widespread use in the adult population. Lung transplantation is the only curative therapy for many types of PAH. Long-term survival is similar with single or bilateral lung transplantation.

Management of Anesthesia

The risk of right-sided heart failure is significantly increased during the perioperative period in patients with PAH. Mechanisms for this include increased RV afterload, hypoxemia, hypotension, and inadequate RV preload. Medications for

PAH should be continued throughout the perioperative period. Continuous infusions of pulmonary vasodilators should be maintained at their usual dosage to prevent rebound pulmonary hypertension. Diuretics may be needed to control edema, but excessive diuresis may dangerously reduce RV preload. Reduction of systemic vascular resistance by inhalational anesthetics or sedatives may be dangerous because of the relatively fixed cardiac output. Hypoxia, hypercarbia, and acidosis must be aggressively controlled because these conditions increase PVR. Maintenance of sinus rhythm is crucial. The atrial "kick" is necessary for adequate right and left ventricular filling.

PREOPERATIVE PREPARATION AND INDUCTION

In patients with newly diagnosed PAH who are not yet receiving long-term therapy, administration of sildenafil or L-arginine preoperatively may be helpful. In patients receiving long-term pulmonary vasodilator therapy, that therapy must be continued. Systems for inhalation of NO or prostacyclin should be available. Sedatives should be used with caution, because respiratory acidosis may increase PVR. Opioids, propofol, thiopental, and depolarizing and nondepolarizing neuromuscular blockers may all be used safely. Ketamine and etomidate may suppress some mechanisms of pulmonary vasorelaxation and should be avoided. Epidural anesthesia has been used for cesarean delivery and other suitable surgical procedures, but very close attention must be paid to intravascular volume and systemic vascular resistance in these situations. It is also important to remember that prostacyclins and NO can inhibit platelet function. If regional anesthesia is to be used, the block must be increased slowly to the required level and with invasive hemodynamic monitoring in place so cardiac parameters can be adjusted promptly.

MONITORING

Central venous catheterization is recommended, although care must be taken in the placement of central venous and pulmonary artery catheters because disruption of sinus rhythm by the catheter or wire can be a critical event. Intraarterial blood pressure monitoring is also recommended.

MAINTENANCE

Inhalational anesthetics, neuromuscular blockers, and opioids, except those associated with histamine release, can be used for maintenance of anesthesia. Hypotension can be corrected with norepinephrine, phenylephrine, or fluids. A potent pulmonary vasodilator such as milrinone, nitroglycerin, NO, or prostacyclin should be available to treat severe pulmonary hypertension should it develop. During mechanical ventilation, fluid balance and ventilator adjustments must be set to prevent a decrease in venous return.

POSTOPERATIVE PERIOD

Patients with PAH are at risk of sudden death in the early postoperative period because of worsening PAH, pulmonary thromboembolism, dysrhythmias, and fluid shifts. These patients must be monitored intensively in the postoperative period to help maintain hemodynamic parameters and oxygenation at acceptable levels. Optimal pain control is an essential component of the postoperative care of these patients.

OBSTETRIC POPULATION

The hemodynamic changes during pregnancy, labor, delivery, and the postpartum period can have a significant impact in patients with pulmonary hypertension.

Forceps delivery to decrease patient effort is recommended. Nitroglycerin should be immediately available at the time of uterine involution, because the return of uterine blood to the central circulation may be poorly tolerated in a parturient with PAH.

KEY POINTS

- Hypertension is a significant risk factor for cardiovascular disease, stroke, and renal disease. Tight control of blood pressure has well-documented beneficial effects. The goal of antihypertensive therapy is to decrease the systemic blood pressure to less than 140/90 mm Hg.

- Hypertensive patients coming for surgery pose management dilemmas for the anesthesiologist. However, the relationship between hypertension and perioperative complications is unclear, and clinical practices vary widely.

- Preoperative evaluation of a patient with essential hypertension should focus on the adequacy of blood pressure control, the antihypertensive drug regimen, and the presence of target organ damage.

- Despite the prevailing desire to render patients normotensive before elective surgery, there is no evidence that the incidence of postoperative complications is increased when hypertensive patients (diastolic blood pressure as high as 110 mm Hg) undergo elective surgery. However, hypertension associated with end-organ damage does increase surgical risk.

- Hypotension requiring vasoconstrictor treatment occurs more often after induction of anesthesia in patients receiving long-term treatment with ACE inhibitors and ARBs than in those in whom such treatment has been discontinued on the day before surgery.

- Direct laryngoscopy and endotracheal intubation may result in a significant increase in blood pressure in patients with essential hypertension, even in those patients who have been treated with antihypertensive drugs and are rendered normotensive preoperatively.

- PAH is hemodynamically defined as a mean pulmonary artery pressure of more than 25 mm Hg at rest.

- Smooth muscle hyperplasia, intimal fibrosis, medial hypertrophy, obliteration of small blood vessels, and neoplastic forms of endothelial cell growth called *plexiform lesions* are all part of the pathophysiology of pulmonary hypertension. In addition, platelet function is enhanced, and in situ thrombosis is a common finding.

■ NO diffuses into vascular smooth muscle, where it activates guanylate cyclase, increasing intracellular cGMP; this reduces the intracellular calcium concentration, which results in smooth muscle relaxation.

■ Calcium channel blockers, prostacyclins, NO, endothelin receptor blockers, and phosphodiesterase inhibitors are all pulmonary vasodilators that are useful in the treatment of patients with PAH. All long-term pulmonary vasodilator therapy must be continued throughout the perioperative period.

■ In the perioperative period, the risk of right-sided heart failure or sudden death is significantly increased in patients with PAH. This may be due to increased RV afterload, inadequate RV preload, hypoxemia, hypotension, dysrhythmias, or pulmonary thromboembolism.

RESOURCES

Aronow WS, Fleg JL, Pepine CJ, et al. ACCF/AHA 2011 expert consensus document on hypertension in the elderly: a report of the American College of Cardiology Foundation Task Force on Clinical Expert Consensus documents developed in collaboration with the American Academy of Neurology, American Geriatrics Society, American Society for Preventive Cardiology, American Society of Hypertension, American Society of Nephrology, Association of Black Cardiologists, and European Society of Hypertension. *J Am Coll Cardiol*. 2011;57:2037-2114.

Chobanian AV, Bakris GL, Black HR, et al. Joint National Committee on Prevention, Detection, Evaluation, and Treatment of High Blood Pressure; National Heart, Lung, and Blood Institute; National High Blood Pressure Education Program Coordinating Committee. Seventh report of the Joint National Committee on Prevention, Detection, Evaluation, and Treatment of High Blood Pressure (JNC 7). *Hypertension*. 2003;42:1206-1252.

Goldman L, Caldera DL. Risks of general anesthesia and elective operation in the hypertensive patient. *Anesthesiology*. 1979;50:285-292.

Hanada S, Kawakami H, Goto T, et al. Hypertension and anesthesia. *Curr Opin Anesth*. 2006;19:315-319.

Humbert M, Sitbon O, Chaouat A, et al. Pulmonary arterial hypertension in France: results from a national registry. *Am J Respir Crit Care Med*. 2006;173:1023-1030.

Marik PE, Varon JV. Perioperative hypertension: a review of current and emerging therapeutic agents. *J Clin Anesth*. 2009;21:220-229.

McLaughlin VV, Archer SL, Badesch DB, et al. American College of Cardiology Foundation Task Force on Expert Consensus Documents; American Heart Association; American College of Chest Physicians; American Thoracic Society, Inc; Pulmonary Hypertension Association: ACCF/AHA 2009 expert consensus document on pulmonary hypertension. *J Am Coll Cardiol*. 2009;53:1573-1619.

Ramakrishna G, Sprung J, Ravi BS, et al. Impact of pulmonary hypertension on the outcomes of noncardiac surgery: Predictors of perioperative morbidity and mortality. *J Am Coll Cardiol*. 2005;45:1691-1699.

Stone JG, Foex P, Sear JW, et al. Risk of myocardial ischaemia during anaesthesia in treated and untreated hypertensive patients. *Br J Anaesth*. 1988;61:675-679.

CHAPTER 6

Heart Failure and Cardiomyopathies

WANDA M. POPESCU ■

HEART FAILURE

Definition

Heart failure is a complex pathophysiologic state characterized by the inability of the heart to fill with or eject blood at a rate appropriate to meet tissue requirements. Symptoms of dyspnea and fatigue and signs of circulatory congestion and/or hypoperfusion are the clinical features of the heart failure syndrome.

Epidemiology and Costs

Heart failure is a major health problem in the United States, affecting about 5.8 million adults. Each year an additional 670,000 patients are diagnosed with heart failure. Heart failure is mainly a disease of the elderly, so aging of the population is contributing to its increased incidence. The incidence of heart failure approaches 10 per 1000 in the population aged 65 or older. Systolic heart failure is more common among middle-aged men because of its association with coronary artery disease. Diastolic heart failure is usually seen in elderly women because of its association with hypertension, obesity, and diabetes after menopause.

Heart failure is the most common Medicare hospital discharge diagnosis. More Medicare dollars are spent on the diagnosis and treatment of heart failure than on any other disease. It is estimated that the annual total direct and indirect cost of heart failure in the United States is $38 billion.

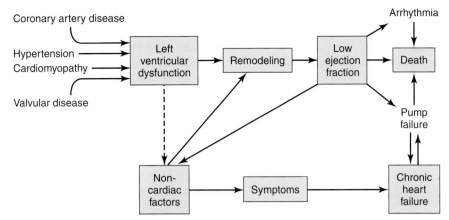

FIGURE 6-1 Left ventricular dysfunction, regardless of cause, results in progressive remodeling of the ventricular chamber leading to dilation and a low ejection fraction. Cardiac dysrhythmias, progressive cardiac failure, and premature death are likely. Non-cardiac factors such as neurohormonal stimulation, vasoconstriction, and renal sodium retention may be stimulated by left ventricular dysfunction and ultimately contribute to remodeling of the left ventricle and to the symptoms (dyspnea, fatigue, edema) considered characteristic of the clinical syndrome of congestive heart failure. *(Adapted from Cohn JN. The management of chronic heart failure.* N Engl J Med. *1996;335:490-498. Copyright 1996 Massachusetts Medical Society. All rights reserved.)*

Etiology

Heart failure is a clinical syndrome arising from diverse causes. The principal pathophysiologic feature of heart failure is the inability of the heart to fill or empty the ventricles. Heart failure is most often a result of (1) impaired myocardial contractility caused by ischemic heart disease or cardiomyopathy, (2) cardiac valve abnormalities, (3) systemic hypertension, (4) diseases of the pericardium, or (5) pulmonary hypertension (cor pulmonale). The most common cause of right ventricular failure is left ventricular (LV) failure.

FORMS OF VENTRICULAR DYSFUNCTION

Heart failure may be described in various ways: systolic or diastolic, acute or chronic, left sided or right sided, high output or low output. Early in the course of heart failure, the various categories may have different clinical and therapeutic implications. Ultimately, however, all forms of heart failure are characterized by high ventricular end-diastolic pressure because of altered ventricular function and neurohormonal regulation.

Systolic and Diastolic Heart Failure

Decreased ventricular systolic wall motion reflects systolic dysfunction, whereas diastolic dysfunction is characterized by abnormal ventricular relaxation and reduced compliance. There are differences in both myocardial architecture and function in systolic and diastolic heart failure, but clinical signs and symptoms cannot reliably differentiate between these two entities.

SYSTOLIC HEART FAILURE

Causes of systolic heart failure include coronary artery disease, dilated cardiomyopathy, chronic pressure overload (aortic stenosis and chronic hypertension), and chronic volume overload (regurgitant valvular lesions and high-output cardiac failure). Coronary disease typically results in regional defects in ventricular contraction, which may become global over time, whereas all other causes of systolic heart failure produce global ventricular dysfunction. Ventricular dysrhythmias are common in patients with LV dysfunction. Patients with left bundle branch block and systolic heart failure are at high risk of sudden death.

A decreased ejection fraction, the hallmark of chronic LV systolic dysfunction, is closely related to the increase in the diastolic volume of the LV (Figure 6-1). Measuring the LV ejection fraction via echocardiography, radionuclide imaging, or ventriculography provides the quantification necessary to document the severity of ventricular systolic dysfunction.

DIASTOLIC HEART FAILURE

Symptomatic heart failure in patients with normal or near-normal LV systolic function is most likely due to diastolic dysfunction. However, diastolic heart failure may co-exist with systolic heart failure. The prevalence of diastolic heart failure is age dependent, increasing from less than 15% in patients younger than 45 years of age to 35% in those between the ages of 50 and 70 to more than 50% in patients older than 70 years. Diastolic heart failure can be classified into four stages. Class I is characterized by an abnormal LV relaxation pattern with normal left atrial pressure. Classes II, III, and IV are characterized by abnormal relaxation as well as reduced LV compliance resulting in an increase in LV end-diastolic pressure (LVEDP). As a compensatory mechanism, the pressure in the left atrium increases so that LV filling can occur despite the increase in LVEDP. Factors that predispose to decreased ventricular distensibility include myocardial edema, fibrosis, hypertrophy, aging, and pressure overload. Ischemic heart disease,

TABLE 6-1   Characteristics of patients with diastolic heart failure and patients with systolic heart failure

Characteristic	Diastolic heart failure	Systolic heart failure
Age	Frequently elderly	Typically 50-70 yr
Sex	Frequently female	More often male
Left ventricular ejection fraction	Preserved, ≥40%	Depressed, ≤40%
Left ventricular cavity size	Usually normal, often with concentric left ventricular hypertrophy	Usually dilated
Chest radiograph	Congestion ± cardiomegaly	Congestion and cardiomegaly
Gallop rhythm present	Fourth heart sound	Third heart sound
Hypertension	+++	++
Diabetes mellitus	+++	++
Previous myocardial infarction	+	+++
Obesity	+++	+
Chronic lung disease	++	0
Sleep apnea	++	++
Dialysis	++	0
Atrial fibrillation	+	+
	Usually paroxysmal	Usually persistent

+, Occasionally associated with; ++, often associated with; +++, usually associated with; 0, no association.

long-standing essential hypertension, and progressive aortic stenosis are the most common causes of diastolic heart failure. In contrast to systolic heart failure, diastolic heart failure affects women more than men. Hospitalization and mortality rates are similar in patients with systolic and with diastolic heart failure. The major differences between systolic and diastolic heart failure are presented in Table 6-1.

Acute and Chronic Heart Failure

Acute heart failure is defined as a change in the signs and symptoms of heart failure requiring emergency therapy. Chronic heart failure is present in patients with long-standing cardiac disease. Typically, chronic heart failure is accompanied by venous congestion, but blood pressure is maintained. In acute heart failure due to a sudden decrease in cardiac output, systemic hypotension is typically present without signs of peripheral edema. Acute heart failure encompasses three clinical entities: (1) worsening chronic heart failure, (2) new-onset heart failure (such as that caused by cardiac valve rupture, large myocardial infarction, or severe hypertensive crisis), and (3) terminal heart failure that is refractory to therapy.

Left-Sided and Right-Sided Heart Failure

Increased ventricular pressures and subsequent fluid accumulation upstream from the affected ventricle produce the clinical signs and symptoms of heart failure. In left-sided heart failure, high LVEDP promotes pulmonary venous congestion. The patient complains of dyspnea, orthopnea, and paroxysmal nocturnal dyspnea, which can evolve into pulmonary edema. Right-sided heart failure causes systemic venous congestion. Peripheral edema and congestive hepatomegaly are the most prominent clinical manifestations. Right-sided heart failure may be caused by pulmonary hypertension or right ventricular myocardial infarction, but the most common cause is left-sided heart failure.

Low-Output and High-Output Heart Failure

The normal *cardiac index* varies between 2.2 and 3.5 L/min/m². It may be difficult to diagnose low-output heart failure, because a patient may have a cardiac index that is nearly normal in the resting state but shows an inadequate response to stress or exercise. The most common causes of low-output heart failure are coronary artery disease, cardiomyopathy, hypertension, valvular disease, and pericardial disease.

Causes of high cardiac output include anemia, pregnancy, arteriovenous fistulas, severe hyperthyroidism, beriberi, and Paget's disease. The ventricles fail not only due to the increased hemodynamic burden, but also due to direct myocardial toxicity (thyrotoxicosis and beriberi) or due to myocardial anoxia caused by severe and prolonged anemia.

PATHOPHYSIOLOGY OF HEART FAILURE

Heart failure is a complex phenomenon at both the clinical and cellular levels. Our understanding of the pathophysiology of heart failure is in evolution. The initiating mechanisms of heart failure are pressure overload (aortic stenosis, essential hypertension), volume overload (mitral or aortic regurgitation), myocardial ischemia or infarction, myocardial inflammatory disease, and restricted diastolic filling (constrictive pericarditis, restrictive myocarditis). In the failing ventricle, various adaptive mechanisms are initiated to help maintain a normal cardiac output. These include (1) increases in stroke volume according to the Frank-Starling relationship; (2) activation of the sympathetic nervous system; (3) alterations in the inotropic state, heart rate, and afterload; and (4) humorally mediated responses. In more advanced stages of heart failure, these mechanisms become maladaptive and ultimately lead to *myocardial remodeling*, which is the key pathophysiologic change responsible for the development and progression of heart failure.

Frank-Starling Relationship

The Frank-Starling relationship describes the increase in stroke volume that accompanies an increase in LV end-diastolic volume and pressure (Figure 6-2). Stroke volume

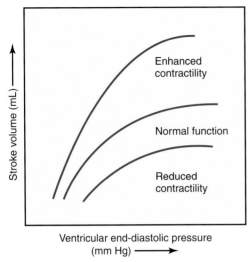

FIGURE 6-2 The Frank-Starling relationship states that stroke volume is directly related to ventricular end-diastolic pressure.

increases because the tension developed by contracting muscle is greater when the resting length of that muscle is increased. Constriction of venous capacitance vessels shifts blood centrally, increases preload, and helps maintain cardiac output by the Frank-Starling relationship. The magnitude of the increase in stroke volume produced by changing the tension of ventricular muscle fibers depends on myocardial contractility. When myocardial contractility is decreased, as in the presence of heart failure, a lesser increase in stroke volume is achieved relative to any given increase in LVEDP.

Activation of the Sympathetic Nervous System

Activation of the sympathetic nervous system promotes arteriolar and venous constriction. Arteriolar constriction serves to maintain systemic blood pressure despite a decrease in cardiac output. Increased venous tone shifts blood from peripheral sites to the central circulation, thereby enhancing venous return and maintaining cardiac output by the Frank-Starling relationship. Furthermore, arteriolar constriction causes redistribution of blood from the kidneys, splanchnic organs, skeletal muscles, and skin to maintain coronary and cerebral blood flow despite an overall decrease in cardiac output. The decrease in renal blood flow activates the renin-angiotensin-aldosterone system (RAAS), which increases renal tubular reabsorption of sodium and water and thus results in an increase in blood volume and ultimately cardiac output by the Frank-Starling relationship. These compensatory responses may be effective in the short term, but they contribute to the deterioration of heart failure in the long term. For example, fluid retention, increased venous return, and increased afterload can impose more work on the failing myocardium, increase myocardial energy expenditure, and further reduce cardiac output and tissue perfusion. Interruption of this vicious circle is the purpose of the current therapeutic strategies for heart failure.

Although heart failure is associated with sympathetic activation, a downregulation of β-adrenergic receptors is observed. Plasma and urinary concentrations of catecholamines are increased in patients in heart failure, and elevated levels correlate with worse clinical outcomes. High plasma levels of norepinephrine are directly cardiotoxic and promote myocyte necrosis and cell death, which lead to ventricular remodeling. Therapy with β-blockers is aimed at decreasing the deleterious effects of catecholamines on the heart.

Alterations in the Inotropic State, Heart Rate, and Afterload

The inotropic state describes myocardial contractility as reflected by the velocity of contraction developed by cardiac muscle. The maximum velocity of contraction is referred to as V_{max}. When the inotropic state of the heart is increased, as in the presence of catecholamines, V_{max} is increased. Conversely, V_{max} is decreased when myocardial contractility is impaired, as in heart failure.

Afterload is the tension the ventricular muscle must develop to open the aortic or pulmonic valve. The afterload presented to the left ventricle is increased in the presence of systemic arteriolar constriction and hypertension. Administration of vasodilating drugs can increase forward LV stroke volume in patients with heart failure.

In the presence of systolic heart failure and low cardiac output, stroke volume is relatively fixed, and any increase in cardiac output depends on an increase in heart rate. Tachycardia is an expected finding in the presence of systolic heart failure with a low ejection fraction and reflects activation of the sympathetic nervous system. In the presence of diastolic heart failure, however, tachycardia can produce a decrease in cardiac output resulting from inadequate ventricular relaxation and filling time. Therefore, heart rate control is an important goal in the treatment of diastolic heart failure.

Humorally Mediated Responses and Biochemical Pathways

As heart failure progresses, various neurohumoral pathways are activated to maintain adequate cardiac output during exercise and ultimately even at rest. Generalized vasoconstriction is initiated via several mechanisms, including increased activity of the sympathetic nervous system and the RAAS, parasympathetic withdrawal, high levels of circulating vasopressin, endothelial dysfunction, and release of inflammatory mediators.

In an attempt to counterbalance these mechanisms, the heart evolves into an "endocrine" organ. This concept emerged more than 20 years ago when the presence of a potent diuretic and vasodilator in the atria of rats was first reported. Atrial natriuretic peptide (ANP) is stored in atrial muscle and released in response to increases in atrial pressure, such as are produced by tachycardia or hypervolemia. B-type natriuretic peptide (BNP) is secreted by both the atrial and ventricular myocardium. In the failing heart, the ventricle becomes the principal site of BNP production. The natriuretic peptides promote blood pressure control and protect the cardiovascular system from the effects of volume and pressure overload. Physiologic effects of the natriuretic peptides include diuresis, natriuresis, vasodilation, antiinflammatory effect, and inhibition of the RAAS and the sympathetic nervous system. Both ANP and BNP inhibit cardiac hypertrophy and fibrosis and therefore limit remodeling. The response to elevated levels of *endogenous* natriuretic peptides is blunted over time in heart failure. However, *exogenous* administration of BNP can be useful in the treatment of acute heart failure. More recently, other protective neurohumoral pathways have been described. Chromogranin A and its derived peptides catestatin and vasostatin appear to counteract the negative myocardial effects of excessive sympathetic stimulation seen in heart failure states.

Myocardial Remodeling

Myocardial remodeling is the result of the various endogenous mechanisms that the body uses to maintain cardiac output. It is the process by which mechanical, neurohormonal, and genetic factors change LV size, shape, and function. The process includes myocardial hypertrophy, myocardial dilation and wall thinning, increased interstitial collagen deposition, myocardial fibrosis, and scar formation resulting from myocyte death. Myocardial hypertrophy represents the compensatory mechanism for chronic pressure overload. The effects of this mechanism are limited because hypertrophied cardiac muscle functions at a lower inotropic state than normal cardiac muscle. Cardiac dilation occurs in response to volume overload and increases cardiac output by the Frank-Starling relationship. However, the increased cardiac wall tension produced by an enlarged ventricular radius is associated with increased myocardial oxygen requirements and decreased pumping efficiency. Ischemic injury is the most common cause of myocardial remodeling and encompasses both hypertrophy and dilation of the left ventricle. Angiotensin-converting enzyme (ACE) inhibitors and aldosterone inhibitors (spironolactone and eplerenone) have been proven to promote a "reverse-remodeling" process. Therefore, they are indicated as first-line therapy for heart failure. Several studies have documented that cardiac resynchronization therapy has beneficial reverse-remodeling effects not only in patients with advanced heart failure, but also in patients with milder forms of disease who exhibit wide QRS complexes.

SIGNS AND SYMPTOMS OF HEART FAILURE

The hemodynamic consequences of heart failure include a decreased cardiac output, increased LVEDP, peripheral vasoconstriction, retention of sodium and water, and decreased oxygen delivery to the tissues with a widened arterial-venous oxygen difference. LV failure results in signs and symptoms of pulmonary edema, whereas right ventricular failure results in systemic venous hypertension and peripheral edema. Fatigue and organ system dysfunction are related to inadequate cardiac output.

Symptoms

Dyspnea reflects increased work of breathing caused by stiffness of the lungs produced by interstitial pulmonary edema. It is one of the earliest subjective findings of LV failure and initially occurs only with exertion. Dyspnea can be quantified by asking the patient how many flights of stairs can be climbed or the distance that can be walked at a normal pace before symptoms begin. Some patients experiencing angina pectoris may interpret substernal discomfort as breathlessness. Dyspnea can be caused by many other diseases, including asthma, chronic obstructive pulmonary disease (COPD), airway obstruction, anxiety, and neuromuscular weakness. Dyspnea related to heart failure will be linked to other supporting evidence, such as a history of orthopnea, paroxysmal nocturnal dyspnea, a third heart sound, rales on physical examination, and elevated BNP levels.

Orthopnea reflects the inability of the failing LV to handle the increased venous return associated with the recumbent position. Clinically, orthopnea is manifested as a dry, nonproductive cough that develops in the supine position and is relieved by sitting up. The orthopneic cough differs from the productive morning cough characteristic of chronic bronchitis and must be differentiated from the cough produced by ACE inhibitors. Paroxysmal nocturnal dyspnea is shortness of breath that awakens a patient from sleep. This symptom must be differentiated from anxiety-provoked hyperventilation or wheezing resulting from accumulation of secretions in patients with chronic bronchitis. Paroxysmal nocturnal dyspnea and wheezing caused by pulmonary congestion (cardiac asthma) are accompanied by radiographic evidence of pulmonary congestion.

Hallmarks of decreased cardiac reserve and low cardiac output include fatigue and weakness at rest or with minimal exertion. During exercise, the failing ventricle is unable to increase its output to deliver adequate amounts of oxygen to muscles. These symptoms, although nonspecific, are very common in patients with heart failure.

Heart failure patients may complain of anorexia, nausea, or abdominal pain related to liver congestion or prerenal azotemia. Decreases in cerebral blood flow may produce confusion, difficulty concentrating, insomnia, anxiety, or memory deficits.

Physical Examination Findings

The classic physical findings of patients with LV failure are tachypnea and the presence of moist rales. These rales may be confined to the lung bases in patients with mild heart failure, or they may be diffuse in those with pulmonary edema. Other findings of heart failure include a resting tachycardia and a third heart sound (S_3 gallop or ventricular diastolic gallop).

This heart sound is produced by blood entering and distending a relatively noncompliant left ventricle. Despite peripheral vasoconstriction, severe heart failure may manifest as *systemic hypotension* with cool and pale extremities. Lip and nail bed cyanosis may be present. A narrow pulse pressure with a high diastolic pressure reflects a decreased stroke volume. Marked weight loss, also known as *cardiac cachexia,* is a sign of severe chronic heart failure. Weight loss is caused by a combination of factors, including an increase in the metabolic rate, anorexia, nausea, decreased intestinal absorption of food because of splanchnic venous congestion, and the presence of high levels of circulating cytokines.

With right-sided heart failure or biventricular failure, jugular venous distention may be present or may be inducible by pressing on the liver (hepatojugular reflux). The liver is typically the first organ to become engorged with blood in the presence of right-sided or biventricular failure. The hepatic engorgement may be associated with right upper quadrant pain and tenderness or even jaundice in severe cases. Pleural effusions (usually right sided) may be present. Bilateral pitting pretibial edema is typically present with right ventricular failure and reflects both venous congestion and sodium and water retention.

DIAGNOSIS OF HEART FAILURE

The diagnosis of heart failure is based on the history, physical examination findings, and results of laboratory and diagnostic tests.

Laboratory Tests

The differential diagnosis of dyspnea continues to be challenging both in the urgent/emergent and in the primary care setting. The use of serum levels of BNP and its associated N-terminal fragment NT-proBNP as biomarkers for heart failure can help in establishing the cause of dyspnea. Plasma BNP levels below 100 pg/mL indicate that heart failure is unlikely (90% negative predictive value). BNP levels in the range of 100 to 500 pg/mL suggest an intermediate probability of heart failure. Levels higher than 500 pg/mL are consistent with the diagnosis of heart failure (90% positive predictive value). An NT-proBNP level of 300 pg/mL appears to be a sensitive cutoff point for detecting dyspnea of cardiac origin. Plasma levels of BNP and NT-proBNP may be affected by other factors such as gender, advanced age, renal function, obesity, pulmonary embolism, and atrial fibrillation and other cardiac tachydysrhythmias. Therefore, the interpretation of BNP levels requires a clinical context.

A complete metabolic profile should be obtained in the evaluation of patients with heart failure. Decreases in renal blood flow may lead to prerenal azotemia characterized by a disproportionate increase in blood urea nitrogen concentration relative to serum creatinine concentration. When moderate liver congestion is present, liver enzyme levels may be mildly elevated, and when liver engorgement is severe, the prothrombin time may be prolonged. Hyponatremia, hypomagnesemia, and hypokalemia may also be present.

Electrocardiography

Patients with heart failure usually have abnormalities on the 12-lead electrocardiogram (ECG). Therefore, this test has a low predictive value for the diagnosis of heart failure. The ECG may show evidence of previous myocardial infarction, LV hypertrophy, conduction abnormalities (left bundle branch block, widened QRS), or various cardiac dysrhythmias, especially atrial fibrillation and ventricular dysrhythmias.

Chest Radiography

Chest radiography (posteroanterior and lateral views) may detect the presence of pulmonary disease, cardiomegaly, pulmonary venous congestion, and interstitial or alveolar pulmonary edema. An early radiographic sign of LV failure and associated pulmonary venous hypertension is distention of the pulmonary veins in the upper lobes of the lungs. Perivascular edema appears as hilar or perihilar haze. The hilus appears large with ill-defined margins. Kerley's lines, which reflect edematous interlobular septae in the upper lung fields (Kerley's A lines), lower lung fields (Kerley's B lines), or basilar regions of the lungs (Kerley's C lines) and produce a honeycomb pattern, may also be present. Alveolar edema produces homogeneous densities in the lung fields, typically in a butterfly pattern. Pleural effusion and pericardial effusion may be observed. Radiographic evidence of pulmonary edema may lag behind the clinical evidence of pulmonary edema by up to 12 hours. Likewise, radiographic patterns of pulmonary congestion may persist for several days after normalization of cardiac filling pressures and resolution of symptoms.

Echocardiography

Echocardiography is the most useful test in the diagnosis of heart failure. Comprehensive two-dimensional echocardiography coupled with Doppler flow examination can assess whether any abnormalities of the myocardium, cardiac valves, or pericardium are present. This examination evaluates LV and RV structure and function (systolic and diastolic) as well as valvular function, and detects the presence of pericardial disease. This information is presented as numerical estimates of ejection fraction, LV size and wall thickness, left atrial size, and pulmonary artery pressures as well as a description of anatomic structures and wall motion. Assessment of diastolic function provides information regarding LV filling and left atrial pressure. A preoperative echocardiographic evaluation provides information useful in guiding perioperative management and serves as a baseline for comparison if the patient's condition changes.

CLASSIFICATION OF HEART FAILURE

Heart failure has been classified in various ways. The most commonly used classification is that of the New York Heart Association (NYHA) and is based on the functional status of the patient at a particular time. Functional status may worsen or improve. The classification is intended for patients who have structural heart disease and symptoms of heart failure. There are four functional classes:

Class I: Ordinary physical activity does not cause symptoms
Class II: Symptoms occur with ordinary exertion
Class III: Symptoms occur with less than ordinary exertion
Class IV: Symptoms occur at rest

This classification is useful because the severity of the symptoms has an excellent correlation with quality of life and survival. However, the American College of Cardiology (ACC) and the American Heart Association (AHA) published the 2005 Guideline Update for the Diagnosis and Management of Chronic Heart Failure and introduced a new classification based on the progression of the disease. This classification stratifies patients into one of four disease stages:

Stage A: Patients at high risk of heart failure but without structural heart disease or symptoms of heart failure
Stage B: Patients with structural heart disease but without symptoms of heart failure
Stage C: Patients with structural heart disease with previous or current symptoms of heart failure
Stage D: Patients with refractory heart failure requiring specialized interventions

This classification is meant to be complementary to the NYHA classification and to be used in guiding therapy.

MANAGEMENT OF HEART FAILURE

Current therapeutic strategies are aimed at reversing the pathophysiologic alterations present in heart failure and at interrupting the vicious circle of maladaptive mechanisms (Figure 6-3). Short-term therapeutic goals in patients with heart failure include relieving symptoms of circulatory congestion, increasing tissue perfusion, and improving quality of life. However, management of heart failure involves more than symptomatic treatment. The processes that contributed to the LV dysfunction may progress independently of the development of symptoms. Therefore, the long-term therapeutic goal is to prolong life by slowing or reversing the progression of ventricular remodeling.

Management of Chronic Heart Failure

Current therapeutic protocols are based on the results of large, adequately powered, randomized trials and on the ACC/AHA and European Society of Cardiology guidelines for the diagnosis and treatment of chronic heart failure. According to these guidelines, treatment options include lifestyle modification, patient and family education, medical therapy, corrective surgery, implantation of cardiac devices, and cardiac transplantation (Figure 6-4).

Lifestyle modifications are aimed at decreasing the risk of heart disease and include smoking cessation, adherence to a healthy diet with moderate sodium restriction, weight control,

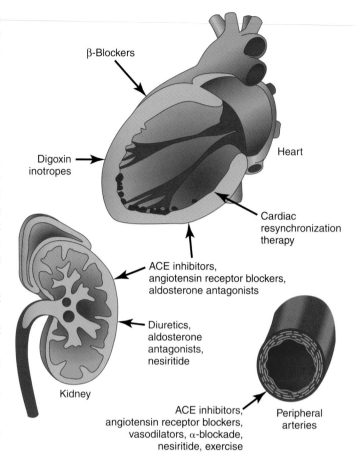

FIGURE 6-3 Primary targets of treatment in heart failure. Treatment options for patients with heart failure affect the pathophysiologic mechanisms that are stimulated in heart failure. Angiotensin-converting enzyme (ACE) inhibitors and angiotensin II receptor blockers decrease afterload by interfering with the renin-angiotensin-aldosterone system, which results in peripheral vasodilation. They also affect left ventricular hypertrophy, remodeling, and renal blood flow. Aldosterone production by the adrenal glands is increased in heart failure. It stimulates renal sodium retention and potassium excretion and promotes ventricular and vascular hypertrophy. Aldosterone antagonists counteract the many effects of aldosterone. Diuretics decrease preload by stimulating natriuresis in the kidneys. Digoxin affects the sodium–potassium–adenosine triphosphatase (Na^+,K^+-ATPase) pump in the myocardial cell, increasing contractility. Inotropes such as dobutamine and milrinone increase myocardial contractility. β-Blockers inhibit the sympathetic nervous system and adrenergic receptors. They slow the heart rate, decrease blood pressure, and have a direct beneficial effect on the myocardium by enhancing reverse remodeling. Selected agents that also block α-adrenergic receptors can cause vasodilation. Vasodilator therapy such as combination therapy with hydralazine and isosorbide dinitrate decreases afterload by counteracting peripheral vasoconstriction. Cardiac resynchronization therapy with biventricular pacing improves left ventricular function and favors reverse remodeling. Nesiritide (B-type natriuretic peptide) decreases preload by stimulating diuresis and decreases afterload by vasodilation. Exercise improves peripheral blood flow by eventually counteracting peripheral vasoconstriction. It also improves skeletal muscle physiology. *(Reproduced with permission from Jessup M, Brozena S. Heart failure.* N Engl J Med. *2003;348:2007-2018. Copyright © 2003 Massachusetts Medical Society. All rights reserved.)*

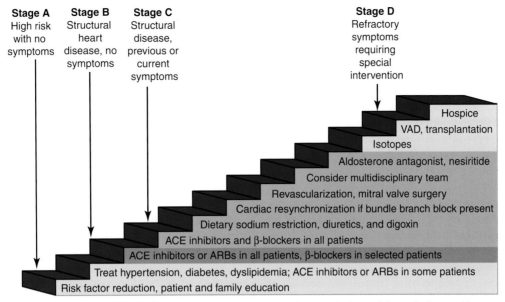

Stage A
High risk with no symptoms

Stage B
Structural heart disease, no symptoms

Stage C
Structural disease, previous or current symptoms

Stage D
Refractory symptoms requiring special intervention

Hospice
VAD, transplantation
Isotopes
Aldosterone antagonist, nesiritide
Consider multidisciplinary team
Revascularization, mitral valve surgery
Cardiac resynchronization if bundle branch block present
Dietary sodium restriction, diuretics, and digoxin
ACE inhibitors and β-blockers in all patients
ACE inhibitors or ARBs in all patients, β-blockers in selected patients
Treat hypertension, diabetes, dyslipidemia; ACE inhibitors or ARBs in some patients
Risk factor reduction, patient and family education

FIGURE 6-4 Stages of heart failure and treatment options for systolic heart failure. Patients with stage A heart failure are at high risk of heart failure but do not yet have structural heart disease or symptoms of heart failure. This group includes patients with hypertension, diabetes, coronary artery disease, previous exposure to cardiotoxic drugs, or a family history of cardiomyopathy. Patients with stage B heart failure have structural heart disease but no symptoms of heart failure. This group includes patients with left ventricular hypertrophy, previous myocardial infarction, left ventricular systolic dysfunction, or valvular heart disease, all of whom would be considered to have New York Heart Association (NYHA) class I symptoms. Patients with stage C heart failure have known structural heart disease and current or previous symptoms of heart failure. Their current symptoms may be classified as NYHA class I, II, III, or IV. Patients with stage D heart failure have refractory symptoms of heart failure at rest despite maximal medical therapy, are hospitalized, and require specialized interventions or hospice care. All such patients would be considered to have NYHA class IV symptoms. *ACE,* Angiotensin-converting enzyme; *ARB,* angiotensin receptor blocker; *VAD,* ventricular assist device. *(Reproduced with permission from Jessup M, Brozena S. Heart failure. N Engl J Med. 2003;348:2007-2018. Copyright © 2003 Massachusetts Medical Society. All rights reserved.)*

exercise, moderation of alcohol consumption, and adequate glycemic control.

Management of Systolic Heart Failure

The major classes of drugs used for medical management of systolic heart failure include inhibitors of the RAAS, β-blockers, diuretics, digoxin, vasodilators, and statins. Most heart failure patients are treated with a combination of drugs. Therapy with ACE inhibitors and β-blockers favorably influences long-term outcome.

INHIBITORS OF THE RENIN-ANGIOTENSIN-ALDOSTERONE SYSTEM

Inhibition of the RAAS can be performed at several levels: by inhibiting the enzyme that converts angiotensin I to angiotensin II, by blocking the angiotensin II receptor, or by blocking the aldosterone receptor.

Angiotensin-Converting Enzyme Inhibitors

ACE inhibitors block the conversion of angiotensin I to angiotensin II. This decreases the activation of the RAAS and decreases the degradation of bradykinin. Beneficial effects include promoting vasodilation, reducing water and sodium reabsorption, and supporting potassium conservation. This class of drugs has been proven to decrease ventricular remodeling and even to potentiate the reverse-remodeling phenomenon. In large clinical trials, ACE inhibitors have consistently been shown to reduce morbidity and mortality in patients at any stage of heart failure. For this reason, they are considered the first line of treatment in heart failure. It appears, however, that the African American population does not derive as much clinical benefit from ACE inhibitor therapy as does the white population. Side effects of ACE inhibitors include hypotension, syncope, renal dysfunction, hyperkalemia, and development of a nonproductive cough and/or angioedema. Treatment with ACE inhibitors should be started at low dosages to avoid significant hypotension. Then the dosage can be gradually increased until the target dosage is reached.

Angiotensin II Receptor Blockers

As their name implies, angiotensin receptor blockers block angiotensin II receptors. The efficacy of these drugs is similar but not superior to that of ACE inhibitors. Currently, angiotensin receptor blockers are recommended only for patients who cannot tolerate ACE inhibitors. In some patients treated with ACE inhibitors, angiotensin levels may gradually return to normal due to alternative pathways of angiotensin production. Such patients may benefit from the addition of an angiotensin receptor blocker to their medical therapy.

Aldosterone Antagonists

In advanced stages of heart failure, there are high circulating levels of aldosterone. Aldosterone stimulates sodium and water retention, hypokalemia, and ventricular remodeling. Aldosterone antagonists reverse all of these effects and therefore improve the cardiovascular milieu in patients with heart failure. There is strong clinical evidence showing reduced mortality and hospitalization rates with use of a low dosage of an aldosterone antagonist in patients with NYHA class III or IV heart failure. More recently, eplerenone has been demonstrated to reduce the rate of death from cardiovascular events and the number of hospitalizations related to heart failure even in patients with NYHA class II heart failure. In patients being treated with aldosterone antagonists renal function and potassium levels should be monitored and the medication dosage adjusted accordingly. Currently it is recommended that aldosterone antagonists be incorporated as first-line therapy in *all* patients with heart failure.

β-BLOCKERS

β-Blockers are used to reverse the harmful effects of sympathetic nervous system activation in heart failure. Clinical trials have consistently shown that use of these drugs reduces morbidity and the number of hospitalizations and improves both quality of life and survival. β-Blockers increase the ejection fraction and decrease ventricular remodeling. ACC/AHA guidelines recommend the use of β-blockers as an integral part of the therapy for heart failure. However, caution must be used when administering β-blockers to patients with reactive airway disease, diabetic patients with frequent hypoglycemic episodes, and patients with bradydysrhythmias or heart block.

DIURETICS

Diuretics can relieve circulatory congestion and its accompanying pulmonary and peripheral edema and do so more rapidly than any other drugs. Symptomatic improvement can be noted within hours. Diuretic-induced decreases in ventricular diastolic pressure will decrease diastolic ventricular wall stress and prevent the persistent cardiac distention that interferes with subendocardial perfusion and negatively affects myocardial metabolism and function. Thiazide and/or loop diuretics are recommended as an essential part of the therapy for heart failure. Potassium and magnesium supplementation may be needed in patients receiving long-term treatment with diuretics to prevent cardiac dysrhythmias. Excessive dosages of diuretics may cause hypovolemia, prerenal azotemia, or an undesirably low cardiac output and are associated with worse clinical outcomes.

DIGITALIS

Digitalis enhances the inotropy of cardiac muscle and decreases sympathetic and RAAS activation. These latter effects are related to the ability of digitalis to restore the inhibitory effects of the cardiac baroreceptors on central sympathetic outflow. It is unclear whether digitalis treatment improves survival, but digoxin may impede the worsening of heart failure and result in fewer hospitalizations. Digitalis can be added to standard therapy when patients are still symptomatic despite treatment with diuretics, ACE inhibitors, and β-blockers. Patients with the combination of atrial fibrillation and heart failure are another subgroup that may benefit from digoxin therapy. Caution should be used when administering this drug to elderly patients or to those with impaired renal function, since these patients are particularly prone to development of digitalis toxicity. Manifestations of digitalis toxicity include anorexia, nausea, blurred vision, and cardiac dysrhythmias. Treatment of toxicity may include reversing hypokalemia, treating cardiac dysrhythmias, administering antidigoxin antibodies, and/or placing a temporary cardiac pacemaker.

VASODILATORS

Vasodilator therapy relaxes vascular smooth muscle, decreases resistance to LV ejection, and increases venous capacitance. In patients with a dilated left ventricle, administration of vasodilators results in increased stroke volume and decreased ventricular filling pressures. African Americans seem to respond very well to vasodilator therapy and show improved clinical outcomes when treated with a combination of hydralazine and nitrates.

STATINS

Because of their antiinflammatory and lipid-lowering effects, statins have been proven to decrease morbidity and mortality in patients with systolic heart failure. Promising studies suggest that patients with diastolic heart failure could derive similar benefits from statin therapy.

Management of Diastolic Heart Failure

The management of systolic heart failure is based on the results of large-scale randomized trials, but the treatment of diastolic heart failure remains mostly empirical. It is generally accepted that the best treatment strategy for diastolic heart failure is prevention. ACC/AHA guidelines recommend that patients at risk of developing diastolic heart failure be preemptively treated. Unfortunately, there are no drugs that selectively improve diastolic distensibility. Current treatment options include consumption of a low-sodium diet, cautious use of diuretics to relieve pulmonary congestion without an excessive decrease in preload, maintenance of normal sinus rhythm at a heart rate that optimizes ventricular filling, and correction of precipitating factors such as acute myocardial ischemia and systemic hypertension. Long-acting nitrates and diuretics may alleviate the symptoms of diastolic heart failure but do not alter the natural history of the disease. Statin therapy early in the course of the disease may play an important role in decreasing ventricular remodeling and reducing disease progression. The general concepts of managing patients with diastolic heart failure are outlined in Table 6-2.

TABLE 6-2 ■ **Management strategies for diastolic heart failure**

Goals	Management strategies
Prevent development of diastolic heart failure by decreasing risk factors	Treatment of coronary artery disease Treatment of hypertension Control of weight gain Treatment of diabetes mellitus
Allow adequate filling time for left ventricle by decreasing heart rate	β-Blockers, calcium channel blockers, digoxin
Control volume overload	Diuretics, long-acting nitrates, consumption of low-sodium diet
Restore and maintain sinus rhythm	Cardioversion, amiodarone, digoxin
Decrease ventricular remodeling	Angiotensin-converting enzyme inhibitors, statins
Correct precipitating factors	Aortic valve replacement Coronary revascularization

TABLE 6-3 ■ **Indications for implantation of a cardioverter-defibrillator for prevention of sudden death**

Cause of heart failure	Condition
Coronary artery disease	Ejection fraction <30% Ejection fraction <40% if electrophysiologic study demonstrates inducible ventricular dysrhythmias
All other causes	After first episode of syncope or aborted ventricular tachycardia/ventricular fibrillation

Surgical Management of Heart Failure

Cardiac resynchronization therapy (CRT) is aimed at patients with heart failure who have a ventricular conduction delay (QRS prolongation on ECG). Such a conduction delay creates a mechanical dyssynchrony that impairs ventricular function and worsens prognosis. CRT, also known as *biventricular pacing,* consists of placement of a dual-chamber cardiac pacemaker (right atrial and ventricular leads) with an additional lead introduced via the coronary sinus into an epicardial coronary vein and advanced until it reaches the lateral wall of the LV. With this lead in place, the heart contracts more efficiently and ejects a larger cardiac output. CRT is recommended for patients with NYHA class III or IV disease with an LV ejection fraction of less than 35% and a QRS duration of 120 to 150 milliseconds. Patients undergoing CRT have fewer symptoms, better exercise tolerance, improved ventricular function, fewer hospitalizations for heart failure, and decreased mortality compared with similar patients receiving pharmacologic therapy alone. The reverse-remodeling process induced by CRT appears to be the main determinant of improved survival in these patients. Unfortunately, this form of therapy fails to produce improvement in about one third of patients.

Implantable cardioverter-defibrillators (ICDs) are used for prevention of sudden death in patients with advanced heart failure. Approximately one half of deaths in heart failure patients are sudden and due to cardiac dysrhythmias. Current recommendations for the use of ICDs in patients at risk of sudden death are listed in Table 6-3. Recent studies have demonstrated that patients treated with a combination of CRT and ICD placement have fewer hospitalizations and better survival rates at 2 years than patients who receive only ICD therapy. However, this advantage comes at the cost of higher device-related complication rates in the first 30 days after implantation.

Part of the overall management of heart failure includes strategies aimed at eliminating the cause of the disease. LV ischemia may be treated with percutaneous coronary interventions or coronary artery bypass surgery. Severe heart failure symptoms in the presence of correctable cardiac valve lesions may be alleviated surgically. Ventricular aneurysmectomy may be useful in patients with large ventricular scars after myocardial infarction. The definitive treatment for heart failure is cardiac transplantation. Currently in the United States 150,000 patients are listed as candidates for cardiac transplantation, but only 2000 hearts are available per year. The limited supply of donors renders this treatment unattainable for most patients.

Patients in the terminal stages of heart failure may benefit from mechanical support of circulation, such as insertion of a pulsatile or nonpulsatile ventricular assist device (VAD) or a total artificial heart. Studies have demonstrated not only increased survival but also improved quality of life in heart failure patients treated with VADs compared with those treated with medical therapy alone. These mechanical pumps take over either partial or total function of the damaged ventricle and facilitate restoration of normal hemodynamics and tissue blood flow. A VAD drains blood returning to the failed side of the heart and pumps it downstream of the failed ventricle. These devices are useful in patients who require temporary ventricular assistance to allow the heart to recover its function, in patients who are awaiting cardiac transplantation (*bridge therapy*), and in patients with advanced heart failure who are not transplant candidates (*destination therapy*). First-generation left ventricular assist devices (LVADs) captured the entire cardiac output and ejected it, in a *pulsatile* fashion, into the ascending aorta as does the native left ventricle. To create pulsatile flow, the device had a complicated mechanism that included valves preventing systolic retrograde blood flow. As a result, the first-generation LVADs were noisy, fairly large, and prone to significant complications related to mechanical pump failure and thromboembolic events. With the advent of modern miniaturization technology and the general acceptance by the medical community that *nonpulsatile* flow can be well tolerated, second and third generations of LVADs have been developed. Second-generation LVADs are axial flow pumps.

Third-generation LVADs are centrifugal electromagnetically powered pumps. These devices generate nonpulsatile flow, are smaller and quieter, and are associated with a lower incidence of thromboembolic events. Therefore they have become an attractive therapeutic option for an increasing number of patients with heart failure.

Patients with fixed pulmonary hypertension requiring biventricular support for extended periods of time may benefit from implantation of a *total artificial heart* as a bridge to transplantation or as destination therapy. The total artificial heart is implanted in the chest in lieu of the native heart. This device generates *pulsatile* flow and consists of two mechanical pumps (each operating as a ventricle) with two valves apiece. The total artificial heart represents the best option for long-term survival in this patient population.

ANESTHETIC CONSIDERATIONS FOR PATIENTS WITH IMPLANTABLE NONPULSATILE VENTRICULAR ASSIST DEVICES

Since more VADs are being inserted, a growing number of patients with VADs will be undergoing noncardiac surgery. To provide optimal care to these patients, the anesthesiologist needs to understand the features of nonpulsatile devices and the potential causes of mishaps that can occur during anesthesia and surgery. The most commonly used VAD in the United States is the HeartMate II (Thoratec Corporation, Pleasanton, Calif.), a second-generation continuous-flow device. The pump is implanted extraperitoneally in the left upper abdomen, draining blood from the LV apex via the inflow cannula and ejecting it into the ascending aorta via the outflow cannula (Figure 6-5). A drive line connects the pump to electrical power as well as to an external console, which displays the pump flows and other system information. The drive line crosses the abdomen and exits the skin in the right upper

quadrant, and this is the site most likely to become infected. However, the drive line should not be prepped with povidone-iodine solutions because this leads to plastic breakdown. Alternatively, the drive line can be draped out of the field.

General anesthetic considerations for patients with VADs include appropriate perioperative management of anticoagulation therapy and cardiac rhythm devices, provision of suitable antibiotic prophylaxis, confirmation that the device is plugged into an electrical outlet, and avoidance of chest compression to prevent dislodgement of cannulae. Use of surgical electrocautery can cause electromagnetic interference with the VAD, which can affect pump flow and induce device reprogramming. Therefore, bipolar cautery should be used when feasible, or the grounding electrode of the monopolar cautery should be placed so as to direct the current away from the VAD generator.

Hemodynamic monitoring of a patient with an implantable nonpulsatile device represents a particular challenge for the anesthesiologist. Neither the noninvasive blood pressure monitor nor the pulse oximeter will provide useful information because there is no pulse. As a substitute for a pulse oximeter, a cerebral oximeter, which does not rely on pulsatile flow, can be used. Intermittent monitoring of oxygen saturation can also be accomplished by arterial blood gas analysis. An intraarterial catheter is required for measurement of *mean* blood pressure. However, because of the lack of pulsatility in the artery, placement of an arterial catheter may be very difficult and is usually facilitated by ultrasonographic guidance. Transesophageal echocardiography represents one of the most useful monitoring techniques for patients with VADs since it provides real-time information regarding volume status, right ventricular function, and inflow-outflow cannulae function.

The three main causes of hypotension occurring in patients with continuous-flow LVADs are decreased preload, right

Continuous-flow LVAD

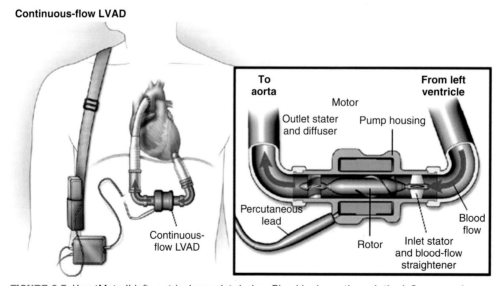

FIGURE 6-5 HeartMate II left ventricular assist device. Blood is drawn through the inflow cannula attached to the ventricular apex into the pump and is ejected into the ascending aorta through the outflow cannula. The percutaneous lead is the drive line, which exits the right side of the abdomen and connects the pump to the external console and power source. *LVAD,* Left ventricular assist device.

ventricular failure, and increased afterload. Intravascular volume optimization is a major concern in patients with all types of VADs, but this is particularly important with nonpulsatile devices, because the continuous drainage of an underfilled left side of the heart will eventually lead to LV *suck-down*. Such a situation results in a dramatic decrease in cardiac output. It can be rapidly diagnosed by transesophageal echocardiography and is treated by temporarily decreasing the pump speed followed by volume expansion. Good right ventricular function is a critical aspect of optimal LVAD flow. Intraoperatively, factors that increase pulmonary vascular resistance (hypercarbia, vasoconstrictor drugs) will impair right ventricular function and thus impede blood flow to the left side of the heart. Both decreases and increases in afterload can significantly impact LVAD flow. Small doses of vasopressor medications that have less impact on pulmonary vascular resistance (e.g., vasopressin) may be successfully used to counteract the decrease in afterload seen with general anesthesia. However, high doses of vasopressors, especially in the face of hypovolemia, will inevitably lead to a decrease in LVAD flow. Excellent communication among the entire perioperative team (anesthesiologist, surgeon, cardiologist, nurses, VAD personnel) is essential for good perioperative outcomes.

Management of Acute Heart Failure

Patients may experience acute heart failure or decompensated chronic heart failure. Anesthesiologists often deal with acute heart failure in patients who undergo emergency surgery or in patients who experience cardiac decompensation during any kind of surgery. Acute heart failure therapy has three phases: the emergency phase, the in-hospital management phase, and the predischarge phase. For the anesthesiologist, the emergency phase is of most interest and is the phase that is addressed here. High ventricular filling pressures, low cardiac output, and hypertension or hypotension characterize the hemodynamic profile of acute heart failure. Traditional therapies include diuretics, vasodilators, inotropic drugs, mechanical assist devices (intraaortic balloon pump, VAD), and emergency cardiac surgery. Newer therapies include calcium sensitizers, exogenous BNP, and nitric oxide synthase inhibitors.

DIURETICS AND VASODILATORS

Loop diuretics can improve symptoms rapidly, but at high doses, they may have deleterious effects on clinical outcomes. It may be more desirable to use a combination of a low dose of loop diuretic and an intravenous vasodilator. Nitroglycerin and nitroprusside reduce LV filling pressure and systemic vascular resistance and increase stroke volume. However, nitroprusside may have a negative impact on clinical outcome in patients with acute myocardial infarction.

INOTROPIC SUPPORT

Positive inotropic drugs have been the mainstay of treatment for patients in cardiogenic shock. The positive inotropic effect is produced via an increase in cyclic adenosine monophosphate (cAMP), which promotes an increase in intracellular calcium levels and thereby an improvement in excitation-contraction coupling. Catecholamines (epinephrine, norepinephrine, dopamine, and dobutamine) do this by direct β-receptor stimulation, whereas phosphodiesterase inhibitors (amrinone, milrinone) block the degradation of cAMP. Side effects of inotropic drugs include tachycardia, increased myocardial oxygen consumption, dysrhythmias, worsening of diastolic heart failure, and downregulation of β receptors. Long-term use of these drugs may result in cardiotoxicity and accelerate myocardial cell death.

CALCIUM SENSITIZERS

Myofilament calcium sensitizers are a new class of positive inotropic drugs that increase contractility without increasing intracellular levels of calcium. Therefore, there is no significant increase in myocardial oxygen consumption or heart rate and no propensity for dysrhythmias. The most widely used medication in this class is levosimendan. It is an *inodilator,* increasing myocardial contractile strength and promoting dilation of systemic, pulmonary, and coronary arteries. It does not worsen diastolic function. Studies have shown that levosimendan may be particularly useful in the setting of myocardial ischemia. Use of levosimendan is included in the European guidelines for treatment of acute heart failure, but the drug is not yet available for use in the United States.

EXOGENOUS B-TYPE NATRIURETIC PEPTIDE

Nesiritide is recombinant BNP that binds to both the A- and B-type natriuretic receptors. By inhibiting the RAAS and sympathetic tone, this natriuretic peptide promotes arterial, venous, and coronary vasodilation, thereby decreasing LVEDP and improving dyspnea. It also induces diuresis and natriuresis, has lusitropic properties, and lacks any prodysrhythmic effects. In many ways its effects are similar to those of nitroglycerin, but nesiritide generally produces less hypotension and more diuresis than nitroglycerin. Nesiritide given *intravenously* has been studied extensively in large clinical trials. Currently it is felt that this drug may not offer advantages over traditional treatments for acute heart failure and may be associated with worsening renal function and perhaps even increased mortality. However, ongoing research is evaluating the use of *subcutaneous* BNP in patients with acute heart failure and an LVEF of less than 35%. The preliminary results are promising and show an increase in cardiac output, decrease in mean arterial pressure, no change in heart rate, a decrease in RAAS activity, and increased diuresis and natriuresis. An oral form of BNP is under investigation.

NITRIC OXIDE SYNTHASE INHIBITORS

The inflammatory cascade stimulated by heart failure results in production of a large amount of nitric oxide in the heart and vascular endothelium. These high levels of nitric oxide have a negative inotropic action and a profound vasodilatory effect that can lead to cardiogenic shock and vascular collapse. Inhibition of nitric oxide synthase should decrease these harmful effects. L-NAME (N^G-nitro-L-arginine methyl ester) is the principal drug in this class currently under investigation.

MECHANICAL DEVICES

If the cause of acute heart failure is an extensive myocardial infarction, the insertion of an intraaortic balloon pump should be considered. The intraaortic balloon pump is a mechanical device inserted via the femoral artery and positioned just below the left subclavian artery. Its balloon inflates in diastole, increasing aortic diastolic blood pressure and coronary perfusion pressure. The balloon deflates in systole, creating a suction effect that enhances LV ejection. Complications of intraaortic balloon pump use include femoral artery or aortic dissection, bleeding, thrombosis, and infection.

In cases of severe cardiogenic shock, emergency insertion of a left and/or right ventricular assist device may be necessary for survival. Percutaneous ventricular assist devices (pVADs) have been developed and successfully inserted in patients with acute heart failure. These devices restore normal hemodynamics and therefore maintain vital organ perfusion. More importantly, these devices allow for unloading of the left side of the heart, thereby reducing LV strain and myocardial work and improving the remodeling process seen in acute heart failure. The pVADs are designed to offer temporary circulatory support in cardiogenic shock for up to 14 days as a transition to recovery or as a bridge to a definitive cardiac procedure (coronary stenting, coronary artery bypass grafting, VAD insertion, or heart transplantation). Trials comparing the efficacy of a pVAD versus an intraaortic balloon pump in patients with severe acute heart failure have demonstrated a better metabolic profile and superior hemodynamic support in patients receiving pVAD therapy but have failed so far to show a decrease in 30-day mortality rates with the use of a pVAD. There are two types of percutaneous devices designed for short-term circulatory support: the Impella system (Abiomed Inc., Danvers, Mass.) and the TandemHeart (CardiacAssist Inc., Pittsburgh, Pa.).

The Impella system consists of a miniaturized axial-flow rotary blood pump that is inserted via the femoral artery and advanced under fluoroscopic or transesophageal echocardiographic guidance until it passes the aortic valve and sits in the LV cavity (Figure 6-6). The pump draws blood continuously from the LV through the distal port and ejects it into the ascending aorta through the proximal port of the device. Depending on the type of system, the pump can generate cardiac outputs of up to 5 L/min. Placement of the Impella device is contraindicated in the presence of a prosthetic aortic valve, severe aortic stenosis or aortic regurgitation, or peripheral vascular disease. Relative contraindications to insertion of the Impella system include thoracoabdominal or abdominal aortic aneurysms or an aortic dissection. In such cases the axillary artery can serve as the insertion site of the

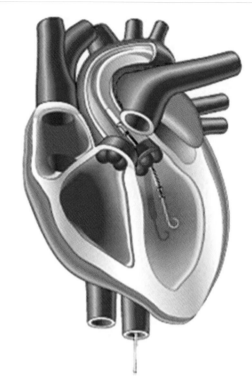

FIGURE 6-6 Impella Recover 2.5 percutaneous ventricular assist device. The pump is percutaneously placed in the femoral artery, advanced through the aortic valve, and situated in the left ventricular cavity. The Impella 5.0 has a similar design.

pump. Possible complications of device use include stroke, aortic valve injury, cardiac tamponade, vascular injury with limb ischemia, and infection. Because of the centrifugal nature of the pump, hemolysis and thrombocytopenia typically develop.

The TandemHeart system is a percutaneous transseptal left atrial–to–femoral arterial circulatory device. The system consists of an extracorporeal centrifugal continuous-flow pump and inflow and outflow cannulae. The inflow cannula is percutaneously placed in the femoral vein, advanced to the right atrium, and then positioned transseptally into the left atrium. The outflow cannula is placed in the femoral artery (Figure 6-7). Oxygenated blood is drained from the left atrium via the inflow cannula and ejected retrograde into the abdominal aorta via the outflow cannula in the femoral artery. This system can generate cardiac outputs similar to those produced by the Impella system. However, optimal functioning of the Tandem-Heart depends on good right ventricular function. In situations of acute right-sided heart failure, the system can be configured as a right-sided VAD, pumping blood from the right-sided atrium into the pulmonary artery. Unique complications of use of this device include paradoxical emboli, a right-to-left intracardiac shunt manifested as hypoxemia, and coronary sinus or right atrial injury with subsequent cardiac tamponade. The most devastating complication is inflow cannula dislodgement

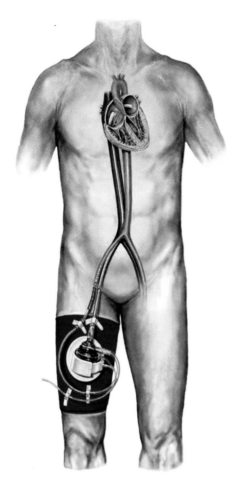

FIGURE 6-7 TandemHeart percutaneous ventricular assist device. The inflow cannula is placed in the femoral vein and advanced into the right atrium. It then pierces the interatrial septum to draw oxygenated blood from the left atrium. The outflow cannula pumps blood retrograde into the aorta via the femoral artery.

with mitral valve entrapment. This situation leads to a sudden decrease in cardiac output and requires immediate diagnosis and cannula repositioning.

Prognosis

Despite advances in therapy, the number of heart failure deaths continues to increase steadily in the United States. Mortality during the first 4 years after the diagnosis of heart failure approaches 40%. Certain factors have been associated with a poor prognosis and include increased blood urea nitrogen and creatinine levels, hyponatremia, hypokalemia, severely depressed ejection fraction, high levels of endogenous BNP, very limited exercise tolerance, and the presence of multifocal premature ventricular contractions. In heart failure patients the prognosis depends on the underlying heart disease and on the presence or absence of a specific precipitating factor. If a correctable cause of heart failure can be effectively eliminated, prognosis improves.

MANAGEMENT OF ANESTHESIA

Preoperative Evaluation and Management

The presence of heart failure has been described as the single most important risk factor for predicting perioperative cardiac morbidity and mortality. In the preoperative period, all precipitating factors for heart failure should be sought and aggressively treated before proceeding with elective surgery.

Patients treated for heart failure are usually taking several medications that may affect anesthetic management. It is generally accepted that diuretics may be discontinued on the day of surgery. Maintaining β-blocker therapy is essential, since many studies have shown that β-blockers reduce perioperative morbidity and mortality. Due to inhibition of the RAAS, ACE inhibitors may put patients at increased risk of intraoperative hypotension. This hypotension can be treated with a sympathomimetic drug such as ephedrine, an α-agonist such as phenylephrine, or vasopressin or one of its analogues. If ACE inhibitors are being used to prevent ventricular remodeling in heart failure patients or kidney dysfunction in diabetic patients, then stopping the medication for 1 day will not significantly alter these effects. However, if ACE inhibitors are being used to treat hypertension, discontinuing therapy the day before or the day of surgery may result in significant hypertension. Angiotensin receptor blockers produce profound RAAS blockade and should be discontinued the day before surgery. Digoxin therapy can be continued until the day of surgery.

Results of recent electrolyte, renal function, and liver function tests and the most recent ECG and echocardiogram should be reviewed.

Intraoperative Management

All types of general anesthetics have been successfully used in patients with heart failure. However, drug dosages may need to be adjusted. Opioids seem to have a particularly beneficial effect in heart failure patients because of their effect on the δ receptor, which inhibits adrenergic activation. Positive pressure ventilation and positive end-expiratory pressure may be beneficial in decreasing pulmonary congestion and improving arterial oxygenation.

Monitoring is based on the complexity of the operation. Intraarterial pressure monitoring is justified when major surgery is required in a patient with heart failure. Monitoring of ventricular filling and fluid status is a more challenging task. Fluid overload during the perioperative period may contribute to the development or worsening of heart failure. Intraoperative use of a pulmonary artery catheter may help in evaluation of optimal fluid loading, but in patients with diastolic heart failure and poor ventricular compliance, accurate assessment of LV end-diastolic volume may be quite difficult. Transesophageal echocardiography may be a better alternative, allowing monitoring of not only ventricular filling but also ventricular wall motion and valvular function. However, transesophageal echocardiography requires trained personnel to perform the study and interpret the results and may not be readily available in all circumstances.

Regional anesthesia is acceptable for suitable operations in heart failure patients. In fact, the modest decrease in systemic vascular resistance secondary to sympathetic blockade may increase cardiac output. However, the decrease in systemic vascular resistance produced by epidural or spinal anesthesia is not always predictable or easy to control. The pros and cons of regional anesthesia must be carefully weighed in heart failure patients.

Special consideration must be given to patients who have undergone cardiac transplantation and now require other surgeries. These patients are receiving long-term immunosuppressive therapy and are at high risk of infection. Strict aseptic technique is necessary when performing any invasive procedure such as central line placement or neuraxial blockade. The transplanted heart is denervated. Therefore, an increase in heart rate can be achieved only by administering direct-acting β-adrenergic agonists such as isoproterenol and epinephrine. An increase in heart rate will *not* occur with administration of atropine or pancuronium. A blunted response to α-adrenergic agonists may also be observed. The transplanted heart increases cardiac output by increasing stroke volume. Therefore, these patients are preload dependent and require adequate intravascular volume. However, diastolic dysfunction can be a result of chronic graft rejection; therefore, intraoperative volume administration decisions must be made with the recognition that adequate preload is a requirement for optimal function of the transplanted heart but excessive fluid administration incurs the risk of pulmonary edema.

Postoperative Management

Patients who have evidence of acute heart failure during surgery should be transferred to an intensive care unit so that invasive monitoring can be continued as long as needed. Pain should be aggressively treated, since its presence and hemodynamic consequences may worsen heart failure. Patients' usual medications should be restarted as soon as possible.

CARDIOMYOPATHIES

The definition of *cardiomyopathies* used by the AHA expert consensus panel in its 2006 document entitled "Contemporary Definition and Classification of the Cardiomyopathies" reads as follows:

> Cardiomyopathies are a heterogeneous group of diseases of the myocardium associated with mechanical and/or electrical dysfunction that usually (but not invariably) exhibit inappropriate ventricular hypertrophy or dilation and are due to a variety of causes that frequently are genetic. Cardiomyopathies either are confined to the heart or are part of generalized systemic disorders, often leading to cardiovascular death or progressive heart failure-related disability.

According to the AHA classification, cardiomyopathies are divided into two major groups: primary cardiomyopathies

TABLE 6-4	Classification of primary cardiomyopathies
Genetic	Hypertrophic cardiomyopathy
	Arrhythmogenic right ventricular cardiomyopathy
	Left ventricular noncompaction
	Glycogen storage disease
	Conduction system disease (Lenègre's disease)
	Ion channelopathies: long QT syndrome, Brugada syndrome, short QT syndrome
Mixed	Dilated cardiomyopathy
	Primary restrictive nonhypertrophic cardiomyopathy
Acquired	Myocarditis (inflammatory cardiomyopathy): viral, bacterial, rickettsial, fungal, parasitic (Chagas's disease)
	Stress cardiomyopathy
	Peripartum cardiomyopathy

and secondary cardiomyopathies. Primary cardiomyopathies are those exclusively (or predominantly) confined to heart muscle. Primary cardiomyopathies can be genetic, acquired, or of mixed origin. Secondary cardiomyopathies demonstrate pathophysiologic involvement of the heart in the context of a multiorgan disorder. Tables 6-4 and 6-5 list the most common cardiomyopathies. It is important to emphasize that the previously used terms *ischemic cardiomyopathy, restrictive cardiomyopathy,* and *obliterative cardiomyopathy* no longer appear in the new classification. The following sections address the cardiomyopathies most often seen by an anesthesiologist: hypertrophic cardiomyopathy, dilated cardiomyopathy, peripartum cardiomyopathy, and secondary cardiomyopathies with restrictive physiology.

Hypertrophic Cardiomyopathy

Hypertrophic cardiomyopathy (HCM) is a complex cardiac disease with unique pathophysiologic characteristics and a great diversity of morphologic, functional, and clinical features. The disease can affect patients of all ages and has a prevalence in the general population approaching 1 in 500. It is the most common genetic cardiovascular disease and is transmitted as an autosomal dominant trait with variable penetrance. The disease is characterized by LV hypertrophy in the absence of any other cardiac disease capable of inducing ventricular hypertrophy, such as hypertension or aortic stenosis. The most common form of HCM presents as hypertrophy of the septum and anterolateral free wall. Histologic features of this disease include hypertrophied myocardial cells and areas of patchy myocardial scarring.

The pathophysiology of HCM is related to the following features: myocardial hypertrophy, dynamic LV outflow tract (LVOT) obstruction, systolic anterior movement of the mitral valve causing mitral regurgitation, diastolic dysfunction, myocardial ischemia, and dysrhythmias. During systole, contraction of the hypertrophied septum accelerates blood flow through the narrow LVOT, which creates a Venturi effect on the anterior leaflet of the mitral valve and induces systolic anterior

TABLE 6-5   Classification of secondary cardiomyopathies

Infiltrative	Amyloidosis Gaucher's disease Hunter's syndrome
Storage	Hemochromatosis Glycogen storage disease Niemann-Pick disease
Toxic	Drugs: cocaine, alcohol Chemotherapy drugs: doxorubicin, daunorubicin, cyclophosphamide Heavy metals: lead, mercury Radiation therapy
Inflammatory	Sarcoidosis
Endomyocardial	Hypereosinophilic (Löffler's) syndrome Endomyocardial fibrosis
Endocrine	Diabetes mellitus Hyperthyroidism or hypothyroidism Pheochromocytoma Acromegaly
Neuromuscular	Duchenne-Becker dystrophy Neurofibromatosis Tuberous sclerosis
Autoimmune	Lupus erythematosus Rheumatoid arthritis Scleroderma Dermatomyositis Polyarteritis nodosa

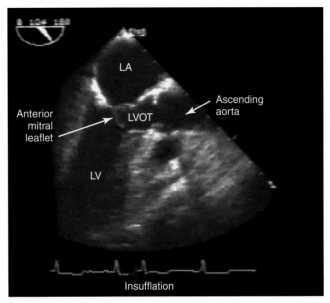

FIGURE 6-8 Two-dimensional echocardiographic image showing the anterior leaflet of the mitral valve abutting the hypertrophied interventricular septum and obstructing the left ventricular outflow tract (LVOT) during systole in a patient with hypertrophic cardiomyopathy. *LA,* Left atrium; *LV,* left ventricle.

movement of the anterior mitral valve leaflet. The presence of this systolic anterior movement accentuates the dynamic LVOT obstruction and causes significant mitral regurgitation (Figure 6-8). LVOT obstruction can be present at rest or can be induced by Valsalva's maneuver. Situations that worsen LVOT obstruction are listed in Table 6-6. With HCM, diastolic dysfunction is seen more often than LVOT obstruction. The hypertrophied myocardium has a prolonged relaxation time and a decreased compliance. Myocardial ischemia is present in patients with HCM, whether or not they have coronary artery disease. Myocardial ischemia is caused by several factors, including abnormal coronary arteries, a mismatch between ventricular mass and coronary artery size, increased LVEDP that compromises coronary perfusion, decreased diastolic filling time, increased oxygen consumption caused by hypertrophy, and the presence of a metabolic derangement in the use of oxygen at the cellular level. Dysrhythmias in patients with HCM result from the disorganized cellular architecture, myocardial scarring, and expanded interstitial matrix. Dysrhythmias are the cause of sudden death in young adults with this cardiomyopathy.

SIGNS AND SYMPTOMS

The clinical course of HCM varies widely. Most patients remain asymptomatic throughout life. Some, however, have symptoms of severe heart failure and others die suddenly. The principal symptoms of HCM are angina pectoris, fatigue or syncope (which may represent aborted sudden death), tachydysrhythmias, and heart failure. Interestingly, lying down often

TABLE 6-6   Factors influencing left ventricular outflow tract obstruction in patients with hypertrophic cardiomyopathy

EVENTS THAT INCREASE OUTFLOW OBSTRUCTION

Increased myocardial contractility
  β-Adrenergic stimulation (catecholamines)
  Digitalis
Decreased preload
  Hypovolemia
  Vasodilators
  Tachycardia
  Positive pressure ventilation
Decreased afterload
  Hypotension
  Vasodilators

EVENTS THAT DECREASE OUTFLOW OBSTRUCTION

Decreased myocardial contractility
  β-Adrenergic blockade
  Volatile anesthetics
  Calcium entry blockers
Increased preload
  Hypervolemia
  Bradycardia
Increased afterload
  Hypertension
  α-Adrenergic stimulation

relieves the angina pectoris of HCM. Presumably, the change in LV size that accompanies this positional change decreases LV outflow obstruction.

Cardiac physical examination may reveal a double apical impulse, gallop rhythm, and cardiac murmurs and thrills. The murmurs can result from LV outflow obstruction or mitral regurgitation and can be confused with aortic or mitral valve disease. The intensity of these murmurs can change markedly with certain maneuvers. For example, Valsalva's maneuver, which increases LV outflow obstruction, will enhance the systolic murmur along the left sternal border. The murmur of mitral regurgitation also intensifies with Valsalva's maneuver. Nitroglycerin and standing (versus lying down) also increase the loudness of these murmurs.

Sudden death is a recognized complication of HCM. The severity of ventricular hypertrophy is directly related to the risk of sudden death. Young individuals with massive hypertrophy, even if they have few or no symptoms, deserve consideration for an intervention to prevent sudden death. Sudden death is especially likely to occur in patients between the ages of 10 and 30 years. For this reason, there is general agreement that young patients with HCM should not participate in competitive sports. Patients with mild hypertrophy are at low risk of sudden death.

DIAGNOSIS

The ECG typically shows signs of LV hypertrophy. In asymptomatic patients, unexplained LV hypertrophy may be the only sign of the disease. The 12-lead ECG shows abnormalities in 75% to 90% of patients with HCM. These abnormalities include high QRS voltage, ST-segment and T-wave alterations, abnormal Q waves resembling those seen with myocardial infarction, and left atrial enlargement. The diagnosis of HCM should also be considered in any young patient whose ECG findings are consistent with previous myocardial infarction, because not all patients with HCM have evidence of LV hypertrophy on their ECGs.

Echocardiography can demonstrate the presence of myocardial hypertrophy. Ejection fraction is usually more than 80%, which reflects the hypercontractile condition of the heart. Echocardiography can also assess the mitral valve apparatus and detect the presence of systolic anterior movement. Color flow Doppler imaging can reveal the presence of LVOT obstruction by demonstrating turbulent flow as well as mitral regurgitation. Pressure gradients across the LVOT can be measured. Echocardiography is also useful in evaluating diastolic function.

Cardiac catheterization allows direct measurement of the increased LVEDP and the pressure gradient between the left ventricle and the aorta. Provocative maneuvers may be required to evoke evidence of LVOT obstruction. Ventriculography characteristically shows cavity obliteration.

The definitive diagnosis of HCM is made by endomyocardial biopsy and DNA analysis, but these diagnostic modalities are usually reserved for patients in whom the diagnosis cannot be otherwise established.

TREATMENT

The diverse clinical and genetic features of HCM make it impossible to define precise guidelines for management (Figure 6-9). However, it is recognized that some patients are at high risk of sudden death and must be treated aggressively. Pharmacologic therapy to improve diastolic filling, reduce LV outflow obstruction, and possibly decrease myocardial

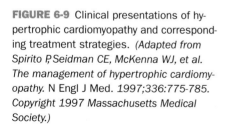

FIGURE 6-9 Clinical presentations of hypertrophic cardiomyopathy and corresponding treatment strategies. *(Adapted from Spirito P, Seidman CE, McKenna WJ, et al. The management of hypertrophic cardiomyopathy. N Engl J Med. 1997;336:775-785. Copyright 1997 Massachusetts Medical Society.)*

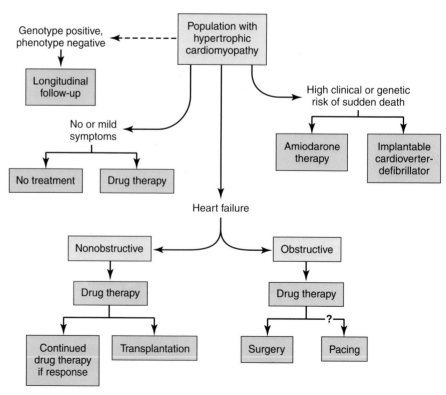

ischemia is the primary means of relieving the signs and symptoms of HCM. Surgery to remove the area of hypertrophy causing outflow tract obstruction is considered in the 5% of patients who have both marked outflow obstruction and severe symptoms unresponsive to medical therapy.

Medical Therapy

β-Blockers and calcium channel blockers have been used extensively to treat HCM. The beneficial effects of β-blockers on dyspnea, angina pectoris, and exercise tolerance are likely due to the resulting decrease in heart rate with consequent prolongation of diastole and a lengthening of the time for passive ventricular filling. β-Blockers can lessen myocardial oxygen requirements and decrease the dynamic outflow tract obstruction during exercise by blunting sympathetic nervous system activity. Similarly, calcium channel blockers, such as verapamil and diltiazem, have beneficial effects on the symptoms of HCM because they improve ventricular filling and decrease myocardial ischemia. Patients who develop congestive heart failure despite treatment with β-blockers or calcium channel blockers may show improvement with the addition of a diuretic. However, because of the presence of diastolic dysfunction and the requirement for relatively high ventricular filling pressures to achieve adequate cardiac output, diuretic administration must be done very cautiously. Patients at high risk of sudden death may require amiodarone therapy or placement of an ICD.

Atrial fibrillation often develops in patients with HCM and is associated with an increased risk of arterial thromboembolism, congestive heart failure, and sudden death. Amiodarone is the most effective antidysrhythmic drug for prevention of paroxysms of atrial fibrillation in these patients. β-Blockers and calcium channel blockers can control the heart rate. Long-term anticoagulation is indicated in those with recurrent or chronic atrial fibrillation.

Surgical Therapy

The small subgroup of patients with HCM who have both large outflow tract gradients (≥50 mm Hg) and severe symptoms of congestive heart failure despite medical therapy are candidates for surgery. There are several surgical strategies. A pacemaker can be placed in an attempt to *desynchronize* the LV during contraction and thereby decrease outflow obstruction. Surgical reduction of the outflow gradient is usually achieved by removing a small amount of cardiac muscle from the ventricular septum (septal myomectomy). Surgery abolishes or greatly reduces the LVOT gradient in most patients. Intraventricular systolic and end-diastolic pressures are markedly reduced, and these changes favorably influence LV filling and myocardial oxygen requirements. Similar results can be obtained by percutaneous cardiac catheterization and selective alcohol injection into the septal perforator arteries. This leads to ischemic injury followed by necrosis of the interventricular septum, which results in relief of the LVOT obstruction. If patients remain symptomatic despite various therapies, a prosthetic mitral valve can be inserted in an attempt to counteract the systolic anterior motion of the mitral leaflet.

The overall annual mortality of patients with HCM is approximately 1%. However, the subset of patients at high risk of sudden death (family history of sudden death or history of malignant ventricular dysrhythmias) have a mortality rate of 5% per year. Only about one fourth of patients diagnosed with HCM will develop signs of LVOT obstruction.

MANAGEMENT OF ANESTHESIA

Management of anesthesia in patients with HCM is directed toward minimizing LVOT obstruction. Any drug or event that decreases myocardial contractility or increases preload or reduces afterload will *improve* LVOT obstruction. Conversely, sympathetic stimulation, hypovolemia, and vasodilation *worsen* LVOT obstruction (see Table 6-6). Intraoperatively, patients with HCM may develop severe hypotension, myocardial ischemia, acute heart failure, and supraventricular or ventricular tachydysrhythmias. Previously unrecognized HCM may become manifest intraoperatively as unexplained hypotension or development of a systolic murmur in association with acute hemorrhage or drug-induced vasodilation.

Preoperative Evaluation and Management

Given the prevalence of HCM in the general population, patients with this disorder will be seen in the operating room with regularity. Patients already diagnosed with this disease should undergo an updated cardiac evaluation before elective surgery. Such evaluation should include a 12-lead ECG and an echocardiogram. Patients taking β-blockers or calcium channel blockers should continue these medications throughout the perioperative period. For patients with an ICD, the unit should be turned off immediately before surgery, an external defibrillator should be readily available in the operating room, and the device should be reactivated in the recovery room.

A more challenging task is detecting patients with HCM in whom the diagnosis has not yet been made. These patients are often young and appear healthy. Every patient should be asked preoperatively about any possible cardiac symptoms or a family history of cardiac disease or sudden death. The presence of a systolic murmur should raise suspicion of a possible diagnosis of HCM. If the ECG shows abnormalities, cardiologic evaluation is prudent.

In patients with HCM, preoperative administration of medication to allay anxiety and its associated activation of the sympathetic nervous system may be advisable. Expansion of intravascular volume during the preoperative period may also be useful in preventing LVOT obstruction and minimizing the adverse effects of positive pressure ventilation on the central blood volume.

Intraoperative Management

Regional or general anesthesia can be selected for patients with HCM as long as the anesthesiologist is aware of the main pathophysiologic mechanisms that trigger LVOT obstruction and develops an anesthetic plan tailored to those specific needs.

Induction of anesthesia with an intravenous drug is acceptable, but the importance of avoiding sudden decreases in systemic vascular resistance and increases in heart rate and contractility must be kept in mind. A modest degree of direct myocardial depression is acceptable. Administration of a volatile anesthetic or β-adrenergic antagonist before direct laryngoscopy can blunt the sympathetic response typically evoked by tracheal intubation. Positive pressure ventilation can significantly decrease preload and predispose a hypovolemic patient to dynamic LVOT obstruction. To help avoid this, smaller tidal volumes and higher respiratory rates should be used and positive end-expiratory pressure should be avoided. Preload reduction and severe hypotension due to LVOT obstruction can also be encountered when abdominal insufflation is performed for laparoscopic surgery. The surgeon should be advised about this possibility, and the abdomen should be insufflated slowly and at pressures not exceeding 15 mm Hg.

Nondepolarizing muscle relaxants that have only minimal effects on the systemic circulation should be used for skeletal muscle relaxation in HCM patients. The increased heart rate that may accompany administration of pancuronium and the histamine release associated with other neuromuscular blockers should be avoided.

Anesthesia should be maintained with drugs that produce mild depression of myocardial contractility and have minimal effects on preload and afterload. A volatile anesthetic in a moderate dose is often used for this purpose.

Invasive monitoring of blood pressure may be helpful. Transesophageal echocardiography during surgery and anesthesia is particularly useful in patients with HCM because of the unique pathophysiology of this disorder. Neither central venous pressure monitoring nor pulmonary artery pressure monitoring can diagnose LVOT obstruction or systolic anterior movement of the mitral valve leaflet, nor do these monitoring techniques give an accurate assessment of LV filling in these patients.

Hypotension that occurs in response to a decrease in preload or afterload should be treated with an α-adrenergic agonist such as phenylephrine. Drugs with β-adrenergic agonist activity, such as ephedrine, dopamine, and dobutamine, are contraindicated because the drug-induced increase in myocardial contractility and heart rate increases LVOT obstruction. Prompt replacement of blood loss and titration of intravenous fluids is important for maintaining preload and blood pressure. However, because of diastolic dysfunction, aggressive fluid replacement may result in pulmonary edema. Vasodilators should not be used to lower blood pressure because the decrease in systemic vascular resistance will accentuate LVOT obstruction.

Maintenance of normal sinus rhythm is very important, because adequate left ventricular filling is dependent on left atrial contraction. Patients who develop intraoperative supraventricular tachydysrhythmias should undergo immediate pharmacologic or electrical cardioversion. A cardioverter-defibrillator must be readily available in the operating room.

β-Blockers such as metoprolol and esmolol are indicated to slow persistently elevated heart rates.

Parturient Patients. Pregnancy is usually well tolerated in patients with HCM despite the pregnancy-induced decrease in systemic vascular resistance and the risk of impaired venous return due to aortocaval compression. Parturient women with HCM may present major anesthetic challenges, because events such as labor pain, which produces catecholamine release, and bearing down (Valsalva's maneuver) may increase LVOT obstruction. There is no evidence that regional anesthesia increases complication rates in parturient patients with HCM undergoing vaginal delivery. Epidural anesthesia has been successfully administered to these patients. Maintenance of euvolemia or slight hypervolemia is helpful. Should hypotension unresponsive to fluid administration occur as a result of regional anesthesia, phenylephrine should be used to increase afterload. Oxytocin must be administered carefully because of its vasodilating properties and compensatory tachycardia, and because of the abrupt inflow of large amounts of blood into the central circulation as a consequence of uterine contraction.

Pulmonary edema has been observed in parturient women with HCM after delivery, a finding that emphasizes the delicate balance in fluid requirements of these patients. Treatment of pulmonary edema in the presence of HCM may include phenylephrine if hypotension is present and esmolol to slow the heart rate, prolong diastolic filling time, and decrease myocardial contractility, all of which will decrease LVOT obstruction. Diuretics, digoxin, and nitrates *cannot* be used to treat pulmonary edema in this setting. They worsen the situation by provoking further LVOT obstruction.

Postoperative Management

Patients with HCM must be vigilantly monitored in the recovery room or intensive care unit in the immediately postoperative period. All factors that stimulate sympathetic activity, such as pain, shivering, anxiety, hypoxia, and hypercarbia, should be eliminated. As in the operating room, maintenance of euvolemia and prompt treatment of hypotension are crucial.

Dilated Cardiomyopathy

Dilated cardiomyopathy is a primary myocardial disease characterized by LV or biventricular dilation, systolic dysfunction, and normal ventricular wall thickness. The etiology of dilated cardiomyopathy is unknown, but it may be genetic or associated with infection such as coxsackievirus B infection. There is a familial transmission pattern in approximately 30% of cases, usually autosomal dominant. Many types of secondary cardiomyopathies have the features of dilated cardiomyopathy. These include the cardiomyopathies associated with alcohol abuse, cocaine abuse, the peripartum state, pheochromocytoma, infectious diseases (human immunodeficiency virus infection), uncontrolled tachycardia, Duchenne's muscular dystrophy, thyroid disease, chemotherapeutic drugs, radiation therapy, hypertension, coronary artery disease, and valvular heart disease. African American men have an increased risk of developing dilated cardiomyopathy. Dilated cardiomyopathy is the most common type of cardiomyopathy, the third most common cause of heart failure, and the most common indication for cardiac transplantation.

SIGNS AND SYMPTOMS

The initial manifestation of dilated cardiomyopathy is usually heart failure. Chest pain on exertion that mimics angina pectoris occurs in some patients. Ventricular dilation may be so marked that functional mitral and/or tricuspid regurgitation occurs. Supraventricular and ventricular dysrhythmias, conduction system abnormalities, and sudden death are common. Systemic embolization is also common as a result of the formation of mural thrombi in dilated and hypokinetic cardiac chambers.

DIAGNOSIS

The ECG often shows ST-segment and T-wave abnormalities and left bundle branch block. Dysrhythmias are common and include ventricular premature beats and atrial fibrillation. Chest radiography may show enlargement of all four cardiac chambers, but LV dilation is the principal morphologic feature.

Echocardiography typically reveals dilation of all four chambers but especially the left ventricle as well as global hypokinesis. Regional wall motion abnormalities may be seen in dilated cardiomyopathy and do not necessarily imply the presence of coronary disease. Mural thrombi can be detected, and valvular regurgitation secondary to annular dilation is a common finding.

Laboratory testing should be performed to eliminate other causes of cardiac dilation such as hyperthyroidism. The findings of coronary angiography are usually normal in patients with dilated cardiomyopathy. Right-sided heart catheterization reveals a high pulmonary capillary wedge pressure, high systemic vascular resistance, and a low cardiac output. Endomyocardial biopsy is not recommended.

TREATMENT

Treatment of dilated cardiomyopathy includes general supportive measures such as adequate rest, weight control, consumption of a low-sodium diet, fluid restriction, abstinence from tobacco and alcohol, and decreased physical activity during periods of cardiac decompensation. Cardiac rehabilitation, if possible, will improve general conditioning.

The medical management of dilated cardiomyopathy is similar to the medical management of chronic heart failure. Patients with dilated cardiomyopathy are at risk of systemic and pulmonary embolization because blood stasis in the hypocontractile cardiac chambers leads to activation of the coagulation cascade. The risk of cardiac embolization is greatest in patients with severe LV dysfunction, atrial fibrillation, a history of thromboembolism, or echocardiographic evidence of intracardiac thrombus. Anticoagulation with warfarin or dabigatran, a direct thrombin inhibitor, is often instituted in patients with dilated cardiomyopathy and symptomatic heart failure.

Asymptomatic, nonsustained ventricular tachycardia is common in patients with dilated cardiomyopathy. However, suppression of this dysrhythmia with drug therapy does not improve survival. Placement of an ICD can decrease the risk of sudden death in patients with heart failure who have survived a previous cardiac arrest (see Table 6-3).

Dilated cardiomyopathy remains the principal indication for cardiac transplantation in adults and children. Patients most likely to benefit from a heart transplant are those formerly vigorous persons younger than 60 years of age who have intractable symptoms of heart failure despite optimal medical therapy.

PROGNOSIS

Symptomatic patients with dilated cardiomyopathy referred to tertiary care medical centers have a 5-year mortality rate of 50%. If the cardiomyopathy involves both the left and right ventricles, the prognosis is even worse. Hemodynamic abnormalities that predict a poor prognosis include an ejection fraction of less than 25%, a pulmonary capillary wedge pressure of more than 20 mm Hg, a cardiac index of less than 2.5 L/min/m^2, systemic hypotension, pulmonary hypertension, and increased central venous pressure. Alcoholic cardiomyopathy is largely reversible if complete abstinence from alcohol is maintained.

MANAGEMENT OF ANESTHESIA

Since dilated cardiomyopathy is a cause of heart failure, the anesthetic management of these patients is the same as that described in the heart failure section of this chapter.

Regional anesthesia may be an alternative to general anesthesia in selected patients with dilated cardiomyopathy. However, the need for anticoagulant therapy may limit this option.

Peripartum Cardiomyopathy

Peripartum cardiomyopathy is a rare, dilated form of cardiomyopathy of unknown cause that arises during the peripartum period, that is, from the third trimester of pregnancy until 5 months after delivery. It occurs in women with no history of heart disease. The estimated incidence of peripartum cardiomyopathy is 1 in 3000 to 1 in 4000 live births. Risk factors include obesity, multiparity, advanced maternal age (>30 years), multifetal pregnancy, preeclampsia, and African American ethnicity. Possible causes of peripartum cardiomyopathy include viral myocarditis, an abnormal immune response to pregnancy, and maladaptive responses to the hemodynamic stresses of pregnancy.

SIGNS AND SYMPTOMS

The signs and symptoms of peripartum cardiomyopathy are those of heart failure: dyspnea, fatigue, and peripheral edema. However, these signs and symptoms are common in the final trimester of pregnancy, and there are no specific criteria for differentiating subtle symptoms of heart failure from normal late pregnancy. Clinical conditions that may mimic heart failure, such as amniotic fluid or pulmonary embolism, should be excluded when considering the diagnosis of peripartum cardiomyopathy.

DIAGNOSIS

The diagnosis of peripartum cardiomyopathy is based on the onset of unexplained LV dysfunction and echocardiographic documentation of a new finding of dilated cardiac chambers with LV systolic dysfunction during the period surrounding parturition.

TREATMENT

The goal of treatment is to alleviate the symptoms of heart failure. Diuretics, vasodilators, and digoxin can be used. ACE inhibitors are teratogenic but can be useful following delivery. During pregnancy, vasodilation is accomplished with hydralazine and nitrates. Intravenous immunoglobulin may have a beneficial effect. Thromboembolic complications are not uncommon, and anticoagulation is often recommended. Heart transplantation may be considered in patients who do not improve over time.

PROGNOSIS

The mortality rate of peripartum cardiomyopathy ranges from 25% to 50%, with most deaths occurring within 3 months of delivery. Death is usually a result of progression of congestive heart failure or sudden death associated with cardiac dysrhythmias or thromboembolic events. The prognosis appears to depend on the degree of normalization of LV size and function within 6 months of delivery.

MANAGEMENT OF ANESTHESIA

The management of anesthesia in parturients with peripartum cardiomyopathy requires assessment of cardiac status and careful planning of the analgesia and/or anesthesia required for delivery. Regional anesthesia may provide a desirable decrease in afterload.

Secondary Cardiomyopathies with Restrictive Physiology

Secondary cardiomyopathies with restrictive physiology are due to systemic diseases that produce myocardial infiltration and severe diastolic dysfunction. The most common of these cardiomyopathies is caused by amyloidosis. Other systemic diseases such as hemochromatosis, sarcoidosis, and carcinoid may produce a similar type of cardiomyopathy. The diagnosis should be considered in patients who have heart failure but no evidence of cardiomegaly or systolic dysfunction. The condition results from increased stiffness of the myocardium caused by the deposition of abnormal substances. Although there is impaired diastolic function and reduced ventricular compliance, systolic function is usually normal. Cardiomyopathies with restrictive physiology must be differentiated from constrictive pericarditis, which has a similar physiology. A clinical history of pericarditis makes the diagnosis of constrictive pericarditis more likely.

SIGNS AND SYMPTOMS

Because cardiomyopathies with restrictive physiology can affect both ventricles, symptoms and signs of left and/or right ventricular failure may be present. In advanced stages of this cardiomyopathy, all the signs and symptoms of heart failure can be present, but there is no cardiomegaly. Amyloid cardiomyopathy often presents with thromboembolic complications. Atrial fibrillation is also common. Cardiac conduction disturbances are particularly common in amyloidosis and sarcoidosis. Over time, this involvement of the conduction system can lead to heart block or ventricular dysrhythmias, resulting in sudden death.

DIAGNOSIS

The ECG may demonstrate conduction abnormalities. The chest radiograph may show signs of pulmonary congestion and/or pleural effusion, but cardiomegaly is absent. Laboratory tests should be employed as needed to diagnose the systemic disease responsible for the cardiac infiltration.

Echocardiography will demonstrate significant diastolic dysfunction and normal systolic function. The atria are enlarged because of the high atrial pressures, but the ventricles are normal in size. In cardiac amyloidosis, the ventricular mass appears speckled, a characteristic sign of amyloid deposition. Various echocardiographic criteria can differentiate secondary cardiomyopathy with restrictive physiology from constrictive pericarditis. Endomyocardial biopsy can elucidate the cause of the infiltrative cardiomyopathy.

TREATMENT

Symptomatic treatment is similar to that for diastolic heart failure. It includes administration of diuretics to treat pulmonary and systemic congestion. Excessive diuresis may decrease ventricular filling pressures and cardiac output and result in hypotension and hypoperfusion. Digoxin must be used with great caution, because it is potentially dysrhythmogenic in patients with amyloidosis. The development of atrial fibrillation with loss of the atrial contribution to ventricular filling may substantially worsen diastolic dysfunction, and a rapid ventricular response may further compromise cardiac output. Maintenance of normal sinus rhythm is extremely important. Because stroke volume tends to be fixed in the presence of cardiomyopathy with restrictive physiology, the onset of bradycardia may precipitate acute heart failure. Significant bradycardia or severe conduction system disease may require implantation of a cardiac pacemaker. With cardiac sarcoidosis, malignant ventricular dysrhythmias are common and may necessitate insertion of an ICD. Anticoagulation may be needed in patients with atrial fibrillation and/or low cardiac output. Cardiac transplantation is *not* a treatment option because myocardial infiltration will recur in the transplanted heart.

PROGNOSIS

The prognosis of secondary cardiomyopathy with restrictive physiology is very poor.

Management of anesthesia for patients with restrictive cardiomyopathy follows the same principles as that for patients with cardiac tamponade (see Chapter 7). Because stroke volume is relatively fixed, it is important to maintain sinus rhythm and to avoid any significant decrease in the heart rate. Maintenance of venous return and intravascular fluid volume is also necessary to maintain an acceptable cardiac output. Anticoagulant therapy will negatively influence the decision to select regional anesthesia.

Cor Pulmonale

Cor pulmonale is right ventricular enlargement (hypertrophy and/or dilation) that may progress to right-sided heart failure. Diseases that induce pulmonary hypertension such as COPD, restrictive lung disease, and respiratory insufficiency of central origin (obesity-hypoventilation syndrome) cause cor pulmonale. It can also result from idiopathic pulmonary artery hypertension, that is, the pulmonary hypertension that occurs in the absence of left-sided heart disease, myocardial disease, congenital heart disease, or any other clinically significant respiratory, connective tissue, or chronic thromboembolic disease. The most common cause of cor pulmonale is COPD.

Cor pulmonale usually occurs in persons older than 50 years of age because of its association with COPD. Men are affected five times more often than women.

PATHOPHYSIOLOGY

The main pathophysiologic determinant of cor pulmonale is pulmonary hypertension. By various mechanisms, chronic lung disease induces an increase in pulmonary vascular resistance. Chronic alveolar hypoxia (PaO_2 <55 mm Hg) is the most important factor in this process. Acute hypoxia, such as seen in exacerbations of COPD or during sleep in patients with obesity-hypoventilation syndrome, causes pulmonary vasoconstriction. Long-standing chronic hypoxia promotes pulmonary vasculature remodeling and an increase in pulmonary vascular resistance. Even mild hypoxemia may result in vascular remodeling, so it appears that other factors are also involved in the development of cor pulmonale.

Because of pulmonary hypertension, the right ventricle has an increased workload, and right ventricular hypertrophy develops. Over time, right ventricular dysfunction occurs, and eventually right ventricular failure is present.

SIGNS AND SYMPTOMS

Clinical manifestations of cor pulmonale may be obscured by the co-existing lung disease. Clinical signs occur late in the course of the disease, and the most prominent is peripheral edema. As right ventricular function deteriorates, dyspnea increases and effort-related syncope can occur. Accentuation of the pulmonic component of the second heart sound, a diastolic murmur due to incompetence of the pulmonic valve, and a systolic murmur due to tricuspid regurgitation connote severe pulmonary hypertension. Evidence of overt right ventricular failure consists of increased jugular venous pressure and hepatosplenomegaly.

DIAGNOSIS

The ECG may show signs of right atrial and right ventricular hypertrophy. Right atrial hypertrophy is suggested by peaked P waves in leads II, III, and aVF (P pulmonale). Right axis deviation and a partial or complete right bundle branch block are often seen with right ventricular hypertrophy. A normal-appearing ECG, however, does not exclude the presence of pulmonary hypertension.

Radiographic signs of cor pulmonale include an increase in the width of the right pulmonary artery and a decrease in pulmonary vascular markings in the lung periphery. On a lateral-projection chest radiograph, right ventricular enlargement is indicated by a decrease in the retrosternal space. However, this is a late sign.

Transesophageal echocardiography can be a very useful diagnostic tool. It can provide quantitative estimates of pulmonary artery pressure, assessment of the size and function of the right atrium and ventricle, and evaluation of the presence and severity of tricuspid or pulmonic regurgitation. *Transthoracic* echocardiography is often difficult to perform in patients with COPD because the hyperinflated lungs impair transmission of the ultrasound waves.

TREATMENT

Treatment of cor pulmonale is geared at reducing the workload of the right ventricle by decreasing pulmonary vascular resistance and pulmonary artery pressure. If the pulmonary artery vasoconstriction has a reversible component, as is likely during an acute exacerbation of COPD, this goal can be achieved by returning the PaO_2, $PaCO_2$, and arterial pH to normal.

Oxygen supplementation to maintain the PaO_2 above 60 mm Hg (oxygen saturation of >90% by pulse oximetry) is useful in both the acute and long-term treatment of right-sided heart failure. Long-term oxygen therapy decreases the mortality of cor pulmonale and improves cognitive function and quality of life.

Diuretics and digitalis may be used to treat right-sided heart failure that does not respond to correction of arterial blood gases. Diuretics must be administered very carefully, because diuretic-induced metabolic alkalosis, which encourages carbon dioxide retention, may aggravate ventilatory insufficiency by depressing the effectiveness of carbon dioxide as a stimulus to breathing. Diuresis can also increase blood viscosity and myocardial work. Digitalis can be used for treatment of atrial fibrillation, but it must be administered very cautiously because the risk of digitalis toxicity is increased in the presence of hypoxemia, acidosis, and electrolyte imbalances. Pulmonary vasodilators, such as sildenafil and bosentan, have been shown to improve the symptoms of cor pulmonale and reduce right ventricular mass as well as right ventricular remodeling.

When cor pulmonale is progressive despite maximum medical therapy, transplantation of one or both lungs or a heart-lung transplantation will provide dramatic relief of cardiorespiratory failure.

PROGNOSIS

The prognosis of patients with cor pulmonale is dependent on the disease responsible for initiating pulmonary hypertension. Patients with COPD in whom arterial oxygenation can be maintained at near-normal levels and whose pulmonary hypertension is mild have a favorable prognosis. Prognosis is poor in patients with severe, irreversible pulmonary hypertension.

MANAGEMENT OF ANESTHESIA

Preoperative preparation of patients with cor pulmonale resulting from chronic lung disease is directed toward (1) eliminating and controlling acute and chronic pulmonary infection, (2) reversing bronchospasm, (3) improving clearance of airway secretions, (4) expanding collapsed or poorly ventilated alveoli, (5) maintaining hydration, and (6) correcting any electrolyte imbalances. Preoperative measurement of arterial blood gases will provide guidelines for perioperative management.

Induction of general anesthesia can be accomplished using any available method or drug. Adequate depth of anesthesia should be present before endotracheal intubation, because this stimulus can elicit reflex bronchospasm in lightly anesthetized patients.

Anesthesia is typically maintained with a volatile anesthetic combined with other drugs. Volatile anesthetics are effective bronchodilators. Large doses of opioids should be avoided because they can contribute to prolonged postoperative ventilatory depression. Muscle relaxants associated with histamine release should also be avoided because of the adverse effect of histamine on airway resistance and pulmonary vascular resistance.

Positive pressure ventilation improves oxygenation, presumably because of better ventilation-perfusion matching. Humidification of inhaled gases helps maintain hydration, liquefaction of secretions, and mucociliary function.

Intraoperative monitoring of patients with cor pulmonale is influenced by the complexity of the surgery. An intraarterial catheter permits frequent determination of arterial blood gas concentrations and subsequent adjustments in the inspired concentration of oxygen. A central venous catheter or pulmonary artery catheter may be useful depending on the surgery. Trend values of right atrial pressure can provide some information about right ventricular function. Direct measurement of pulmonary artery pressure helps determine the time to treat pulmonary hypertension and the response to treatment. Transesophageal echocardiography is an alternative method for monitoring right ventricular function and fluid status. However, the need for trained personnel and expensive equipment prevents this monitoring modality from being universally available.

Regional anesthetic techniques can be used in appropriate situations in patients with cor pulmonale, but regional anesthesia is best avoided for operations that require high levels of sensory and motor block. Loss of function of the accessory muscles of respiration may be very deleterious in patients with pulmonary disease. In addition, any decrease in systemic vascular resistance in the presence of fixed pulmonary hypertension can produce a very significant degree of systemic hypotension.

The respiratory and cardiovascular status of a patient with cor pulmonale must be vigilantly monitored in the postoperative period, and any factors that exacerbate pulmonary hypertension, such as hypoxia and hypercarbia, must be avoided. Oxygen therapy should be maintained as needed.

KEY POINTS

■ Heart failure is a complex pathophysiologic state in which the heart is unable to fill with or eject blood at a rate appropriate to tissue requirements. Heart failure is characterized by specific symptoms (dyspnea and fatigue) and signs of circulatory congestion or hypoperfusion.

■ In the United States 5.8 million people have heart failure, and this imposes a great financial burden on the health care system.

■ The principal pathophysiologic derangement in the development and progression of heart failure is ventricular remodeling. The principal treatment goals in heart failure patients are avoiding or decreasing the degree of ventricular remodeling and promoting reverse remodeling. Therapies proven to be of value in this regard include ACE inhibitors, β-blockers, aldosterone inhibitors, and CRT.

■ The management of acute heart failure includes the use of low-dose loop diuretics in combination with vasodilators, positive inotropic drugs, exogenous BNP, and/or insertion of mechanical devices.

■ HCM is the most common genetic cardiac disorder. Its pathophysiology is related to the development of LVOT obstruction and ventricular dysrhythmias that can cause sudden death.

■ Factors that induce LVOT obstruction in HCM include hypovolemia, tachycardia, an increase in myocardial contractility, and a decrease in afterload. Outflow tract obstruction is managed by maintaining hydration, increasing afterload (phenylephrine), and decreasing heart rate and myocardial contractility (β-blockers and calcium channel blockers).

■ Dilated cardiomyopathy is the most common form of cardiomyopathy and the second most common cause of heart failure. The treatment and anesthetic implications are similar to those for chronic heart failure.

■ Cor pulmonale is right ventricular enlargement (hypertrophy and/or dilation) that may progress to right-sided heart failure. It is caused by diseases that promote development of pulmonary hypertension.

■ The most important pathophysiologic determinant of the development of pulmonary hypertension and cor pulmonale in patients with chronic lung disease is alveolar hypoxia. The best available treatment to improve the prognosis in these patients is long-term oxygen therapy.

RESOURCES

Armstrong PW. Aldosterone antagonists—last man standing? *N Engl J Med.* 2011;364:79-80.

Gheorghiade M, Zannad F, Sopko G, et al. International Working Group on Acute Heart Failure Syndromes: Acute heart failure syndromes: current state and framework for future research. *Circulation.* 2005;112:3958-3968.

Groban L, Butterworth J. Perioperative management of chronic heart failure. *Anesth Analg.* 2006;103:57-75.

Hunt SA, Abraham WT, Chin MH, et al. ACC/AHA 2005 guideline update for the diagnosis and management of chronic heart failure in the adult: a report of the American College of Cardiology/American Heart Association Task Force on Practice Guidelines (Writing Committee to Update the 2001 Guidelines for the Evaluation and Management of Heart Failure): developed in collaboration with the American College of Chest Physicians and the International Society for Heart and Lung Transplantation: endorsed by the Heart Rhythm Society. *Circulation.* 2005;112:154-235.

Jessup M, Brozena S. Heart failure. *N Engl J Med.* 2003;348:2007-2018.

Maron BJ, Towbin JA, Thiene G, et al. Contemporary definition and classification of the cardiomyopathies: an American Heart Association scientific statement from the Council on Clinical Cardiology, Heart Failure and Transplantation Committee; Quality of Care and Outcomes Research and Functional Genomics and Transplantational Biology Interdisciplinary Working Groups; and Council on Epidemiology and Prevention. *Circulation.* 2006;113:1807-1816.

Poliac LC, Barron ME, Maron BJ. Hypertrophic cardiomyopathy. *Anesthesiology.* 2006;104:183-192.

Pulido JN, Park SJ, Rihal CS. Percutaneous left ventricular assist devices: clinical uses, future applications, and anesthetic considerations. *J Cardiothorac Vasc Anesth.* 2010;24:478-486.

Rauch H, Motsch J, Böttiger BW. Newer approaches to the pharmacologic management of heart failure. *Curr Opin Anesthesiol.* 2006;19:75-81.

Swedberg K, Cleland J, Dargie H, et al. Guidelines for the diagnosis and treatment of chronic heart failure: executive summary (update 2005): the Task Force for the Diagnosis and Treatment of Chronic Heart Failure of the European Society of Cardiology. *Eur Heart J.* 2005;26:1115-1140.

Thunberg CA, Gaitan BD, Arabia FA, et al. Ventricular assist devices today and tomorrow. *J Cardiothorac Vasc Anesth.* 2010;24:656-680.

Weitzenblum E. Chronic cor pulmonale. *Heart.* 2003;89:225-230.

Yan AT, Yan RT, Liu PP. Narrative review: pharmacotherapy for chronic heart failure: evidence from recent clinical trials. *Ann Intern Med.* 2005;142:132-145.

CHAPTER 7

Pericardial Diseases and Cardiac Trauma

RAJ K. MODAK ■

Although the etiology of pericardial diseases is diverse, the resulting clinical and pathologic manifestations are similar. The three most frequent responses to pericardial injury are characterized as acute pericarditis, pericardial effusion, and constrictive pericarditis. Cardiac tamponade may present whenever pericardial fluid accumulates under pressure. Management of anesthesia in patients with pericardial disease is facilitated by an understanding of the alterations in cardiovascular function produced by pericardial disease.

ACUTE PERICARDITIS

Viral infection is often presumed to be the cause of acute pericarditis when it occurs as a primary illness (Table 7-1). Most cases of acute pericarditis follow a transient and uncomplicated clinical course, and thus this entity is often termed *acute benign pericarditis*. Acute benign pericarditis is unaccompanied by either a substantial pericardial effusion or cardiac tamponade and rarely progresses to constrictive pericarditis.

Pericarditis can also occur after myocardial infarction. It most commonly appears 1 to 3 days following a transmural myocardial infarction as a result of the interaction between the healing necrotic myocardium and the pericardium. Dressler's syndrome is a delayed form of acute pericarditis that may follow acute myocardial infarction. It can occur weeks to months after the initial myocardial event. It is thought that Dressler's syndrome is the result of an autoimmune process that is initiated by the entry of necrotic myocardium into the circulation, where it acts as an antigen. Acute pericarditis occurs more commonly in adult men 20 to 50 years of age.

Diagnosis

The clinical diagnosis of acute pericarditis is based on the presence of chest pain, a pericardial friction rub, and changes on the electrocardiogram (ECG). The chest pain is typically acute in onset and is described as a severe pain localized over the anterior chest. This pain typically worsens with inspiration, which helps to distinguish it from pain caused by myocardial ischemia. Patients often report relief when changing position from being supine to sitting forward. Low-grade fever and sinus tachycardia are also common. Auscultation of the chest often reveals a friction rub, especially when the symptoms are acute. These high-pitched scratchy sounds occur when volumes in the heart undergo the most dramatic changes, such as during early ventricular filling and ventricular ejection. Pericardial friction rubs are related to the cardiac cycle; this makes it possible to differentiate these sounds from pleural rubs, which are related to inspiration.

Inflammation of the superficial myocardium is the most likely explanation for the diffuse changes seen on the ECG. Classically, the ECG changes associated with acute pericarditis evolve through four stages. Stage I is characterized by diffuse ST-segment elevation and PR-segment depression. In stage II, the ST and PR segments normalize. Stage III shows widespread

TABLE 7-1 ■ Causes of acute pericarditis and pericardial effusion

Infection
  Viral
  Bacterial
  Fungal
  Tuberculous
Myocardial infarction (Dressler's syndrome)
Trauma or cardiotomy
Metastatic disease
Drugs
Mediastinal radiation
Systemic disease
  Rheumatoid arthritis
  Systemic lupus erythematosus
  Scleroderma

T-wave inversions. And stage IV is characterized by normalization of the T waves. The early ST elevations are usually present in all leads, but in post–myocardial infarction pericarditis, the changes may be more localized. The diffuse distribution and the absence of reciprocal ST-segment depressions distinguish these changes from the ECG changes of myocardial infarction. Depression of the PR segment seen on the ECG reflects superficial injury of the atrial myocardium and may be the earliest sign of acute pericarditis. ECG changes are seen in 90% of patients with acute pericarditis. However, a clear evolution of ECG changes through the four stages described earlier is noted in only approximately 60% of all patients with acute pericarditis. Patients with uremic pericarditis frequently do not have these typical ECG abnormalities of pericarditis. Acute pericarditis in the absence of an associated pericardial effusion does not alter cardiac function.

Treatment

Salicylates or other nonsteroidal antiinflammatory drugs may be useful for decreasing pericardial inflammation. Aspirin is most commonly prescribed, although ketorolac has also been used successfully. Symptomatic relief of the pain of acute pericarditis can also be provided by oral analgesics such as codeine. In some settings, relief may be achieved with the use of colchicine. Corticosteroids such as prednisone can also relieve the symptoms of acute pericarditis. However, their use early in the course of acute pericarditis is associated with an increased incidence of relapse after discontinuation of the drug. Therefore, steroid therapy is usually reserved for cases that do not respond to conventional therapy.

Relapsing Pericarditis

Acute pericarditis resulting from any cause may follow a recurrent or chronic relapsing course. Relapsing pericarditis has two clinical presentations: incessant and intermittent. *Incessant pericarditis* is diagnosed in patients in whom discontinuation of or attempts to wean from antiinflammatory drugs nearly always result in a relapse within a period of 6 weeks or less. *Intermittent pericarditis* occurs in patients who have symptom-free intervals of longer than 6 weeks without drug treatment. In many patients, the symptoms of relapsing pericarditis include weakness, fatigue, and headache, and are associated with chest discomfort. Although relapsing pericarditis is uncomfortable, it is rarely life threatening. Treatment may include the standard therapies for acute pericarditis and/or corticosteroids (prednisone) or immunosuppressive drugs such as azathioprine.

Pericarditis after Cardiac Surgery

Postcardiotomy syndrome presents primarily as acute pericarditis. The cause of this syndrome may be infective or autoimmune, and it may follow blunt or penetrating trauma, hemopericardium, or epicardial pacemaker implantation. Most commonly, it is seen in patients undergoing cardiac surgery in which pericardiotomy was performed. The incidence of postcardiotomy syndrome associated with cardiac surgery is between 10% and 40%. It is more common in pediatric patients. The risk is lower after cardiac transplantation, presumably because of the immunosuppressed state. Cardiac tamponade is a rare complication of postcardiotomy syndrome, with an incidence ranging from 0.1% to 6%. The treatment of postcardiotomy syndrome is similar to that of other forms of acute pericarditis.

PERICARDIAL EFFUSION AND CARDIAC TAMPONADE

Pericardial fluid may accumulate in the pericardial sac with virtually any form of pericardial disease. The pathophysiologic effects of a pericardial effusion reflect whether or not the fluid is under pressure. Cardiac tamponade occurs when the pressure of the fluid in the pericardial space impairs cardiac filling. Common causes of atraumatic and traumatic pericardial effusion are listed in Table 7-1. In up to 20% of cases, the cause of the pericardial effusion is unknown. Neoplastic pericardial effusion is a common cause of cardiac tamponade in nonsurgical patients.

Pericardial fluid may be classified as transudative or exudative. Serosanguineous (exudative) fluid is typically seen when the pericardial disease is due to cancer, tuberculosis, or radiation exposure. Serosanguineous pericardial effusion also occurs in patients with end-stage renal disease. Traumatic injury usually presents as hemopericardium. Perforation of the heart and subsequent cardiac tamponade may also result from insertion of central venous catheters or pacemaker wires.

Signs and Symptoms

The signs and symptoms of a pericardial effusion depend on its size and duration (acute versus chronic). The pericardial space normally holds 15 to 50 mL of pericardial fluid. This fluid is an ultrafiltrate of plasma that comes from the visceral pericardium. Native pericardial fluid lubricates the heart and

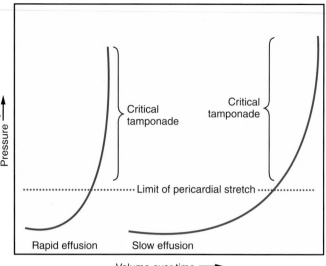

FIGURE 7-1 Pericardial pressure-volume curves are shown in which the intrapericardial volume increases slowly or rapidly over time. On the left, rapidly increasing pericardial fluid quickly exceeds the limit of pericardial stretch, which causes a steep increase in pericardial pressure. On the right, a slower rate of pericardial filling takes longer to exceed the limit of pericardial stretch because there is more time for the pericardium to stretch and for compensatory mechanisms to become activated. *(From Spodick DH. Acute cardiac tamponade. N Engl J Med. 2003;349:684-690. Copyright 2003 Massachusetts Medical Society, with permission.)*

facilitates normal cardiac motion within the pericardial sac. Acute changes in pericardial volume as small as 100 mL may result in increased intrapericardial pressure and development of cardiac tamponade. Conversely, large volumes can be accommodated if the pericardial effusion develops gradually. In this context, the pressure-volume relationship is altered, and cardiac tamponade may not develop because the pericardium stretches to accommodate the volume of the effusion (Figure 7-1). The development of a chronic pericardial effusion in this setting can result in effusion volumes in excess of 2 L. If the pressure in the pericardium remains low, large effusions can be tolerated without significant signs and symptoms. However, as pericardial pressure increases, the right atrial pressure increases in parallel, so that the right atrial pressure becomes an accurate reflection of the intrapericardial pressure. At this point, signs and symptoms of cardiac tamponade may develop.

CARDIAC TAMPONADE

Cardiac tamponade presents as a spectrum of hemodynamic abnormalities of varying severity, rather than as an all-or-none phenomenon. Symptoms of large pericardial effusions reflect compression of adjacent anatomic structures, specifically the esophagus, trachea, and lung. In this situation, common symptoms include anorexia, dyspnea, cough, and chest pain. Symptoms such as dysphagia, hiccups, and hoarseness may indicate higher pressure on the adjacent tissues.

Two important physical signs of cardiac tamponade and constrictive pericarditis were described by Dr. Adolf Kussmaul in 1873. *Kussmaul's sign* is distention of the jugular veins during inspiration. *Pulsus paradoxus* was described by Kussmaul as "a pulse simultaneously slight and irregular, disappearing during inspiration and returning on expiration." The modern definition of pulsus paradoxus is a decrease in systolic blood pressure of more than 10 mm Hg during inspiration (Figure 7-2). This hemodynamic change reflects selective impairment of diastolic filling of the left ventricle. Pulsus paradoxus is observed in approximately 75% of patients with acute cardiac

tamponade, but in only about 30% of patients with chronic pericardial effusion. Kussmaul's sign and pulsus paradoxus both reflect dyssynchrony or opposing responses of the right and left ventricles to filling during the respiratory cycle. Another term for this occurrence is *ventricular discordance.*

Beck's triad consists of distant heart sounds, increased jugular venous pressure, and hypotension. Beck's triad is observed in one third of patients with acute cardiac tamponade. Another triad consisting of quiet heart sounds, increased central venous pressure, and ascites has been described in patients with chronic pericardial effusion. More commonly, symptomatic patients with chronic pericardial effusion exhibit sinus tachycardia, jugular venous distention, hepatomegaly, and peripheral edema. Ewart's sign, in which there is an area of bronchial breath sounds and dullness to percussion, is an uncommon sign of pericardial effusion. It is caused by compression of the left lower lobe by the pericardial effusion. When this sign is present, it is observed at the inferior angle of the left scapula.

Depending on the severity of cardiac tamponade, systemic blood pressure may be decreased or maintained in the normal range. Central venous pressure is almost always increased. Activation of the sympathetic nervous system reflects an attempt to maintain cardiac output and blood pressure by tachycardia and peripheral vasoconstriction. Cardiac output is maintained as long as central venous pressure exceeds right ventricular end-diastolic pressure. A progressive increase in intrapericardial pressure, however, eventually results in equalization of right atrial pressure and right ventricular end-diastolic pressure. Ultimately, the increased intrapericardial pressure leads to impaired diastolic filling of the heart, decreased stroke volume, and hypotension (Table 7-2).

Cardiac tamponade may be the cause of low cardiac output syndrome during the early postoperative period after cardiac surgery. Cardiac tamponade may occur as a complication of various invasive procedures in the cardiac catheterization laboratory and intensive care unit. Acute cardiac tamponade may also be due to hemopericardium caused by aortic dissection, penetrating cardiac trauma, or acute myocardial infarction.

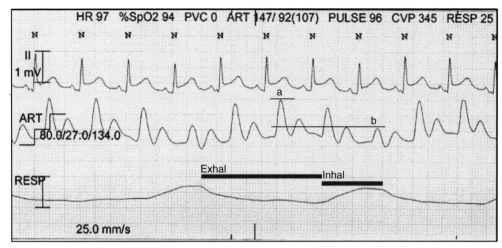

FIGURE 7-2 Cyclical systolic pressure variation during tidal breathing is normal. In the presence of cardiac tamponade, the arterial blood pressure decreases more than 10 mm Hg (a→b) from exhalation (*Exhal*) to inhalation (*Inhal*) as a reflection of a concomitant decrease in left ventricular stroke volume. This contrasts with the opposite response observed during inspiration in the absence of cardiac tamponade, which accounts for its designation as a paradoxical pulse (pulsus paradoxus). *(From Binks A, Soar J, Cranshaw J. Pulsus paradoxus and pericardial effusion. Resuscitation. 2006;68[2]:177-178.)*

TABLE 7-2	Signs and symptoms of cardiac tamponade

Increased central venous pressure
Pulsus paradoxus
Equalization of cardiac filling pressures
Hypotension
Decreased voltage on the electrocardiogram
Activation of the sympathetic nervous system

LOCULATED PERICARDIAL EFFUSIONS

Loculated pericardial effusion may selectively compress one or more cardiac chambers producing a localized cardiac tamponade. This localization is most frequently observed after cardiac surgery, when blood accumulates behind the sternum and selectively compresses the right ventricle and right atrium. A similar response may be seen following anterior chest wall trauma. Transesophageal echocardiography is superior to transthoracic echocardiography for demonstrating a localized pericardial effusion.

Diagnosis

Echocardiography is the most accurate and practical method for diagnosing pericardial effusion and cardiac tamponade. Because of this, echocardiography fulfills the class I recommendations by the 2003 Task Force of the American Society of Echocardiography, American College of Cardiology, and the American Heart Association for the evaluation of all patients with suspected pericardial disease. Echocardiography can detect pericardial effusions of as little as 20 mL. The measurement of the echo-free space between the heart and pericardium allows easy assessment of effusion size and may also provide information about the cause of the effusion. Computed tomography (CT) and magnetic resonance imaging (MRI) are also useful in detecting both pericardial effusion and pericardial thickening. The ECG may demonstrate low voltage in the presence of a large effusion. Chest radiography often shows a characteristic "water bottle heart." However, this is a nonspecific sign for pericardial effusion. Pericardiocentesis may be useful for diagnosing metastatic disease or infection.

Echocardiography, although definitive for diagnosing pericardial effusion, cannot always confirm the presence of cardiac tamponade. However, a finding of early diastolic inward wall motion of the right atrium or right ventricle ("collapse"), reflecting similar intracavitary and intrapericardial pressure, is suggestive of the presence of cardiac tamponade. Echocardiography can also demonstrate ventricular discordance. Pulsed wave Doppler examination of peak mitral and tricuspid inflow velocities will show a decrease in mitral flow and an increase in tricuspid flow during inspiration if tamponade is present. Ventricular septal deviation toward the left can also be seen during inspiration. With cardiac tamponade, the pressures within the cardiac chambers will eventually equilibrate. Clinically, this can be confirmed by right-sided heart catheterization. Pulmonary artery occlusion pressure and pulmonary artery diastolic pressure (both estimates of left atrial pressure and left ventricular end-diastolic pressure), right atrial pressure, and right ventricular end-diastolic pressure will be nearly equal.

Treatment

Mild cardiac tamponade can be managed conservatively in some patients. However, removal of fluid is required for definitive treatment and should be performed when central venous pressure is increased. Pericardial fluid may be removed by pericardiocentesis or by surgical techniques, which include subxiphoid pericardiostomy, thoracoscopic pericardiostomy, and thoracotomy with pericardiostomy. Removal of even a small amount of pericardial fluid can result in a dramatic decrease in intrapericardial pressure.

Temporizing measures likely to help maintain stroke volume until definitive treatment of cardiac tamponade can be instituted include expanding intravascular volume, administering catecholamines to increase myocardial contractility, and correcting metabolic acidosis. Expansion of intravascular fluid volume can be achieved by infusion of either colloid or crystalloid solution. However, improvement in hemodynamic function may be limited, and pericardiocentesis should not be delayed.

Continuous intravenous infusion of a catecholamine such as isoproterenol may be an effective temporizing measure for increasing myocardial contractility and heart rate. Atropine may be necessary to treat the bradycardia that results from vagal reflexes evoked by the increased intrapericardial pressure. Dopamine infusion, which increases systemic vascular resistance, can also be employed to treat cardiac tamponade. As with intravascular fluid replacement, pericardiocentesis should never be delayed in deference to drug therapy.

Correction of metabolic acidosis is essential when considering the management of a cardiac tamponade. Metabolic acidosis resulting from low cardiac output should be treated to correct the myocardial depression seen with severe acidosis and to improve the inotropic effects of catecholamines.

Management of Anesthesia

General anesthesia and positive pressure ventilation in the presence of a hemodynamically significant cardiac tamponade can result in *life-threatening hypotension*. This hypotension may be due to anesthesia-induced peripheral vasodilation, direct myocardial depression, or decreased venous return caused by the increased intrathoracic pressure associated with positive pressure ventilation. Pericardiocentesis *performed under local anesthesia* is often preferred for the initial management of hypotensive patients with cardiac tamponade. After the hemodynamic status is improved by percutaneous pericardiocentesis, general anesthesia and positive pressure ventilation can be instituted to permit surgical exploration and more definitive treatment of the cardiac tamponade. Induction and maintenance of anesthesia with ketamine or a benzodiazepine in combination with nitrous oxide is often used. The circulatory effects of pancuronium are particularly useful for producing skeletal muscle relaxation in these patients. Intraoperative monitoring typically includes intraarterial and central venous pressure monitoring.

In cases in which it is not possible to relieve the cardiac tamponade before induction of anesthesia, the principal goals of anesthetic induction are maintenance of adequate cardiac output and blood pressure. Anesthesia-induced decreases in myocardial contractility, systemic vascular resistance, and heart rate must be avoided. Increased intrathoracic pressure caused

by straining or coughing during induction or by mechanical ventilation may further decrease venous return. Some advocate preparing and draping for incision before induction of anesthesia and endotracheal intubation. This would allow for the shortest possible time from the adverse hemodynamic consequences related to the anesthetic and mechanical ventilation and the surgical relief of the tamponade. Ketamine is useful for induction and maintenance of anesthesia because it increases myocardial contractility, systemic vascular resistance, and heart rate. Induction of anesthesia with a benzodiazepine followed by maintenance with nitrous oxide plus fentanyl (or another synthetic narcotic), combined with pancuronium for skeletal muscle relaxation, has also been used successfully. Continuous monitoring of blood pressure and central venous pressure should be initiated before induction of anesthesia. Administration of intravenous fluids and/or continuous infusion of a catecholamine may be useful for maintaining cardiac output until the cardiac tamponade is relieved by surgical drainage. After release of a severe tamponade, there is often a significant swing in blood pressure from hypotension to *hypertension*. This change should be anticipated and appropriate treatment should be prompt, especially if the cause of the tamponade is an aortic hematoma, dissection, or aneurysm that could be significantly compromised by hypertension.

CONSTRICTIVE PERICARDITIS

Constrictive pericarditis is most often idiopathic or the result of previous cardiac surgery or exposure to radiotherapy. Tuberculosis may also cause constrictive pericarditis. *Chronic constrictive pericarditis* is characterized by fibrous scarring and adhesions that obliterate the pericardial space, creating a rigid shell around the heart. Calcification may develop in long-standing cases. *Subacute constrictive pericarditis* is more common than chronic calcific pericarditis, and the resulting constriction in this situation is fibroelastic.

Signs and Symptoms

Pericardial constriction typically presents with symptoms and signs because of a combination of increased central venous pressure and low cardiac output. Symptoms of pericardial constriction include decreased exercise tolerance and fatigue. Jugular venous distention, hepatic congestion, ascites, and peripheral edema are signs of pericardial constriction that mimic right ventricular failure. Pulmonary congestion is usually absent. Increases in and eventual equalization of right atrial pressure, right ventricular end-diastolic pressure, and pulmonary artery occlusion pressure are features that occur in the presence of both constrictive pericarditis and cardiac tamponade. As pericardial pressure increases, right atrial pressure increases in parallel, and therefore the central venous pressure is an accurate reflection of intrapericardial pressure. Atrial dysrhythmias (atrial fibrillation or flutter) are often seen in patients with chronic constrictive pericarditis and presumably reflect involvement of the sinoatrial node by the disease process.

Constrictive pericarditis is similar to cardiac tamponade in that both conditions impede diastolic filling of the heart and result in an increased central venous pressure and ultimately a decreased cardiac output. Diagnostic signs, however, differ in the two conditions. Pulsus paradoxus is a regular feature of cardiac tamponade but is often absent in constrictive pericarditis. Kussmaul's sign (increased central venous pressure during inspiration) occurs more frequently in patients with constrictive pericarditis than in those with cardiac tamponade. An early diastolic sound (pericardial knock) is often heard in patients with constrictive pericarditis but does not occur in cardiac tamponade. A prominent *y* descent of the jugular venous pressure waveform (Friedreich's sign) reflects rapid right ventricular filling in early diastole that is seen with constrictive pericarditis. This rapid early diastolic filling is also detected by a dip in early diastolic pressure. The ventricle is completely filled by the end of the rapid filling phase, and a period of constant ventricular volume, known as *diastasis,* persists for the remainder of diastole. Corresponding to this prolonged diastasis, ventricular diastolic pressure remains unchanged for the latter two thirds of diastole. This pattern of ventricular diastolic pressure in constrictive pericarditis is referred to as the *square root sign* or *dip-and-plateau* morphology (Figure 7-3, *A*).

Diagnosis

Constrictive pericarditis is difficult to diagnose, and its signs and symptoms are therefore often erroneously attributed to liver disease or idiopathic pericardial effusion. The clinical diagnosis of constrictive pericarditis depends on the confirmation of an increased central venous pressure without other signs or symptoms of heart disease. Heart size and lung fields appear normal on chest radiographs. However, pericardial calcification can be seen in 30% to 50% of cases. The ECG may display only minor, nonspecific abnormalities. Echocardiography can be quite helpful in many instances by demonstrating abnormal septal motion and pericardial thickening that suggests the presence of constrictive pericarditis. Transesophageal echocardiography, CT of the chest, and MRI are superior to transthoracic echocardiography for demonstrating pericardial thickening. As with cardiac tamponade, ventricular discordance is a feature of constrictive pericarditis. Pulsed wave Doppler studies often demonstrate an exaggerated respiratory variation in mitral and tricuspid diastolic flow velocities. Cardiac catheterization reveals characteristic abnormalities, including increased central venous pressure, nondilated and normally contracting right and left ventricles, near equilibration of right- and left-sided cardiac filling pressures, and a dip-and-plateau waveform in the right ventricle (see Figure 7-3). Many features considered characteristic of constrictive pericarditis may also be present in patients with restrictive cardiomyopathy, but several features help to distinguish these two entities (Table 7-3). Ventricular discordance is a feature of constrictive pericarditis but not of restrictive cardiomyopathy. Kussmaul's sign and pulsus paradoxus are present in constrictive pericarditis but absent in restrictive cardiomyopathy. Two echocardiographic techniques can also help in this evaluation. Pulsed wave Doppler ultrasonography demonstrates ventricular discordance in constrictive pericarditis. Tissue Doppler ultrasonography can be used to interrogate the motion of the mitral valve annulus. In restrictive cardiomyopathy, the motion of the mitral annulus is restricted. In constrictive pericarditis, the motion of the mitral annulus is normal. Cardiac catheterization can demonstrate ventricular discordance by allowing simultaneous recording of right and left ventricular systolic pressures. If discordance is present, right ventricular peak systolic pressure increases on inspiration, whereas left ventricular peak pressure decreases. This observation of ventricular discordance indicates the presence of constrictive pericarditis rather than restrictive cardiomyopathy.

Treatment

Constrictive pericarditis that develops as a complication of acute pericarditis will occasionally resolve spontaneously. In most

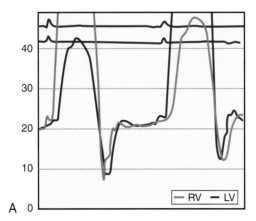
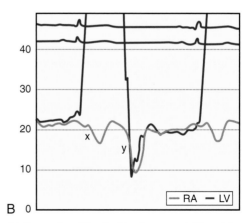

FIGURE 7-3 Pressure recordings in a patient with constrictive pericarditis. **A,** Simultaneous right ventricular (RV) and left ventricular (LV) pressure tracings with equalization of diastolic pressure as well as dip-and-plateau morphology. **B,** Simultaneous right atrial (RA) and LV pressure with equalization of RA and LV diastolic pressure. Note the prominent *y* descent. *(From Vaitkus PT, Cooper KA, Shuman WP, et al. Images in cardiovascular medicine: constrictive pericarditis.* Circulation. *1996;93:834-835, with permission.)*

TABLE 7-3 ■ Features useful for differentiating constrictive pericarditis from restrictive cardiomyopathy

Feature	Constrictive pericarditis	Restrictive cardiomyopathy
Medical history	Previous pericarditis, cardiac surgery, trauma, radiotherapy, connective tissue disease	No such history
Mitral or tricuspid regurgitation	Usually absent	Often present
Ventricular septal movement with respiration	Movement toward left ventricle on inspiration	Little movement toward left ventricle
Respiratory variation in mitral and tricuspid flow velocity	>25% in most cases	<15% in most cases
Equilibration of diastolic pressures in all cardiac chambers	Within 5 mm Hg in nearly all cases	Present in only a small proportion of cases
Respiratory variation of ventricular peak systolic pressures	Right and left ventricular peak systolic pressures are out of phase (discordant)	Right and left ventricular peak systolic pressures are in phase
Magnetic resonance imaging/computed tomography	Show pericardial thickening in most cases	Rarely show pericardial thickening
Endomyocardial biopsy	Normal or nonspecific findings	Amyloid present in some cases

Adapted from Hancock EW. Differential diagnosis of restrictive cardiomyopathy and constrictive pericarditis. *Heart.* 2001;86:343-349.

patients, however, the definitive treatment of constrictive pericarditis consists of surgical removal of the adherent constricting pericardium. This procedure may result in considerable bleeding from the epicardial surface of the heart. Cardiopulmonary bypass may occasionally be needed to facilitate pericardial stripping, especially if hemorrhage is difficult to control. Unlike the treatment of cardiac tamponade, in which hemodynamic improvement occurs immediately, surgical removal of constricting pericardium is not followed by an immediate improvement in cardiac output or a reduction in right atrial pressure. Typically, right atrial pressure returns to normal within 3 months of surgery. The absence of immediate hemodynamic improvement may be due to disuse atrophy of myocardial muscle fibers or persistent constrictive effects from sclerotic epicardium that is not removed with the pericardium. Inadequate long-term relief after surgical removal of constricting pericardium may reflect associated myocardial disease, especially in patients with radiation-induced pericardial disease.

Management of Anesthesia

Anesthetic drugs and techniques that minimize changes in heart rate, systemic vascular resistance, venous return, and myocardial contractility should be selected. Combinations of opioids, benzodiazepines, and nitrous oxide with or without low doses of volatile anesthetics are appropriate for maintenance of anesthesia. Muscle relaxants with minimal circulatory effects are the best choices, although the modest increase in heart rate observed with the administration of pancuronium is also acceptable. Preoperative optimization of intravascular volume is essential. When hemodynamic compromise (hypotension) resulting from increased intrapericardial pressure is present before surgery, management of anesthesia is as described for cardiac tamponade.

Invasive monitoring of arterial and central venous pressure is helpful, because removal of adherent pericardium may be a tedious and long operation and is often associated with significant fluid and blood losses. Cardiac dysrhythmias are common and presumably reflect direct mechanical irritation of the heart. Intravenous administration of fluids and blood products will be necessary to treat the significant fluid and blood losses associated with pericardiectomy.

Postoperative ventilatory insufficiency may necessitate continued mechanical ventilation. Cardiac dysrhythmias and low cardiac output may require treatment during the postoperative period.

PERICARDIAL AND CARDIAC TRAUMA

Blunt injuries to the chest can result in cardiovascular injury. The severity of this injury may be as mild as bruising or as severe as death within minutes. There may be serious cardiovascular injury despite the lack of obvious external signs of trauma. Trauma, especially that caused by motor vehicle crashes, is the primary cause of blunt chest injury. In automobile accidents, rapid deceleration of the chest as it impacts the steering wheel serves as the main mechanism of injury. Sudden deceleration from speeds as low as 20 mph can result in serious injury. Soft mobile tissues can be crushed by their impact on the sternum and ribs. Shear forces on internal thoracic structures may result in tears to fragile tissues. Injuries to the aorta include aortic hematoma, dissection, and rupture. The pericardium can be lacerated or ruptured, and the heart can herniate through the pericardial defect. The heart itself can be contused or ruptured or suffer damage to its internal structures (valves) or to its blood supply. Because of its location immediately below the sternum, the right ventricle is more likely than the left ventricle to be seriously injured. Blood from aortic or cardiac injury can fill the pericardial space causing cardiac tamponade. Pulmonary contusion may also result from blunt chest trauma and can manifest as hypoxemia, consolidation on chest radiograph, or pleural effusion. Hemorrhage into the tracheobronchial tree may accompany pulmonary contusion.

Pericardial Trauma

Autopsy studies indicate that pericardial lacerations are common in persons sustaining severe chest wall injuries due to rapid deceleration. Lacerations can be limited to the pericardium or can involve adjacent structures such as the pleura and diaphragm. Pericardial-pleural tears can result in cardiac herniation and strangulation. The diaphragmatic portion of the pericardium may rupture when the diaphragm is injured, and this can result in herniation of the bowel into the pericardial sac or herniation of the heart into the abdomen. Left-sided herniations occur more frequently than right-sided ones.

Small herniations may manifest as impaired cardiac filling or ischemia if coronary blood flow becomes impaired. Larger herniations can result in strangulation of the heart by impaired ventricular filling and ejection.

DIAGNOSIS

The nonspecific signs and symptoms of pericardial rupture and cardiac herniation make the diagnosis difficult. Suspicion of pericardial trauma or pericardial rupture should be raised when unexplained alterations in heart rate and blood pressure occur after initial resuscitation, especially if a sternal fracture and/or multiple rib fractures are present. Palpation and auscultation can reveal an abnormal location of the heart. Mediastinal air on a chest radiograph should be investigated further to rule out pneumopericardium, which could indicate the presence of a pericardial laceration. Rarely, chest radiography or CT shows evidence of cardiac herniation. Two characteristic CT findings include the *collar sign* and *empty pericardial sac sign*. The collar sign is a tomographically observable waist around the strangled portion of the heart through the pericardial defect. The empty pericardial sac sign appears on CT scan as air outlining the empty pericardium as a result of displacement of the heart into the hemithorax.

TREATMENT

Minor injury or a small pericardial laceration can often go unnoticed. These patients may develop an "idiopathic" pericarditis with or without pericardial effusion. Severe lacerations associated with hemodynamic instability and cardiac herniation require emergency thoracotomy. However, initiation of mechanical ventilation may precipitate hemodynamic collapse. Cardiac output should be maintained by fluids and/or inotropic drugs as needed until the herniation is released.

Myocardial Contusion

SIGNS AND SYMPTOMS

The symptoms of myocardial contusion typically include chest pain and palpitations. The chest pain can resemble angina pectoris but is not relieved by nitroglycerin. Dysrhythmias frequently complicate myocardial contusion, but cardiac failure is uncommon.

DIAGNOSIS

The presence of chest pain and ECG changes, especially in young patients, should prompt questions regarding recent chest trauma that might have seemed trivial at the time of its occurrence. ECG changes include ST-T wave abnormalities, supraventricular and ventricular dysrhythmias, and AV nodal dysfunction. However, diffuse nonspecific ST-T wave abnormalities are commonly noted in trauma patients, even in the absence of myocardial contusion.

Cardiac contusions can be recognized by transthoracic or transesophageal echocardiography, which may demonstrate impaired ventricular wall motion, valvular regurgitation, or pericardial effusion. Wall motion abnormalities usually resolve within a few days.

Serum concentrations of creatine kinase and its MB fraction increase but are often difficult to interpret because of the release of creatine kinase from injured skeletal muscles. However, the cardiac biomarkers troponin I and T can provide specific information about myocardial injury.

TREATMENT

The treatment of a myocardial contusion is directed toward improving the symptoms and anticipating possible complications. Life-threatening dysrhythmias can occur within the first 24 to 48 hours after injury. Severely contused hearts may also require hemodynamic support. Patients with a severe myocardial contusion may have other injuries that require emergent surgical intervention. Invasive hemodynamic monitoring together with ECG monitoring is prudent in this situation. Anesthetic drugs that depress myocardial function should be avoided. A cardioverter-defibrillator and medications for dysrhythmia management should be immediately available.

Commotio Cordis

Commotio cordis describes a syndrome in which a blunt injury directly over the heart causes a malignant ventricular dysrhythmia that, if left untreated, leads to death. It is not a new medical phenomenon but was first described in 1557. However, awareness of this syndrome has increased due to the occurrence of sports-related injuries in which healthy athletes have been observed to sustain a single focal, high-impact injury to the chest over the heart. One of the most common scenarios is that of a baseball player struck in the chest by a ball. The injured player instantly falls down dead or may take a few steps before the cardiac insult is realized. Other sports in which similar injuries have been reported are hockey and lacrosse. About 25% of commotio cordis cases are not sports related but occur due to brawls, falls, or motor vehicle crashes. In the last 15 years, the National Commotio Cordis Registry has recorded 224 cases.

The mechanism of this injury is not well understood. However, some use the term *mechano-electric coupling* to describe the process. The ventricles of the heart are sensitive to ventricular dysrhythmias within a 10- to 20-millisecond window during ventricular repolarization. On ECG, this period occurs on the T wave and is called the *vulnerable period.* A focused mechanical injury during this small window of time could stretch cardiac fibers and cause an unsynchronized impulse, a *mechanical* R-on-T phenomenon. Cellular membrane instability may play a role in commotio cordis. This was demonstrated in animal studies in which a colchicine-treated group developed ventricular fibrillation more frequently than a control group after a focused precordial injury. The colchicine was believed to disrupt the cellular cytoskeleton of cardiac cell membranes, which increased the likelihood of an impact-induced dysrhythmia.

Treatment for commotio cordis is rapid defibrillation. Because of this, the syndrome must be recognized and rapid defibrillation must be available. Public awareness programs and the availability of rapid-response teams and automatic external defibrillators at sporting events are already making an impact on the survival of individuals sustaining this injury.

KEY POINTS

■ Most cases of acute pericarditis are due to viral infection and follow a transient and uncomplicated clinical course. Therefore, this disease process is often termed *acute benign pericarditis.*

■ Postcardiotomy syndrome presents primarily as acute pericarditis. It may follow blunt or penetrating trauma, hemopericardium, or epicardial pacemaker implantation. However, it is most commonly seen after cardiac surgery in which pericardiotomy was performed.

■ The pathophysiologic effects of a pericardial effusion depend on whether the fluid is under increased pressure or not. Cardiac tamponade occurs when the pressure of the fluid in the pericardial space impairs cardiac filling.

■ Pulsus paradoxus is defined as a decrease in systolic blood pressure of more than 10 mm Hg during inspiration. This hemodynamic change reflects impairment of diastolic filling of the left ventricle. Pulsus paradoxus represents dyssynchrony or opposing responses of the right and left ventricles to filling during the respiratory cycle. Another term for this occurrence is *ventricular discordance.*

■ Cardiac output is maintained during cardiac tamponade as long as central venous pressure exceeds right ventricular end-diastolic pressure, but a progressive increase in intrapericardial pressure will eventually result in equalization of right atrial pressure and right ventricular end-diastolic pressure. Ultimately, the increased intrapericardial pressure leads to impaired diastolic filling of the heart, decreased stroke volume, and hypotension.

■ Temporizing measures likely to help maintain stroke volume until definitive treatment of cardiac tamponade is undertaken include expanding intravascular volume, administering catecholamines to increase myocardial contractility, and correcting metabolic acidosis.

■ Removal of pericardial fluid is the definitive treatment of cardiac tamponade and should be performed when central venous pressure is increased. Pericardial fluid may be removed by percutaneous pericardiocentesis or by surgical techniques. Removal of even a small amount of pericardial fluid can result in a dramatic decrease in intrapericardial pressure.

■ Pericardiocentesis under local anesthesia is often preferred for the initial management of hypotensive patients with cardiac tamponade. After the hemodynamic status has been improved by percutaneous pericardiocentesis, general anesthesia and positive pressure ventilation can be instituted to permit surgical exploration and more definitive treatment of the tamponade.

■ Many features considered characteristic of constrictive pericarditis may also be present in patients with restrictive cardiomyopathy, but several characteristics help to distinguish between these two entities. Kussmaul's sign and pulsus paradoxus are present with constrictive pericarditis but are not associated with restrictive cardiomyopathy. Ventricular discordance is a feature of constrictive pericarditis but not of restrictive cardiomyopathy.

■ Trauma, especially motor vehicle trauma, is the primary cause of blunt chest injury. Rapid deceleration of the chest as it impacts the steering wheel serves as the main mechanism of cardiovascular injury. Injuries to the aorta include aortic hematoma, dissection, and rupture. The pericardium can be lacerated or ruptured, and the heart can herniate through the pericardial defect. The heart itself can be contused or ruptured, or suffer damage to its internal structures (valves) or blood supply. Because it is immediately below the sternum, the right ventricle is more likely than the left ventricle to be seriously injured.

■ Commotio cordis is a syndrome in which a focused high-impact injury to the chest results in a malignant ventricular dysrhythmia and sudden death.

RESOURCES

Ariyarajah V, Spodick DH. Acute pericarditis: diagnostic cues and common electrocardiographic manifestations. *Cardiol Rev.* 2007;15(1):24-30.

Asher CR, Klein AL. Diastolic heart failure: restrictive cardiomyopathy, constrictive pericarditis, and cardiac tamponade: clinical and echocardiographic evaluation. *Cardiol Rev.* 2002;10:218-229.

Hancock EW. Differential diagnosis of restrictive cardiomyopathy and constrictive pericarditis. *Heart.* 2001;86:343-349.

Hoit BD. Pericardial disease and pericardial tamponade. *Crit Care Med.* 2007;35(8 suppl):S355-364.

Imazio M, Brucato A, Derosa FG, et al. Aetiological diagnosis in acute and recurrent pericarditis: when and how. *J Cardiovasc Med (Hagerstown).* 2009;10(3):217-230.

Little WC, Freeman GL. Pericardial disease. *Circulation.* 2006;113:1622-1632.

Maron BJ, Estes NAM. Commotio cordis. *N Engl J Med.* 2010;362:917-927.

Singh KE, Baum VC. The anesthetic management of cardiovascular trauma. *Curr Opin Anaesthesiol.* 2011;24(1):98-103.

Sybrandy KC, Cramer MJ, Burgersdijk C. Diagnosing cardiac contusion: old wisdom and new insights. *Heart.* 2003;89:485-489.

Verhaert D, Gabriel RS, Johnston D, et al. The role of multimodality imaging in the management of pericardial disease. *Circ Cardiovasc Imaging.* 2010;3(3):333-343.

CHAPTER 8

Vascular Disease

LORETA GRECU ■
ROBERT B. SCHONBERGER ■

DISEASES OF THE THORACIC AND ABDOMINAL AORTA

Diseases of the aorta are most often aneurysmal. Occlusive disease is more likely to occur in peripheral arteries. The aorta and its major branches are affected by two abnormalities that may be present simultaneously or occur at different stages of the same disease process (Table 8-1). An *aneurysm* is a dilation of all three layers of an artery. The most common definition is a 50% increase in diameter compared with normal. Arterial diameter depends on age, gender, and body habitus. Aneurysms may occasionally produce symptoms because of compression of surrounding structures, but rupture with exsanguination is the most dreaded complication, since only approximately 25% of patients who experience rupture of an abdominal aortic aneurysm survive. Aneurysms of the aorta may involve the ascending or descending portions of the thoracic aorta or the abdominal aorta.

Dissection of an artery occurs when blood enters the medial layer. The media of large arteries is made up of organized lamellar units that decrease in number with distance from the heart. The initiating event of an aortic dissection is a tear in the intima. Blood surges through the intimal tear into an extraluminal channel called the *false lumen*. Blood in the false lumen can reenter the true lumen anywhere along the course of the dissection. The origins of aortic branch arteries arising

153

TABLE 8-1   Comparison between aortic aneurysms and dissections

	Aortic aneurysm	Aortic dissection
Definition	Dilatation of aortic layers	Blood entry into the media
False lumen	No	Yes
Predisposing factors	HTN, atherosclerosis, age, male sex, smoking, family history of aneurysms	HTN, atherosclerosis, preexisting aneurysm, inflammatory diseases, collagen diseases, family history of aortic dissection, aortic coarctation, bicuspid aortic valve, Turner's syndrome, CABG, previous aortic valve replacement, cardiac catheterization, crack cocaine use, trauma
Symptoms	May be asymptomatic or present with pain mostly due to compression of adjacent structures or vessels	Severe sharp pain in the posterior chest or back pain
Diagnosis	CXR, echocardiography, CT, MRI, angiography	For patients in unstable condition, echocardiography; after patient's condition is medically stabilized, imaging can include CT, CXR, aortography, MRI, echocardiography.
Management	Elective surgical repair, whether thoracic or abdominal, for diameter of >6 cm or rapidly enlarging aneurysms with >10 mm growth over 6 mo for thoracic and diameter of >5.5 cm or >5 mm increase for abdominal; endovascular repair recommended due to better patient outcomes, especially in patients at high risk, although no randomized trial data exist	*Type A dissection:* Acute surgical emergency; as accurate diagnosis is made, patient will require acute medical management to decrease blood pressure and aortic wall stress. *Type B dissection:* If uncomplicated, medical management can be pursued.

CABG, Coronary artery bypass grafting; *CT,* Computed tomography; *CXR,* chest radiography; *HTN,* hypertension; *MRI,* magnetic resonance imaging.

from the area involved in the dissection may be compromised and the aortic valve rendered incompetent. This sequence of events occurs over minutes to hours. A delay in diagnosis or treatment can be fatal.

ANEURYSMS AND DISSECTION OF THE THORACIC AORTA

Incidence

The incidence of descending thoracic aneurysms is 5.9 to 10.4 per 100,000 person-years, and rupture occurs at a rate of 3.5 per 100,000 person-years. Although it is commonly accepted that the threshold for repair is a diameter of 6 cm or larger, one must be aware of the possibility of synchronous aneurysms involving the ascending aorta or arch, which occur in approximately 10% of patients. Dissection of the aorta can originate anywhere along the length of the aorta, but the most common points of origin are in the thorax, in the ascending aorta just above the aortic valve and just distal to the origin of the left subclavian artery near the insertion of the ligamentum arteriosum.

Etiology

The most frequently implicated factors in the development of aortic aneurysmal disease are hypertension, atherosclerosis, older age, male sex, family history of aneurysmal disease, and smoking. Causes of aortic dissection are deceleration injuries resulting from blunt trauma and use of crack cocaine, and iatrogenic dissection may occur secondary to aortic cannulation including cardiac catheterization, cross-clamping, aortic manipulation, or arterial incision for surgical procedures

such as aortic valve replacement, bypass grafting, or aneurysm operations. Systemic hypertension is a factor that can be implicated in both genetic and nongenetic causes. Aortic dissection is more common in men, but there is also an association with pregnancy. Approximately half of all aortic dissections in women younger than 40 years of age occur during pregnancy, usually in the third trimester.

Thoracic aortic aneurysms and dissections associated with known genetic syndromes are well described. These inherited diseases of blood vessels include both conditions affecting large arteries such as the aorta and those involving the microvasculature. Four major inherited disorders are known to affect major arteries. These are Marfan's syndrome, Ehlers-Danlos syndrome, bicuspid aortic valve, and nonsyndromic familial aortic dissection. Although it was once believed that mutant connective tissue proteins corrupted proteins from the normal allele (dominant negative effect) in combination with normal wear and tear, it is now known that matrix proteins, in addition to showing specific mechanical properties, have important roles in the homeostasis of the smooth muscle cells that produce them. Matrix proteins play a key metabolic function because of their ability to sequester and store bioactive molecules, and participate in their precisely controlled activation and release. In the inherited disorders associated with aortic dissection, loss of this function (biochemical rather than mechanical) is thought to alter smooth muscle cell homeostasis. The end result is a change in matrix metabolism that causes structural weakness in the aorta.

Marfan's syndrome is one of the most prevalent hereditary connective tissue disorders. Its inheritance pattern is autosomal dominant. Marfan's syndrome is caused by mutations in the fibrillin-1 gene. Fibrillin is an important connective tissue protein in the capsule of the ocular lens, arteries, lung, skin, and dura mater. Fibrillin mutations can result in disease manifestations in each of these tissues. Because fibrillin is an integral part of elastin, the recognition of the mutations in fibrillin led to the assumption that the clinical manifestations of Marfan's syndrome in the aorta were secondary to an inherent weakness of the aortic wall exacerbated by aging. However, histologic studies of the aortas of Marfan's syndrome patients also demonstrate abnormalities in matrix metabolism that can result in matrix destruction.

Although the genetics of thoracic aortic aneurysm disease in patients with Marfan's syndrome are well documented, less is known about familial patterns of aneurysm occurrence not associated with any particular collagen or vascular disease. Up to 19% of people with thoracic aortic aneurysm and dissection do not have syndromes traditionally considered to predispose them to aortic disease. However, these individuals often have several relatives with thoracic aortic aneurysm disease, which suggests a strong genetic predisposition.

Ehlers-Danlos syndrome represents a group of connective tissue disorders associated with skin fragility, easy bruisability, and osteoarthritis. There are several forms of the syndrome, but an increased risk of premature death occurs only in Ehlers-Danlos syndrome type IV. This vascular form of Ehlers-Danlos syndrome is caused by mutations in the type III procollagen gene. Type III collagen is abundant in the intestine and arterial walls. The alteration in type III collagen associated with Ehlers-Danlos syndrome type IV accounts for the most common clinical presentation of these patients, which is arterial dissection or intestinal rupture.

Bicuspid aortic valve is the most common congenital anomaly resulting in aortic dilation/dissection. It occurs in 1% of the general population. Histologic studies show elastin degradation in the aorta just above the aortic valve. Echocardiography shows that aortic root dilation is common even in younger patients with bicuspid aortic valve. Bicuspid aortic valve clusters in families and is found in approximately 9% of first-degree relatives of affected individuals.

Nonsyndromic familial aortic dissection and aneurysm is found in approximately 20% of patients referred for repair of thoracic aneurysm or dissection. Affected families do not meet the clinical criteria for Marfan's syndrome and do not have biochemical abnormalities in type III collagen. In most of these families, the inheritance pattern appears to be dominant with variable penetrance. At least three chromosomal regions have so far been mapped in families with nonsyndromic thoracic aortic aneurysm disease. The specific biochemical abnormalities predisposing to thoracic aortic aneurysm disease remain to be identified.

Classification

Aortic aneurysms can be classified morphologically as either fusiform or saccular. In fusiform aneurysm there is a uniform dilation involving the entire circumference of the aortic wall, whereas a saccular aneurysm is an eccentric dilation of the aorta that communicates with the main lumen by a variably sized neck. Aneurysms can also be classified based on the pathologic features of the aortic wall (e.g., atherosclerosis or cystic medial necrosis).

Arteriosclerosis is the primary lesion associated with aneurysms in the infrarenal abdominal aorta, thoracoabdominal aorta, and descending thoracic aorta. Aneurysms affecting the ascending aorta are primarily the result of lesions that cause degeneration of the aortic media, a pathologic process termed *cystic medial necrosis.*

Aneurysms of the thoracoabdominal aorta may also be classified according to their anatomic location. Two classifications widely used for aortic dissection are the *DeBakey* and *Stanford classifications* (Figure 8-1). The DeBakey classification includes types I to III. In type I, the intimal tear originates in the ascending aorta and the dissection involves the ascending aorta, arch, and variable lengths of the descending thoracic and abdominal aorta. In DeBakey type II, the dissection is confined to the ascending aorta. In type III, the dissection is confined to the descending thoracic aorta (type IIIa) or extends into the abdominal aorta and iliac arteries (type IIIb). The Stanford classification describes thoracic aneurysms as type A or B. Type A includes all cases in which the ascending aorta is involved by the dissection, with or without involvement of the arch or descending aorta. Type B includes all cases in which the ascending aorta is not involved.

Signs and Symptoms

Many patients with thoracic aortic aneurysms are asymptomatic at the time of presentation, and the aneurysm is detected during testing for other disorders. Symptoms resulting from thoracic aneurysm typically reflect impingement of the aneurysm on adjacent structures. Hoarseness results from stretching of the left recurrent laryngeal nerve. Stridor is due to compression of the trachea. Dysphagia is due to compression of the esophagus. Dyspnea results from compression of the lungs. Plethora and edema result from compression of the superior vena cava. Patients with ascending aortic aneurysms associated with dilation of the aortic valve annulus may have signs of aortic regurgitation and congestive heart failure.

Acute, severe, sharp pain in the anterior chest, the neck, or between the shoulder blades is the typical presenting symptom of thoracic aortic dissection. The pain may migrate as the dissection advances along the aorta. Patients with aortic dissection often appear as if they are in shock (vasoconstricted), yet the systemic blood pressure may be quite elevated. Patients who have severe hypotension or even shock at presentation have a worse prognosis. Hypotension at presentation is more common with proximal dissections. Other symptoms and signs of acute aortic dissection, such as diminution or absence of peripheral pulses, reflect occlusion of branches of the aorta and may be followed by inadequate treatment because of falsely low blood pressure measurements. Neurologic complications of aortic dissection may include stroke caused by occlusion of a carotid artery, ischemic peripheral neuropathy

DeBakey Classification			Stanford Classification	
Type I	Type II	Type III	Type A	Type B
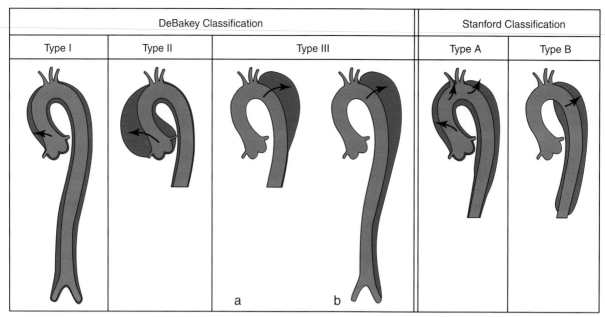		a b		

FIGURE 8-1 The two most widely used classifications of aortic dissection. The DeBakey classification includes three types: in type I, the intimal tear usually originates in the proximal ascending aorta and the dissection involves the ascending aorta and variable lengths of the aortic arch and descending thoracic and abdominal aorta; in type II, the dissection is confined to the ascending aorta; in type III, the dissection is confined to the descending thoracic aorta (type IIIa) or extends into the abdominal aorta and iliac arteries (type IIIb). The Stanford classification has two types: type A includes all cases in which the ascending aorta is involved by the dissection, with or without involvement of the arch or the descending aorta; type B includes cases in which the ascending aorta is not involved. *(From Kouchoukos NT, Dougenis D. Surgery of the thoracic aorta.* N Engl J Med. *1997;336:1876-1888. Copyright 1997 Massachusetts Medical Society with permission.)*

associated with ischemia of an arm or a leg, and paraparesis or paraplegia caused by impairment of the blood supply to the spinal cord. Myocardial infarction may reflect occlusion of a coronary artery. Gastrointestinal ischemia may occur. Renal artery obstruction is manifested by an increase in serum creatinine concentration. Retrograde dissection into the sinus of Valsalva with rupture into the pericardial space leading to cardiac tamponade is a major cause of death. Approximately 90% of patients with acute dissection of the ascending aorta who are not treated surgically die within 3 months.

Diagnosis

Widening of the mediastinum on chest radiograph may be diagnostic of a thoracic aortic aneurysm. However, enlargement of the ascending aorta may be confined to the retrosternal area, so the aortic silhouette can appear normal. Computed tomography (CT) and magnetic resonance imaging (MRI) can be used to diagnose thoracic aortic disease, but in acute aortic dissection, the diagnosis is most rapidly and safely made using echocardiography with color Doppler imaging. Although transthoracic echocardiography is the mainstay in evaluation of the heart, including evaluation for complications of dissection like aortic insufficiency, pericardial effusions, and impaired regional left ventricular function, it is of somewhat limited value in assessment of the distal ascending, transverse, and descending aorta. Transesophageal echocardiography, on the other hand, plays an essential role in diagnosing aortic dissection because it is both highly sensitive and specific (98% and 95%,

respectively), has the advantage of using portable equipment, and can be performed as a single study, especially in patients in unstable condition. Angiography of the aorta may be required for patients undergoing elective surgery on the thoracic aorta so that the complete extent of the dissection and the location of all compromised aortic branches can be defined.

Preoperative Evaluation

Because myocardial ischemia or infarction, respiratory failure, renal failure, and stroke are the principal causes of morbidity and mortality associated with surgery of the thoracic aorta, preoperative assessment of the function of the corresponding organ systems is needed. Assessment for the presence of myocardial ischemia, previous myocardial infarction, valvular dysfunction, and heart failure is important in performing risk stratification and in planning maneuvers for risk reduction. A preoperative percutaneous coronary intervention or coronary artery bypass grafting may be indicated in some patients with ischemic heart disease. Adjustment of drugs for manipulation of preload and afterload may be very advantageous in those with heart failure or significant aortic regurgitation.

Cigarette smoking and the presence of chronic obstructive pulmonary disease are important predictors of respiratory failure after thoracic aorta surgery. Spirometric tests of lung function and arterial blood gas analysis may better define this risk. Reversible airway obstruction and pulmonary infection should be treated with bronchodilators, antibiotics, and chest physiotherapy. Smoking cessation is very desirable.

The presence of preoperative renal dysfunction is the single most important predictor of the development of acute renal failure after surgery on the thoracic aorta. Preoperative hydration and avoidance of hypovolemia, hypotension, low cardiac output, and nephrotoxic drugs during the perioperative period are important to decrease the likelihood of postoperative renal failure.

Duplex imaging of the carotid arteries or angiography of the brachiocephalic and intracranial arteries may be performed preoperatively in patients with a history of stroke or transient ischemic attacks. Patients with severe stenosis of one or both common or internal carotid arteries could be considered for carotid endarterectomy before elective surgery on the thoracic aorta.

Indications for Surgery

Thoracic aortic aneurysm repair is an elective procedure considered when aneurysm size exceeds a diameter of 5 cm. This size limit may be raised somewhat for patients with a significant family history, a previous diagnosis of any of the hereditable diseases that affect blood vessels, or an aneurysm growth rate of 10 mm or more per year. A number of important technical advances have decreased the risk of surgery on the thoracic aorta. These advances include the use of adjuncts such as distal aortic perfusion, profound hypothermia with circulatory arrest, monitoring of evoked potentials in the brain and spinal cord, and cerebrospinal fluid drainage, as well as the rapid increase in endovascular procedures for aortic repairs.

Ascending and aortic arch dissection requires emergent or urgent surgery. Descending thoracic aortic dissection is generally associated with better survival than a dissection involving the ascending aorta and is rarely treated with urgent surgery.

TYPE A DISSECTION

The International Registry of Acute Aortic Dissection is a consortium of 21 large referral centers around the world. Data of this registry have shown that the in-hospital mortality rate of patients with ascending aortic dissection is approximately 27% in those who undergo timely and successful surgery. This is in contrast to an in-hospital mortality rate of 56% in those treated medically. Other independent predictors of in-hospital death include older age, visceral ischemia, hypotension, renal failure, cardiac tamponade, coma, and pulse deficits.

Long-term survival rate (i.e., survival at 1 to 3 years after hospital discharge) is 90% to 96% in the surgically treated group and 69% to 89% in those treated medically who survive the initial hospitalization. Thus, aggressive medical treatment and imaging surveillance of patients who, for various reasons, are unable to undergo surgery appears prudent.

Ascending Aorta

All patients with acute dissection involving the ascending aorta should be considered candidates for surgery. The most commonly performed procedures are replacement of the ascending aorta and aortic valve with a composite graft (a Dacron graft containing a prosthetic valve) or replacement of the ascending aorta and resuspension of the aortic valve.

Aortic Arch

In patients with acute aortic arch dissection, resection of the aortic arch (i.e., the segment of aorta that extends from the origin of the innominate artery to the origin of the left subclavian artery) is indicated. Surgery on the aortic arch requires cardiopulmonary bypass, profound hypothermia, and a period of circulatory arrest. With current techniques, a period of circulatory arrest of 30 to 40 minutes at a body temperature of 15° to 18° C can be tolerated by most patients. Focal and diffuse neurologic deficits are the major complications associated with replacement of the aortic arch. These occur in 3% to 18% of patients.

TYPE B DISSECTION: DESCENDING THORACIC AORTA

For patients with degenerative or chronic aneurysms, elective resection is advisable if the aneurysm exceeds 5 to 6 cm in diameter or if symptoms are present.

Patients with an acute but uncomplicated type B aortic dissection who have normal hemodynamics, no periaortic hematoma, and no branch vessel involvement at presentation can be treated with medical therapy. Such therapy consists of (1) intraarterial monitoring of systemic blood pressure and urinary output and (2) administration of drugs to control blood pressure and the force of left ventricular contraction. Short-acting β-blockers like esmolol and nitroprusside are commonly used for this purpose. This patient population has an in-hospital mortality rate of 10%. Long-term survival rate with medical therapy only is approximately 60% to 80% at 4 to 5 years and 40% to 50% at 10 years.

Surgery is indicated for patients with type B aortic dissection who have signs of impending rupture (persistent pain, hypotension, left-sided hemothorax); ischemia of the legs, abdominal viscera, or spinal cord; and/or renal failure. Surgical treatment of distal aortic dissection is associated with a 29% in-hospital mortality rate.

UNIQUE RISKS OF SURGERY

Surgical resection of thoracic aortic aneurysms can be associated with a number of serious, even life-threatening complications. There is the risk of spinal cord ischemia (anterior spinal artery syndrome) with resulting paraparesis or paraplegia. Cross-clamping and unclamping the aorta introduces the potential for adverse hemodynamic responses such as myocardial ischemia and heart failure. Hypothermia, an important neuroprotective maneuver, can be responsible for the development of coagulopathy. Renal insufficiency or renal failure occurs in up to 30% of patients. Approximately 6% of patients will require hemodialysis. Pulmonary complications are common; the incidence of respiratory failure approaches 50%. Cardiac complications are the leading cause of mortality.

Anterior Spinal Artery Syndrome

Cross-clamping the thoracic aorta can result in ischemic damage to the spinal cord (Figure 8-2). The frequency of spinal cord injury ranges from 0.2% after elective infrarenal

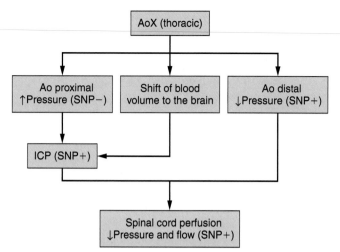

FIGURE 8-2 Spinal cord blood flow and perfusion pressure during thoracic aortic occlusion, with or without sodium nitroprusside (SNP) infusion. The arrows represent the response to aortic cross-clamping (AoX) per se. ↑, Increased; ↓, decreased; *Ao*, aorta; *ICP*, intracranial pressure; *SNP+*, the effects enhanced by SNP infusion; *SNP−*, the effects counteracted by SNP infusion. *(Adapted from Gelman S. The pathophysiology of aortic cross-clamping and unclamping. Anesthesiology. 1995;82:1026-1060. © 1995, Lippincott Williams & Wilkins.)*

abdominal aortic aneurysm repair to 8% in elective thoracic aortic aneurysm repair to 40% in the setting of acute aortic dissection or rupture involving the descending thoracic aorta. Manifestations of anterior spinal artery syndrome include flaccid paralysis of the lower extremities and bowel and bladder dysfunction. Sensation and proprioception are spared.

Spinal Cord Blood Supply. The spinal cord is supplied by one anterior spinal artery and two posterior spinal arteries (see Figure 8-2). The anterior spinal artery begins at the fusion of branches of both vertebral arteries and relies on reinforcement of its blood supply by six to eight radicular arteries, the largest and most important of which is the great radicular artery of Adamkiewicz. Multiple levels of the spinal cord do not receive feeding radicular branches, which leaves watershed areas that are particularly susceptible to ischemic injury. These areas are in jeopardy during aortic occlusion or hypotension. Damage can also result from surgical resection of the artery of Adamkiewicz (because the origin is unknown) or exclusion of the origin of the artery by the cross-clamp. In this situation, not only is the anterior spinal artery blood flow reduced directly, but the potential for collateral blood flow to the spinal cord is also reduced because aortic pressure distal to the cross-clamp is very low.

Risk Factors. The risk of paraplegia during thoracic aortic surgery is determined by the interaction of four factors: (1) the decrease in spinal cord blood flow, (2) the rate of neuronal metabolism, (3) postischemia reperfusion, and (4) blow flow after reperfusion. The duration of aortic cross-clamping is critical in determining the risk of paraplegia. A brief period

of thoracic aortic cross-clamping (<30 minutes) is usually tolerated. If cross-clamp time is more than 30 minutes, the risk of spinal cord ischemia is significant, and use of techniques for spinal cord protection is indicated. These include partial circulatory assistance (left atrium–to–femoral artery bypass), reimplantation of critical intercostal arteries when possible, cerebrospinal fluid drainage, maintenance of proximal hypertension during cross-clamping, reduction of spinal cord metabolism by moderate hypothermia (30° to 32° C) including spinal cooling, avoidance of hyperglycemia, and the use of mannitol, corticosteroids, and/or calcium channel blockers.

There is debate regarding the incidence of spinal cord ischemia after endovascular repair. Although some studies report an incidence similar to that with open aortic surgery, others showed a lower rate with endovascular repair. Nevertheless the incidence seems to be directly correlated with the severity of aortic disease. The theoretical reason is that although the respective vessel may be taken out of circulation, with endovascular repair as opposed to open repair, there is no dissection of other vessels that may represent important collateral flow, which ensures secularization of the spinal cord.

Hemodynamic Responses to Aortic Cross-Clamping

Thoracic aortic cross-clamping and unclamping are associated with severe hemodynamic and homeostatic disturbances in virtually all organ systems because of the decrease in blood flow distal to the aortic clamp and the substantial increase in blood flow above the level of aortic occlusion. There is a substantial increase in systemic blood pressure and systemic vascular resistance with no significant change in heart rate. A reduction in cardiac output usually accompanies these changes. Systemic hypertension is attributed to increased impedance to aortic outflow (increased afterload). In addition, there is blood volume redistribution caused by collapse and constriction of the venous vasculature distal to the aortic cross-clamp. An increase in preload results. Evidence of this blood volume redistribution can be seen as an increase in filling pressures (central venous pressure, pulmonary capillary occlusion pressure, left ventricular end-diastolic pressure). Substantial differences in the hemodynamic response to aortic cross-clamping can be seen at different levels of clamping: thoracic, supraceliac, and infrarenal. Changes in mean arterial pressure, end-diastolic and end-systolic left ventricular area and ejection fraction, and wall motion abnormalities may be assessed by transesophageal echocardiography or pulmonary artery catheterization and are minimal during infrarenal aortic cross-clamping but dramatic during intrathoracic aortic cross-clamping. Some of these differences result in part from different patterns of blood volume redistribution. Preload may not increase if the aorta is clamped distal to the celiac artery because the blood volume from the distal venous vasculature may be redistributed into the splanchnic circulation. For the increase in afterload and preload to be tolerated, an increase in myocardial contractility and an autoregulatory increase in coronary blood flow are required. If coronary blood flow and myocardial contractility cannot increase, left ventricular dysfunction is likely. Indeed, echocardiography often indicates abnormal wall motion of the left ventricle during aortic cross-clamping, which suggests the presence of myocardial ischemia. Hemodynamic responses to aortic cross-clamping are blunted in patients with aortoiliac occlusive disease.

Pharmacologic interventions intended to offset the hemodynamic effects of aortic cross-clamping, especially clamping of the thoracic aorta, are related to the effects of the administered drug on arterial and/or venous capacitance. For example, vasodilators such as nitroprusside and nitroglycerin often reduce the clamp-induced decrease in cardiac output and ejection fraction. The most plausible explanation for this effect is a drug-induced decrease in systemic vascular resistance and afterload, and increased venous capacitance.

It is important, however, to recognize that perfusion pressures distal to the aortic cross-clamp are decreased and are directly dependent on proximal aortic pressure, that is, the pressure above the level of aortic clamping. Blood flow to tissues distal to aortic occlusion (kidneys, liver, spinal cord) occurs through collateral vessels or through a shunt. It decreases dramatically during aortic clamping. Blood flow to vital organs distal to the aortic clamp depends on perfusion pressure and not on cardiac output or intravascular volume.

Clinically, drugs and volume replacement must be adjusted to maintain distal aortic perfusion pressure even if that results in an increase in blood pressure proximal to the clamp. Strategies for myocardial preservation during and after aortic cross-clamping include decreasing afterload and normalizing preload, coronary blood flow, and contractility. Modalities such as placement of temporary shunts, reimplantation of arteries supplying distal tissues (spinal cord), and hypothermia may influence the choice of drugs and end points of treatment.

Cross-clamping of the thoracic aorta just distal to the left subclavian artery is associated with severe decreases (approximately 90%) in spinal cord blood flow and renal blood flow, glomerular filtration rate, and urinary output. Infrarenal aortic cross-clamping is associated with a large increase in renal vascular resistance and a decrease (approximately 30%) in renal blood flow. Renal dysfunction results from renal hypoperfusion. Renal failure following aortic surgery is almost always due to acute tubular necrosis. Ischemia-reperfusion insults to the kidneys play a central role in the pathogenesis of this renal failure.

Cross-clamping of the thoracic aorta is associated not only with a decrease in distal aortic–anterior spinal artery pressure but also with an increase in cerebrospinal fluid pressure. Presumably, intracranial hypertension resulting from systemic hypertension above the clamp produces redistribution of blood volume and engorgement of the intracranial compartment (intracranial hypervolemia). This results in a redistribution of cerebrospinal fluid into the spinal fluid space and a decrease in the compliance of the spinal fluid space. Cerebrospinal fluid drainage may increase spinal cord blood flow and decrease the incidence of neurologic complications.

Pulmonary damage associated with aortic cross-clamping and unclamping is reflected by an increase in pulmonary vascular resistance (particularly with unclamping of the aorta), an increase in pulmonary capillary membrane permeability, and development of pulmonary edema. The mechanisms involved may include pulmonary hypervolemia and the effects of various vasoactive mediators.

Aortic cross-clamping is associated with formation and release of hormonal factors (caused by activation of the sympathetic nervous system and the renin-angiotensin-aldosterone system) and other mediators (prostaglandins, oxygen-free radicals, complement cascade). These mediators may aggravate or blunt the harmful effects of aortic cross-clamping and unclamping. Overall, injury to the spinal cord, lungs, kidneys, and abdominal viscera is principally due to ischemia and subsequent reperfusion injury caused by the aortic cross-clamp (local effects) and/or the release of mediators from ischemic and reperfused tissues (distant effects).

Hemodynamic Responses to Aortic Unclamping

Unclamping of the thoracic aorta is associated with substantial decreases in systemic vascular resistance and systemic blood pressure. Cardiac output may increase, decrease, or remain unchanged. Left ventricular end-diastolic pressure decreases, and myocardial blood flow increases. Gradual release of the aortic clamp is recommended to allow time for volume replacement and to slow the washout of the vasoactive and cardiodepressant mediators from ischemic tissues.

The principal causes of unclamping hypotension include (1) central hypovolemia caused by pooling of blood in reperfused tissues; (2) hypoxia-mediated vasodilation, which causes an increase in vascular capacitance in the tissues below the level of aortic clamping; and (3) accumulation of vasoactive and myocardial-depressant metabolites in these tissues. Vasodilation and hypotension may be further aggravated by the transient increase in carbon dioxide release and oxygen consumption in these tissues following unclamping. Correction of metabolic acidosis does not significantly influence the degree of hypotension following aortic unclamping.

Management of Anesthesia

Management of anesthesia in patients undergoing thoracic aortic aneurysm resection requires consideration of monitoring systemic blood pressure, neurologic function, and intravascular volume and planning the pharmacologic interventions and hemodynamic management that will be needed to control hypertension during the period of aortic cross-clamping. Proper monitoring is more important than the selection of anesthetic drugs in these patients.

MONITORING OF BLOOD PRESSURE

Surgical repair of a thoracic aortic aneurysm requires aortic cross-clamping just distal to the left subclavian artery or between the left subclavian artery and the left common carotid artery. Therefore, blood pressure monitoring must be via an artery in the right arm, since occlusion of the aorta can prevent measurement of blood pressure in the left arm. Monitoring blood pressure both above (right radial artery) and below (femoral artery) the aneurysm is less commonly done but may be useful. This approach permits assessment of cerebral, renal, and spinal cord perfusion pressure during cross-clamping.

Blood flow to tissues below the aortic cross-clamp is dependent on perfusion pressure rather than on preload and cardiac output. Therefore, during cross-clamping of the thoracic aorta, proximal aortic pressures should be maintained as high as the heart can safely withstand unless other modalities (such as temporary shunts or hypothermia) are implemented. Sympathomimetic or vasodilator drugs may be needed to adjust perfusion pressure above and below the level of the aortic cross-clamp. A common recommendation is to maintain mean arterial pressure near 100 mm Hg above the cross-clamp and above 50 mm Hg in the areas distal to the cross-clamp.

The use of vasodilators to treat hypertension above the level of the aortic cross-clamp must be balanced against the likelihood of a decrease in perfusion pressure in the tissues below the clamp. Indeed, nitroprusside may decrease spinal cord perfusion pressure, both by decreasing distal aortic pressure and by increasing cerebrospinal fluid pressure as a result of cerebral vasodilation (see Figure 8-2). It is prudent to limit the use of drugs that decrease proximal aortic pressure and cause cerebral vasodilation. Use of temporary shunts to bypass the occluded thoracic aorta (proximal aorta–to–femoral artery or left atrium–to–femoral artery shunts) may be considered when attempting to maintain renal and spinal cord perfusion. Partial cardiopulmonary bypass is another option to maintain distal aortic perfusion.

MONITORING OF NEUROLOGIC FUNCTION

Somatosensory evoked potentials and electroencephalography are monitoring methods for evaluating central nervous system viability during the period of aortic cross-clamping. Unfortunately, intraoperative monitoring of somatosensory evoked potentials is not completely reliable for detecting spinal cord ischemia during aortic surgery, because somatosensory evoked potential monitoring reflects dorsal column (sensory tract) function. Ischemic changes in anterior spinal cord function (motor tracts) are not detected. Monitoring of motor evoked potentials would indicate anterior spinal cord function but is impractical since it prohibits use of neuromuscular blocking drugs. Spinal cooling with epidural instillation of iced saline during cross-clamping in thoracic aneurysm surgery has been employed successfully for many years in some institutions across the United States on the basis that lowering the spinal cord temperature directly will improve the recovery of potentially poorly perfused tissues after reimplantation of patent critical intercostal vessels by the surgeon. Nevertheless, spinal drainage has been used to decrease pressure around the spinal cord and avoid ischemia in a confined space if the spinal cord dilates after adequate perfusion is reestablished. The cerebrospinal fluid pressure is also maintained at a value of less than 10 cm H_2O in the days immediately after surgery for the same reason, namely, that an increase in pressure in the spinal canal may decrease perfusion to the spinal cord and impair motor function. Another method that can be useful is atriofemoral bypass to maintain distal aortic perfusion.

MONITORING OF CARDIAC FUNCTION

During operations on the thoracic aorta, transesophageal echocardiography can provide valuable information about the presence of atherosclerosis in the thoracic aorta, the competence of cardiac valves, ventricular function, the adequacy of myocardial perfusion, and the intravascular volume status. A pulmonary artery catheter provides data that may complement the information obtained from transesophageal echocardiography.

MONITORING OF INTRAVASCULAR VOLUME AND RENAL FUNCTION

Optimization of systemic hemodynamics, including circulating blood volume, represents the most effective measure for protecting the kidneys from the ischemic effects produced by aortic cross-clamping. Use of diuretics such as mannitol before aortic clamping may also be useful. Mannitol improves renal cortical blood flow and glomerular filtration rate. Endothelial swelling is decreased, and an osmotic diuresis occurs.

Renal protection is achieved by direct instillation of renal preservation fluid (4° C lactated Ringer's solution with 25 g of mannitol per liter and 1 g methylprednisolone per liter) and can be administered directly by the surgeon into the renal artery.

In the future, specific antagonists of hormonal and humoral factors that are formed and released from ischemic tissues during and after the period of aortic cross-clamping may become available to prevent or ameliorate vital organ ischemia.

INDUCTION AND MAINTENANCE OF ANESTHESIA

Induction of anesthesia and tracheal intubation must minimize undesirable increases in systemic blood pressure, which could exacerbate an aortic dissection or rupture an aneurysm. Use of a double-lumen endobronchial tube permits collapse of the left lung and facilitates surgical exposure during resection of a thoracic aneurysm.

General anesthesia can be maintained with volatile anesthetics and/or opioids. General anesthesia may cause some reduction in cerebral metabolic rate, which may be particularly desirable during this surgery. The choice of neuromuscular blocking drug may be influenced by the dependence of a particular drug on renal clearance.

Postoperative Management

Posterolateral thoracotomy is among the most painful of surgical incisions because major muscles are transected and ribs are removed. In addition, chest tube insertion sites can be very painful. Amelioration of pain is essential to ensure patient comfort and to facilitate coughing and maneuvers designed to prevent atelectasis. Pain relief is commonly provided by neuroaxial opioids and/or local anesthetics. Intrathecal or epidural catheters providing intermittent or continuous infusion of analgesic medications can be adapted to provide an element of patient-controlled analgesia as well. Inclusion of local anesthetic drugs in these solutions may produce sensory and motor anesthesia and delay recognition of anterior spinal artery syndrome. Moreover, when a neurologic deficit is recognized, the epidural drug may be implicated as the cause of the paraplegia. If neuraxial analgesia is used in the period immediately after surgery, opioids are preferred over local anesthetics to prevent masking of anterior spinal artery syndrome.

Patients recovering from thoracic aortic aneurysm resection are at risk of developing cardiac, pulmonary, and renal failure during the immediately postoperative period. In the majority of clinical series, postoperative pulmonary complications are the most common, representing 25% to 45% of cases. Cerebrovascular accidents may result from air or thrombotic emboli that occur during surgical resection of the diseased aorta. Patients with co-existing cerebrovascular disease may be more vulnerable to the development of new central nervous system complications. Spinal cord injury may manifest during the period immediately after surgery as paraparesis or flaccid paralysis. Delayed appearance of paraplegia (12 hours to 21 days postoperatively) has been associated with postoperative hypotension in patients with severe atherosclerotic disease in whom marginally adequate collateral circulation to the spinal cord is present.

Systemic hypertension is not uncommon and may jeopardize the integrity of the surgical repair and/or predispose to myocardial ischemia. The role of pain in the development of hypertension must be considered. Institution of antihypertensive therapy with drugs such as nitroglycerin, nitroprusside, and labetalol may be appropriate. Some patients benefit from concomitant administration of β-blockers to attenuate manifestations of a hyperdynamic circulation.

ANEURYSMS OF THE ABDOMINAL AORTA

Abdominal aortic aneurysms have traditionally been viewed as resulting from atherosclerosis. This atherosclerosis involves several highly interrelated processes, including lipid disturbances, platelet activation, thrombosis, endothelial dysfunction, inflammation, oxidative stress, vascular smooth muscle cell activation, altered matrix metabolism, remodeling, and genetic factors. Atherosclerosis represents a response to vessel wall injury caused by processes such as infection, inflammation, increased protease activity within the arterial wall, genetically regulated defects in collagen and fibrillin, and mechanical factors. The primary event in the development of an abdominal aortic aneurysm is proteolytic degradation of the extracellular matrix proteins elastin and collagen. Various proteolytic enzymes, including matrix metalloproteinases, play critical roles during degradation and remodeling of the aortic wall. Oxidative stress, lymphocytic and monocytic infiltration with immunoglobulin deposition in the aortic wall, and biomechanical wall stress also contribute to the

formation and rupture of aneurysms. A familial component has also been identified, because 12% to 19% of first-degree relatives (usually men) of a patient with an abdominal aortic aneurysm will develop an aneurysm. Specific genetic markers and biochemical changes that produce this pathologic condition remain to be elucidated.

Diagnosis

Abdominal aortic aneurysms are usually detected as asymptomatic, pulsatile abdominal masses. Abdominal ultrasonography is a very sensitive test for the detection of abdominal aortic aneurysms. CT is also very sensitive and is more accurate than ultrasonography in estimating aneurysm size.

Improvements in CT technology, such as the advent of helical CT and CT angiography, have increased the role of CT imaging in the evaluation and treatment of abdominal aortic aneurysms. Helical CT provides excellent three-dimensional anatomic detail and is particularly useful for evaluating the feasibility of endovascular stent graft repair of the aneurysm.

MRI is useful for accurate measurement of aneurysm size and evaluation of relevant vascular anatomy without the need for the use of ionizing radiation or contrast medium.

Treatment

Surgery is usually recommended for abdominal aortic aneurysms larger than 5.5 cm in diameter. This recommendation is based on clinical studies indicating that the risk of rupture within a 5-year period is 25% to 41% for aneurysms larger than 5 cm. Smaller aneurysms are less likely to rupture. Patients with aneurysms of less than 5.0 cm in diameter should be followed with serial ultrasonography. These recommendations are only guidelines. Each patient must be evaluated for the presence of risk factors for accelerated aneurysm growth and rupture, such as tobacco use and family history. If the abdominal aortic aneurysm expands by more than 0.6 to 0.8 cm per year, repair is usually recommended. Surgical risk and overall health are also part of the evaluation to determine the timing of aneurysm repair. Endovascular aneurysm repair is an alternative to surgical repair.

Preoperative Evaluation

Co-existing medical conditions, especially coronary artery disease, chronic obstructive pulmonary disease, and renal dysfunction, are important to identify preoperatively in an attempt to minimize postoperative complications. Myocardial ischemia or infarction is responsible for most postoperative deaths following elective abdominal aortic aneurysm resection. Other postoperative cardiac events include cardiac dysrhythmias and congestive heart failure. Preoperative evaluation of cardiac function might include exercise or pharmacologic stress testing with or without echocardiography or radionuclide imaging. Severe reductions in vital capacity and forced expiratory volume in 1 second and abnormal renal function may mitigate against abdominal aortic aneurysm resection or significantly increase the risk of elective aneurysm repair.

Rupture of an Abdominal Aortic Aneurysm

The classic triad (hypotension, back pain, and a pulsatile abdominal mass) is present in only approximately half of patients who have a ruptured abdominal aortic aneurysm. Renal colic, diverticulitis, and gastrointestinal hemorrhage may be confused with a ruptured abdominal aortic aneurysm.

Most abdominal aortic aneurysms rupture into the left retroperitoneum. Although hypovolemic shock may be present, exsanguination may be prevented by clotting and the tamponade effect of the retroperitoneum. Euvolemic resuscitation may be deferred until the aortic rupture is surgically controlled in the operating room, because euvolemic resuscitation and the resultant increase in blood pressure without surgical control of bleeding may lead to loss of retroperitoneal tamponade, further bleeding, hypotension, and death.

Patients in unstable condition who have a suspected ruptured abdominal aortic aneurysm require immediate operation and control of the proximal aorta without preoperative confirmatory testing or optimal volume resuscitation.

Management of Anesthesia

Management of anesthesia for resection of an abdominal aortic aneurysm requires consideration of commonly associated medical conditions in this patient group: ischemic heart disease, hypertension, chronic obstructive pulmonary disease, diabetes mellitus, and renal dysfunction. Monitoring of intravascular volume and cardiac, pulmonary, and renal function is essential during the perioperative period. Systemic blood pressure is monitored continuously by an intraarterial catheter. Pulmonary artery catheterization is indicated in most patients, because it is not always possible to predict whether central venous pressure will parallel left ventricular filling pressure, particularly in patients with previous myocardial infarction, angina pectoris, or congestive heart failure. If appropriate personnel and equipment are available, echocardiography can be very useful for evaluating the cardiac response to aortic cross-clamping and unclamping, and assessing left ventricular filling volume and regional and global myocardial function. Urine output is monitored continuously.

No single anesthetic drug or technique is ideal for all patients undergoing elective abdominal aortic aneurysm repair. Combinations of volatile anesthetics and/or opioids are commonly used with or without nitrous oxide. Continuous epidural anesthesia combined with general anesthesia may offer advantages by decreasing overall anesthetic drug requirements, attenuating the increased systemic vascular resistance associated with aortic cross-clamping, and facilitating postoperative pain management. Nevertheless, there is no evidence that the combination of epidural anesthesia and general anesthesia decreases postoperative cardiac or pulmonary morbidity compared with general anesthesia alone in high-risk patients who undergo aortic surgery. Postoperative epidural analgesia may favorably influence the postoperative course, however. Administration of anticoagulants during abdominal aortic surgery raises the controversial issue of placement of an epidural catheter and the remote risk of epidural hematoma formation.

Patients undergoing abdominal aortic aneurysm repair usually experience significant fluid and blood losses. Administration of a combination of balanced salt and colloid solutions (and blood if needed) guided by appropriate monitoring of cardiac and renal function facilitates maintenance of adequate intravascular volume, cardiac output, and urine formation. Balanced salt and/or colloid solutions should be infused during aortic cross-clamping to build up an intravascular volume reserve and thereby minimize unclamping hypotension. If urinary output is decreased despite adequate fluid and blood replacement, diuretic therapy with mannitol or furosemide might be considered. The efficacy of low-dose dopamine in preserving renal function during abdominal aortic aneurysm surgery is unproven.

Infrarenal aortic cross-clamping and unclamping are significant events during abdominal aortic surgery. The anticipated consequences of abdominal aortic cross-clamping include increased systemic vascular resistance (afterload) and decreased venous return (see the earlier section on the hemodynamic responses to aortic cross-clamping). Often myocardial performance and circulatory parameters remain acceptable after the aorta is clamped at an infrarenal level. An alteration in anesthetic depth or infusion of vasodilators may be necessary in some patients to maintain myocardial performance at acceptable levels.

Hypotension may occur when the aortic cross-clamp is removed (see the earlier section on hemodynamic responses to aortic unclamping). Prevention of unclamping hypotension and maintenance of a stable cardiac output can often be achieved by volume loading to pulmonary capillary occlusion pressures higher than normal before the cross-clamp is removed. Likewise, gradual opening of the aortic cross-clamp may minimize the decrease in systemic blood pressure by allowing some pooled venous blood to return to the central circulation. The washout of acid metabolites from ischemic areas below the cross-clamp when the clamp is released plays a much less important role than central hypovolemia in producing unclamping hypotension, and sodium bicarbonate pretreatment does not reliably blunt unclamping hypotension. If hypotension persists for more than a few minutes after removal of the cross-clamp, the presence of unrecognized bleeding or inadequate volume replacement must be considered. Echocardiography at this time may be particularly helpful in determining the adequacy of volume replacement and cardiac function.

Postoperative Management

Patients recovering from abdominal aortic aneurysm repair are at risk of developing cardiac, pulmonary, and renal dysfunction during the postoperative period. Assessment of graft patency and lower-extremity blood flow is important. Adequate pain control accomplished with either neuraxial opioids or patient-controlled analgesia is very important in facilitating early tracheal extubation.

Systemic hypertension is common during the postoperative period and may be more likely in patients with preoperative hypertension. Overzealous intraoperative hydration and/or postoperative hypothermia with compensatory vasoconstriction may exacerbate postoperative hypertension. Postoperative hypertension should be treated either by eliminating the specific cause if identified or by initiating antihypertensive therapy. Preoperative administration of clonidine may attenuate hypertension during the postoperative period.

ENDOVASCULAR AORTIC ANEURYSM REPAIR

Endovascular placement of intraluminal stent grafts to treat patients with aneurysms of the descending thoracic aorta may be particularly useful in the elderly and in those with co-existing medical conditions such as hypertension, chronic obstructive pulmonary disease, and renal insufficiency that would significantly increase the risks associated with conventional operative treatment. Endovascular treatment of aortic aneurysms is achieved by transluminal placement of one or more stent graft devices across the longitudinal extent of the lesion. The prosthesis bridges the aneurysmal sac to exclude it from high-pressure aortic blood flow, thereby allowing for sac thrombosis around the stent and possible remodeling of the aortic wall. Endovascular repair offers the benefit of aneurysm exclusion without causing the significant physiologic changes that occur during cross-clamping (see earlier discussion).

Currently, endovascular aneurysm repair of the intrathoracic aorta has been focused on the descending thoracic aorta, that is, the portion distal to the left subclavian artery. Endovascular repair of the thoracic aorta poses several unique challenges compared with endovascular repair of the abdominal aorta. First, the hemodynamic forces are significantly more severe and place greater mechanical demands on thoracic endografts. The potential for device migration, kinking, and late structural failure is an important concern. Second, greater flexibility is required of thoracic devices to conform to the natural curvature of the proximal descending aorta and to lesions with tortuous morphology. Third, because larger devices are necessary to accommodate the diameter of the thoracic aorta, arterial access is more problematic. Fourth, as with conventional open thoracic aneurysm repair, paraplegia remains a potential complication of the endovascular approach despite the absence of aortic cross-clamping. Fifth, visceral and renal ischemia still can occur if the celiac axis is occluded by the graft.

Over the past decade, many endovascular devices to repair abdominal aortic aneurysms have been developed (Figure 8-3). Endovascular repair involves gaining access to the lumen of the abdominal aorta, usually via small incisions over the femoral vessels. Although each device has unique features, all employ the same basic structural design. The endovascular devices are composed of a metal stent (made of nitinol, stainless steel, or Elgiloy) covered with fabric (polyester or polytetrafluoroethylene). There are two types of devices: unibody and modular. The unibody type comes in one piece and is easier to deploy, but requires contralateral occlusion and bypass grafting. The modular devices are composed of more than one piece and the components are deployed through both groin areas. Since there is so much variability in patient anatomy, it is difficult to find a single graft that will be adequate to cover an aneurysm. That is the reason why most surgeons use multipart grafts that interlock and provide a better fit.

The literature on thoracic stent grafting consists mostly of reports of small- to medium-sized case series with short- to medium-term follow-up. All these studies show a common pattern of outcomes. Overall, successful device deployment is achieved in 85% to 100% of cases and perioperative mortality ranges from 0% to 14%, falling within or below elective surgery mortality rates of 5% to 20%. Outcomes have improved over time with accumulated technical expertise, technologic advances in the devices, and improved patient selection criteria. Current reported experience with thoracic stent grafting demonstrates successful deployment in 87% of cases, 30-day mortality of 1.9% to 2.1% in elective cases, and paraplegia and endoleak rates of 4% to 9%. Survival at 1, 5, and 8 years is 82%, 49%, and 27%, respectively. Therefore, mortality at 3 or 4 years is nearly identical in patients receiving stent grafts and in those undergoing open aneurysm repair. Other authors describe an approximately 98% rate of freedom from aneurysm rupture at 9 years in a cohort of 817 patients undergoing stenting, but a high rate of death (47% survival at 8 years) from comorbid medical diseases, especially cardiovascular events, even though patients were evaluated preoperatively with stress testing and revascularization was performed if needed. There are no randomized studies comparing endovascular repair with the open procedure. Nevertheless, the overall trend is that endovascular procedures are associated with lower perioperative mortality, and the endovascular approach offers patients shorter hospital stay, quicker rehabilitation, and longer average number of months lived resulting from the decrease in preoperative mortality. Even if the results of the open procedure are more durable, it is associated with major postoperative complications; therefore, with the development of new types of grafts, the endovascular approach will most probably become the primary method of aortic aneurysmal repair when anatomic conditions are optimal.

Complications

Complications associated with endografts include endoleaks; vascular injury during graft deployment; inadequate fixation and sealing of the graft to the wall, which may lead to migration of the graft; stent frame fractures; and breakdown of graft material. After the graft has been deployed, the aneurysm eventually will thrombose and decrease in diameter.

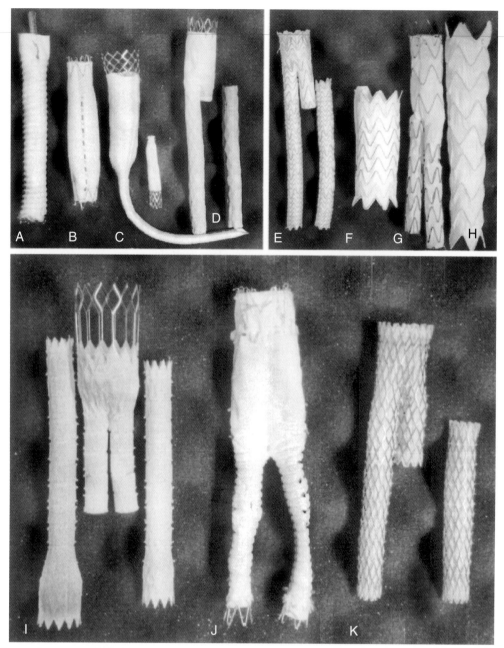

FIGURE 8-3 Endovascular stent graft devices. **A,** Parodi graft. **B,** EVT Endograft. **C,** Investigator ESG. **D,** Boston Scientific Vanguard stent graft. **E,** W.L. Gore Excluder stent graft. **F,** W.L. Gore thoracic stent graft. **G,** Medtronic/World Medical Talent abdominal aortic stent graft. **H,** Medtronic/World Medical Talent thoracic aortic stent graft. **I,** Teramed/Cordis abdominal aortic stent graft. **J,** Guidant Ancure stent graft. **K,** Medtronic AneuRx stent graft. *(From Marin ML, Hollier LH, Ellozy SH, et al. Endovascular stent graft repair of abdominal and thoracic aortic aneurysms: a ten-year experience with 817 patients. Ann Surg. 2003;238:586-595.)*

There are several types of endoleaks. Type I occurs in approximately 0% to 10% of aortic aneurysms repairs, commonly at the proximal or distal stent attachment site. Some authors recommend subclassification of these endoleaks into type IA proximal and type IB distal. Type I endoleaks are serious and require expeditious intervention, since they represent a direct communication between the aneurysm sac and aortic blood flow. Treatment options include transcatheter coil or glue embolization, balloon angioplasty, placement of endovascular graft extensions, and open surgical repair. Type II endoleaks are the most common with an incidence of 10% to 25% and are described as collections of contrast outside the graft but within the aneurysm because of flow from patent collateral branch vessels, usually originating from inferior mesenteric and lumbar arteries. Management is controversial because spontaneous resolution occurs in 30% to 100% of cases, but if the aneurysm sac is expanding then these endoleaks must be repaired, either via a transarterial approach or by direct translumbar endoleak puncture. Type III endoleaks represent leakage into the aneurysm from tears in the graft fabric or stent graft fractures. Type IV endoleak is a diagnosis of exclusion, and these leaks are due to flow through the pores of the graft material.

Device migration is one of the most common causes of a need for secondary intervention, because if such migration is left unmanaged, it may lead to endoleaks, aneurysm expansion, and rupture.

Reinterventions are part of late complications and, although minor, are more common after endovascular repair (9% of cases) than after open repair (1.7%); however, repeat laparotomy and hospitalizations are more common after open surgical repair (9.7% vs. 4.1%). Most practitioners do not consider the requirement for a secondary intervention to represent a failure. Nevertheless, patients must be aware that they will require life-long surveillance.

Several other important aspects must be considered by the surgeon in evaluating for endovascular repair in addition to aneurysm diameter and rate of increase. For example, the so-called landing zones, represented by the proximal and distal seal zones, must be at least 2 cm in length to ensure adequate fixation of the graft.

Although endovascular repair does not require a period of aortic clamping, the possibility of spinal cord ischemia still exists because of exclusion of important intercostal arteries. There is no role for epidural cooling, but spinal drainage may offer some benefits in individuals at high risk. These may include patients with prior aortic repair (usually infrarenal), those with aortic dissections, and those with stable aortic ruptures. In patients in unstable condition the drain may be placed postoperatively.

Several centers report occlusion of the left subclavian artery without any apparent side effects. However, a report of the Eurostar registry indicated that patients who had occlusion of the left subclavian artery experienced a higher incidence of paraplegia, so some surgeons are now performing elective pre-aneurysm repair of the left subclavian artery.

Consideration of the risk of intraabdominal ischemia is an important aspect, especially when the celiac artery is occluded by the graft. Although this is not the optimal course, the superior mesenteric artery may provide adequate collateral flow, especially if the gastroduodenal artery is patent, but there is no exact method to determine if this will be adequate.

Bifurcated grafts are under development that will be used in the near future to achieve aneurysm exclusion with preservation of flow to important vessels such as the celiac and renal arteries when the aneurysms involves their origins.

More complicated hybrid operations such as an elephant trunk procedure and endovascular completion can be performed with minimal mortality.

Anesthetic Management

General or regional anesthesia is acceptable for endovascular aneurysm repair. Monitoring consists of at least intravascular blood pressure and urine output monitoring. The potential need for conversion to an open aneurysm repair must always be kept in mind. Large-bore intravenous access and availability

of blood are still important concerns. Spinal drain placement is a consideration for thoracic aneurysm repair after discussion with the surgeon (see earlier discussion). Maintenance of euvolemia and normotension are important.

Administration of heparin and verification of activated clotting time are still the mainstay, as in any other vascular procedure.

Postoperative Management

Postoperative management depends on numerous physiologic and procedural variables. Commonly, patients undergoing higher thoracic aortic repair will be cared for in an intensive care unit until all perioperative concerns have been resolved, including the possibility of ischemia, acidosis, ongoing respiratory failure, and cardiac problems. Patients undergoing lower abdominal aortic repair still must be followed closely with particular attention to the development or worsening of renal dysfunction, even if it is transitory because of intravenous dye administration.

CAROTID ARTERY DISEASE AND STROKE

Cerebrovascular accidents (strokes) are characterized by sudden neurologic deficits resulting from ischemic or hemorrhagic events. Carotid artery disease is an important contributor to stroke risk. Anesthesiologists frequently manage anesthesia in patients with carotid diseases, both for carotid surgery and for other surgical procedures.

Epidemiology and Risk Factors

In the United States, approximately 3% of adults have experienced a stroke. It is the leading cause of disability and the third leading cause of death in the United States. Strokes are classified as either ischemic (most commonly thrombotic or embolic in origin) or hemorrhagic (secondary to vascular malformation, trauma, or coagulopathy). Approximately 87% of all strokes are ischemic. Transient ischemic attacks are a subset of self-limited ischemic strokes and present as a sudden, focal neurologic deficit that resolves within 24 hours. Transient ischemic attacks often herald an impending ischemic stroke, and individuals experiencing transient ischemic attacks have a 10 times greater risk of subsequent stroke than age- and sex-matched populations.

Neurologic deficits following intracranial arterial occlusion are often extensive, reflecting the large areas of brain supplied by the major arteries and their branches. Six months after an ischemic stroke, fully one quarter of survivors over 65 years of age will be institutionalized.

Major risk factors for stroke are listed in Table 8-2. Although anesthesiologists may play a role in educating patients with modifiable health risk factors such as smoking or hypertension, the anesthetic management of patients who have already developed cerebrovascular disorders, including advanced carotid disease, is a common challenge for the specialty.

TABLE 8-2 ■ Factors predisposing to stroke

INHERITED RISK FACTORS

Age

Prior history of stroke

Family history of stroke

Black race

Male gender

Sickle cell disease

MODIFIABLE RISK FACTORS

Elevated blood pressure

Smoking

Diabetes

Carotid artery disease

Atrial fibrillation

Heart failure

Hypercholesterolemia

Obesity or physical inactivity

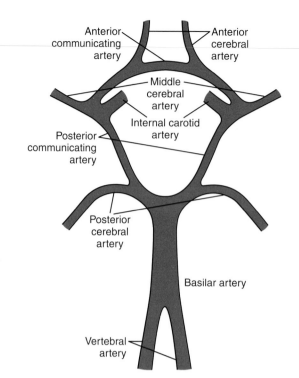

FIGURE 8-4 Cerebral circulation and the circle of Willis. The cerebral blood supply comes from the vertebral arteries (arising from the subclavian arteries) and the internal carotid arteries (arising from the common carotid arteries).

Cerebrovascular Anatomy

The blood supply to the brain (20% of cardiac output) is brought through the neck via two pairs of blood vessels: the internal carotid arteries and the vertebral arteries, which join into the basilar artery (Figure 8-4). These vessels join in the circle of Willis to form major intracranial blood vessels (anterior cerebral arteries, middle cerebral arteries, posterior cerebral arteries). Occlusion of a specific major intracranial artery results in a constellation of predictable clinical neurologic deficits.

The major branches of the vertebral arteries are the arteries to the spinal cord and the posteroinferior cerebellar arteries that supply the inferior cerebellum and lateral medulla. The two vertebral arteries then unite to form the basilar artery. Occlusion of the vertebral arteries or basilar artery results in signs and symptoms that depend on the level of the infarction. The basilar artery terminates by dividing into two posterior cerebral arteries, which supply the medial temporal lobe, occipital lobe, and parts of the thalamus.

Diagnostic Tests

Conventional angiography can demonstrate acute vascular occlusion from a thrombus or embolus lodged in the vascular tree. The vasculature can also be visualized noninvasively by CT angiography and magnetic resonance angiography. In addition to identifying ischemic stroke, these modalities can also identify aneurysms or arteriovenous malformations that may be the precipitant for hemorrhagic stroke. Transcranial Doppler ultrasonography can provide indirect evidence of major vascular occlusion and offers the advantage of real-time bedside monitoring in patients undergoing thrombolytic therapy.

In the evaluation of ischemic stroke or transient ischemic attack, auscultation of the carotid arteries may identify a bruit. Carotid ultrasonography can quantify carotid stenosis and

may rarely identify a dissection. Carotid stenosis most commonly occurs at the bifurcation of the internal and external carotid arteries because of the tendency for turbulent flow at this branch point. Even in the presence of known carotid stenosis, workup of an intracranial embolic event includes evaluation for cardiac sources of emboli such as intraluminal thrombi (secondary to heart failure or atrial fibrillation), valvular vegetations, or paradoxical emboli in the setting of a patent foramen ovale.

Treatment of Stroke

The U.S. Food and Drug Administration has approved intravenous administration of recombinant tissue plasminogen activator within 3 hours of stroke onset, once the diagnosis of ischemic stroke is established and in the absence of contraindications. The American Heart Association has subsequently expanded that recommended window to 4.5 hours. In qualifying patients, the number needed to treat with recombinant tissue plasminogen activator for one additional favorable outcome is approximately 10. Some stroke centers with access to interventional neuroradiology may offer intraarterial thrombolysis or endovascular clot removal, particularly in cases of persistent thrombus. As a treatment modality, low-frequency transcranial ultrasound–mediated thrombolysis has also been investigated in adjunctive treatment of middle cerebral artery occlusion.

Regardless of thrombolytic efforts, the importance of evaluating for and avoiding hypoxia is paramount, as are the control of glycemic derangements, hyperthermia, hypotension, severe hypertension, and unstable arrhythmias. Specific hemodynamic goals for patients with acute stroke undergoing thrombolysis or neuroradiologic procedures depend on a variety of patient-specific factors, but the overarching need to preserve or restore perfusion of at-risk brain tissue is universal. Outside the acute setting, medical management of strokes in general overlaps with the medical management of carotid stenosis discussed in the next section.

Carotid Endarterectomy

Surgical treatment of symptomatic carotid artery stenosis greatly decreases the risk of stroke compared with medical management in men with severe carotid stenosis (70% to 99% luminal stenosis) and modestly reduces stroke risk in those with 50% to 69% luminal narrowing. Strokes and transient ischemic attacks caused by carotid stenosis occur as a result of atheroembolic phenomena or hemodynamically significant pressure drops across the stenosis in the absence of sufficient collateral cerebral blood flow.

The advisability of surgical treatment for asymptomatic carotid disease varies based on the expected periprocedural risk and associated patient comorbid conditions. The absolute risk reduction in stroke is small (approximately 1% per year for the first few years) but is higher with longer-term follow-up. A suggested guideline has been to recommend surgery for asymptomatic carotid disease only for patients and at centers for which the expected periprocedural complication rates are 3% or less. In patients foregoing surgical treatment, optimal medical therapy includes smoking cessation, antiplatelet therapy, aggressive blood pressure control, physical activity, and both dietary and pharmacologic lipid-lowering strategies. Hypoglycemic medications for diabetic patients as well as angiotensin-converting enzyme inhibitors are also beneficial.

PREOPERATIVE EVALUATION

In addition to undergoing a neurologic evaluation, patients scheduled for carotid endarterectomy should be examined for significant comorbid conditions, particularly cardiovascular disease. Perioperative myocardial infarction is a major cause of morbidity and mortality following carotid endarterectomy, and predisposing coronary artery disease is highly prevalent among patients with cerebrovascular occlusive disease. The reported incidence of perioperative myocardial infarction in this population depends on the threshold and method of surveillance but was 2.3% among symptomatic patients who underwent endarterectomy in the Carotid Revascularization Endarterectomy versus Stenting Trial (CREST).

Chronic essential hypertension is a common finding in patients with cerebrovascular disease. It is useful to establish the usual range of blood pressure for each patient preoperatively to provide a guide for acceptable perfusion pressures during anesthesia and surgery. Intraoperative stability of chronically elevated blood pressure may be critical for maintenance of collateral blood flow through the stenotic cranial vasculature, especially during cross-clamping of the carotid artery. The effect of a change in head position on cerebral function should also be ascertained. Extreme head rotation, flexion, or extension in patients with co-existing vertebral or carotid artery disease could lead to angulation or compression of the artery. Recognition of this response preoperatively allows hazardous head positions to be avoided while patients are anesthetized.

Patients with known severe coronary artery disease and severe carotid occlusive disease present a clinical dilemma. A staged surgical approach in which carotid endarterectomy is performed first could result in significant morbidity or mortality from cardiac causes. On the other hand, performing coronary revascularization first is associated with a high incidence of stroke. Insufficient evidence exists to make general guidelines, and the timing of surgical procedures should instead be individualized based on the severity and symptomatic profile of each patient.

MANAGEMENT OF ANESTHESIA

Anesthetic management for carotid endarterectomy mandates careful control of heart rate, blood pressure, pain, and stress responses so that organ perfusion is maintained in patients with a high preoperative risk of cardiac and cerebral ischemic events. In addition, at the conclusion of surgery, the goal should be to awaken the patient sufficiently for a neurologic examination.

Carotid endarterectomy can be performed under regional or general anesthesia. Regional anesthesia via cervical plexus blockade allows a patient to remain awake to facilitate neurologic assessment during carotid artery cross-clamping. During establishment of the block, care should be taken to avoid vascular puncture that would obscure the surgical field or that could unlodge microemboli.

Appropriate sedation during surgical preparation and draping allows many otherwise anxious patients to tolerate the procedure quite well when a regional anesthetic technique under regional blockade is used. If general anesthesia is selected, the focus should be on maintenance of hemodynamic stability and prompt emergence to allow immediate assessment of neurologic status in the operating room.

Appropriate blood pressure management is important during carotid endarterectomy and is made more crucial because of the abnormal cerebral autoregulation present in many of these patients. Elevated blood pressure during cross-clamping may facilitate collateral blood flow but after surgery may predispose to hematoma formation. Vasopressors or vasodilators are often needed to maintain an appropriate perfusion pressure during the various stages of the procedure. Surgical manipulation of the carotid sinus may cause marked alterations in heart rate and blood pressure.

It is generally accepted that changes in regional cerebral blood flow associated with changes in $Paco_2$ are unpredictable in these patients. Therefore, maintenance of normocarbia is generally recommended.

Monitoring usually includes placement of an intraarterial catheter. As with any major vascular surgery, patients with poor left ventricular function and/or severe coronary artery disease might require a central venous or pulmonary artery catheter or transesophageal echocardiography, but this is rarely necessary. The hemodynamic goals for cerebral and coronary perfusion are similar, and achievement of these goals will benefit both organ systems. If central venous cannulation is pursued, particular care must be taken during contralateral jugular venous access attempts to prevent inadvertent arterial or venous puncture, which could cause a hematoma that compromises collateral blood flow during carotid cross-clamping.

When carotid endarterectomy is performed under general anesthesia, monitoring for cerebral ischemia, hypoperfusion, and cerebral emboli should be strongly considered. The principal reason to monitor cerebral function in these patients is to identify patients who would benefit from use of a carotid artery shunt during carotid cross-clamping as well as to guide hemodynamic management in patients who require increased cerebral perfusion pressure. The standard electroencephalogram is a sensitive indicator of inadequate cerebral perfusion during carotid cross-clamping, and perioperative neurologic complications correlate with intraoperative electroencephalographic changes indicating cerebral ischemia. However, the utility of electroencephalographic monitoring during carotid endarterectomy is limited by several factors: (1) electroencephalography may not detect subcortical or small cortical infarcts, (2) false-negative results are not uncommon (patients with previous strokes or transient ischemic attacks have a high incidence of false-negative test results), and (3) the electroencephalogram can be affected not only by cerebral ischemia but also by changes in temperature, blood pressure, and depth of anesthesia. Somatosensory-evoked potential monitoring can detect specific changes produced by decreased regional cerebral blood flow, but it can be difficult to determine whether these changes are due to anesthesia, hypothermia, changes in blood pressure, or cerebral ischemia. Stump pressure (internal carotid artery back pressure) is a poor indicator of the adequacy of cerebral perfusion. Transcranial Doppler ultrasonography allows continuous monitoring for blood flow velocity and the occurrence of microembolic events. It can be used to determine the need for shunt placement, to recognize shunt malfunction, and to manage postoperative hyperperfusion.

In situations in which general anesthesia is chosen and cerebral perfusion monitoring is unavailable, an alternative approach is to insert shunts in all patients, but placement of the shunt can itself predispose to an increased embolic load. Overall, awake neurologic assessment is the simplest, most cost-effective, and most reliable method of cerebral function monitoring during carotid endarterectomy.

POSTOPERATIVE MANAGEMENT AND COMPLICATIONS

In the period immediately after carotid endarterectomy, patients must be observed for cardiac, airway, and neurologic complications. These include hypertension or hypotension, myocardial ischemia or infarction, development of significant soft tissue edema or a hematoma in the neck, and the onset of neurologic signs and symptoms that signal a new stroke or acute thrombosis at the endarterectomy site.

Hypertension is frequently observed during the immediately postoperative period, often in patients with co-existing essential hypertension. The increase in blood pressure often reaches a maximum 2 to 3 hours after surgery and may persist for 24 hours. Hypertension should be treated to avoid the hazards of cerebral edema, myocardial ischemia, and hematoma formation. The incidence of new neurologic deficits is increased threefold in patients who are hypertensive postoperatively. Continuous infusion of short-acting drugs such as nitroprusside, nitroglycerin, or clevidipine and the use of longer-acting drugs such as hydralazine or labetalol are options for blood pressure control. The mechanism of this postoperative hypertension may be related to altered activity of the carotid sinus or loss of carotid sinus function resulting from denervation during surgery.

Hypotension is also commonly observed during the period immediately after surgery. This hypotension can be explained based on carotid sinus hypersensitivity. The carotid sinus, previously shielded by atheromatous plaque, is now able to perceive blood pressure oscillations more clearly and goes through a period of hyperresponsiveness to these stimuli. Hypotension resulting from carotid sinus hypersensitivity is usually treated with vasopressors such as phenylephrine. It typically resolves within 12 to 24 hours.

Nerve dysfunction is possible after carotid endarterectomy, but most injuries are transient. Patients should be examined for evidence of hypoglossal, recurrent laryngeal, or superior laryngeal nerve injury. Such injury may produce difficulty swallowing or protecting the airway and could result in aspiration.

Carotid body denervation can also occur after carotid artery surgery and impair the cardiac and ventilatory responses to hypoxemia. This can be clinically significant after bilateral carotid endarterectomy or with administration of narcotics.

Endovascular Treatment of Carotid Disease

The technique of carotid artery stenting continues to evolve as an alternative to carotid endarterectomy. The major complication of carotid stenting is stroke as a result of microembolization of atherosclerotic material into the cerebral circulation during the procedure. Embolic protection devices for use during carotid stenting have been developed, but the technology has so far failed to reduce endovascular stroke risk to that seen with the surgical approach. Nevertheless, endovascular approaches carry a lower risk of myocardial infarction, and if embolic protection devices are improved, stenting may one day reemerge as a more widespread alternative to surgery.

Data comparing surgical and endovascular approaches comes from several studies. The Carotid Revascularization Endarterectomy versus Stenting Trial (CREST) demonstrated an increased risk of stroke and decreased risk of myocardial infarction in endovascular treatment compared with endarterectomy, but the investigators also found that periprocedural stroke was more devastating to quality of life than myocardial infarction. The Stent-Supported Percutaneous Angioplasty of the Carotid Artery versus Endarterectomy (SPACE) trial also showed increased rates of ischemic stroke or death within 30 days after an endovascular repair compared with a surgical procedure. As a result of this evidence, surgical endarterectomy for symptomatic carotid stenosis remains the recommended treatment for most patients.

PERIPHERAL ARTERIAL DISEASE

Peripheral arterial disease results in compromised blood flow to the extremities. Chronic impairment of blood flow to the extremities is most often due to atherosclerosis, whereas arterial embolism is most likely to be responsible for acute arterial occlusion (Table 8-3). Vasculitis may also be responsible for compromised peripheral blood flow.

Chronic Arterial Insufficiency

The most widely accepted definition of peripheral arterial insufficiency is an ankle-brachial index of less than 0.9. The ankle-brachial index is calculated as the ratio of the systolic blood pressure at the ankle to the systolic blood pressure in the brachial artery. An ankle-brachial index of less than 0.9 correlates extremely well with angiogram-positive disease.

The characteristics of peripheral atherosclerosis resemble those of atherosclerosis seen in the aorta, coronary arteries, and extracranial cerebral arteries. The prevalence of peripheral atherosclerosis increases with age, exceeding 70% in individuals older than 75 years of age. Peripheral arterial disease has been estimated to reduce quality of life in approximately 2 million symptomatic Americans, and millions more without claudication are likely to experience peripheral arterial disease–associated impairment. Among patients who have claudication, 80% have femoropopliteal stenosis, 40% have tibioperoneal stenosis, and 30% have lesions in the aorta or iliac arteries.

Atherosclerosis is a systemic disease. Consequently, patients with peripheral arterial disease have a three to five times overall greater risk of cardiovascular ischemic events such as myocardial infarction, ischemic stroke, and death than do those without this disease. Critical limb ischemia is associated with a very high intermediate-term morbidity and mortality, due mostly to a high incidence of cardiovascular events in these patients. Associated cardiovascular ischemic events are much more frequent than actual ischemic limb events.

RISK FACTORS

Risk factors associated with the development of peripheral atherosclerosis are similar to those related to ischemic heart disease: older age, family history, smoking, diabetes mellitus, hypertension, obesity, and dyslipidemia. The risk of significant peripheral arterial disease and claudication is doubled in smokers compared with nonsmokers, and continued cigarette smoking increases the risk of progression from stable claudication to severe limb ischemia and amputation.

TABLE 8-3 ■ Peripheral vascular diseases

Chronic peripheral arterial occlusive disease (atherosclerosis)
    Distal abdominal aorta or iliac arteries
    Femoral arteries
    Subclavian steal syndrome
    Coronary-subclavian steal syndrome
Acute peripheral arterial occlusive disease (embolism)
Systemic vasculitis
    Takayasu's arteritis
    Thromboangiitis obliterans
    Wegener's granulomatosis
    Temporal arteritis
    Polyarteritis nodosa
Other vascular syndromes
    Raynaud's phenomenon
    Kawasaki's disease

SIGNS AND SYMPTOMS

Intermittent claudication and rest pain are the principal symptoms of peripheral arterial disease. Intermittent claudication occurs when the metabolic requirements of exercising skeletal muscles exceed oxygen delivery. Rest pain occurs when the arterial blood supply does not meet even the minimal nutritional requirements of the affected extremity. Even minor trauma to an ischemic foot may produce a nonhealing skin lesion.

Decreased or absent arterial pulses are the most reliable physical findings associated with peripheral arterial disease. Bruits auscultated in the abdomen, pelvis, or inguinal area and decreased femoral, popliteal, posterior tibial, or dorsalis pedis pulses may indicate the anatomic site of arterial stenosis. Less commonly, reduced lower extremity pulses may be the presenting sign of undiagnosed aortic coarctation. Signs of chronic leg ischemia include subcutaneous atrophy, hair loss, coolness, pallor, cyanosis, and dependent redness. Patients may report relief with hanging the affected extremity over the edge of the bed, a move that increases hydrostatic pressure in the arterioles of the affected limb.

DIAGNOSIS

Doppler ultrasonography and the resulting pulse volume waveform are used to identify arterial vessels with stenotic lesions. In the presence of severe ischemia, the arterial waveform may be entirely absent. The ankle-brachial index is a quantitative means of assessing the presence and severity of peripheral arterial stenosis. A ratio of less than 0.9 is associated with claudication, a ratio of less than 0.4 with rest pain, and a ratio of less than 0.25 with ischemic ulceration or impending gangrene. Duplex ultrasonography can identify areas of plaque formation and calcification as well as blood flow abnormalities caused by arterial stenoses. Transcutaneous oximetry can be used to assess the severity of skin ischemia in patients with peripheral arterial disease. The normal transcutaneous oxygen tension of a resting foot is approximately 60 mm Hg. It may be less than 40 mm Hg in patients with skin ischemia. Results of noninvasive tests and clinical evaluation are usually sufficient for the diagnosis of peripheral arterial disease. MRI and contrast angiography are used to guide endovascular intervention or surgical bypass.

TREATMENT

Medical therapy for peripheral arterial disease includes exercise programs and treatment or modification of risk factors for atherosclerosis. Supervised exercise training programs can improve the walking capacity of patients with peripheral arterial disease even though no change in ankle-brachial index can be demonstrated. Patients who stop smoking have a more favorable prognosis than those who continue to smoke. Aggressive lipid-lowering therapy slows the progression of peripheral atherosclerosis, and treatment of diabetes mellitus can slow microvascular disease progression.

Treatment of hypertension results in a reduction in stroke and cardiovascular morbidity. Although β-adrenergic antagonists are a mainstay for patients who have experienced myocardial infarction, their use solely as an antihypertensive agent has fallen out of favor. In patients with peripheral arterial disease, β-adrenergic antagonists have been theorized to evoke potentially harmful peripheral cutaneous vasoconstriction, but randomized trials enrolling patients with both coronary artery disease and peripheral arterial disease have failed to show worsening of claudication or other measures of arterial insufficiency. In sum, patients with severe arterial insufficiency benefit from effective blood pressure control because cardiovascular and stroke risk are reduced, but the presence of peripheral arterial insufficiency does not in itself govern the choice of an antihypertensive agent.

Revascularization procedures are indicated in patients with disabling claudication, ischemic rest pain, or impending limb loss. The prognosis of the limb is determined by the extent of arterial disease, the severity of limb ischemia, and the feasibility and rapidity of restoring arterial circulation. In patients with chronic arterial occlusive disease and continuous progression of symptoms (i.e., development of new wounds, rest pain, or gangrene), the prognosis is very poor unless revascularization can be accomplished. In patients who experience acute occlusive events resulting from arterial embolism in an extremity with little underlying arterial disease, the long-term prognosis of the limb is related to the rapidity and completeness of revascularization before the onset of irreversible ischemic tissue or nerve damage.

Revascularization can be achieved by endovascular interventions or surgical reconstruction. Percutaneous transluminal angioplasty of iliac arteries has a high initial success rate that is further improved by selective stent placement. Femoral and popliteal artery percutaneous transluminal angioplasty has lower success rates than iliac artery percutaneous transluminal angioplasty; however, stent placement has improved superficial femoral artery patency substantially.

Despite improvement in long-term outcome after percutaneous transluminal angioplasty and stenting of peripheral vessels, restenosis remains a significant problem, particularly in long lesions, small-diameter vessels, and recurrently stenotic lesions. Current therapies focus on the use of mechanical devices, stents, stent grafts, vascular irradiation, and drugs, although none of these approaches has yet become a definitive treatment.

The operative procedures used for vascular reconstruction depend on the location and severity of the peripheral arterial stenosis. Aortobifemoral bypass is a surgical procedure used to treat aortoiliac disease. Intraabdominal aortoiliac reconstructive surgery may not be feasible in patients with severe comorbid conditions. However, in these patients, axillobifemoral bypass can circumvent the abdominal aorta and achieve revascularization of both legs. Femorofemoral bypass can be performed in patients with unilateral iliac artery obstruction. Infrainguinal bypass procedures using saphenous vein grafts or synthetic grafts include femoropopliteal and tibioperoneal reconstruction. Amputation is frequently necessary for patients with advanced limb ischemia in whom revascularization is not possible or has failed. Lumbar sympathectomy is occasionally used to treat critical limb ischemia in cases of persistent vasospasm.

MANAGEMENT OF ANESTHESIA

Management of anesthesia for surgical revascularization of the lower extremities incorporates principles similar to those described earlier for the management of patients undergoing abdominal aortic aneurysm repair. For example, the principal risk during reconstructive peripheral vascular surgery is myocardial ischemia. The increased incidence of perioperative myocardial infarction and cardiac death in patients with peripheral arterial disease is due to the high prevalence of coronary artery disease in this patient population. Mortality following revascularization surgery is usually a result of myocardial infarction in patients with preoperative evidence of ischemic heart disease.

Because patients with claudication are usually unable to perform an exercise stress test, pharmacologic stress testing with or without echocardiography or nuclear imaging is helpful to determine the presence and severity of ischemic heart disease preoperatively in patients with multiple cardiac risk factors. Depending on the severity of coronary artery disease and claudication, treatment of the ischemic heart disease by percutaneous coronary intervention or coronary artery bypass grafting may be considered before revascularization surgery is performed. In American College of Cardiology/American Heart Association (ACC/AHA) guidelines, unstable angina is considered an active cardiac condition requiring treatment or optimization before nonemergent surgery. However, in patients with anatomically significant but *stable* coronary artery disease, vascular surgery can proceed, and mortality and morbidity outcomes are similar to those in patients who undergo coronary artery revascularization before elective vascular surgery.

Perioperative heart rate control (usually with carefully titrated β-blockers) in vascular surgery patients at high risk reduces the incidence of myocardial ischemia. The ACC/AHA guidelines on perioperative β-blocker therapy recommend β-blockade for patients at intermediate and high risk who are undergoing vascular surgery. For patients with low cardiac risk who are undergoing vascular surgery, β-blockers may still be considered. Both acute withdrawal of β-blockers and initiation of high-dose β-blocker therapy on the day of surgery are associated with increased mortality.

The choice of anesthetic technique must be individualized for each patient. Regional anesthesia and general anesthesia each offer specific advantages and disadvantages. Patient preference for general anesthesia, patient factors such as obesity or previous spine surgery, and use of antiplatelet or anticoagulant drugs may increase the risks associated with use of a regional technique. Regional anesthesia may also be poorly tolerated in patients with severe dementia but may reduce the risk of postoperative delirium compared with general anesthesia. Epidural or spinal anesthesia offers the advantages of increased graft blood flow, postoperative analgesia, less activation of the coagulation system, and fewer postoperative respiratory complications. Intraoperative heparinization is not, in itself, a contraindication to epidural anesthesia, but risk of bleeding may increase when the patient is also taking other anticoagulants or antiplatelet agents. If epidural catheter placement is attempted, it should occur at least 1 hour before intraoperative heparinization. In addition, before placement of the catheter is attempted, the surgical team should be consulted regarding the possible need to delay the procedure in the event of a bloody tap.

General anesthesia may be necessary when procedures are expected to require long operative hours or when vein harvesting from the upper extremities is needed. There is no strong evidence to suggest an advantage of one particular type of general anesthetic agent over another. The possible benefits of using inhalation anesthetics in patients with high cardiac risk resulting from the cardiac preconditioning effects of these agents are the subject of ongoing investigations.

During aortoiliac or aortofemoral surgery, infrarenal aortic cross-clamping is associated with fewer hemodynamic derangements than higher aortic cross-clamping. Likewise, the hemodynamic changes associated with unclamping the abdominal aorta are less with infrarenal aortic cross-clamping. Because of the comparatively benign effects of infrarenal clamping, many practitioners place a central venous pressure catheter in lieu of a pulmonary artery catheter in these patients, especially in the absence of symptomatic left ventricular dysfunction. Monitoring of left ventricular function and intravascular volume may also be facilitated by the use of transesophageal echocardiography.

Heparin is commonly administered before application of a vascular cross-clamp to decrease the risk of thromboembolic complications. However, distal embolization may still occur to any downstream vascular bed, including to the bowel or kidneys. Administration of heparin does not obviate the importance of surgical care when manipulating and clamping an atherosclerotic artery to minimize the likelihood of distal embolization. Spinal cord damage associated with surgical revascularization of the legs is extremely unlikely, and special monitoring for this complication is not generally pursued.

POSTOPERATIVE MANAGEMENT

Postoperative management includes provision of analgesia, treatment of fluid and electrolyte derangements, and maintenance of oxygenation, ventilation, heart rate, and blood pressure to reduce the incidence of myocardial ischemia or infarction. As with the choice of intraoperative anesthetics, there is no strong evidence to recommend a particular postoperative medication regimen, as long as the goal of patient stability and comfort is achieved.

Subclavian Steal Syndrome

Occlusion of the subclavian or innominate artery proximal to the origin of the vertebral artery may result in reversal of flow through the ipsilateral vertebral artery into the distal subclavian artery (Figure 8-5). This reversal of flow diverts blood from the brain to supply the arm (subclavian steal syndrome). Symptoms of central nervous system ischemia (syncope, vertigo, ataxia, hemiplegia) and/or arm ischemia are

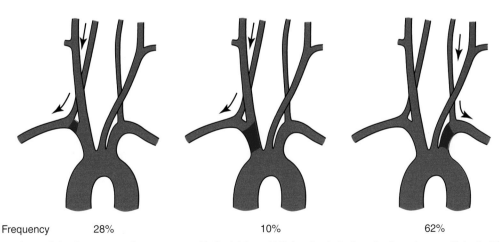

| Frequency | 28% | 10% | 62% |

FIGURE 8-5 Comparison of the frequency of occurrence of left, right, and bilateral subclavian steal syndrome. *(Adapted from Heidrich H, Bayer O. Symptomatology of the subclavian steal syndrome.* Angiology. *1969;20:406-413.)*

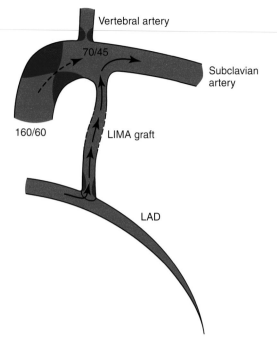

FIGURE 8-6 Coronary-subclavian steal syndrome. Development of subtotal stenosis of the left subclavian artery may produce reversal of flow through a patent internal mammary graft (LIMA), which thereby diverts flow destined for the left anterior descending (LAD) coronary artery. *(Adapted from Martin JL, Rock P. Coronary-subclavian steal syndrome: anesthetic implications and management in the perioperative period. Anesthesiology. 1988;68:933-936.)*

usually present. Extreme neck movements or exercise of the ipsilateral arm may accentuate these hemodynamic changes and may cause neurologic symptoms. There is often an absent or diminished pulse in the ipsilateral arm, and systolic blood pressure is often found to be 20 mm Hg lower in that arm. A bruit may be heard over the subclavian artery. Stenosis of the left subclavian artery is responsible for this syndrome in most patients. Subclavian endarterectomy may be curative.

Coronary-Subclavian Steal Syndrome

A rare complication of using the left internal mammary artery for coronary revascularization is coronary-subclavian steal syndrome. This syndrome occurs when proximal stenosis in the left subclavian artery produces reversal of blood flow through the patent internal mammary artery graft (Figure 8-6). This steal syndrome is characterized by angina pectoris and a 20-mm Hg or more decrease in systolic blood pressure in the ipsilateral arm. Angina pectoris associated with coronary-subclavian steal syndrome requires surgical bypass grafting.

Acute Arterial Occlusion

Acute arterial occlusion differs from the gradual development of arterial occlusion caused by atherosclerosis and is frequently the result of cardiogenic embolism. Systemic emboli may arise from a left atrial thrombus in the setting of atrial

fibrillation or less commonly from an atrial myxoma. Left ventricular thrombi may develop after myocardial infarction or in the setting of dilated cardiomyopathy. Other cardiac causes of systemic emboli are valvular heart disease, prosthetic heart valves, infective endocarditis, and paradoxical emboli from a patent foramen ovale. Noncardiac causes of acute arterial occlusion include atheroemboli from an upstream artery, plaque rupture, and hypercoagulability derangements. Aortic dissection and trauma can acutely occlude an artery by disrupting the integrity of the vessel lumen.

SIGNS AND SYMPTOMS
Acute arterial occlusion in an extremity presents with signs of limb ischemia: intense pain, paresthesias, and motor weakness distal to the site of arterial occlusion. There is loss of a palpable peripheral pulse, cool skin, and sharply demarcated skin color changes (pallor or cyanosis) distal to the arterial occlusion. Large embolic fragments often lodge at an arterial bifurcation such as the aortic bifurcation or the femoral artery bifurcation.

DIAGNOSIS
Noninvasive tests can provide additional evidence of peripheral arterial occlusion and reveal the severity of the ischemia, but such testing should not delay definitive treatment. Arteriography may be used to define the site of acute arterial occlusion and the appropriateness of revascularization surgery.

TREATMENT
Surgical embolectomy is used to treat acute systemic embolism, typically thromboembolism, to a large peripheral artery. Embolectomy is rarely feasible for atheromatous embolism, because the atheromatous material usually fragments into very small pieces. However, if the primary source of atheroembolism is identified and amenable to surgical exposure, it may be resectable. Once the diagnosis of acute arterial embolism is confirmed, anticoagulation with heparin is initiated to prevent propagation of the thrombus. Intraarterial thrombolysis with urokinase or recombinant tissue plasminogen activator may restore vascular patency in acutely occluded arteries and synthetic bypass grafts. The clinical outcome is highly dependent on the rapidity of revascularization. Amputation is necessary in some patients.

MANAGEMENT OF ANESTHESIA
Management of anesthesia in patients undergoing surgical treatment of acute arterial occlusion resulting from a systemic embolism is similar to that in patients with chronic peripheral arterial disease.

Raynaud's Phenomenon

Raynaud's phenomenon is episodic vasospastic ischemia of the digits. It affects women more often than men. Raynaud's phenomenon is characterized by digital blanching or cyanosis in association with cold exposure or sympathetic activation. Vasodilation with hyperemia is often seen after rewarming and reestablishment of blood flow. The disorder is categorized as

TABLE 8-4 ■ Secondary causes of Raynaud's phenomenon

CONNECTIVE TISSUE DISEASES
Scleroderma
Systemic lupus erythematosus
Rheumatoid arthritis
Dermatomyositis

PERIPHERAL ARTERIAL OCCLUSIVE DISEASE
Atherosclerosis
Thromboangiitis obliterans
Thromboembolism
Thoracic outlet syndrome

NEUROLOGIC SYNDROMES
Carpal tunnel syndrome
Reflex sympathetic dystrophy
Cerebrovascular accident
Intervertebral disc herniation

TRAUMA
Cold thermal injury (frostbite)
Percussive injury (vibrating tools)

DRUGS
β-Adrenergic antagonists
Tricyclic antidepressants
Antimetabolites
Ergot alkaloids
Amphetamines

either primary (also called *Raynaud's disease*) or as secondary when it is associated with other diseases. Associated diseases include many immunologic disorders, most often scleroderma or systemic lupus erythematosus (Table 8-4). Raynaud's disease is typically bilateral and occurs most frequently as a mild condition in many young adult women. Secondary Raynaud's phenomenon tends to be unilateral and may be the first symptom in patients who develop scleroderma, although the systemic disease may not become apparent until years later.

DIAGNOSIS

The primary diagnosis of Raynaud's phenomenon is based on history and physical examination findings. When the clinical diagnosis of Raynaud's phenomenon is made, it may lead to workup for associated inflammatory diseases. Measurement of the erythrocyte sedimentation rate and titers of antinuclear antibodies, rheumatoid factor, cryoglobulins, and cold agglutinins can be useful to define specific secondary causes of Raynaud's phenomenon. Angiography is not necessary to diagnose this disorder but may be useful if digital ischemia is due to atherosclerosis or thrombosis and revascularization is being considered.

Raynaud's phenomenon sometimes appears as part of the constellation of symptoms seen with the scleroderma subtype known as *CREST syndrome*. *CREST* is an acronym for *s*ubcutaneous *c*alcinosis, *R*aynaud's phenomenon, *e*sophageal

dysmotility, *s*clerodactyly (scleroderma limited to the fingers), and *t*elangiectasia.

TREATMENT

Primary and secondary Raynaud's phenomena are usually managed conservatively by protecting the hands and feet from exposure to cold. Pharmacologic intervention including calcium channel blockade or α-blockade may be helpful in some patients. In rare instances, surgical sympathectomy is considered for treatment of persistent, severe digital ischemia.

MANAGEMENT OF ANESTHESIA

There are no specific recommendations as to the choice of drugs to produce general anesthesia in patients with Raynaud's phenomenon. Increasing the ambient temperature of the operating room and maintaining normothermia are basic considerations. Noninvasive blood pressure measurement techniques may be strongly considered to avoid any arterial compromise of potentially affected extremities.

Regional anesthesia is acceptable for peripheral operations in patients with Raynaud's phenomenon, but it may be prudent not to include epinephrine in the local anesthetic solution to avoid undesirable vasoconstriction.

PERIPHERAL VENOUS DISEASE

Common peripheral venous diseases encountered in patients undergoing surgery include superficial thrombophlebitis, deep vein thrombosis, and chronic venous insufficiency. The most important associated complication of deep vein thrombosis is pulmonary embolism, a leading cause of perioperative morbidity and mortality.

The major factors predisposing to venous thrombosis, classically referred to as *Virchow's triad*, are routinely encountered in the perioperative period: (1) venous stasis (due to immobility), (2) hypercoagulability (due to inflammation and acute surgical stress), and (3) disruption of vascular endothelium (due to perioperative trauma). Table 8-5 expands on Virchow's triad to include more recently appreciated risk factors such as the use of oral contraceptives.

Superficial Thrombophlebitis and Deep Vein Thrombosis

Thrombosis of deep or superficial peripheral veins is particularly common among surgical patients, occurring in approximately 50% of patients undergoing total hip replacement. Most of these thromboses are subclinical and resolve completely when mobility is restored. Although deep and superficial venous thromboses may co-exist, isolated deep thrombosis may be distinguished from superficial venous thrombosis based on history, physical examination findings, and results of confirmatory ultrasonography.

Superficial venous thrombosis of a saphenous vein or its tributary often occurs in association with intravenous therapy,

TABLE 8-5 ■ **Factors predisposing to thromboembolism**

Venous stasis
   Recent surgery
   Trauma
   Lack of ambulation
   Pregnancy
   Low cardiac output (congestive heart failure, myocardial
     infarction)
   Stroke
Abnormality of the venous wall
   Varicose veins
   Drug-induced irritation
Hypercoagulable state
   Surgery
   Estrogen therapy (oral contraceptives)
   Cancer
   Deficiencies of endogenous anticoagulants
     (antithrombin III, protein C, protein S)
   Stress response associated with surgery
   Inflammatory bowel disease
History of previous thromboembolism
Morbid obesity
Advanced age

varicose veins, or systemic vasculitis and causes localized pain and superficial inflammation along the path of the involved vein. Superficial thrombophlebitis is rarely associated with pulmonary embolism. The intense inflammation that accompanies superficial thrombophlebitis rapidly leads to total venous occlusion. Typically, the vein can be palpated as a cordlike structure surrounded by an area of erythema, warmth, and edema.

Deep vein thrombosis is more often associated with generalized pain of the affected extremity, tenderness, and unilateral limb swelling, but diagnosis based on clinical signs alone is unreliable. Doppler ultrasonography with vein compression is highly sensitive for detecting proximal vein thrombosis (popliteal or femoral vein) but less sensitive for detecting calf vein thrombosis (Figure 8-7). Venography and impedance plethysmography are also potential diagnostic modalities.

Most postoperative venous thrombi arise in the lower legs, often in the low-flow soleal sinuses and in large veins draining the gastrocnemius muscle. However, in approximately 20% of patients, thrombi originate in more proximal veins. Left untreated, deep vein thromboses can extend into larger and more proximal veins, and such extension is associated with subsequent fatal pulmonary emboli.

PREVENTION OF VENOUS THROMBOEMBOLISM

Clinical Risk Factors

Assessment of clinical risk factors identifies patients who can benefit from prophylactic measures aimed at reducing the risk of development of deep vein thrombosis (Table 8-6). Patients at low risk require only minimal prophylactic measures, such as early postoperative ambulation and the use of compression stockings, which augment propulsion of blood from the ankles to the knees. The risk of deep vein thrombosis may be much higher in patients older than age 40 who are undergoing operations lasting longer than 1 hour, especially orthopedic surgery on the lower extremities, pelvic or abdominal surgery, and surgery that requires a prolonged convalescence period with bed rest or limited mobility. The presence of cancer also increases the risk of thrombotic complications.

Subcutaneous heparin in doses of 5000 units administered twice or three times daily reduces deep vein thrombosis risk, as does the use of intermittent external pneumatic compression devices (see Table 8-6).

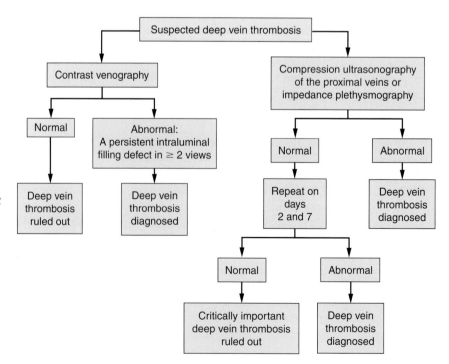

FIGURE 8-7 Steps in the diagnosis of deep vein thrombosis. *(Adapted from Ginsberg JS. Management of venous thromboembolism. N Engl J Med. 1996;335:1816-1828. Copyright 1996 Massachusetts Medical Society.)*

TABLE 8-6 ■ Risk and predisposing factors for the development of deep vein thrombosis after surgery or trauma

Associated conditions	Low risk	Moderate risk	High risk
General surgery	<40 yr old Operation <60 min	>40 yr old Operation >60 min	>40 yr old Operation >60 min Previous deep vein thrombosis Previous pulmonary embolism Extensive trauma Major fractures
Orthopedic surgery			Knee or hip replacement
Trauma			Extensive soft tissue injury Major fractures Multiple trauma sites
Medical conditions	Pregnancy	Postpartum period Myocardial infarction Congestive heart failure	Stroke
Incidence of deep vein thrombosis without prophylaxis	2%	10%-40%	40%-80%
Incidence of symptomatic pulmonary embolism	0.2%	1%-8%	5%-10%
Incidence of fatal pulmonary embolism	0.002%	0.1%-0.4%	1%-5%
Recommended steps to minimize deep vein thrombosis	Graduated compression stockings Early ambulation	External pneumatic compression Subcutaneous heparin Intravenous dextran	External pneumatic compression Subcutaneous heparin Intravenous dextran or vena cava filter Warfarin

Adapted from Weinmann EE, Salzman EW. Deep-vein thrombosis. *N Engl J Med.* 1994;331:1630-1642.

Regional Anesthesia

The incidence of postoperative deep vein thrombosis and pulmonary embolism in patients undergoing total knee or total hip replacement can be substantially decreased (20% to 40%) by using epidural or spinal anesthesia techniques instead of general anesthesia. Postoperative epidural analgesia does not augment this benefit but may allow earlier ambulation, which can reduce the risk of deep vein thrombosis.

Presumably, the beneficial effects of regional anesthesia compared with general anesthesia are due to (1) vasodilation, which maximizes venous blood flow; and (2) the ability to provide excellent postoperative analgesia and early ambulation.

TREATMENT OF DEEP VEIN THROMBOSIS

Anticoagulation is the first-line treatment for all patients with a diagnosis of deep vein thrombosis. Therapy is initiated with heparin (unfractionated or low-molecular-weight heparin) because this drug produces an immediate anticoagulant effect. Heparin has a narrow therapeutic window, and the response of individual patients can vary considerably. Advantages of low-molecular-weight heparin over unfractionated heparin include a longer half-life, a more predictable dose response without the need for serial assessment of activated partial thromboplastin time, and a lower risk of bleeding complications. Disadvantages include increased cost and the lack of availability of a rapid reversal agent.

Therapy with warfarin, an oral vitamin K antagonist, is initiated during heparin treatment and adjusted to achieve a prothrombin time yielding an international normalized ratio between 2 and 3. Heparin is discontinued when warfarin has achieved its therapeutic effect. Oral anticoagulants may be continued for 3 to 6 months or longer. Inferior vena cava filters may be inserted into patients who experience recurrent pulmonary embolism despite adequate anticoagulant therapy or in whom anticoagulation is contraindicated.

Thrombophilia workup should be considered for patients with deep vein thrombosis. Laboratory abnormalities associated with initial and recurrent venous thrombosis or embolism include the presence of factor V Leiden and congenital deficiencies of antithrombin III, protein C, protein S, or plasminogen. Congenital resistance to activated protein C and increased levels of antiphospholipid antibodies are also associated with venous thromboembolism. A family history of unexplained venous thrombosis is often present.

Complications of Anticoagulation

The most obvious complication of anticoagulant therapy is bleeding. Frequent monitoring of activated partial thromboplastin time in patients receiving intravenous heparin is necessary due to the variability in dose response.

A frequently encountered complication of unfractionated heparin administration is heparin-induced thrombocytopenia (HIT). HIT is classically divided into two types. HIT type

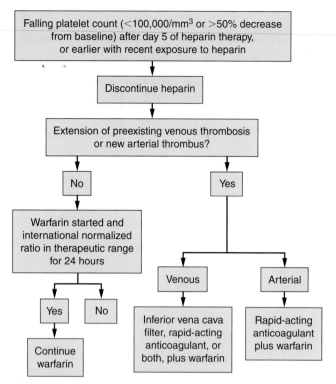

FIGURE 8-8 Steps in the management of patients with venous thromboembolism and heparin-induced thrombocytopenia. *(Adapted from Ginsberg JS. Management of venous thromboembolism. N Engl J Med. 1996;335:1816-1828. Copyright 1996 Massachusetts Medical Society.)*

TABLE 8-7 ■ Signs and symptoms of Takayasu's arteritis
CENTRAL NERVOUS SYSTEM
Vertigo
Visual disturbances
Syncope
Seizures
Cerebral ischemia or infarction
CARDIOVASCULAR SYSTEM
Multiple occlusions of peripheral arteries
Ischemic heart disease
Cardiac valve dysfunction
Cardiac conduction defects
LUNGS
Pulmonary hypertension
Ventilation/perfusion mismatch
KIDNEYS
Renal artery stenosis
MUSCULOSKELETAL SYSTEM
Ankylosing spondylitis
Rheumatoid arthritis

1 is a benign thrombocytopenia seen soon after initiation of heparin therapy (within the first few days) that resolves spontaneously and does not preclude continued treatment with heparin. In HIT type 1, thrombocytopenia is mild, generally staying above 100,000 platelets/mm³. In contrast, HIT type 2 is an immune-mediated phenomenon occurring in 1% to 3% of patients receiving unfractionated heparin. HIT type 2 is caused by antibodies to the heparin–platelet factor 4 complex and leads to severe thrombocytopenia and platelet activation that causes microvascular thrombosis. Identification of thrombosis in the setting of HIT type 2 necessitates treatment with a direct thrombin inhibitor such as argatroban or lepirudin to prevent further thrombosis. The diagnosis of HIT type 2 is based on the presence of heparin antibodies along with a positive result on a platelet serotonin-release assay. Such a diagnosis mandates avoidance of all future heparin exposure (Figure 8-8).

SYSTEMIC VASCULITIS

Inflammatory diseases of the vasculature form a diverse and numerous group of ailments with characteristic presentations that are often grouped by the size of the vessels at the primary site of clinically apparent abnormalities. Large artery vasculitides include Takayasu's arteritis and temporal (or giant cell) arteritis. In contrast, Kawasaki's disease is a vasculitis affecting

medium-sized arteries, most prominently the coronary arteries. Medium and small artery vasculitides include thromboangiitis obliterans, Wegener's granulomatosis, and polyarteritis nodosa. In addition, vasculitis can be a feature of connective tissue diseases such as systemic lupus erythematosus and rheumatoid arthritis, which are discussed in other chapters.

Takayasu's Arteritis

Takayasu's arteritis is a rare, idiopathic, chronic, progressive occlusive vasculitis that causes narrowing, thrombosis, or aneurysms of the aorta and its primary branches. It has alternative names such as *pulseless disease, occlusive thromboaortopathy,* and *aortic arch syndrome.* The disease occurs most often in Asian women younger than age 40. Takayasu's arteritis is usually diagnosed based on contrast angiography, CT, or MRI of the aortic arch and its branches.

SIGNS AND SYMPTOMS

Clinical signs and symptoms of Takayasu's arteritis occur as a consequence of progressive obliteration of the lumen of the aorta and its main branches (Table 8-7). Decreased perfusion of the brain because of involvement of the carotid arteries may manifest as vertigo, visual disturbances, seizures, or a stroke with hemiparesis or hemiplegia. Hyperextension of the head may decrease carotid blood flow further in these patients. Indeed, these patients often hold their heads in flexed ("drooping") positions to prevent syncope. Involvement of the subclavian arteries can lead to loss of arm pulses. Bruits are often audible over a stenotic carotid or subclavian artery.

Vasculitis of the pulmonary arteries occurs in approximately 50% of patients and can manifest as pulmonary hypertension. Ventilation/perfusion abnormalities owing to occlusion of small pulmonary arteries may contribute to hypoxemia. Myocardial ischemia may reflect inflammation of the coronary arteries. Cardiac valves and the cardiac conduction system may also be involved. Renal artery stenosis can lead to both decreased renal function and development of renovascular hypertension. Ankylosing spondylitis and rheumatoid arthritis may accompany this syndrome.

TREATMENT

Takayasu's arteritis is treated with glucocorticoids. Patients whose arteritis is resistant to this therapy may also benefit from methotrexate or azathioprine therapy. Anticoagulants or antiplatelet drugs may be administered to select patients. Hypertension may respond well to treatment with calcium channel blockers or angiotensin-converting enzyme inhibitors. Life-threatening or incapacitating arterial occlusions are sometimes amenable to percutaneous or surgical intervention.

MANAGEMENT OF ANESTHESIA AND MONITORING

Takayasu's arteritis may be encountered incidentally in patients coming for surgery or obstetric care or in patients undergoing vascular surgery, such as carotid endarterectomy. Management of anesthesia must consider the drugs used to treat this syndrome as well as the multiple organ systems involved by this vasculitis. For example, long-term corticosteroid therapy likely results in suppression of adrenocortical function and suggests the need for supplemental corticosteroid administration during the perioperative period. During the preoperative evaluation, it is useful to establish the effect of changes in head position on cerebral function. For instance, hyperextension of the head during direct laryngoscopy and tracheal intubation could compromise blood flow through the carotid or vertebral arteries.

No recommendations can be made regarding regional versus general anesthesia that are specifically related to Takayasu's arteritis. Regardless of the technique or drugs selected to produce anesthesia, adequate arterial perfusion pressure must be maintained during the perioperative period. Decreases in systemic blood pressure caused by either decreased cardiac output or reduced systemic vascular resistance must be recognized promptly and treated as needed. Excessive hyperventilation should be avoided because of its effect on an already stenotic cerebral vasculature. In patients with significant compromise of carotid artery blood flow, intraoperative electroencephalographic monitoring may be useful for detecting cerebral ischemia.

Patients with systemic vascular diseases should be assessed to determine whether blood pressure measurements can be obtained noninvasively in the upper extremities given the narrowing of the subclavian and brachial arterial lumens. If necessary, intraarterial cannulation of arteries can be considered, but few data are available assessing the safety of arterial cannulation in the presence of this inflammatory process. Either femoral or radial pressure monitoring can be considered depending on patient-specific pathologic features.

Temporal (Giant Cell) Arteritis

Temporal arteritis is inflammation of the arteries of the head and neck, manifesting most often as headache, scalp tenderness, or jaw claudication. This diagnosis is suspected in any patient older than age 50 complaining of a unilateral headache. Superficial branches of the temporal arteries are often tender and enlarged. Arteritis of branches of the ophthalmic artery may lead to ischemic optic neuritis and unilateral blindness. Indeed, prompt initiation of treatment with corticosteroids is indicated in patients with visual symptoms to prevent blindness. Evidence of arteritis on a biopsy specimen of the temporal artery is present in approximately 90% of patients.

Kawasaki's Disease

Kawasaki's disease (mucocutaneous lymph node syndrome) occurs primarily in children and manifests as fever, conjunctivitis, inflammation of the mucous membranes, swollen erythematous hands and feet, truncal rash, and cervical lymphadenopathy. Subsequently, a vasculitis develops that often affects the coronary arteries and other medium-sized muscular arteries, which may develop focal segmental destruction. Coronary artery aneurysms develop in approximately 20% to 25% of affected children. Causes of Kawasaki's disease continue to be investigated. Once the diagnosis is established, urgent treatment with gamma globulin and aspirin is initiated and reduces substantially the proportion of patients developing coronary aneurysms. Management of anesthesia in these patients should consider the possibility of intraoperative myocardial ischemia. Peripheral nerve blockade to provide a sympathectomy to inflamed peripheral arteries has been reported but has not been systematically evaluated.

Thromboangiitis Obliterans (Buerger's Disease)

Thromboangiitis obliterans is an inflammatory vasculitis leading to occlusion of small and medium-sized arteries and veins in the extremities. The disease is most prevalent in men, and the onset is typically before age 45. The most important predisposing factor is tobacco use. The disorder has been identified as an autoimmune response triggered when nicotine is present. The traditional diagnosis of Buerger's disease is based on five criteria: smoking history, onset before age 50, infrapopliteal arterial occlusive disease, upper limb involvement or phlebitis migrans, and the absence of risk factors for atherosclerosis other than smoking. The diagnosis of thromboangiitis obliterans is confirmed by biopsy of active vascular lesions.

SIGNS AND SYMPTOMS

Involvement of extremity arteries causes forearm, calf, or foot claudication. Severe ischemia of the hands and feet can cause rest pain, ulcerations, and skin necrosis. Raynaud's phenomenon is commonly associated with thromboangiitis obliterans, and cold exacerbates the symptoms. Periods of vasospasm may alternate with periods of quiescence. Migratory superficial vein thrombosis develops in approximately 40% of patients.

TREATMENT

The most effective treatment for patients with thromboangiitis obliterans is smoking cessation. Surgical revascularization is not usually feasible because of the involvement of small distal blood vessels. There is no proven effective drug therapy, and the efficacy of platelet inhibitors, anticoagulants, and thrombolytic therapy is not established. Recently, gene therapy with vascular endothelial growth factor was found to be helpful in healing ischemic ulcerations and relieving rest pain. Cyclophosphamide therapy has been tried because of the autoimmune nature of the disease.

MANAGEMENT OF ANESTHESIA

Management of anesthesia in the presence of thromboangiitis obliterans requires avoidance of events that might damage already ischemic extremities. Positioning and padding of pressure points must be meticulous. The operating room ambient temperature should be warm, and inspired gases should be warmed and humidified to maintain normal body temperature. When feasible, systemic blood pressure should be measured noninvasively rather than by intraarterial means. Co-existing pulmonary and cardiac disease are considerations in these cigarette smokers.

Regional or general anesthetic techniques can be used in these patients. If regional anesthesia is selected, it may be prudent to omit epinephrine from the local anesthetic solution to avoid any possibility of accentuating vasospasm.

Wegener's Granulomatosis

Wegener's granulomatosis is characterized by the formation of necrotizing granulomas in inflamed blood vessels in the central nervous system, airways, lungs, cardiovascular system, and kidneys (Table 8-8). Patients may have sinusitis, pneumonia, or renal failure at presentation. The laryngeal mucosa may be replaced by granulation tissue that leads to narrowing of the glottic opening or subglottic stenosis. Vasculitis may result in occlusion of pulmonary vessels. There may be a seemingly random interstitial distribution of pulmonary granulomas with surrounding infection and hemorrhage. Progressive renal failure is the most frequent cause of death in patients with Wegener's granulomatosis. Tests for antineutrophil cytoplasmic antibodies (ANCAs) yield positive results in Wegener's granulomatosis as well as in several other vasculitides, including Churg-Strauss syndrome and microscopic polyangiitis. Treatment of Wegener's granulomatosis with cyclophosphamide and glucocorticoids can produce dramatic remissions. Methotrexate and rituximab have also been used as initial treatment. Once remission is achieved, azathioprine or methotrexate maintenance therapy is usually continued to prevent relapse.

Management of anesthesia in patients with Wegener's granulomatosis requires an appreciation of the widespread organ system involvement in this disease. The potential depressant effects of cyclophosphamide on the immune system and the association of hemolytic anemia and leukopenia with

TABLE 8-8 ■ Signs and symptoms of Wegener's granulomatosis
CENTRAL NERVOUS SYSTEM
Cerebral aneurysms
Peripheral neuropathy
RESPIRATORY TRACT AND LUNGS
Sinusitis
Laryngeal stenosis
Epiglottic destruction
Ventilation/perfusion mismatch
Pneumonia
Hemoptysis
Bronchial destruction
CARDIOVASCULAR SYSTEM
Cardiac valve destruction
Disturbances of cardiac conduction
Myocardial ischemia
KIDNEYS
Hematuria
Azotemia
Renal failure

administration of this drug should be considered. Cyclophosphamide may also decrease plasma cholinesterase activity, but prolonged skeletal muscle paralysis after administration of succinylcholine has not been described.

Avoidance of trauma during direct laryngoscopy is important, since bleeding from granulomas and dislodgment of friable ulcerated tissue can occur. A smaller than expected endotracheal tube may be required if the glottic opening or trachea is narrowed by granulomatous changes. Suctioning of the airway may be required to remove necrotic debris. The likely presence of pulmonary disease emphasizes the need for supplemental oxygen during the perioperative period. Arteritis that involves peripheral vessels may obviate placement of an indwelling arterial catheter to monitor blood pressure or limit the frequency of arterial punctures to obtain samples for blood gas analysis.

A careful neurologic examination should be performed before the decision is made to recommend regional anesthesia to a patient with Wegener's granulomatosis. The choice and doses of neuromuscular blocking drugs may be influenced by the magnitude of renal dysfunction, and myocardial-depressant effects of anesthetics may be exaggerated in patients with associated cardiac disease. Preoperative electrocardiography may also detect conduction abnormalities.

Churg-Strauss Syndrome

Churg-Strauss syndrome is a vasculitis of small and medium-sized vessels. It is associated with inflammation of the respiratory tract with symptoms of rhinitis and asthma as well as eosinophilia. Cardiac, renal, neurologic, and gastrointestinal manifestations may also be prominent. This syndrome usually responds well to glucocorticoid therapy followed by maintenance immunosuppressant therapy.

Patients with severe disease may come for nasal polypectomy or placement of myringotomy tubes and may present an anesthetic challenge because of the presence of reactive airway disease.

Polyarteritis Nodosa

Polyarteritis nodosa is an ANCA-negative vasculitis that sometimes occurs in association with hepatitis B, hepatitis C, or hairy cell leukemia. Males more frequently contract this disease than females. Small and medium-sized arteries are involved, with inflammatory changes resulting in glomerulonephritis, myocardial ischemia, peripheral neuropathy, and seizures. The lung vasculature is generally not affected. Hypertension is common and presumably reflects renal disease. Renal failure is the most common cause of death. Human immunodeficiency virus–associated vasculitis may present in a similar fashion.

The diagnosis of polyarteritis nodosa depends on histologic evidence of vasculitis on biopsy specimens and demonstration of characteristic aneurysms on arteriography. Treatment is empirical and usually includes corticosteroids and cyclophosphamide, removal of offending drugs, and treatment of underlying diseases such as cancer.

Management of anesthesia in patients with polyarteritis nodosa should take into consideration the likelihood of coexisting renal disease, cardiac disease, and systemic hypertension. Supplemental corticosteroids may be appropriate in patients who have been receiving these drugs as treatment for this disease.

KEY POINTS

■ Cardiac complications are the leading cause of perioperative morbidity and mortality in patients undergoing noncardiac surgery. Compared with the general surgical population, the incidence of these complications is higher in patients undergoing vascular surgery. Vascular surgery patients have a higher incidence of coronary artery disease and are at a particularly high risk of perioperative myocardial infarction. However, the risk of perioperative cardiac complications differs based on the type of vascular surgery performed. For example, peripheral vascular procedures actually carry a higher rate of cardiovascular complications than central vascular procedures such as aortic aneurysm repair. The recent trend toward endovascular management of aortic and peripheral vascular disease may change cardiovascular risk substantially.

■ Atherosclerosis is a systemic disease. Patients with peripheral arterial disease have a three to five times greater risk of cardiovascular ischemic events such as myocardial infarction, ischemic stroke, and death than those without this

disease. Critical limb ischemia is associated with a very high intermediate-term morbidity and mortality resulting from cardiovascular events.

■ Aortic cross-clamping and unclamping are associated with significant hemodynamic disturbances because of the decrease in blood flow distal to the aortic clamp and the increase in blood flow proximal to the level of aortic occlusion. There is also a substantial increase in systemic blood pressure. The hemodynamic response to aortic cross-clamping differs depending on the level of clamping: thoracic, supraceliac, or infrarenal.

■ Perfusion pressures distal to the aortic cross-clamp are decreased and are directly dependent on the pressure above the level of aortic clamping to aid in blood flow through collateral vessels or through a shunt. Blood flow to vital organs distal to the aortic clamp depends on perfusion pressure and not on cardiac output or intravascular volume.

■ Aortic cross-clamping is associated with formation and release of hormonal factors (activation of the sympathetic nervous system and the renin-angiotensin-aldosterone system) and other mediators (prostaglandins, oxygen-free radicals, complement cascade). Overall, injury to the spinal cord, lungs, kidneys, and abdominal viscera is principally due to ischemia and subsequent reperfusion injury caused by the aortic cross-clamp (local effects) and/or to release of mediators from ischemic and reperfused tissues (distant effects).

■ The principal causes of unclamping hypotension are (1) central hypovolemia caused by pooling of blood in reperfused tissues, (2) hypoxia-mediated vasodilation causing an increase in vascular capacitance in the tissues below the level of aortic clamping, and (3) accumulation of vasoactive and myocardial-depressant metabolites in these tissues.

■ Data from transcranial Doppler and carotid duplex ultrasonography studies suggest that carotid artery stenosis with a residual luminal diameter of 1.5 mm (70% to 75% stenosis) represents the point at which a pressure drop occurs across the stenosis, that is, the point at which the stenosis becomes hemodynamically significant. Therefore, if collateral cerebral blood flow is not adequate, transient ischemic attacks and ischemic infarction can occur.

■ Both hypertension and hypotension may be observed frequently during the period immediately after carotid endarterectomy.

■ Acute arterial occlusion is typically caused by cardiogenic embolism. Systemic emboli may arise from a mural thrombus in the left ventricle that develops because of myocardial infarction or dilated cardiomyopathy. Other cardiac causes of systemic emboli are valvular heart disease, prosthetic heart valves, infective endocarditis, left atrial myxoma, atrial fibrillation, and atheroemboli from the aorta and iliac or femoral arteries.

■ Thromboangiitis obliterans is an inflammatory vasculitis leading to occlusion of small and medium-sized arteries and veins in the extremities.

■ Patients at low risk for deep vein thrombosis require only minimal prophylactic measures, such as early postoperative ambulation and use of compression stockings. The risk of deep vein thrombosis may be much higher in patients older than age 40 who are undergoing operations lasting longer than 1 hour, especially orthopedic surgery on the lower extremities, pelvic or abdominal surgery, and surgery that requires a prolonged convalescence with bed rest or limited mobility. The presence of cancer also increases the risk of thrombotic complications. Subcutaneous heparin (minidose heparin) and intermittent external pneumatic compression of the legs help to prevent deep vein thrombosis in patients at moderate risk following abdominal and orthopedic surgery.

■ Endovascular repair of aortic lesions is a relatively new technique for which data on long-term outcomes and randomized trials are lacking, but the significant improvement in perioperative mortality together with development of new grafts and devices has started a new era in vascular surgery. Carotid and peripheral arterial endovascular procedures have emerged as alternative, less invasive methods of arterial repair.

RESOURCES

Asymptomatic Carotid Surgery Trial (ACST) Collaborative Group. Prevention of disabling and fatal strokes by successful carotid endarterectomy in patients without recent neurological symptoms: randomized controlled trial. *Lancet.* 2004;363:1491-1502.

Baum RA, Stavropoulos W, Fairman RM, et al. Endoleaks after endovascular repair of abdominal aortic aneurysms. *J Vasc Interv Radiol.* 2003;14:1111-1117.

Brott TG, Hobson RW II, Howard G, et al. Stenting versus endarterectomy for treatment of carotid-artery stenosis. *Erratum. N Engl J Med.* 2010;363(5):498:*N Engl J Med.* 2010;363(2):198. *N Engl J Med.* 363;11-23.

Chaturvedi S, Bruno A, Feasby T, et al. Carotid endarterectomy—an evidence-based review: report of the Therapeutics and Technology Assessment Subcommittee of the American Academy of Neurology. *Neurology.* 2005;65:794-801.

Conrad MF, Cambria RP. Contemporary management of descending thoracic and thoracoabdominal aortic aneurysms: endovascular versus open. *Circulation.* 2008;117:841-852.

Cremonesi A, Setacci C, Angelo Bignamini A, et al. Carotid artery stenting: first consensus document of the ICCS-SPREAD Joint Committee. *Stroke.* 2006;37:2400-2409.

European Carotid Surgery Trialists' Collaborative Group. MRC European Carotid Surgery Trial: interim results for symptomatic patients with severe (70-99%) or with mild (0-29%) carotid stenosis. *Lancet.* 1991;337:1235-1243.

EVAR trial participants. Endovascular aneurysm repair versus open repair in patients with abdominal aortic aneurysm (EVAR trial 1): randomised controlled trial. *Lancet.* 2005;365:2179-2186.

EVAR trial participants. Endovascular aneurysm repair and outcome in patients unfit for open repair of abdominal aortic aneurysm (EVAR trial 2): randomised controlled trial. *Lancet.* 2005;365:2187-2192.

Freeman A, Shulman S. Kawasaki disease: summary of the American Heart Association guidelines. *Am Fam Physician.* 2006;74:1441-1448.

Geerts WH, Heit JA, Clagett GP, et al. Prevention of venous thromboembolism. *Chest.* 2001;119:S132-S175.

Gelman S. The pathophysiology of aortic cross-clamping and unclamping. *Anesthesiology.* 1995;82:1026-1060.

Hirsch AT, Haskal ZJ, Hertzer NR, et al. ACC/AHA 2005 practice guidelines for the management of patients with peripheral arterial disease (lower extremity, renal, mesenteric, and abdominal aortic): a collaborative report from the American Association for Vascular Surgery/Society for Vascular Surgery, Society for Cardiovascular Angiography and Interventions, Society for Vascular Medicine and Biology, Society of Interventional Radiology, and the ACC/AHA Task Force on Practice Guidelines (Writing Committee to Develop Guidelines for the Management of Patients with Peripheral Arterial Disease): endorsed by the American Association of Cardiovascular and Pulmonary Rehabilitation; National Heart, Lung, and Blood Institute; Society for Vascular Nursing; TransAtlantic Inter-Society Consensus; and Vascular Disease Foundation. *Circulation.* 2006;113:e463-e654.

Jonker FHW, Verhagen HJM, Linn PH, et al. Outcomes of endovascular repair of ruptured descending thoracic aortic aneurysms. *Circulation.* 2010;121:2718-2723.

Katzen BT, Dake MD, MacLean AA, et al. Endovascular repair of abdominal and thoracic aortic aneurysms. *Circulation.* 2005;112:1663-1675.

Kouchoukos NT, Dougenis D. Surgery of the thoracic aorta. *N Engl J Med.* 1997;336:1876-1888.

Longo DL, Kasper DL, Fauci AS, et al. *Harrison's principles of internal medicine,* 18th ed. New York, NY. McGraw-Hill; 2008.

Marin ML, Hollier LH, Ellozy SH, et al. Endovascular stent graft repair of abdominal and thoracic aortic aneurysms. A ten-year experience with 817 patients. *Ann Surg.* 2003;238:586-595.

McFalls EO, Ward HB, Moritz TE, et al. Coronary artery revascularization before elective major vascular surgery. *N Engl J Med.* 2004;351:2795-2804.

Meyers PM, Schumacher HC, Connolly ES, Jr., Current status of endovascular stroke treatment. *Circulation.* 123: 2591-2601.

Norris EJ, Beattie C, Perler BA, et al. Double masked randomized trial comparing alternate combinations of intraoperative anesthesia and postoperative analgesia in abdominal aortic surgery. *Anesthesiology.* 2001;95:1054-1067.

North American Symptomatic Carotid Endarterectomy Trial Collaborators. Beneficial effect of carotid endarterectomy in symptomatic patients with high-grade carotid stenosis. *N Engl J Med.* 1991;325:445-453.

Pleis JR, Ward BW, Lucas JW. Summary health statistics for U. S. adults: National Health Interview Survey, 2009. National Center for Health Statistics. *Vital Health Stat.* 2010;10.

Sharrock NE, Ranawat CS, Urquhart B, et al. Factors influencing deep vein thrombosis after total hip arthroplasty under epidural anesthesia. *Anesth Analg.* 1993;76:765-771.

Trimarchi S, Nienaber CA, Rampoldi V, et al. Role and results of surgery in acute type B aortic dissection: insights from the International Registry of Acute Aortic Dissection (IRAD). *Circulation.* 2006;114:357-364.

Tsai TT, Evangelista A, Nienaber CA, et al. Long-term survival in patients presenting with type A acute aortic dissection. Insights from the International Registry of Acute Aortic Dissection (IRAD). *Circulation.* 2006;114(suppl I): I-350-I-356.

Veith FJ, Lachat M, Mayer D, et al. Collected world and single center experience with endovascular treatment of ruptured abdominal aortic aneurysms. *Ann Surg.* 2009;250:818-824.

Yadav JS, Wholey MH, Kuntz RE, et al. Protected carotid-artery stenting versus endarterectomy in high-risk patients. *N Engl J Med.* 2004;351:1493-1501.

CHAPTER 9

Respiratory Diseases

SHARIF AL-RUZZEH ■
VIJI KURUP ■

Patients with preoperative respiratory diseases are at increased risk of perioperative respiratory complications. There is increasing awareness of the importance of postoperative pulmonary complications in contributing to morbidity, mortality, and increased hospital length of stay. Pulmonary complications also play an important part in determining long-term mortality after surgery. Modification of disease severity and optimization of the patient's condition before surgery significantly decrease the incidence of these complications.

Respiratory diseases can be divided into the following groups for discussion of their influence on anesthetic management: acute upper respiratory tract infection, asthma, chronic obstructive pulmonary disease, acute respiratory failure, restrictive lung disease, pulmonary embolism, and lung transplantation.

ACUTE UPPER RESPIRATORY TRACT INFECTION

Every year approximately 25 million patients visit their doctors with an uncomplicated upper respiratory tract infection (URI). The common cold syndrome results in about 20 million days of absence from work and 22 million days of absence from school. It is likely, then, that there will be a population of patients scheduled for elective surgery who have an active URI.

Infectious (viral or bacterial) nasopharyngitis accounts for approximately 95% of all URIs, with the most common responsible viruses being rhinovirus, coronavirus, influenzavirus, parainfluenza virus, and respiratory syncytial virus. Noninfectious nasopharyngitis is allergic and vasomotor in origin.

Signs and Symptoms

Patients with nasopharyngitis present with a broad spectrum of signs and symptoms. Sneezing, runny nose, and a history of allergies point to an allergic cause. When nasopharyngitis is associated with infection, there is usually a history of fever, purulent nasal discharge, productive cough, fever, and malaise. On examination, the patient may be tachypneic or wheezing or show signs of toxicity.

Diagnosis

The diagnosis of a URI is usually based on clinical signs and symptoms. Although viral cultures and laboratory tests are available to confirm the diagnosis, they lack sensitivity and are impractical in a busy clinical setting.

Management of Anesthesia

PREOPERATIVE

Most studies regarding the effects of URI on postoperative complications have involved pediatric patients. There is evidence to show an increased incidence of respiratory complications in patients with a history of copious secretions, endotracheal intubation, prematurity, parental smoking, nasal congestion, and reactive airway disease and in those undergoing airway surgery. Those with clear systemic signs of infection such as fever, purulent rhinitis, productive cough, and rhonchi who are undergoing elective surgery, particularly airway surgery, are at considerable risk of perioperative adverse events. Consultation with the surgeon regarding the urgency of the case must be undertaken. A patient who has had a URI for days or weeks and is in stable or improving condition can be safely managed without postponing surgery. Delaying surgery does not reduce the incidence of adverse respiratory events if the patient undergoes anesthesia within 4 weeks of the URI. Airway hyperreactivity may require 6 weeks or more to abate. The economic and practical aspects of canceling surgery should be taken into consideration before a decision is made to postpone surgery.

Viral infections, particularly during the infectious phase, can cause morphologic and functional changes in the respiratory epithelium. The relationship between epithelial damage, viral infection, airway reactivity, and anesthesia remains unclear. Tracheal mucociliary flow and pulmonary bactericidal activity can be decreased by general anesthesia. It is possible that positive pressure ventilation may help in spreading infection from the upper to the lower respiratory tract. The immune response of the body is altered by surgery and anesthesia. A reduction in B-lymphocyte numbers, T-lymphocyte responsiveness, and antibody production may be associated with anesthesia, but the clinical significance of this remains to be elucidated.

INTRAOPERATIVE

The anesthetic management of a patient with a URI should include adequate hydration, reducing secretions, and limiting manipulation of a potentially sensitive airway. Use of a laryngeal mask airway (LMA) may be a good alternative to endotracheal intubation to reduce the risk of bronchospasm from airway manipulation. The role of prophylactic administration of bronchodilators to reduce the incidence of perioperative bronchospasm has not been clearly established.

POSTOPERATIVE

Reported adverse respiratory events in patients with URIs include bronchospasm, laryngospasm, airway obstruction, postintubation croup, desaturation, and atelectasis. Long-term complications from general anesthesia in patients with URIs have not been demonstrated. Intraoperative and immediately postoperative hypoxemia is common and amenable to treatment with supplemental oxygen.

ASTHMA

Asthma is a disease characterized by chronic airway inflammation, reversible expiratory airflow obstruction in response to various stimuli, and bronchial hyperreactivity. Data from the American Academy of Allergy, Asthma and Immunology indicate that an estimated 300 million people worldwide have asthma, and the prevalence is increasing. Some 250,000 deaths each year are attributed to the disease. The prevalence of asthma in adult women was 23% greater than the rate in men in 2006.

Signs and Symptoms

Asthma is an episodic disease with acute exacerbations interspersed with symptom-free periods. Most attacks are short-lived, lasting minutes to hours, and clinically the patient seems to recover completely after an attack. However, there can be a phase in which the patient experiences some degree of airway obstruction daily. This phase can be mild, with or without superimposed severe episodes, or much more serious, with significant obstruction persisting for days or weeks. Status asthmaticus is defined as life-threatening bronchospasm that persists despite treatment. When patient history is elicited, attention should be paid to factors associated with increased risk, such as previous intubation or admission to the intensive care unit (ICU), two or more hospitalizations for asthma in the past year, and the presence of co-existing diseases. Clinical manifestations of asthma include wheezing, productive or nonproductive cough, dyspnea, chest discomfort or tightness that may lead to air hunger, and eosinophilia.

Pathogenesis

Asthma is a heterogeneous disease, and genetic (atopic) and environmental factors such as viruses, occupational exposure, and allergens contribute to its initiation and continuance.

Stimuli provoking an episode of asthma are summarized in Table 9-1.

Features that support the allergen-induced immunologic model of the etiology of asthma include the following: (1) Atopy is the single greatest risk factor for the development of asthma. (2) A personal and/or family history of allergic diseases such as rhinitis, urticaria, and eczema is often present. (3) There is usually a positive wheal-and-flare skin reaction to intradermal injection of extracts of airborne antigens. (4) Serum immunoglobulin E levels are increased and/or there is a positive response to provocative tests involving the inhalation of specific antigens. (5) Evidence of a genetic linkage between high total serum immunoglobulin E levels and atopy has been observed.

An alternative explanation for the characteristic features of asthma is abnormal autonomic regulation of neural function, specifically an imbalance between excitatory (bronchoconstrictor) and inhibitory (bronchodilator) neural input. It is likely that chemical mediators released from mast cells interact with the autonomic nervous system. Some chemical mediators can stimulate airway receptors to trigger reflex bronchoconstriction, whereas other mediators sensitize bronchial smooth muscle to the effects of acetylcholine. In addition, stimulation of muscarinic receptors can facilitate mediator release from mast cells, providing a positive feedback loop for sustained inflammation and bronchoconstriction.

TABLE 9-1 ■ Stimuli provoking symptoms of asthma
Allergens
Pharmacologic agents: aspirin, β-antagonists, some nonsteroidal antiinflammatory drugs, sulfiting agents
Infections: respiratory viruses
Exercise: the attacks typically follow exertion rather than occurring during it
Emotional stress: endorphins and vagal mediation

Diagnosis

SPIROMETRY

Forced expiratory volume in 1 second (FEV_1) and maximum mid-expiratory flow (MMEF) rate are direct measures of the severity of expiratory airflow obstruction (Figure 9-1 and Tables 9-2 and 9-3).* These measurements provide objective data that can be used to assess the severity and monitor the course of an exacerbation of asthma. The typical asthmatic patient who comes to the hospital for treatment has an FEV_1 that is less than 35% of normal and a MMEF that is 20% or less of normal. Flow-volume loops show characteristic downward scooping of the expiratory limb of the loop. Flow-volume loops in which the inhaled or exhaled portion of the loop is flat help distinguish wheezing caused by airway obstruction (foreign body, tracheal stenosis, mediastinal tumor) from asthma (Figures 9-2 and 9-3). During moderate to severe asthmatic attacks, the functional residual capacity (FRC) may increase substantially, but total lung capacity usually remains within the normal range. Diffusing capacity for carbon monoxide is not changed. Bronchodilator responsiveness can provide supporting evidence when asthma is suspected on clinical grounds. In patients with expiratory airflow obstruction, an increase in airflow after inhalation of a bronchodilator suggests asthma. Abnormalities in pulmonary function test results may persist for several days after an acute asthmatic attack despite the absence of symptoms. Since asthma is an episodic illness, its diagnosis may be suspected even when results of pulmonary function tests are normal.

ARTERIAL BLOOD GAS ANALYSIS

Mild asthma is usually accompanied by a normal Pao_2 and $Paco_2$. Tachypnea and hyperventilation observed during an acute asthmatic attack do not reflect arterial hypoxemia but

---

*FEV_1 is a spirometric test. MMEF is the peak rate of expiratory flow taken from a flow-volume curve. It is usually measured clinically by a peak flow meter.

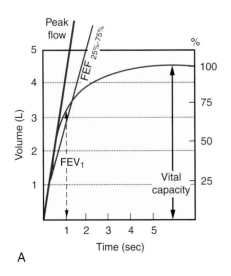

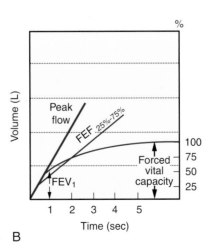

FIGURE 9-1 Spirographic changes of a healthy subject (**A**) and a patient in bronchospasm (**B**). The forced expiratory volume in 1 second (FEV_1) is typically less than 80% of the vital capacity in the presence of obstructive airway disease. Peak flow and maximum mid-expiratory flow rate ($FEF_{25\%-75\%}$) are also decreased in these patients (**B**). *(Adapted from Kingston HGG, Hirshman CA. Perioperative management of the patient with asthma. Anesth Analg. 1984;63:844-855.)*

A   B

TABLE 9-2 ■ Classification of asthma based on severity of expiratory airflow obstruction

Severity	FEV$_1$ (% predicted)	FEF$_{25\%-75\%}$ (% predicted)	Pao$_2$ (mm Hg)	Paco$_2$ (mm Hg)
Mild (asymptomatic)	65-80	60-75	>60	<40
Moderate	50-64	45-59	>60	<45
Marked	35-49	30-44	<60	>50
Severe (status asthmaticus)	<35	<30	<60	>50

Adapted from Kingston HGG, Hirshman CA. Perioperative management of the patient with asthma. *Anesth Analg.* 1984;63:844-855.
FEF$_{25\%-75\%}$, Forced expiratory flow at 25% to 75% of forced vital capacity; *FEV$_1$*, forced expiratory volume in 1 sec.

TABLE 9-3 ■ Most useful spirometric tests of lung function

Forced expiratory volume in 1 sec (FEV$_1$): The volume of air that can be forcefully exhaled in 1 sec. Values of between 80% and 120% of the predicted value are considered normal.

Forced vital capacity (FVC): The volume of air that can be exhaled with maximum effort after a deep inhalation. Normal values are ~3.7 L in females and ~4.8 L in males.

Ratio of FEV$_1$ to FVC: This ratio in healthy adults is 75% to 80%.

Forced expiratory flow at 25%-75% of vital capacity (FEF$_{25\%-75\%}$): A measurement of airflow through the midpoint of a forced exhalation.

Maximum voluntary ventilation (MVV): The maximum amount of air that can be inhaled and exhaled within 1 min. For the comfort of the patient, the volume is measured over a 15-sec time period and the results are extrapolated to obtain a value for 1 min expressed as liters per minute. Average values for males and females are 140-180 and 80-120 L/min, respectively.

Diffusing capacity (Dlco): The volume of a substance (carbon monoxide, or CO) transferred across the alveoli into blood per minute per unit of alveolar partial pressure. CO is rapidly taken up by hemoglobin. Its transfer is therefore limited mainly by diffusion. A single breath of 0.3% CO and 10% helium is held for 20 sec. Expired partial pressure of CO is measured. Normal value is 17-25 mL/min/mm Hg.

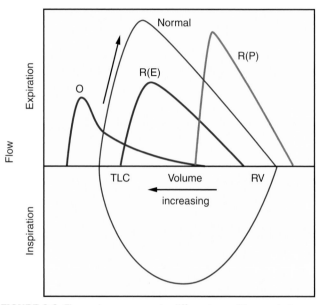

FIGURE 9-2 Flow-volume curves in different conditions: obstructive disease, O; extraparenchymal restrictive disease with limitation in inspiration and expiration, R(E); and parenchymal restrictive disease, R(P). Forced expiration is plotted for all conditions; forced inspiration is shown only for the normal curve. By convention, lung volume increases to the left on the abscissa. The arrow alongside the normal curve indicates the direction of expiration from total lung capacity (TLC) to residual volume (RV). *(Adapted from Weinberger SE. Disturbances of respiratory function. In: Fauci B, Braunwald E, Isselbacher KJ, et al, eds. Harrison's Principles of Internal Medicine. 14th ed. New York, NY: McGraw-Hill; 1998.)*

rather neural reflexes in the lungs. Hypocarbia and respiratory alkalosis are the most common arterial blood gas findings in the presence of asthma. As the severity of expiratory airflow obstruction increases, the associated ventilation/perfusion mismatching may result in a Pao$_2$ of less than 60 mm Hg while breathing room air. The Paco$_2$ is likely to increase when the FEV$_1$ is less than 25% of the predicted value. Fatigue of the skeletal muscles necessary for breathing may also contribute to the development of hypercarbia.

CHEST RADIOGRAPHY AND ELECTROCARDIOGRAPHY

Chest radiographs may demonstrate hyperinflation of the lungs. They can also be useful in diagnosing pneumonia or congestive heart failure, which may be confused with asthma. The electrocardiogram (ECG) may show evidence of acute right heart failure and ventricular irritability during an asthmatic attack.

The differential diagnosis of asthma includes viral tracheobronchitis, sarcoidosis, rheumatoid arthritis with bronchiolitis, and extrinsic compression (thoracic aneurysm, mediastinal neoplasm) or intrinsic compression (epiglottitis, croup) of the upper airway. Upper airway obstruction produces a characteristic flow-volume loop (see Figure 9-3). A history of recent trauma, surgery, or tracheal intubation may be present in patients with upper airway obstruction mimicking asthma. Congestive heart failure and pulmonary embolism may cause dyspnea and wheezing. Wheezing in association with pulmonary edema has been characterized as "cardiac asthma." Improvement after inhaled bronchodilator administration does not exclude cardiac asthma as the cause of wheezing.

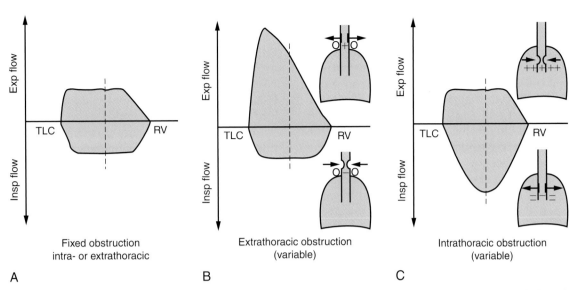

FIGURE 9-3 Flow-volume curves in fixed and variable obstruction. **A,** Fixed obstruction, intrathoracic or extrathoracic. **B,** Extrathoracic obstruction (variable). **C,** Intrathoracic obstruction (variable). *Exp,* Expiratory; *Insp,* inspiratory; *RV,* residual volume; *TLC,* total lung capacity. *(Adapted from Benumof J, ed. Anesthesia for Thoracic Surgery. 2nd ed. Philadelphia, PA: Saunders; 1995.)*

TABLE 9-4 ■ **Pharmacologic agents used in the treatment of asthma**

Class	Drug	Actions	Adverse effects
Antiinflammatory drugs	Corticosteroids: beclomethasone, triamcinolone, flunisolide, fluticasone, budesonide	Decrease airway inflammation, reduce airway hyperresponsiveness	Dysphonia, myopathy of laryngeal muscles, oropharyngeal candidiasis
	Cromolyn	Inhibits mediator release from mast cells, stabilizes membranes	
	Leukotriene modifiers: zafirlukast, pranlukast, montelukast, zileuton	Reduce synthesis of leukotrienes by inhibiting 5-lipoxygenase enzyme	Minimal
Bronchodilators	β-Adrenergic agonists: albuterol, metaproterenol, salmeterol	Stimulate β_2-receptors of tracheobronchial tree	Tachycardia, tremors, dysrhythmias, hypokalemia
	Anticholinergics: ipratropium, atropine, glycopyrrolate	Decrease vagal tone by blocking muscarinic receptors in airway smooth muscle	Dry mouth, cough, blurred vision
Methylxanthines	Theophylline	Increases cyclic adenosine monophosphate levels by inhibiting phosphodiesterase, blocks adenosine receptors, releases endogenous catecholamines	Disrupted sleep cycle, nervousness, nausea, vomiting, anorexia, headache, dysrhythmias

Treatment

Historically, treatment of asthma has been directed at preventing and controlling bronchospasm with bronchodilator drugs. However, recognition of the consistent presence of airway inflammation in patients with asthma has resulted in a change in pharmacologic therapy. The emphasis now is on preventing and controlling bronchial inflammation. Bronchodilator therapy does not influence inflammatory changes in the airways and could mask underlying inflammation by relieving symptoms and allowing continued exposure to allergens. The various drugs used to treat asthma are listed in Table 9-4.

Asthma treatment has two components. The first is the use of "controller" treatments, which modify the airway environment so that acute airway narrowing occurs less frequently. Controller treatments include inhaled and systemic corticosteroids, theophylline, and antileukotrienes. The other component of asthma treatment is the use of "reliever" or rescue agents for acute bronchospasm. Reliever treatments include β-adrenergic agonists and anticholinergic drugs. Albuterol is the inhaled β_2-agonist that is most commonly used. Levalbuterol, the *R*-enantiomer of albuterol, has been used in emergency medicine and appears to be effective at half the dose of racemic albuterol.

Anticholinergic agents such as ipratropium have a relatively slow onset of action and can be used along with short-acting β_2-agonists to produce a prolonged bronchodilatory effect.

If oral corticosteroids are needed, the usual treatment is prednisone 40 to 80 mg/day given in a single dose or in two divided doses. Traditionally aminophylline was a mainstay in the treatment of asthma. However, it appears that the addition of intravenous aminophylline to therapy with inhaled β-agonists in adult patients with acute asthma provides no additional benefit and is associated with an increased frequency of adverse effects. Routine use of antibiotics, aggressive hydration, and administration of mucolytics are not recommended for acute exacerbations of asthma.

Serial determination of pulmonary function test values is useful for monitoring the response to treatment. When the FEV_1 improves to about 50% of normal, patients usually have minimal or no symptoms.

STATUS ASTHMATICUS

Status asthmaticus is defined as bronchospasm that does not resolve despite treatment and is considered life threatening. Emergency treatment of status asthmaticus consists of intermittent or continuous administration of β$_2$-agonists by inhalation using a metered-dose inhaler or a nebulizer. β$_2$-Agonists can be administered every 15 to 20 minutes for several doses without significant adverse hemodynamic effects, although patients may experience unpleasant sensations resulting from adrenergic overstimulation. Continuous rather than intermittent administration of β$_2$-agonists by nebulizer may be more effective for delivery of these drugs to relieve airway spasm. Intravenous corticosteroids are administered early in treatment, because it takes several hours for their effect to appear. The corticosteroids most commonly selected are (1) cortisol 2 mg/kg IV followed by 0.5 mg/kg/hr by infusion, and (2) methylprednisolone 60 to 125 mg IV every 6 hours. Supplemental oxygen is administered to help maintain arterial oxygen saturation above 90%. Other drugs used in intractable cases include magnesium sulfate and oral leukotriene inhibitors. Studies of the use of intravenous magnesium sulfate indicate that it may significantly improve lung function and reduce rates of hospital admission in children. The National Asthma Education and Prevention Program Expert Panel and the Global Initiative for Asthma have the most recent evidence-based guidelines for treatment of asthma.

Measurements of lung function can be very helpful in assessing the severity of status asthmaticus and the response to treatment. Patients whose FEV_1 or peak expiratory flow rate is decreased to 25% of normal or less are at risk of the development of hypercarbia and respiratory failure. The presence of hypercarbia ($Paco_2 > 50$ mm Hg) despite aggressive antiinflammatory and bronchodilator therapy is a sign of respiratory fatigue that requires tracheal intubation and mechanical ventilation. The pattern of mechanical ventilation is particularly important in the patient with status asthmaticus. Because of the bronchoconstriction, high peak airway pressures may be required to deliver acceptable tidal volumes. High gas flows allow for a shorter inspiratory time and a longer time for exhalation. The expiratory phase must be prolonged to allow for complete exhalation and to prevent self-generated or intrinsic positive end-expiratory pressure (auto-PEEP). To prevent barotrauma, some recommend a degree of permissive hypercarbia. When the FEV_1 or peak expiratory flow rate improves to 50% of normal or more, patients usually have minimal or no symptoms. At this point, the frequency and intensity of bronchodilator therapy can be decreased, and weaning from mechanical ventilation can ensue.

When a patient's status asthmaticus is resistant to therapy, it is likely that the expiratory airflow obstruction is caused predominantly by airway edema and intraluminal secretions. Indeed, patients with status asthmaticus are at risk of asphyxia due to the presence of mucus-plugged airways. In rare circumstances, when life-threatening status asthmaticus persists despite aggressive pharmacologic therapy, it may be necessary to consider general anesthesia to produce bronchodilation. Halothane, enflurane, isoflurane, and sevoflurane have all been described as effective bronchodilators in this situation.

Management of Anesthesia

The occurrence of clinically significant "severe" bronchospasm has been reported in 0.2% to 4.2% of all procedures involving general anesthesia performed in asthmatic patients. Factors that are more significant in predicting the occurrence of severe bronchospasm include the type of surgery (risk is higher with upper abdominal surgery and oncologic surgery) and the proximity of the most recent asthmatic attack to the date of surgery.

Several pathophysiologic mechanisms could explain the contribution of general anesthesia to increased airway resistance. Among these are depression of the cough reflex, impairment of mucociliary function, reduction of palatopharyngeal muscle tone, depression of diaphragmatic function, and an increase in the amount of fluid on the airway wall. In addition, direct mechanical airway stimulation by endotracheal intubation, parasympathetic nervous system activation, and/or release of neurotransmitters of pain such as substance P and neurokinins may play a role.

PREOPERATIVE

Preoperative evaluation of patients with asthma requires an assessment of disease severity, the effectiveness of current pharmacologic management, and the potential need for additional therapy before surgery. The goal of preoperative evaluation is to formulate an anesthetic plan that prevents or blunts expiratory airflow obstruction.

Preoperative evaluation begins with taking a clinical history to elicit the severity and characteristics of the patient's asthma (Table 9-5). On physical examination, the general appearance of the patient and any use of accessory muscles of respiration should be noted. Auscultation of the chest to detect wheezing or crepitations is important. Blood eosinophil counts often parallel the degree of airway inflammation, and airway hyperreactivity provides an indirect assessment of the current status of the disease. Pulmonary function tests (especially FEV_1) performed before and after bronchodilator

TABLE 9-5 ■ Characteristics of asthma to be evaluated preoperatively

Age at onset
Triggering events
Hospitalization for asthma
   Frequency of emergency department visits
   Need for intubation and mechanical ventilation
Allergies
Cough
Sputum characteristics
Current medications
Anesthetic history

therapy may be indicated in patients scheduled for major surgery. A reduction in FEV$_1$ or forced vital capacity (FVC) of less than 70%, as well as an FEV$_1$/FVC ratio that is less than 65% of predicted values, is usually considered a risk factor for perioperative complications.

Chest physiotherapy, antibiotic therapy, and bronchodilator therapy during the preoperative period can often improve reversible components of asthma. Measurement of arterial blood gases is indicated if there is any question about the adequacy of ventilation or oxygenation.

The use of anticholinergic drugs should be individualized, and it should be kept in mind that these drugs can increase the viscosity of airway secretions. Intramuscular doses of anticholinergic drugs such as those used for preanesthetic medication are unlikely to decrease airway resistance.

Antiinflammatory and bronchodilator therapy should be continued until the time of anesthesia induction. Supplementation with stress-dose corticosteroids may be indicated before major surgery if hypothalamic-pituitary-adrenal suppression by drugs used to treat asthma is a possibility. However, hypothalamic-pituitary-adrenal suppression is very unlikely with inhaled corticosteroids. In selected patients, a preoperative course of oral corticosteroids may be useful.

Patients should be free of wheezing and have a peak expiratory flow of more than 80% of predicted or at the level of the patient's personal best value before surgery.

INTRAOPERATIVE

During induction and maintenance of anesthesia in asthmatic patients, airway reflexes must be suppressed to avoid bronchoconstriction in response to mechanical stimulation of hyperreactive airways. Stimuli that do not ordinarily evoke airway responses can precipitate life-threatening bronchoconstriction in patients with asthma.

Because it avoids instrumentation of the airway and tracheal intubation, regional anesthesia is an attractive option when the operative site is suitable for this. Concerns that high sensory levels of anesthesia will lead to sympathetic blockade and consequent bronchospasm are unfounded.

When general anesthesia is selected, induction of anesthesia is most often accomplished with an intravenous induction drug. The incidence of wheezing is higher in asthmatic patients receiving thiopental for induction than in those given propofol. Thiopental itself does not cause bronchospasm, but it may inadequately suppress upper airway reflexes so airway instrumentation may trigger bronchospasm. The mechanism of propofol's relative bronchodilating effect is unknown. Ketamine can produce smooth muscle relaxation and contribute to decreased airway resistance, especially in patients who are actively wheezing. However, ketamine increases airway secretions.

After the patient is rendered unconscious, the lungs are often ventilated for a time with a gas mixture containing a volatile anesthetic. The goal is to establish a depth of anesthesia that depresses hyperreactive airway reflexes sufficiently to permit tracheal intubation without precipitating bronchospasm. The lesser pungency of halothane and sevoflurane (compared with isoflurane and desflurane) may decrease the likelihood of coughing, which can trigger bronchospasm. An alternative method to suppress airway reflexes before intubation is the intravenous or intratracheal injection of lidocaine (1 to 1.5 mg/kg) 1 to 3 minutes before endotracheal intubation.

Opioids should be administered to suppress the cough reflex and to achieve deep anesthesia. However, prolongation of opioid effects can cause postoperative respiratory depression. Remifentanil (continuous IV infusion at 0.05 to 0.1 mcg/kg/min) may be particularly useful because it is ultra–short-acting and does not accumulate. All opioids have some histamine-releasing effects, but fentanyl and analogous agents can be used safely in asthmatic patients. The administration of opioids during intubation can prevent increased airway resistance, but muscle rigidity caused by opioid administration can decrease lung compliance and impair ventilation. Opioid-induced muscle rigidity can be decreased by the combined use of intravenous anesthetics and neuromuscular blocking agents.

Insertion of a laryngeal mask airway is less likely to result in bronchoconstriction than insertion of an endotracheal tube. Therefore, use of a laryngeal mask airway may be a better method of airway management in asthmatic patients who are not at risk of reflux or aspiration. After endotracheal intubation, it may be difficult to differentiate light anesthesia from bronchospasm as the cause of a decrease in pulmonary compliance. Administration of neuromuscular blocking drugs relieves the difficulty of ventilation resulting from light anesthesia but has no effect on bronchospasm.

Intraoperatively, the desirable level of arterial oxygenation and carbon dioxide removal is usually provided by mechanical ventilation. In asthmatic patients, a slow inspiratory flow rate produces optimal distribution of ventilation relative to perfusion. Sufficient time for exhalation is necessary to prevent air trapping. Humidification and warming of inspired gases may be especially useful in patients with exercise-induced asthma, in whom bronchospasm is presumably due to transmucosal loss of heat. Liberal administration of fluids during the perioperative period is important for maintaining adequate hydration and ensuring the presence of less viscous airway secretions that can be removed more easily.

Skeletal muscle relaxation is usually provided with non-depolarizing muscle relaxants. Drugs with limited ability to evoke the release of histamine should be selected.

Theoretically, antagonism of neuromuscular blockade with anticholinesterase drugs can precipitate bronchospasm secondary to stimulation of postganglionic cholinergic receptors in airway smooth muscle. Such bronchospasm does not predictably occur after administration of anticholinesterase drugs, probably because of the protective bronchodilating effects provided by the simultaneous administration of anticholinergic drugs.

At the conclusion of surgery, it is prudent to remove the endotracheal tube while anesthesia is still sufficient to suppress hyperreactive airway reflexes, a technique referred to as "deep extubation." When it is deemed unwise to extubate the trachea before the patient is fully awake, suppressing airway reflexes and/or the risk of bronchospasm by administration of intravenous lidocaine or pretreatment with inhaled bronchodilators should be considered.

Intraoperative Bronchospasm

Intraoperatively, bronchospasm is often due to factors other than asthma (Table 9-6). Treatment with bronchodilator drugs should not be instituted until causes of wheezing such as mechanical obstruction of the breathing circuit, the airway, or the endotracheal tube are considered. Bronchospasm resulting from asthma may respond to deepening of the anesthetic with a volatile agent. If bronchospasm persists, then β_2-agonist therapy should be considered.

If bronchospasm persists despite β_2-agonist therapy and deep general anesthesia, corticosteroid administration may be necessary. It must be recognized that several hours may pass before the therapeutic effects of corticosteroids become apparent.

Emergency surgery in the asthmatic patient introduces a conflict between protection of the airway in someone at risk of aspiration and the possibility of triggering bronchospasm. In addition, there may be insufficient time to optimize bronchodilator therapy before surgery. Regional anesthesia may be preferable if the site of surgery is suitable.

TABLE 9-6 ▪ Differential diagnosis of intraoperative bronchospasm and wheezing

Mechanical obstruction of endotracheal tube
  Kinking
  Secretions
  Overinflation of the tracheal tube cuff
Inadequate depth of anesthesia
  Active expiratory efforts
  Decreased functional residual capacity
Endobronchial intubation
Pulmonary aspiration
Pulmonary edema
Pulmonary embolus
Pneumothorax
Acute asthmatic attack

CHRONIC OBSTRUCTIVE PULMONARY DISEASE

Chronic obstructive pulmonary disease (COPD) is a common condition mainly related to smoking. The burden of the disease is increasing, and it is projected that by 2020, COPD will rank fifth among diseases worldwide. COPD causes 100,000 deaths per year in the United States. Patients with COPD pose a challenge to the anesthesiologist, because intraoperative and postoperative pulmonary complications are more common in this population, and COPD can lead to increased length of hospital stay and mortality.

COPD is characterized by the progressive development of airflow limitation that is not fully reversible. COPD causes (1) pathologic deterioration in elasticity or "recoil" within the lung parenchyma, which normally maintains the airways in an open position; (2) pathologic changes that decrease the rigidity of the bronchiolar wall and thus predispose them to collapse during exhalation; (3) an increase in gas velocity in narrowed bronchioli, which lowers the pressure inside the bronchioli and further favors airway collapse; (4) active bronchospasm and obstruction resulting from increased pulmonary secretions; and (5) destruction of lung parenchyma, enlargement of air sacs, and development of emphysema.

The risk factors for development of COPD are (1) cigarette smoking; (2) respiratory infection; (3) occupational exposure to dust, especially in coal mining, gold mining, and the textile industry; and (4) genetic factors such as α_1-antitrypsin deficiency.

Signs and Symptoms

Physical findings vary with the severity of COPD, and during the early stages of the disease, the physical examination may yield normal findings. As expiratory airflow obstruction increases in severity, tachypnea and a prolonged expiratory phase are evident. Breath sounds are likely to be decreased, and expiratory wheezes are common.

Diagnosis

A chronic productive cough, progressive exercise limitation, and expiratory airflow obstruction are characteristic of COPD (Table 9-7). Although these symptoms are nonspecific, a diagnosis of COPD is likely if the patient has smoked cigarettes for a long period. Patients with predominantly chronic bronchitis have a chronic productive cough, whereas patients with predominantly emphysema report dyspnea. Patients with emphysema experience dyspnea during the activities of daily living when the FEV_1 is less than 40% of the normal value. Orthopnea is often present in patients with advanced COPD, especially if there are substantial airway secretions. The orthopnea of COPD may be difficult to differentiate from that resulting from congestive heart failure. Transient periods of sputum discoloration occur in association with respiratory tract infection. Wheezing is common with mucus accumulation in the airways and may mimic asthma. The combination of chronic bronchitis and reversible bronchospasm is referred to as *asthmatic bronchitis*.

PULMONARY FUNCTION TESTS

Results of pulmonary function tests reveal a decrease in the FEV_1/FVC ratio and an even greater decrease in the forced expiratory flow between 25% and 75% of vital capacity ($FEF_{25\%-75\%}$). Measurement of lung volumes may reveal an increased residual volume and normal to increased FRC and total lung capacity (Figure 9-4). Slowing of expiratory airflow and gas trapping behind prematurely closed airways

are responsible for the increase in residual volume. The pathophysiologic "advantage" of an increased residual volume and FRC in patients with COPD is an enlarged airway diameter and increased elastic recoil for exhalation. The cost is the greater work of breathing at the higher lung volumes.

CHEST RADIOGRAPHY

Radiographic abnormalities may be minimal, even in the presence of severe COPD. Hyperlucency due to arterial vascular deficiency in the lung periphery and hyperinflation (flattening of the diaphragm with loss of its normal domed appearance and a very vertical cardiac silhouette) suggest the diagnosis of emphysema. If bullae are present, the diagnosis of emphysema is certain. However, only a small percentage of patients with emphysema have bullae. Computed tomography (CT) of the chest can also be useful for diagnosing emphysema. Chronic bronchitis is rarely diagnosed by chest radiography.

GLOBAL INITIATIVE FOR CHRONIC OBSTRUCTIVE LUNG DISEASE CLASSIFICATION/SEVERITY GRADING

The Global Initiative for Chronic Obstructive Lung Disease (GOLD) works with health care professionals and public health officials around the world to raise awareness of COPD and to improve prevention and treatment of this lung disease. GOLD was launched in 1997 in collaboration with the National Heart, Lung, and Blood Institute of the U.S. National Institutes of Health and the World Health Organization. GOLD developed a classification/severity grading system that is now commonly used by physicians around the world (Table 9-8).

TABLE 9-7 ▪ **Comparative features of chronic obstructive pulmonary disease**

Feature	Chronic bronchitis	Emphysema
Mechanism of airway obstruction	Decreased airway lumen due to mucus and inflammation	Loss of elastic recoil
Dyspnea	Moderate	Severe
FEV_1	Decreased	Decreased
Pao_2	Marked decrease ("blue bloater")	Modest decrease ("pink puffer")
$Paco_2$	Increased	Normal to decreased
Diffusing capacity	Normal	Decreased
Hematocrit	Increased	Normal
Cor pulmonale	Marked	Mild
Prognosis	Poor	Good

FEV_1, Forced expiratory volume in 1 sec.

TABLE 9-8 ▪ **Spirometric classification of the severity of COPD based on postbronchodilator FEV_1 measurements**

Stage	Characteristics
0: At risk	Normal spirometric findings Chronic symptoms (cough, sputum production)
I: Mild COPD	$FEV_1/FVC < 70\%$ $FEV_1 \geq 80\%$ predicted, with or without chronic symptoms (cough, sputum production)
II: Moderate COPD	$FEV_1/FVC < 70\%$ $50\% \leq FEV_1 < 80\%$ predicted, with or without chronic symptoms (cough, sputum production)
III: Severe COPD	$FEV_1/FVC < 70\%$ $30\% \leq FEV_1 < 50\%$ predicted, with or without chronic symptoms (cough, sputum production)
IV: Very severe COPD	$FEV_1/FVC < 70\%$ $FEV_1 < 30\%$ predicted or $FEV_1 < 50\%$ predicted plus chronic respiratory failure, i.e., $Pao_2 < 60$ mm Hg and/or $Pco_2 > 50$ mm Hg

Adapted from Global Initiative for Chronic Obstructive Lung Disease. Global strategy for the diagnosis, management and prevention of COPD: update 2010. http://www.goldcopd.com.
COPD, Chronic obstructive pulmonary disease; *FEV₁*, forced expiratory volume in 1 sec; *FVC*, forced vital capacity.

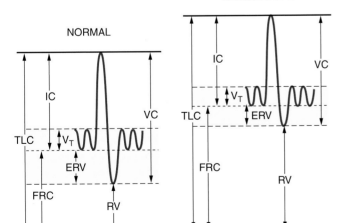

FIGURE 9-4 Lung volumes in chronic obstructive pulmonary disease compared with normal values. In the presence of obstructive lung disease, the vital capacity (VC) is normal to decreased, the residual volume (RV) and functional residual capacity (FRC) are increased, the total lung capacity (TLC) is normal to increased, and the RV/TLC ratio is increased. *ERV,* Expiratory reserve volume; *IC,* inspiratory capacity; *V_T,* tidal volume.

Treatment

Treatment of COPD is designed to relieve existing symptoms and slow the progression of the disease.

CESSATION OF SMOKING AND OXYGEN SUPPLEMENTATION

Smoking cessation and long-term oxygen administration are the two important therapeutic interventions that can alter the natural progression of COPD. Smoking cessation causes the symptoms of chronic bronchitis to diminish or entirely disappear, and it eliminates the accelerated loss of lung function observed in those who continue to smoke. Long-term oxygen administration (home oxygen therapy) is recommended if the Pao_2 is less than 55 mm Hg, the hematocrit is more than 55%, or there is evidence of cor pulmonale. The goal of supplemental oxygen administration is to achieve a Pao_2 between 60 and 80 mm Hg. This goal can usually be accomplished by delivering oxygen through a nasal cannula at 2 L/min. Ultimately, the flow rate of oxygen is titrated as needed according to arterial blood gas or pulse oximetry measurements. Relief of arterial hypoxemia with supplemental oxygen administration is more effective than any known drug therapy in decreasing pulmonary vascular resistance and pulmonary hypertension and in preventing erythrocytosis.

DRUG THERAPY

Bronchodilators are the mainstay of drug therapy for COPD. Bronchodilators cause only a small increase in FEV_1 but may alleviate symptoms by decreasing hyperinflation and dyspnea. They may thus improve exercise tolerance, despite the fact that there is little improvement in spirometric measurements. An additional benefit of β_2-agonists may be fewer infections, since these drugs decrease the adhesion of bacteria such as *Haemophilus influenzae* to airway epithelial cells. COPD is often more effectively treated by anticholinergic drugs than by β_2-agonists. This is in contrast to asthma, in which β_2-agonists are usually more effective. Inhaled corticosteroids are widely prescribed for COPD. Intermittent administration of broad-spectrum antibiotics is indicated for acute episodes of increased dyspnea associated with excessive or purulent sputum production. Annual vaccination against influenza is beneficial. Administration of pneumococcal vaccine is also recommended. Exacerbations of COPD may be due to viral infection of the upper respiratory tract or may be noninfective, so antibiotic treatment is not always warranted. Diuretic therapy may be considered for patients with cor pulmonale and right ventricular failure with peripheral edema. Diuretic-induced chloride depletion may produce a hypochloremic metabolic alkalosis that depresses the ventilatory drive and may aggravate chronic carbon dioxide retention. Physical training programs can increase the exercise capacity of patients with COPD despite the absence of detectable effects on the FEV_1. However, prompt deconditioning occurs when the exercise program is abandoned.

LUNG VOLUME REDUCTION SURGERY

Lung volume reduction surgery may be considered in selected patients with emphysema who have regions of overdistended, poorly functioning lung tissue. Surgical removal of these overdistended areas allows more normal areas of the lung to expand and improves not only lung function but quality of life. Lung volume reduction surgery is performed by either a median sternotomy or video-assisted thoracoscopic surgery (VATS) approach. The proposed mechanisms for improvement in lung function after this surgery include (1) an increase in elastic recoil, which increases expiratory airflow; (2) a decrease in the degree of hyperinflation, which results in improved diaphragmatic and chest wall mechanics; and (3) a decrease in the inhomogeneity of regional ventilation and perfusion, which results in improved alveolar gas exchange and increased effectiveness of ventilation. Currently research is under way to examine nonsurgical approaches for achieving benefits similar to those provided by lung volume reduction surgery.

Management of anesthesia for lung volume reduction surgery includes use of a double-lumen endobronchial tube to permit lung separation, avoidance of nitrous oxide, and avoidance of excessive positive airway pressure. Monitoring of central venous pressure as a guide to fluid management is unreliable in this situation.

Management of Anesthesia

PREOPERATIVE

The history and physical examination findings of patients with COPD provide a more accurate assessment of the likelihood of postoperative pulmonary complications than pulmonary function test results or measurement of arterial blood gases. A history of poor exercise tolerance, chronic cough, or unexplained dyspnea combined with diminished breath sounds, wheezing, and a prolonged expiratory phase predicts an increased risk of postoperative pulmonary complications. Preoperative preparation of patients with COPD includes smoking cessation, treatment of bronchospasm, and eradication of bacterial infection.

Pulmonary Function Testing

The value of routine preoperative pulmonary function testing remains controversial. The results of pulmonary function tests and arterial blood gas analysis can be useful for predicting pulmonary function following lung resection, but they do not reliably predict the likelihood of postoperative pulmonary complications after nonthoracic surgery. Clinical findings (smoking, diffuse wheezing, productive cough) are more predictive of pulmonary complications than spirometric results. Patients with mild pulmonary disease undergoing peripheral surgery do not require pulmonary function tests. If doubt exists, simple spirometry with measurement of FEV_1 is sufficient.

Even patients defined as high risk by spirometry (FEV_1 < 70% of predicted, FEV_1/FVC ratio < 65%) or arterial blood gas analysis ($Paco_2$ > 45 mm Hg) can undergo surgery, including lung resection, with an acceptable risk of postoperative pulmonary complications. Pulmonary function tests should be viewed as a management tool to optimize preoperative pulmonary function but not as a means to predict risk. Indications for a preoperative pulmonary evaluation (which may include consultation with a pulmonologist and/or performance of pulmonary function tests) typically include (1) hypoxemia on room air or the need for home oxygen therapy without a known cause, (2) a bicarbonate concentration of more than 33 mEq/L or P_{CO_2} of more than 50 mm Hg in a patient whose pulmonary disease has not been previously evaluated, (3) a history of respiratory failure resulting from a problem that still exists, (4) severe shortness of breath attributed to respiratory disease, (5) planned pneumonectomy, (6) difficulty in assessing pulmonary function by clinical signs, (7) the need to distinguish among potential causes of significant respiratory compromise, (8) the need to determine the response to bronchodilators, and (9) suspected pulmonary hypertension.

Right ventricular function should be carefully assessed by clinical examination and echocardiography in patients with advanced pulmonary disease.

Ventilatory function is quantified under static conditions by measuring lung volumes and under dynamic conditions by measuring flow rates. In assessing lung function, expiratory flow rates can be plotted against lung volumes to produce flow-volume curves. When flow rates during inspiration are added to these curves, flow-volume loops are obtained. The flow rate is zero at total lung capacity before the start of expiration. Once forced expiration begins, the peak flow rate is achieved rapidly and flow rate then falls in a linear fashion as the lung volume decreases to residual volume. During maximal inspiration from residual volume to total lung capacity, the inspiratory flow is most rapid at the midpoint of inspiration, so that the inspiratory curve is U-shaped.

In patients with COPD, there is a decrease in the expiratory flow rate at any given lung volume. The expiratory curve is concave upward due to uniform emptying of the airways. The residual volume is increased because of air trapping (see Figure 9-2).

Evaluation of Risk Factors for Postoperative Pulmonary Complications

The major risk factors for the development of postoperative pulmonary complications are shown in Table 9-9. Obesity and mild to moderate asthma have not been shown to be independent risk factors. An algorithm for reducing pulmonary complications in patients undergoing noncardiothoracic surgery is shown in Figure 9-5.

Risk-Reduction Strategies

Strategies to decrease the incidence of postoperative pulmonary complications include preoperative, intraoperative, and postoperative interventions (Table 9-10).

Smoking Cessation. Approximately 20% of American adults smoke, of whom 5% to 10% will annually undergo

TABLE 9-9	**Major risk factors associated with postoperative pulmonary complications**

PATIENT RELATED

Age > 60 yr
American Society of Anesthesiologists class higher than II
Congestive heart failure
Preexisting pulmonary disease (chronic obstructive pulmonary disease)
Cigarette smoking

PROCEDURE RELATED

Emergency surgery
Abdominal or thoracic surgery, head and neck surgery, neurosurgery, vascular/aortic aneurysm surgery
Prolonged duration of anesthesia (> 2.5 hr)
General anesthesia

TEST PREDICTORS

Albumin level of < 3.5 g/dL

Adapted from Smetana GW, Lawrence VA, Cornell JE. Preoperative pulmonary risk stratification for noncardiothoracic surgery. A systematic review for the American College of Physicians. *Ann Intern Med.* 2006;144:581-595.

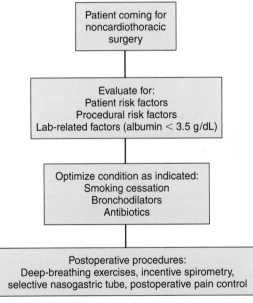

FIGURE 9-5 Algorithm for decreasing pulmonary complications in patients undergoing noncardiothoracic surgery. *(Adapted from Qaseem A, Snow V, Fitterman N, et al. Risk assessment for and strategies to reduce perioperative pulmonary complications for patients undergoing noncardiothoracic surgery: a guideline from the American College of Physicians. Ann Intern Med. 2006;144:575-580.)*

general anesthesia and/or surgery. These times of exposure to general anesthesia and/or surgery offer a window of opportunity for a smoking cessation intervention by a health care provider or other individual. This person can be the surgeon, the anesthesiologist, the nurse, or even a member of an active patient group or community group, who should

TABLE 9-10 ◼ Risk-reduction strategies to decrease the incidence of postoperative pulmonary complications

PREOPERATIVE

Encourage cessation of smoking for at least 6 wk
Treat evidence of expiratory airflow obstruction
Treat respiratory infection with antibiotics
Initiate patient education regarding lung volume expansion maneuvers

INTRAOPERATIVE

Use minimally invasive surgery (endoscopic) techniques when possible
Consider regional anesthesia
Avoid surgical procedures likely to last longer than 3 hr

POSTOPERATIVE

Institute lung volume expansion maneuvers (voluntary deep breathing, incentive spirometry, continuous positive airway pressure)
Maximize analgesia (neuraxial opioids, intercostal nerve blocks, patient-controlled analgesia)

Adapted from Smetana GW. Preoperative pulmonary evaluation. *N Engl J Med*. 1999;340:937-944. Copyright 1999 Massachusetts Medical Society.

TABLE 9-11 ◼ Effects of smoking on different organ systems

CARDIAC EFFECTS OF SMOKING

Smoking is a risk factor for development of cardiovascular disease.
Carbon monoxide decreases oxygen delivery and increases myocardial work.
Smoking releases catecholamines and causes coronary vasoconstriction.
Smoking decreases exercise capacity.

RESPIRATORY EFFECTS OF SMOKING

Smoking is the major risk factor for development of chronic pulmonary disease.
Smoking decreases mucociliary activity.
Smoking results in hyperreactive airways.
Smoking decreases pulmonary immune function.

OTHER ORGAN SYSTEM EFFECTS

Smoking impairs wound healing.

encourage the patient to stop smoking temporarily before the surgery or, preferably, permanently. The intervention can be carried out at the surgical clinic or anesthetic preadmission testing clinic, via phone calls by nurses or health care workers, or in a letter indicating the risks of postoperative complications caused by continued smoking. Recent evidence shows that the earlier the intervention before surgery, the more effective it is in reducing the postoperative complications and maintaining abstinence. Cigarette smoking is the single most important risk factor for the development of COPD and death caused by lung disease. The effects of smoking on different organ systems are described in Table 9-11. Smoking cessation is strongly encouraged by the U.S. Public Health Service (http://www.surgeongeneral.gov/tobacco). It recommends systematically identifying all tobacco users who come in contact with the health care system to urge and help them to quit smoking. The American Society of Anesthesiologists also has a Stop Smoking Initiative and provides resources to help practitioners encourage smoking cessation (http://www.asahq.org/For-Members/Clinical-Information/ASA-Stop-Smoking-Initiative.aspx).

Among smokers, predictive factors for the development of pulmonary complications are a lower diffusing capacity than predicted and a smoking history of more than 60 pack-years. Those who have smoked more than 60 pack-years have double the risk of any pulmonary complication and triple the risk of pneumonia compared with those who have smoked less than 60 pack-years. Smoking cessation causes the symptoms of chronic bronchitis to diminish or disappear and eliminates the accelerated loss of lung function observed in those who continue to smoke.

Anesthesiologists who practice pain medicine also have the opportunity to encourage smoking cessation in their patients. Among adults with chronic pain, smoking is associated with higher levels of pain, greater levels of depression and anxiety, worse physical functioning, and use of larger amounts of prescription opioids. However, it is not known how smoking cessation might affect pain symptoms.

ACUTE EFFECTS OF SMOKING CESSATION

SHORT-TERM EFFECTS. The adverse effects of carbon monoxide on oxygen-carrying capacity and of nicotine on the cardiovascular system are short-lived. The elimination half-life of carbon monoxide is approximately 4 to 6 hours when breathing room air. Within 12 hours after cessation of smoking the Pao_2 at which hemoglobin is 50% saturated with oxygen (P_{50}) increases from 22.9 to 26.4 mm Hg, and the plasma levels of carboxyhemoglobin decrease from 6.5% to approximately 1%. Carbon monoxide may have negative inotropic effects. Despite the favorable effects on plasma carboxyhemoglobin concentration, short-term abstinence from cigarettes has not been proven to decrease the incidence of postoperative pulmonary complications. The sympathomimetic effects of nicotine on the heart are transient, lasting only 20 to 30 minutes.

INTERMEDIATE-TERM EFFECTS. Cigarette smoking causes mucus hypersecretion, impairment of mucociliary transport, and narrowing of small airways. In contrast to the rapid favorable effect of short-term abstinence from smoking on carboxyhemoglobin concentrations, improved ciliary and small airway function and decreased sputum production occur slowly over a period of weeks after smoking cessation. Cigarette smoking may interfere with normal immune responses and could interfere with the ability of smokers to respond to pulmonary infection following anesthesia and surgery. A decrease in postoperative pulmonary complications resulting from smoking cessation is thought to be related to the physiologic improvement in ciliary action, macrophage activity, and small airway function, as well as a decrease in sputum production. However, these changes take weeks to months to occur. Return of normal immune function requires at least 6 weeks of abstinence from smoking. Some components of cigarette smoke stimulate hepatic enzymes. As with immune responses, it may take 6 weeks or longer for hepatic enzyme activity to return to normal following cessation of smoking.

The optimal timing of smoking cessation before surgery to reduce postoperative pulmonary complications remains unclear, but many suggest it to be around 4 to 8 weeks. Smokers scheduled for surgery in less than 4 weeks should be advised to quit and should be offered effective interventions, including behavioral support and pharmacotherapy, to help achieve this goal. Despite the clear advantages of long-term smoking cessation, there can be disadvantages to smoking cessation in the immediate preoperative period. These include an increase in sputum production, patient fear of the inability to handle stress, nicotine withdrawal, and symptoms including irritability, restlessness, sleep disturbances, and depression.

Countless methods have been devised to aid in smoking cessation. Most involve some form of counseling and pharmacotherapy. Nicotine replacement therapy, with various delivery systems including patches, inhalers, nasal sprays, lozenges, and gum, is generally well tolerated. The major side effect is local irritation at the site of drug delivery. The atypical antidepressant bupropion in a sustained-release formulation can also aid in smoking cessation. The drug is typically started 1 to 2 weeks before smoking is stopped.

Nutritional Status. Poor nutritional status with a low serum albumin level (<3.5 mg/dL) is a powerful predictor of postoperative pulmonary complications in COPD patients. Malnutrition can increase the risk of prolonged postoperative air leaks in patients after lung surgery.

INTRAOPERATIVE

Regional Anesthesia

Regional anesthesia is suitable for operations that do not invade the peritoneum and for surgical procedures performed on the extremities. Lower intraabdominal surgery can also be performed using a regional technique. General anesthesia is the usual choice for upper abdominal and intrathoracic surgery. The choice of anesthetic technique or specific anesthetic drugs does not seem to alter the incidence of postoperative pulmonary complications. Studies in patients with COPD suggest that there is a higher incidence of postoperative respiratory failure in patients who undergo general anesthesia, but whether this reflects the nature and complexity of the surgery and/or the operative site, or the selection of anesthetic drugs or technique is unclear. Whether there is a relationship between the duration of anesthesia and the incidence of postoperative pulmonary complications is controversial. Some suggest that operations lasting longer than 3 hours are more likely to be associated with postoperative pulmonary complications.

Regional anesthesia via peripheral nerve blockade such as an axillary blockade carries a lower risk of pulmonary complications than either spinal or general anesthesia. Regional anesthesia is a useful choice in patients with COPD only if large doses of sedative and anxiolytic drugs will not be needed. It must be appreciated that COPD patients can be extremely sensitive to the ventilatory depressant effects of sedative drugs. Elderly patients may be especially susceptible. Often small doses of a benzodiazepine such as midazolam, in increments of 1 to 2 mg IV, can be administered without producing undesirable degrees of ventilatory depression. Use of regional anesthetic techniques that produce sensory anesthesia above T6 is not recommended, because such high blocks can impair the ventilatory functions requiring active exhalation; this affects parameters such as expiratory reserve volume, peak expiratory flow, and maximum minute ventilation. Clinically, this is manifested as an inadequate cough.

General Anesthesia

General anesthesia is often accomplished with volatile anesthetics. Volatile anesthetics are useful because of the ability of these drugs (especially desflurane and sevoflurane) to be rapidly eliminated. Residual ventilatory depression during the early postoperative period is thereby minimized. Volatile anesthetics are also known to cause bronchodilation and have been used to treat bronchospasm in status asthmaticus. Desflurane, however, may cause irritation of the bronchi and increased airway resistance, so there may be an advantage to choosing a less irritating agent such as sevoflurane for induction and emergence in cases of severe airway reactivity. Emergence from anesthesia with inhalational agents can be prolonged significantly, especially in patients with significant airway obstruction, because air trapping also traps inhalational agents as they flood out of the body's compartments into the lungs. An alternative is total intravenous anesthesia with propofol. A short-acting analgesic such as remifentanil can be used to relieve the irritation of the endotracheal tube sufficiently so that the required level of propofol can be diminished considerably and the attendant risk of hypotension is reduced.

Nitrous oxide can be administered in combination with a volatile anesthetic. When nitrous oxide is used, there is the potential for passage of this gas into pulmonary bullae. This could lead to enlargement or even rupture of the bullae, resulting in development of a pneumothorax. Another potential disadvantage of nitrous oxide is the limitation on the inspired oxygen concentration that it imposes. It is important to remember that inhaled anesthetics may attenuate regional hypoxic pulmonary vasoconstriction and produce more intrapulmonary shunting. Increasing the fraction of inspired oxygen (FIO_2) may be necessary to offset this loss of hypoxic pulmonary vasoconstriction.

Opioids may be less useful than inhaled anesthetics for maintenance of anesthesia in patients with COPD because they can be associated with prolonged ventilatory depression as a result of their slow rate of metabolism or elimination. Even the duration of ventilatory depression produced by drugs such as thiopental and midazolam may be prolonged in patients with COPD compared with healthy individuals. A high inspired concentration of nitrous oxide might be used to ensure amnesia when opioids are used for maintenance of anesthesia. This may be difficult to achieve if a high F_{IO_2} is also required.

An endotracheal tube bypasses most of the natural airway humidification system, so humidification of inspired gases and use of low gas flows are needed to keep airway secretions moist.

Controlled mechanical ventilation is useful for optimizing oxygenation in patients with COPD who are undergoing operations requiring general anesthesia. Tidal volumes of 6 to 8 mL/kg combined with slow inspiratory flow rates minimize the likelihood of turbulent airflow and help maintain optimal ventilation/perfusion matching. Slow respiratory rates (6 to 10 breaths per minute) provide sufficient time for complete exhalation to occur, which is particularly important if air trapping is to be minimized. Slow rates also allow sufficient time for venous return and are less likely to be associated with undesirable degrees of hyperventilation. The phenomenon of air trapping or dynamic hyperinflation is enhanced when positive pressure ventilation is applied and insufficient expiratory time is allowed. This contributes to increased intrathoracic pressure, impedes venous return, and transmits the elevated intrathoracic pressure to the pulmonary artery. An increase in pulmonary vascular resistance can lead to right ventricular strain. Hyperinflated lungs may exert direct pressure on the heart, limiting its ability to expand fully during diastole even with adequate preload. Shift of the ventricular septum and ventricular interdependence due to the shared pericardium may cause a distended right ventricle to impinge on the filling of the left ventricle.

Air trapping can be detected during mechanical ventilation intraoperatively by the following methods:

1. Capnography shows that the carbon dioxide concentration does not plateau but is still upsloping at the time of the next breath. This indicates that there is still admixture of air from dead space reducing the carbon dioxide concentration.
2. Direct measurement of flow may be displayed graphically by the ventilator, showing that the expiratory flow has not reached baseline (zero) before initiation of the next breath.
3. Direct measurement of the resulting PEEP can be performed using more advanced ventilators that are capable of an expiratory hold.
4. The patient can simply be disconnected from the ventilator briefly and observed to see whether the blood pressure increases significantly as PEEP is eliminated.

The hazard of pulmonary barotrauma in the presence of bullae should be appreciated, particularly when high positive airway pressures are required to provide adequate ventilation If spontaneous breathing is permitted during anesthesia in patients with COPD, it should be appreciated that the ventilatory depression produced by volatile anesthetics may be greater in these patients than in individuals without COPD.

POSTOPERATIVE

Prophylaxis against the development of postoperative pulmonary complications is based on maintaining adequate lung volumes, especially FRC, and facilitating an effective cough. Identification of the FRC as the most important lung volume during the postoperative period provides a specific goal for therapy.

Lung Expansion Maneuvers

Lung expansion maneuvers (deep breathing exercises, incentive spirometry, chest physiotherapy, positive pressure breathing techniques) are of proven benefit for preventing postoperative pulmonary complications in patients at high risk. These techniques decrease the risk of atelectasis by increasing lung volumes. All regimens seem to be efficacious in decreasing the frequency of postoperative pulmonary complications by approximately twofold compared with no therapy. Incentive spirometry is simple and inexpensive and provides objective goals for and monitoring of patient performance. Patients are given a particular inspired volume as a goal to achieve and hold. This provides sustained lung inflation, which is important for reexpanding collapsed alveoli. The major disadvantage of incentive spirometry is the need for patient cooperation to accomplish the treatment. Providing education in lung expansion maneuvers before surgery decreases the incidence of pulmonary complications to a greater degree than beginning education after surgery.

Intermittent positive pressure breathing can decrease the incidence of postoperative pulmonary complications, but its complexity has resulted in a decline in its use. Continuous positive airway pressure is reserved for the prevention of postoperative pulmonary complications in patients who are not able to perform deep-breathing exercises or incentive spirometry. Nasal positive airway pressure can also minimize the expected decrease in lung volumes after surgery.

Postoperative neuraxial analgesia with opioids may permit early tracheal extubation. The sympathetic blockade, muscle weakness, and loss of proprioception that are produced by local anesthetics are not produced by neuraxial opioids. Therefore, early ambulation is possible. Ambulation serves to increase FRC and improve oxygenation, presumably by improving ventilation/perfusion matching. Neuraxial opioids may be especially useful after intrathoracic and upper abdominal surgery. Breakthrough pain may require treatment with systemic opioids administered by bolus or via patient-controlled analgesia. Sedation may accompany neuraxial opioid administration, and delayed respiratory depression can be seen, especially when poorly lipid-soluble opioids such as morphine are used.

The quality of neuraxial analgesia (epidural or spinal) may be superior to that provided by parenteral administration of opioids, but it has not been possible to document that neuraxial analgesia decreases the incidence of clinically significant postoperative pulmonary complications or is superior to parenteral opioids in this regard. Postoperative neuraxial analgesia is recommended after high-risk thoracic, abdominal, and major vascular surgery. Intermittent or continuous intercostal nerve blockade may be an alternative if neuraxial analgesia is ineffective or technically difficult.

Mechanical Ventilation

Continued mechanical ventilation during the immediately postoperative period may be necessary in patients with severe COPD who have undergone major abdominal or intrathoracic surgery. Patients with preoperative FEV_1/FVC ratios of less than 0.5 or with a preoperative $PaCO_2$ of more than 50 mm Hg are likely to need some postoperative mechanical ventilation. If the $PaCO_2$ has been increased for a long period, it is important not to correct the hypercarbia too quickly, because this will result in a metabolic alkalosis that can be associated with cardiac dysrhythmias and central nervous system irritability and even seizures.

When continued mechanical ventilation is necessary, FiO_2 and ventilator settings should be adjusted to keep the PaO_2 between 60 and 100 mm Hg and the $PaCO_2$ in a range that maintains the arterial pH (pHa) at 7.35 to 7.45. Reduction of the respiratory rate or the I:E ratio allows more time for exhalation and thus reduces the likelihood of air trapping. However, this may also lower the tidal volume and minute ventilation and exacerbate hypercapnia, hypoxia, and acidosis. Pulmonary vascular resistance may increase and can lead to right ventricular strain. Electrolyte shifts resulting from acidemia can cause cardiac dysrhythmias in patients with COPD or asthma. Extubation of the high-risk patient to continuous positive airway pressure or bilevel positive airway pressure may reduce the work of breathing and air trapping. However, use of positive airway pressure in the setting of an unprotected airway raises concern about insufflation of the stomach and the risk of vomiting and aspiration. Treatment with sympathomimetic bronchodilators such as albuterol and inhaled anticholinergics such as ipratropium may improve airflow if a reactive component of air trapping is present.

Chest Physiotherapy

A combination of chest physiotherapy and postural drainage plus deep-breathing exercises taught during the preoperative period may decrease the incidence of postoperative pulmonary complications. Presumably, vibrations produced on the chest wall by physiotherapy result in dislodgment of mucus plugs from peripheral airways. Appropriate positioning facilitates elimination of loosened mucus.

LESS COMMON CAUSES OF EXPIRATORY AIRFLOW OBSTRUCTION

Expiratory airflow obstruction occurs, although less often, in conditions other than chronic bronchitis and emphysema.

Bronchiectasis

Bronchiectasis is a chronic suppurative disease of the airways that, if sufficiently widespread, may cause expiratory airflow obstruction similar to that seen in COPD. Despite the availability of antibiotics, bronchiectasis is an important cause of chronic productive cough with purulent sputum and accounts for a significant number of cases of massive hemoptysis.

PATHOPHYSIOLOGY

Bronchiectasis is characterized by the localized, irreversible dilation of a bronchus caused by destructive inflammatory processes involving the bronchial wall. Mycobacterial or other bacterial infections are presumed to be responsible for most cases of bronchiectasis. The most important consequence of bronchiectatic destruction of airways is an increased susceptibility to recurrent or persistent bacterial infection, which reflects impaired mucociliary activity and pooling of mucus in dilated airways. Once bacterial superinfection is established, it is nearly impossible to eradicate, and daily expectoration of purulent sputum persists.

DIAGNOSIS

The history of a chronic cough productive of purulent sputum is highly suggestive of bronchiectasis. Clubbing of the fingers occurs in most patients with significant bronchiectasis and is a valuable diagnostic clue, especially since this change is not characteristic of COPD. Pulmonary function changes vary considerably and range from no change to alterations characteristic of COPD or restrictive lung disease. Computed tomography provides excellent images of bronchiectatic airways and can be used to confirm the presence and extent of the disease.

TREATMENT

Bronchiectasis is treated by administration of antibiotics and postural drainage. Results of periodic sputum cultures guide antibiotic selection. *Pseudomonas* is the most common organism cultured. Mild hemoptysis can be controlled with appropriate antibiotic therapy. However, massive hemoptysis (>200 mL over a 24-hour period) may require surgical resection of the involved lung segment or selective bronchial arterial embolization. Postural drainage is useful to assist in expectoration of secretions that pool distal to the diseased airways. Chest physiotherapy with chest percussion and vibration is another aid for bronchopulmonary drainage. Surgical resection has played a declining role in the management of bronchiectasis in the modern antibiotic era and is considered only in the rare instance in which severe symptoms persist or recurrent complications occur.

MANAGEMENT OF ANESTHESIA

Before elective surgery, the pulmonary status of patients with bronchiectasis is optimized by antibiotic therapy and postural drainage. Airway management might include use of a double-lumen endobronchial tube to prevent spillage of purulent sputum into normal areas of the lungs. Instrumentation of the nares should be avoided because of the high incidence of chronic sinusitis in these patients.

Cystic Fibrosis

Cystic fibrosis is an autosomal recessive disorder. It affects an estimated 30,000 persons in the United States.

PATHOPHYSIOLOGY

The cause of cystic fibrosis is a mutation in a single gene on chromosome 7 that encodes the cystic fibrosis transmembrane conductance regulator. The result of this mutation is defective chloride ion transport in epithelial cells in the lungs, pancreas, liver, gastrointestinal tract, and reproductive organs. Decreased chloride transport is accompanied by decreased transport of sodium and water, which results in dehydrated, viscous secretions that are associated with luminal obstruction as well as destruction and scarring of various exocrine glands. Pancreatic insufficiency, meconium ileus at birth, diabetes mellitus, obstructive hepatobiliary tract disease, and azoospermia are often present, but the primary cause of morbidity and mortality in patients with cystic fibrosis is chronic pulmonary infection.

DIAGNOSIS

The presence of a sweat chloride concentration higher than 80 mEq/L plus the characteristic clinical manifestations (cough, chronic purulent sputum production, exertional dyspnea) or family history of the disease confirms the diagnosis of cystic fibrosis. Chronic pansinusitis is almost universal. The presence of normal sinuses on radiographic examination is strong evidence that cystic fibrosis is not present. Malabsorption with a response to pancreatic enzyme treatment is evidence of the exocrine insufficiency associated with cystic fibrosis. Obstructive azoospermia confirmed by testicular biopsy is also strong evidence of cystic fibrosis. Bronchoalveolar lavage typically shows a high percentage of neutrophils, a sign of airway inflammation. COPD is present in virtually all adult patients with cystic fibrosis and follows a relentless course.

TREATMENT

Treatment of cystic fibrosis is similar to that for bronchiectasis and is directed toward alleviation of symptoms (mobilization and clearance of lower airway secretions and treatment of pulmonary infection) and correction of organ dysfunction (pancreatic enzyme replacement).

Clearance of Airway Secretions

The abnormal viscoelastic properties of the sputum in patients with cystic fibrosis lead to sputum retention resulting in airway obstruction. The principal nonpharmacologic approach to enhancing clearance of pulmonary secretions is chest physiotherapy with postural drainage. High-frequency chest compression with an inflatable vest and airway oscillation with a flutter valve are alternative methods of physiotherapy that are less time consuming and do not require trained personnel.

Bronchodilator Therapy

Bronchial reactivity to histamine and other provocative stimuli is greater in patients with cystic fibrosis than in individuals without the disease. Bronchodilator therapy is considered if patients have an increase of 10% or more in FEV_1 in response to an inhaled bronchodilator.

Reduction in Viscoelasticity of Sputum

The abnormal viscosity of airway secretions is due primarily to the presence of neutrophils and their degradation products. DNA released from neutrophils forms long fibrils that contribute to the viscosity of the sputum. Recombinant human deoxyribonuclease I (dornase alfa [Pulmozyme]) can cleave this DNA and increase the clearance of sputum in these patients.

Antibiotic Therapy

Patients with cystic fibrosis have periodic exacerbations of pulmonary infection that are recognized primarily by an increase in symptoms and in sputum production. Antibiotic therapy is based on identification and susceptibility testing of bacteria isolated from the sputum. In patients in whom cultures yield no pathogens, bronchoscopy to remove lower airway secretions may be indicated. Many patients with cystic fibrosis are given long-term maintenance antibiotic therapy in hope of suppressing chronic infection and the development of bronchiectasis.

MANAGEMENT OF ANESTHESIA

Management of anesthesia in patients with cystic fibrosis follows the same principles as outlined for patients with COPD and bronchiectasis. Elective surgical procedures should be delayed until optimal pulmonary function can be ensured by controlling bronchial infection and facilitating removal of airway secretions. Vitamin K treatment may be necessary if hepatic function is poor or if absorption of fat-soluble vitamins from the gastrointestinal tract is impaired. Maintenance of anesthesia with volatile anesthetics permits the use of high inspired concentrations of oxygen, decreases airway resistance by decreasing bronchial smooth muscle tone, and decreases the responsiveness of hyperreactive airways. Humidification of inspired gases, hydration, and avoidance of anticholinergic drugs are important to maintain secretions in a less viscous state. Frequent tracheal suctioning may be necessary.

Primary Ciliary Dyskinesia

Primary ciliary dyskinesia is characterized by congenital impairment of ciliary activity in respiratory tract epithelial cells and sperm tails (spermatozoa are alive but immobile). As a result of impaired ciliary activity in the respiratory tract, chronic sinusitis, recurrent respiratory infections, and bronchiectasis develop. Not only is there infertility in males, but fertility is decreased in females since oviducts also have ciliated epithelium. The triad of chronic sinusitis, bronchiectasis, and situs inversus is known as *Kartagener's syndrome.* It is speculated that the normal asymmetrical positioning of body organs is dependent on normal ciliary function of the embryonic epithelium. In the absence of normal ciliary function, placement of organs to the left or the right is random. As expected, approximately one half of patients with congenitally nonfunctioning cilia manifest situs inversus. Isolated dextrocardia is almost always associated with congenital heart disease.

Preoperative preparation is directed at treating active pulmonary infection and determining whether any significant organ inversion is present. In the presence of dextrocardia, it is necessary to reverse the ECG leads to permit accurate interpretation. Inversion of the great vessels is a reason to select the left internal jugular vein for central venous cannulation. Uterine displacement in parturient women is logically to the right in these patients. Should a double-lumen endobronchial tube be considered, it is necessary to appreciate the altered anatomy introduced by pulmonary inversion. In view of the high incidence of sinusitis, nasopharyngeal airways should be avoided.

Bronchiolitis Obliterans

Bronchiolitis is a disease of childhood and is most often the result of infection with respiratory syncytial virus. Bronchiolitis obliterans is a rare cause of COPD in adults. The process may accompany viral pneumonia, collagen vascular disease (especially rheumatoid arthritis), and inhalation of nitrogen dioxide (silo filler's disease), or it may be a sequela of graft-versus-host disease after bone marrow transplantation. Bronchiolitis obliterans with organizing pneumonia (BOOP) is a clinical entity that shares certain features of interstitial lung disease and bronchiolitis obliterans. Treatment of bronchiolitis obliterans is usually ineffective, although corticosteroids may be administered in an attempt to suppress inflammation involving the bronchioles. BOOP, however, does respond well to corticosteroid therapy. Symptomatic improvement may accompany the use of bronchodilators.

Tracheal Stenosis

Tracheal stenosis typically develops after prolonged endotracheal intubation. Tracheal mucosal ischemia that may progress to destruction of cartilaginous rings and subsequent circumferential constricting scar formation is minimized by the use of high-volume, low-pressure cuffs on endotracheal tubes. Infection and hypotension may also contribute to events that culminate in tracheal stenosis.

DIAGNOSIS

Tracheal stenosis becomes symptomatic when the lumen of the adult trachea is decreased to less than 5 mm in diameter. Symptoms may not develop until several weeks after tracheal extubation. Dyspnea is prominent even at rest. These patients must use accessory muscles of respiration during all phases of the breathing cycle and must breathe slowly. Peak expiratory flow rates are decreased. Stridor is usually audible. Flow-volume loops display flattened inspiratory and expiratory curves (see Figure 9-3, *A*). Tomograms of the trachea demonstrate tracheal narrowing.

MANAGEMENT OF ANESTHESIA

Tracheal dilation is useful in some patients, but surgical resection of the stenotic tracheal segment with primary reanastomosis is often required. Translaryngeal endotracheal intubation is accomplished. After surgical exposure, the distal normal trachea is opened and a sterile cuffed tube is inserted and attached to the anesthetic circuit. Maintenance of anesthesia with volatile anesthetics is useful for ensuring maximum inspired concentrations of oxygen. High-frequency ventilation is helpful in selected patients. Anesthesia for tracheal resection may be facilitated by the addition of helium to the inspired gases. This decreases the density of the gases and may improve flow through the area of tracheal narrowing.

RESTRICTIVE LUNG DISEASE

Restrictive pulmonary diseases include both acute and chronic intrinsic pulmonary disorders as well as extrinsic (extrapulmonary) disorders involving the pleura, chest wall, diaphragm, and neuromuscular function (Table 9-12). Restrictive lung disease is characterized by decreases in all lung volumes, decreased lung compliance, and preservation of expiratory flow rates (Figure 9-6).

Pulmonary Edema

ACUTE INTRINSIC RESTRICTIVE LUNG DISEASE

Pulmonary edema is due to leakage of intravascular fluid into the interstitium of the lungs and into the alveoli. Acute pulmonary edema can be caused by increased capillary pressure (hydrostatic or cardiogenic pulmonary edema) or by increased capillary permeability. Pulmonary edema typically manifests as bilateral symmetrical opacities on chest radiography. A perihilar distribution (butterfly pattern) of the lung opacity is common. However, this pattern of lung opacity is more commonly seen with increased capillary pressure than with increased capillary permeability. The presence of air bronchograms on chest radiography suggests increased-permeability pulmonary edema. Cardiogenic pulmonary edema is characterized by extreme dyspnea, tachypnea, and signs of sympathetic nervous system activation (hypertension, tachycardia, diaphoresis) that may be more pronounced than in patients with increased-permeability pulmonary edema. Pulmonary edema caused by increased capillary permeability is characterized by a high concentration of protein and secretory products in the edema fluid. Diffuse alveolar damage is typically present with the increased-permeability pulmonary edema associated with acute respiratory distress syndrome (ARDS).

TABLE 9-12 ■ Causes of restrictive lung disease

ACUTE INTRINSIC RESTRICTIVE LUNG DISEASE (PULMONARY EDEMA)

Acute respiratory distress syndrome
Aspiration
Neurogenic problems
Opioid overdose
High altitude
Reexpansion of collapsed lung
Upper airway obstruction (negative pressure)
Congestive heart failure

CHRONIC INTRINSIC RESTRICTIVE LUNG DISEASE (INTERSTITIAL LUNG DISEASE)

Sarcoidosis
Hypersensitivity pneumonitis
Eosinophilic granuloma
Alveolar proteinosis
Lymphangioleiomyomatosis
Drug-induced pulmonary fibrosis

DISORDERS OF THE CHEST WALL, PLEURA, AND MEDIASTINUM

Deformities of the costovertebral skeletal structures
   Kyphoscoliosis
   Ankylosing spondylitis
Deformities of the sternum
Flail chest
Pleural effusion
Pneumothorax
Mediastinal mass
Pneumomediastinum
Neuromuscular disorders
   Spinal cord transection
   Guillain-Barré syndrome
   Neuromuscular Transmission
   Muscular dystrophies

OTHER

Obesity
Ascites
Pregnancy

ASPIRATION

Aspirated acidic gastric fluid is rapidly distributed throughout the lung and produces destruction of surfactant-producing cells and damage to the pulmonary capillary endothelium. As a result, there is atelectasis and leakage of intravascular fluid into the lungs, producing capillary permeability pulmonary edema. The clinical picture is similar to that of ARDS. Arterial hypoxemia is typically present. In addition, there may be tachypnea, bronchospasm, and acute pulmonary hypertension. Chest radiographs may not demonstrate evidence of aspiration pneumonitis for 6 to 12 hours after the event. Evidence of aspiration, when it does appear, is most likely to be in the right lower lobe if the patient aspirated while in the supine position.

Measurement of gastric fluid pH is useful since it reflects the pH of the aspirated fluid. Measurement of tracheal aspirate pH is of no value because the aspirated gastric fluid is rapidly diluted by airway secretions. The aspirated gastric fluid is also rapidly distributed to peripheral lung regions, so lung lavage is not useful unless there has been aspiration of particulate material.

Aspiration pneumonitis is best treated by delivery of supplemental oxygen and PEEP. Bronchodilation may be needed to relieve bronchospasm. There is no evidence that prophylactic antibiotics decrease the incidence of pulmonary infection or alter outcome. Corticosteroid treatment of aspiration pneumonitis is controversial. Despite the absence of confirmatory evidence that corticosteroids are beneficial, some practitioners treat aspiration pneumonitis with very large dosages of methylprednisolone or dexamethasone.

NEUROGENIC PROBLEMS

Neurogenic problems develop in a small proportion of patients experiencing acute brain injury. Typically, this form of pulmonary edema occurs minutes to hours after central nervous system injury and may manifest during the perioperative period. There is a massive outpouring of sympathetic impulses from the injured central nervous system that results in generalized

FIGURE 9-6 Lung volumes in restrictive lung disease compared with normal values. *ERV,* Expiratory reserve volume; *FRC,* functional residual capacity; *IC,* inspiratory capacity; *RV,* residual volume; *TLC,* total lung capacity; *VC,* vital capacity; *V_T*, tidal volume.

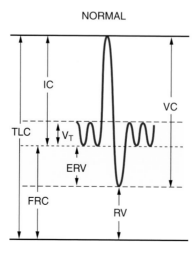
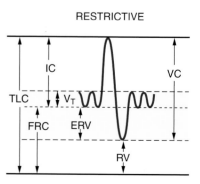

vasoconstriction and a shift of blood volume into the pulmonary circulation. Presumably, increased pulmonary capillary pressure leads to transudation of fluid into the interstitium and alveoli. Pulmonary hypertension and hypervolemia can also injure blood vessels in the lungs.

The association of pulmonary edema with a recent central nervous system injury should suggest the diagnosis of neurogenic pulmonary edema. The principal entity in the differential diagnosis is aspiration pneumonitis. Unlike neurogenic pulmonary edema, chemical pneumonitis resulting from aspiration frequently persists longer and is often complicated by secondary bacterial infection.

OPIOID OVERDOSE

Acute noncardiogenic pulmonary edema can occur after administration of a number of drugs, especially opioids (heroin) and cocaine. High-permeability pulmonary edema is suggested by high protein concentrations in the pulmonary edema fluid. Cocaine can also cause pulmonary vasoconstriction, acute myocardial ischemia, and myocardial infarction. There is no evidence that administration of naloxone speeds resolution of opioid-induced pulmonary edema. Treatment of patients who develop drug-induced pulmonary edema is supportive and may include tracheal intubation for airway protection and mechanical ventilation.

HIGH-ALTITUDE PULMONARY EDEMA

High-altitude pulmonary edema may occur at heights ranging from 2500 to 5000 m and is influenced by the rate of ascent to that altitude. The onset of symptoms is often gradual but typically occurs within 48 to 72 hours at high altitude. Fulminant pulmonary edema may be preceded by the less severe symptoms of acute mountain sickness. The cause of this high-permeability pulmonary edema is presumed to be hypoxic pulmonary vasoconstriction, which increases pulmonary vascular pressures. Treatment includes administration of oxygen and prompt descent from the high altitude. Inhalation of nitric oxide may improve oxygenation.

REEXPANSION OF COLLAPSED LUNG

Rapid expansion of a collapsed lung may lead to pulmonary edema in that lung. The risk of reexpansion pulmonary edema after relief of a pneumothorax or pleural effusion is related to the amount of air or liquid that was present in the pleural space (>1 L increases the risk), the duration of collapse (>24 hours increases the risk), and the rapidity of reexpansion. High protein concentrations in the edema fluid suggest that enhanced capillary membrane permeability is important in the development of this form of pulmonary edema. Treatment of reexpansion pulmonary edema is supportive.

UPPER AIRWAY OBSTRUCTION (NEGATIVE-PRESSURE)

Negative-pressure pulmonary edema may follow relief of acute upper airway obstruction (postobstructive pulmonary edema) caused by postextubation laryngospasm, epiglottitis, tumors, obesity, hiccups, or obstructive sleep apnea in *spontaneously breathing* patients. The time to onset of pulmonary edema after relief of airway obstruction ranges from a few minutes to as long as 2 to 3 hours. Tachypnea, cough, and failure to maintain oxygen saturation above 95% are common presenting signs and may be confused with pulmonary aspiration or pulmonary embolism. It is possible that many cases of postoperative oxygen desaturation are due to unrecognized negative-pressure pulmonary edema.

The pathogenesis of negative-pressure pulmonary edema is related to the development of high negative intrapleural pressure by vigorous inspiratory efforts against an obstructed upper airway. High negative intrapleural pressure decreases the interstitial hydrostatic pressure, increases venous return, and increases left ventricular afterload. In addition, such negative pressure leads to intense sympathetic nervous system activation, hypertension, and central displacement of blood volume. Together these factors produce acute pulmonary edema by increasing the transcapillary pressure gradient.

Maintenance of a patent upper airway and administration of supplemental oxygen are sufficient treatment, because this form of pulmonary edema is typically transient and self-limited. Mechanical ventilation may occasionally be needed for a brief period of time. Hemodynamic monitoring reveals normal right and left ventricular function. Central venous pressure and pulmonary artery occlusion pressure are normal. Radiographic evidence of this form of pulmonary edema resolves within 12 to 24 hours.

MANAGEMENT OF ANESTHESIA

Preoperative

Elective surgery should be delayed in patients with acute pulmonary edema, and every effort must be made to optimize cardiorespiratory function. Large pleural effusions may need to be drained. Persistent hypoxemia may require mechanical ventilation and PEEP. Hemodynamic monitoring may be useful in both the assessment and treatment of pulmonary edema.

Intraoperative

Patients with pulmonary edema are critically ill. Intraoperative management should be a continuation of critical care management and include a plan for intraoperative ventilator management. The best way to ventilate patients with acute respiratory failure and restrictive lung disease has not been determined. However, because the pathophysiology is similar to that of acute lung injury and because there is the risk of hemodynamic compromise and barotrauma with the use of large tidal volumes and high airway pressures, it is reasonable to ventilate with low tidal volumes (e.g., 6 mL/kg) with a compensatory increase in ventilatory rate (14 to 18 breaths per minute) while attempting to keep the end-inspiratory plateau pressure at less than 30 cm H_2O. Typical anesthesia ventilators may not be adequate for patients with severe ARDS, and more sophisticated ICU ventilators may occasionally be needed. Patients with restrictive lung disease typically breathe rapidly and shallowly, so tachypnea is likely during the weaning process and should not be used as the sole reason for delaying extubation if gas exchange and results of other assessments are satisfactory.

Chronic Intrinsic Restrictive Lung Disease (Interstitial Lung Disease)

Interstitial disease is characterized by changes in the intrinsic properties of the lungs, most often caused by pulmonary fibrosis. This produces a chronic restrictive form of lung disease. Pulmonary hypertension and cor pulmonale develop as progressive pulmonary fibrosis results in the loss of pulmonary vasculature. Dyspnea is prominent and breathing is rapid and shallow.

SARCOIDOSIS

Sarcoidosis is a systemic granulomatous disorder that involves many tissues but has a predilection for intrathoracic lymph nodes and the lungs. Most patients have no symptoms at the time of presentation, and the disease is identified only because of abnormal findings on chest radiographs. Patients may have respiratory symptoms such as dyspnea and cough. Ocular sarcoidosis may produce uveitis; myocardial sarcoidosis may produce conduction defects and dysrhythmias. The most common form of neurologic involvement in sarcoidosis is unilateral facial nerve palsy. Endobronchial sarcoid is common. Laryngeal sarcoidosis occurs in up to 5% of patients and may interfere with the passage of adult-size tracheal tubes. Cor pulmonale may develop. Hypercalcemia occurs in fewer than 10% of patients but is a classic manifestation of sarcoidosis.

Mediastinoscopy may be necessary to provide lymph node tissue for the diagnosis of sarcoidosis. Angiotensin-converting enzyme activity is increased in patients with sarcoidosis, presumably due to production of this enzyme by cells within the granuloma. However, this increase in angiotensin-converting enzyme activity does not have useful diagnostic or prognostic significance. Corticosteroids are administered to suppress the manifestations of sarcoidosis and to treat the hypercalcemia.

HYPERSENSITIVITY PNEUMONITIS

Hypersensitivity pneumonitis is characterized by diffuse interstitial granulomatous reactions in the lungs after inhalation of dust containing fungi, spores, and animal or plant material. Signs and symptoms of hypersensitivity pneumonitis include the onset of dyspnea and cough 4 to 6 hours after inhalation of the antigens. This is followed by leukocytosis, eosinophilia, and often arterial hypoxemia. Chest radiographs show multiple pulmonary infiltrates. Repeated episodes of hypersensitivity pneumonitis may lead to pulmonary fibrosis.

EOSINOPHILIC GRANULOMA

Pulmonary fibrosis accompanies the disease process known as *eosinophilic granuloma* (histiocytosis X). No treatment has been shown to be beneficial for this disease.

ALVEOLAR PROTEINOSIS

Pulmonary alveolar proteinosis is a disease of unknown etiology characterized by the deposition of lipid-rich proteinaceous material in the alveoli. Dyspnea and arterial hypoxemia are the typical clinical manifestations. This process may occur independently or in association with chemotherapy, acquired immunodeficiency syndrome, or inhalation of mineral dusts. Although spontaneous remission may occur, treatment of severe cases requires whole-lung lavage to remove alveolar material and improve macrophage function. Lung lavage in patients with hypoxemia may further decrease the level of oxygenation. Airway management during anesthesia for lung lavage includes placement of a double-lumen endobronchial tube to facilitate lavage of each lung and optimize oxygenation during lavage.

LYMPHANGIOLEIOMYOMATOSIS

Lymphangioleiomyomatosis is the proliferation of smooth muscle in airways, lymphatics, and blood vessels that occurs in females of reproductive age. Pulmonary function test results show restrictive and obstructive lung disease with a decrease in diffusing capacity. Lymphangioleiomyomatosis presents clinically as progressive dyspnea, hemoptysis, recurrent pneumothorax, and pleural effusions. Nearly all lymphangioleiomyomatosis cells express progesterone receptors. Progesterone or tamoxifen can be used for treatment, but there is progressive deterioration in pulmonary function, and most patients die within 10 years of the onset of symptoms.

MANAGEMENT OF ANESTHESIA

Preoperative

Patients usually have dyspnea and nonproductive cough. Cor pulmonale may be present. Coarse breath sounds with crepitations are heard on auscultation. A chest radiograph may show a ground glass or nodular pattern. Arterial blood gas analysis reveals hypoxemia with normocarbia. Pulmonary function tests show restrictive ventilatory defects, and carbon monoxide diffusing capacity is decreased. A vital capacity of less than 15 mL/kg indicates severe pulmonary dysfunction. Infection should be treated, secretions cleared, and smoking stopped preoperatively.

Intraoperative

Patients with interstitial lung disease tolerate apneic periods very poorly because of their small FRC and low oxygen stores. General anesthesia, the supine position, and controlled ventilation all contribute to further decreases in FRC. Alterations in FRC and the risk of hypoxia continue into the postoperative period. Uptake of inhaled anesthetics is faster in these patients because of the small FRC. Peak airway pressures should be kept as low as possible to minimize the risk of barotrauma.

Disorders of the Chest Wall, Pleura, and Mediastinum

Chronic extrinsic restrictive lung disease is most often due to disorders of the thoracic cage (chest wall) that interfere with lung expansion (Table 9-12). The lungs are compressed and lung volumes are reduced. The work of breathing is increased because of the abnormal mechanical properties of the chest and the increased airway resistance that results from decreased lung volumes. Any thoracic deformity may cause compression of the pulmonary vasculature and lead to right ventricular dysfunction. Recurrent pulmonary infection resulting from poor cough dynamics may lead to the development of COPD.

DEFORMITIES OF THE COSTOVERTEBRAL SKELETAL STRUCTURES

The two basic types of costovertebral skeletal deformity are scoliosis (lateral curvature with rotation of the vertebral column) and kyphosis (anterior flexion of the vertebral column), which are most commonly present in combination as kyphoscoliosis. Idiopathic kyphoscoliosis accounts for 80% of cases. It commonly begins during late childhood or early adolescence and may progress in severity during the years of rapid skeletal growth. Mild to moderate kyphoscoliosis (scoliotic angle of <60 degrees) is associated with minimal to mild restrictive ventilatory defects. Dyspnea may occur during exercise, but as the skeletal deformity worsens, the vital capacity declines and dyspnea becomes a common complaint with even moderate exertion. Severe deformities (scoliotic angle of >100 degrees) may lead to chronic alveolar hypoventilation, hypoxemia, secondary erythrocytosis, pulmonary hypertension, and cor pulmonale. Respiratory failure is most likely in patients with kyphoscoliosis associated with a vital capacity of less than 45% of the predicted value and a scoliotic angle of more than 110 degrees. Compression of underlying lung tissue results in an increased alveolar-arterial oxygen difference. Patients with severe kyphoscoliosis are at increased risk of developing pneumonia and hypoventilation when exposed to central nervous system depressant drugs. Supplemental oxygen therapy augmented by nocturnal ventilatory support may be useful.

DEFORMITIES OF THE STERNUM

Deformities of the sternum and costochondral articulations are characterized by pectus excavatum (inward concavity of the lower sternum) and pectus carinatum (outward protuberance of the upper, middle, or lower sternum). In most patients with pectus excavatum, there are no significant functional limitations. Lung volumes and cardiovascular function are preserved. Surgical correction is indicated when the sternal deformity is accompanied by evidence of pulmonary restriction or cardiovascular dysfunction.

FLAIL CHEST

Multiple rib fractures, especially when they occur in a parallel vertical orientation, can produce a flail chest characterized by paradoxical inward movement of the unstable portion of the thoracic cage while the remainder of the thoracic cage moves outward during inspiration. The flail portion of the chest then moves outward with exhalation. The pathophysiology of a flail chest can also result from dehiscence of a median sternotomy. Tidal volumes are diminished because the region of the lung associated with the chest wall abnormality paradoxically increases its volume during exhalation and deflates during

inspiration. The result is progressive hypoxemia and alveolar hypoventilation. Treatment of a flail chest includes positive pressure ventilation until a definitive stabilization procedure can be carried out or the rib fractures are stabilized.

PLEURAL EFFUSION

Pleural effusion is most often confirmed by chest radiography when blunting of the costophrenic angle is seen with as little as 25 to 50 mL of pleural fluid. Larger amounts of fluid produce a characteristic homogeneous opacity that forms a concave meniscus with the chest wall. Ultrasonography and CT are also useful in evaluating a pleural effusion. In patients with congestive heart failure, pleural fluid may collect in the interlobular fissure as an interlobular effusion. Various types of fluid may accumulate in the pleural space, including blood (hemothorax), pus (empyema), lipids (chylothorax), and serous liquid (hydrothorax). All these conditions have an identical radiographic appearance.

Pleural effusion is diagnosed and treated by thoracentesis. The pleural fluid can be either transudative or exudative, and the distinction points to potential diagnoses and the need for further evaluation. Bloody pleural effusion is common in patients with malignant disease, trauma, or pulmonary infarction.

PNEUMOTHORAX

Pneumothorax is the presence of gas in the pleural space caused by disruption of either the parietal pleura (external penetrating injury) or visceral pleura (tear or rupture in the lung parenchyma). When the gas originates in the lung, the rupture may occur in the absence of known lung disease (simple pneumothorax) or as a result of parenchymal disease (secondary pneumothorax). Idiopathic spontaneous pneumothorax occurs most often in tall, thin males 20 to 40 years of age and is due to rupture of apical subpleural blebs. Smoking cigarettes increases the risk of primary spontaneous pneumothorax 20-fold. Most episodes of spontaneous pneumothorax occur while patients are at rest. Exercise or airline travel does not increase the likelihood of spontaneous pneumothorax.

MEDIASTINAL MASS

In the evaluation of mediastinal widening, contrast-enhanced CT can distinguish between vascular structures, soft tissues, and calcifications. Lymphoma, thymoma, teratoma, and retrosternal goiter are common causes of an anterior mediastinal mass. Large mediastinal tumors may be associated with progressive airway obstruction, loss of lung volumes, pulmonary artery or cardiac compression, and superior vena cava obstruction.

Superior vena cava syndrome is a constellation of signs that develops in patients with a mediastinal tumor that obstructs venous drainage in the upper thorax. Increased venous pressure leads to (1) dilation of collateral veins in the thorax and neck; (2) edema and cyanosis of the face, neck, and upper chest; (3) edema of the conjunctiva; and (4) evidence of increased intracranial pressure, including headache and altered mental status. Dyspnea is common. Cancer accounts for nearly all cases of superior vena cava syndrome.

MEDIASTINITIS

Acute mediastinitis usually results from bacterial contamination after esophageal perforation. Symptoms include chest pain and fever. It is treated with broad-spectrum antibiotics and surgical drainage.

PNEUMOMEDIASTINUM

Pneumomediastinum may follow a tear in the esophagus or tracheobronchial tree or alveolar rupture, although it most often occurs without a known cause. Spontaneous pneumomediastinum has been observed after recreational cocaine use. Symptoms of retrosternal chest pain and dyspnea are typically abrupt in onset and usually follow exaggerated breathing efforts (cough, emesis, Valsalva's maneuver). Subcutaneous emphysema may be extensive in the neck, arms, abdomen, and scrotum. Gas in the mediastinum may decompress into the pleural space leading to pneumothorax, usually on the left. The diagnosis of pneumomediastinum is established by chest radiography. Spontaneous pneumomediastinum resolves without specific therapy. When pneumomediastinum is a result of organ rupture, surgical drainage and repair may be necessary.

BRONCHOGENIC CYSTS

Bronchogenic cysts are fluid- or air-filled cysts arising from the primitive foregut that are lined with respiratory epithelium. They are usually located in the mediastinum or in the lung parenchyma. These cysts may be asymptomatic, the focus of recurrent pulmonary infection, or the cause of life-threatening airway obstruction. Cysts located in the mediastinum are more likely to be filled with fluid than air and are usually not in direct communication with the airways. These masses cause symptoms of airway compression as they grow. Surgical excision may be necessary.

Theoretical concerns in patients with bronchogenic cysts include the hazards related to nitrous oxide administration and the use of positive pressure ventilation. Nitrous oxide can diffuse into air-filled bronchogenic cysts and cause their expansion, with associated life-threatening respiratory or cardiovascular compromise. Institution of positive pressure ventilation may have a ball-valve effect, particularly in cysts that extrinsically compress the tracheobronchial tree, resulting in air trapping. Despite these concerns, clinical experience confirms that nitrous oxide and positive pressure ventilation often may be safely used in patients with bronchogenic cysts.

NEUROMUSCULAR DISORDERS

Neuromuscular disorders that interfere with the transfer of central nervous system input to the skeletal muscles necessary for inspiration and exhalation can result in restrictive lung disease. Abnormalities of the spinal cord, peripheral nerves, neuromuscular junction, or skeletal muscles may result in restrictive pulmonary defects characterized by an inability to generate normal respiratory pressures. In contrast to the mechanical disorders of the thoracic cage, in which an effective cough is typically preserved, the expiratory muscle weakness characteristic of neuromuscular disorders prevents generation of sufficient expiratory airflow velocity to provide a forceful cough. The extreme example is cervical spinal cord injury in which paralysis of abdominal and intercostal muscles severely decreases the ability to cough. Acute respiratory failure is likely when atelectasis associated with pneumonia (caused by retained secretions resulting from an ineffective cough) occurs or depressant drugs are administered. Patients with neuromuscular disorders are somewhat dependent on the state of wakefulness to maintain adequate ventilation. During sleep, hypoxemia and hypercapnia may develop and contribute to the development of cor pulmonale. Vital capacity is an important indicator of the total impact of a neuromuscular disorder on ventilation.

Spinal Cord Transection

Breathing is maintained solely or predominantly by the diaphragm in quadriplegic patients (transection must be at or below C4 or the diaphragm is paralyzed). Because the diaphragm is active only during inspiration, cough—which requires activity by expiratory muscles, including those of the abdominal wall—is almost totally absent. Intercostal muscles are required to stabilize the upper rib cage against inward collapse when negative intrathoracic pressure is produced by descent of the diaphragm. With diaphragmatic breathing, there is a paradoxical inward motion of the upper thorax during inspiration. The result is a diminished tidal volume. When quadriplegic patients are placed in the upright position, the weight of the abdominal contents pulls on the diaphragm, and the absence of abdominal muscle tone results in less efficient function of the diaphragm. Abdominal binders serve to replace lost abdominal muscle tone and may be useful whenever tidal volume decreases in the upright posture. Quadriplegic patients have mild degrees of bronchial constriction caused by the parasympathetic tone that is unopposed by sympathetic activity from the spinal cord. Use of anticholinergic bronchodilating drugs can reverse this abnormality. Respiratory failure almost never occurs in quadriplegic patients in the absence of complications such as pneumonia.

Guillain-Barré Syndrome

Respiratory insufficiency that requires mechanical ventilation occurs in 20% to 25% of patients with Guillain-Barré syndrome. Ventilatory support is needed, on average, for 2 months. A small number of patients have persistent skeletal muscle weakness and are susceptible to recurring episodes of respiratory failure in association with pulmonary infection.

Disorders of Neuromuscular Transmission

Myasthenia gravis is the most common of the disorders affecting neuromuscular transmission that may result in respiratory failure. Myasthenic syndrome (Eaton-Lambert syndrome) may be confused with myasthenia gravis. Prolonged skeletal muscle paralysis or weakness may occur following administration of nondepolarizing neuromuscular blocking drugs.

Muscular Dystrophy

Patients with pseudohypertrophic (Duchenne's) muscular dystrophy, myotonic dystrophy, and other forms of muscular dystrophy are predisposed to pulmonary complications and respiratory failure. Chronic alveolar hypoventilation caused by inspiratory muscle weakness may develop. Expiratory muscle weakness impairs cough, and accompanying weakness of the swallowing muscles may lead to pulmonary aspiration of gastric contents. As with all neuromuscular syndromes, central nervous system depressant drugs should be avoided or administered in minimal dosages when necessary. Nocturnal ventilation with noninvasive techniques such as nasal intermittent positive pressure or external negative pressure ventilation may be useful.

DIAPHRAGMATIC PARALYSIS

In the absence of respiratory complications, neuromuscular disorders rarely progress to the point of hypercapnic respiratory failure unless diaphragmatic weakness or paralysis is present. Thus, quadriplegic patients who have preserved phrenic nerve and diaphragmatic function are unlikely to develop respiratory failure in the absence of pneumonia or administration of central nervous system depressant drugs. In the supine position, patients with diaphragmatic paralysis may develop a ventilatory pattern similar to that seen with a flail chest (abdominal contents push the diaphragm into the chest). In the upright posture these patients experience a significant increase in vital capacity and improved oxygenation and ventilation. Most cases of unilateral diaphragmatic paralysis are the result of neoplastic invasion of the phrenic nerve. In the absence of associated pleuropulmonary disease, most adult patients with unilateral diaphragmatic paralysis remain asymptomatic, and the defect is detected as an incidental finding on chest radiography. In contrast, infants are more dependent on bilateral diaphragmatic function for adequate respiratory function. In these patients and in symptomatic adults, plication of the hemidiaphragm may be necessary to prevent flail motion of the thoracic cage.

Transient diaphragmatic dysfunction may occur after abdominal surgery. Lung volumes are decreased, the alveolar-arterial oxygen difference increases, and respiratory frequency increases. These changes may be caused by irritation of the diaphragm, which causes reflex inhibition of phrenic nerve activity. As a result of postoperative diaphragmatic dysfunction, atelectasis and arterial hypoxemia may occur. Incentive spirometry may alleviate these abnormalities.

DISORDERS OF THE PLEURA AND MEDIASTINUM

Disorders of the pleura and mediastinum may contribute to mechanical changes that interfere with optimal lung expansion.

Pleural Fibrosis

Pleural fibrosis may follow hemothorax, empyema, or surgical pleurodesis for the treatment of recurrent pneumothorax. Despite obliteration of the pleural space, functional restrictive lung abnormalities remain but are usually minor. Surgical decortication to remove thick fibrous pleura is technically difficult and is considered only if the restrictive lung disease is symptomatic.

TENSION PNEUMOTHORAX

Tension pneumothorax develops when gas enters the pleural space during inspiration and is prevented from escaping during exhalation. The result is a progressive increase in the amount of air trapped under increasing pressure (tension). Tension pneumothorax occurs in fewer than 2% of patients experiencing an idiopathic spontaneous pneumothorax, but it is a common manifestation of rib fractures, insertion of central lines, and barotrauma in patients undergoing mechanical ventilation. Dyspnea, hypoxemia, and hypotension may be severe. Immediate evacuation of gas through a needle or a small-bore catheter placed into the second anterior intercostal space may be lifesaving.

Signs and Symptoms. Dyspnea is always present with a pneumothorax. Most patients also have ipsilateral chest pain and cough. Arterial hypoxemia, hypotension, and hypercarbia may occur. Physical findings are often subtle, which emphasizes the importance of considering this diagnosis whenever dyspnea and chest pain occur acutely. Tachycardia is the most common physical finding. In patients with a large pneumothorax, the findings on physical examination of the affected side may include decreased chest wall movement, hyperresonance to percussion, and decreased or absent breath sounds.

Treatment. Treatment of a symptomatic pneumothorax requires evacuation of air from the pleural space by aspiration through a small-bore plastic catheter or placement of a chest tube. Aspiration of a pneumothorax followed by catheter removal is successful in 70% of patients with a small to moderate-sized primary spontaneous pneumothorax. When the pneumothorax is small (<15% of the volume of the hemithorax) and symptoms are absent, observation may suffice. Oxygen supplementation accelerates the reabsorption of air in the pleural space. A continued air leak from the lung requires chest tube placement. Most air leaks resolve within 7 days. Complications of chest tube drainage include pain, pleural infection, hemorrhage, and pulmonary edema related to lung reexpansion. Recurrent pneumothoraces may require surgical intervention including chemical pleurodesis.

MANAGEMENT OF ANESTHESIA

Preoperative

Preoperative evaluation of patients with mediastinal tumors includes chest radiography, measurement of a flow-volume loop, chest imaging studies, and clinical evaluation for evidence of tracheobronchial compression. The size of the mediastinal mass and the degree of tracheal compression can be established by CT, and this study is a useful predictor of whether airway difficulties during anesthesia are to be expected. Flexible fiberoptic bronchoscopy under topical anesthesia may also be useful for evaluating airway obstruction. Interestingly, the severity of preoperative pulmonary symptoms bears no relationship to the degree of respiratory compromise that can be encountered during anesthesia. Indeed, a number of asymptomatic patients have developed unexpected airway obstruction during anesthesia. Preoperative radiation therapy should be considered whenever possible. In symptomatic patients requiring a diagnostic tissue biopsy, a local anesthetic technique, if feasible, is best. Patients with mediastinal tumors may be asymptomatic while awake yet develop airway obstruction during anesthesia in the supine position. During anesthesia, the tumor may increase in size because of venous engorgement, and its position may shift somewhat. As a result, it may compress the airway, the vena cava, the pulmonary artery, or the atria and create life-threatening hypoxemia, hypotension, or even cardiac arrest.

Intraoperative

Restrictive lung disease does not influence the choice of drugs used for induction or maintenance of anesthesia. Drugs with prolonged respiratory-depressant effects that may persist into the postoperative period should be avoided. A high index of suspicion for the presence of a pneumothorax and the need to avoid or discontinue nitrous oxide must be maintained. Regional anesthesia can be considered for peripheral operations, but it must be appreciated that involvement of sensory levels above T10 can be associated with impairment of the respiratory muscle activity needed by patients with restrictive lung disease to maintain acceptable ventilation. Mechanical ventilation during the intraoperative period facilitates optimal oxygenation and ventilation. Since the lungs are poorly compliant, increased inspiratory pressures may be necessary. Postoperative mechanical ventilation is often required in patients with significantly impaired pulmonary function. Restrictive lung disease contributes to the risk of postoperative pulmonary complications.

The method of induction of anesthesia and tracheal intubation in the presence of mediastinal tumors depends on the preoperative assessment of the airway. External edema associated with superior vena cava syndrome may be accompanied by similar edema inside the mouth and hypopharynx. If edema resulting from caval obstruction is severe, it may be necessary to establish intravenous access in the legs rather than in the arms. A central venous or pulmonary artery catheter can be inserted through the femoral vein. Invasive blood pressure monitoring should be considered. Symptomatic patients may need to be in the sitting position to breathe adequately. If so, anesthetic induction in this position may proceed after the airway has been secured. Topical anesthesia of the airway with or without sedation can be used to facilitate fiberoptic laryngoscopy. In very young patients, an inhalation induction with maintenance of spontaneous ventilation may be necessary. If severe airway obstruction occurs, it can be alleviated

by placing the patient in the lateral or prone position. Spontaneous ventilation throughout surgery is recommended whenever possible. Worsening of superior vena cava syndrome may occur as a result of generous intraoperative fluid replacement. Diuretics may decrease the tumor volume, but the reduction in preload in these patients with already compromised venous return may result in significant hypotension. Surgical bleeding is often increased due to an increased central venous pressure.

Postoperative

Postoperatively, tumor swelling as a result of partial resection or biopsy may increase airway obstruction and require reintubation of the trachea.

DIAGNOSTIC PROCEDURES IN PATIENTS WITH LUNG DISEASE

Fiberoptic bronchoscopy has generally replaced rigid bronchoscopy for visualizing the airways and obtaining samples for culture, cytologic examination, and biopsy. Pneumothorax occurs in 5% to 10% of patients after transbronchial lung biopsy and in 10% to 20% of patients after percutaneous needle biopsy of peripheral lung lesions. The principal contraindication to pleural biopsy is a coagulopathy.

Mediastinoscopy is performed under general anesthesia through a small transverse incision just above the suprasternal notch. Blunt dissection along the pretracheal fascia is performed, which permits biopsy of paratracheal lymph nodes to the level of the carina. Complications include pneumothorax, mediastinal hemorrhage, venous air embolism, and injury to the recurrent laryngeal nerve leading to hoarseness and vocal cord paralysis. The mediastinoscope can also exert pressure against the right innominate artery, causing loss of pulses in the right arm and compromise of right carotid artery blood flow.

RESPIRATORY FAILURE

Acute Respiratory Failure

Respiratory failure is the inability to provide adequate arterial oxygenation and/or elimination of carbon dioxide.

DIAGNOSIS

Acute respiratory failure is considered to be present when the Pao_2 is less than 60 mm Hg despite oxygen supplementation and in the absence of a right-to-left intracardiac shunt. In the presence of acute respiratory failure, $Paco_2$ can be increased, unchanged, or decreased depending on the relationship of alveolar ventilation to metabolic production of carbon dioxide. A $Paco_2$ higher than 50 mm Hg in the absence of respiratory compensation for metabolic alkalosis is consistent with the diagnosis of acute respiratory failure.

Acute respiratory failure is distinguished from chronic respiratory failure based on the relationship of $Paco_2$ to pHa. Acute respiratory failure is typically accompanied by abrupt increases in $Paco_2$ and by corresponding decreases in pHa.

In the presence of chronic respiratory failure, pHa is usually between 7.35 and 7.45 despite an increased $Paco_2$. This normal pHa reflects renal compensation for the respiratory acidosis via renal tubular reabsorption of bicarbonate.

Respiratory failure is often accompanied by a decrease in FRC and lung compliance. Increased pulmonary vascular resistance and pulmonary hypertension are likely to develop if respiratory failure persists.

Acute/Adult Respiratory Distress Syndrome (ARDS)

ARDS is caused by an inflammatory injury to the lung and is manifested clinically as acute hypoxemic respiratory failure.

EPIDEMIOLOGY AND PATHOGENESIS

Clinical disorders and risk factors associated with the development of ARDS include events that cause direct lung injury as well as those that lead to indirect injury to the lungs in the setting of a systemic process (Table 9-13). Overall, sepsis is associated with the highest risk of progression of acute lung injury to ARDS. The acute phase of ARDS manifests as the rapid onset of respiratory failure accompanied by arterial hypoxemia refractory to treatment and radiographic findings indistinguishable from those of cardiogenic pulmonary edema. There is an influx of protein-rich edema fluid into the alveoli as a result of increased alveolar capillary membrane permeability. There is evidence of neutrophil-mediated lung injury. Proinflammatory cytokines may be produced locally in the lungs. This acute phase usually resolves completely, but in some patients, it may progress to fibrosing alveolitis with persistent arterial hypoxemia and decreased pulmonary compliance. The recovery or resolution phase of ARDS is characterized by gradual resolution of the hypoxemia and improved lung compliance. Typically, the radiographic abnormalities resolve completely.

SIGNS AND SYMPTOMS

Arterial hypoxemia resistant to treatment with supplemental oxygen is usually the first sign. Radiographic signs may appear before symptoms develop. Patients usually have a normal pulmonary capillary wedge pressure. Pulmonary hypertension can occur due to pulmonary artery vasoconstriction and obliteration of portions of the pulmonary capillary bed and, when severe, can cause right-sided heart failure. Death from ARDS is most often a result of sepsis or multiple organ failure rather than respiratory failure, although some deaths can be directly related to lung injury.

DIAGNOSIS

The diagnosis of ARDS is dependent on the presentation of acute refractory hypoxemia, diffuse infiltrates on chest radiograph consistent with pulmonary edema, and a pulmonary capillary wedge pressure of less than 18 mm Hg. The Pao_2/Fio_2 ratio is typically less than 200 mm Hg. A less severe form of ARDS is acute lung injury, which has a similar presentation, but the Pao_2/Fio_2 ratio is less than 300 mm Hg. An algorithm for clinical differentiation of cardiogenic and noncardiogenic pulmonary edema is shown in Figure 9-7.

TREATMENT

Treatment of acute respiratory failure is directed at initiating specific therapies that support oxygenation and ventilation. The three principal goals in the management of acute respiratory failure are (1) correcting hypoxemia, (2) removing excess carbon dioxide, and (3) securing a patent upper airway.

Improved supportive care of patients with acute lung injury and ARDS may contribute to improved survival rates (Table 9-14). There should be a thorough search for the underlying cause, with particular attention paid to the possibility of a treatable infection such as sepsis or pneumonia. Prevention or early treatment of nosocomial infection is critical. Adequate nutrition should be provided, preferably through the use of enteral feedings. Prevention of gastrointestinal bleeding and thromboembolism is important. At the present time, routine use of surfactant therapy or inhaled nitric oxide is not recommended. However, in the future, strategies that hasten

TABLE 9-13	Clinical disorders associated with acute lung injury and acute respiratory distress syndrome

DIRECT LUNG INJURY

Pneumonia
Aspiration of gastric contents
Pulmonary contusion
Fat emboli
Near drowning
Inhalational injury

INDIRECT LUNG INJURY

Sepsis
Trauma associated with shock
Multiple blood transfusions
Cardiopulmonary bypass
Drug overdose
Acute pancreatitis

TABLE 9-14	Treatment of acute respiratory failure

Oxygen supplementation
Tracheal intubation
Mechanical ventilation
Positive end-expiratory pressure
Optimization of intravascular fluid volume
Diuretic therapy
Inotropic support
Glucocorticoid therapy (?)
Removal of secretions
Control of infection
Nutritional support
Administration of inhaled β-adrenergic agonists

?, Questionable efficacy.

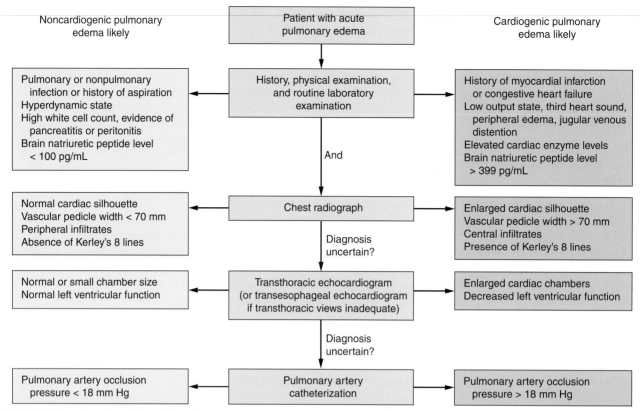

FIGURE 9-7 Algorithm for clinical differentiation between cardiogenic and noncardiogenic pulmonary edema. *(Adapted from Ware LB, Matthay MA. Acute pulmonary edema.* N Engl J Med. *2005;353:2788-2796. Copyright Massachusetts Medical Society, 2005.)*

the resolution phase of ARDS, including the ability to remove alveolar fluid and sustain improvements in oxygenation, may become as important as traditional ventilatory management. Inhaled β-agonists may be of value in removal of pulmonary edema fluid, stimulating the secretion of surfactant and even exerting antiinflammatory effects that may help restore the proper vascular permeability to the lungs.

Tracheal Intubation and PEEP Therapy

The initial steps in the treatment of patients with acute respiratory failure and ARDS who cannot be adequately oxygenated are endotracheal intubation and mechanical ventilation. Inspired oxygen concentrations are adjusted to maintain the Pa_{O_2} between 60 and 80 mm Hg. The higher tidal volumes (12 to 15 mL/kg) used in the past for treatment of ARDS are associated with decreased pulmonary compliance and can result in alveolar overdistention and barotrauma. The risk of barotrauma can be lessened by adjustment of tidal volumes so that increases in peak airway pressure do not exceed 35 to 40 cm H_2O. Ideal tidal volume is determined by assessing lung mechanics rather than by measuring arterial blood gases.

Application of PEEP is one of the most effective ways to improve oxygenation in patients with ARDS. PEEP helps prevent alveolar collapse at end expiration and thereby increases lung volumes (especially FRC), improves ventilation/perfusion matching, and decreases the magnitude of right-to-left intrapulmonary shunting. PEEP does not decrease the

amount of extravascular lung water or prevent the formation of pulmonary edema fluid. However, edema fluid is likely to be redistributed to the interstitial lung regions, which causes previously flooded alveoli to become ventilated.

Application of PEEP is indicated when high concentrations of inspired oxygen ($FI_{O_2} > 0.5$) are needed for prolonged periods to maintain an acceptable Pa_{O_2} and may introduce the risk of oxygen toxicity. It is possible that PEEP may decrease the shear stress associated with the opening and closing of alveoli in ARDS. The lowest level of PEEP necessary to achieve acceptable oxygenation at nontoxic oxygen concentrations should be employed. High levels of PEEP decrease cardiac output and increase the incidence of barotrauma. The level of PEEP that results in optimal pulmonary compliance is usually similar to the level associated with optimal oxygenation. PEEP is typically added in increments of 2.5- to 5.0-cm H_2O until the Pa_{O_2} is at least 60 mm Hg with an FI_{O_2} of less than 0.5. Most patients show maximal improvement in oxygen transport and pulmonary compliance with levels of PEEP below 15 cm H_2O. Excessive levels of PEEP can decrease the Pa_{O_2} by overdistending alveoli and compressing the capillaries surrounding these alveoli, and shunting more blood to less ventilated areas.

An important adverse effect of PEEP is decreased cardiac output resulting from interference with venous return and leftward displacement of the interventricular septum, which restricts left ventricular filling. The decrease in cardiac output caused by PEEP is exaggerated in the presence of hypovolemia.

Replacement of intravascular fluid volume and administration of inotropic drugs may offset the effects of PEEP on venous return and improve myocardial contractility. A pulmonary artery catheter is useful for monitoring the adequacy of intravascular fluid replacement, myocardial contractility, and tissue oxygenation in patients being treated with PEEP. Measurement of pulmonary artery occlusion pressures may be complicated by transmission of PEEP (intraalveolar pressure) to the pulmonary capillaries, which causes an erroneous interpretation of pulmonary artery occlusion pressure.

Inverse-ratio ventilation is characterized by an inspiratory time that exceeds the expiratory time; that is, the inspiratory/expiratory ratio is greater than 1. This is accomplished by adding an end-inspiratory pause to maintain the alveolar pressure briefly at the plateau level. Arterial oxygenation may be improved without increasing minute ventilation or PEEP. Risks of inverse-ratio ventilation include barotrauma and hypotension caused by development of auto-PEEP as a result of the shortened expiratory time. Although inverse-ratio ventilation may improve oxygenation in some patients with ARDS, prospective studies have not confirmed a benefit in most patients.

Fluid and Hemodynamic Management

The rationale for restricting fluids in patients with acute lung injury and ARDS is to decrease the magnitude of the pulmonary edema. Pulmonary artery occlusion pressures below 15 mm Hg may reflect inadequate intravascular fluid volume. Urine outputs of 0.5 to 1.0 mL/kg/hr are consistent with an adequate cardiac output and intravascular fluid volume. Diuresis using furosemide may be effective in reversing some effects of excessive fluid administration as evidenced by improved oxygenation and resolution of pulmonary infiltrates. Measurement of central venous pressure is not a reliable guide for monitoring intravascular fluid volume in patients with ARDS.

A reasonable goal of fluid therapy is to maintain the intravascular fluid volume at the lowest level consistent with adequate organ perfusion as assessed by metabolic acid-base balance and renal function. If organ perfusion cannot be maintained after restoration of intravascular fluid volume, as in patients with septic shock, treatment with vasopressors may be necessary to improve organ perfusion pressures and normalize tissue oxygen delivery.

Corticosteroids

Despite the recognized role of inflammation in acute lung injury and ARDS, the value of corticosteroid administration early in the course of the disease remains unproven. Corticosteroids may have value in treatment of the later fibrosing alveolitis phase of ARDS or as rescue therapy in patients with severe ARDS that is not resolving.

Removal of Secretions

Optimal removal of airway secretions is facilitated by adequate hydration and humidification of inspired gases. Tracheal suctioning, chest physiotherapy, and postural drainage may also enhance secretion removal. Fiberoptic bronchoscopy may be indicated to remove thicker accumulated secretions that are contributing to atelectasis.

Control of Infection

Control of infection using specific antibiotic therapy based on sputum culture and sensitivity testing is a valuable adjunct in the management of ARDS. However, the use of prophylactic antibiotics is not recommended because this practice leads to overgrowth with resistant organisms. Not uncommonly, the earliest evidence of infection in patients with ARDS is a further deterioration in pulmonary function.

Nutritional Support

Nutritional support is important to prevent skeletal muscle weakness. Hypophosphatemia may contribute to skeletal muscle weakness and to the poor contractility of the diaphragm that may accompany acute respiratory failure and ARDS. Increased carbohydrate intake, such as that associated with hyperalimentation, increases the respiratory quotient and thereby increases the production of carbon dioxide, which necessitates greater alveolar ventilation. In the severely compromised patient, meeting this need for greater ventilation might not be possible without mechanical support of ventilation.

Mechanical Support of Ventilation

Supplemental oxygen can be provided to spontaneously breathing patients using a nasal cannula, Venturi mask, nonrebreathing mask, or T-piece. These devices seldom provide inspired oxygen concentrations higher than 50% and therefore are of value only in correcting the hypoxemia resulting from mild to moderate ventilation/perfusion mismatching. When these methods of oxygen delivery fail to maintain the Pao_2 above 60 mm Hg, continuous positive airway pressure by face mask can be tried. Continuous positive airway pressure may increase lung volumes by opening collapsed alveoli and decreasing right-to-left intrapulmonary shunting. A disadvantage of continuous positive airway pressure by face mask is that the tight mask fit required may increase the risk of aspiration should the patient vomit. Maintenance of the Pao_2 above approximately 60 mm Hg is adequate because hemoglobin saturation with oxygen is >90% at this level. In some patients, it is necessary to perform tracheal intubation and institute mechanical ventilation to maintain acceptable oxygenation and ventilation. Typical devices that provide positive pressure ventilation include volume-cycled and pressure-cycled ventilators.

Volume-Cycled Ventilation. Volume-cycled ventilation provides a fixed tidal volume, and inflation pressure is the dependent variable. A pressure limit can be set, and when inflation pressure exceeds this value, a pressure relief valve prevents further gas flow. This valve prevents the development of dangerously high peak airway and alveolar pressures and warns that a change in pulmonary compliance has occurred. Large increases in peak airway pressure may reflect worsening pulmonary edema, development of a pneumothorax, kinking of the tracheal tube, or the presence of mucus plugs in the tube or large airways. Tidal volume is maintained despite small changes in peak airway pressure. This is in contrast to pressure-cycled ventilation. A disadvantage of volume-cycled ventilation is the inability of these devices to compensate for leaks in the delivery system. The primary modalities of ventilation using volume-cycled ventilation are assist-control ventilation and synchronized intermittent mandatory ventilation (Figure 9-8).

ASSIST-CONTROL VENTILATION. In the control mode, a preset respiratory rate ensures that a patient receives a predetermined number of mechanically delivered breaths even if there are no inspiratory efforts. In the assist mode, however, if

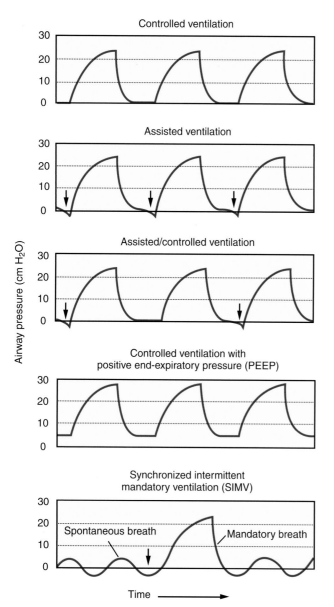

the patient can create some negative airway pressure, a breath at the preset tidal volume will be delivered.

SYNCHRONIZED INTERMITTENT MANDATORY VENTILATION. The synchronized intermittent mandatory ventilation (SIMV) technique allows patients to breathe spontaneously at any rate and tidal volume while a defined minute ventilation is provided by the ventilator. The gas delivery circuit is modified to provide sufficient gas flow for spontaneous breathing and to permit periodic mandatory breaths that are synchronous with the patient's inspiratory efforts. Theoretical advantages of SIMV compared with assist-control ventilation include continued use of respiratory muscles, lower mean airway and mean intrathoracic pressure, prevention of respiratory alkalosis, and improved patient-ventilator coordination.

Pressure-Cycled Ventilation. Pressure-cycled ventilation provides gas flow into the lungs until a preset airway pressure is reached. Tidal volume is the dependent variable. Tidal volume varies with changes in lung compliance and airway resistance.

Management of Patients Receiving Mechanical Support of Ventilation. Critically ill patients who require mechanical ventilation may benefit from continuous infusion of sedative drugs to treat anxiety and agitation and to facilitate coordination with ventilator-delivered breaths. Inadequate sedation or agitation can lead to life-threatening problems such as self-extubation, acute deterioration in gas exchange, and barotrauma. The need for neuromuscular blockade is reduced by the optimum use of sedation. However, when acceptable sedation without hemodynamic compromise cannot be achieved, it may be necessary to produce skeletal muscle paralysis to ensure appropriate ventilation and oxygenation.

SEDATION. Benzodiazepines, propofol, and narcotics are the drugs most commonly administered to decrease anxiety, produce amnesia, increase patient comfort, and provide analgesia during mechanical ventilation. Newer approaches to mechanical ventilation involving the use of permissive hypercapnia ($Paco_2$ may reach 50 mm Hg) can cause substantial discomfort and necessitate deep sedation. Continuous infusion of drugs rather than intermittent injection provides a more constant and desirable level of sedative effect. Daily interruption of sedative infusions to allow the patient to "awaken" may facilitate evaluation of mental status and ultimately shorten the period of mechanical ventilation. Continuous infusion of propofol is uniquely attractive for this purpose, because the brief context-sensitive half-life of this drug is not influenced by the duration of the infusion, and rapid awakening is predictable. Prompt recovery from the effects of a remifentanil infusion also is not affected by the duration of the intravenous drug infusion.

PARALYSIS. When sedation is inadequate or hypotension accompanies the administration of drugs used for sedation, the use of nondepolarizing neuromuscular blocking drugs to produce skeletal muscle relaxation may be necessary to permit optimal mechanical ventilation. The dependence of

FIGURE 9-8 Tidal volume and airway pressures produced by various modes of ventilation delivered through an endotracheal tube. Arrows indicate initiation of a spontaneous breath by the patient, who triggers the ventilator to deliver a mechanically assisted breath.

certain of these drugs on renal clearance should be considered. It is better to use intermittent rather than continuous skeletal muscle paralysis to allow periodic assessment of the adequacy of sedation and the need for ongoing paralysis. Monitoring of neuromuscular blockade and titration of muscle relaxant doses so that a twitch response remains present is prudent. A risk of prolonged drug-induced skeletal muscle paralysis is accentuation of the diffuse polyneuropathy that may accompany critical illness.

COMPLICATIONS

Infection

In mechanically ventilated patients with acute respiratory failure, tracheal intubation is the single most important predisposing factor for development of nosocomial pneumonia (ventilator-associated pneumonia). The major pathogenic mechanism is microaspiration of contaminated secretions around the tracheal tube cuff. Diagnosis of pneumonia in the presence of acute respiratory failure may be difficult, since fever and pulmonary infiltrates may already be present in association with the cause of the acute respiratory failure.

Nosocomial sinusitis is strongly related to the presence of a nasotracheal tube. Treatment of nosocomial sinusitis includes administration of antibiotics, replacement of nasal tubes with oral tubes, and use of decongestants and head elevation to facilitate sinus drainage.

Alveolar Overdistention

Alveolar overdistention resulting from large tidal volumes (10 to 12 mL/kg) and high airway pressures (>50 cm H_2O) may result in alveolar rupture and alveolar hemorrhage. In the presence of acute lung injury and ARDS, a ventilator-delivered breath preferentially follows the path of least resistance and travels to better-aerated regions of the lungs, which puts the alveoli there at risk of overdistention. These alveoli may collapse and reopen repeatedly, and this could be responsible for ventilator-induced lung injury. A gentler form of mechanical ventilation using tidal volumes of 5 to 8 mL/kg and airway pressures not exceeding 30 cm H_2O may be indicated for treating acute respiratory failure and ARDS. However, use of this form of ventilation may require acceptance of some degree of hypercarbia and respiratory acidosis and often a Pao_2 of less than 60 mm Hg.

Permissive hypercapnia or controlled hypoventilation may accompany the reduction in tidal volume and airway pressure designed to minimize or prevent alveolar overdistention. The increased respiratory drive associated with permissive hypercapnia causes discomfort, which makes deep sedation, skeletal muscle paralysis, or both necessary. Permissive hypercapnia is not recommended in patients with increased intracranial pressure, cardiac dysrhythmias, or pulmonary hypertension.

Barotrauma

Barotrauma may present as subcutaneous emphysema, pneumomediastinum, pulmonary interstitial emphysema, pneumoperitoneum, pneumopericardium, arterial gas embolism, or tension pneumothorax. These examples of extraalveolar air almost always reflect dissection or passage of air from overdistended and ruptured alveoli. Infection increases the risk of barotrauma, presumably by weakening pulmonary tissue. Tension pneumothorax is the most common life-threatening manifestation of ventilator-induced barotrauma. Hypotension, worsening hypoxemia, and increased airway pressure suggest the presence of a tension pneumothorax.

Atelectasis

Atelectasis is a common cause of hypoxemia that develops during mechanical ventilation. Migration of the tracheal tube into the left or right main bronchus or development of mucus plugs should be considered when abrupt worsening of oxygenation occurs in the absence of hypotension. Arterial hypoxemia resulting from atelectasis is not responsive to an increase in Fio_2. Other causes of sudden hypoxemia in mechanically ventilated patients include tension pneumothorax and pulmonary embolism, but in contrast to atelectasis, these are usually accompanied by hypotension. Bronchoscopy may be necessary to remove mucus plugs responsible for persistent atelectasis.

Critical Illness Myopathy

Patients who undergo mechanical ventilation for treatment of acute respiratory failure are at risk of neuromuscular weakness that persists long after the cause of the respiratory failure has resolved. A common cause of diffuse skeletal muscle weakness is *polyneuropathy of critical illness,* an axonal disorder that occurs in the presence of sepsis and multiple organ system failure. Prolonged administration of nondepolarizing neuromuscular blocking drugs may contribute to the development of an acute myopathy, particularly in patients who undergo concomitant therapy with corticosteroids. The duration of drug-induced paralysis rather than the specific neuromuscular blocker used seems to be more important in the development of persistent weakness. Decreased clearance of active metabolites of nondepolarizing neuromuscular blocking drugs resulting from renal and/or hepatic dysfunction is also a consideration when persistent weakness follows prolonged administration of these drugs.

MONITORING OF TREATMENT

Monitoring the progress of the treatment of acute respiratory failure includes evaluation of pulmonary gas exchange (arterial and venous blood gases, pHa) and cardiac function (cardiac output, cardiac filling pressures, intrapulmonary shunt). A pulmonary artery catheter is useful for performing many of these measurements.

Weaning from the Ventilator

Mechanical ventilatory support can be withdrawn when a patient can maintain oxygenation and carbon dioxide elimination without assistance. When determining whether the patient can be safely weaned from mechanical ventilation and will tolerate extubation, important considerations are that the patient be alert and cooperative and able to tolerate a trial of spontaneous ventilation without excessive tachypnea, tachycardia, or respiratory distress. Some of the guidelines that have been proposed for indicating the feasibility of discontinuing mechanical ventilation include (1) vital capacity of more than 15 mL/kg, (2) alveolar-arterial oxygen difference of less than 350 cm H_2O while breathing 100% oxygen, (3) Pao_2 of more than 60 mm Hg with Fio_2 of less than 0.5, (4) negative inspiratory pressure of more than −20 cm H_2O, (5) normal pHa, (6) respiratory rate of less than 20 breaths per minute, and (7) dead-space ventilation/tidal volume ratio (V_D/V_T) of less than 0.6. Breathing at rapid rates and with low tidal volumes usually signifies an inability to tolerate extubation. Ultimately, the decision to attempt withdrawal of mechanical ventilation is individualized and considers not only pulmonary function but also the presence of co-existing abnormalities.

When a patient is ready for a trial of withdrawal from mechanical support of ventilation, three options may be considered: (1) synchronized intermittent mandatory ventilation, which allows spontaneous breathing amid progressively fewer mandatory breaths per minute until the patient is breathing unassisted; (2) intermittent trials of total removal of mechanical support and breathing through a T-piece; and (3) use of decreasing levels of pressure-support ventilation. Overall, correcting the underlying condition responsible for the need for mechanical support of ventilation seems to be more important for successful extubation than the weaning method. Deterioration in oxygenation after withdrawal of mechanical ventilation may reflect progressive alveolar collapse, which can be responsive to treatment with continuous positive airway pressure rather than reinstitution of mechanical ventilation. Presumably continuous positive airway pressure helps maintain FRC.

Several things may interfere with successful withdrawal from mechanical ventilation and extubation. Excessive workload on the respiratory muscles imposed by hyperinflation, copious secretions, bronchospasm, increased lung water, or increased carbon dioxide production from fever or parenteral nutrition greatly decreases the likelihood of successful tracheal extubation. Use of noninvasive ventilation as a bridge to discontinuation of mechanical ventilation may occasionally be considered. This involves early extubation with immediate application of a form of noninvasive ventilation. This method of weaning may be associated with a decreased incidence of

nosocomial pneumonia, a shorter ICU stay, and a reduction in mortality. However, noninvasive ventilation may impair the ability to clear airway secretions if the patient does not have a good cough, and there may be inadequate control of minute ventilation. Careful patient selection is required if this modality is being considered.

Tracheal Extubation

Tracheal extubation should be considered when patients tolerate 30 minutes of spontaneous breathing with a continuous positive airway pressure of 5 cm H_2O without deterioration in arterial blood gas concentrations, mental status, or cardiac function. The Pao_2 should remain above 60 mm Hg with an Fio_2 of less than 0.5. Likewise, the $Paco_2$ should remain less than 50 mm Hg, and the pHa should remain above 7.30. Additional criteria for tracheal extubation include the need for less than 5 cm H_2O PEEP, spontaneous breathing rates of less than 20 breaths per minute, and vital capacity of more than 15 mL/kg. Patients should be alert with active laryngeal reflexes and the ability to generate an effective cough and clear secretions. Protective glottic closure function may be impaired following tracheal extubation, which results in an increased risk of aspiration.

Oxygen Supplementation

Oxygen supplementation is often needed after tracheal extubation. This need reflects the persistence of ventilation/perfusion mismatching. Weaning from supplemental oxygen is accomplished by gradually decreasing the inspired concentration of oxygen, as guided by measurements of Pao_2 and monitoring of oxygen saturation by pulse oximetry.

Oxygen Exchange and Arterial Oxygenation

Adequacy of oxygen exchange across alveolar-capillary membranes is reflected by the Pao_2. The efficacy of this exchange is paralleled by the differences between the calculated Pao_2 and measured Pao_2. Calculation of $Pao_2 − Pao_2$ is useful for evaluating the gas-exchange function of the lungs and for distinguishing among the various causes of arterial hypoxemia (Table 9-15).

Significant desaturation of arterial blood occurs only when the Pao_2 is less than 60 mm Hg. Ventilation/perfusion mismatching, right-to-left intrapulmonary shunting, and

TABLE 9-15   Mechanisms of arterial hypoxemia

Mechanism	Pao_2	$Paco_2$	$Pao_2−Pao_2$	Response to Supplemental Oxygen
Low inspired oxygen concentration (altitude)	Decreased	Normal to decreased	Normal	Improved
Hypoventilation (drug overdose)	Decreased	Increased	Normal	Improved
Ventilation/perfusion mismatching (COPD, pneumonia)	Decreased	Normal to decreased	Increased	Improved
Right-to-left intrapulmonary shunt (pulmonary edema)	Decreased	Normal to decreased	Increased	Poor to none
Diffusion impairment (pulmonary fibrosis)	Decreased	Normal to decreased	Increased	Improved

COPD, Chronic pulmonary obstructive disease; $Pao_2−Pao_2$, alveolar-arterial difference in partial pressure of oxygen.

hypoventilation are the principal causes of arterial hypoxemia. Increasing the inspired oxygen concentration is likely to improve Pao_2 in all these conditions, with the exception of a significant right-to-left intrapulmonary shunt.

Compensatory responses to arterial hypoxemia vary. As a general rule, these responses are stimulated by an acute decrease in Pao_2 below 60 mm Hg. Compensatory responses are also present in chronic hypoxemia when the Pao_2 is less than 50 mm Hg. These responses to arterial hypoxemia include (1) carotid body–induced increase in alveolar ventilation, (2) regional pulmonary artery vasoconstriction (hypoxic pulmonary vasoconstriction) to divert pulmonary blood flow away from hypoxic alveoli, and (3) increased sympathetic nervous system activity to enhance tissue oxygen delivery by increasing cardiac output. With chronic hypoxemia, there is also an increase in red blood cell mass to improve the oxygen-carrying capacity of the blood.

Carbon Dioxide Elimination

The adequacy of alveolar ventilation relative to the metabolic production of carbon dioxide is reflected by the $Paco_2$ (Table 9-16). The efficacy of carbon dioxide transfer across alveolar-capillary membranes is reflected by V_D/V_T. This ratio indicates areas in the lungs that receive adequate ventilation but inadequate or no pulmonary blood flow. Ventilation to these alveoli is described as "wasted ventilation" or dead-space ventilation. Normally, the V_D/V_T is less than 0.3, but it may increase to 0.6 or more when there is an increase in dead-space ventilation. An increased V_D/V_T occurs in the presence of acute respiratory failure, a decrease in cardiac output, and pulmonary embolism.

Hypercarbia is defined as a $Paco_2$ of more than 45 mm Hg. Permissive hypercapnia is the strategy of allowing $Paco_2$ to increase to up to 55 mm Hg in spontaneously breathing patients to avoid or delay the need for tracheal intubation and mechanical ventilation. Symptoms and signs of hypercarbia depend on the rate of increase and the ultimate level of $Paco_2$. Acute increases in $Paco_2$ are associated with increased cerebral blood flow and increased intracranial pressure. Extreme increases in $Paco_2$ to more than 80 mm Hg may result in central nervous system depression.

Mixed Venous Partial Pressure of Oxygen

The mixed venous partial pressure of oxygen (Pvo_2) and the arterial-venous oxygen difference ($Cao_2 - Cvo_2$) reflect the overall adequacy of the oxygen transport system (cardiac output) relative to tissue oxygen extraction. For example, a decrease in cardiac output that occurs in the presence of unchanged tissue oxygen consumption causes Pvo_2 to decrease and $Cao_2 - Cvo_2$ to increase. These changes reflect the continued extraction of the same amount of oxygen by the tissues during a time of decreased tissue blood flow. A Pvo_2 of less than 30 mm Hg or a $Cao_2 - Cvo_2$ higher than 6 mL/dL indicates the need to increase cardiac output to facilitate tissue oxygenation. A pulmonary artery catheter permits sampling of mixed venous blood, measurement of Pvo_2, and calculation of Cvo_2.

Arterial pH

Measurement of pHa is necessary to detect acidemia or alkalemia. Metabolic acidosis predictably accompanies arterial hypoxemia and inadequate delivery of oxygen to tissues. Acidemia caused by respiratory or metabolic derangements is associated with dysrhythmias and pulmonary hypertension.

Alkalemia is often associated with mechanical hyperventilation and diuretic use, which lead to loss of chloride and potassium ions. The incidence of dysrhythmias may be increased by metabolic or respiratory alkalosis. The presence of alkalemia in patients recovering from acute respiratory failure can delay or prevent successful weaning from mechanical ventilation because of the compensatory hypoventilation that will occur in an effort to correct the pH disturbance.

Intrapulmonary Shunt

Right-to-left intrapulmonary shunting occurs when there is perfusion of alveoli that are not ventilated. The net effect is a decrease in Pao_2, reflecting dilution of oxygen in blood exposed to ventilated alveoli with blood containing little oxygen coming from unventilated alveoli. Calculation of the shunt fraction provides a reliable assessment of ventilation/perfusion matching and serves as a useful estimate of the response to various therapeutic interventions during treatment of acute respiratory failure.

Physiologic shunt normally comprises 2% to 5% of the cardiac output. This degree of right-to-left intrapulmonary shunting reflects the passage of pulmonary arterial blood directly to the left side of the circulation through the bronchial and thebesian veins. It should be appreciated that determination of the shunt fraction in a patient breathing less than 100% oxygen reflects the contribution of ventilation/perfusion mismatching and right-to-left intrapulmonary shunting. Calculation of the shunt fraction from measurements obtained when the patient breathes 100% oxygen eliminates the contribution of ventilation/perfusion mismatching.

PULMONARY THROMBOEMBOLISM

Surgery predisposes patients to pulmonary thromboembolism even as late as 1 month postoperatively. Despite significant advances in the prophylaxis and diagnosis of deep venous

TABLE 9-16 ■ **Mechanisms of hypercarbia**

Mechanism	$Paco_2$	V_D/V_T	$Pao_2 - Pao_2$
Drug overdose	Increased	Normal	Normal
Restrictive lung disease (kyphoscoliosis)	Increased	Normal to increased	Normal to increased
Chronic obstructive pulmonary disease	Increased	Increased	Increased
Neuromuscular disease	Increased	Normal to increased	Normal to increased

$Pao_2 - Pao_2$, Alveolar-arterial difference in partial pressure of oxygen; V_D/V_T, dead-space ventilation/tidal volume ratio.

thrombosis, the mortality and recurrence rate of pulmonary embolism remain high. The clinical presentation of acute pulmonary thromboembolism ranges from shock or sustained hypotension to mild dyspnea. Pulmonary embolism may even be asymptomatic and diagnosed by imaging procedures performed for other purposes. Depending on the clinical presentation, the case fatality rate for acute pulmonary embolism ranges from 1% to 60%. Anticoagulation is the mainstay of therapy for pulmonary embolism.

Diagnosis

Accurate detection of pulmonary embolism remains difficult, and the differential diagnosis is extensive (Table 9-17). Pulmonary embolism can accompany or mimic other cardiopulmonary illnesses. Clinical manifestations of pulmonary embolism are nonspecific, and the diagnosis is often difficult to establish on clinical grounds alone (Table 9-18). The most consistent symptom of acute pulmonary embolism is acute dyspnea. Pleuritic or substernal chest pain, cough, or hemoptysis suggest pulmonary infarction resulting from an embolism near the pleural surface. Tachypnea and tachycardia are the most common signs of pulmonary embolism

but are nonspecific. Other physical findings include wheezing, fever, rales, a pleural rub, a loud pulmonic component of the second heart sound, a right ventricular lift, and bulging neck veins. Arterial blood gas values can be normal or demonstrate arterial hypoxemia and hypocapnia (from stimulation of airway irritant receptors that causes hyperventilation), but this is not specific to pulmonary embolism. In the presence of a patent foramen ovale or atrial septal defect, paradoxical embolization may occur and interatrial right-to-left shunting of blood may cause severe hypoxemia. ECG findings in the majority of patients with acute pulmonary embolism include ST-T wave changes and right axis deviation. Peaked P waves, atrial fibrillation, and right bundle branch block may be present if the pulmonary embolism is sufficiently large to cause acute cor pulmonale. The principal utility of the ECG is to help distinguish between pulmonary embolism and acute myocardial infarction or other alternative diagnoses.

Transthoracic echocardiography may be particularly useful in critically ill patients suspected of having pulmonary embolism and can help identify right ventricular pressure overload as well as myocardial infarction, aortic dissection, and pericardial tamponade, which can mimic pulmonary embolism. Transesophageal echocardiography may show acute dilation of the right atrium and right ventricle, pulmonary hypertension, and occasionally even thrombus in the main pulmonary arteries.

Manifestations of pulmonary embolism during anesthesia are nonspecific and often transient. Changes suggestive of pulmonary embolism during anesthesia include unexplained arterial hypoxemia, hypotension, tachycardia, and bronchospasm. The ECG and central venous pressure may indicate the onset of pulmonary hypertension and right ventricular dysfunction.

Capnography will demonstrate a decrease in end-tidal carbon dioxide tension. This represents an increase in dead-space ventilation.

Laboratory testing that aids in the diagnosis of acute pulmonary embolism includes the D-dimer test. A positive D-dimer test result means that a pulmonary embolism is possible. A negative D-dimer result strongly suggests that thromboembolism is absent. The negative predictive value of the D-dimer test is above 99%. Troponin levels may be elevated and may represent right ventricular myocyte damage caused by acute right ventricular strain.

Spiral CT scanning with contrast is useful for diagnosing both acute and chronic pulmonary embolism and has replaced ventilation-perfusion scanning in many centers. It is most useful in detecting clots in the main, lobar, and segmental pulmonary arteries and is much less sensitive in detecting emboli in smaller blood vessels. However, it is these larger emboli that are most important clinically.

Pulmonary arteriography is the gold standard for the diagnosis of pulmonary embolism. It is used when pulmonary embolism must be diagnosed or excluded and other preliminary testing has yielded inconclusive results.

TABLE 9-17 ■ Differential diagnosis of pulmonary embolism

Myocardial infarction
Pericarditis
Congestive heart failure
Chronic obstructive pulmonary disease
Pneumonia
Pneumothorax
Pleuritis
Thoracic herpes zoster
Anxiety/hyperventilation syndrome
Thoracic aorta dissection
Rib fractures

TABLE 9-18 ■ Signs and symptoms of pulmonary embolism

Sign/Symptom	Incidence (%)
Acute dyspnea	75
Tachypnea (>20 breaths/min)	70
Pleuritic chest pain	65
Rales	50
Nonproductive cough	40
Tachycardia (>100 beats/min)	30
Accentuation of pulmonic component of second heart sound	25
Hemoptysis	15
Fever (38°-39° C)	10
Homans's sign	5

Ventilation-perfusion lung scanning and ultrasonography of leg veins are other noninvasive tests that can aid in the diagnosis of deep venous thrombosis and/or pulmonary embolism.

The initial assessment of the clinical probability of pulmonary embolism is based on clinical judgment. Patients are considered to be in hemodynamically unstable condition if they are in shock or have a systolic blood pressure of less than 90 mm Hg or a decrease in blood pressure of more than 40 mm Hg for longer than 15 minutes in the absence of new-onset dysrhythmias, hypovolemia, or sepsis. In cases in which spiral CT is not available or in patients with renal failure or allergy to contrast dye, the use of ventilation-perfusion scanning is the best alternative. However, spiral CT should be performed when the patient's condition has stabilized if doubts remain about clinical management. In patients who are candidates for percutaneous embolectomy, conventional pulmonary angiography can be performed to confirm the diagnosis of pulmonary embolism immediately before the embolectomy procedure.

Treatment

Treatment options for acute pulmonary embolism include anticoagulation, thrombolytic therapy, inferior vena caval filter placement, and surgical embolectomy.

Heparin remains the cornerstone of treatment for acute pulmonary embolism. An intravenous bolus of unfractionated heparin (5000 to 10,000 units) followed by a continuous intravenous infusion should be administered immediately to any patient considered to have a high clinical likelihood of pulmonary embolism. An alternative is low-molecular-weight heparin given subcutaneously. The optimal duration of anticoagulation for pulmonary embolism remains uncertain, but it is known that a treatment period of 6 months is associated with many fewer recurrences than a treatment period of 6 weeks. This extended period of anticoagulation is usually accomplished with warfarin in a dosage that maintains an international normalized ratio of 2.0 to 3.0.

Patients who cannot undergo anticoagulation, experience significant bleeding while being treated with anticoagulants, or have recurrent pulmonary emboli despite receiving anticoagulant therapy may require insertion of a vena cava filter to prevent lower-extremity thrombi from becoming pulmonary emboli. The use of vena cava filters should be reserved for patients with contraindications to anticoagulant treatment. Retrievable vena cava filters may be an option for patients with presumed time-limited contraindications to anticoagulant therapy or for patients requiring procedures that are associated with both a risk of bleeding and a risk of pulmonary embolism.

Thrombolytic therapy may be considered to hasten dissolution of pulmonary emboli, especially if there is hemodynamic instability or severe hypoxemia. Hemorrhage is the principal adverse effect of thrombolytic therapy, and so this treatment is contraindicated in patients at high risk of bleeding.

The hypotension caused by a pulmonary embolism may require treatment with inotropes such as dopamine and dobutamine or a vasoconstrictor such as norepinephrine. A pulmonary vasodilator may be needed to help control pulmonary hypertension. Tracheal intubation and mechanical ventilation may be necessary. Analgesics to treat the pain associated with pulmonary embolism are important but must be administered very carefully because of the underlying cardiovascular instability. Pulmonary artery embolectomy is reserved for patients who have a massive pulmonary embolism that is unresponsive to medical therapy and who cannot receive thrombolytic therapy.

Management of Anesthesia

Management of anesthesia for the surgical treatment of life-threatening pulmonary embolism is designed to support vital organ function and to minimize anesthetic-induced myocardial depression. Patients typically arrive in the operating room intubated and mechanically ventilated, often with a high FiO_2. Monitoring of intraarterial pressure and cardiac filling pressures is necessary. Right atrial filling pressure can be a guide to intravenous fluid administration aimed at optimizing right ventricular filling pressure and stroke volume in the presence of a marked increase in right ventricular afterload. It may be necessary to support cardiac output with inotropic drugs. Catecholamines such as dopamine and dobutamine may increase myocardial contractility but have little effect on pulmonary vascular resistance. The phosphodiesterase inhibitors amrinone and milrinone increase myocardial contractility and are excellent pulmonary artery vasodilators. This combination of effects may be particularly useful in this situation.

Induction and maintenance of anesthesia must avoid any accentuation of arterial hypoxemia, systemic hypotension, or pulmonary hypertension. Anesthesia can be maintained with any drug or combination of drugs that does not produce significant myocardial depression. Nitrous oxide is not a likely selection, because of the need to administer high concentrations of oxygen and the potential for this drug to increase pulmonary vascular resistance. A nondepolarizing neuromuscular blocking drug that does not release histamine is best.

Removal of embolic fragments from the distal pulmonary artery may be facilitated by the application of positive pressure while the surgeon applies suction through the arteriotomy in the main pulmonary artery. Although the cardiopulmonary status of these patients is perilous before surgery, significant hemodynamic improvement usually occurs postoperatively.

FAT EMBOLISM

The syndrome of fat embolism typically appears 12 to 72 hours after long-bone fractures, especially fractures of the femur or tibia. Fat embolism syndrome has also been observed in association with acute pancreatitis, cardiopulmonary bypass, parenteral infusion of lipids, and liposuction. The triad of hypoxemia, mental confusion, and petechiae in patients with tibia or femur fractures should arouse suspicion of fat embolism. Associated pulmonary dysfunction may be limited to arterial hypoxemia, which is always present, or it may progress from tachypnea to acute respiratory distress syndrome. Central nervous system dysfunction ranges from confusion to seizures and coma. Petechiae, especially over the neck, shoulders, and chest, occur in at least 50% of patients with clinical evidence of fat embolism and are thought to be caused by embolic fat rather than by thrombocytopenia or other disorders of coagulation. An increased serum lipase concentration or the presence of lipiduria is suggestive of fat embolism but may also occur after trauma in the absence of a fat embolism. Significant fever and tachycardia are often present. Magnetic resonance imaging can show the characteristic cerebral lesions during the acute stage of fat embolism syndrome.

The source of fat producing a fat embolism is most likely disruption of the adipose architecture of the bone marrow. The pathophysiology of fat embolism syndrome relates to obstruction of blood vessels by fat particles and the deleterious effects of free fatty acids released from the fat particles as a result of lipase activity. These free fatty acids can cause an acute, diffuse vasculitis, especially of the cerebral and pulmonary vasculature. Treatment of fat embolism syndrome includes management of acute respiratory distress syndrome and immobilization of long-bone fractures. Prophylactic administration of corticosteroids to patients at risk may be useful, but the efficacy of corticosteroids for treatment of the established syndrome has not been documented. Conceptually, corticosteroids could decrease the incidence of fat embolism syndrome by limiting the endothelial damage caused by free fatty acids.

LUNG TRANSPLANTATION

Indications

The four principal approaches to lung transplantation are (1) single-lung transplantation, (2) bilateral sequential lung transplantation, (3) heart-lung transplantation, and (4) transplantation of lobes from living donors. Table 9-19 lists the typical indications for lung transplantation.

The presence of cor pulmonale is not an indication for heart-lung transplantation, because recovery of right ventricular function is typically rapid and complete after lung

---

TABLE 9-19 ■ Indications for lung transplantation

Chronic obstructive pulmonary disease
Cystic fibrosis
Idiopathic pulmonary fibrosis
Primary pulmonary hypertension
Bronchiectasis
Eisenmenger's syndrome

Adapted from Singh H, Bossard RF. Perioperative anaesthetic considerations for patients undergoing lung transplantation. *Can J Anaesth.* 1997;44:284-299.

---

transplantation alone. In patients with pulmonary hypertension, high vascular resistance in the remaining native lung requires the allograft to handle nearly the entire cardiac output. This could result in reperfusion pulmonary edema and poor allograft function in the period immediately after surgery. Fibrotic lung disease responds well to single-lung transplantation because both ventilation and perfusion are distributed preferentially to the transplanted lung. Bilateral sequential lung transplantation involves the sequential performance of two single-lung transplants at one time. In the absence of severe pulmonary hypertension, cardiopulmonary bypass can usually be avoided by ventilating the contralateral lung during each implantation. The primary indications for double-lung transplantation are cystic fibrosis and other forms of bronchiectasis. Immunosuppression is initiated intraoperatively and continued for life.

Anesthetic Considerations

MANAGEMENT OF ANESTHESIA FOR LUNG TRANSPLANTATION

Management of anesthesia for lung transplantation invokes the same principles followed when pneumonectomy is performed.

Preoperative

Physiologically, patients selected for lung transplantation most often have restrictive lung disease and a large $P_{AO_2} - P_{aO_2}$. These patients generally have irreversible and progressive pulmonary disease. (Malignancy is regarded as a contraindication to transplantation because of the risk of cancer recurrence with immunosuppression.) Mild to moderate degrees of pulmonary hypertension and some degree of right-sided heart failure are often present. Smokers should have quit smoking at least 6 to 12 months before transplantation. The ability of the right ventricle to maintain an adequate stroke volume in the presence of the acute increase in pulmonary vascular resistance produced by clamping the pulmonary artery before the native lung is removed needs to be assessed. Evaluation of oxygen dependence and steroid use, hematologic and biochemical analyses, and tests of lung and other major organ system function are also required.

Intraoperative

Posterolateral thoracotomy is performed for single-lung transplantation and bilateral anterothoracosternotomy for bilateral or sequential single-lung transplantation. Cardiopulmonary bypass may be needed if cardiac or respiratory instability develops during the procedure. The lung with poorer perfusion is removed in single-lung transplantation. Monitoring includes placement of intraarterial and pulmonary artery catheters. Pulmonary artery pressure monitoring is especially important. During surgery, care must be taken to make sure that the pulmonary artery catheter is withdrawn from the pulmonary artery to be stapled and refloated to the nonoperative lung. Transesophageal echocardiographic monitoring can be used to evaluate right and left ventricular function and fluid balance. There are no specific recommendations regarding drugs for induction and maintenance of anesthesia and skeletal muscle paralysis for lung transplantation. Drug-induced histamine release is undesirable, and drug-induced bronchodilation is useful.

The trachea is intubated with a double-lumen endobronchial tube, and its proper placement is verified by fiberoptic bronchoscopy. Possible intraoperative problems include arterial hypoxemia, especially during one-lung ventilation. Continuous positive airway pressure to the nondependent lung, PEEP to the dependent lung, or some form of differential lung ventilation may be needed to minimize intrapulmonary shunting. Severe pulmonary hypertension and right ventricular failure can occur when the pulmonary artery is clamped. Infusion of a pulmonary vasodilator such as prostacyclin or inhalation of nitric oxide may be helpful for controlling pulmonary hypertension. In extreme cases, support with partial cardiopulmonary bypass is required. Connection of the donor lung to the recipient is usually performed in the sequence of pulmonary veins to the left atrium, then anastomosis of the pulmonary artery, and finally anastomosis of the bronchus.

Postoperative

Postoperative mechanical ventilation is continued as needed. The principal causes of mortality with lung transplantation are bronchial dehiscence and respiratory failure due to sepsis or rejection. The denervation of the donor lung deprives patients of normal cough reflexes from the lower airways and predisposes to the development of pneumonia. In the absence of rejection, pulmonary function test results can be normal.

MANAGEMENT OF ANESTHESIA IN LUNG TRANSPLANT RECIPIENTS

Anesthetic management in patients requiring surgery following lung transplantation should focus on (1) the function of the transplanted lung, (2) the possibility of rejection or infection in the transplanted lung, (3) the effect of immunosuppressive therapy on other organ systems and the effect of other organ system dysfunction on the transplanted lung, (4) the disease in the native lung, and (5) the planned surgical procedure and its likely effects on the lungs.

PREOPERATIVE

Evaluation before surgery includes obtaining a history suggestive of rejection or infection, auscultation of the lungs (normally clear), and evaluation of the results of pulmonary function tests, arterial blood gas analyses, and chest radiographs. If rejection or infection is suspected, elective surgery should be postponed. The side effects of immunosuppressive drugs should be noted. Hypertension and renal dysfunction related to cyclosporine therapy are present in many patients.

Because transplanted lungs may have ongoing rejection that can adversely affect pulmonary function, it is recommended that spirometry be performed preoperatively. It may be difficult to differentiate between chronic rejection and infection.

With chronic rejection, the FEV_1, vital capacity, and total lung capacity decrease and arterial blood gas values show an increased alveolar-arterial oxygen gradient, but carbon dioxide retention is rare. Bronchiolitis obliterans usually presents as a nonproductive cough developing after the third month following transplantation. Symptoms can mimic those of URI and include fever and fatigue. Dyspnea occurs within months and is followed by a clinical course similar to that of COPD. Chest radiographs show peribronchial and interstitial infiltrates.

Premedication is acceptable if pulmonary function is adequate. Hypercarbia is common during the early posttransplantation period. This could be exacerbated by opioid administration. Antisialagogues can be useful, since secretions can be excessive. Supplemental corticosteroids may be needed for long, stressful surgical procedures. A major cause of morbidity and mortality in transplant recipients is infection. Prophylactic antibiotics are indicated, and strict aseptic technique is required for placement of intravascular catheters. Lung denervation has limited effects on the pattern of breathing, but bronchial hyperreactivity and bronchoconstriction are common. Denervation ablates afferent sensation below the level of the tracheal anastomosis. Patients lose the cough reflex and are prone to retention of secretions and silent aspiration. Response to carbon dioxide rebreathing is normal.

INTRAOPERATIVE

Because lung transplant recipients lack a cough reflex below the tracheal anastomosis, they do not clear secretions unless they are awake. Because of the diminished cough reflex, the potential for bronchoconstriction, and the increased risk of pulmonary infection, it is recommended that regional anesthesia be selected whenever possible. Epidural and spinal anesthesia are acceptable. However, depression of intercostal muscle function may have special implications in these patients. Any nerve blockade procedure carries a risk of introducing infection. The importance of using sterile technique in this high-risk population cannot be overemphasized. Fluid preloading before spinal or epidural anesthesia may be risky in patients with a transplanted lung, because disruption of the lymphatic drainage in the transplanted lung causes interstitial fluid accumulation. This is particularly problematic during the early posttransplantation period.

In heart-lung transplant recipients, fluid management may be particularly challenging, because the heart requires adequate preload to maintain cardiac output, but the lungs have a lower than normal threshold for developing pulmonary edema. In this situation, invasive monitoring may be very useful, but the benefits must be balanced against the risk of infection. Transesophageal echocardiography can be useful for monitoring volume status and cardiac function. If a central venous catheter is inserted via the internal jugular vein, it is prudent to select the internal jugular vein on the side of the native lung. Cardiac denervation is another consideration in patients who have undergone heart-lung transplantation. These patients may develop intraoperative bradycardia that does not respond to administration of atropine. Epinephrine and/or isoproterenol may be required to increase the heart rate.

An important goal of anesthetic management is prompt recovery of adequate respiratory function and early tracheal extubation. Volatile anesthetics are well tolerated, and use of nitrous oxide is acceptable in the absence of bullous disease. Immunosuppressive drugs may interact with neuromuscular blocking drugs, and the impaired renal function caused by immunosuppressive drugs may prolong the effects of certain muscle relaxants. The effects of nondepolarizing neuromuscular blockers are routinely antagonized pharmacologically, because even minimal residual weakness can compromise ventilation in these patients.

When an endotracheal tube is positioned, it is best to place the cuff just beyond the vocal cords to minimize the risk of traumatizing the tracheal anastomosis. Inadvertent endobronchial intubation of the native or transplanted lung must be avoided. If the surgical procedure requires use of a double-lumen endobronchial tube, it is preferable to place the endobronchial portion of the tube in the native bronchus, so as to avoid contact with the tracheal anastomosis. In patients with a single lung transplant, positive pressure ventilation may be complicated by differences in lung compliance between the native and transplanted lung.

Physiologic Effects

Single or bilateral lung transplantation in patients with end-stage lung disease can dramatically improve lung function. Peak improvement is usually achieved within 3 to 6 months. Arterial oxygenation rapidly returns to normal, and supplemental oxygen is no longer needed. In patients with pulmonary vascular disease, both single and bilateral lung transplantation result in immediate and sustained normalization of pulmonary vascular resistance and pulmonary artery pressure. This is accompanied by a prompt increase in cardiac output and a gradual remodeling of the right ventricle with a decrease in ventricular wall thickness. Exercise capacity improves sufficiently to permit most lung transplant patients to resume an active lifestyle.

The innervation of the lung, the lymphatic drainage of the lung, and the bronchial circulation are disrupted when the donor pneumonectomy is performed. The principal effect of lung denervation is loss of the cough reflex, which places patients at risk of aspiration and pulmonary infection. Mucociliary clearance is impaired during the early postoperative period. Lymphatic drainage disrupted by transection of the trachea and bronchi may be reestablished during the first few weeks postoperatively. Often a blunted ventilatory response to carbon dioxide persists even though pulmonary function improves. Denervation of the heart is another consideration in patients undergoing heart-lung transplantation.

COMPLICATIONS

Mild transient pulmonary edema is common in a newly transplanted lung. In some patients, however, pulmonary edema is sufficiently severe to cause a form of acute respiratory failure termed *primary graft failure.* The diagnosis is confirmed by the appearance of infiltrates on chest radiographs and severe hypoxemia during the first 72 hours postoperatively. Treatment is supportive and includes mechanical ventilation. Mortality is high.

Dehiscence of the bronchial anastomosis mandates immediate surgical correction or retransplantation. Stenosis of the bronchial anastomosis is the most common airway complication and typically occurs several weeks after transplantation. Evidence of clinically significant airway stenosis includes focal wheezing, recurrent lower respiratory tract infection, and suboptimal pulmonary function.

The rate of infection in lung transplant recipients is several times higher than that in recipients of other transplanted organs and is most likely related to exposure of the allograft to the external environment. Bacterial infection of the lower respiratory tract is the most common manifestation of pulmonary infection. A ubiquitous organism acquired by inhalation is *Aspergillus,* which frequently colonizes the airways of lung transplant recipients. However, clinical infection with *Aspergillus* develops in only a small number of these patients.

Acute rejection of a lung allograft is a common event and is usually seen during the first 100 days following transplantation. Clinical manifestations are nonspecific and include malaise, low-grade fever, dyspnea, impaired oxygenation, and leukocytosis. Transbronchial lung biopsy is needed for a definitive diagnosis. Treatment of acute rejection consists of intravenous methylprednisolone. Most patients have a prompt clinical response, although histologic evidence of rejection may persist even in the absence of clinical symptoms and signs.

Chronic rejection is manifested as bronchiolitis obliterans, a fibroproliferative process that targets the small airways and leads to submucosal fibrosis and luminal obliteration. Bronchiolitis obliterans is uncommon during the first 6 months following transplantation, but its incidence exceeds 60% in patients who survive at least 5 years. The onset of this syndrome is insidious and is characterized by dyspnea, cough, and colonization of the airways with *Pseudomonas aeruginosa,* which produces recurrent bouts of purulent tracheobronchitis. The overall prognosis is poor. Retransplantation is the only definitive treatment for severe bronchiolitis obliterans.

KEY POINTS

■ Surgical patients with preexisting respiratory disease are at increased risk of respiratory complications both during and after surgery.

■ The anesthetic management of a patient with a recent URI should be focused on reducing secretions and limiting manipulation of a potentially hyperresponsive airway.

■ Asthma treatment has two components. The first is the use of controller treatments, which modify the airway environment so that acute airway narrowing occurs less frequently. The second is the use of reliever or rescue agents for acute bronchospasm. Reliever treatments include β-adrenergic agonists and anticholinergic drugs.

- In asthmatic patients, the goal during induction and maintenance of anesthesia is to depress airway reflexes sufficiently to avoid bronchoconstriction in response to mechanical stimulation of the airway.
- Cessation of smoking and long-term oxygen therapy are two important therapeutic interventions that may favorably alter the natural progression of COPD associated with hypoxemia.
- Pulmonary function tests have limited value in predicting the likelihood of postoperative pulmonary complications, and the results of pulmonary function tests alone should not be used to deny patients surgery.
- Patients with COPD need to be ventilated at slow respiratory rates to allow sufficient time for exhalation to occur. This minimizes the risk of air trapping and auto-PEEP.
- In patients with COPD, prophylaxis against the development of postoperative pulmonary complications is based on restoring diminished lung volumes, especially FRC, and facilitating production of an effective cough to remove airway secretions.
- The most effective treatment for aspiration pneumonitis is delivery of supplemental oxygen and initiation of PEEP.
- Treatment options for acute pulmonary embolism include anticoagulation, thrombolytic therapy, inferior vena cava filter placement, and surgical embolectomy.
- The principal effect of lung denervation as a result of lung transplantation is loss of the cough reflex, which places patients at risk of aspiration and pulmonary infection.
- In heart-lung transplant recipients, fluid management is a challenge because the heart requires adequate preload to maintain cardiac output, but the lungs have a low threshold for developing pulmonary edema.

RESOURCES

Agnelli G, Becattini C. Acute pulmonary embolism. *N Engl J Med.* 2010; 363:266-274.

Arcasoy SM, Kotloff RM. Lung transplantation. *N Engl J Med.* 1999; 340:1081-1091.

Barrera R, Shi W, Amar D, et al. Smoking and timing of cessation: impact on pulmonary complications after thoracotomy. *Chest.* 2005;127:1977-1983.

Burns KE, Adhikari NK, Keenan SP, et al. Use of non-invasive ventilation to wean critically ill adults off invasive ventilation: meta-analysis and systematic review. *BMJ.* 2009;338:b1574.

Kostopanagiotou GMDP, Smyrniotis VMDP, Arkadopoulos NMD, et al. Anesthetic and perioperative management of adult transplant recipients in nontransplant surgery. *Anesth Analg.* 1999;89:613-622.

Lazarus SC. Emergency treatment of asthma. *N Engl J Med.* 2010; 363(8):755-764.

Qaseem A, Snow V, Fitterman N, et al. Risk assessment for and strategies to reduce perioperative pulmonary complications for patients undergoing noncardiothoracic surgery: a guideline from the American College of Physicians. *Ann Intern Med.* 2006;144:575-580.

Sadovnikoff N. Anesthesia for patients with severe chronic obstructive pulmonary disease. *Curr Opin Anaesthesiol.* 2010;23:18-24.

Smetana GW, Lawrence VA, Cornell JE. Preoperative pulmonary risk stratification for noncardiothoracic surgery: a systematic review for the American College of Physicians. *Ann Intern Med.* 2006;144:581-595.

Thomsen T, Villebro N, Møller AM. Interventions for preoperative smoking cessation. *Cochrane Database Syst Rev.* 2010(7):CD002294.

Ware LB, Matthay MA. Acute pulmonary edema. *N Engl J Med.* 2005; 353:2788-2796.

Yamakage M, Iwasaki S, Namiki A. Guideline-oriented perioperative management of patients with bronchial asthma and chronic obstructive pulmonary disease. *J Anesth.* 2008;22:412-428.

Diseases Affecting the Brain

JEFFREY J. PASTERNAK ■
WILLIAM L. LANIER, JR. ■

Patients with diseases affecting the brain and central nervous system may undergo surgery to treat the neurologic condition or surgery unrelated to the nervous system disease. Regardless of the reason for surgery, co-existing nervous system diseases often have important implications for the selection of anesthetic drugs, techniques, and monitoring methods. Concepts of cerebral protection and resuscitation assume unique importance in these patients. This chapter reviews these issues and also discusses various diseases of the retina and optic nerve.

CEREBRAL BLOOD FLOW, BLOOD VOLUME, AND METABOLISM

Generally, cerebral blood flow (CBF) is governed by cerebral metabolic rate, cerebral perfusion pressure (CPP, defined as the difference between the mean arterial pressure [MAP] and intracranial pressure [ICP]), arterial blood carbon dioxide ($Paco_2$) and oxygen (Pao_2) tensions, the influence of various drugs, and intracranial abnormalities. CBF is normally autoregulated, that is, constant over a given range of perfusion pressures. In a healthy adult, CBF is approximately 50 mL/100 g brain tissue per minute over a CPP range of 50 to 150 mm Hg.

Normal cerebral metabolic rate, generally measured as rate of oxygen consumption ($CMRO_2$), is 3.0 to 3.8 mL O_2/100 g brain tissue per minute. It can be decreased by temperature reductions and various anesthetic agents and increased by temperature increases and seizures.

Anesthetic and intensive care management of neurologically impaired patients relies heavily on manipulation of intracranial volume and pressure. These, in turn, are influenced by cerebral blood volume (CBV) and CBF. CBF and CBV do not always change in parallel. For example, vasodilatory anesthetics and hypercapnia may produce parallel increases in CBF and CBV. Conversely, moderate systemic hypotension can produce a reduction in CBF but, as a result of compensatory vessel dilation, an increase in CBV. Similarly, partial occlusion of an intracranial artery such as occurs in embolic stroke may reduce regional CBF. However, vessel dilation distal to the occlusion, which is an attempt to restore circulation, can produce an increase in CBV.

Arterial Carbon Dioxide Partial Pressure

Variations in $Paco_2$ produce corresponding changes in CBF (Figure 10-1). As a guideline, CBF (normally approximately 50 mL/100 g brain tissue per minute) increases by 1 mL/100 g per minute for every 1 mm Hg increase in $Paco_2$. A similar decrease occurs during hypocarbia, so that CBF is decreased by approximately 50% when $Paco_2$ is acutely reduced to 20 mm Hg. The impact of $Paco_2$ on CBF is mediated by variations in the pH of the cerebrospinal fluid (CSF) around the walls of arterioles. Decreased CSF pH causes cerebral vasodilation, and increased CSF pH results in vasoconstriction. $Paco_2$ can also modulate CBV. The extent of CBV reduction is dependent on the anesthetic being used. In general, vasoconstricting anesthetics tend to attenuate the effects of $Paco_2$ on CBV.

The ability of hypocapnia to acutely decrease CBF, CBV, and ICP is fundamental to the practice of clinical neuroanesthesia. Concern that cerebral hypoxia due to vasoconstriction can occur when the $Paco_2$ is lowered to less than 20 mm Hg has not been substantiated. The ability of hypocapnia to decrease CBV, and thus ICP, is attenuated by the return of CSF pH to normal after prolonged periods of hypocapnia. This reduces the effectiveness of induced hypocapnia as a means of long-term control of intracranial hypertension. This adaptive change, which reflects active transport of bicarbonate ions into or from the CSF, requires approximately 6 hours to return the CSF pH to normal.

Arterial Oxygen Partial Pressure

Decreased Pao_2 does not significantly affect CBF until a threshold value of approximately 50 mm Hg is reached (see Figure 10-1). Below this threshold, there is abrupt cerebral vasodilation, and CBF increases. Furthermore, the combination of arterial hypoxemia and hypercarbia exert synergistic effects.

Cerebral Perfusion Pressure and Cerebral Autoregulation

The ability of the brain to maintain CBF at constant levels despite changes in CPP is known as *autoregulation* (see Figure 10-1). Autoregulation is an active vascular response characterized by (1) arterial constriction when the blood pressure is increased, and (2) arterial dilation in response to decreases in systemic blood pressure. For example, in normotensive patients, the lower limit of CPP associated with autoregulation is believed to be approximately 50 mm Hg, although the exact value is controversial. Below this threshold, cerebral blood vessels are maximally vasodilated and CBF decreases. CBF becomes directly related to CPP—that is, it becomes pressure-dependent blood flow. Indeed, at a CPP of 30 to 45 mm Hg, symptoms of cerebral ischemia may appear in the form of nausea, dizziness, and slow cerebration. Autoregulation of CBF also has an upper limit above which the flow becomes directly proportional to the CPP. This upper limit of autoregulation in normotensive patients is believed to be a CPP of approximately 150 mm Hg. Above this pressure, the cerebral blood vessels are maximally constricted. If CPP increases further, then CBF increases and becomes pressure dependent. This results in overdistention of the cerebral blood vessels, and as a result, fluid may be forced across the blood vessel walls into the brain tissue, producing cerebral edema.

Autoregulation of CBF is altered in the presence of chronic hypertension. Specifically, the autoregulation curve is displaced to the right, so that pressure dependence of CBF occurs at a higher CPP at both the upper and lower thresholds of autoregulation. The adaptation of cerebral blood vessels to increased blood pressure requires some time. Indeed, acute hypertension, as seen in children with acute-onset glomerulonephritis or in patients with short-duration pregnancy-induced

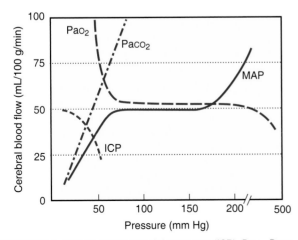

FIGURE 10-1 Impact of intracranial pressure (ICP), Pao_2, $Paco_2$, and mean arterial pressure (MAP) on cerebral blood flow.

hypertension, often produces signs of central nervous system dysfunction at MAP values that are well tolerated in chronically hypertensive patients. Similarly, an acute hypertensive response associated with direct laryngoscopy or surgery may cause a breakdown of autoregulation in previously normotensive patients. The lower limit of autoregulation is also shifted upward in chronically hypertensive patients, so that decreases in systemic blood pressure that would be tolerated in normotensive patients are not well tolerated in these individuals. Therefore, rapid lowering of blood pressure with the use of a vasodilating drug to population-normal values in patients who are chronically hypertensive can precipitate a stroke. Gradual decreases in systemic blood pressure over time resulting from antihypertensive drug therapy can improve the tolerance of the brain to hypotension as the autoregulation curve shifts back toward a more normal position.

Autoregulation of CBF may be lost or impaired under a variety of conditions, including the presence of intracranial tumors or head trauma and the administration of volatile anesthetics. The loss of autoregulation in the blood vessels surrounding intracranial tumors reflects acidosis leading to maximum vasodilation, so that blood flow becomes pressure dependent.

Venous Blood Pressure

Increases in the brain's venous blood pressure can influence CBF either directly or indirectly. Directly, increased brain venous pressure contributes to reductions in arterial/venous pressure gradients. Indirectly, increases in brain venous blood pressure increase CBV and ICP (see the section on intracranial pressure later), which in turn reduces CPP. If these changes in brain venous blood pressure are not compensated for by an increase in MAP, the CPP reduction will produce the expected effects on CBF.

Venous pressure increases emanating from the central circulation—that is, central venous pressure (CVP)—are variably transmitted to the brain depending on whether the patient's position is horizontal (maximal CBV increase) or head up (minimal CBV increase). In contrast, venous blood pressure increases emanating from the neck or skull base are more effectively translated to the brain. Regardless of its origin, an increase in brain venous pressure can contribute to increased brain bulk during intracranial surgery and impede the surgeon's access to the target brain areas.

Causes of increased brain venous pressure include venous sinus thrombosis and jugular compression resulting from improper neck positioning, such as extreme flexion or rotation. Superior vena cava syndrome can cause long-term increases in brain venous pressure. With coughing, increases in intrathoracic pressure result in transient increases in CVP. However, if a coughing or bucking patient is tracheally intubated, the glottis is stented open by the endotracheal tube, and the effects of a cough or buck on CVP will be different from those in a nonintubated patient. CVP will transiently increase during forced exhalation, but transiently decrease during forced inhalation, which results in no meaningful change in CVP over an entire coughing or bucking cycle. In such a setting, ICP can still increase, but this increase would be due to increases in CBF and CBV resulting from muscle afferent–mediated stimulation of the brain, a mechanism shared by succinylcholine-induced increases in ICP.

Anesthetic Drugs

Under normal physiologic conditions, changes in $CMRO_2$ usually lead to concomitant changes in CBF, a phenomenon known as *CBF-CMRO₂ coupling*. In contrast, volatile anesthetics, such as isoflurane, sevoflurane, and desflurane, particularly when administered in concentrations greater than 0.6 to 1.0 minimum alveolar concentration (MAC), are often potent direct cerebral vasodilators that produce dose-dependent increases in CBF despite concomitant decreases in cerebral metabolic oxygen requirements. Below 1 MAC, volatile anesthetics alter CBF minimally, in part because any direct effects of the anesthetics are counterbalanced by $CMRO_2$ coupling. When volatile anesthetic–induced $CMRO_2$ depression is maximized, concomitant with maximal depression of cerebral electrical activity, larger dosages of volatile anesthetic will continue to dilate cerebral blood vessels. This can lead to increases in CBF, CBV, and possibly ICP. With halothane, which at clinically relevant dosages does not induce the extent of $CMRO_2$ depression that is seen with other volatile anesthetics (isoflurane, sevoflurane, desflurane), direct vasodilatory effects predominate, which results in greater increases in CBV at equipotent doses compared with other commonly used volatile agents. This can lead to increased ICP, which makes halothane a less than ideal volatile anesthetic agent for neurosurgical procedures in which CBV and ICP management is critical. With all volatile anesthetics arterial hypocapnia helps to minimize increases in CBV that might accompany administration of these drugs at normocarbia. These same CBV- and ICP-attenuating effects can also be achieved by administration of supplemental cerebral vasoconstricting anesthetics such as thiopental or propofol.

In contrast to volatile anesthetics, nitrous oxide has less effect on CBF and does not appear to interfere with autoregulation. The exact effects of nitrous oxide on human cerebral hemodynamics remain elusive, probably because of a wide range of interspecies differences in the MAC of nitrous oxide as well as the invariable presence of other drugs used to maintain general anesthesia in human studies. The initiation of nitrous oxide administration after closure of the dura may contribute to the development of a tension pneumocephalus, since there is likely to be air in the intracranial vault following dural closure and nitrous oxide has greater solubility in air than nitrogen. This leads to an increase in the size and pressure of the air pocket. Clinically, tension pneumocephalus usually presents as delayed emergence from general anesthesia after craniotomy.

Like the volatile anesthetics, ketamine is considered to be a cerebral vasodilator. In contrast to volatile anesthetics and possibly ketamine, barbiturates, etomidate, propofol, and opioids are cerebral vasoconstrictors, provided the patient is not permitted to develop respiratory depression and hypercapnia. Drugs that produce cerebral vasoconstriction predictably decrease CBV and ICP.

Propofol and barbiturates such as thiopental are potent cerebral vasoconstrictors capable of decreasing CBF, CBV, and ICP. Opioids are also cerebral vasoconstrictors, assuming that opioid-induced ventilatory depression is controlled and no increase in $Paco_2$ is allowed.

Administration of nondepolarizing neuromuscular blocking drugs does not meaningfully alter ICP. However, muscle relaxation may help prevent acute increases in ICP resulting from movement or coughing during direct laryngoscopy. Neuromuscular blocker–induced histamine release, as occurs with atracurium, D-tubocurarine, and metocurine, could theoretically produce cerebral vasodilation and an associated increase in CBV and ICP, particularly if large doses of these drugs are administered rapidly. The use of succinylcholine in the setting of increased ICP may temporarily raise ICP. The mechanism for this effect is most likely increases in muscle afferent activity, a process somewhat independent of visible muscle fasciculations. This can lead to cerebral arousal (which can be seen on electroencephalography [EEG]) and corresponding increases in CBF and CBV. These cerebral effects of succinylcholine can be attenuated or prevented by prior induction of deep anesthesia with a cerebral vasoconstricting anesthetic.

INCREASED INTRACRANIAL PRESSURE

The intracranial and spinal vault contains neural tissue (brain and spinal cord), blood, and CSF, and is enclosed by the dura mater and bone. The pressure within this space is referred to as the *intracranial pressure* (ICP). Under normal conditions, brain tissue, intracranial CSF, and intracranial blood have a combined volume of approximately 1200 to 1500 mL, and normal ICP is usually 5 to 15 mm Hg. Any increase in one component of intracranial volume must be offset by a decrease in another component to prevent an increase in ICP. Normally, changes in one component are well compensated for by other components, but eventually a point can be reached at which even a small change in intracranial contents results in a large change in ICP (Figure 10-2). This condition is known as *increased intracranial elastance*. Since ICP is one of the determinants of CPP, homeostatic mechanisms work to increase MAP to help support CPP despite increases in ICP, but eventually compensatory mechanisms can fail and cerebral ischemia will result.

Factors leading to alterations in CSF flow or its absorption into the vasculature can often lead to increased ICP. CSF is produced by two mechanisms: (1) ultrafiltration and secretion by the cells of the choroid plexus, and (2) the passage of water, electrolytes, and other substances across the blood–brain barrier. CSF is, therefore, a direct extension of the extracellular fluid compartment of the central nervous system. CSF is produced at a constant rate of 500 to 600 mL/day in adults and is

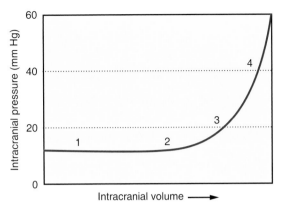

FIGURE 10-2 Intracranial elastance curve depicting the impact of increasing intracranial volume on intracranial pressure (ICP). As intracranial volume increases from point 1 to point 2, ICP does not increase because cerebrospinal fluid is shifted from the cranium into the spinal subarachnoid space. Patients on the rising portion of the curve (point 3) can no longer compensate for increases in intracranial volume; the ICP begins to increase and is likely to be associated with clinical symptoms. Additional increases in intracranial volume at this point (point 3), as produced by anesthetic drug–induced increases in cerebral blood volume, can precipitate abrupt increases in ICP (point 4).

contained within the ventricular system of the brain, the central canal of the spinal cord, and the subarachnoid space, as well as the extracellular compartment of the central nervous system. CSF is absorbed from microscopic arachnoid villi and macroscopic arachnoid granulations within the dura mater and bordering venous sinusoids and sinuses.

It is important to note that the intracranial vault is considered to be compartmentalized. Specifically, there are various meningeal barriers within the intracranial vault that functionally separate the contents: the falx cerebri (a reflection of dura mater that separates the two cerebral hemispheres) and the tentorium cerebelli (a reflection of dura mater that lies rostral to the cerebellum and marks the border between the supratentorial and infratentorial spaces). Increases in the contents of one region of brain may cause regional increases in ICP, and in extreme instances, the contents of that compartment can move, or herniate, into a different compartment. Various types of herniation syndromes are categorized based on the region of brain affected (Figure 10-3). Herniation of cerebral hemispheric contents under the falx cerebri is referred to as *subfalcine herniation*. Typically, this condition leads to compression of branches of the anterior cerebral artery and is evident on radiographic imaging as midline shift. Herniation of the supratentorial contents past the tentorium cerebelli is referred to as *transtentorial herniation*, in which evidence of brainstem compression occurs in a rostral to caudal manner, resulting in altered consciousness, defects in gaze and afferent ocular reflexes, and, finally, hemodynamic and respiratory compromise followed by death. The uncus (i.e., the medial portion of the temporal lobe) may herniate over the tentorium cerebelli, which results in a subtype of transtentorial

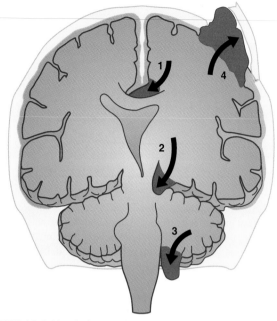

FIGURE 10-3 Herniation syndromes. An increase in the contents of the supratentorial space caused by masses, edema, or hematoma can lead to (1) herniation of the cingulate gyrus under the falx, or subfalcine herniation; (2) herniation of contents over the tentorium cerebelli, or transtentorial herniation; (3) herniation of the cerebellar tonsils out through the foramen magnum; and (4) herniation of brain contents out of a traumatic defect in the cranial cavity. *(Adapted from Fishman RA. Brain edema.* N Engl J Med. *1975;293:706-711.)*

herniation referred to as *uncal herniation*. A specific sign is ipsilateral oculomotor nerve dysfunction, because the oculomotor nerve is compressed against the brainstem; this results in pupillary dilatation, ptosis, and lateral deviation of the affected eye, which occurs before evidence of brainstem compression and death. Herniation of the cerebellar tonsils can occur in the setting of elevated infratentorial pressure, which leads to extension of these cerebellar structures through the foramen magnum. Typical signs are those indicating medullary dysfunction, including cardiorespiratory instability and subsequently death.

Nonspecific signs and symptoms of increased ICP include headache, nausea, vomiting, and papilledema. As ICP increases and cerebral perfusion is limited, decreased levels of consciousness and possibly coma can be observed. Acute increases in ICP may not be tolerated as well as chronic intracranial hypertension.

Increased ICP is often diagnosed clinically based on the symptoms described earlier, by radiographic means, and by direct measurement of ICP. Typically, computed tomography (CT) or magnetic resonance imaging (MRI) will help identify the cause of an increase in ICP. For example, a large mass or hematoma may be evident. If aqueductal stenosis is present, the third, but not fourth, ventricle is enlarged.

Several methods are currently available to measure and monitor ICP. The choice of technique depends on the clinical situation. Pressure transducers can be placed under aseptic conditions into the subdural space (known as a *subdural bolt*), brain parenchyma, or ventricle. This last technique, also known as a *ventriculostomy*, has the advantage that, in addition to pressure monitoring, it allows for withdrawal of CSF. This is a major benefit, since the drainage system can be organized so that CSF will only drain if the ICP is above a selected value. Such an approach allows some control over ICP. A second advantage of ventriculostomy is that CSF can be easily obtained for laboratory analysis. A lumbar subarachnoid catheter is another available modality. It offers advantages similar to those of ventriculostomy in that CSF can be withdrawn or allowed to passively drain if the ICP increases above a set value. The disadvantage of a lumbar subarachnoid catheter compared with ventriculostomy is that, because of the compartmentalization of the intracranial contents, lumbar CSF pressure may not accurately reflect ICP in all circumstances. In certain clinical settings, such as a brain tumor, there is also a risk of tonsillar herniation when CSF is drained using the lumbar subarachnoid approach.

A normal ICP waveform is pulsatile and varies with the cardiac impulse and spontaneous breathing. The mean ICP should remain below 15 mm Hg. Abrupt increases in ICP to as high as 100 mm Hg observed during continuous monitoring are characterized as *plateau waves*. During these dramatic increases in ICP, patients may become symptomatic and manifest evidence of inadequate cerebral perfusion. Spontaneous hyperventilation or changes in mental status may occur. Anxiety and painful stimulation can initiate abrupt increases in ICP.

Methods to Decrease Intracranial Pressure

Methods to decrease ICP include elevation of the head; hyperventilation; CSF drainage; administration of hyperosmotic drugs, diuretics, corticosteroids, and cerebral vasoconstricting anesthetics such as barbiturates and propofol; and surgical decompression. It is not possible to reliably identify the level of ICP that will interfere with regional CBF or alter cerebral function and well-being in individual patients. Therefore, a frequent recommendation is to treat any sustained increase in ICP that exceeds 20 mm Hg. Treatment may be indicated even when the ICP is less than 20 mm Hg if the appearance of occasional plateau waves suggests the presence of increased intracranial elastance.

Posture is important for ensuring optimal venous drainage from the brain. For example, elevating the patient's head to approximately 30 degrees above heart level encourages venous outflow from the brain and lowers ICP. Extreme flexion or rotation of the head can obstruct the jugular veins and restrict venous outflow from the brain. The head-down position must be avoided since this position can increase ICP.

Hyperventilation, and hence lowering of the $Paco_2$, is an effective method for rapidly reducing ICP. In adults a frequent recommendation is to maintain the $Paco_2$ near 30 to 35 mm Hg. Lowering the $Paco_2$ more than this may not meaningfully decrease ICP further, but may result in adverse changes in systemic physiology. The optimal $Paco_2$-related reduction in ICP is influenced by whether or not the patient is receiving a vasodilating or vasoconstricting anesthetic. However, regardless of the anesthetic used, the effects of hyperventilation will diminish with time and wane after 6 to 12 hours. When prolonged hyperventilation is discontinued, rebound increases in ICP are a potential problem, especially if normocapnia is rapidly restored.

Draining of CSF from the lateral cerebral ventricles or the lumbar subarachnoid space decreases intracranial volume and ICP. Lumbar CSF drainage via a catheter is usually reserved for operations in which surgical exposure is difficult, such as surgery on the pituitary gland or an intracranial aneurysm. Lumbar CSF drainage is not routinely used for the treatment of baseline intracranial hypertension, particularly that related to mass lesions, because of the fear that pressure gradients induced by drainage could result in cerebral herniation. If the cause of increased ICP is chronic, shunting of CSF from an intracranial ventricle is preferred. For long-term treatment, CSF is typically drained to the right atrium (ventriculoatrial shunt) or the peritoneal cavity (ventriculoperitoneal shunt).

Infusion of hyperosmotic drugs such as mannitol is effective in decreasing ICP. These drugs produce transient increases in the osmolarity of plasma, which act to draw water from tissues, including the brain. With osmotic diuretics, diuresis and a reduction in systemic blood volume, similar to that occurring with loop diuretics, are important secondary effects. When mannitol or any other diuretic is administered, care should be taken to avoid significant hypovolemia. Excessive fluid losses can result in hypotension and jeopardize maintenance of adequate CPP. In addition, urinary losses of electrolytes, particularly potassium, may occur, and thus careful monitoring and replacement are required. Moreover, an intact blood-brain barrier is necessary so that mannitol can exert maximum beneficial effects on brain size. If the blood-brain barrier is disrupted, these drugs may cross into the brain, causing cerebral edema and increases in brain size. The brain eventually adapts to sustained increases in plasma osmolarity, so long-term use of hyperosmotic drugs results in reduced effectiveness.

Mannitol is ideally administered in doses of 0.25 to 0.5 g/kg IV over 15 to 30 minutes. Larger initial doses have little incremental effect on ICP, but may predispose the patient to rebound increases in ICP. Hence, it is better to give an initial dose of 0.25 to 0.5 g/kg IV and, if the desired effect is not achieved, either administer another dose or switch to another type of therapy. Under ideal conditions, treatment with mannitol results in removal of approximately 100 mL of water from the brain. After mannitol administration, decreases in ICP are seen within 30 minutes, with maximum effects occurring within 1 to 2 hours. Urine output can reach 1 to 2 L within an hour after administration of mannitol. Appropriate infusion of crystalloid and colloid solutions may be necessary to prevent adverse changes in plasma electrolyte concentrations and intravascular fluid volume caused by the brisk diuresis. On the other hand, mannitol can initially increase intravascular

fluid volume, which emphasizes the need to carefully monitor patients who have limited cardiac reserve or congestive heart failure. Mannitol has direct vasodilating properties. Interestingly, mannitol can transiently contribute to increased CBV and ICP in individuals with normal ICP, but in those with intracranial hypertension, mannitol will *not* further increase ICP. The duration of the hyperosmotic effects produced by mannitol is approximately 6 hours.

Loop diuretics, particularly furosemide, have been used to decrease ICP. Furosemide is particularly useful in patients with evidence of increased intravascular fluid volume and pulmonary edema and in patients who, because of various co-existing diseases such as congestive heart failure or nephrotic syndrome, would not tolerate the initial increase in intravascular volume associated with mannitol use. In these patients furosemide will promote diuresis and systemic dehydration and improve arterial oxygenation along with causing a concomitant decrease in ICP. Furosemide affects plasma osmolarity much less than mannitol, but it can also produce hypokalemia.

Corticosteroids, such as dexamethasone or methylprednisolone, are effective in lowering ICP caused by the development of localized vasogenic cerebral edema around brain tumors. The precise mechanism of action is unknown but may involve stabilization of capillary membranes and decreased production of CSF. Patients with brain tumors often exhibit improved neurologic status and disappearance of headache within 12 to 36 hours after initiation of corticosteroid therapy. Corticosteroids are also effective in treating increased ICP in patients with pseudotumor cerebri (benign intracranial hypertension). On the other hand, corticosteroids are *not* effective in reducing ICP in some other forms of intracranial hypertension, such as closed head injury. Corticosteroids can increase blood glucose concentration, which may adversely affect outcome if ongoing cerebral ischemia is present. Because of this, corticosteroids should not be administered for the nonspecific treatment of increased ICP.

Barbiturates in high dosages are particularly effective in treating increased ICP that develops after an acute head injury. Propofol may also be useful in this situation. However, patients receiving prolonged propofol infusions, particularly pediatric patients, should be monitored for drug-associated metabolic acidosis, which can be fatal.

Specific Causes of Increased Intracranial Pressure

Increased ICP is typically a sign of an underlying intracranial pathologic process. Therefore, one should seek the cause of increased ICP in addition to instituting treatment. Causes of increased ICP are many. Tumors can lead to increased ICP either (1) directly because of their size, (2) indirectly by causing edema in normal surrounding brain tissue, or (3) by causing obstruction of CSF flow, as is commonly seen with tumors involving the third ventricle. Intracranial hematomas can cause increased ICP in a manner similar to mass lesions. Blood in the CSF, as is seen in subarachnoid hemorrhage, may lead to obstruction of CSF reabsorption at the arachnoid villi and granulations, and may further exacerbate increased ICP. Infection, such as meningitis or encephalitis, can lead to edema or obstruction of CSF reabsorption. Some causes of intracranial hypertension not discussed elsewhere in this chapter are described in the following sections.

AQUEDUCTAL STENOSIS

Stenotic central nervous system lesions that impede CSF flow can lead to increased ICP. Aqueductal stenosis, one of the more common causes of obstructive hydrocephalus, is caused by congenital narrowing of the cerebral aqueduct that connects the third and fourth ventricles. Obstructive hydrocephalus can present during infancy when the narrowing is severe. Lesser obstruction results in slowly progressive hydrocephalus, which may not be evident until adulthood. Symptoms of aqueductal stenosis are the same as those seen with other forms of intracranial hypertension. Seizure disorders are present in approximately one third of these patients. CT is useful to confirm the presence of obstructive hydrocephalus. Symptomatic aqueductal stenosis is treated by ventricular shunting. Management of anesthesia for ventricular shunt placement must focus on managing intracranial hypertension.

BENIGN INTRACRANIAL HYPERTENSION

Benign intracranial hypertension (pseudotumor cerebri) is a syndrome characterized by ICP higher than 20 mm Hg, normal CSF composition, normal sensorium, and absence of local intracranial lesions. This disorder typically occurs in obese women with menstrual irregularities. CT scan indicates a normal or even small cerebral ventricular system. Headaches and bilateral visual disturbances typically occur. Of note, symptoms may be exaggerated during pregnancy. Interestingly, no identifiable cause of increased ICP is found in most patients. The prognosis is usually excellent.

Acute treatment of benign intracranial hypertension includes removal of 20 to 40 mL of CSF via a needle or catheter placed in the lumbar subarachnoid space, as well as the administration of acetazolamide to decrease CSF formation. Patients also respond to treatment with corticosteroids. The principal indication for treatment is loss of visual acuity. Treatment may involve repeated lumbar punctures to remove CSF, which also facilitates measurement of ICP. Interestingly, continued leakage of CSF through the dural puncture site may be therapeutic. Long-term administration of acetazolamide can result in acidemia, which presumably reflects inhibition of hydrogen ion secretion by renal tubules. Surgical therapy, most often insertion of a lumboperitoneal shunt, is indicated only after medical therapy has failed and the patient's vision has begun to deteriorate. Optic nerve sheath fenestration is another surgical alternative to CSF shunting.

Anesthesia management for lumboperitoneal shunt placement involves avoiding exacerbation of intracranial hypertension and ensuring an adequate CPP. Hypoxia and hypercarbia must be rigorously avoided. Spinal anesthesia may be beneficial in parturient women, since continued leakage of CSF is acceptable. In the presence of a lumboperitoneal shunt, there is a theoretical possibility that local anesthetic solution injected into the subarachnoid space could escape into the peritoneal cavity, which could result in inadequate anesthesia. Therefore, general anesthesia may be a more logical choice in this patient population.

NORMAL PRESSURE HYDROCEPHALUS

Normal pressure hydrocephalus usually presents as the triad of dementia, gait changes, and urinary incontinence that develops over a period of weeks to months. The mechanism is thought to be related to compensated but impaired CSF absorption from a previous insult such as subarachnoid hemorrhage, meningitis, or head trauma. In most cases, however, the cause is never identified. Lumbar puncture usually reveals normal or low CSF pressure, yet CT or MRI will often demonstrate large ventricles. Treatment typically involves drainage of CSF via ventriculoperitoneal or ventriculoatrial shunting.

INTRACRANIAL TUMORS

Intracranial tumors may be classified as primary (those arising from the brain and its coverings) or metastatic. Tumors can originate from virtually any cell type within the central nervous system. Supratentorial tumors are more common in adults and often present with headache, seizures, or new neurologic deficits, whereas infratentorial tumors are more common in children and often present with obstructive hydrocephalus and ataxia. Treatment and prognosis depend on both the tumor type and location. Treatment may consist of surgical resection or debulking, chemotherapy, or radiation. Gamma Knife irradiation differs from traditional radiation therapy in that multiple radiation sources are used, and because the tumor is addressed from multiple angles, radiation to the tumor can be maximized while the radiation dose to any single area of surrounding brain tissue can be diminished. Such treatment can also be accomplished with the use of radiation produced by a linear accelerator.

Tumor Types

ASTROCYTOMA

Astrocytes are the most prevalent neuroglial cells in the central nervous system and give rise to many types of infratentorial and supratentorial tumors. Well-differentiated (low-grade) gliomas are the least aggressive class of astrocyte-derived tumors. They often are found in young adults with new-onset seizures. Imaging generally shows minimal enhancement with contrast. Surgical or radiation treatment of low-grade gliomas usually results in symptom-free long-term survival.

Pilocytic astrocytomas usually affect children and young adults. They often arise in the cerebellum (cerebellar astrocytoma), cerebral hemispheres, hypothalamus, or optic pathways (optic glioma). The tumor usually appears as a contrast-enhancing, well-demarcated lesion with minimal to no surrounding edema. Because of its benign pathologic characteristics, prognosis following surgical resection is generally very good. However, the location of the lesion, such as within the brainstem, may preclude resection.

Anaplastic astrocytomas are poorly differentiated, usually appear as a contrast-enhancing lesion on imaging because of disruption of the blood-brain barrier, and generally evolve into glioblastoma multiforme. Treatment involves resection, radiation, or chemotherapy. Prognosis is intermediate between that for low-grade gliomas and glioblastoma multiforme.

Glioblastoma multiforme (grade IV glioma) accounts for 30% of all primary brain tumors in adults. Imaging usually reveals a ring-enhancing lesion reflecting central necrosis and surrounding edema. Because of microscopic infiltration of normal brain by tumor cells, resection alone is usually inadequate. Instead, treatment generally consists of surgical debulking combined with chemotherapy and radiation and is aimed at palliation, not cure. Despite treatment, life expectancy may be measured in weeks.

OLIGODENDROGLIOMA

Oligodendrogliomas arise from myelin-producing cells within the central nervous system and account for only 6% of primary intracranial tumors. Classically, seizures predate the appearance of tumor on imaging, often by many years. Calcifications within the tumor are common and are visualized on CT imaging. The tumor usually consists of a mixture of both oligodendrocytic and astrocytic cells. Treatment and prognosis depend on the pathologic features. Initial treatment involves resection, since early in the course, the tumor typically consists of primarily oligodendrocytic cells, which are radioresistant. Because of the presence of astrocytic cells, these tumors commonly behave more like anaplastic astrocytomas or glioblastoma multiforme later in their course.

EPENDYMOMA

Arising from cells lining the ventricles and central canal of the spinal cord, ependymomas commonly present in childhood and young adulthood. Their most common location is the floor of the fourth ventricle. Symptoms include obstructive hydrocephalus, headache, nausea, vomiting, and ataxia. Treatment consists of resection and radiation. Tumor infiltration into surrounding tissues may preclude complete resection. Prognosis depends on the completeness of resection.

PRIMITIVE NEUROECTODERMAL TUMOR

Primitive neuroectodermal tumor represents a diverse class of tumors including retinoblastoma, medulloblastoma, pineoblastoma, and neuroblastoma, all believed to arise from primitive neuroectodermal cells. Medulloblastoma is the most common pediatric primary malignant brain tumor and may disseminate via the CSF to the spinal cord. The presentation of medulloblastoma is similar to that of ependymoma. Treatment usually involves a combination of resection and radiation given the tumor's high radiosensitivity. Prognosis is very good in children if treatment leads to disappearance of both tumor on MRI and tumor cells within the CSF.

MENINGIOMA

Meningiomas are usually extraaxial (arising outside of the brain proper), slow-growing, well-circumscribed, benign tumors arising from arachnoid cap cells, not the dura mater. Because of their slow growth, they can be very large at the time of diagnosis. They can occur anywhere arachnoid cap cells exist, but are most common near the sagittal sinus, falx cerebri, and cerebral convexity. Tumors are usually apparent on plain radiographs and CT scans as a result of the presence of calcifications. On MRI and conventional angiography, these tumors are often seen to receive their blood supply from the *external* carotid artery. Surgical resection is the mainstay of treatment. Prognosis is usually excellent. However, some tumors may be recurrent and require additional resection. Malignant meningiomas are rare.

PITUITARY TUMOR

Pituitary adenomas usually arise from cells of the anterior pituitary gland. They may occur along with tumors of the parathyroid glands and pancreatic islet cells as part of multiple endocrine neoplasia type I. These tumors are usually divided into functional (i.e., hormone-secreting) and nonfunctional types. The former usually present as an endocrinologic disturbance related to the hormone secreted by the tumor. Functional tumors are usually smaller (<1 cm in diameter) at the time of diagnosis; hence, they are often called *microadenomas*. Macroadenomas are usually nonfunctional, present with symptoms related to their mass (i.e., headache or visual changes resulting from compression of the optic chiasm), and are larger at the time of diagnosis, usually greater than 1 cm in diameter. Panhypopituitarism may be caused by either tumor type because of compression of normally functioning pituitary gland tissue. Pituitary tumors may also present as *pituitary apoplexy,* which is characterized by the abrupt onset of headache, visual changes, ophthalmoplegia, and altered mental status secondary to hemorrhage, necrosis, or infarction within the tumor. These tumors can also invade the cavernous sinus or internal carotid artery or compress various cranial nerves, causing an array of symptoms. Treatment depends on tumor type. Prolactinomas are often initially treated medically with bromocriptine. Surgical resection via the transsphenoidal approach or open craniotomy can be curative for most pituitary tumors.

ACOUSTIC NEUROMA

Usually the result of a benign schwannoma involving the vestibular component of cranial nerve VIII within the internal auditory canal, an acoustic neuroma typically occurs as a single mass. However, bilateral tumors may occur as part of neurofibromatosis type 2. Common presenting symptoms include hearing loss, tinnitus, and disequilibrium. Larger tumors, which grow out of the internal auditory canal and into the cerebellopontine angle, may cause symptoms related to compression of a cranial nerve, especially the facial nerve, or compression of the brainstem. Treatment usually consists of surgical resection with or without radiation therapy. Surgery generally involves intraoperative cranial nerve monitoring with electromyography or brainstem auditory evoked potentials. Prognosis is usually very good; however, recurrence of tumor is not uncommon.

CENTRAL NERVOUS SYSTEM LYMPHOMA

Central nervous system lymphoma is a rare tumor that can arise as a primary brain tumor, also known as a *microglioma*, or via metastatic spread from a systemic lymphoma. Primary central nervous system lymphoma can occur anywhere within the brain but is most common in supratentorial locations, especially in deep gray matter or the corpus callosum. Primary central nervous system lymphoma is thought to be associated with a variety of systemic disorders, including systemic lupus erythematosus, Sjögren's syndrome, rheumatoid arthritis, immunosuppressed states, and infection with Epstein-Barr virus. Symptoms depend on the location of the tumor. Diagnosis is made by imaging as well as biopsy. During biopsy, it may be reasonable to wait to administer corticosteroids, such as dexamethasone, until after pathologic specimens have been obtained, since these tumors may be very sensitive to steroids. Indeed, steroid-associated tumor lysis before a biopsy is performed may result in failure to obtain an adequate sample to make the diagnosis. The mainstay of treatment is chemotherapy (including intraventricularly delivered drugs) and whole-brain radiation. Prognosis is poor despite treatment.

METASTATIC TUMOR

Metastatic brain tumors originate most often from primary sites in the lung or breast. Malignant melanoma, hypernephroma, and carcinoma of the colon are also likely to spread to the brain. Metastatic brain tumor is the likely diagnosis when more than one intracranial lesion is present. Because of abnormal angiogenesis in metastatic lesions, these tumors tend to bleed more during resection than other central nervous system tumors.

Management of Anesthesia

Management of anesthesia during tumor resection procedures can be challenging, since patients may be of any age and a variety of operative positioning issues may arise. Furthermore, some procedures may be conducted with electrophysiologic monitoring, which may have implications for anesthetic drug choices and the use of muscle relaxants. Some procedures may even be performed in awake patients to facilitate resection of a mass located near an eloquent region of brain, such as the motor cortex. Major goals during anesthesia include (1) maintaining adequate cerebral perfusion and oxygenation of normal brain, (2) optimizing operative conditions to facilitate resection, (3) ensuring a rapid emergence from anesthesia at the conclusion of the procedure to facilitate neurologic assessment, and (4) accommodating intraoperative electrophysiologic monitoring if needed.

PREOPERATIVE MANAGEMENT

Preoperative evaluation of a patient with an intracranial tumor is directed toward identifying the presence or absence of increased ICP. Symptoms of increased ICP include nausea and vomiting, altered level of consciousness, mydriasis and decreased reactivity of pupils to light, papilledema, bradycardia, systemic hypertension, and breathing disturbances. Evidence of midline shifts (>0.5 cm) on CT or MRI suggests the presence of increased ICP.

Patients with an intracranial pathologic process may be extremely sensitive to the central nervous system depressant effects of opioids and sedatives. Drug-induced hypoventilation can lead to accumulation of arterial carbon dioxide and further increase ICP. Likewise, drug-induced sedation can mask alterations in the level of consciousness that accompany intracranial hypertension. On the other hand, preoperative sedation can unmask subtle neurologic deficits that may not usually be apparent. This is thought to result from an increased sensitivity of injured neurons to the depressant effects of various anesthetic and sedative agents. Considering all the potential adverse effects of preoperative medication, it is prudent to use premedication very sparingly. Preoperative administration of depressant drugs should be avoided in patients with diminished levels of consciousness. In alert adult patients with intracranial tumors, benzodiazepines in small doses can provide anxiety relief without meaningfully affecting ventilation. The decision to administer an anticholinergic drug or histamine 2 receptor antagonist is not influenced by the presence or absence of increased ICP.

INDUCTION OF ANESTHESIA

Anesthesia induction is typically achieved with drugs such as thiopental, etomidate, or propofol that produce a rapid, reliable onset of unconsciousness without increasing ICP. This can be followed by a nondepolarizing muscle relaxant to facilitate tracheal intubation. Administration of succinylcholine may be associated with a modest transient increase in ICP. Mechanical hyperventilation is initiated with the goal of decreasing $Paco_2$ to about 35 mm Hg. Adequate depth of anesthesia and profound skeletal muscle paralysis should be achieved before laryngoscopy to avoid the noxious stimulation or patient movement that can abruptly increase CBF, CBV, and ICP.

Direct laryngoscopy should be accomplished during profound skeletal muscle paralysis as confirmed by a nerve stimulator. Additional doses of intravenous anesthetic drugs, lidocaine 1.5 mg/kg IV, esmolol, or potent short-acting opioids may help blunt the response to laryngoscopy or other forms of intraoperative stimulation such as placement of pinions or skin incision.

Abrupt, sustained increases in systemic blood pressure, particularly in areas of impaired cerebral vasomotor tone, may be accompanied by undesirable increases in CBF, CBV, and ICP and precipitate cerebral edema. Sustained hypotension must also be avoided to prevent brain ischemia. Positive end-expiratory pressure has a highly variable effect on ICP. Hence, it should be used with caution, and attention must be paid to changes in ICP, MAP, and CPP as a result of this intervention.

MAINTENANCE OF ANESTHESIA

Maintenance of anesthesia in patients undergoing surgical resection of supratentorial brain tumors is often achieved by combining drugs of various classes, including nitrous oxide, volatile anesthetics, opioids, barbiturates, and propofol. Although modest cerebrovascular differences can be demonstrated with different combinations of drugs, there is no evidence that any particular combination is significantly different from another or superior in terms of effects on ICP and short-term patient outcome.

The use of nitrous oxide is controversial if there is any potential for venous air embolism (e.g., in operations performed with patients in the sitting position). Despite theoretical concerns, however, the actual incidence of venous air embolism in sitting patients is not influenced by nitrous oxide use. Once a venous air embolism has been detected, nitrous oxide use must be discontinued because of the concern that the embolus volume will expand and exacerbate the physiologic consequences of the embolus. Both nitrous oxide and potent volatile anesthetics have the potential to increase CBV and ICP as a result of direct cerebral vasodilation. However, low concentrations of volatile anesthetics (0.6 to 1.0 MAC) may be useful for preventing or treating increases in blood pressure related to noxious surgical stimulation. Administration of peripheral vasodilating drugs, such as nitroprusside or nitroglycerin, may increase CBV and ICP despite accompanying decreases in systemic blood pressure. This, in turn, can dramatically reduce CPP, which is dependent on both MAP and ICP. For this reason, vasodilating drugs should be used only after craniotomy and opening of the dura.

Spontaneous movement by patients undergoing surgical resection of brain tumors must be prevented. Such movement could result in an increase in intracranial volume and ICP, increased surgical bleeding (making surgical exposure difficult), or direct injury to the head and brain from pinions or surgical instrumentation. Therefore, in addition to adequate depth of anesthesia, skeletal muscle paralysis is typically maintained during intracranial surgery.

FLUID THERAPY

Relatively iso-osmolar solutions (e.g., 0.9% sodium chloride, lactated Ringer's solution) do not adversely affect brain water or edema formation provided the blood–brain barrier is intact, and they are used in modest amounts. In contrast, free water in hypo-osmolar solutions, such as 0.45% sodium chloride, is rapidly distributed throughout body water, including brain water, and may adversely affect ICP management. Hyper-osmolar solutions, such as 3% sodium chloride, initially tend to decrease brain water by increasing the osmolarity of plasma. Regardless of the crystalloid solution selected, any solution administered in large amounts can increase CBV and ICP in patients with brain tumors. Therefore, the rate of fluid infusion should be titrated to maintain euvolemia, and measures should be taken to avoid hypervolemia. Intravascular fluid volume depletion caused by blood loss during surgery should be corrected with packed red blood cells or colloid solutions supplemented with balanced salt solutions. Glucose-containing solutions should be avoided or used with caution, since hyperglycemia in the setting of central nervous system ischemia will exacerbate neuronal injury and worsen outcome.

MONITORING

The insertion of an intraarterial catheter is useful for continuous monitoring of blood pressure and blood sampling as needed. Capnography can facilitate ventilation and $Paco_2$ management as well as detect venous air embolism (see the section on the sitting position and venous air embolism). Continuous ICP monitoring, although not routine, can be of significant value. Nasopharyngeal or esophageal temperature is monitored to prevent hyperthermia or uncontrolled hypothermia. A bladder catheter has utility in managing perioperative fluid balance. It is necessary if drug-induced diuresis is planned; if the patient has diabetes insipidus, syndrome of inappropriate secretion of antidiuretic hormone, or other aberration of salt or water physiology; or if a lengthy surgical procedure is anticipated and bladder distention is a concern.

Intravenous access with large-bore catheters should be obtained, given the likelihood of bleeding and the need for transfusion or rapid administration of fluids. Central venous catheterization can be useful for both intravenous access and monitoring of fluid status. Central venous cannulation, with the tip of a multiorifice catheter placed at the junction of the superior vena cava and right atrium, also has utility as a means to aspirate intracardiac air following venous air embolism should this occur during surgery performed with the patient in the sitting position. Transesophageal echocardiography can also be useful for procedures in the sitting position to identify intravenous air and help assess cardiac function. Pulmonary artery catheterization should be considered in patients with cardiac disease.

A peripheral nerve stimulator is helpful for monitoring the persistence of drug-induced skeletal muscle paralysis. One must be aware that when paresis or paralysis of an extremity is associated with the brain tumor, the paretic extremity will show resistance (decreased sensitivity) to nondepolarizing muscle relaxants compared with a normal extremity (Figure 10-4). Therefore, monitoring of skeletal muscle paralysis on the paretic limb may provide misleading information. For example, the response to nerve stimulation may be erroneously interpreted as inadequate skeletal muscle paralysis. Likewise, at the conclusion of surgery, the nerve stimulator response could be interpreted as indicating better recovery from neuromuscular blockade than actually exists. These altered muscle responses to neuromuscular blockers likely reflect the proliferation of acetylcholine-responsive cholinergic receptors that can occur after denervation.

Monitoring of electrocardiographic (ECG) activity is necessary to detect responses related to intracranial tumors or surgery. ECG changes can reflect increased ICP or, more importantly, surgical retraction or manipulation of the brainstem or cranial nerves. Indeed, the cardiovascular centers, respiratory control areas, and nuclei of the lower cranial nerves lie in close proximity in the brainstem. Manipulation of the brainstem may produce systemic hypertension and bradycardia or hypotension and tachycardia. Cardiac dysrhythmias range from acute sinus arrhythmia to ventricular premature beats or ventricular tachycardia.

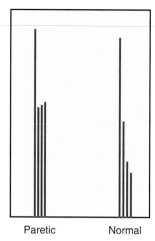

Paretic   Normal

FIGURE 10-4 In a surgical patient with mild residual hemiparesis after stroke, the train-of-four ratio recorded from the paretic arm (0.6) is higher than that recorded from the normal arm (0.3), which reflects resistance of the paretic arm to the effects of nondepolarizing muscle relaxants. *(Adapted from Moorthy SS, Hilgenberg JC. Resistance to nondepolarizing muscle relaxants in paretic upper extremities of patients with residual hemiplegia.* Anesth Analg. *1980;59:624-627.)*

POSTOPERATIVE MANAGEMENT

Ideally, the effects of anesthetics and muscle relaxants should be dissipated or pharmacologically reversed at the conclusion of surgery. This facilitates immediate monitoring of neurologic status and recognition of any adverse events related to the surgery. It is important to have patients awaken with little reaction to the presence of the endotracheal tube. Intraoperative use of narcotics and other drugs that suppress tracheal reflexes, such as lidocaine, may aid in attenuating the physiologic responses to the presence of the tube and facilitate optimal timing of extubation. However, it must be appreciated that the local anesthetic lidocaine also has general anesthetic properties and can produce central nervous system depression. If consciousness was depressed preoperatively or new neurologic deficits are anticipated as a result of the surgery, it may be best to delay tracheal extubation until return of airway reflexes is confirmed and spontaneous ventilation is sufficient to prevent carbon dioxide retention. Hypothermia may be a cause of slow postoperative awakening. Other causes of delayed emergence from anesthesia include residual neuromuscular block, residual effects of drugs with sedative effects (i.e., narcotics, benzodiazepines, volatile anesthetics), or a primary central nervous system event such as ischemia, hematoma, or tension pneumocephalus.

Following general anesthesia, a preexisting neurologic deficit may be exacerbated by the sedative effects of anesthetic drugs, which makes a subtle preoperative deficit appear more severe. This *differential awakening* is thought to be due to increased sensitivity of injured neurons to the depressant effects of anesthetic agents. Often, these deficits will disappear and neurologic function will return to its baseline state with time. Any persistent new deficit that does not quickly resolve must be further investigated.

SITTING POSITION AND VENOUS AIR EMBOLISM

Craniotomy to remove a supratentorial tumor is usually performed with the patient in the supine position with the head elevated 10 to 15 degrees to facilitate cerebral venous drainage. Infratentorial tumors have more unusual patient positioning requirements and may be performed with the patient in the lateral, prone, or sitting position.

The sitting position deserves special attention since it has a variety of implications for management of anesthesia. The sitting position is often used for exploration of the posterior cranial fossa, and it may be employed to resect intracranial tumors, clip aneurysms, decompress cranial nerves, or implant electrodes for cerebellar stimulation. In addition, it may be used for surgery on the cervical spine and posterior cervical musculature. Advantages of the sitting position include excellent surgical exposure and enhanced cerebral venous and CSF drainage, which minimizes blood loss and reduces ICP. These advantages are offset by the decreases in systemic blood pressure and cardiac output produced by this position, and the potential hazard of venous air embolism. For these reasons, the lateral or prone position is often selected as an alternative. However, as long as no contraindication to the sitting position exists, such as a patent foramen ovale, the outcome of patients undergoing surgery in the sitting position is similar or superior to that of patients placed in other positions.

If the sitting position is used, one should account for the effect of hydrostatic pressure gradients on CPP. Specifically, CPP should reflect correction for the hydrostatic pressure difference between the heart and the brain. This is generally accomplished by measuring blood pressure via an intraarterial catheter and referencing the pressure transducer to the vertical height of the external auditory meatus, which approximates the position of the circle of Willis. Lack of correction for hydrostatic pressure may put the patient at undue risk of cerebral hypoperfusion, since the measured systemic blood pressure, but not necessarily the true pressure at the level of the brain, will be greater if the transducer is referenced at the level of the heart.

Venous air embolism is a potential hazard whenever the operative site is above the level of the heart, so that pressure in the exposed veins is subatmospheric. Although this complication is most often associated with neurosurgical procedures, venous air embolism may also occur during operations involving the neck, thorax, abdomen, and pelvis and during open heart surgery, repair of liver and vena cava lacerations, obstetric and gynecologic procedures, and total hip replacement. Patients undergoing intracranial surgery are at increased risk not only because the operative site is above the level of the heart but also because veins in the skull may not collapse when cut, owing to their attachment to bone or dura. Indeed, the cut edge of cranial bone, including that associated with burr holes, is a common site for the entry of air into veins.

When air enters the right atrium and ventricle, there is interference with right-sided cardiac output and blood flow into the pulmonary artery. Air that eventually enters the pulmonary artery may trigger pulmonary edema and reflex bronchoconstriction. Death is usually secondary to an air lock in the right ventricular outflow tract that causes right-sided cardiac output to plummet, acute cor pulmonale to develop, and hypoxemia to occur from the combined cardiac and pulmonary insults.

Small quantities of air can sometimes pass through pulmonary vessels to reach the coronary and cerebral circulations. Large quantities of air can travel directly to the systemic circulation through right-to-left intracardiac shunts created by a patent foramen ovale or septal defects. This passage of air from the right to left circulation is known as *paradoxical air embolism.* Basically a venous embolism becomes an arterial embolism. A known patent foramen ovale or other cardiac defects that could result in a right-to-left shunt are relative contraindications to use of the sitting position.

Fatal cerebral embolism subsequent to entrainment of systemic venous air has occurred even in the absence of identifiable shunts or intracardiac defects. This may occur because of failure of contrast echocardiography to detect an existing patent foramen ovale or septal defect. There are many theoretical reasons for this failure of detection. One is that Valsalva or other provocative maneuvers are not always successful in mimicking the physiologic changes that occur during general anesthesia and true venous air embolism, and for this reason may underestimate the potential for venous air to pass from the right to the left circulation. Paradoxical air embolism can occur even in the absence of any detectable elevation of right atrial pressure compared with left atrial pressure. This happens as a result of small differences in the timing of contraction of the various heart chambers. As a result, pressure gradients transiently reverse, which makes a shunt bidirectional. An extremely brief right-to-left shunting could introduce a few air bubbles into the left cardiac chambers and lead to severe consequences if those bubbles were to embolize to the brain. Also, various anesthetic drugs may diminish the ability of the pulmonary circulation to filter out air emboli and thus facilitate the passage of venous air emboli through the pulmonary vasculature to the systemic circulation.

The use of the sitting position inherently predisposes neurosurgical patients to paradoxical air embolism, because the normal interatrial pressure gradient frequently becomes reversed in this position. When the likelihood of venous air embolism is increased, it is useful, but not mandatory, to place a right atrial catheter before beginning surgery. Death caused by paradoxical air embolism results from obstruction of the coronary arteries by air, which leads to myocardial ischemia and ventricular fibrillation. Neurologic damage may follow air embolism to the brain.

Early detection of venous air embolism is important for successful treatment. A Doppler ultrasonographic transducer placed over the right cardiac structures is one of the most sensitive detectors of intracardiac air. Indeed, the small amount of air detected by the transducer is often clinically unimportant. However, this transducer cannot provide information regarding the volume of air that has entered the venous circulation. Transesophageal echocardiography, by comparison, is useful for both detecting and quantifying intracardiac air. A sudden decrease in end-tidal $Paco_2$ may reflect increased alveolar dead space and/or diminished cardiac output resulting from air embolism. An increase in right atrial and pulmonary artery pressure can reflect acute cor pulmonale and correlates with abrupt decreases in end-tidal carbon dioxide concentration. Although $ETco_2$ changes are less sensitive indicators of the presence of air than the findings of Doppler ultrasonography or transesophageal echocardiography, they reflect the size of the venous air embolism. Increased end-tidal nitrogen concentration can identify and partially quantify the presence of venous air embolism. Changes in end-tidal nitrogen concentration may precede decreased end-tidal $Paco_2$ or increased pulmonary artery pressures. During controlled ventilation, sudden attempts by the patient to initiate spontaneous breaths (gasp reflex) may be the first indication of venous air embolism. Hypotension, tachycardia, cardiac dysrhythmias, and cyanosis are late signs of venous air embolism. Certainly detection of the characteristic mill wheel murmur, as heard through an esophageal stethoscope, is a late sign of catastrophic venous air embolism.

Once a venous air embolism is detected, the surgeon should flood the operative site with fluid, apply occlusive material to all bone edges, and attempt to identify any other sources of air entry such as perforation of a venous sinus. Aspiration of air should be attempted through the right atrial catheter. The ideal location for the tip of the right atrial catheter is controversial, but evidence suggests that the junction of the superior vena cava with the right atrium is preferable, because this position appears to provide the most rapid aspiration of air. Multiorifice right atrial catheters permit aspiration of larger amounts of air than do single-orifice catheters. Because of its small lumen and slow speed of blood return, a pulmonary artery catheter is not very useful for aspirating air but may provide additional evidence that venous air embolism has occurred. Administration of nitrous oxide is promptly discontinued to avoid increasing the size of any venous air bubbles. Indeed, elimination of nitrous oxide from the inhaled gases after detection of a venous air embolism often results in decreased pulmonary artery pressures. Pure oxygen is substituted for nitrous oxide. Direct jugular venous compression may increase venous pressure at the surgical site entraining air, but the use of positive end-expiratory pressure to accomplish this same effect has not been shown to be of value.

Extreme hypotension from massive air embolism may require support of the blood pressure using sympathomimetic drugs with inotropic and vasoconstrictive properties. Bronchospasm is treated with β_2-adrenergic agonists delivered by aerosol. Although the traditional admonition is to treat venous air embolism by placing the patient in the lateral position with the right chest uppermost, this is rarely possible or safe during intracranial surgery. It is likely that attempting to attain this patient position would lose valuable time that would be better spent aspirating air and supporting the circulation.

After successful treatment of small or modest venous air embolism, the surgical procedure can be resumed. However, the decision to reinstitute administration of nitrous oxide must be individualized. If nitrous oxide is not used, maintenance of an adequate depth of anesthesia requires administration of larger doses of volatile or intravenous anesthetics. If nitrous oxide is added to the inhaled gases, it is possible that residual air in the circulation could again produce symptoms.

Hyperbaric therapy may be useful in the treatment of both severe venous air embolism and paradoxical air embolism. Transfer of patients to a hyperbaric chamber in an attempt to decrease the size of air bubbles and improve blood flow is likely to be helpful only if the transfer can be accomplished within 8 hours.

The postoperative complications that may occur after posterior fossa craniotomy include apnea due to hematoma formation, tension pneumocephalus, and cranial nerve injuries. Macroglossia is also a possibility and is presumably due to impaired venous and lymphatic drainage from the tongue. This is sometimes associated with excessive neck flexion and may be influenced by the simultaneous use of multiple oral instruments (e.g., endotracheal tube, oral airway, esophageal stethoscope, transesophageal echocardiography probe).

DISORDERS RELATED TO VEGETATIVE BRAIN FUNCTION

Coma

Coma is a state of profound unconsciousness produced by drugs, disease, or injury affecting the central nervous system. It is usually caused by dysfunction of regions of the brain that are responsible for maintaining consciousness, such as the pontine reticular activating system, midbrain, or cerebral hemispheres. The causes of coma are many and can be divided into two groups: structural lesions (i.e., tumor, stroke, abscess, intracranial bleeding) and diffuse disorders (i.e., hypothermia, hypoglycemia, hepatic or uremic encephalopathy, postictal state following seizures, encephalitis, drug effects). The most common means used to assess the overall severity of coma is the Glasgow Coma Scale (Table 10-1).

The initial management of any comatose patient involves establishing a patent airway and ensuring the adequacy of oxygenation, ventilation, and circulation. One should then attempt to determine the cause of coma. This attempt should begin with obtaining a medical history from family members or caretakers, if possible, and conducting a physical examination followed by diagnostic studies. Blood pressure and heart rate are important because they might suggest a cause such as hypothermia. Respiratory patterns can also aid in diagnosis. Irregular breathing patterns may reflect an abnormality at a specific site in the central nervous system (Table 10-2). Ataxic breathing is characterized by a completely random pattern of tidal volumes that results from the disruption of medullary neural pathways by trauma, hemorrhage, or compression by tumors. Lesions in the pons may result in apneustic breathing characterized by prolonged end-inspiratory pauses maintained for as long as 30 seconds. Occlusion of the basilar artery

TABLE 10-1 Glasgow Coma Scale	
Response	**Score**
EYE OPENING	
Spontaneous	4
To speech	3
To pain	2
Nil	1
BEST MOTOR RESPONSE	
Obeys	6
Localizes	5
Withdraws (flexion)	4
Abnormal flexion	3
Extensor response	2
Nil	1
VERBAL RESPONSES	
Oriented	5
Confused conversation	4
Inappropriate words	3
Incomprehensible sounds	2
Nil	1

TABLE 10-2 Abnormal patterns of breathing		
Abnormality	**Pattern**	**Site of lesion/ condition**
Ataxic (Biot's breathing)	Unpredictable sequence of breaths varying in rate and tidal volume	Medulla
Apneustic breathing	Gasps and prolonged pauses at full inspiration	Pons
Cheyne-Stokes breathing	Cyclic crescendo-decrescendo tidal volume pattern interrupted by apnea	Cerebral hemispheres Congestive heart failure
Central neurogenic hyperventilation	Marked hyperventilation	Cerebral thrombosis or embolism
Posthyperventilation apnea	Awake apnea following moderate decreases in $Paco_2$	Frontal lobes

leading to pontine infarction is a common cause of apneustic breathing. Cheyne-Stokes breathing is characterized by breaths of progressively increasing and then decreasing tidal volume (crescendo-decrescendo pattern), followed by periods of apnea lasting 15 to 20 seconds. This pattern of breathing may reflect brain injury in the cerebral hemispheres or basal ganglia, or may be due to arterial hypoxemia and congestive heart failure. In the presence of congestive heart failure, the delay in circulation time from the pulmonary capillaries to the carotid bodies

TABLE 10-3 ▪ Neurologic findings on compression of the brainstem during transtentorial herniation

Region of compression	Pupillary examination	Response to oculocephalic or cold caloric testing	Gross motor findings
Diencephalon	Small pupils (2 mm) reactive to light	Normal	Purposeful, semipurposeful, or decorticate (flexor) posturing
Midbrain	Midsize pupils (5 mm) unreactive to light	May be impaired	Decerebrate (extensor) posturing
Pons or medulla oblongata	Midsize pupils (5 mm) unreactive to light	Absent	No response

Adapted from Aminoff MJ, Greenberg DA, Simon RP. *Clinical Neurology*. 3rd ed. Stamford, CT: Appleton & Lange; 1996:291.
In the early stages, the diencephalon (i.e., hypothalamic region) is compressed. Small pupils are the result of interrupted sympathetic innervation from hypothalamic compression. Reflex eye movements are intact, and motor responses may be purposeful or semipurposeful (i.e., localized to painful stimuli) early in the course but may progress to decerebrate posturing in response to stimuli. During midbrain compression, oculomotor nerve dysfunction leads to loss of the pupillary response to light. As the midbrain nuclei of cranial nerves that innervate extraocular muscles (i.e., oculomotor and trochlear) become affected, there is impaired response to oculocephalic and cold caloric testing. Further, decerebrate posturing is seen at this stage. As compression progresses to affect the pons or medulla oblongata, pupils are unresponsive, response to testing of reflexes involving eye movement is absent, and the patient is generally unresponsive to stimuli.

is presumed to be responsible for Cheyne-Stokes breathing. Central neurogenic hyperventilation is most often due to acute neurologic insults that are associated with cerebral thrombosis, embolism, or closed head injury. Hyperventilation is spontaneous and may be so severe that the $Paco_2$ is decreased to less than 20 mm Hg. The basic neurologic examination can be the key to diagnosis and should, at a minimum, include examination of the pupils and pupillary responses to light, function of the extraocular muscles via reflexes, and gross motor responses in the extremities (Table 10-3).

Under normal conditions, pupils are usually 3 to 4 mm in diameter and equal bilaterally, and react briskly to light, but approximately 20% of the general population normally have physiologic anisocoria, that is, a slight (<1 mm) difference in the diameters of the pupils. Compression of the diencephalon or thalamic structures leads to small (2 mm) but reactive pupils, probably resulting from interruption of descending sympathetic fibers. Unresponsive midsize pupils (5 mm) usually indicate midbrain compression. A fixed and dilated pupil (>7 mm) usually indicates oculomotor nerve compression and can be seen in herniation as well as either anticholinergic or sympathomimetic drug intoxication. Pinpoint pupils (1 mm) usually indicate opioid or organophosphate intoxication, focal pontine lesions, or neurosyphilis.

Evaluation of the function of the extraocular muscles allows testing of brainstem function via assessment of the function of the oculomotor, trochlear, and abducens nerves (cranial nerves III, IV, and VI). In the comatose patient, this testing can be performed by means of passive head rotation (oculocephalic reflex or doll's eye maneuver) or by cold water irrigation of the tympanic membrane (oculovestibular reflex or cold caloric testing). In unresponsive patients with normal brainstem function, oculocephalic maneuvers will produce full conjugate horizontal eye movements. Eliciting the oculovestibular reflex will result in tonic conjugate eye movements toward the side of cold water irrigation of the external auditory canal. Unilateral oculomotor nerve or midbrain lesions will result in failed adduction but intact contralateral abduction. Complete absence of responses can indicate pontine lesions or diffuse disorders.

Evaluation of motor responses to painful stimuli can also be helpful in localizing the cause of coma. Patients with mild to moderate diffuse brain dysfunction above the level of the diencephalon will usually react with purposeful or semipurposeful movements toward the painful stimulus. Unilateral reactions may indicate unilateral lesions such as stroke or tumor. Decorticate responses to pain consist of flexion of the elbow, adduction of the shoulder, and extension of the knee and ankle and are usually indicative of diencephalic dysfunction. Decerebrate responses consist of extension of the elbow, internal rotation of the forearm, and leg extension and imply more severe brain dysfunction. Patients with pontine or medullary lesions often exhibit no response to painful stimuli.

In cases in which the cause of coma is unknown, useful discriminatory laboratory tests include levels of serum electrolytes and glucose level to assess for disorders of sodium and glucose. Liver and renal function tests help to evaluate for hepatic or uremic encephalopathy. Drug and toxicology screens may help to identify exogenous intoxicants. A complete blood count and results of coagulation studies may suggest the risk of intracranial bleeding from thrombocytopenia or coagulopathy. CT or MRI may reveal a structural cause such as tumor or stroke. A lumbar puncture can be performed if meningitis or subarachnoid hemorrhage is suspected.

Outcomes for patients in comatose states depend on many factors but are usually related to the cause and extent of injury to brain tissue.

MANAGEMENT OF ANESTHESIA

Comatose patients may be brought to the operating suite either for treatment of the cause of the coma (e.g., burr hole drainage of an intracranial hematoma) or for treatment of injuries related to the comatose state (e.g., bone fractures caused by a motor vehicle accident in an intoxicated patient). It is important for the anesthesia provider to be aware of the likely cause of the coma, since anesthetic management will vary depending on the cause as well as the type of planned surgery. Primary overall goals should be to safely establish an airway, provide adequate cerebral perfusion and oxygenation, and optimize operating conditions. Careful attention should be paid to avoiding increases in ICP during stimulating events. Treatments should be instituted to decrease elevations in baseline ICP. Intracranial monitoring may be helpful. Intraarterial catheterization is useful for blood pressure optimization as well as management of hyperventilation, if needed. Anesthetic agents that increase ICP, such as halothane and ketamine, should be avoided, but other potent volatile agents such as isoflurane, sevoflurane, and desflurane, used at low doses (<1 MAC) in combination with intravenous cerebral vasoconstrictive anesthetics, are acceptable. Nitrous oxide should be avoided if the patient has known or suspected pneumocephalus (e.g., after recent intracranial surgery, basilar skull fracture). Administration of nondepolarizing muscle relaxants helps to facilitate tracheal intubation and patient positioning; however, succinylcholine is best avoided, since it may transiently increase ICP.

Brain Death and Organ Donation

Brain death is defined as the permanent cessation of total brain function. The traditional criteria used to define brain death, which are an adaptation of the original Harvard criteria established in 1968, are as follows:

Coma of an established and irreversible cause. All listed tests and assessments of reflexes should be performed after all possible reversible causes of coma have been ruled out.

    a. Lack of spontaneous movement, with the recognition that spinal reflexes may remain intact.

    b. Lack of all cranial nerve reflexes and function. This includes the failure of heart rate to increase by more than 5 beats per minute in response to intravenously, and preferably centrally, administered 0.04 mg/kg atropine, which suggests loss of vagal nuclear—and thus tonic vagal nerve—function.

    c. Positive result on an apnea test indicating lack of function of the respiratory control nuclei in the brainstem. The test is performed by initially ensuring a $Paco_2$ of 40 ± 5 mm Hg and an arterial pH of 7.35 to 7.45. The patient is then ventilated with 100% oxygen for longer than 10 minutes. Then, while vital signs are monitored and the trachea is insufflated with 100% oxygen, mechanical ventilation is discontinued for 10 minutes. Arterial blood gas values are obtained at 5 and 10 minutes following the cessation of mechanical ventilation and the patient is observed for signs of spontaneous respiration. Given that hypercarbia ($Paco_2 > 60$ mm Hg) is a potent stimulus for ventilation, if no respiratory activity is noted, the result of the apnea test is deemed positive.

Other confirmatory test results include isoelectricity demonstrated by EEG and absence of CBF as demonstrated by various techniques, including transcranial Doppler ultrasonography, cerebral angiography, and magnetic resonance angiography.

Following the establishment of the diagnosis of brain death and discussions with the immediate family, legal guardian, or next of kin, the decision is made either to withdraw artificial means of support or to proceed to organ retrieval if that was the wish of the patient or is the desire of the family or legal guardian.

MANAGEMENT OF ANESTHESIA

The major goal when patients diagnosed with brain death undergo surgery for multiorgan retrieval is to attempt to optimize oxygenation and perfusion of the organs to be retrieved. It is important to be aware of the various physiologic sequelae of brain death, because it is useful to direct management of physiologic parameters with the needs of the organ recipient, not the donor, in mind. Because of loss of central hemodynamic regulatory mechanisms—that is, the presence of neurogenic shock—brain-dead patients are often hypotensive. Hypovolemia caused by diabetes insipidus, third space losses, or drugs can contribute to hypotension. Aggressive fluid resuscitation should be considered, with efforts made to avoid hypervolemia, which could lead to pulmonary edema, cardiac distention, or hepatic congestion. Vasoconstrictive drugs should be avoided when considering pharmacologic treatment of hypotension. Inotropic agents are preferred for this. Dopamine and dobutamine should be first-line agents for the treatment of hypotension in euvolemic patients, with low-dose epinephrine as a second-line agent. For those in whom the heart is to be retrieved, catecholamine doses should be minimized because of the theoretical risk of catecholamine-induced cardiomyopathy. ECG abnormalities such as ST-segment and T-wave changes, as well as dysrhythmias, can occur. Possible causes include electrolyte abnormalities, loss of vagal nerve function, increased ICP, and cardiac contusion (if death was trauma related). Dysrhythmias should be treated pharmacologically or by electrical pacing.

Hypoxemia can occur as a result of diminished cardiac output or multiple pulmonary factors such as aspiration, edema, contusion, or atelectasis. Inspired oxygen concentration and ventilatory parameters should be adjusted in an attempt to maintain normoxia and normocapnia. Excessive positive end-expiratory pressure should be avoided because of its effect on cardiac output as well as the risk of barotrauma in the setting of possible trauma-related lung injury. Oxygen delivery to tissues should be optimized by treating coagulopathy and anemia with blood products.

Diabetes insipidus frequently occurs in brain-dead patients and, if not treated, can lead to hypovolemia, hyperosmolality, and electrolyte abnormalities that could contribute to hypotension and cardiac dysrhythmias. Treatment should initially include volume replacement with hypotonic solutions titrated to volume status and electrolyte concentrations. In severe cases, patients may need inotropic support, and either vasopressin (0.04 to 0.1 units/hr IV) or desmopressin (0.3 mcg/kg IV) to treat the diabetes insipidus. Because of its vasoconstrictive properties, vasopressin use should be minimized to avoid end-organ ischemia. A vasodilator such as nitroprusside may

TABLE 10-4 ▪ Characteristics of stroke subtypes

Parameter	Systemic hypoperfusion	Embolism	Thrombosis	Subarachnoid hemorrhage	Intracerebral hemorrhage
Risk factors	Hypotension Hemorrhage Cardiac arrest	Smoking Ischemic heart disease Peripheral vascular disease Diabetes mellitus White race and male gender	Smoking Ischemic heart disease Peripheral vascular disease Diabetes mellitus White race and male gender	Often none Hypertension Coagulopathy Drugs Trauma	Hypertension Coagulopathy Drugs Trauma
Onset	Parallels risk factors	Sudden	Often preceded by a transient ischemic attack	Sudden, often during exertion	Gradually progressive
Signs and symptoms	Pallor Diaphoresis Hypotension	Headache	Headache	Headache Vomiting Transient loss of consciousness	Headache Vomiting Decreased level of consciousness Seizures
Imaging	CT (hypodensity) MRI	CT (hypodensity) MRI	CT (hypodensity) MRI	CT (hyperdensity) MRI	CT (hyperdensity) MRI

Adapted from Caplan LR. Diagnosis and treatment of ischemic stroke. *JAMA.* 1991;266:2413-2418.
CT, Computed tomography; *MRI,* magnetic resonance imaging.

be administered with the vasopressin to avoid vasopressin-induced hypertension and vasoconstriction in end organs.

Because of loss of temperature-regulatory mechanisms, brain-dead patients tend to become poikilothermic and may require aggressive measures to avoid hypothermia. Although mild hypothermia possibly provides some degree of organ protection, it can also result in cardiac dysrhythmias, coagulopathy, and reduced oxygen delivery to tissue, thus causing harm to the organs to be retrieved. A good rule of thumb for the management of patients for organ donation is the rule of 100s: systolic blood pressure greater than 100 mm Hg, urine output greater than 100 mL/hr, PaO_2 greater than 100 mm Hg, and hemoglobin level greater than 100 g/L.

CEREBROVASCULAR DISEASE

Stroke is characterized by sudden neurologic deficits resulting from ischemia (88% of cases) or hemorrhage (12% of cases) (Table 10-4). Ischemic strokes are described by the area of the brain affected and the etiologic mechanism. Hemorrhagic strokes are classified as intracerebral (15%) or subarachnoid (85%).

Stroke is the third leading cause of death in the United States and the leading cause of major disability. The pathogenesis of stroke differs among ethnic groups. Extracranial carotid artery disease and heart disease–associated embolism more commonly cause ischemic stroke in non-Hispanic whites, whereas intracranial thromboembolic disease is more common in African Americans. Women have lower stroke rates than men at all ages until age 75 years and older. Stroke rates are at their highest after age 75. Overall, stroke-related mortality has decreased over the past several decades, probably because of better control of co-existing diseases such as hypertension and diabetes,

smoking cessation, and greater awareness of stroke and its risk factors.

Other disorders of the cerebrovascular system include atherosclerotic disease of the carotid artery, cerebral aneurysm, arteriovenous malformation, and moyamoya disease.

Cerebrovascular Anatomy

Blood supply to the brain (20% of cardiac output) is via two pairs of vessels: the internal carotid arteries and the vertebral arteries (Figure 10-5). These vessels join on the inferior surface of the brain to form the circle of Willis, which, under ideal circumstances, provides collateral circulation to multiple areas of the brain. Unfortunately, all of the elements of an intact circle of Willis are present in only about a third of people. Only 20% to 25% of people have a functionally normal circle of Willis in which no component is absent or hypoplastic. Each internal carotid artery gives rise to an anterior cerebral artery and continues on to become a middle cerebral artery. These vessels arising from the carotid arteries comprise the *anterior circulation* and ultimately supply the frontal, parietal, and lateral temporal lobes; the basal ganglia; and most of the internal capsule. The vertebral arteries each give rise to a posterior-inferior cerebellar artery before converging at the level of the pons to form the basilar artery. The basilar artery generally gives rise to two anterior-inferior and two superior cerebellar arteries before dividing to become the paired posterior cerebral arteries. Vessels that receive their predominant blood supply from this vertebral-basilar system comprise the *posterior circulation* and typically supply the brainstem, occipital lobes, cerebellum, medial portions of the temporal lobes, and most of the thalamus. The anterior and posterior circulations communicate via the posterior communicating artery,

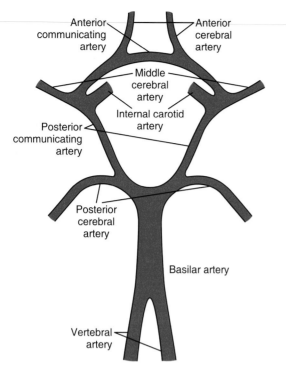

FIGURE 10-5 Cerebral circulation and circle of Willis. The cerebral blood supply is from the vertebral arteries (arising from the subclavian arteries) and the internal carotid arteries (arising from the common carotid arteries).

TABLE 10-5	Clinical features of cerebrovascular occlusive syndromes
Occluded artery	**Clinical features**
Anterior cerebral artery	Contralateral leg weakness
Middle cerebral artery	Contralateral hemiparesis and hemisensory deficit (face and arm more than leg)
	Aphasia (dominant hemisphere)
	Contralateral visual field defect
Posterior cerebral artery	Contralateral visual field defect
	Contralateral hemiparesis
Penetrating arteries	Contralateral hemiparesis
	Contralateral hemisensory deficits
Basilar artery	Oculomotor deficits and/or ataxia with crossed sensory and motor deficits
Vertebral artery	Lower cranial nerve deficits and/or ataxia with crossed sensory deficits

Adapted from Morgenstern LB, Kasner SE. Cerebrovascular disorders. *Sci Am Med*. 2000:1-15.

and the left and right anterior cerebral arteries communicate via the anterior communicating artery. Occlusion of specific arteries distal to the circle of Willis results in predictable clinical neurologic deficits (Table 10-5).

Acute Ischemic Stroke

Patients who experience the sudden onset of neurologic dysfunction or describe neurologic signs and symptoms evolving over minutes to hours are most likely experiencing a stroke. A transient ischemic attack is a sudden vascular-related focal neurologic deficit that resolves promptly (within 24 hours). A transient ischemic attack is not considered a separate entity but rather evidence of an impending ischemic stroke. Stroke represents a medical emergency, and the prognosis depends on the time elapsed from the onset of symptoms to thrombolytic intervention if thrombosis is the cause of the symptoms. Patients who receive early treatment to restore cerebral perfusion have better outcomes.

Systemic hypertension is the most significant risk factor for acute ischemic stroke, and long-term treatment of systolic or diastolic hypertension dramatically reduces the risk of a first stroke. Cigarette smoking, hyperlipidemia, diabetes mellitus, excessive alcohol consumption, and increased serum homocysteine concentrations are also associated with increased risk of acute ischemic stroke.

In patients with suspected stroke, the brain should be imaged using noncontrast CT, which reliably distinguishes

acute intracerebral hemorrhage from ischemia. This distinction is important, because treatment of hemorrhagic stroke is substantially different from treatment of ischemic stroke. CT is relatively insensitive to ischemic changes during the first few hours after a stroke, but is very sensitive for detection of intracranial bleeding.

Conventional angiography is useful for demonstrating arterial occlusion. The vasculature can also be visualized noninvasively using CT or magnetic resonance angiography. Alternatively, transcranial Doppler ultrasonography can provide indirect evidence of major vascular occlusion and offers the advantage of real-time bedside monitoring in patients undergoing thrombolytic therapy.

Acute ischemic stroke most likely reflects embolism occurring as a result of a cardiac cause, for example, atrial fibrillation, ventricular akinesis following myocardial infarction, dilated cardiomyopathy, valvular heart disease, large vessel atherothromboembolism (from atherosclerotic narrowing, especially at major arterial branch points such as the carotid bifurcation), or small vessel occlusive disease (lacunar infarction). Patients with long-standing diabetes mellitus or systemic hypertension are most likely to experience acute ischemic stroke resulting from small vessel occlusive disease. Echocardiography is useful for evaluating the presence of anatomic or vascular anomalies that could result in embolization.

MANAGEMENT OF ACUTE ISCHEMIC STROKE

Aspirin is often recommended as initial therapy in patients with an acute ischemic stroke and for the prevention of recurrent stroke. Intravenous recombinant tissue plasminogen activator is used in patients who meet specific eligibility requirements and in whom treatment can be initiated within 3 hours of the onset of acute symptoms. Direct infusion of thrombolytic drugs (prourokinase or recombinant tissue plasminogen activator) into occluded blood vessels is a potential alternative or adjunctive therapy to intravenous administration of recombinant tissue plasminogen activator. Despite advances in the treatment of acute ischemic stroke, most patients will have residual neurologic dysfunction. The initial stroke severity is a strong predictor of outcome, and early evidence of recovery is a good prognostic sign.

Management of the airway, oxygenation, ventilation, systemic blood pressure, blood glucose concentration, and body temperature are part of the overall medical management of acute ischemic stroke. In the most critically ill stroke patients, cerebral edema and increased ICP may complicate the clinical course. The expanding infarction may cause focal or diffuse mass effects that typically peak 2 to 5 days following stroke onset. Large hemispheric strokes may be characterized by *malignant middle cerebral artery syndrome,* in which the edematous infarcted tissue causes compression of the anterior and posterior cerebral arteries and results in secondary infarctions. Similarly, infarction of the cerebellum may result in basilar artery compression and brainstem ischemia. Mortality rates for both middle cerebral artery syndrome and infarction of the cerebellum approach 80%.

Surgical decompression has a role in a small number of stroke patients. Craniotomy with cerebellar resection is a lifesaving intervention for acute cerebellar stroke because it prevents secondary brainstem and vascular compression. Malignant middle cerebral artery syndrome may be amenable to treatment with hemicraniectomy.

Respiratory function must be evaluated promptly in all stroke patients. Ventilatory drive is usually intact except after medullary or massive hemispheric infarction. The ability to protect the lungs against aspiration may be impaired in the acute setting, so that endotracheal intubation is necessary. In most patients, however, supplemental oxygen administration without endotracheal intubation is sufficient to maintain arterial oxygen saturation at more than 95%.

Maintenance of adequate blood pressure is critically important, because blood flow to ischemic regions is dependent on CPP. Systemic hypertension is common at the time of initial stroke presentation, and rapid lowering of blood pressure can impair CBF and worsen the ischemic injury. Hypertension often gradually decreases during the first few days following an acute stroke. Antihypertensive drug therapy such as small intravenous doses of labetalol may be used when necessary to maintain the systemic blood pressure at less than 185/110 mm Hg in an attempt to lessen myocardial work and irritability. Appropriate intravascular volume replacement in patients with acute stroke improves cardiac output and cerebral perfusion. Hypervolemic hemodilution may be considered in an attempt to increase CBF while decreasing blood viscosity without causing a significant decrease in oxygen delivery.

Hyperglycemia appears to parallel poor outcomes in patients experiencing acute ischemic stroke. During periods of cellular hypoxia or anoxia, as occur with stroke, glucose is metabolized to lactic acid, which results in tissue acidosis and increased tissue injury. Normalization of blood glucose concentration is recommended, using insulin when appropriate. Parenteral administration of glucose should be avoided.

Based on animal data, hypothermia may improve outcome following acute ischemic stroke as a result of its ability to decrease neuronal oxygen demands, cerebral edema, and neurotransmitter toxicity. There are few human studies evaluating the effectiveness of hypothermia for the reduction of morbidity and mortality from acute stroke. Use of hypothermia in this setting continues to be controversial. However, it is certain that fever must be avoided in patients with acute stroke. Even a mild increase in body temperature can be deleterious. Normothermia should be maintained in acute ischemic stroke patients using antipyretics or cooling blankets as necessary.

Prophylaxis to prevent deep vein thrombosis is initiated early in the treatment of patients experiencing acute ischemic stroke. Heparin 5000 units SC every 12 hours is the most common intervention. Patients with acute hemorrhage who cannot be given heparin are treated with pneumatic compression stockings.

Acute Hemorrhagic Stroke

Acute hemorrhagic stroke results from either intracerebral hemorrhage or subarachnoid hemorrhage.

INTRACEREBRAL HEMORRHAGE

Intracerebral hemorrhage is four times more likely than ischemic stroke to cause death. It is notably a problem in African Americans. Acute hemorrhagic stroke cannot be reliably distinguished from ischemic stroke based on clinical criteria alone. A noncontrast CT evaluation is needed to detect the presence of bleeding. The estimated volume of extravasated blood and the level of consciousness are the two most reliable predictors of outcome. Patients with intracerebral hemorrhage often deteriorate clinically as cerebral edema worsens during the first 24 to 48 hours following the acute bleed. Late hematoma evacuation is ineffective in decreasing mortality. The efficacy of earlier surgical evacuation of a hematoma to decrease ischemic injury and edema to the surrounding tissue remains unclear. Intravenous administration of recombinant activated factor VII within 4 hours of onset of symptoms has been shown not only to decrease hematoma volume, but possibly to improve clinical outcome. Intraventricular hemorrhage is a particularly ominous form of intracranial hemorrhage because the blood will occlude CSF drainage. Prompt ventricular drainage should be performed to treat any signs of hydrocephalus. Sedation (with propofol infusion, barbiturates, or benzodiazepines), with or without drug-induced skeletal muscle paralysis, is often helpful in managing patients who require endotracheal intubation. An ICP monitor is often recommended for patients who are obtunded. Blood pressure management in patients who experience intracerebral hemorrhage is controversial because there is concern about decreasing CPP in those with increased ICP. In patients with co-existing essential hypertension, a goal may be to keep the MAP at less than 130 mm Hg.

SUBARACHNOID HEMORRHAGE AND INTRACRANIAL ANEURYSMS

Spontaneous subarachnoid hemorrhage most commonly results from rupture of an intracranial aneurysm. Various pathologic conditions such as hypertension, coarctation of the aorta, polycystic kidney disease, fibromuscular dysplasia, and the occurrence of cerebral aneurysms in first-degree relatives are associated with the presence of cerebral aneurysms. The risk of aneurysm rupture depends on the size of the aneurysm, with a 6% risk of rupture during the first year in aneurysms of at least 25 mm in diameter. Other risk factors for rupture include hypertension, cigarette smoking, cocaine abuse, female sex, and use of oral contraceptives.

Patients may also have unruptured aneurysms. A common presentation of an unruptured aneurysm is the development of a new focal neurologic deficit. The cause of this new deficit may be either a mass effect from an expanding aneurysm that compresses normal neurologic structures or small emboli to the distal cerebral circulation from a thrombus contained within the aneurysm. Headache caused by mass effect can occur. New-onset seizures can indicate an unruptured aneurysm and are thought to result from the formation of a glial scar (gliosis) in brain parenchyma adjacent to the aneurysm. Unruptured aneurysms may also be identified incidentally on cerebral imaging performed for unrelated reasons. The annual risk of rupture of an aneurysm depends on its diameter. For aneurysms smaller than 10 mm in diameter, the annual risk of rupture is approximately 0.05%, and for those larger than 10 mm in diameter, annual rupture risk is 1%. Aneurysm diameter is not static; thus, although smaller aneurysms may be followed with serial imaging, larger aneurysms are often considered for surgery.

The diagnosis of subarachnoid hemorrhage is based on clinical symptoms ("worst headache of my life") and CT demonstration of subarachnoid blood. MRI is not as sensitive as CT for detecting acute hemorrhage, especially with thin layers of subarachnoid blood, although this technique may be useful for demonstrating subacute or chronic subarachnoid hemorrhage or infarction after CT findings have returned to normal. In addition to severe headache, the rapid onset of photophobia, stiff neck, decreased level of consciousness, and focal neurologic changes suggest subarachnoid hemorrhage. Prompt establishment of the diagnosis followed by treatment of the aneurysm can decrease morbidity and mortality. Two of the most common methods used to grade the severity of subarachnoid hemorrhage are the Hunt and Hess classification and the World Federation of Neurologic Surgeons grading system (Table 10-6). These grading systems are useful because they help predict severity and outcome and can be used as metrics to evaluate the efficacy of various therapies.

Changes in the ECG are common following subarachnoid hemorrhage, typically ST-segment depression and T-wave inversion. These changes are most often noted within 48 hours

TABLE 10-6 ■ Common grading systems for subarachnoid hemorrhage

HUNT & HESS CLASSIFICATION

Score	Neurologic finding	Mortality
0	Unruptured aneurysm	0%-2%
1	Ruptured aneurysm with minimal headache and no neurologic deficits	2%-5%
2	Moderate to severe headache, no deficit other than cranial nerve palsy	5%-10%
3	Drowsiness, confusion, or mild focal motor deficit	5%-10%
4	Stupor, significant hemiparesis, early decerebration	25%-30%
5	Deep coma, decerebrate rigidity	40%-50%

WORLD FEDERATION OF NEUROLOGIC SURGEONS GRADING SYSTEM

Score	Glasgow Coma Scale score	Presence of Major Focal Deficit
0		Intact, unruptured aneurysm
1	15	No
2	13 or 14	No
3	13 or 14	Yes
4	7-12	Yes or no
5	3-6	Yes or no

Adapted from Lam AM. Cerebral aneurysms: anesthetic considerations. In: Cottrell JE, Smith DS, eds. *Anesthesia and Neurosurgery*. 4th ed. St Louis, MO: Mosby; 2001.

after the hemorrhage and have been attributed to catecholamine release. This same catecholamine release may result in cardiac dysrhythmias and may also be responsible for producing pulmonary edema. Echocardiography has demonstrated temporary depression of myocardial contractility, independent of coronary artery disease, in patients with subarachnoid hemorrhage. Of note, apical cardiac function may be preserved, a phenomenon attributed to the paucity of sympathetic innervation at the cardiac apex.

Treatment of subarachnoid hemorrhage involves localizing the aneurysm with conventional or magnetic resonance angiography and surgically excluding the aneurysmal sac from the intracranial circulation while preserving its parent artery. Outcome is optimal when surgical treatment is performed within the first 72 hours after bleeding. Placing a clip across the neck of the intracranial aneurysm is the most definitive surgical treatment. For larger or fusiform aneurysms that lack a definitive neck, surgical options include wrapping the exterior of the aneurysm or aneurysm trapping. In aneurysm trapping a clip is placed on the artery both proximal and distal to the aneurysm after the artery distal to the aneurysm has been bypassed, usually by means of the superficial temporal artery. Endovascular techniques that involve placing soft metallic coils in the lumen of an aneurysm may be an alternative to surgical therapy but may not be an option for the treatment of all aneurysms, specifically those with a large neck or those that lack a neck. Because of the immense morbidity and mortality associated with surgical treatment of basilar tip aneurysms, endovascular treatment is preferred in this situation.

Surgery is often delayed in patients with severe symptoms such as coma. In these patients, other options, including interventional radiographic procedures, may be used. Anticonvulsants are administered should seizure activity occur. Systemic blood pressure is controlled, in recognition that hypertension increases the risk of rebleeding. Hydrocephalus is common after subarachnoid hemorrhage and is treated with ventricular drainage. Any change in mental status must be promptly evaluated by CT to look for signs of rebleeding or hydrocephalus.

Following subarachnoid hemorrhage with or without surgical or endovascular treatment of the aneurysm, an important goal is prevention of vasospasm (intracranial arterial narrowing) and its consequences. Development of vasospasm can be triggered by many mechanisms, the most important of which is the contact of free hemoglobin with the abluminal surface of cerebral arteries. Not surprisingly, the incidence and severity of vasospasm correlate with the amount of subarachnoid blood seen on CT. Vasospasm typically occurs 3 to 15 days after subarachnoid hemorrhage. For this reason, daily transcranial Doppler ultrasonographic examinations may be performed to detect vasospasm. If vasospasm is identified, *triple H therapy* (*h*ypertension, *h*ypervolemia, passive *h*emodilution) is initiated. Colloid and crystalloid therapy can be used, and pressor support may be needed. Administration of nimodipine, a calcium channel blocker, has been shown to improve outcome when initiated on the first day and continued for 21 days after subarachnoid hemorrhage, which presumably reflects a protective effect from the consequences of vasospasm. This benefit of nimodipine occurs without angiographic evidence of vessel luminal enlargement. Cerebral angiographic techniques can also be employed to dilate vasospastic arteries mechanically (via balloons) or chemically (via intraarterial administration of papaverine).

MANAGEMENT OF ANESTHESIA

The goals of anesthesia during intracranial aneurysm surgery are to limit the risk of aneurysm rupture, prevent cerebral ischemia, and facilitate surgical exposure.

The goal during the induction of anesthesia is to prevent any increase in the transmural pressure of the aneurysmal sac, which could increase the risk of aneurysm rupture. Therefore, significant increases in systemic blood pressure must be avoided. In those patients with cerebral aneurysms *without* increased ICP and in those with unruptured aneurysms, it is reasonable to avoid excessive *decreases* in ICP before dural opening so as not to decrease the tamponading force on the external surface of the aneurysm. Hyperventilation then should be avoided. Patients who have increased ICP before surgery present a challenge because they may not tolerate a decrease in MAP to protect against aneurysm rupture without developing cerebral ischemia. Patients with vasospasm also present a quandary because systemic hypertension may improve flow through vasospastic vessels but may increase the risk of aneurysm rebleeding. Aneurysm clipping during the period in which the patient is at high risk of vasospasm is associated with increased mortality. Therefore, in patients with vasospasm who require anesthetic care, CPP should be kept elevated to maintain blood flow through vasospastic arteries.

Monitoring of the blood pressure via an intraarterial catheter is desirable to ensure the adequacy of blood pressure control during direct laryngoscopy and at other times of noxious stimulation. Prophylaxis against significant hypertension during direct laryngoscopy may be accomplished by administration of esmolol, lidocaine, propofol, barbiturates, or short-acting opioids. Loss of consciousness is achieved with intravenous administration of thiopental, propofol, or etomidate. Nondepolarizing neuromuscular blocking drugs are most often selected to facilitate endotracheal intubation.

Placement of a CVP catheter may be useful because of the likely presence of hypovolemia, the large intraoperative fluid shifts associated with osmotic and loop diuretics, the potential for intraoperative aneurysm rupture, and the need for fluid resuscitation. A pulmonary artery catheter or transesophageal echocardiography may be considered when patients have known cardiac disease. Electrophysiologic monitoring (EEG, somatosensory or motor-evoked potentials) may be helpful to identify intraoperative cerebral ischemia, but its complexity during this surgery limits its routine use.

The goals of anesthesia maintenance include providing a depth of anesthesia appropriate to the level of surgical stimulation, facilitating surgical exposure through optimal brain relaxation, maintaining CPP, reducing transmural pressure in the aneurysm during clipping of the aneurysm, and prompt awakening of the patient at the end of the procedure to permit immediate neurologic assessment. Drugs, fluid, and blood must be immediately available to manage resuscitation should the aneurysm rupture intraoperatively. The risk of intraoperative rupture is approximately 7%, and rupture most commonly occurs during the late stages of surgical dissection. Anesthetic management of rupture consists of aggressive volume resuscitation to maintain normovolemia combined with controlled hypotension (e.g., with nitroprusside) to temporarily limit hemorrhage and permit the neurosurgeon to gain control of the aneurysm.

If temporary clipping of the feeding vessel is used to gain control of a ruptured aneurysm, the systemic blood pressure can be returned to normal or even slightly elevated levels to improve collateral blood flow while the vessel is obstructed by the occlusion clip.

Anesthesia is typically maintained with volatile anesthetics (isoflurane, desflurane, sevoflurane) with or without the addition of nitrous oxide, which may be supplemented with intermittent (fentanyl) or continuous (remifentanil) infusion of opioids. Alternatively, a total intravenous anesthetic technique (propofol and short-acting opioid) can be used. Cerebral vasoconstricting anesthetics such as barbiturates and propofol help reduce brain volume and, in the case of barbiturates and possibly propofol, may provide some degree of neuronal protection against ischemia. Muscle paralysis is critical to prevent movement during aneurysm clipping.

In view of the current trend toward earlier surgical intervention in patients with subarachnoid hemorrhage due to rupture of an intracranial aneurysm, it is likely that many patients will have brain edema. Therefore, optimization of brain relaxation is an important part of anesthetic maintenance, and combinations of lumbar CSF drainage, mild hyperventilation, administration of loop and/or osmotic diuretics, and proper positioning to facilitate cerebral venous drainage can help to optimize surgical exposure. Intraoperative fluid administration is guided by blood loss, urine output, and measurement of cardiac filling pressures. Normovolemia is the goal, which is best achieved by intravenous administration of balanced salt solutions. Intravenous solutions containing glucose are *not* recommended because of fear of exacerbating neuronal injury. Current best evidence suggests no benefit to intraoperative hypothermia in patients undergoing aneurysm clipping. However, hyperthermia must be avoided because it increases $CMRO_2$ and CBV.

Traditionally, drug-induced controlled hypotension has been used to decrease transmural pressure in the aneurysm and thereby decrease the risk of aneurysm rupture during microscopic isolation and clipping. Controlled hypotension is used less often now than before because of concerns about the impairment of autoregulation that follows subarachnoid hemorrhage, unpredictable cerebrovascular responses to drug-induced hypotension, and the risk of global ischemia. As an alternative to drug-induced hypotension, *regional controlled hypotension* produced by placing a vascular clamp on the parent artery supplying the aneurysm provides protection against aneurysm rupture without incurring the risk of global cerebral ischemia. Ideally, temporary occlusion of the parent artery does not exceed 10 minutes. If longer periods of occlusion are needed, the administration of metabolism-suppressing anesthetics, particularly barbiturates, might provide protection against regional cerebral ischemia and infarction. However, the utility and efficacy of this intervention remains controversial. During temporary clamping of the feeding vessel, systemic blood pressure should be maintained toward the higher end of the normal blood pressure range to encourage collateral circulation.

At the conclusion of the surgical procedure, prompt emergence from anesthesia is desirable to facilitate immediate neurologic evaluation of the patient. The use of short-acting inhaled and intravenous anesthetic drugs makes prompt awakening more likely. However, incremental doses of antihypertensive drugs such as labetalol or esmolol may be needed as the patient emerges from anesthesia. Lidocaine may be administered intravenously to suppress airway reflexes and the response to the presence of the endotracheal tube. Tracheal extubation immediately after surgery is acceptable and encouraged in patients who are awake with adequate spontaneous ventilation and protective upper airway reflexes. Patients who were obtunded preoperatively are likely to require continued intubation and mechanical ventilation during the postoperative period. Patients who experience intraoperative rupture of an intracranial aneurysm may recover slowly and benefit from postoperative airway and ventilatory support.

Neurologic status is assessed at frequent intervals in the postanesthesia care unit or intensive care unit. Patients may manifest delayed emergence from anesthesia or focal neurologic deficits after intracranial aneurysm resection, and it may be difficult to distinguish between drug-induced causes (e.g., differential awakening) and surgical causes (e.g., ischemic or mechanical brain injury). The appearance of a new *focal* deficit should raise suspicion of a surgical cause, since anesthetic drugs would be expected to cause primarily global effects. Inequality of pupils that was not present preoperatively is also likely to reflect a surgical event. CT or angiography may be necessary if the patient does not awaken promptly. Successful surgical therapy may be followed by delayed neurologic deficits (hours to days later) resulting from cerebral vasospasm. This, in turn, requires aggressive therapy, including hypertension, hypervolemia, passive hemodilution, or invasive radiographic interventions.

The anesthetic goals for patients undergoing angiographically guided cerebral aneurysm coil placement are similar to those for patients undergoing aneurysm clip placement. Typically, coil placement procedures are performed using sedation or general anesthesia. The principal advantage of sedation is that intraprocedural neurologic assessment can be performed. However, patient movement during the procedure poses the risk of aneurysm rupture or coil dislodgment resulting in coil embolization. For this reason, general anesthesia is preferred during coil placement. Anesthetic goals include ICP control, maintenance of adequate cerebral perfusion without excessive hypertension, and facilitation of a rapid postprocedural assessment of neurologic function.

Arteriovenous Malformation

Arteriovenous malformations (AVMs) are abnormal collections of blood vessels in which multiple direct arterial-to-venous connections exist without intervening capillaries. There is also no neural tissue within the nidus. AVMs typically represent high-flow, low-resistance shunts, with vascular intramural pressure being less than systemic arterial pressure. Thus, rupture does not appear to be clinically associated with acute or chronic hypertension. These malformations are believed to be congenital and commonly present in adulthood as either hemorrhage or new-onset seizures. The exact cause of AVM-associated seizures is unknown but has been attributed to either steal (e.g., shunting of blood away from normal brain tissue toward the low-resistance AVM) or gliosis due to hemosiderin deposits from previous hemorrhage. Most AVMs are supratentorial. AVMs are associated with a 4% to 10% incidence of cerebral aneurysm. AVMs presenting in the neonatal or childhood period usually involve the vein of Galen, and presenting symptoms include hydrocephalus or macrocephaly and prominence of forehead veins, as well as evidence of a high-output cardiac state or heart failure. Diagnosis is made by either MRI or angiography.

TABLE 10-7 ■ Spetzler-Martin arteriovenous malformation (AVM) grading system

Graded feature	Points assigned
Nidus size	
Small (<3 cm)	1
Medium (3-6 cm)	2
Large (>6 cm)	3
Eloquence of adjacent brain*	
Noneloquent	0
Eloquent	1
Pattern of venous drainage	
Superficial only	0
Deep only or deep and superficial	1

SURGICAL OUTCOME BASED ON SPETZLER-MARTIN AVM GRADE

Grade	Percent of patients with no postoperative neurologic deficit
1	100
2	95
3	84
4	73
5	69

Adapted from Spetzler RF, Martin NA. A proposed grading system for arteriovenous malformations. *J Neurosurg.* 1986;65:476-483.
Points assigned in the three categories are added together to form a grade.
*Eloquent brain includes the sensory, motor, language, and visual areas as well as the hypothalamus, thalamus, internal capsule, brainstem cerebellar peduncles, and deep nuclei.

Before the advent of focused, high-dose radiation and selective cerebral angiography, treatment of AVMs was associated with a high morbidity and mortality. Currently, treatment may involve a combination of surgical resection, highly focused (Gamma Knife) irradiation, and/or angiographically guided embolization. With smaller AVMs, patients may respond completely to radiation or embolization therapy. With larger AVMs, however, these two techniques are typically used as adjunctive therapy before surgery to decrease the size of the AVM nidus and reduce both the complexity and risks of surgery. Prognosis and perioperative outcome can be estimated using the Spetzler-Martin AVM grading system, which classifies the AVM based on three features (Table 10-7).

Other types of intracranial AVMs include venous angiomas, cavernous angiomas, capillary telangiectasias, and arteriovenous fistulas.

VENOUS ANGIOMA

Venous angiomas or malformations consist of tufts of veins. Often, they are occult lesions found during cerebral angiography or MRI performed to evaluate other disease states. Rarely will a venous angioma present as either hemorrhage or new-onset seizures. These are low-flow, low-pressure lesions and usually contain intervening brain parenchyma within the nidus; they are therefore treated only if bleeding or intractable seizures occur.

CAVERNOUS ANGIOMA

Cavernous angiomas, also known as *cavernous hemangiomas* or *cavernomas,* are benign lesions consisting of vascular channels without large feeding arteries or large veins. Brain parenchyma is not found within the nidus of the lesion. These low-flow, well-circumscribed lesions often present as new-onset seizures but occasionally manifest as hemorrhage. They may be seen on CT or MRI scans and typically appear as a flow void on cerebral angiographs. Treatment involves surgical resection of symptomatic lesions. They do not respond to irradiation nor are they amenable to embolization, since they are angiographically silent.

CAPILLARY TELANGIECTASIA

Capillary telangiectasias are low-flow, enlarged capillaries and are probably one of the least understood vascular lesions in the central nervous system. They are angiographically silent and difficult to diagnose antemortem. The risk of hemorrhage is low except for lesions occurring in the brainstem. They are often found incidentally at autopsy and are often associated with other disorders, including Osler-Weber-Rendu syndrome and Sturge-Weber syndrome. These lesions are not treatable.

ARTERIOVENOUS FISTULA

Arteriovenous fistulas are direct communications between arteries and veins without an intervening nidus of smaller blood vessels. They commonly occur between meningeal vessels within the dura mater or between the carotid artery and venous sinuses within the cavernous sinus. Some arteriovenous fistulas are thought to occur spontaneously. Many others are associated with a previous traumatic injury or, in the case of carotid-cavernous fistulas, with previous (presumably silent) rupture of an intracavernous carotid artery aneurysm. Dural arteriovenous fistulas commonly present with pulsatile tinnitus or headache. An occipital bruit can be appreciated in 24% of these cases since the occipital artery is a common arterial feeder of an arteriovenous fistula. Treatment options include angiographically guided embolization or surgical ligation. Surgical treatment is associated with a risk of rapid and significant blood loss.

Patients with carotid-cavernous arteriovenous fistulas often have orbital or retro-orbital pain, arterialization of the conjunctiva, or visual changes. Diagnosis is made by magnetic resonance or conventional angiography. Embolization is usually an effective treatment option.

MANAGEMENT OF ANESTHESIA

Surgical resection of low-flow vascular malformations such as venous angiomas and cavernous angiomas is generally associated with fewer intraoperative and postoperative complications than resection of high-flow vascular lesions such as AVMs and arteriovenous fistulas. AVMs often involve multiple feeding and draining vessels, unlike arteriovenous fistulas, which involve a single feeding and a single draining vessel, so surgical resection of AVMs can pose great clinical challenges during resection and postoperative care.

Preoperatively, a patient with an intracranial vascular malformation should be evaluated for evidence of cerebral ischemia or increased ICP. The nature of the malformation, including size, location, mechanism of venous drainage, presence of associated aneurysms, and any prior treatment, should be elicited, since these factors may help in anticipating perioperative complications. Medications, including antiepileptic drugs if the patient has a concurrent seizure disorder, should be administered preoperatively. Patients who underwent preoperative angiography may experience fluid and electrolyte abnormalities secondary to the administration of hypertonic contrast material.

In addition to standard monitoring, an intraarterial catheter may be placed before induction of anesthesia. Blood pressure control throughout anesthesia, surgery, and the postoperative period is critical, since hypotension may result in ischemia in hypoperfused areas and hypertension may increase the risk of rupture of an associated aneurysm, exacerbate intraoperative bleeding, or worsen intracranial hypertension. For embolization or surgical resection of a vascular malformation in an eloquent region of brain, monitored anesthesia care is an attractive option. In cases requiring general anesthesia, a hemodynamically stable induction is desirable, although AVMs—unlike cerebral aneurysms—are unlikely to hemorrhage during anesthesia induction, even with moderate increases in blood pressure. Thiopental, propofol, and etomidate are all effective and safe induction agents. Muscle relaxation should be accomplished with a nondepolarizing neuromuscular blocking agent, since succinylcholine may induce further increases in ICP as well as cause hyperkalemia if motor deficits are present. Techniques to blunt the hemodynamic responses to stimulating events such as laryngoscopy, pinion placement, and incision should be used as needed. These may include the administration of lidocaine, esmolol, or nitroprusside or deepening of the anesthetic state with either higher concentrations of volatile anesthetics, small doses of intravenous anesthetics, short-acting opioids, or intravenous lidocaine.

Given the risk of severe and rapid *intraoperative* hemorrhage, especially with AVMs and arteriovenous fistulas, adequate intravenous access is essential. Further, central venous access may be useful in some cases to monitor volume status or to allow rapid administration of large volumes of fluids or blood products. Monitoring via a pulmonary artery catheter or transesophageal echocardiography can be useful in patients with cardiac disease.

In cases of large or high-flow vascular malformations, frequent communication with the surgeon is of paramount importance, because impressions of the lesions and the surgical and anesthetic requirements for safe resection may change during the operation. This is due, in part, to somewhat less than definitive imaging assessment preoperatively or changing surgical requirements during various stages of resection of a large, complex lesion. Hemodynamic stability, optimal surgical conditions, and rapid emergence from anesthesia at the end of surgery are appropriate goals when selecting anesthetic maintenance medications. Both intravenous and volatile anesthetic–based techniques are appropriate.

Hypotonic and glucose-containing solutions should be avoided, since the former can exacerbate cerebral edema and the latter can worsen the outcome of neurologic ischemia. Mild hyperventilation ($Paco_2$ of 30 to 35 mm Hg) will help facilitate surgical exposure. Lumbar CSF drainage may also help to decrease intracranial volume and improve exposure. Cerebral edema can be a significant problem during AVM treatment. Because AVMs represent high-flow, low-resistance vascular lesions, as arterial feeders are ligated during resection or embolization, blood flow is directed toward the surrounding brain tissue. These surrounding blood vessels may have experienced a chronic reduction in vascular resistance to compete with the AVM, so development of cerebral edema is quite possible. Treatment of cerebral edema may include moderate hyperventilation as a temporizing measure, administration of diuretics such as mannitol and furosemide, and blood pressure reduction. In extreme cases, high-dose barbiturate or propofol anesthesia or temporary craniectomy with postoperative ventilatory support may be useful.

Most patients respond quite well to surgical resection, and emergence from anesthesia should be smooth and rapid. Agents such as β-adrenergic antagonists as well as lidocaine or nitroprusside can be used to control short-term hypertension during emergence. Prompt neurologic assessment should follow emergence.

Moyamoya Disease

Progressive stenosis of intracranial vessels with the secondary development of an anastomotic capillary network is the hallmark of moyamoya disease. *Moyamoya* is the Japanese term for "puff of smoke" and refers to the angiographic finding of a cluster of small abnormal blood vessels. There seems to be a familial tendency toward the development of this disease, but it may be seen following head trauma or in association with other disorders such as neurofibromatosis, tuberous sclerosis, and fibromuscular dysplasia. Affected arteries have a thickened intima and a thin media. Since similar pathologic findings may be found in other organs, central nervous system abnormalities may be manifestations of a systemic disease. Intracranial aneurysms occur with increased frequency in those with moyamoya disease. Symptoms of ischemia, such as transient ischemic attacks and cerebral infarcts, are common initial findings in children, whereas hemorrhagic complications are usually the presenting symptoms in adults. The diagnosis is typically made by conventional or magnetic resonance angiography, which demonstrates a cluster of small abnormal blood vessels. Conventional MRI and CT imaging will show a tissue void or hemorrhage.

Medical treatment is aimed at decreasing ischemic symptoms and usually consists of a combination of vasodilators and anticoagulants. Surgical options include direct anastomosis of the superficial temporal artery to the middle cerebral artery (also known as an *extracranial-intracranial bypass*) or other indirect revascularization procedures, which may be combined with an extracranial-intracranial bypass. These techniques include laying the temporalis muscle directly on the brain surface and suturing the superficial temporal artery to the dura mater. Even with treatment, the overall prognosis is not good. Only about 58% of patients ever attain normal neurologic function.

MANAGEMENT OF ANESTHESIA

Preoperative assessment of the patient with moyamoya disease should involve documentation of preexisting neurologic deficits, a history of hemorrhage, or the concurrent presence of an intracranial aneurysm. Anticoagulant or antiplatelet drug therapy should be discontinued, if possible, to avoid bleeding complications intraoperatively.

The goals of induction and maintenance of anesthesia include (1) ensuring hemodynamic stability, because hypotension could lead to ischemia in the distribution of the abnormal vessels and hypertension may cause hemorrhagic complications; (2) avoiding factors that lead to cerebral or peripheral vasoconstriction, such as hypocapnia or phenylephrine, which can compromise blood flow in the feeding or recipient vessels; and (3) facilitating a rapid emergence from anesthesia so that neurologic function can be assessed. In addition to standard monitoring, intraarterial catheterization is essential to rapidly assess changes in blood pressure. If possible, this should be done before induction of anesthesia to help ensure a hemodynamically stable induction sequence. Central venous catheterization is not essential, but can be useful to guide fluid management and can also provide access for administering vasoactive agents or blood products. Any intravenous induction agent can be used safely. Inhalational induction with sevoflurane is an option for children. Succinylcholine should be used with caution in patients with preexisting neurologic deficits resulting from the risk of hyperkalemia. Hemodynamic responses to stimulating events should be blunted. A volatile anesthetic–based technique may have the theoretical advantage of enhancing cerebral vasodilation. Excessive hyperventilation should be avoided because of its cerebral vasoconstrictive effect. Hypovolemia should be treated with colloid or crystalloid solutions. Dopamine and ephedrine are reasonable options for the pharmacologic treatment of hypotension because they will avoid the adverse effects on the cerebral vasculature that can result from the use of a pure vasoconstrictor. Anemia should be avoided to prevent ischemia in already compromised brain regions.

Postoperative complications include stroke, seizure, and hemorrhage. Any of these may present as delayed awakening or a new neurologic deficit.

TRAUMATIC BRAIN INJURY

Traumatic brain injury is the leading cause of disability and death in young adults in the United States. Brain injury may result from both closed head injury and penetrating injuries caused by bullets or other foreign objects. Associated injuries, including cervical spine injury and thoracoabdominal trauma, frequently accompany acute head injury. Brain injury can be further exacerbated by systemic conditions related to trauma, including hypotension and hypoxia related to excessive bleeding, pulmonary contusion, aspiration, or adult respiratory distress syndrome.

Initial management of patients with acute head injury includes immobilization of the cervical spine, establishment of a patent airway, protection of the lungs from aspiration of gastric contents, and maintenance of brain perfusion by treatment of hypotension. The most useful diagnostic procedure, in terms of simplicity and rapidity, is CT, which should be performed as soon as possible. CT has greatly facilitated identification of epidural or subdural hematomas. Routine CT may not be needed in patients with minor head trauma who meet the following criteria: no headache or vomiting, younger than 60 years of age, no intoxication, no deficits in short-term memory, no physical evidence of trauma above the clavicles, and no seizures.

It is not unusual for patients with traumatic brain injury who initially are in stable condition and awake or in light coma to deteriorate suddenly. Delayed hematoma formation or cerebral edema is often responsible for these changes. Uncontrolled brain swelling that is not responding to conventional management may also cause sudden neurologic deterioration. Delayed secondary injury at the cellular level is an important contributor to brain swelling and subsequent irreversible brain damage.

The Glasgow Coma Scale provides a reproducible method for assessing the seriousness of brain injury and for following neurologic status (see Table 10-1). Head injury patients with scores of less than 8 are by definition in coma, and approximately 50% of these patients die or remain in vegetative states. The type of head injury and patient age are important determinants of outcome when Glasgow Coma Scale scores are low. For example, patients with acute subdural hematoma have a poorer prognosis than do patients with diffuse brain contusion injury. Mortality in children with severe head injury is lower than that in adults.

Perioperative Management

Perioperative management of patients with acute head trauma must consider the risks of ongoing injury to the brain as well as co-existing injuries affecting organs and structures other than the brain. CBF is usually initially reduced and then gradually increases with time. Factors contributing to poor outcome in head injury patients are increased ICP and MAPs of less than 70 mm Hg. Normal autoregulation of CBF is often impaired in patients with acute head injury, but carbon dioxide reactivity is usually preserved. Control of increased ICP with mannitol or furosemide is indicated, and in some patients craniectomy may be necessary. Hyperventilation, although effective in controlling ICP, may contribute to cerebral ischemia in patients with head injury, and for this reason, the common recommendation is to *avoid hyperventilation* as a routine treatment. Barbiturate coma may be useful in some patients to control intracranial hypertension when other measures have failed. In adults, induced mild hypothermia in patients with acute head injury has not been shown to improve outcome. Administration of hypertonic saline and mannitol may decrease brain volume. Associated lung injuries may impair oxygenation and ventilation in these patients and necessitate mechanical ventilation. Neurogenic pulmonary edema may also contribute to acute pulmonary dysfunction. The exact mechanism of neurogenic pulmonary edema is unknown, but it may be related to hyperactivity of the sympathetic nervous system resulting in alterations in Starling forces in the lung that ultimately result in pulmonary edema. Coagulopathy occurs in head injury patients and may be enhanced by hypothermia and the need for massive blood transfusion. Disseminated intravascular coagulation can occur following severe head injury and is perhaps related to the release of brain thromboplastin into the systemic circulation. Brain thromboplastin is known to activate the coagulation cascade. Replacement of clotting factors may be necessary.

Management of Anesthesia

Patients with traumatic brain injury may require anesthesia for neurosurgical interventions such as hematoma drainage, decompressive craniectomy for cerebral edema, or spinal stabilization. Anesthesia may also be required for the treatment of a variety of nonneurologic problems such as the repair of limb fractures and intraabdominal injuries. Management of anesthesia must include efforts to optimize CPP, minimize the occurrence of cerebral ischemia, and avoid drugs and techniques that could increase ICP. CPP should be maintained above 70 mm Hg if possible, and hyperventilation should *not* be used unless it is needed as a temporizing measure to control ICP. During surgical evacuation of acute epidural or subdural hematomas, systemic blood pressure may decrease precipitously at the time of surgical decompression and require aggressive management. Patients with severe head injury may experience impaired oxygenation and ventilation that complicates management during the intraoperative period. Adequate fluid resuscitation and replacement are important. Hypertonic crystalloid solutions, such as 3% saline, increase the plasma osmotic pressure and thus remove water from the brain's interstitial space. Hypotonic crystalloid solutions are avoided because they decrease plasma osmotic pressure and increase cerebral edema. Glucose-containing solutions must be avoided unless specifically indicated, such as for the treatment of laboratory-diagnosed hypoglycemia.

INDUCTION AND MAINTENANCE OF ANESTHESIA

In patients in hemodynamically stable condition, induction of anesthesia with intravenous induction drugs and nondepolarizing muscle relaxants is acceptable. Fiberoptically guided intubation or tracheostomy should be considered in patients

for whom there is concern either that tracheal intubation via direct laryngoscopy cannot be performed safely or that a neurologic deficit may be further exacerbated (e.g., in cases of cervical spine fracture) and in patients who already show evidence of airway compromise. In moribund patients, the establishment of a safe and effective airway takes priority over concerns about anesthetic drug selection, since drugs may not be needed. One must be aware of the possibility of hidden extracranial injuries (e.g., bone fractures, pneumothorax) that may lead to problems such as extensive blood loss or perturbations in ventilation and circulation. Maintenance of anesthesia often includes continuous infusions of intravenous drugs or low-dose volatile anesthetics with the goal of optimizing CPP and preventing increases in ICP. Nitrous oxide should be avoided because of the risk of pneumocephalus and concern for nonneurologic injuries such as pneumothorax. Low-dose sevoflurane may be desirable because of its relatively minimal impairment of cerebral autoregulation, although low-dose isoflurane is also a good choice. If acute brain swelling develops, correctable causes such as hypercapnia, arterial hypoxemia, hypertension, and venous obstruction must be considered and corrected if present. Intraarterial monitoring of blood pressure is very useful, but time constraints may limit the use of CVP or pulmonary artery catheter monitoring.

POSTOPERATIVE PERIOD

During the postoperative period, it is common to maintain skeletal muscle paralysis to facilitate mechanical ventilation. Continuous monitoring of ICP is also useful in many patients.

Hematomas

Hematoma formation can result from head trauma. Typically, four major types of intracranial hematomas are described based on their location: epidural, subarachnoid, subdural, and intraparenchymal.

EPIDURAL HEMATOMA

Epidural hematoma results from arterial bleeding into the space between the skull and the dura. The cause is usually a tear in a meningeal artery, and this may be associated with a skull fracture. Classically, patients experience loss of consciousness in association with the head injury, followed by return of consciousness and a variable lucid period. Hemiparesis, mydriasis, and bradycardia then suddenly develop a few hours after the head injury, reflecting uncal herniation and brainstem compression. If an epidural hematoma is suspected, treatment entails prompt drainage.

TRAUMATIC SUBARACHNOID HEMATOMA

Blood in the subarachnoid space most commonly follows rupture of an intracranial aneurysm. However, it can also be seen after trauma and is usually caused by bleeding from cortical blood vessels. It has been found in up to 40% of patients who have moderate or severe head injury. These lesions can evolve over time because of further bleeding. Like subarachnoid hemorrhage associated with aneurysm rupture, these hematomas are also associated with the development of cerebral vasospasm.

SUBDURAL HEMATOMA

Subdural hematoma results from laceration or tearing of bridging veins that bleed into the space between the dura and arachnoid. Examination of CSF reveals clear fluid, since subdural blood does not typically have access to the subarachnoid CSF. Diagnosis of a subdural hematoma is confirmed by CT. Head trauma is the most common cause of a subdural hematoma. Patients may view the causative head trauma as trivial or may even have forgotten it. This presentation is especially prevalent in elderly patients. Occasionally, subdural hematoma formation is spontaneous, such as in patients receiving hemodialysis or those being treated with anticoagulants.

Signs and symptoms of a subdural hematoma characteristically evolve gradually over several days (in contrast to epidural hematomas) because the hematoma is due to slow venous bleeding. Headache is a universal complaint. Drowsiness and obtundation are characteristic findings, but the magnitude of these changes may fluctuate from hour to hour. Lateralizing neurologic signs eventually occur, manifesting as hemiparesis, hemianopsia, or language disturbances. Elderly patients may have unexplained progressive dementia.

Conservative medical management of subdural hematomas may be acceptable for patients whose condition stabilizes, but surgical evacuation of the clot is desirable in most patients. The prognosis of subarachnoid hemorrhage is poor if coma develops. Most subdural hematomas can be drained via burr holes; the procedure can be performed under either general anesthesia, local anesthesia, or monitored anesthesia care. If the subdural hematoma is particularly large, is chronic, or consists of clotted blood, drainage may require craniotomy. Because a subdural hematoma is usually caused by venous bleeding, normocapnia is desirable following evacuation of the hematoma to allow for a larger brain volume, which may help to tamponade any sites of venous bleeding.

INTRAPARENCHYMAL HEMATOMA

An abnormal collection of blood located within the brain tissue proper is referred to as an *intraparenchymal hematoma*. These lesions can be difficult to treat because of their location and because they often acutely increase in size. Conservative management is usually initiated unless the size or rate of growth of the hematoma is likely to cause brain herniation.

CONGENITAL ANOMALIES OF THE BRAIN

Congenital anomalies of the central nervous system result from defects in the development or architecture of the nervous system. Often a hereditary pattern is responsible. Pathologic processes may be diffuse or may involve only those neurons that are anatomically and functionally related.

Chiari's Malformation

Chiari's malformation refers to a group of disorders consisting of congenital displacement of the cerebellum. A Chiari I malformation consists of downward displacement of the cerebellar tonsils over the cervical spinal cord, whereas a Chiari II malformation is downward displacement of the cerebellar vermis. This is often associated with a meningomyelocele. Chiari III malformations are extremely rare and represent displacement of the cerebellum into an occipital encephalocele.

Signs and symptoms of Chiari I malformation can appear at any age. The most common complaint is occipital headache, often extending into the shoulders and arms, with corresponding cutaneous dysesthesias. Pain is aggravated by coughing or moving the head. Visual disturbances, intermittent vertigo, and ataxia are prominent symptoms. Signs of syringomyelia are present in approximately 50% of patients with this disorder. Chiari II malformations usually present in infancy with obstructive hydrocephalus plus lower brainstem and cranial nerve dysfunction.

Treatment of Chiari's malformation consists of surgical decompression by freeing of adhesions and enlargement of the foramen magnum. Management of anesthesia must consider the possibility of increases in ICP as well as significant intraoperative blood loss, especially in the case of Chiari II malformations.

Tuberous Sclerosis

Tuberous sclerosis (Bourneville's disease) is an autosomal dominant disease characterized by mental retardation, seizures, and facial angiofibromas. Pathologically, tuberous sclerosis can be viewed as a condition in which a constellation of benign hamartomatous lesions and malformations occur in virtually every organ of the body. Brain lesions include cortical tubers and giant cell astrocytomas. Cardiac rhabdomyoma, although rare, is the most common benign cardiac tumor associated with tuberous sclerosis. Both echocardiography and MRI are useful for detecting cardiac tumors. An association of Wolff-Parkinson-White syndrome with tuberous sclerosis has been described. Co-existing angiomyolipomas and cysts of the kidney may result in renal failure. Oral lesions such as nodular tumors, fibromas, or papillomas may be present on the tongue, palate, pharynx, and larynx. The prognosis for patients with tuberous sclerosis depends on the organ systems involved and ranges from no symptoms to life-threatening complications.

Anesthesia management must consider the likely presence of mental retardation and a seizure disorder requiring antiepileptic drugs. Upper airway abnormalities must be identified preoperatively. Cardiac involvement may be associated with intraoperative cardiac dysrhythmias. Impaired renal function may have implications when selecting drugs that depend on renal clearance mechanisms. Although experience is limited, these patients seem to respond normally to inhaled and intravenous drugs, including opioids.

Von Hippel–Lindau Disease

Von Hippel–Lindau disease is a familial disease transmitted by an autosomal dominant gene with variable penetrance. It is characterized by retinal angiomas, hemangioblastomas, and central nervous system (typically cerebellar) and visceral tumors. Although these tumors are benign, they can cause symptoms resulting from pressure on surrounding structures or bleeding. The incidence of pheochromocytoma, renal cysts, and renal cell carcinoma is increased in this syndrome. These patients may require intracranial surgery for resection of hemangioblastomas.

Management of anesthesia in patients with von Hippel–Lindau disease must consider the possible presence of a pheochromocytoma. Preoperative treatment with antihypertensive drugs is indicated if a pheochromocytoma is identified. The possibility of spinal cord hemangioblastomas may limit the use of spinal anesthesia, although epidural anesthesia has been described for cesarean section. Exaggerated hypertension, especially during direct laryngoscopy or sudden changes in the intensity of surgical stimulation, may require intervention with esmolol, labetalol, sodium nitroprusside, or a combination of these drugs.

Neurofibromatosis

Neurofibromatosis is due to an autosomal dominant mutation. Both sexes are equally affected. Expressivity is variable, but penetrance of the trait is virtually 100%. Manifestations are categorized as classic (von Recklinghausen's disease), acoustic, or segmental.

The diversity of clinical features of neurofibromatosis emphasizes the protean nature of this disease (Table 10-8). One feature common to all cases is progression of the disease over time.

Café au lait spots (abnormal cutaneous pigmentation) are present in almost every affected individual. Six or more spots larger than 1.5 cm in diameter are considered diagnostic of neurofibromatosis. Café au lait spots are usually present at birth and continue to increase in number and size during the first decade of life. They can vary in size from 1 mm to more than 15 cm. The distribution of the spots is random, except that very few are present on the face. Although they have an adverse cosmetic effect, café au lait spots pose no direct threat to health.

Neurofibromas nearly always involve the skin, but they can also occur in the deeper peripheral nerves and nerve roots and in or on viscera or blood vessels innervated by the autonomic nervous system. These neurofibromas may be nodular and discrete or diffuse with extensive interdigitations into surrounding tissues. Although neurofibromas are histologically benign, functional compromise and cosmetic disfigurement may result from their presence. The airway may be compromised when neurofibromas develop in the laryngeal, cervical, or mediastinal regions. Neurofibromas may be highly vascular. Pregnancy or puberty can lead to increases in their number and size.

Intracranial tumors occur in 5% to 10% of patients with neurofibromatosis and account for a major portion of the morbidity and mortality of this disease. The bilateral presence of acoustic neuromas in patients with café au lait spots establishes the diagnosis of neurofibromatosis.

Congenital pseudoarthrosis—that is, a spontaneous fracture that progresses to nonunion—is commonly encountered in neurofibromatosis. The tibia is involved most often, with the radius the next most frequent site. Typically only a single site is involved in any one patient. The severity of pseudoarthrosis ranges from an asymptomatic radiographic presentation to a severe nonunion requiring limb amputation. Kyphoscoliosis occurs in approximately 2% of patients with neurofibromatosis. Cervical and thoracic vertebrae are most often involved. Paravertebral neurofibromas are often present, but their role, if any, in the development of kyphoscoliosis is unclear. Untreated, kyphoscoliosis often progresses, leading to cardiorespiratory and neurologic compromise. Short stature is a recognized feature of neurofibromatosis.

There is an increased incidence of cancer in patients with neurofibromatosis. Commonly associated cancers include neurofibrosarcoma, malignant schwannoma, Wilms' tumor, rhabdomyosarcoma, and leukemia.

Endocrine disorders can be associated with neurofibromatosis. These include pheochromocytoma, disturbances in sexual development, medullary thyroid carcinoma, and hyperparathyroidism. Pheochromocytomas occur with a frequency of less than 1% in adults with neurofibromatosis and are not seen in children with neurofibromatosis.

Intellectual impairment occurs in about 40% of patients with neurofibromatosis. Mental retardation is less frequent than learning disabilities. The intellectual handicap is usually apparent by school age and does not progress over time. Seizures may complicate neurofibromatosis and may be idiopathic or reflect the presence of intracranial tumors.

Treatment of neurofibromatosis consists of drug therapy as needed to treat symptoms, such as antiepileptic drugs, and appropriately timed surgery. Surgical removal of cutaneous neurofibromas is reserved for those lesions that are particularly disfiguring or cause functional problems. Progressive kyphoscoliosis is best treated with surgical stabilization. Nervous

---

TABLE 10-8 ■ Manifestations of neurofibromatosis

Café au lait spots
Neurofibromas (cutaneous, neural, vascular)
Intracranial tumor
Spinal cord tumor
Pseudarthrosis
Kyphoscoliosis
Short stature
Cancer
Endocrine abnormalities
Learning disability
Seizures

system involvement or associated endocrine dysfunction may also require surgery.

MANAGEMENT OF ANESTHESIA

Management of anesthesia in patients with neurofibromatosis includes consideration of the many clinical presentations of this disease. The possible presence of a pheochromocytoma should be considered during the preoperative evaluation. Signs of increased ICP may reflect expanding intracranial tumors. Airway patency may be jeopardized by expanding laryngeal neurofibromas. Patients with neurofibromatosis and scoliosis are likely to have cervical spine defects that could influence positioning for direct laryngoscopy and the subsequent surgical procedure. Responses to muscle relaxants are variable. These patients have been described as both sensitive and resistant to succinylcholine and sensitive to nondepolarizing muscle relaxants. Selection of regional anesthesia must consider the possible future development of neurofibromas involving the spinal cord. Epidural analgesia is an effective method for producing analgesia during labor and delivery.

DEGENERATIVE DISEASES OF THE BRAIN

Degenerative diseases of the central nervous system usually involve neuronal malfunction or loss within specific anatomic regions and represent a diverse group of disease states.

Alzheimer's Disease

Alzheimer's disease is a chronic neurodegenerative disorder. It is the most common cause of dementia in patients older than 65 years of age and the fourth most common cause of disease-related death in patients older than age 65. Diffuse amyloid-rich senile plaques and neurofibrillary tangles are the hallmark pathologic findings. There are also changes in synapses and in the activity of several major neurotransmitters, especially involving acetylcholine and central nervous system nicotinic receptors. Two types of Alzheimer's disease have been described: early onset and late onset. Early-onset Alzheimer's disease usually presents before age 60 and appears to be due to missense mutations in several genes. These mutations have an autosomal dominant mode of transmission. Late-onset Alzheimer's disease usually develops after age 60, and genetic factors appear to play a relatively minor role in the risk of developing this disorder. In both forms of the disease, patients typically develop progressive cognitive impairment that can consist of problems with memory as well as apraxia, aphasia, and agnosia. Definitive diagnosis is usually made on postmortem examination. The antemortem diagnosis of Alzheimer's disease is one of exclusion. There is currently no cure for Alzheimer's disease, and treatment focuses on control of symptoms. Pharmacologic options include cholinesterase inhibitors such as tacrine, donepezil, rivastigmine, and galantamine. Drug therapy should be combined with nonpharmacologic therapy including caregiver education and family support. Even with treatment, the prognosis for patients with Alzheimer's disease is poor.

Patients with Alzheimer's disease may come for a variety of surgical interventions that are common in the elderly population. Patients are often confused and sometimes uncooperative, which makes monitored anesthesia care or regional anesthesia challenging. There is no one single anesthetic technique or drug that is ideal in this group of patients. Shorter-acting sedative-hypnotic drugs, anesthetic agents, and narcotics are preferred since they allow a more rapid return to baseline mental status. One should be aware of potential drug interactions, especially prolongation of the effect of succinylcholine and relative resistance to nondepolarizing muscle relaxants resulting from the use of cholinesterase inhibitors.

Parkinson's Disease

Parkinson's disease is a neurodegenerative disorder of unknown cause. Increasing age is the single most important risk factor in the development of this disease. However, association between Parkinson's disease and manganese exposure in welders and a variety of genetic associations has recently been identified. There is a characteristic loss of dopaminergic fibers normally present in the basal ganglia, and as a result, regional dopamine concentrations are depleted. Dopamine is presumed to inhibit the rate of firing of the neurons that control the extrapyramidal motor system. Depletion of dopamine results in diminished inhibition of these neurons and unopposed stimulation by acetylcholine.

The classic triad of major signs of Parkinson's disease consists of skeletal muscle tremor, rigidity, and akinesia. Skeletal muscle rigidity first appears in the proximal muscles of the neck. The earliest manifestations may be loss of associated arm swings when walking and absence of head rotation when turning the body. There is facial immobility manifested by infrequent blinking and by a paucity of emotional expressions. Tremors are characterized as rhythmic, alternating flexion and extension of the thumbs and other digits (pill-rolling tremor). Tremors are more prominent during rest and tend to disappear during voluntary movement. Seborrhea, oily skin, diaphragmatic spasms, and oculogyric crises are frequent. Dementia and depression are often present.

Treatment of Parkinson's disease is designed to increase the concentration of dopamine in the basal ganglia or to decrease the neuronal effects of acetylcholine. Replacement therapy with the dopamine precursor levodopa combined with administration of a decarboxylase inhibitor, which prevents peripheral conversion of levodopa to dopamine and optimizes the amount of levodopa available to enter the central nervous system, is the standard medical treatment. Indeed, levodopa is the most effective treatment for Parkinson's disease, and early treatment with this drug prolongs life. Levodopa is associated with a number of side effects, including dyskinesias and psychiatric disturbances. The increased myocardial contractility and heart rate seen in treated patients may reflect increased levels of circulating dopamine converted from levodopa. Orthostatic hypotension may be prominent in treated patients. Gastrointestinal side effects of levodopa therapy include nausea and vomiting, most likely caused by stimulation of the medullary chemoreceptor trigger zone.

Amantadine, an antiviral agent, is reported to help control the symptoms of Parkinson's disease. The mechanism for its effect is not fully understood. The type B monoamine oxidase inhibitor selegiline can also help control the symptoms of Parkinson's disease by inhibiting the catabolism of dopamine in the central nervous system. Selegiline has an advantage over nonspecific monoamine oxidase inhibitors because it is not associated with the occurrence of tyramine-related hypertensive crises.

Surgical treatment of Parkinson's disease is reserved for patients with disabling and medically refractory symptoms. Stimulation of the various nuclei within the basal ganglia via an implanted deep brain stimulating device can relieve or help to control tremor. Pallidotomy is associated with significant improvement in levodopa-induced dyskinesias, although the improvement may be short-lived. Fetal tissue transplantation for treatment of Parkinson's disease is based on the demonstration that implanted embryonic dopaminergic neurons can survive in recipients. The effectiveness of this treatment is not currently known.

Deep brain stimulator placement is often done in an awake patient. However, in certain circumstances, such as in patients with developmental delay or those with severe claustrophobia, the procedure is performed under general anesthesia. The procedure begins with placement of a rigid head frame, followed by MRI to allow for coordinate determination relative to fiduciary markers on the head frame. The deep brain electrode is then advanced through a burr hole, often with microelectrode recordings taken, since specific nuclei differ in their spontaneous firing patterns. The target tissue is then stimulated via the electrode to determine if clinical symptoms abate. Following successful brain lead placement, a generator pack is implanted below the clavicle or in the abdomen. Of note, deep brain stimulation is currently under investigation for treatment of a variety of other disorders, such as Hallervorden-Spatz disease, depression, and eating disorders.

MANAGEMENT OF ANESTHESIA

Management of anesthesia in patients with Parkinson's disease requires an understanding of how this disease is treated. The elimination half-time of levodopa and the dopamine it produces is brief, so interruption of drug therapy for more than 6 to 12 hours can result in an abrupt loss of therapeutic effects. Abrupt drug withdrawal can also lead to skeletal muscle rigidity, which can interfere with ventilation. Therefore, levodopa therapy, including the usual morning dose on the day of surgery, must be continued throughout the perioperative period. Oral levodopa can be administered approximately 20 minutes before induction of anesthesia, and the dose may be repeated intraoperatively and postoperatively via an orogastric or nasogastric tube as needed.

The possibility of hypotension and cardiac dysrhythmias must be considered, and butyrophenones (e.g., droperidol, haloperidol) must be available to antagonize the effects of dopamine in the basal ganglia. Acute dystonic reactions following administration of alfentanil might indicate an opioid-induced decrease in central dopaminergic transmission. The use of ketamine is controversial because of the possible provocation of exaggerated sympathetic nervous system responses, but ketamine has been administered safely to patients treated with levodopa. The choice of a muscle relaxant is not influenced by the presence of Parkinson's disease.

Patients undergoing deep brain stimulator implantation may have been told by the surgeon to refrain from taking the usual morning dose of levodopa to facilitate the return of tremors and enhance sensitivity in detecting the efficacy of deep brain stimulation during the procedure. If that is the case, then establishment of intravenous access may prove challenging in an extremity with a significant tremor. Patients should receive minimal sedation during lead placement to prevent interference with microelectrode recordings and clinical assessment. Since γ-aminobutyric acid (GABA) is a common neurotransmitter involved in the normal circuitry of the basal ganglia, anesthetic agents with significant effects on GABA, such as propofol and benzodiazepines, can alter the characteristic microelectrode recordings of specific nuclei and should be avoided. Sedative agents such as opioids and dexmedetomidine are more satisfactory alternatives. Excessive sedation should be avoided not only to minimize difficulty obtaining neurologic assessments, but more importantly to avoid respiratory depression in a patient in whom there is little access to the airway because of the presence of a head frame. A variety of airway management devices (e.g., fiberoptic bronchoscope, laryngeal mask airway) should be readily available should airway compromise become an issue intraoperatively.

Lead placement can be a long procedure, so care should be taken to position the patient properly and comfortably. Proper padding should be placed at sites that may be prone to pressure injury.

The procedure is performed with the patient in the sitting position, so there is a risk of air embolism. Precordial Doppler ultrasonographic monitoring can help identify air entrainment. If venous air embolism and oxygen desaturation occur, the patient should *not* be encouraged to take a deep breath, because this can lower intrathoracic pressure and cause the entrainment of even more air. Instead, the surgeon should flood the field with saline and attempt to identify and treat the site of air entrainment. In more severe cases, the patient should be placed supine and hemodynamic support instituted.

Other potential complications of deep brain stimulation placement include hypertension, seizures, and bleeding. Hypertension should be treated to avoid increasing the risk of intracranial hemorrhage. Seizures often spontaneously abate, but very small doses of a barbiturate, propofol, or a benzodiazepine may be required to terminate their activity despite the potentially suppressive effect of administration of these drugs on microelectrode recordings. The effect of these drugs on ventilatory drive must also be appreciated and minimized. A sudden alteration of consciousness could indicate intracranial hemorrhage. Hemorrhage would require aggressive management, such as emergent removal of the head frame, endotracheal intubation, and craniotomy after imaging.

Hallervorden-Spatz Disease

Hallervorden-Spatz disease is a rare autosomal recessive disorder of the basal ganglia. It follows a slowly progressive course from its onset during late childhood to death in approximately 10 years. No specific laboratory tests are diagnostic for this condition, and no effective treatment is known. Dementia, dystonia with torticollis, and scoliosis are commonly present. Dystonic posturing often disappears with the induction of general anesthesia. However, skeletal muscle contractures and bony changes that accompany this chronic disease can cause immobility of the temporomandibular joint and cervical spine, even in the presence of deep general anesthesia or drug-induced skeletal muscle paralysis.

Management of anesthesia must consider the possibility that these patients may not be able to be positioned optimally for tracheal intubation. Noxious stimulation caused by attempted awake tracheal intubation can intensify dystonia, so an inhalation induction with maintenance of spontaneous ventilation is a common choice. Administration of succinylcholine is potentially dangerous, since skeletal muscle wasting and diffuse axonal changes in the brain that involve upper motor neurons could accentuate the release of potassium. However, safe use of succinylcholine has been reported. Required skeletal muscle relaxation is best provided by deep general anesthesia or administration of nondepolarizing neuromuscular blockers. Emergence from anesthesia is predictably accompanied by return of dystonic posturing.

Huntington's Disease

Huntington's disease is a degenerative disease of the central nervous system characterized by marked atrophy of the caudate nucleus and, to a lesser degree, the putamen and globus pallidus. Biochemical abnormalities include deficiencies in the basal ganglia of acetylcholine (and its synthesizing enzyme choline acetyltransferase) and GABA. Selective loss of GABA can decrease inhibition of the dopamine nigrostriatal system. Huntington's disease is transmitted as an autosomal dominant trait, but its delayed appearance at 35 to 40 years of age interferes with effective genetic counseling. Identification of the genetic defect may be useful for disease risk prediction in those who have inherited the defective gene.

Manifestations of Huntington's disease consist of progressive dementia combined with choreoathetosis. Chorea is usually considered the first sign of Huntington's disease. This is the reason for the former designation of this disease as *Huntington's chorea*. Behavioral changes such as depression, aggressive outbursts, and mood swings may precede the onset of involuntary movements by several years. Involvement of the pharyngeal muscles makes these patients susceptible to pulmonary aspiration. The disease progresses over several years, and accompanying mental depression makes suicide a frequent cause of death. The duration of Huntington's disease from clinical onset to death averages 17 years.

Treatment of Huntington's disease is symptomatic and is directed at decreasing the choreiform movements. Haloperidol and other butyrophenones may be administered to control the chorea and emotional lability associated with the disease. The most useful therapy for controlling involuntary movements is drugs that interfere with the neurotransmitter effects of dopamine either by antagonizing dopamine (haloperidol, fluphenazine) or by depleting dopamine stores (reserpine, tetrabenazine).

Experience in the management of anesthesia in patients with Huntington's chorea is too limited to allow recommendation of specific anesthetic drugs or techniques. Preoperative sedation using butyrophenones such as droperidol or haloperidol may be helpful in controlling choreiform movements. The increased likelihood of pulmonary aspiration must be considered. Use of nitrous oxide and volatile anesthetics is acceptable. Thiopental, succinylcholine, and mivacurium have been administered without adverse effects, but decreased plasma cholinesterase activity with prolonged responses to succinylcholine has been observed. It has been suggested that these patients may be sensitive to the effects of nondepolarizing muscle relaxants.

Torticollis

Torticollis is thought to result from disturbances in basal ganglia function. The most common mode of presentation is spasmodic contraction of nuchal muscles, which may progress to involvement of limb and girdle muscles. Hypertrophy of the sternocleidomastoid muscles may be present. Spasm may involve the muscles of the vertebral column, leading to lordosis, scoliosis, and impaired ventilation. Treatment is not very effective, but bilateral anterior rhizotomy at C1 and C3, with a sectioning of the spinal accessory nerve, may be attempted. This operation may cause postoperative paralysis of the diaphragm, resulting in respiratory distress. Selective peripheral denervation of affected cervical musculature is another surgical option. There are no known problems influencing the selection of anesthetic drugs, but spasm of nuchal muscles can interfere with maintenance of a patent upper airway before institution of skeletal muscle paralysis. Awake tracheal intubation may be necessary if chronic skeletal muscle spasm has led to fixation of the cervical vertebrae. Surgery may be performed with the patient in the sitting position. If so, anesthetic considerations related to use of the sitting position and the potential for venous air embolism will come into play.

The sudden appearance of torticollis after administration of anesthetic drugs has been reported. Administration of diphenhydramine 25 to 50 mg IV produces a dramatic reversal of this drug-induced torticollis.

Transmissible Spongiform Encephalopathies

The human transmissible spongiform encephalopathies are Creutzfeldt-Jakob disease (CJD), kuru, Gerstmann-Sträussler-Scheinker syndrome, and fatal familial insomnia. These noninflammatory diseases of the central nervous system are caused by transmissible slow-acting infectious protein pathogens known as *prions*. Prions differ from viruses in that they lack RNA and DNA and fail to produce a detectable immune reaction. Transmissible spongiform encephalopathies are diagnosed on the basis of clinical and neuropathologic findings, including the presence of diffuse or focal clustered small round vacuoles that may become confluent. Familial progressive subcortical gliosis and some inherited thalamic dementias may also be spongiform encephalopathies. Bovine spongiform encephalopathy (mad cow disease) is a transmissible spongiform encephalopathy that occurs in animals. Infectivity of skeletal muscles, milk, and blood has not been detected.

CJD is the most common transmissible spongiform encephalopathy, with an estimated incidence of one case per million worldwide. Transmission of the prion and the development of clinical disease are still poorly understood. In fact, a significant proportion of the population are probably carriers of the CJD prion, but most do not develop clinical disease. Approximately 10% to 15% of patients with CJD have a family history of the disease, so both infectious and genetic factors probably play a role in disease development. The time interval between infection and development of symptoms is measured in months to years. The disease develops by accumulation of an abnormal protein thought to act as a neurotransmitter in the central nervous system. This prion protein is encoded by a specific gene, and sporadic and random mutations result in variants of CJD. Rapidly progressive dementia with ataxia and myoclonus suggests the diagnosis, although confirmation usually requires brain biopsy because there are no reliable noninvasive diagnostic tests. Alzheimer's disease poses the most difficult differential diagnosis. Unlike in toxic and metabolic disorders, myoclonus is rarely present at the onset of CJD, and seizures, when they occur, are a late phenomenon. No vaccines or treatments are effective.

Universal infection precautions are recommended when caring for patients with CJD, but other precautions are not necessary. Handling of CSF calls for special precautions (use of double gloves and protective glasses, specimen labeling as "infectious"), since CSF has been the only body fluid shown to result in transmission to primates. Performance of biopsies and autopsies requires similar precautions. The main risk of transmitting CJD is during brain biopsy for diagnostic confirmation of the disease. Instruments used should be disposable or should be decontaminated by soaking in sodium hypochlorite or autoclaving.

Human-to-human transmission has occurred inadvertently in association with surgical procedures (corneal transplantation, stereotactic procedures with previously used electrodes, procedures with contaminated neurosurgical instruments, and human cadaveric dura mater transplantation). Transmission also has been attributed to treatment with human-derived growth hormone and gonadotropic hormones. Although the injection or transplantation of human tissues may result in transmission of infectious prions, the hazards of transmission through human blood are debatable, since this disease is not observed more frequently in individuals with hemophilia than in the general population. Nevertheless, transfusion of blood from individuals known to be infected is not recommended.

Management of anesthesia includes the use of universal infection precautions, disposable equipment, and sterilization of any reusable equipment using sodium hypochlorite. Surgery in patients known or suspected to be infected might be better performed at the end of the day to allow thorough cleansing of equipment and the operating room before the next use. The number of personnel participating in anesthesia and surgery is kept to a minimum, and all should wear protective gowns, gloves, and face masks with transparent visors to protect the eyes. Since a proportion of the general population are probably carriers of the prion thought to cause CJD and both infectious and genetic factors play a role in the development of clinical symptoms, the likelihood of developing CJD after coming in contact with a CJD prion is probably very low. However, standard precautionary measures still should be taken.

Multiple Sclerosis

Multiple sclerosis is an autoimmune disease affecting the central nervous system that seems to occur in genetically susceptible persons. There is a high rate of concordance among twins and an increased risk in individuals who have a first-degree relative with the disease. There are also geographic associations with this disease, which reaches its highest incidence in northern Europe, southern Australia, and North America. However, no clear genetic, environmental, or infectious causes have yet been identified. There is also no clear understanding of the immunopathogenic processes that determine the sites of tissue damage in the central nervous system, the variations in natural history, and the severity of disability caused by this disease.

Pathologically, multiple sclerosis is characterized by diverse combinations of inflammation, demyelination, and axonal damage in the central nervous system. The loss of myelin covering the axons is followed by formation of demyelinative plaques. Peripheral nerves are not affected by multiple sclerosis.

Clinical manifestations of multiple sclerosis reflect its multifocal involvement. The course may be subacute, with relapses followed by remissions, or the course may be chronic and progressive. Manifestations of multiple sclerosis reflect the sites of demyelination in the central nervous system and spinal cord. For example, inflammation of the optic nerves (optic neuritis) causes visual disturbances, involvement of the cerebellum leads to gait disturbances, and lesions of the spinal cord cause limb paresthesias and weakness as well as urinary incontinence and impotence. Optic neuritis is characterized by diminished visual acuity and defective pupillary reaction to light. Ascending spastic paresis of the skeletal muscles is often prominent. Intramedullary disease of the cervical cord is suggested by an electrical sensation that runs down the back into the legs in response to flexion of the neck (Lhermitte's sign). Typically, symptoms develop over the course of a few days, remain stable for a few weeks, and then improve. Because remyelination probably does not occur in the central nervous system, remission of symptoms most likely results from correction of transient chemical and physiologic disturbances that have interfered with nerve conduction in the areas of demyelination. Increases in body temperature can also cause exacerbation of symptoms due to further alterations in nerve conduction in regions of demyelination. There is an increased incidence of seizure disorders in patients with multiple sclerosis.

The course of multiple sclerosis is characterized by exacerbations and remissions at unpredictable intervals over a period of several years. Symptoms eventually persist during remissions, leading to severe disability from visual failure, ataxia, spastic skeletal muscle weakness, and urinary incontinence. However, in some patients the disease remains benign, with infrequent, mild episodes of demyelination, followed by prolonged remissions. The onset of multiple sclerosis after 35 years of age is typically associated with slow disease progression.

The diagnosis of multiple sclerosis can be established with different degrees of confidence—that is, probable or definite—on the basis of clinical features alone or clinical features in combination with oligoclonal immunoglobulin abnormalities in the CSF, prolonged latency of evoked potentials reflecting slowing of nerve conduction resulting from demyelination, and signal changes in white matter seen on cranial MRI.

No treatment is curative for multiple sclerosis, so treatment is directed at symptom control and slowing of disease progression. Corticosteroids, the principal treatment for acute relapses of multiple sclerosis, have immunomodulatory and antiinflammatory effects that restore the blood–brain barrier, decrease edema, and possibly improve axonal conduction. Treatment with corticosteroids shortens the duration of a relapse and accelerates recovery, but whether the overall degree of recovery or progression of the disease is altered is not known. Interferon-β is the treatment of choice for patients with relapsing-remitting multiple sclerosis. The most common side effect of interferon-β therapy is transient influenza-like symptoms for 24 to 48 hours after injection. Slight increases in serum aminotransferase concentrations, leukopenia, or anemia may be present, and co-existing depression may be exaggerated. Glatiramer acetate is a mixture of random synthetic polypeptides synthesized to mimic myelin basic protein. This drug is an alternative to interferon-β and is most useful in patients who become resistant to interferon-β treatment caused by serum interferon-β–neutralizing activity. Mitoxantrone is an immunosuppressive drug that functions by inhibiting lymphocyte proliferation. Because of severe cardiac toxicity, its use is limited to patients with rapidly progressive multiple sclerosis. Azathioprine is a purine analogue that depresses both cell-mediated and humoral immunity. Treatment with this drug may decrease the rate of relapses in multiple sclerosis but has no effect on the progression of disability. Azathioprine is considered when patients show no response to therapy with interferon-β or glatiramer acetate. Low-dose methotrexate is relatively nontoxic and inhibits both cell-mediated and humoral immunity due to its antiinflammatory effects. Patients with secondary progressive multiple sclerosis may benefit from treatment with this drug.

MANAGEMENT OF ANESTHESIA

Management of anesthesia in patients with multiple sclerosis must consider the impact of surgical stress on the natural progression of the disease. Regardless of the anesthetic technique or drugs selected for use during the perioperative period, it is possible that symptoms and signs of multiple sclerosis will be exacerbated postoperatively. This may be due to factors such as infection and fever. Any increase in body temperature, even of as little as 1° C, can cause an exacerbation of multiple sclerosis. It is possible that increased body temperature results in complete block of conduction in demyelinated nerves. The unpredictable cycle of clinical exacerbations and remissions that are inherent in multiple sclerosis might lead to erroneous conclusions that there are cause-and-effect relationships between disease severity and drugs or events occurring during the perioperative period.

The changing and unpredictable neurologic presentation of patients with multiple sclerosis during the perioperative period must be appreciated when regional anesthetic techniques are selected. Indeed, spinal anesthesia has been implicated in postoperative exacerbations of multiple sclerosis, whereas exacerbations of the disease after epidural anesthesia or peripheral nerve blockade have not been described. The mechanism by which spinal anesthesia might differ in this regard from epidural anesthesia is unknown, but it might involve local anesthetic neurotoxicity. Specifically, it is speculated that the demyelination associated with multiple sclerosis renders the spinal cord more susceptible to the neurotoxic effects of local anesthetics. Epidural anesthesia may carry less risk than spinal anesthesia because the concentration of local anesthetics in the white matter of the spinal cord is lower than after spinal anesthesia. Nevertheless, both epidural anesthesia and spinal anesthesia have been used in parturient women with multiple sclerosis.

General anesthesia is the most frequently used technique in patients with multiple sclerosis. There are no unique interactions between multiple sclerosis and the drugs used to provide general anesthesia, and there is no evidence to support use of one inhaled or injected anesthetic drug over another. When selecting muscle relaxants, one should consider the possibility of exaggerated release of muscle potassium, causing hyperkalemia, following administration of succinylcholine to these patients. Prolonged responses to the paralyzing effects of nondepolarizing muscle relaxants would be consistent with co-existing skeletal muscle weakness and decreased skeletal muscle mass. However, resistance to the effects of nondepolarizing muscle relaxants has been observed, which perhaps reflects the proliferation of extrajunctional cholinergic receptors characteristic of upper motor neuron lesions.

Corticosteroid supplementation during the perioperative period may be indicated in patients being treated long term with these drugs. Efforts must be made to recognize and prevent even a modest increase in body temperature, since this change may exacerbate symptoms. Periodic neurologic evaluation during the postoperative period is useful for detection of exacerbations.

Postpolio Sequelae

Poliomyelitis is caused by an enterovirus that initially infects the reticuloendothelial system. In a minority of patients, the virus enters the central nervous system and preferentially targets motor neurons in the brainstem and anterior horn of the spinal cord. The worldwide incidence of poliomyelitis has significantly decreased since the institution of vaccination against this disease. Because poliomyelitis is so rare at this time in the United States, a clinician will see patients with postpolio sequelae much more commonly than those with acute polio. Postpolio sequelae manifest as fatigue, skeletal muscle weakness, joint pain, cold intolerance, dysphagia, and sleep and breathing problems (i.e., obstructive sleep apnea), which presumably reflect neurologic damage from the original poliovirus infection. Poliovirus may damage the reticular activating system; this accounts for the fact that these individuals may exhibit exquisite sensitivity to the sedative effects of anesthetics as well as delayed awakening from general anesthesia. Sensitivity to nondepolarizing muscle relaxants is common. Severe back pain following surgery may be due to co-existing skeletal muscle atrophy and scoliosis. Postoperative shivering may be profound, since these individuals are very sensitive to cold. Postoperative pain perception may be abnormal, possibly because of poliovirus damage to endogenous opioid-secreting cells in the brain and spinal cord. Outpatient surgery may not be appropriate for many postpolio patients since they are at increased risk of complications, especially those related to respiratory muscle weakness and dysphagia.

SEIZURE DISORDERS

Seizures are caused by transient, paroxysmal, and synchronous discharge of groups of neurons in the brain. Seizure is one of the most common neurologic disorders and may occur at any age. More than 10% of the population will experience a seizure at some time during their lives. Clinical manifestations depend on the location and number of neurons involved in the seizure discharge and its duration. Transient abnormalities of brain function, such as occur with hypoglycemia, hyponatremia, hyperthermia, and drug toxicity, typically result in a single seizure. Treatment of the underlying disorder is usually curative. *Epilepsy* is defined as recurrent seizures resulting from congenital or acquired factors (e.g., cerebral scarring) and affects approximately 0.6% of the population.

Seizures are grossly classified based on two factors: loss of consciousness and focus of seizure activation. Simple seizures involve no loss of consciousness, whereas altered levels of consciousness are seen in complex seizures. Partial seizures appear to originate from a limited population of neurons in a single hemisphere, whereas generalized seizures appear to involve diffuse activation of neurons in both cerebral hemispheres. A partial seizure may initially be evident in one region of the body and may subsequently become generalized, involving both hemispheres, a process known as the *jacksonian march.*

MRI is the preferred method for studying brain structure in patients with epilepsy. Standard EEG is used to identify the location(s) of seizure foci as well as to characterize their electrical properties. The use of videography in addition to EEG allows simultaneous documentation of electrical and clinical seizure activity. Electrocorticography, in which electrodes are surgically placed directly on the cerebral cortex, not only permits more accurate focus identification but also allows mapping of electrical events in relation to identifiable brain surface anatomy, a feature that is valuable during surgical resection. Stimulation of various electrocorticographic electrodes can also help identify eloquent brain areas before seizure focus resection, so that those areas can be avoided during surgery.

Pharmacologic Treatment

Seizures are treated with antiepileptic drugs, starting with a single drug and achieving seizure control by increasing the dosage as necessary. Drug combinations may be considered when monotherapy fails. Changes in drug dosage are guided by clinical response (antiseizure effects vs. side effects) rather than by serum drug concentrations. Monitoring of serum drug levels is usually not necessary for patients who are experiencing adequate seizure control without evidence of toxicity. Effective antiepileptic drugs appear to decrease neuronal excitability or enhance neuronal inhibition. Drugs effective for the treatment of *partial* seizures include carbamazepine, phenytoin, eslicarbazepine, and valproate. *Generalized* seizure disorders can be managed with carbamazepine, phenytoin, valproate, barbiturates, gabapentin, levetiracetam, or lamotrigine. Except for gabapentin, all of the useful antiepileptic drugs are metabolized in the liver before undergoing renal excretion. Gabapentin appears to undergo no in vivo metabolism and is excreted unchanged by the kidneys. Carbamazepine, phenytoin, and barbiturates cause enzyme induction, and long-term treatment with these drugs can alter the rate of their own metabolism as well as that of other drugs. Pharmacokinetic and pharmacodynamic drug interactions are considerations in patients being treated with antiepileptic drugs.

Dose-dependent neurotoxic effects are the most common adverse effects of antiepileptic drugs. All antiepileptic drugs can cause depression of cerebral function with symptoms of sedation.

Phenytoin has many side effects, including hypotension, cardiac dysrhythmias, gingival hyperplasia, and aplastic anemia. It is associated with various cutaneous manifestations, including erythema multiforme and Stevens-Johnson syndrome. Extravasation or intraarterial injection of phenytoin can induce significant vasoconstriction resulting in purple glove syndrome, which can lead to skin necrosis, compartment syndrome, and gangrene. These side effects make fosphenytoin, a phosphorylated prodrug that does not share the same toxicity profile as phenytoin, a more attractive option for intravenous antiepileptic administration.

Valproate produces hepatic failure in approximately 1 in every 10,000 recipients. The mechanism of this hepatotoxicity is unknown, but it may represent an idiosyncratic hypersensitivity reaction. Pancreatitis has also been observed during valproate therapy. Long-term use of valproate is associated with increased surgical bleeding, especially in children. The mechanism is currently unknown but might involve a combination of thrombocytopenia and valproate-induced decreases in von Willebrand factor and factor VIII.

Carbamazepine can cause diplopia, dose-related leukopenia, and hyponatremia (which is usually clinically unimportant) as well as alterations in the hepatic metabolism of various drugs.

Adverse hematologic reactions associated with antiepileptic drugs range from mild anemia to aplastic anemia and are most commonly associated with the use of carbamazepine, phenytoin, and valproate.

Surgical Treatment

Surgical treatment of seizure disorders is considered in patients whose seizures do not respond to antiepileptic drugs or who cannot tolerate the side effects of pharmacologic therapy. Surgery is now being performed much earlier than in the past, particularly in young patients, to avoid social isolation resulting from medication side effects and persistent seizures. Partial seizures may respond to resection of a pathologic region within the brain such as a tumor, hamartoma, or scar tissue. Corpus callosotomy may help to prevent the generalization of partial seizures to the opposite hemisphere. Finally, hemispherectomy is sometimes needed for persistent catastrophic seizures.

In preparation for surgery, the seizure focus is first located by imaging and functional studies. MRI is the imaging modality of choice, especially for detection of mesial temporal sclerosis, a common cause of complex partial seizures. Nuclear medicine–based modalities, such as positron emission tomography (PET) and single-photon emission computed tomography (SPECT), may demonstrate alterations in metabolism or abnormal blood flow in regions of the brain. Video-EEG monitoring can assist in correlating electrical activity and clinical manifestations of seizures.

Electrocorticography, as mentioned earlier, involves placement of electrodes either as a grid directly on the brain surface or deeper within the brain. Electrocorticography offers many advantages over surface EEG recordings, such as increased precision in seizure focus determination, the ability to monitor deep regions of cortex, and the ability to stimulate regions of brain to map eloquent regions. Electrocorticography can be performed during the same surgical procedure as cortical resection or electrodes can be placed during one procedure and the patient allowed to return on a different day for seizure focus resection. In the latter case, video monitoring and mapping with grids in place can increase the accuracy of identifying the specific seizure focus for resection.

A more conservative surgical approach to medically intractable seizures involves the implantation of a left vagal nerve stimulator. The left side is chosen because the right vagal nerve usually has significant cardiac innervation, which could lead to severe bradyarrhythmias. The mechanism by which vagal nerve stimulation produces its effects is unclear. Patients tolerate this treatment well except for the occurrence of hoarseness in some cases, which reflects the vagal innervation of the larynx.

Status Epilepticus

Status epilepticus is a life-threatening condition that manifests as continuous seizure activity or two or more seizures occurring in sequence without recovery of consciousness between them.

The goal of treatment of status epilepticus is prompt establishment of venous access and subsequent pharmacologic suppression of seizure activity combined with support of the airway, ventilation, and circulation. Hypoglycemia can be ruled out as a cause within minutes using rapid bedside glucose assessment techniques. If hypoglycemia is present, it can be corrected by intravenous administration of 50 mL of 50% glucose solution. Routine glucose administration before confirmation of hypoglycemia is potentially dangerous, since hyperglycemia can exacerbate brain injury. Tracheal intubation may be needed to protect the airway and/or optimize oxygen delivery and ventilation. Muscle relaxants should be avoided if muscle movement, rather than electrophysiologic monitoring, is the principal method for assessing therapy effectiveness. Administration of an antiepileptic anesthetic, such as propofol or thiopental, will temporarily halt seizure activity during tracheal intubation. Monitoring of arterial blood gas levels and pH may be useful for confirming the adequacy of oxygenation and ventilation. Metabolic acidosis is a common sequela of ongoing seizure activity. Intravenous administration of sodium bicarbonate may be needed to treat extreme acid-base abnormalities. Hyperthermia occurs frequently during status epilepticus and necessitates active cooling.

Management of Anesthesia

Management of anesthesia in patients with seizure disorders includes considering the impact of antiepileptic drugs on organ function and the effect of anesthetic drugs on seizures. Sedation produced by antiepileptic drugs may have additive effects with that produced by anesthetic drugs, and enzyme induction by antiepileptic drugs may alter the pharmacokinetics and pharmacodynamics of anesthetic drugs.

When selecting anesthetic induction and maintenance drugs, one must consider their effects on central nervous system electrical activity. Methohexital administration can activate epileptic foci and has been recommended as a method for delineating these foci during electrocorticography in patients undergoing surgical treatment of epilepsy. Alfentanil, ketamine, enflurane, isoflurane, and sevoflurane can cause epileptiform spike-and-wave EEG activity in patients without a history of seizures, but they are also known to suppress epileptiform and epileptic activity. Seizures and opisthotonos have been observed in rare cases after propofol anesthesia, which suggests caution when administering this drug to patients with known seizure disorders. In selection of muscle relaxants, the central nervous system–stimulating effects of laudanosine, a proconvulsant metabolite of atracurium and cisatracurium, may merit consideration. Various antiepileptic drugs, specifically phenytoin and carbamazepine, shorten the duration of action of nondepolarizing muscle relaxants through both pharmacokinetic and pharmacodynamic means. Topiramate may be the cause of unexplained metabolic acidosis, given its ability to inhibit carbonic anhydrase.

It seems reasonable to avoid administering potentially epileptogenic drugs to patients with epilepsy. Instead, thiobarbiturates, opioids, and benzodiazepines are preferred. Isoflurane, desflurane, and sevoflurane seem to be acceptable choices in patients with seizure disorders. Regardless of the anesthetic drugs used, it is important to maintain treatment with the preoperative antiepileptic drugs throughout the perioperative period.

During intraoperative electrocorticography, monitoring is aimed at identifying *interictal* epileptiform activity, that is, the characteristic patterns of electrical activity that occur in the time between seizures. Many anesthetic agents, such as benzodiazepines, volatile anesthetics, and anesthetic doses of barbiturates and propofol, can significantly suppress epileptiform activity, which renders electrocorticographic monitoring difficult or impossible. During the monitoring period, anesthesia should be managed with agents such as narcotics, nitrous oxide, droperidol, diphenhydramine, and possibly dexmedetomidine. If epileptiform activity remains suppressed or is inadequate for analysis, high-dose short-acting opioids (e.g., alfentanil 50 mcg/kg as an intravenous bolus), or small intravenous boluses of methohexital (0.3 mg/kg) or etomidate (0.05 to 0.1 mg/kg) can serve to enhance epileptiform activity. Careful attention to maintaining muscle paralysis during this part of the procedure is important. When the preoperative discussion is held and informed consent is obtained, the patient should be made aware that anesthetic techniques used to improve the quality of electrophysiologic recordings may also increase the risk of awareness during anesthesia.

Despite general anesthesia and muscle relaxation, patients may still exhibit seizure activity. This may manifest as unexplained abrupt changes in heart rate and blood pressure with or without overt clonic movement, depending on the degree of muscle paralysis. Increases in carbon dioxide production from increased brain and muscle metabolism will be reflected in an increased end-tidal carbon dioxide concentration and may result in patient respiratory efforts. Seizures can be terminated by the administration of a barbiturate, propofol, or a benzodiazepine that is titrated to seizure cessation. Seizures can also be rapidly terminated by the direct application of cold saline to the brain surface. This is a very useful technique in procedures performed in awake patients, because it avoids

the use of drugs that could potentially produce somnolence, hypoventilation, airway obstruction, or apnea.

NEURO-OCULAR DISORDERS

Disorders involving the visual system discussed in this section are limited to those affecting the retina, optic nerve, and intracranial optic system. Degenerative diseases involving this part of the visual system include Leber's optic atrophy, retinitis pigmentosa, and Kearns-Sayer syndrome. The most common cause of new-onset blindness during the postoperative period is ischemic optic neuropathy. Other causes of postoperative visual defects are cortical blindness, retinal artery occlusion, and ophthalmic vein obstruction.

Leber's Optic Atrophy

Leber's optic atrophy, or Leber's hereditary optic neuropathy, is characterized by degeneration of the retina and atrophy of the optic nerves culminating in blindness. This disorder was the first human disorder for which a mitochondrial pattern of inheritance was definitively described. This rare disorder usually presents as loss of central vision in adolescence or early adulthood and is often associated with other neuropathologic conditions, including multiple sclerosis and dystonia.

Retinitis Pigmentosa

Retinitis pigmentosa refers to a genetically and clinically heterogeneous group of inherited retinopathies characterized by degeneration of the retina. These debilitating disorders collectively represent a common form of human visual handicap, with an estimated prevalence of approximately 1 in 3000. Examination of the retina shows areas of pigmentation, particularly in the peripheral regions. Vision is lost from the periphery of the retina toward the center until total blindness occurs.

Kearns-Sayer Syndrome

Kearns-Sayer syndrome is characterized by retinitis pigmentosa associated with progressive external ophthalmoplegia, typically manifesting before 20 years of age. Cardiac conduction abnormalities, ranging from bundle branch block to complete atrioventricular heart block, are common. Complete heart block can occur abruptly, leading to sudden death. Generalized degeneration of the central nervous system has been observed. This finding and the often increased concentration of protein in the CSF suggest a viral etiology. Although Kearns-Sayer syndrome is rare, it is possible that patients with this disorder will require anesthesia for insertion of implantable cardiac pacemakers.

Management of anesthesia requires a high index of suspicion for, and preparation to treat, third-degree atrioventricular heart block. Transthoracic pacing capability must be available. Experience is too limited to recommend specific drugs for induction and maintenance of anesthesia. Presumably,

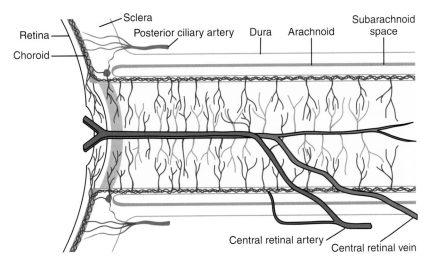

FIGURE 10-6 Blood supply to retina and optic nerve. Note the greater supply to the anterior portion of the optic nerve via the central retinal artery. Blood flow to the posterior portion of the optic nerve is supplied by pial perforators and is much less than blood flow to the anterior segment. *(Adapted from Hayreh SS. Anatomy and physiology of the optic nerve head.* Trans Am Acad Ophthalmol Otolaryngol. *1974;78:240-254.)*

the response to succinylcholine and nondepolarizing muscle relaxants is not altered, since this disease does not involve the neuromuscular junction.

Ischemic Optic Neuropathy

Ischemic optic neuropathy should be suspected in patients who complain of visual loss during the first week following surgery of any form. Ischemic injury to the optic nerve can result in loss of both central and peripheral vision.

The optic nerve can be functionally divided into an anterior and a posterior segment based on differences in blood supply (Figure 10-6). Blood supply to the anterior portion is derived from both the central retinal artery and small branches of the ciliary artery. In contrast, blood supply to the posterior segment of the optic nerve is derived from small branches of the ophthalmic and central retinal arteries. Baseline blood flow to the posterior segment of the optic nerve is significantly less than that to the anterior segment. Because of this difference, ischemic events in the anterior and posterior segments of the optic nerve are associated with different risk factors and physical findings. However, the prognosis, in terms of improvement of vision, is poor in either case. If ischemic optic neuropathy is suspected, urgent ophthalmologic consultation should be obtained so that other treatable causes of perioperative blindness can be ruled out.

ANTERIOR ISCHEMIC OPTIC NEUROPATHY

The visual loss associated with *anterior ischemic optic neuropathy* is due to infarction within the watershed perfusion zones between the small branches of the short posterior ciliary arteries. The usual presentation is a sudden, painless, monocular visual deficit varying in severity from a slight decrease in visual acuity to blindness. Asymptomatic optic disk swelling may be the earliest sign. A congenitally small optic disk is often present. The prognosis varies, but the most common outcome is minimal recovery of visual function.

The *nonarteritic form* of anterior ischemic optic neuropathy is more likely than the arteritic form to manifest during the

postoperative period. It is usually attributed to decreased oxygen delivery to the optic disk in association with hypotension and/or anemia. This form of visual loss has been associated with hemorrhagic hypotension (e.g., from gastrointestinal hemorrhage), anemia, cardiac surgery, head and neck surgery, cardiac arrest, and hemodialysis. It may also occur spontaneously. *Arteritic* anterior ischemic optic neuropathy, which is less common than the nonarteritic form, is associated with inflammation and thrombosis of the short posterior ciliary arteries. The diagnosis is confirmed by demonstration of giant cell arteritis on a biopsy sample from the temporal artery. High-dose corticosteroids are used to treat arteritic anterior ischemic optic neuropathy and to provide prophylaxis against disease manifestation in the contralateral eye.

POSTERIOR ISCHEMIC OPTIC NEUROPATHY

Posterior ischemic optic neuropathy presents as acute loss of vision and visual field defects similar to those in anterior ischemic optic neuropathy. It is presumed to be caused by decreased oxygen delivery to the posterior portion of the optic nerve between the optic foramen and the point of entry of the central retinal artery. Spontaneous occurrence is less frequent than with anterior ischemic optic neuropathy. However, posterior ischemic optic neuropathy is more common than anterior ischemic optic neuropathy as a cause of visual loss in the perioperative period. There may be no abnormal ophthalmoscopic findings initially, which reflects retrobulbar involvement of the optic nerve. Mild disk edema is present after a few days, and CT of the orbits may reveal enlargement of the intraorbital optic nerve.

The etiology of *postoperative ischemic optic neuropathy* appears to be multifactorial and may include hypotension, anemia, congenital absence of the central retinal artery, altered optic disk anatomy, air embolism, venous obstruction, and infection. It has been described following prolonged spine surgery performed in the prone position, cardiac surgery, radical neck dissection, and hip arthroplasty. Associated nonsurgical, but potentially contributory, factors include cardiac arrest, acute treatment of malignant hypertension, blunt trauma, and severe anemia. It has been hypothesized that the risk of posterior ischemic optic neuropathy may be reduced by avoiding anemia, hypotension, excessive fluid administration, and excessive use of vasopressors, but such speculation has not been proven.

Cortical Blindness

Cortical blindness may follow profound hypotension or circulatory arrest/cardiac arrest as a result of hypoperfusion and infarction of watershed areas in the parietal or occipital lobes. This form of blindness has been observed after many different kinds of surgical procedures, such as cardiac surgery, craniotomy, laryngectomy, and cesarean section, and can result from air or particulate emboli during cardiopulmonary bypass. Cortical blindness is characterized by loss of vision but retention of pupillary reactions to light and normal findings on funduscopic examination. Patients may not be aware of focal vision loss, which usually improves with time. The presence of abnormalities in the parietal or occipital lobes on CT or MRI scans confirms the diagnosis.

Retinal Artery Occlusion

Central retinal artery occlusion presents as painless monocular blindness. It is due to occlusion of a branch of the retinal artery. Visual field defects are often severe initially but, unlike with ischemic optic neuropathy, improve with time. Ophthalmoscopic examination reveals a pale edematous retina. Unlike ischemic optic neuropathy, central retinal artery occlusion is often caused by emboli from an ulcerated atherosclerotic plaque in the ipsilateral carotid artery. Many retinal artery occlusions are due to emboli during open heart surgery, and these resolve promptly. Vasospasm or thrombosis may also cause central retinal artery occlusion following radical neck surgery complicated by hemorrhage and hypotension. The condition can also occur following intranasal injection of α-adrenergic agonists. Stellate ganglion block improves vision in some patients.

Ophthalmic Venous Obstruction

Obstruction of venous drainage from the eyes may occur intraoperatively when patient positioning results in external pressure on the orbits. Placement in the prone position and use of headrests during neurosurgical procedures require careful attention to ensure that the eyeballs and orbits are free from external compression. Ophthalmoscopic examination reveals engorgement of the veins and edema of the macula.

KEY POINTS

- Major goals when providing anesthesia care for patients undergoing neurologic surgery include maintenance of adequate cerebral oxygen delivery, optimization of operative conditions, and facilitation of a rapid, smooth emergence from anesthesia to allow for immediate assessment of neurologic function.

- In the perioperative period, factors affecting CBF include Pao_2 and $Paco_2$, systemic blood pressure, cerebral autoregulation, cerebral venous pressure, and various drugs.

- Major techniques to decrease ICP include head elevation, hyperventilation, CSF drainage, and administration of hyperosmotic drugs, diuretics, corticosteroids, and cerebral vasoconstrictors.

- Venous air embolism can occur in a variety of circumstances, most commonly in patients who are placed in the sitting position. Techniques available to monitor for the entrainment of air include precordial Doppler ultrasonography, transesophageal echocardiography, and measurement of end-tidal oxygen and nitrogen content. Treatment includes discontinuation of nitrous oxide administration, flooding of the surgical field with fluid, aspiration of air via a central venous catheter, and hemodynamic support.

- Succinylcholine should be used with caution in patients with neurologic diseases because of its potential to produce a transient increase in ICP and because of the risk of hyperkalemia in the setting of denervating diseases that cause an upregulation of acetylcholine receptors at the neuromuscular junction.

RESOURCES

Adams H, Adams R, Del Zoppo G, et al. Guidelines for the early management of patients with ischemic stroke: 2005 guidelines update a scientific statement from the Stroke Council of the American Heart Association/American Stroke Association. *Stroke.* 2005;36:916-923.

Bederson JB, Connolly Jr ES, Batjer HH, et al. Guidelines for the management of aneurysmal subarachnoid hemorrhage: a statement for healthcare professionals from a special writing group of the Stroke Council, American Heart Association. *Stroke.* 2009;40:994-1025.

Brott TG, Hobson RW, Howard G, et al. Stenting versus endarterectomy for treatment of carotid artery stenosis. *N Engl J Med.* 2010;363:11-23.

Browne TR, Holmes GL. Epilepsy. *N Engl J Med.* 2001;344:1145-1151.

Lee LA, Roth S, Posner KL, et al. The American Society of Anesthesiologists Postoperative Visual Loss Registry: analysis of 93 spine surgery cases with postoperative visual loss. *Anesthesiology.* 2006;105:652-659.

Leipzig TJ, Morgan J, Horner TG, et al. Analysis of intraoperative rupture in the surgical treatment of 1694 saccular aneurysms. *Neurosurgery.* 2005;56:455-468.

Lukovits TG, Goddeau Jr RP. Critical care of patients with acute ischemic and hemorrhagic stroke: update on recent evidence and international guidelines. *Chest.* 2011;139:694-700.

Mayer SA, Brun NC, Begtrup K, et al. Recombinant activated factor VII for acute intracerebral hemorrhage. *N Engl J Med.* 2005;352:777-785.

Mendelow AD, Gregson BA, Fernandes HM, et al. Early surgery versus initial conservative treatment in patients with spontaneous supratentorial intracerebral haematomas in the International Surgical Trial in Intracerebral Haemorrhage (STICH): a randomised trial. *Lancet.* 2005;365:387-397.

Practice advisory for perioperative visual loss associated with spine surgery: a report by the American Society of Anesthesiologists Task Force on Perioperative Blindness. *Anesthesiology.* 2006;104:1319-1328.

Todd MM, Hindman BJ, Clarke WR, et al. Mild intraoperative hypothermia during surgery for intracranial aneurysm. *N Engl J Med.* 2005;352:135-145.

Wass CT, Lanier WL. Glucose modulation of ischemic brain injury: review and clinical recommendations. *Mayo Clin Proc.* 1996;71:801-812.

CHAPTER 11

Spinal Cord Disorders

JEFFREY J. PASTERNAK ■

WILLIAM L. LANIER, JR. ■

The most common cause of acute spinal cord injury is trauma. However, various disease processes, including tumors and congenital and degenerative diseases of the spinal cord and vertebral column, can also cause cord injury.

ACUTE SPINAL CORD INJURY

The mobility of the cervical spine makes it vulnerable to injury, especially hyperextension injury, during impact accidents. It is estimated that cervical spine injury occurs in 1.5% to 3.0% of all major trauma victims. About 4% to 5% of patients with traumatic head injury have a concurrent injury to the spine, typically occurring in the upper cervical spine (i.e., C1 to C3). Trauma can also injure the thoracic and lumbar spinal cord segments.

The clinical manifestations of acute spinal cord injury depend on both the extent and the site of injury. Acute spinal cord injury initially produces flaccid paralysis, with loss of sensation below the level of injury. The extent of injury is commonly described in terms of the American Spinal Injury Association (ASIA) classification system (Table 11-1), which characterizes the injury in terms of both motor and sensory impairment (Table 11-2 and Figure 11-1). A score of A indicates a "complete" injury in which all motor and sensory function is lost below the level of the lesion, including function at the lower sacral segments of S4 and S5, which is determined by assessing rectal tone and sensation. Scores of B through D are assigned to "incomplete" lesions in which some degree of spinal cord integrity is maintained below the level of injury. A score of E indicates normal spinal cord function.

The extent of physiologic effects from spinal cord injury depends on the level of injury, with the most severe physiologic derangements occurring with injury to the cervical cord and lesser perturbations occurring with more caudal cord injuries. Reductions in blood pressure are common, especially with cervical cord injury, and are influenced by (1) loss of sympathetic nervous system activity and a decrease in systemic vascular resistance, and (2) bradycardia resulting from loss of the T1-T4 sympathetic innervation to the heart. Hypotension can also occur with thoracic and lumbar cord injuries, although typically it is less severe than with cervical injuries. These hemodynamic perturbations are collectively known as *spinal shock* and typically last 1 to 3 weeks. With cervical and upper thoracic cord injury, the major cause of morbidity and mortality is alveolar hypoventilation combined with an inability to clear bronchial secretions. Respiratory muscles are not affected with lumbar and low thoracic injuries, so minimal respiratory impairment can be expected with these injuries. Aspiration of gastric contents, pneumonia, and pulmonary embolism are constant threats during spinal shock.

Cervical spine radiographs are obtained for a large percentage of patients who come for treatment of various forms of trauma caused by fear that occult cervical spine injuries will be missed. However, the probability of cervical spine injury is minimal in patients who meet the following five criteria: (1) no midline cervical spine tenderness, (2) no focal neurologic deficits, (3) normal sensorium, (4) no intoxication, and (5) no painful distracting injury. Patients who meet these criteria do *not* require routine imaging studies to rule out occult cervical spine injury.

An estimated two thirds of trauma patients have multiple injuries that can interfere with cervical spine evaluation.

Evaluation ideally includes computed tomography or magnetic resonance imaging, but imaging may not be practical in some cases because of the risk of transporting patients in unstable condition. For this reason, standard radiographic views of the cervical spine, often taken with a portable x-ray machine, are frequently relied upon to evaluate for the presence of cervical spine injury and associated instability. For cervical spine imaging to be useful, the entire cervical spine (including the body of the first thoracic vertebra) must be visible. Images are analyzed for alignment of the vertebrae (lateral view) and presence of fractures (all views), and disk and soft tissue spaces are evaluated. The sensitivity of plain radiographs for detecting cervical spine injury is less than 100%, and so the likelihood of cervical spine injury must be interpreted in conjunction with other clinical signs and symptoms and risk factors. If there is any doubt, it is prudent to treat all acute cervical spine injuries as potentially unstable.

Treatment of a cervical fracture or dislocation entails immediate immobilization to limit neck flexion and extension. Soft neck collars have little effect in limiting neck flexion or neck extension. Hard neck collars limit neck flexion and extension by only about 25%. Immobilization and traction provided by halo-thoracic devices are most effective in preventing cervical spine movement. During direct laryngoscopy, manual in-line stabilization (in which an assistant's hands are placed on each side of the patient's face with the fingertips resting on the mastoid process and application of downward pressure against a firm table surface to hold the head immobile in a neutral position) is recommended to help minimize

TABLE 11-1   American Spinal Injury Association Impairment Scale

Category	Description	Definition
A	Complete	No motor function below level of lesion or in sacral segments S4 and S5
B	Incomplete	Sensory but not motor function is preserved below neurologic level and includes S4-S5 segments
C	Incomplete	Motor function is preserved below level of injury and more than half of key muscles below neurologic level have a grade less than 3
D	Incomplete	Motor function is preserved below level of injury and more than half of key muscles below neurologic level have a grade of 3 or more
E	Normal	Sensory and motor function are intact

TABLE 11-2   Major muscle innervations

Muscle	Action	Roots	Nerve
Serratus anterior	Anterior movement of shoulder	C5, C6, C7	Long thoracic
Rhomboids	Scapula adduction	C4, C5	Dorsal scapular
Deltoid	Arm abduction	C5, C6	Axillary
Biceps brachii	Forearm flexion and supination	C5, C6	Musculocutaneous
Flexor carpi ulnaris	Hand flexion	C7, C8, T1	Ulnar
Adductor pollicis	Thumb adduction	C8, T1	Ulnar
Pronator teres	Forearm pronation	C6, C7	Median
Abductor pollicis	Thumb metacarpal abduction	C8, T1	Median
Triceps brachii	Forearm extension	C6, C7, C8	Radial
Extensor carpi radialis	Hand extension	C5, C6	Radial
Iliopsoas	Hip flexion	L1, L2, L3	Femoral
Quadriceps femoris	Knee extension	L2, L3, L4	Femoral
Adductor longus	Thigh adduction	L2, L3, L4	Obturator
Gluteus medius	Thigh abduction and medial rotation	L4, L5, S1	Superior gluteal
Gluteus maximus	Thigh abduction	L5, S1, S2	Inferior gluteal
Biceps femoris	Leg flexion	L5, S1, S2	Sciatic
Tibialis anterior	Foot dorsiflexion	L4, L5, S1	Deep peroneal
Tibialis posterior	Foot plantar flexion	L4, L5	Tibial
Gastrocnemius	Knee flexion and foot plantar flexion	S1, S2	Tibial
Soleus	Foot plantar flexion	S1, S2	Tibial
Rectal sphincter	Rectal sphincter contraction	S2, S3, S4	Pudendal

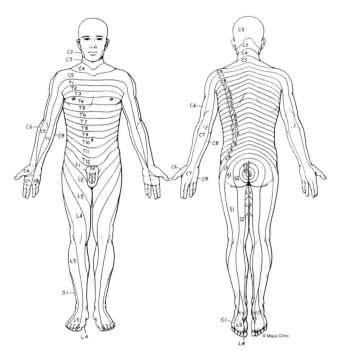

FIGURE 11-1 Anterior and posterior sensory dermatomes. *(By permission of the Mayo Foundation for Medical Education and Research. All rights reserved.)*

cervical spine flexion and extension. Cervical spine movement during direct laryngoscopy is likely to be concentrated in the occipito-atlanto-axial area, which suggests an increased risk of spinal cord injury at this level in vulnerable patients, even with the use of in-line stabilization.

Not only can movement of the neck in the presence of cervical spine injury cause mechanical deformation of the spinal cord, but there is an even greater risk that neck motion that elongates the cord will compromise the blood supply to the spinal cord by narrowing the longitudinal blood vessels. In fact, maintenance of perfusion pressure may be of more importance than positioning for prevention of spinal cord injury in the presence of cervical spine injury.

Management of Anesthesia

Patients with acute spinal cord injury often require special precautions during airway management. When direct laryngoscopy is performed, neck movement must be minimized and hypotension avoided so that spinal cord perfusion pressure can be maintained. However, fear of possible spinal cord compression must not prevent necessary airway interventions. Extensive clinical experience supports the use of direct laryngoscopy for orotracheal intubation provided that (1) maneuvers are taken to stabilize the head during the procedure and thus to avoid hyperextension of the neck, and (2) prior evaluation of the airway did not suggest the likelihood of any associated technical difficulties.

Awake fiberoptic laryngoscopy under topical anesthesia is an alternative to direct laryngoscopy if the patient is

cooperative and airway trauma—with associated blood, secretions, and anatomic deformities—does not preclude visualization with the fiberscope. It is important to remember that coughing during topical anesthetization of the airway and fiberoptic intubation may result in cervical spine movement. It is reasonable to have an assistant maintain manual in-line stabilization of the cervical spine during *all* airway manipulations. Alternative methods to secure the airway include rapid-sequence or non–rapid-sequence induction of general anesthesia with intravenous anesthetics and a muscle relaxant. However, induction of general anesthesia should precede tracheal intubation only in those patients in whom the clinician anticipates effective ventilation of the lungs by mask should initial attempts at endotracheal intubation fail. Intubation under general anesthesia can be performed using a standard laryngoscope, a videolaryngoscope, a fiberoptic bronchoscope, or any other airway device depending on the clinician's experience and the patient's anatomic requirements. When the cervical spine is unstable or there is a strong suspicion of cervical spine injury, it is important to proceed carefully because neck hyperextension could further damage the spinal cord. However, there is no evidence of increased neurologic morbidity after elective or emergency orotracheal intubation of anesthetized or awake patients who have an unstable cervical spine if appropriate steps are taken to minimize neck movement. Awake tracheostomy is reserved for the most challenging airway conditions, in which neck injury, combined with facial fractures or other severe anomalies of airway anatomy, makes securing the airway by nonsurgical means difficult or unsafe. Airway management in the presence of cervical spine injury should be dictated by common sense, not dogmatic approaches. Certainly, clinical experience supports the safety of a variety of airway management techniques.

The absence of compensatory sympathetic nervous system responses in patients with cervical or high thoracic spinal cord injury makes these patients particularly vulnerable to dramatic decreases in blood pressure following changes in body position, blood loss, or positive pressure ventilation. To minimize these effects, liberal intravenous infusion of crystalloid solutions may be necessary to fill the intravascular space, which has been compromised by vasodilation. Acute blood loss should be treated promptly. Electrocardiographic abnormalities are common during the acute phase of spinal cord injury, especially with cervical cord injuries. Breathing is best managed by mechanical ventilation, since abdominal and intercostal muscle weakness or paralysis is exacerbated by general anesthesia and increases the likelihood of respiratory failure with ensuing hypoxemia and hypercapnia. Body temperature should be monitored and manipulated, because patients tend to become poikilothermic in dermatomes below the level of the spinal cord lesion. Maintenance of anesthesia is targeted at ensuring physiologic stability and facilitating tolerance of the endotracheal tube. Volatile and intravenous anesthetics are both satisfactory. Nitrous oxide should be used with great caution, if at all, given concerns for co-existing trauma and air entrainment in closed spaces, as can occur with basilar skull fracture or rib fracture. Nitrous oxide could contribute to expansion of pneumocephalus or pneumothorax. Arterial hypoxemia is common following spinal cord injury, which emphasizes the need for continuous pulse oximetry and oxygen supplementation.

Muscle relaxant use should be based on the operative site and the level of spinal cord injury. If muscle relaxants are necessary, the sympathomimetic effects of pancuronium makes this drug an attractive choice, but other nondepolarizing muscle relaxants can be used safely. Succinylcholine does not provoke excessive release of potassium during the first few hours after spinal cord injury. The benefits of succinylcholine, which include rapid onset of action and short duration of paralysis must, as always, be weighed against potential side effects. Use of a nondepolarizing relaxant, with mask ventilation while cricoid pressure is employed, is another alternative to airway management during anesthetic induction and before laryngoscopy. A nondepolarizing relaxant may also facilitate patient positioning.

CHRONIC SPINAL CORD INJURY

Sequelae of chronic spinal cord injury include impaired alveolar ventilation, cardiovascular instability manifested as autonomic hyperreflexia, chronic pulmonary and genitourinary tract infections, anemia, and altered thermoregulation (Table 11-3). Injuries that occur more rostral along the spinal cord tend to have more significant systemic effects. Chronic urinary tract infection reflects the inability to empty the bladder completely and predisposes to calculus formation. As a result, renal failure may occur and is a common cause of death in patients with chronic spinal cord injury. Prolonged immobility leads to osteoporosis, skeletal muscle atrophy, and decubitus ulcers. Immobility can also predispose patients to deep venous thrombosis, so prophylactic measures such as use of compression stockings, low-dose anticoagulant therapy, and insertion of inferior vena cava filters may be indicated. Pathologic fractures can occur when these patients are moved. Pressure points should be well protected and padded to minimize the likelihood of trauma to the skin and the development of decubitus ulcers.

Depression and chronic pain are common problems following spinal cord injury. Nerve root pain is localized at or near the level of injury. Visceral pain is produced by distention of the bladder or bowel. Phantom body pain can occur in areas of complete sensory loss. As a result of depression and/or pain, these patients are often treated with antidepressants and analgesics, including opioids, that require attention when anesthetic management is planned.

Several weeks after acute spinal cord injury, spinal cord reflexes gradually return, and patients enter a more chronic stage characterized by overactivity of the sympathetic nervous system and involuntary skeletal muscle spasms. Baclofen, which potentiates the inhibitory effects of γ-aminobutyric acid, is useful for treating spasticity. Abrupt cessation of baclofen therapy, as may occur with hospitalization for an unrelated problem, may result in dramatic withdrawal

TABLE 11-3	Early and late complications in patients with spinal cord injury
Complication	**Incidence (%)**
2 YEARS AFTER INJURY	
Urinary tract infection	59
Skeletal muscle spasticity	38
Chills and fever	19
Decubitus ulcer	16
Autonomic hyperreflexia	8
Skeletal muscle contractures	6
Heterotopic ossification	3
Pneumonia	3
Renal dysfunction	2
Postoperative wound infection	2
30 YEARS AFTER INJURY	
Decubitus ulcers	17
Skeletal muscle or joint pain	16
Gastrointestinal dysfunction	14
Cardiovascular dysfunction	14
Urinary tract infection	14
Infectious disease or cancer	11
Visual or hearing disorders	10
Urinary retention	8
Male genitourinary dysfunction	7
Renal calculi	6

reactions, including seizures. Diazepam and other benzodiazepines also facilitate the inhibitory effects of γ-aminobutyric acid and may have utility in the management of a patient receiving baclofen. Spasticity refractory to pharmacologic suppression may require surgical treatment via dorsal rhizotomy or myelotomy, but usually implantation of a spinal cord stimulator or subarachnoid baclofen pump will be undertaken before rhizotomy is considered.

Spinal cord injury at or above the fifth cervical vertebra may result in apnea caused by denervation of the diaphragm (C3 to C5 innervation). When function of the diaphragm is intact, the tidal volume is likely to remain adequate, but the ability to cough and clear secretions from the airway is often impaired because of a decreased expiratory reserve volume resulting from denervation of intercostal and abdominal muscles. Indeed, acute spinal cord injury at the cervical level is accompanied by marked decreases in vital capacity. Arterial hypoxemia is a consistent early finding following cervical spinal cord injury. Tracheobronchial suctioning has been associated with bradycardia and even cardiac arrest in these patients, so it is important to optimize arterial oxygenation before suctioning the airway.

Management of Anesthesia

Anesthetic management in patients with chronic spinal cord injury should focus on preventing autonomic hyperreflexia. When general anesthesia is selected, administration of muscle relaxants is useful to facilitate tracheal intubation and prevent reflex skeletal muscle spasms in response to surgical stimulation. Nondepolarizing muscle relaxants are the primary choice in this circumstance, since succinylcholine is likely to provoke hyperkalemia, particularly during the initial 6 months after spinal cord injury. Indeed, it seems reasonable to avoid the use of succinylcholine in patients with a spinal cord injury of longer than 24 hours' duration.

The anesthesiologist must be aware of the potential for altered hemodynamics, especially with cervical and high thoracic cord lesions. These can manifest as wide alterations in both blood pressure and heart rate. In chronically immobile patients, the index of suspicion for pulmonary thromboembolism, which can manifest as alterations in hemodynamics and oxygenation, must be high. If intercostal muscle function is impaired, patients may be at high risk of postoperative hypoventilation and may have an impaired cough and a corresponding accumulation of secretions. Baclofen and benzodiazepines should be continued throughout the perioperative period to avoid withdrawal symptoms.

AUTONOMIC HYPERREFLEXIA

Autonomic hyperreflexia appears following spinal shock and in association with return of spinal cord reflexes. This reflex response can be initiated by cutaneous or visceral stimulation below the level of spinal cord injury. Surgery and distention of a hollow viscus such as the bladder or rectum are common stimuli.

Stimulation below the level of spinal cord injury initiates afferent impulses that enter the spinal cord (Figure 11-2). Because of reflexes entirely within the spinal cord itself, these impulses elicit an increase in sympathetic nervous system activity along the splanchnic outflow tract. In neurologically intact individuals, this outflow would be modulated by inhibitory impulses from higher centers in the central nervous system, but in the presence of a spinal cord lesion, this outflow is isolated from inhibitory impulses from above, so generalized *vasoconstriction* occurs *below* the level of the spinal cord injury.

Hypertension and reflex bradycardia are the hallmarks of autonomic hyperreflexia. Stimulation of the carotid sinus is the cause of the bradycardia. Reflex cutaneous *vasodilation* occurs *above* the level of the spinal cord injury. Nasal stuffiness reflects this vasodilation. Patients may complain of headache and blurred vision, which indicate severe hypertension. These increases in blood pressure can result in cerebral, retinal, or subarachnoid hemorrhage as well as increased operative blood loss. Loss of consciousness and seizures may also occur, and cardiac dysrhythmias are often present. Pulmonary edema reflects acute left ventricular failure resulting from dramatically increased afterload.

The incidence of autonomic hyperreflexia depends on the level of spinal cord injury. Approximately 85% of patients with lesions above T6 exhibit this reflex. It is unlikely to be associated with spinal cord lesions below T10 (Figure 11-3). Since the greater, lesser, and least splanchnic nerves typically receive

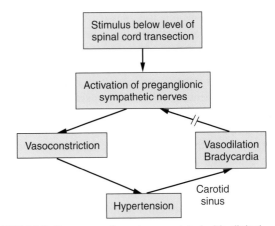

FIGURE 11-2 Sequence of events associated with clinical manifestations of autonomic hyperreflexia. Because the efferent impulses from the brain that produce compensatory vasodilation (in response to increased baroreceptor activity) cannot reach the neurologically isolated portion of the spinal cord, unmodulated vasoconstriction develops below the level of the spinal cord injury, resulting in systemic hypertension.

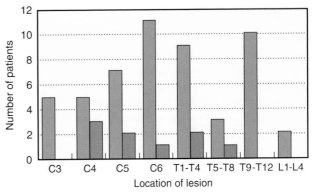

FIGURE 11-3 Incidence of autonomic hyperreflexia in patients with spinal cord injury undergoing extracorporeal shock wave lithotripsy. This reflex did not occur in any patient with an injury below T9. Blue bars show the distribution of lesion sites in all patients with spinal cord injury (n = 52); orange bars show the lesion sites in the subset of patients developing autonomic hyperreflexia (n = 9). *(Adapted from Stowe DF, Bernstein JS, Madsen KE, et al. Autonomic hyperreflexia in spinal cord injured patients during extracorporeal shock wave lithotripsy. Anesth Analg. 1989;68:788-791.)*

innervation from T5 to T9, T10 and T11, and T12, respectively, loss of input from higher centers to these nerves and to the sympathetic chain will place larger regions of the body at risk of exaggerated autonomic reflexes. Spinal cord lesions above T5 and T6 will completely isolate the splanchnic nerves from higher centers of control, whereas spinal cord lesions at lumbar levels of the cord will leave the peripheral sympathetic nervous system intact.

Management of patients at risk should begin with efforts to *prevent* the development of autonomic hyperreflexia. Patients who have no history of this reflex are still at risk of its occurrence during surgery, simply because of the intense stimuli that surgery can produce. Before surgical or other stimulation is initiated in locations that lack sensory innervation, general, neuraxial, or regional anesthesia should be instituted. Epidural anesthesia has been described for the treatment of autonomic hyperreflexia provoked by uterine contractions during labor. However, epidural anesthesia may be less effective than spinal anesthesia in preventing autonomic hyperreflexia because of its relative sparing of the sacral segments and lesser block density. Blocking afferent pathways with topical local anesthetics applied to the urethra for a cystoscopic procedure does *not* prevent autonomic hyperreflexia, because this form of anesthesia does not block the bladder muscle proprioceptors that are stimulated by bladder distention.

Regardless of the anesthesia technique selected, vasodilator drugs having a short half-life (e.g., sodium nitroprusside) should be readily available to treat sudden-onset severe hypertension. Persistence of hypertension requires continuous infusion of vasodilators, perhaps supplemented with longer-acting drugs such as hydralazine. It is important to note that autonomic hyperreflexia may first manifest postoperatively when the effects of the anesthetic drugs begin to wane.

SPINAL CORD TUMORS

Spinal cord tumors can be divided into two broad categories. *Intramedullary* tumors are located within the spinal cord and account for approximately 10% of tumors affecting the spinal column. Gliomas and ependymomas account for the vast majority of intramedullary tumors. *Extramedullary* tumors can be either intradural or extradural. Neurofibromas and meningiomas account for most of the intradural tumors. Metastatic lesions, usually from lung, breast, or prostate cancer or myeloma, are the most common extradural lesions. Other mass lesions of the spinal cord, including abscesses and hematomas, share many of the clinical signs and symptoms of tumors.

Spinal cord tumors typically present with symptoms of cord compression. Pain is a common finding and is usually aggravated by coughing or straining. Motor symptoms and sphincter disturbances may occur. Sometimes spinal tenderness may be present. Diagnosis is usually based on symptoms and imaging of the spinal cord. Magnetic resonance imaging is the technique of choice. Treatment and prognosis depend on the nature of the lesion, and treatment may include corticosteroids, radiation therapy, chemotherapy, or surgical decompression or excision.

Management of Anesthesia

Management of anesthesia involves ensuring adequate spinal cord oxygenation and perfusion. This is achieved by maintaining Pao_2 at sufficient levels and by avoiding hypotension and anemia. Specifics of management will depend on the level of the lesion and the extent of neurologic impairment.

Tumors involving the cervical spinal cord may influence the approach used to secure the airway. Significant motion of the cervical spine could lead to further cord compromise via compression and decreased cord perfusion. With any form of disease that places the cervical spine at risk of new injury, airway

management should be similar to that discussed for the management of acute spinal cord injury. This may include in-line stabilization during laryngoscopy with either a standard laryngoscope or videolaryngoscope or awake fiberoptic intubation. If the approach to patient management is uncertain, it is useful, before administering sedatives or narcotics, to have the patient placed in position for airway management (e.g., on the operating room table) and then to move carefully through the anticipated variations of head and neck movements before actual airway manipulation or induction of anesthesia is carried out. Elicitation or exacerbation of symptoms upon movement should tip the clinician toward fiberoptic laryngoscopy (with the head held in neutral position) or other options that are less likely to cause movement with its potential for harm to the spinal cord. Use of a light wand or videolaryngoscope may facilitate intubation of the trachea without significant neck extension.

Safe resection of a tumor may require the use of intraoperative electrophysiologic monitoring of neurologic function. Electromyography, somatosensory-evoked potential monitoring, and motor-evoked potential monitoring have a variety of anesthetic implications. The preferred approach may vary from institution to institution.

Succinylcholine should be used with caution in patients with spinal cord tumors given the risk of associated hyperkalemia. Neuromuscular monitoring with train-of-four stimulation should be performed on a neurologically intact extremity. Upper motor neuron impairment may lead to upregulation of acetylcholine receptors, which makes an affected extremity more resistant to nondepolarizing blockade. If there are significant concerns regarding the possibility of altered responsiveness to neuromuscular blockade because of tumor-induced spinal cord dysfunction, then train-of-four monitoring on the facial nerve may be a reasonable option. One should be careful to monitor evoked muscle twitches, not direct muscle stimulation.

INTERVERTEBRAL DISK DISEASE

Low back pain ranks second only to upper respiratory tract disease as the most common reason for office visits to physicians. An estimated 70% of adults experience low back pain at some time in their lives. Among chronic conditions, low back pain is the most common cause of limitation of activity in patients younger than 45 years of age. Primary or metastatic cancer is the most common systemic disease affecting vertebral bodies, but it accounts for fewer than 1% of all episodes of low back pain.

One of the most common causes of back pain is intervertebral disk disease. The intervertebral disk is composed of a compressible nucleus pulposus surrounded by a fibrocartilaginous annulus fibrosis. The disk acts as a shock absorber between vertebral bodies. Trauma or degenerative processes lead to changes in the intervertebral disk. Nerve root or spinal cord compression results when the nucleus pulposus protrudes through the annulus fibrosis. With compression of a single nerve root, patients usually complain of pain in a single dermatomal distribution or localized muscle weakness. Spinal cord compression can lead to complex sensory, motor, and autonomic symptoms at and below the level of the insult. Computed tomography or magnetic resonance imaging confirms the diagnosis and the location of intervertebral disk herniation.

Cervical Disk Disease

Lateral protrusion of a cervical disk usually occurs at the C5-6 or C6-7 intervertebral spaces. Protrusion can be secondary to trauma or can occur spontaneously. Symptoms are commonly aggravated by coughing. The same symptoms can be due to osteophytes that compress nerve roots in the intervertebral foramina.

Initial treatment of cervical disk protrusion is typically conservative and includes rest, pain control, and possibly epidural administration of steroids. Surgical decompression is necessary if symptoms do not abate with conservative treatment or if there is significant motor involvement.

MANAGEMENT OF ANESTHESIA

The primary initial concern in the perioperative care of patients with cervical spine disease is airway management. The clinician should base the approach to airway management on the medical history, physical examination findings, review of radiologic studies, and discussion with the surgeon. Direct laryngoscopy can be considered if the patient shows no significant exacerbation of neurologic symptoms with neck movement (especially neck extension), spinal instability, or other airway abnormalities. The use of a videolaryngoscope or an assistant to manually maintain neck neutrality can be considered. If there is any significant concern that laryngoscopy may induce spinal cord compromise, awake fiberoptic intubation followed by a brief neurologic examination after successful tube placement should be considered.

In cervical spine procedures performed via an anterior approach, retraction of the airway structures to attain access to the cervical spine may result in injury to the ipsilateral recurrent laryngeal nerve. Many cases of nerve injury are asymptomatic, but injury may manifest as hoarseness, stridor, or, less frequently, frank airway compromise postoperatively. Injury may be due either to direct compression of or traction on the recurrent laryngeal nerve, or compression of nerve fibers within the airway. Such compression of nerve fibers may be caused either (1) by the endotracheal tube itself, since it is rigidly held in place by an inflated cuff and also fixed at the mouth; or (2) directly by the inflated cuff. Because of this it is common practice following airway retraction to let air out of the endotracheal tube cuff and then reinflate the cuff to the point at which no air leak is noted.

Lumbar Disk Disease

The most common sites for lumbar disk protrusion are the L4-5 and L5-S1 intervertebral spaces. Disk protrusion at both sites produces low back pain, which radiates down the posterior and lateral aspect of the thighs and calves (sciatica). The exact pattern and distribution of symptoms depend on the spinal level and nerve roots affected. A history of trauma, often viewed as trivial by the patient, is commonly associated with the sudden onset of back pain and signals disk protrusion. Back pain is aggravated by coughing or stretching of the sciatic nerve as, for example, by straight-leg raising. These mechanical signs help distinguish disk protrusion from peripheral nerve disorders. For example, diabetes mellitus–associated peripheral neuropathy may share the symptoms, but not the signs, of a ruptured lumbar disk.

Treatment of acute lumbar disk protrusion has historically included bed rest, analgesics, and centrally acting "muscle relaxants." Patients with acute low back pain who continue ordinary activities within the limits permitted by the pain have a more rapid recovery than those who stay on bed rest or perform back-mobilizing exercises. When neurologic symptoms persist despite conservative medical management, surgical laminectomy or microdiskectomy can be considered to decompress the affected nerve roots. Epidural steroids (e.g., triamcinolone, methylprednisolone) are an alternative to surgery in select patients. These drugs act by decreasing inflammation and edema around the nerve roots. Suppression of the hypothalamic-pituitary-adrenal axis is a consideration in patients treated with oral steroids and may have implications for anesthetic management. Although epidural steroid injections may provide short-term alleviation of symptoms caused by sciatica, this treatment offers no significant functional benefit nor does it decrease the need for surgery.

CONGENITAL ANOMALIES AND DEGENERATIVE DISEASES OF THE VERTEBRAL COLUMN

Spina bifida occulta is a common form of congenital vertebral column disease. Spondylosis and spondylolisthesis are forms of degenerative vertebral column diseases. It is not uncommon for multiple types of degenerative changes to occur concomitantly, which leads to more rapid progression of neurologic symptoms and the need for surgical intervention.

Spina bifida occulta (incomplete formation of a single lamina in the lumbosacral spine without other abnormalities) is a congenital defect that is present in an estimated 20% of individuals. It usually produces no symptoms and is often discovered as an incidental finding on radiographic examination during evaluation of some other unrelated disease process. Because there are no associated abnormalities, an increased risk with spinal anesthesia is not expected, and large numbers of these patients have undergone spinal anesthesia safely. There is a variant of spina bifida occulta known as *occult spinal dysraphism* in which the bony defect may involve more than one lamina. A significant number of these defects are associated with a tethered spinal cord—that is, the spinal cord ends below the L2-3 interspace—and this may be responsible for progressive neurologic symptoms. Up to 50% of individuals with a tethered spinal cord have cutaneous manifestations overlying the anomaly, including tufts of hair, hyperpigmented areas, cutaneous lipomas, and skin dimples. Performance of spinal anesthesia in patients with a tethered spinal cord may increase the risk of cord injury.

Spondylosis is a common acquired disorder that leads to osteophyte formation and degenerative disk disease. The term *spondylosis* is used synonymously with *spinal stenosis.* There is narrowing of the spinal canal and compression of the spinal cord by transverse osteophytes or nerve root compression by bony spurs in the intervertebral foramina. Spinal cord dysfunction can also reflect ischemia of the spinal cord caused by bony compression of the spinal arteries. Symptoms typically develop insidiously after age 50. With cervical spondylosis, neck pain and radicular pain in the arms and shoulders are accompanied by sensory loss and skeletal muscle wasting. Later, sensory and motor signs may appear in the legs producing an unsteady gait. Lumbar spondylosis usually leads to radicular pain and muscle wasting in the lower extremities. Sphincter disturbances are uncommon regardless of the location of spondylosis. Radiographs of the spine often demonstrate osteoarthritic changes, but these changes correlate poorly with neurologic symptoms. Surgery may be necessary to arrest progression of the symptoms, especially if there is evidence of motor loss.

Spondylolisthesis refers to anterior subluxation of one vertebral body on another. This most commonly occurs at the lumbosacral junction. Radicular symptoms usually involve the nerve root inferior to the pedicle of the anteriorly subluxed vertebra. Treatment includes analgesics, antiinflammatory medications, and physical therapy if low back pain is the only symptom. Surgery is reserved for patients who have myelopathy, radiculopathy, or neurogenic claudication.

CONGENITAL ANOMALIES AND DEGENERATIVE DISEASES OF THE SPINAL CORD

Syringomyelia

Syringomyelia, also known as *syrinx,* is a disorder in which there is cystic cavitation of the spinal cord. The condition is often congenital, but it can also occur following spinal cord trauma or in association with various neoplastic conditions such as gliomas. Rostral extension into the brainstem is called *syringobulbia.* Two main forms of syringomyelia occur depending on whether there is communication of the cystic regions with the subarachnoid space or central canal. In communicating syringomyelia, either there is only dilation of the central canal of the cord, known as *hydromyelia,* or there is communication between the abnormal cystic lesions in the spinal cord proper and the cerebrospinal fluid spaces. Communicating syringomyelia is usually associated with either a history of basilar arachnoiditis or Chiari's malformation. In contrast, the presence of cysts that have no connection to the cerebrospinal fluid spaces is called *noncommunicating syringomyelia* and is often associated with a history of trauma, neoplasms, or arachnoiditis.

Signs and symptoms of congenital syringomyelia usually begin during the third or fourth decade of life. Early complaints are those of sensory impairment involving pain and temperature sensation in the upper extremities. This reflects destruction of pain and temperature neuronal pathways that cross within the spinal cord near the central canal. As cavitation of the spinal cord progresses, destruction of lower motor neurons ensues, with the development of skeletal muscle weakness and wasting and loss of reflexes. Thoracic scoliosis may result from weakness of paravertebral muscles. Syringobulbia is characterized by paralysis of the palate, tongue, and vocal cords, and loss of sensation over the face. Magnetic resonance imaging is the preferred procedure to diagnose syringomyelia.

There is no known treatment that is effective in arresting the progressive degeneration of the spinal cord or medulla. Surgical procedures designed to restore normal cerebrospinal fluid flow have not been predictably effective.

Management of anesthesia in patients with syringomyelia or syringobulbia should consider the neurologic deficits associated with this disease. Thoracic scoliosis can contribute to ventilation/perfusion mismatching. Lower motor neuron disease with skeletal muscle wasting suggests the possibility that hyperkalemia can develop after administration of succinylcholine. Exaggerated responses to nondepolarizing muscle relaxants can be observed. Thermal regulation may be impaired. The selection of drugs for induction and maintenance of anesthesia is not influenced by this disease. With syringobulbia, any decrease in or absence of protective airway reflexes may influence the timing of endotracheal tube removal postoperatively.

Amyotrophic Lateral Sclerosis

Amyotrophic lateral sclerosis (ALS) is a degenerative disease involving (1) the lower motor neurons in the anterior horn gray matter of the spinal cord, and (2) the corticospinal tracts, that is, the primary descending upper motor neurons. Therefore, this disease process produces both upper and lower motor neuron degeneration. It most commonly affects men 40 to 60 years of age. When the degenerative process is limited to the motor cortex of the brain, the disease is called *primary lateral sclerosis;* limitation to the brainstem nuclei is known as *pseudobulbar palsy.* Werdnig-Hoffmann disease resembles ALS except that it occurs during the first 3 years of life. Although the cause of ALS is unknown, occasionally a genetic pattern is present. A viral etiology is also under consideration.

Signs and symptoms of ALS reflect upper and lower motor neuron dysfunction. Electromyographically, dysfunction sometimes resembles that of myasthenia gravis. Frequent initial manifestations include skeletal muscle atrophy, weakness, and fasciculations, often beginning in the intrinsic muscles of the hands. With time, atrophy and weakness involve most of the skeletal muscles, including the tongue, pharynx, larynx, and chest. Early symptoms of bulbar involvement include fasciculations of the tongue plus dysphagia, which leads to pulmonary aspiration. The ocular muscles are spared. Autonomic nervous system dysfunction can be manifested as orthostatic hypotension and resting tachycardia. An inability to control emotional responses is characteristic. Complaints of cramping and aching sensations, particularly in the legs, are common. Plasma creatine kinase concentrations are normal, which distinguishes this disease from chronic polymyositis.

Carcinoma of the lung has been associated with ALS. ALS has no known treatment, and death is likely within 6 years after the onset of clinical symptoms, usually resulting from respiratory failure.

General anesthesia in patients with ALS may be associated with exaggerated respiratory depression. ALS patients are also vulnerable to hyperkalemia following administration of succinylcholine as a result of lower motor neuron disease, and these patients may show prolonged responses to nondepolarizing muscle relaxants. Bulbar involvement with dysfunction of pharyngeal muscles may predispose to pulmonary aspiration. There is no evidence that any specific anesthetic drug or combination of drugs is ideal in these patients. Regional anesthesia is usually avoided because of fear of exacerbating disease symptoms, but epidural anesthesia has been used successfully in patients with ALS without neurologic exacerbation or impairment of pulmonary function.

Friedreich's Ataxia

Friedreich's ataxia is an autosomal recessive condition characterized by degeneration of the spinocerebellar and pyramidal tracts. Cardiomyopathy is present in 10% to 50% of patients with this disease. Kyphoscoliosis, producing a progressive deterioration in pulmonary function, is seen in nearly 80% of affected individuals. Ataxia is the typical presenting symptom. Dysarthria, nystagmus, skeletal muscle weakness and spasticity, and diabetes mellitus may be present. Friedreich's ataxia is usually fatal by early adulthood, most often because of heart failure.

Management of anesthesia in patients with Friedreich's ataxia is similar to that described for patients with ALS. If cardiomyopathy is present, the negative inotropic effects of anesthetic drugs must be considered when selecting a technique. Although experience is limited, the response to muscle relaxants seems normal. Kyphoscoliosis may make epidural anesthesia technically difficult. Spinal anesthesia has been used successfully. The likelihood of postoperative ventilatory failure may be increased, especially in the presence of kyphoscoliosis.

KEY POINTS

■ The extent of physiologic effects from spinal cord injury depends on the level of injury, with the most severe physiologic derangements occurring with injury to the cervical cord. Hypotension is a result of (1) loss of sympathetic nervous system activity and a decrease in systemic vascular resistance and (2) bradycardia resulting from loss of the T1-T4 sympathetic innervation to the heart. These hemodynamic changes are collectively known as *spinal shock* and typically last 1 to 3 weeks.

■ Major goals in caring for patients who have spinal cord disease or are undergoing surgical procedures involving the spinal cord or vertebral column are maintenance of adequate oxygen delivery, optimization of operative conditions, and facilitation of a rapid, smooth emergence from anesthesia to allow immediate assessment of neurologic function.

■ Succinylcholine should be used with caution in patients with spinal cord injury because of the potential risk of hyperkalemia in the setting of diseases that cause an upregulation of acetylcholine receptors at the neuromuscular junction.

■ In acute spinal cord injury, care must be taken during airway manipulation to avoid excessive neck movement. Succinylcholine can be used without significant risk of hyperkalemia in the first few hours following spinal cord injury.

■ Sequelae of chronic spinal cord injury include impaired alveolar ventilation, cardiovascular instability manifested as autonomic hyperreflexia, chronic pulmonary and genitourinary tract infections, anemia, and altered thermoregulation.

■ Patients with cervical and thoracic spinal cord injuries are at risk of developing autonomic hyperreflexia in response to various stimuli, including surgery, bowel distention, and bladder distention. Autonomic hyperreflexia can be prevented by either general or spinal anesthesia, since both methods are effective in blocking the afferent limb of the pathway. Use of topical anesthesia for cystoscopic procedures does not prevent autonomic hyperreflexia, and epidural anesthesia is not reliably effective in preventing autonomic hyperreflexia.

■ Spinal cord tumors can be divided into two broad categories. *Intramedullary* tumors are located within the spinal cord and account for approximately 10% of tumors affecting the spinal column. Gliomas and ependymomas account for the vast majority of intramedullary tumors. *Extramedullary* tumors can be either intradural or extradural. Neurofibromas and meningiomas account for most of the intradural tumors. Metastatic lesions, usually from lung, breast, or prostate cancer or myeloma, are the most common causes of extradural lesions.

■ Low back pain ranks second only to upper respiratory tract disease as the most common reason for office visits to physicians. An estimated 70% of adults experience low back pain at some time in their lives.

RESOURCES

Hindman BJ, Palecek JP, Posner KL, et al. Cervical spinal cord, root, and bony spine injuries: a closed claims analysis. *Anesthesiology*. 2011;114:782-795.

Hoffman JR, Mower WR, Wolfson AB, et al. Validity of a set of clinical criteria to rule out injury to the cervical spine in patients with blunt trauma. National Emergency X-Radiography Utilization Study Group. *N Engl J Med*. 2000;343:94-99.

Jung A, Schramm J. How to reduce recurrent laryngeal nerve palsy in anterior cervical spine surgery: a prospective observational study. *Neurosurgery*. 2010;67:10-15.

Lennarson PJ, Smith D, Todd MM, et al. Segmental cervical spine motion during orotracheal intubation of the intact and injured spine with and without external stabilization. *J Neurosurg*. 2000;92:201-206.

Loftus RW, Yeager MP, Clark JA, et al. Intraoperative ketamine reduces perioperative opiate consumption in opiate-dependent patients with chronic back pain undergoing back surgery. *Anesthesiology*. 2010;113:639-646.

Lotto ML, Banoub M, Schubert A. Effects of anesthetic agents and physiologic changes on intraoperative motor evoked potentials. *J Neurosurg Anesthesiol*. 2004;16:32-42.

Diseases of the Autonomic and Peripheral Nervous Systems

JEFFREY J. PASTERNAK ■
WILLIAM L. LANIER, JR. ■

Autonomic Disorders
  Shy-Drager Syndrome
  Orthostatic Intolerance Syndrome
  Glomus Tumors of the Head and Neck
  Carotid Sinus Syndrome
  Hyperhidrosis
Diseases of the Peripheral Nervous System
  Idiopathic Facial Paralysis (Bell's Palsy)
  Trigeminal Neuralgia (Tic Douloureux)
  Glossopharyngeal Neuralgia
  Charcot-Marie-Tooth Disease
  Brachial Plexus Neuropathy
  Guillain-Barré Syndrome (Acute Idiopathic Polyneuritis)
  Entrapment Neuropathies
  Diseases Associated with Peripheral Neuropathies
  Perioperative Peripheral Neuropathies
Key Points

The peripheral nervous system consists of nerve elements outside the brain and spinal cord. It contains both peripheral nerves and elements of the autonomic nervous system. Disorders of the autonomic nervous system can result in significant hemodynamic changes as well as abnormal responses to drugs that work via adrenergic receptors. Diseases affecting peripheral nerves often have implications for perioperative patient management, including the choice of muscle relaxants and control of neuropathic pain.

AUTONOMIC DISORDERS

Shy-Drager Syndrome

Shy-Drager syndrome belongs to a group of heterogeneous disorders known as *multiple-system atrophy*. Multiple-system atrophy includes three conditions that, in years past, were thought to be unrelated: striatonigral degeneration, olivopontocerebellar atrophy, and Shy-Drager syndrome. The hallmark of multiple-system atrophy is degeneration and dysfunction of diverse central nervous system structures such as the basal ganglia, cerebellar cortex, locus ceruleus, pyramidal tracts, inferior olives, vagal motor nucleus, and spinocerebellar tracts. The extent of the differential degeneration in these structures dictates signs and symptoms. Shy-Drager syndrome is characterized by autonomic dysfunction and degeneration of the locus ceruleus, intermediolateral column of the spinal cord, and peripheral autonomic neurons. Other regions of the central nervous system described earlier may also be affected, but to a lesser degree. Specifically, striatonigral degeneration and olivopontocerebellar atrophy may also be present in patients with Shy-Drager syndrome, resulting in parkinsonism and ataxia. Idiopathic orthostatic hypotension, rather than Shy-Drager syndrome, is thought to be present when autonomic nervous system dysfunction occurs in the absence of central nervous system degeneration.

Signs and symptoms of Shy-Drager syndrome include orthostatic hypotension, urinary retention, bowel dysfunction, and impotence. Postural hypotension, when severe, can produce syncope. Plasma norepinephrine concentrations fail to show a normal increase after standing or exercise. Pupillary reflexes may be sluggish and control of breathing abnormal. Further evidence of autonomic nervous system dysfunction is noted by the failure of baroreceptor reflexes to produce an increase in heart rate or vasoconstriction in response to hypotension.

Treatment of orthostatic hypotension is symptomatic and includes use of elastic stockings, consumption of a high-sodium diet to expand intravascular fluid volume, and administration of vasoconstricting α_1-adrenergic agonists such as midodrine or α_2-adrenergic antagonists such as yohimbine. These drugs facilitate continued release of norepinephrine from postganglionic adrenergic neurons. Patients with

Shy-Drager syndrome have an ominous prognosis, with death usually occurring within 8 years of diagnosis. Death is generally a result of cerebral ischemia from prolonged hypotension.

MANAGEMENT OF ANESTHESIA

Preoperative evaluation may disclose orthostatic hypotension and the absence of the beat-to-beat variability in heart rate that should be associated with deep breathing. Management of anesthesia should focus on the decreased autonomic nervous system activity and hemodynamic aberrations that will occur in response to changes in body position, positive airway pressure, and acute blood loss. The negative inotropic effects of anesthetic drugs should also be considered.

Despite the obvious vulnerability of these patients to adverse perioperative events, most tolerate general and regional anesthesia without undue risk. The keys to management include continuous monitoring of the systemic blood pressure and prompt correction of hypotension. Crystalloid or colloid solutions can be infused to treat the hypotension. If vasopressors are needed, a direct-acting vasopressor such as phenylephrine is preferred, because these patients may have an exaggerated response to indirect-acting drugs that provoke the release of norepinephrine. Small doses of phenylephrine should be used initially until the response can be assessed, because the upregulated expression of α-adrenergic receptors in this disease of chronic relative autonomic denervation can produce an exaggerated response to even a small dose of drug. A continuous infusion of phenylephrine may be used to maintain systemic blood pressure during general anesthesia if needed. Spinal or epidural anesthesia can be considered, although the risk of hypotension demands diligence and caution. Volatile anesthetics can diminish cardiac contractility and result in exaggerated hypotension, because absent carotid sinus activity will impair the usual compensatory responses to a decreased cardiac output such as vasoconstriction or tachycardia. Bradycardia, which contributes to hypotension, is best treated with atropine or glycopyrrolate. Signs of light anesthesia may be less apparent in these patients because the sympathetic nervous system is less responsive to noxious stimulation. Administration of a muscle relaxant that has little or no effect on hemodynamics, such as vecuronium, is preferred. The dose and rate of administration of thiopental or propofol must be adjusted to accommodate for the patient's diminished ability to tolerate hypotension. Conversely, an accentuated blood pressure increase is a theoretical possibility following ketamine administration.

Orthostatic Intolerance Syndrome

Orthostatic intolerance syndrome is a chronic idiopathic disorder of primary autonomic system dysfunction characterized by episodic or postural tachycardia occurring independently of alterations in blood pressure. It manifests physiologic responses similar to those of other entities including postural tachycardia syndrome, effort syndrome, hyperdynamic β-adrenergic state, hyperdynamic orthostatic tachycardia, idiopathic hypovolemia, irritable heart, mitral valve prolapse syndrome, and neurocirculatory asthenia. Orthostatic intolerance syndrome is most often observed in young women. Symptoms include palpitations, tremulousness, light-headedness, fatigue, and syncope. The pathophysiology is unclear, although possible explanations include enhanced sensitivity of β_1-adrenergic receptors, hypovolemia, excessive venous pooling during standing, primary dysautonomia, and lower extremity sympathetic denervation.

Medical treatment of patients with orthostatic intolerance syndrome includes increasing intravascular fluid volume (increased sodium and water intake, administration of mineralocorticoids) to increase venous return. Long-term administration of α_1-adrenergic agonists such as midodrine may compensate for the decreased sympathetic activity in the legs and blunt heart rate responses to standing.

MANAGEMENT OF ANESTHESIA

Management of anesthesia in patients with orthostatic intolerance syndrome includes preoperative administration of crystalloid solutions to expand intravascular fluid volume. Low-dose phenylephrine infusions may be cautiously administered, with the recognition that lower extremity sympathetic nervous system denervation may cause upregulation of α_1-adrenergic receptors and contribute to receptor hypersensitivity. The combination of volume expansion and low-dose phenylephrine infusion should be sufficient to augment venous return, maintain blood pressure, and decrease autonomic nervous system lability in the presence of vasodilating anesthetic drugs or techniques. β-Blockers may be used to blunt tachycardia if needed, but care must be taken to avoid excessive hypotension. Neuraxial opioids may be quite useful for postoperative pain management.

Glomus Tumors of the Head and Neck

Glomus tumors are paragangliomas that arise embryologically from neural crest cells. These tumors develop in the head and neck within neuroendocrine tissues that lie along the carotid artery, aorta, glossopharyngeal nerve, and middle ear. They are rarely malignant. Tumor location determines signs and symptoms, which most often reflect middle ear and cranial nerve invasion. Unilateral pulsatile tinnitus, conductive hearing loss, aural fullness, and a bluish red mass behind the tympanic membrane are characteristic of middle ear involvement. Facial paralysis, dysphonia, hearing loss, and pain are characteristic of cranial nerve invasion. Recurrent aspiration, dysphagia, and upper airway obstruction may also accompany cranial nerve involvement. Invasion of the posterior fossa may obstruct the aqueduct of Sylvius, causing hydrocephalus. It is common for glomus tumors to invade the internal jugular vein.

Glomus tumors can secrete a variety of substances. The most common is norepinephrine, so that symptoms are produced mimicking those of a pheochromocytoma. Cholecystokinin secretion is thought to play a role in the high incidence of postoperative ileus following tumor resection. Release of serotonin or kallikrein can cause carcinoid-like symptoms such as bronchoconstriction, diarrhea, headache, flushing, and hypertension. Release of histamine or bradykinin can cause bronchoconstriction and hypotension.

Small glomus tumors are most often treated with radiation or embolization, either as a primary treatment or as adjunctive treatment before surgery. Surgery is recommended if bony destruction is present. Preoperative determination of serum concentrations of norepinephrine and catecholamine metabolites may be useful to determine if a pheochromocytoma-like condition is present. However, unlike some pheochromocytomas, glomus tumors do not secrete epinephrine because they lack the transferase necessary to convert norepinephrine to epinephrine. Phenoxybenzamine or prazosin may be administered preoperatively to lower blood pressure and facilitate volume expansion in patients with increased serum norepinephrine concentrations. Patients with increased serum 5-hydroxyindoleacetic acid (5-HIAA) concentration, especially those with symptoms resembling those of carcinoid syndrome, should receive octreotide preoperatively.

MANAGEMENT OF ANESTHESIA

Anesthetic management can be a formidable challenge in these patients. Risks include catecholamine secretion producing exaggerated hemodynamic changes, serotonin secretion producing signs of carcinoid syndrome, aspiration after tumor resection caused by cranial nerve dysfunction, impaired gastric emptying caused by vagal nerve dysfunction, the threat of venous air embolism, and massive blood loss. Histamine and bradykinin released during surgical manipulation can cause profound hypotension. Cranial nerve deficits (vagus, glossopharyngeal, hypoglossal nerves) may be present preoperatively or may occur as a result of tumor resection. Airway obstruction is a risk after cranial nerve injury resulting from unilateral vocal cord paralysis. In adults this does not usually result in complete airway obstruction by itself, but could produce airway obstruction in combination with airway edema or laryngeal distortion.

Invasive arterial and venous pressure monitoring is indicated, and urinary output should be monitored with a urinary bladder catheter. Given the risk of pheochromocytoma-like and carcinoid-like signs occurring intraoperatively, drugs used to treat both hypertension (e.g., sodium nitroprusside, phentolamine) and carcinoid-like signs (e.g., octreotide) should be immediately available.

Venous air embolism is a risk, especially if the internal jugular vein is opened to remove tumor. It is also a risk if excision of a tumor that has invaded temporal bone results in exposure of veins that cannot collapse because of bony attachments. Appropriate monitoring to detect venous air is indicated when venous air embolism is considered a risk. Sudden, unexplained cardiovascular collapse and death during resection of these tumors may reflect the presence of a venous air or tumor embolism. If the surgeon finds it necessary to identify the facial nerve, skeletal muscle paralysis should be avoided

so that a visible twitch response to direct neural stimulation can be obtained. The choice of anesthetic drugs is not uniquely influenced by the presence of glomus tumors, although the potential adverse effects of nitrous oxide have implications if venous air embolism occurs.

Carotid Sinus Syndrome

Carotid sinus syndrome is an uncommon entity caused by exaggeration of normal activity of the baroreceptors in response to mechanical stimulation. For example, stimulation of the carotid sinus by external massage, which in normal individuals produces modest decreases in heart rate and systemic blood pressure, can produce syncope in those with carotid sinus syndrome. Affected individuals have an increased incidence of peripheral vascular disease. Carotid sinus syndrome is a recognized although transient complication following carotid endarterectomy.

Two distinct cardiovascular responses may be noted in the presence of carotid sinus hypersensitivity. In approximately 80% of affected individuals, a cardioinhibitory reflex, mediated by the vagus nerve, produces profound bradycardia. In approximately 10% of affected individuals, a vasodepressor reflex mediated by inhibition of vasomotor tone produces decreases in systemic vascular resistance and profound hypotension. The remaining 10% exhibit components of both reflexes.

Carotid sinus syndrome may be treated with drugs, an artificial cardiac pacemaker, or ablation of the carotid sinus. The use of anticholinergic and vasopressor drugs is limited by their adverse effects, and they are rarely effective in patients with vasodepressor or mixed forms of carotid sinus hypersensitivity. Because most patients have the cardioinhibitory type of carotid sinus syndrome, implantation of an artificial cardiac pacemaker is the usual treatment. Denervation of the carotid sinus may be attempted in patients in whom the vasodepressor reflex response is refractory to cardiac pacing. Since the glossopharyngeal nerve provides the afferent limb of the reflex that produces symptoms in carotid sinus syndrome, block of this nerve may be an alternative therapy in patients refractory to cardiac pacing or drug therapy. The nerve is approached with a stimulating needle as it passes anterior to the styloid process. Successful identification of its location is noted when the patient complains of vague sensations in the region supplied by this nerve (e.g., external ear and pharynx) upon electrical nerve stimulation. Typically a test blockade is performed first with local anesthetic. If the desired effect of reduced symptomatology with carotid massage is obtained, then the nerve can be ablated with alcohol.

MANAGEMENT OF ANESTHESIA

Anesthetic management in patients with carotid sinus syndrome is often complicated by hypotension, bradycardia, and cardiac dysrhythmias. Infiltration of a local anesthetic–containing solution around the carotid sinus before dissection usually improves hemodynamic stability, but may interfere with determination of the completeness of the ablation.

Hyperhidrosis

Hyperhidrosis is a rare disorder in which individuals produce an excessive amount of sweat. The disorder can be either primary (idiopathic) or secondary to other conditions such as hyperthyroidism, pheochromocytoma, hypothalamic disorders (including that following central nervous system trauma), spinal cord injury, parkinsonism, or menopause. The disorder results from overactivity of sudomotor nerve fibers innervating eccrine sweat glands. The location of excess sweat production in secondary hyperhidrosis depends on the specific cause. Patients with primary hyperhidrosis often complain of excess sweat production in the palms of the hands and axillae, which often leads to social embarrassment. Conservative treatments include topical astringents such as potassium permanganate or tannic acid, or antiperspirants. Although these sudomotor nerve fibers belong to the sympathetic nervous system, the primary neurotransmitter in sweat glands is acetylcholine. Patients may respond to anticholinergic agents or to botulinum toxin injections. Botulinum toxin temporarily blocks the nerves that stimulate sweating. Severe cases may require surgical sympathectomy.

MANAGEMENT OF ANESTHESIA

The sympathetic chain is most commonly accessed in the thoracic cavity via video-assisted thoracoscopy. Bilateral hyperhidrosis will require bilateral sympathectomy, which can be performed during two separate operations but more commonly is done during a single procedure. Each thoracic cavity will need to be accessed, so one-lung ventilation will be required and is facilitated by placement of a double-lumen endotracheal tube. Successful sympathectomy will produce vasodilation in the ipsilateral upper extremity, documented by an immediate increase in temperature of 1° C or more in that extremity. Therefore, cutaneous temperature monitoring on a finger or palm is necessary before sectioning of the sympathetic chain to determine baseline and postlesion temperatures. In otherwise healthy patients, this surgery can be performed as an outpatient procedure. Patients often have minimal pain postoperatively, which responds well to opioids and nonsteroidal antiinflammatory drugs. Common surgical complications include infection, Horner's syndrome, and a compensatory hyperhidrosis elsewhere (e.g., trunk or lower extremity).

DISEASES OF THE PERIPHERAL NERVOUS SYSTEM

Idiopathic Facial Paralysis (Bell's Palsy)

Idiopathic facial paralysis is characterized by the rapid onset of motor weakness or paralysis of all the muscles innervated by the facial nerve. Onset is typically noted on arising in the morning and looking into a mirror. Additional symptoms can include the loss of taste sensation over the anterior two thirds of the tongue as well as hyperacusis and diminished salivation and lacrimation. There is no cutaneous sensory loss because the trigeminal nerve, not the facial nerve, supplies sensory innervation to the face. The cause of idiopathic facial paralysis is presumed to be inflammation and edema of the facial nerve, most often in the facial canal in the temporal bone. A virus, perhaps herpes simplex virus, may be the cause. Indeed, the onset of this cranial mononeuropathy is often preceded by a viral prodrome. During pregnancy, there is an increased incidence of idiopathic facial paralysis. The presence of idiopathic facial paralysis does not influence the choice of anesthetic technique.

Spontaneous recovery usually occurs in approximately 12 weeks. If no recovery is seen in 16 to 20 weeks, the clinical signs and symptoms are probably *not* due to idiopathic facial paralysis. Prednisone (1 mg/kg orally daily for 5 to 10 days, depending on the extent of facial nerve paralysis) can dramatically relieve pain and decrease the likelihood of complete denervation of the facial nerve. If blinking is not possible, the patient's affected eye should be covered to protect the cornea from dehydration.

Surgical decompression of the facial nerve may be needed for persistent or severe cases of idiopathic facial paralysis or for facial paralysis secondary to trauma. Paralysis of the facial nerve can reflect a stretch injury produced by excessive traction on the angle of the mandible during maintenance of the upper airway in unconscious patients. Uveoparotid fever (Heerfordt's syndrome) is a variant of sarcoidosis characterized by bilateral anterior uveitis, parotitis, and low-grade fever as well as the presence of facial nerve paralysis in 50% to 70% of patients. Facial nerve paralysis associated with postoperative uveoparotid fever may be erroneously attributed to mechanical pressure over the nerve during general anesthesia.

Trigeminal Neuralgia (Tic Douloureux)

Trigeminal neuralgia is characterized by the sudden onset of brief but intense unilateral facial pain triggered by local sensory stimuli to the affected side of the face. Trigeminal neuralgia can be diagnosed purely on the basis of clinical signs and symptoms. Patients report brief, stabbing pain or clusters of stabbing pain in the face or mouth that are restricted to one or more divisions of the trigeminal nerve, most often the mandibular division (Figure 12-1). Trigeminal neuralgia most often develops in otherwise healthy individuals during late middle age. The appearance of this neuralgia at an earlier age should arouse suspicion of multiple sclerosis. The pathophysiology of the pain associated with trigeminal neuralgia is uncertain. However, compression of the nerve root by a blood vessel is sometimes the cause. The most common blood vessel causing such compression is a branch of the superior cerebellar artery. Antiepileptic drugs are useful for treating trigeminal neuralgia. The anticonvulsant carbamazepine is the drug treatment of choice, but baclofen and lamotrigine are also effective. Surgical therapy (selective radiofrequency destruction of trigeminal nerve fibers, transection of the sensory root of the trigeminal nerve, microsurgical decompression of the

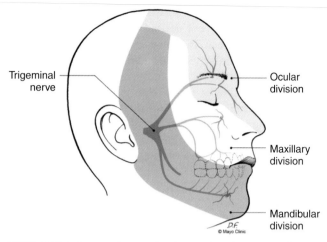

FIGURE 12-1 Sensory innervation by the three branches of the trigeminal nerve. *(By permission of the Mayo Foundation for Medical Education and Research. All rights reserved.)*

trigeminal nerve root) is recommended for individuals who develop pain refractory to drug therapy.

Patients undergoing surgery may experience bradycardia caused by activation of the trigeminocardiac reflex. In patients having microsurgical decompression, placement of a retractor to gain access to the root of the trigeminal nerve can stretch the vestibulocochlear nerve (cranial nerve VIII), which can potentially result in hearing loss. Therefore, intraoperative monitoring of brainstem auditory evoked potentials may be used to assess the integrity of cranial nerve VIII. Because brainstem auditory-evoked potentials can be suppressed by anesthetic drugs, an anesthetic technique that minimizes such suppression should be used. The potential enzyme-inducing effects of anticonvulsant drugs must be considered when predicting drug effects. Carbamazepine can also cause altered hepatic function and produce leukopenia and thrombocytopenia.

Glossopharyngeal Neuralgia

Glossopharyngeal neuralgia is characterized by episodes of intense pain in the throat, neck, tongue, and ear. Swallowing, chewing, coughing, or talking can trigger the pain. This neuralgia may also be associated with severe bradycardia and syncope, presumably because of the close association of the glossopharyngeal and vagus nerves, especially the branch of the glossopharyngeal nerve carrying afferent impulses from the carotid sinus (Hering's nerve). Hypotension, seizures caused by cerebral ischemia, and even cardiac arrest may occur in some patients.

Glossopharyngeal neuralgia is usually idiopathic but has been described in patients with cerebellopontine angle vascular anomalies and tumors, vertebral and carotid artery occlusive disease, arachnoiditis, and extracranial tumors arising in the area of the pharynx, larynx, and tonsils. The diagnosis of glossopharyngeal neuralgia is supported by pain in the distribution of the glossopharyngeal nerve and relief of this pain by topical anesthesia of the oropharynx at the tonsillar pillar.

In the absence of pain, cardiac symptoms associated with glossopharyngeal neuralgia may be confused with sick sinus syndrome or carotid sinus syndrome. Sick sinus syndrome can be discounted by the absence of characteristic changes on the electrocardiogram. Failure of carotid sinus massage to produce cardiac symptoms rules out carotid sinus hypersensitivity. Glossopharyngeal nerve blockade is useful for differentiating glossopharyngeal neuralgia from atypical trigeminal neuralgia. This nerve blockade does not, however, differentiate glossopharyngeal neuralgia from carotid sinus syndrome, because afferent pathways of both syndromes are mediated by the glossopharyngeal nerve.

Glossopharyngeal neuralgia–associated cardiac symptoms should be aggressively treated because there is a risk of sudden death. Cardiovascular symptoms are treated acutely with atropine, isoproterenol, a cardiac pacemaker, or a combination of these modalities. Pain associated with this syndrome is managed by administration of anticonvulsant drugs such as carbamazepine and phenytoin. Prevention of cardiovascular symptoms and predictable pain relief can be achieved by intracranial surgical transection of the glossopharyngeal nerve and the upper two roots of the vagus nerve. Although permanent pain relief is possible after repeated glossopharyngeal nerve blockade, this neuralgia is sufficiently life-threatening to justify intracranial transection of the nerve in patients who do not respond to medical therapy.

MANAGEMENT OF ANESTHESIA

Preoperative evaluation of patients with glossopharyngeal neuralgia is directed at assessing cardiac status and intravascular fluid volume. Hypovolemia may be present since these patients avoid oral intake and its associated pharyngeal stimulation in an attempt to avoid triggering the pain attacks. In addition, drooling can contribute to fluid losses. A preoperative history of syncope or documented bradycardia concurrent with an episode of pain introduces the possible need for transcutaneous cardiac pacing or placement of a transvenous cardiac pacemaker before induction of anesthesia. Continuous monitoring of electrocardiographic activity and of blood pressure via an intraarterial catheter is useful. Topical anesthesia of the oropharynx with lidocaine is helpful to prevent bradycardia and hypotension, which may occur in response to pharyngeal stimulation during direct laryngoscopy. Intravenous administration of atropine or glycopyrrolate before initiation of laryngoscopy may be useful in some patients.

Cardiovascular changes should be expected in response to surgical manipulation during intracranial transection of the glossopharyngeal and vagus nerve roots. Bradycardia and hypotension are likely during manipulation of the vagus nerve. Anticholinergic drugs should be immediately available to treat these vagally mediated responses. Hypertension, tachycardia, and ventricular premature beats may occur after surgical transection of the glossopharyngeal nerve and the upper two roots of the vagus nerve because of the sudden loss of sensory input from the carotid sinus. Hypertension is usually transient but can persist into the postoperative period. In this setting, hydralazine may be useful. Experience is too limited to permit recommendations for specific anesthetic drugs or muscle relaxants. The possible development of vocal cord paralysis after vagal nerve transection should be considered if airway obstruction follows tracheal extubation.

Charcot-Marie-Tooth Disease

The most common inherited cause of chronic motor and sensory peripheral neuropathy, Charcot-Marie-Tooth disease type 1A (CMT1A), also called *peroneal muscle disease,* has an estimated incidence of 1 in 2500 individuals. An autosomal dominant mode of inheritance is most common but an X-linked variant is known to exist. This disorder manifests as distal skeletal muscle weakness, wasting, and loss of tendon reflexes, which becomes evident by the middle teenage years. Classically, this neuropathy is described as being restricted to the lower one third of the legs, producing foot deformities (high pedal arches and talipes) and peroneal muscle atrophy ("stork-leg" appearance). The disease may slowly progress to include wasting of the quadriceps muscles and the muscles of the hands and forearms. Mild to moderate stocking-glove sensory loss occurs in many patients. Pregnancy may precipitate exacerbations of CMT.

Treatment of CMT1A is limited to supportive measures, including splinting, tendon transfers, and various arthrodeses. Although life span is not decreased, many individuals with CMT1A experience long-term disability.

MANAGEMENT OF ANESTHESIA

Management of anesthesia in patients with CMT1A should focus on the response to neuromuscular blocking drugs and the possibility of postoperative respiratory failure resulting from weakness of the respiratory muscles. Cardiac manifestations attributed to this neuropathy, including conduction disturbances, atrial flutter, and cardiomyopathy, are seen occasionally. Drugs known to trigger malignant hyperthermia have been used safely in patients with CMT. The response to neuromuscular blocking drugs seems to be normal in patients with CMT1A. It may be reasonable to avoid succinylcholine because of theoretical concerns about exaggerated potassium release in individuals with neuromuscular diseases. However, succinylcholine has been used safely in some patients without producing hyperkalemia or triggering malignant hyperthermia. Use of epidural anesthesia for labor has been described.

Brachial Plexus Neuropathy

Brachial plexus neuropathy (idiopathic brachial neuritis, Parsonage-Turner syndrome, shoulder-girdle syndrome) is characterized by the acute onset of severe pain in the upper arm. The pain is typically most severe at the onset of the neuropathy. As the pain diminishes, patchy paresis or paralysis of the skeletal muscles innervated by branches of the brachial plexus appears. Skeletal muscle wasting, particularly involving the shoulder girdle and arm, is common. Brachial plexus

neuropathy is more common on the right side, although nerve involvement and pain are bilateral in 10% to 30% of affected individuals, with both sides becoming involved either simultaneously or sequentially. Although this neuropathy seems to have a predilection for the upper trunks of the brachial plexus (axillary, suprascapular, long thoracic nerves), it may involve other nerves in the upper extremity. An estimated 70% of patients have involvement of the axillary nerve. Secondary causes of brachial plexus neuropathy include trauma to the neck or upper limb. In neonates, shoulder dystocia during delivery is another cause of brachial plexus neuropathy.

Electrophysiologic studies are valuable in diagnosing brachial plexus neuropathy and demonstrating the multifocal pattern of denervation. Muscle fibrillations and slowing of nerve conduction velocity are observed. The skeletal muscles most often affected, in decreasing order, are the deltoid, supraspinatus, infraspinatus, serratus anterior, biceps, and triceps. The diaphragm may also be affected. Sensory disturbances occur in most patients, but tend to be minimal and generally disappear over time. The incidence of this neuropathy is two to three times higher in males than in females. Overall, recovery may take 2 to 3 years but is nearly always complete. The annual incidence of brachial plexus neuropathy is estimated at 1.64 cases per 100,000.

Nerve biopsy findings in individuals with hereditary brachial plexus neuropathy and Parsonage-Turner syndrome suggest an inflammatory-immune pathogenesis. Autoimmune neuropathies may also occur during the postoperative period independent of the site of surgery. It is possible that the stress of surgery activates an unidentified dormant virus in the nerve roots, a circumstance that would be similar to the onset of herpes zoster after surgery. In addition, strenuous exercise or pregnancy may be inciting events for brachial plexus neuropathy.

Guillain-Barré Syndrome (Acute Idiopathic Polyneuritis)

Guillain-Barré syndrome is characterized by sudden onset of skeletal muscle weakness or paralysis that typically begins in the legs and spreads cephalad over the ensuing days to involve the arms, trunk, and face. With the virtual elimination of poliomyelitis, this syndrome has become the most common cause of acute generalized paralysis, with an annual incidence of 0.75 to 2.0 cases per 100,000. Bulbar involvement typically manifests as bilateral facial paralysis. Difficulty swallowing because of pharyngeal muscle weakness and impaired ventilation because of intercostal muscle paralysis are the most serious signs of this process. Because of lower motor neuron involvement, paralysis is flaccid, and corresponding tendon reflexes are diminished. Sensory disturbances (e.g., paresthesias) generally precede the onset of paralysis and are most prominent in the distal extremities. Pain often exists in the form of headache, backache, or tenderness of skeletal muscles to deep pressure.

Autonomic nervous system dysfunction is a prominent finding in patients with Guillain-Barré syndrome and is usually manifested as fluctuations in blood pressure, sudden profuse diaphoresis, peripheral vasoconstriction, resting tachycardia, and cardiac conduction abnormalities. Orthostatic hypotension may be so severe that elevating the patient's head onto a pillow may lead to syncope. Thromboembolism may occur due to immobility. Sudden death associated with this disease is most likely caused by autonomic nervous system dysfunction.

Complete spontaneous recovery from acute idiopathic polyneuritis can occur within a few weeks if segmental demyelination is the predominant pathologic process. Axonal degeneration (as detected by electromyographic screening) may result in slower recovery that takes several months and leaves some residual weakness. The mortality rate associated with Guillain-Barré syndrome is 3% to 8%, and death is most often a result of sepsis, acute respiratory failure, pulmonary embolism, or cardiac arrest.

The diagnosis of Guillain-Barré syndrome is based on clinical signs and symptoms (Table 12-1), supported by findings of an increased protein concentration in the cerebrospinal fluid. Cerebrospinal fluid cell counts typically remain within the normal range. This syndrome develops after respiratory or gastrointestinal infection in approximately half of patients, which hints that the cause may be related to either a viral or mycoplasma infection.

Treatment of Guillain-Barré syndrome is symptomatic. Vital capacity is monitored, and when it decreases to less than 15 mL/kg, mechanical support of ventilation is initiated. Arterial blood gas measurements help in assessing the adequacy of ventilation and oxygenation. Pharyngeal muscle weakness, even in the absence of ventilatory failure, may require insertion of a cuffed endotracheal tube or tracheostomy to protect the lungs from aspiration of secretions or gastric fluid. Autonomic nervous system dysfunction may require treatment of hypertension or hypotension. Corticosteroids are not useful. Plasma exchange or infusion of gamma globulin may benefit some patients.

MANAGEMENT OF ANESTHESIA

Abnormal autonomic nervous system function and the presence of lower motor neuron lesions are the major factors to consider in developing an anesthetic plan for patients with Guillain-Barré syndrome. Compensatory cardiovascular responses may be absent, so that profound hypotension occurs in response to changes in posture, blood loss, or positive airway pressure. Conversely, noxious stimulation, such as direct laryngoscopy, can cause exaggerated increases in blood pressure. Because of these unpredictable changes in blood pressure, it may be prudent to monitor blood pressure continuously with an intraarterial catheter. Patients may also exhibit exaggerated responses to indirect-acting vasopressors, probably as a result of upregulation of postsynaptic receptors.

Succinylcholine should not be administered because there is a risk of excessive potassium release from denervated skeletal muscles. A nondepolarizing muscle relaxant with minimal circulatory effects, such as cisatracurium or vecuronium, may be used if needed. Even if a patient is breathing spontaneously before surgery, it is likely that mechanical ventilation will be necessary during the postoperative period.

Entrapment Neuropathies

Entrapment neuropathies occur at anatomic sites where peripheral nerves pass through narrow passages (e.g., median nerve and carpal tunnel at the wrist, ulnar nerve and cubital tunnel at the elbow) that make compression a possibility. Peripheral nerves are probably more sensitive to compressive (ischemic) injury in patients who also have generalized polyneuropathies such as those that occur with diabetes mellitus or hereditary peripheral neuropathies. A peripheral nerve may also be more susceptible to compression if the same fibers have been partially damaged proximally (*double crush hypothesis*). For example, spinal nerve root compression (cervical radiculopathy) may increase the vulnerability of nerve fibers to injury at distal entrapment sites, such as the carpal tunnel at the wrist. Osteoarthritis could also explain symptoms attributed to the double crush phenomenon. Peripheral nerve damage resulting from compression depends on the severity of the compression and the anatomy of the nerve. In most instances, the outermost nerve fibers—that is, those that innervate more proximal tissues—are more vulnerable to ischemia from compression than the fibers lying more deeply in the nerve bundle. This differing damage to individual fascicles in a peripheral nerve makes it difficult to localize the site of nerve injury precisely, although nerve conduction studies can be helpful. Focal demyelination of nerve fibers causes slowing or blocking of nerve impulse conduction through the damaged area. Electromyographic studies are adjuncts to nerve conduction studies and can show patterns characteristic of denervation and subsequent reinnervation of muscle fibers by surviving axons.

CARPAL TUNNEL SYNDROME

Carpal tunnel syndrome is the most common entrapment neuropathy. It results from compression of the median nerve between the transverse carpal ligament and the carpal bones

---

TABLE 12-1 ■ Diagnostic criteria for Guillain-Barré syndrome

FEATURES REQUIRED FOR DIAGNOSIS

Progressive bilateral weakness in legs and arms
Areflexia

FEATURES STRONGLY SUPPORTING THE DIAGNOSIS

Progression of symptoms over 2-4 wk
Symmetry of symptoms
Mild sensory symptoms or signs (a definitive sensory level makes diagnosis doubtful)
Cranial nerve involvement (especially bilateral facial weakness)
Spontaneous recovery beginning 2-4 wk after progression ceases
Autonomic nervous system dysfunction
Absence of fever at onset
Increased concentrations of protein in the cerebrospinal fluid

at the wrist. This compression neuropathy most often occurs in otherwise healthy women (three times more frequently than in men) and is often bilateral, although the dominant hand is typically involved first. Patients describe repeated episodes of pain and paresthesias in the wrist and hand following the distribution of the median nerve (thumb and index and middle fingers), often occurring during sleep or upon awakening. Population-based studies reveal that approximately 3% of adults have symptomatic electrodiagnostically confirmed carpal tunnel syndrome.

The exact cause of carpal tunnel syndrome is unknown, but affected individuals often engage in occupations that require repetitive movements of the hands and fingers. Nerve conduction studies are the definitive method for confirming the diagnosis. In previously asymptomatic patients who acquire symptoms of carpal tunnel syndrome shortly after an unrelated surgery, it is likely that accumulation of third space fluid resulting in increased tissue pressure caused compression of the nerve. In such patients, subsequent neurologic examination and neurophysiologic testing often find asymptomatic evidence of preexisting carpal tunnel syndrome. Pregnancy and associated peripheral edema may also precipitate the initial manifestations of carpal tunnel syndrome. Cervical radiculopathy may produce similar symptoms unilaterally but rarely bilaterally.

Immobilizing the wrist with a splint is a common treatment for carpal tunnel syndrome that is likely to be transient (pregnancy) or caused by a medically treatable disease (hypothyroidism, acromegaly). Injection of corticosteroids into the carpal tunnel may relieve symptoms but is seldom curative. Definitive treatment of carpal tunnel syndrome is decompression of the median nerve by surgical division of the transverse carpal ligament.

Compression of the ulnar nerve after it passes through the condylar groove and enters the cubital tunnel results in clinical symptoms considered typical of ulnar nerve neuropathy. It may be difficult to differentiate clinical symptoms of ulnar nerve neuropathy caused by compression in the condylar groove from symptoms related to entrapment in the cubital tunnel. Surgical treatment of cubital tunnel entrapment syndrome (by tunnel decompression and transposition of the nerve) may be helpful in relieving symptoms, but may also make symptoms worse, perhaps by interfering with the nerve's blood supply.

MERALGIA PARESTHETICA

The lateral femoral cutaneous nerve, a pure sensory nerve, can become entrapped as it crosses under the inguinal ligament near the attachment of the ligament to the anterior superior iliac spine. Patients complain of burning pain down the lateral thigh, but may also have sensory loss in that region and possibly point tenderness at the site of entrapment. Meralgia paresthetica often occurs in overweight individuals and is exacerbated by wearing tight-fitting garments, such as belts. It may also occur following abdominal surgery or iliac crest bone graft harvesting, during pregnancy, or in conditions involving fluid overload such as ascites or congestive heart failure. Treatment is usually conservative since meralgia paresthetica tends to regress spontaneously. Treatment options include weight loss, removal of offending garments, elimination of activities involving hip flexion, topical cooling and administration of nonsteroidal analgesics. Refractory cases may require local anesthetic and corticosteroid injections at the site of entrapment and possible surgical decompression.

Diseases Associated with Peripheral Neuropathies

DIABETES MELLITUS

Diabetes mellitus is commonly associated with peripheral polyneuropathies. The incidence of this problem increases with the duration of the diabetes and perhaps the degree of hypoinsulinemia. The etiology of diabetic neuropathy is multifactorial and may include microvascular damage resulting in neuronal ischemia; formation of glycosylated intraneuronal proteins; activation of protein kinase C; inhibition of glutathione, which increases reactive oxygen species; and activation of the sorbitol-aldose reductase pathway. Neurons in this latter pathway (like retinal and renal cells), do not require insulin to allow intracellular entry of glucose. The increased intracellular glucose is converted to sorbitol via aldose reductase, and since sorbitol cannot cross cell membranes, this results in increased intracellular osmolarity, cellular osmotic stress, and subsequent neuronal dysfunction.

Up to 7.5% of patients with non–insulin-dependent diabetes mellitus have clinical neuropathy at the time that their diabetes is diagnosed. Electrophysiologic studies show evidence of denervation and reduced nerve conduction velocity. The most common neuropathy is distal, symmetrical, and predominantly sensory. The principal manifestations are unpleasant tingling, numbness, burning, and aching in the lower extremities; skeletal muscle weakness; and distal sensory loss. Occasionally, an isolated sciatic neuropathy suggests the presence of a herniated intervertebral disc. Sciatic neuropathy in patients with diabetes mellitus is not associated with pain in response to straight-leg raising, which distinguishes this peripheral neuropathy from lumbar disk disease. In diabetic neuropathy, discomfort is prominent at night and is often relieved by walking. Symptoms often progress and may extend to the upper extremities. Impotence, urinary retention, gastroparesis, resting tachycardia, and postural hypotension are common and reflect autonomic nervous system dysfunction. For reasons that are not understood, the peripheral nerves of patients with diabetes mellitus are more vulnerable to ischemia resulting from compression or stretch injury such as may occur during intraoperative and postoperative positioning.

ALCOHOL ABUSE

Polyneuropathy of chronic alcoholism is nearly always associated with nutritional and vitamin deficiencies. Symptoms characteristically begin in the lower extremities, with pain and numbness in the feet. Weakness and tenderness of the intrinsic muscles of the feet, loss of the Achilles tendon reflex, and hypalgesia in a stocking-glove distribution are early manifestations. Restoration of a proper diet, abstinence from alcohol, and multivitamin therapy promote slow but predictable resolution of the neuropathy.

VITAMIN B₁₂ DEFICIENCY

The earliest neurologic symptoms of vitamin B_{12} deficiency resemble the neuropathy typically seen in patients who abuse alcohol. Paresthesias in the legs with sensory loss in a stocking distribution plus absent Achilles tendon reflexes are characteristic findings. Similar neurologic findings have been reported in dentists who experience long-term exposure to nitrous oxide and in individuals who habitually inhale nitrous oxide for nonmedical purposes. Nitrous oxide is known to inactivate certain vitamin B_{12}–dependent enzymes, which could lead to symptoms of altered nerve function.

UREMIA

Distal polyneuropathy with sensory and motor components often occurs in the extremities of patients with chronic renal failure. Symptoms tend to be more prominent in the legs than in the arms. Presumably, metabolic abnormalities are responsible for the axonal degeneration and segmental demyelination that accompany the neuropathy. Slowing of nerve conduction has been correlated with increased plasma concentrations of parathyroid hormone and myoinositol, a component of myelin. Improved nerve conduction velocity often occurs within a few days after renal transplantation. However, hemodialysis is ineffective in reversing this polyneuropathy.

CANCER

Peripheral sensory and motor neuropathies occur in patients with a variety of malignancies, especially those involving the lung, ovary, and breast. Polyneuropathy that develops in elderly patients should always arouse suspicion of undiagnosed cancer. Myasthenic (Eaton-Lambert) syndrome may be observed in patients with carcinoma of the lung. This paraneoplastic syndrome results from the abnormal production of an antibody against presynaptic calcium channels located on cholinergic neurons. As a result of calcium channel blockade, decreased quantities of acetylcholine are released from nerve terminals at the neuromuscular junction, which results in weakness. Myasthenic syndrome is associated with increased sensitivity to both depolarizing and nondepolarizing neuromuscular blocking drugs. Invasion of the lower trunks of the brachial plexus by tumors in the apex of the lungs (Pancoast's syndrome) produces arm pain, paresthesias, and weakness of the hands and arms.

COLLAGEN VASCULAR DISEASES

Collagen vascular diseases are commonly associated with peripheral neuropathies. These occur most often in systemic lupus erythematosus, polyarteritis nodosa, rheumatoid arthritis, and scleroderma. Detection of multiple mononeuropathies suggests vasculitis of nerve trunks and should stimulate a search for the presence of a collagen vascular disease.

SARCOIDOSIS

Sarcoidosis is a disorder of unknown etiology in which noncaseating granulomas occur in multiple organ systems, most commonly the lung, lymphatics, bone, liver, and nervous system. Polyneuropathy resulting from the presence of granulomatous lesions in peripheral nerves is a frequent finding. Unilateral or bilateral facial nerve paralysis may result from sarcoid involvement of this nerve in the parotid gland and is often one of the first manifestations of sarcoidosis.

ACQUIRED IMMUNODEFICIENCY SYNDROME–ASSOCIATED NEUROPATHY

Peripheral neuropathy is common in patients with acquired immunodeficiency syndrome (AIDS) but not in patients with human immunodeficiency virus infection without AIDS. AIDS-associated neuropathy is typically a distal symmetric polyneuropathy, and patients complain of numbness, tingling, and sometimes pain in their feet. There may be loss of vibratory sensation and light touch. Although the exact cause is unclear, infection with cytomegalovirus or *Mycobacterium avium-intracellulare,* lymphomatous invasion of peripheral nerves, or adverse effects of antiretroviral medication may be responsible.

Perioperative Peripheral Neuropathies

Perioperative neuropathies have been described following a variety of surgical procedures and affecting a multitude of nerves. Although such neuropathies were originally thought to be primarily the result of errors in patient positioning during surgery, epidemiologic data suggest that in most circumstances, preexisting aberrations of patient anatomy and physiology predispose the patient to this kind of injury. Intraoperative positioning must still be considered as contributory in many instances, but other critical factors including obesity, bony abnormalities, edema formation, metabolic derangements, and the failure of sedated, pain-free patients to frequently reposition themselves in bed postoperatively (and hence a failure to relieve pressure on individual nerves) may also be involved. Ulnar neuropathy is the most common perioperative neuropathy, typically affecting obese males who undergo abdominal or pelvic procedures. Symptoms of ulnar neuropathy do not typically present until at least 48 hours after surgery, and patients are often found to have *contralateral* nerve conduction dysfunction, which indicates a predisposition to this injury. Postoperative brachial plexus neuropathy may initially be mistaken for ulnar neuropathy and appears to be associated with brachial plexus stretch resulting from sternal retraction during median sternotomy, placement in steep Trendelenburg's position, and prone positioning with shoulder abduction and contralateral head rotation. Lower extremity neuropathies are most common following procedures performed in the lithotomy position and usually affect the common peroneal nerve where it may become compressed by a leg holder in this position as the nerve crosses over the fibular head. Sciatic and femoral neuropathy may also be associated with lithotomy positioning, but these are seen much less often than peroneal neuropathy.

Management of patients who develop perioperative peripheral neuropathies begins with (1) taking a history and performing a physical examination, which should focus on identifying risk factors for or a history of neuropathy; (2) determining whether the deficit is sensory, motor, or mixed; and (3) documenting the distribution of the deficit. Most sensory deficits resolve within 5 days, so if the deficit is purely sensory, expectant management is suggested. Since motor fibers tend to be located deeper within nerves, the presence of a motor deficit suggests a more extensive injury. In this situation, a neurology consultation is warranted.

KEY POINTS

■ When caring for patients with diseases affecting the autonomic nervous system, one must carefully monitor for and be prepared to treat significant changes in heart rate and blood pressure.

■ In the setting of autonomic disorders, changes in catecholamine release and adrenergic receptor density may occur. Therefore, one should titrate the dosage of direct-acting adrenergic agonists and avoid the use of indirect-acting adrenergic agonists.

■ Succinylcholine should be used with caution in patients with neurologic diseases affecting the peripheral nervous system because of the risk of hyperkalemia resulting from upregulation of acetylcholine receptors at the neuromuscular junction.

■ Some diseases affecting the peripheral nervous system may be associated with significant neuropathic pain. Both narcotic and nonnarcotic pain management options should be considered.

RESOURCES

Lupski JR, Chance PF, Garcia CA. Inherited primary peripheral neuropathies. Molecular genetics and clinical implications of CMT1A and HNPP. *JAMA*. 1993;270:2326-2330.

Ropper AH. The Guillain-Barré syndrome. *N Engl J Med*. 1992;326:1130-1136.

Scrivani SJ, Mathews ES, Maciewicz RJ. Trigeminal neuralgia. *Oral Surg Oral Med Oral Pathol Oral Radiol Endod*. 2005;100:527-538.

Warner MA. Perioperative neuropathies. *Mayo Clin Proc*. 1998;73:567-574.

CHAPTER 13

Diseases of the Liver and Biliary Tract

ZOLTAN G. HEVESI ■
MICHAEL HANNAMAN ■

The overall frequency of clinically significant liver disease is relatively low in the surgical patient population. However, the complexity of derangements in hepatic function necessitates an in-depth understanding of this topic. The liver plays a central role in the functioning of several body systems, such as the activity of the gastrointestinal tract; metabolic activities, including the synthesis and degradation or detoxification of essential compounds; the pharmacokinetics of anesthetic and anesthesia adjuncts; and hemostasis. It is thus desirable that an anesthesiologist be familiar with the various hepatic pathophysiologic conditions and anticipate the consequences of liver dysfunction.

ASSESSMENT OF LIVER FUNCTION

The initial presentation of most hepatic abnormalities typically involves symptoms of malaise or flulike symptoms followed by the development of jaundice. Thus laboratory testing is essential to assess the cause and the severity of the illness.

TABLE 13-1 ■ Causes of hepatic dysfunction based on liver function test results

Hepatic dysfunction	Bilirubin	Aminotransferase enzymes	Alkaline phosphatase	Causes
Prehepatic	Increased unconjugated fraction	Normal	Normal	Hemolysis Hematoma resorption Bilirubin overload from blood transfusion
Intrahepatic (hepatocellular)	Increased conjugated fraction	Markedly increased	Normal to slightly increased	Viral infection Drugs Alcohol Sepsis Hypoxemia Cirrhosis
Posthepatic (cholestatic)	Increased conjugated fraction	Normal to slightly increased	Markedly increased	Biliary tract stones or tumors Sepsis

Bilirubin

Bilirubin is the degradation product of hemoglobin and myoglobin. Unconjugated bilirubin formed in the periphery is transported to the liver, where it is conjugated to monoglucuronides and diglucuronides by the action of the enzyme glucuronosyl transferase. This greatly increases the water solubility of bilirubin, which enhances its elimination from the body while simultaneously decreasing its ability to cross biologic membranes, including the blood-brain barrier. *Unconjugated hyperbilirubinemia* occurs with an increase in bilirubin production, decreased hepatic uptake of bilirubin, or decreased conjugation of bilirubin. *Conjugated hyperbilirubinemia* occurs with decreased canalicular transport of bilirubin, acute or chronic hepatocellular dysfunction, or obstruction of the bile ducts (Table 13-1).

Normally, total bilirubin concentration is less than 1 mg/dL. A serum bilirubin concentration of 3 mg/dL results in scleral icterus and a level above 4 mg/dL causes overt jaundice.

Aminotransferases

Alanine aminotransferase (ALT) and aspartate aminotransferase (AST) are enzymes involved in hepatic gluconeogenesis. ALT is a cytoplasmic enzyme that is highly specific to the liver, but the cytoplasmic and mitochondrial isoenzymes of AST are present in extrahepatic tissues as well. Frequently, hepatocellular injury results in the release of aminotransferases and leads to significantly increased serum levels of these enzymes. The AST/ALT ratio can be a useful measurement. When levels of both enzymes are elevated, a ratio of less than 1 is characteristic of nonalcoholic steatohepatitis. A ratio between 2 and 4 is typical of alcoholic liver disease, and a ratio of more than 4 is distinctive of Wilson's disease.

Alkaline Phosphatase

Increases in serum alkaline phosphatase lack specificity as a diagnostic test for liver disease because its isoenzymes are present in plasma membranes throughout the body. However, in cholestatic disorders, an increased alkaline phosphatase concentration may indicate the bile salt–induced damage of hepatocyte membranes. Alkaline phosphatase has a serum half-life of approximately 1 week, so the level remains elevated for several days after resolution of biliary obstruction.

International Normalized Ratio

Prolongation of the international normalized ratio (INR) shows strong correlation with deteriorating hepatic function and has a reliable predictive value for survival of patients with liver disease. It is, of course, not a complete indicator of hemostatic function. It can indicate impairment of hepatic synthetic function of coagulation factors, but evaluation of the entire coagulation cascade requires other testing.

Albumin

Albumin is the most abundant plasma protein. It is synthesized exclusively by hepatocytes and accounts for about 15% of all the protein synthesized by the liver. Albumin concentration is a major determinant of countless metabolic processes and the bioavailability of a wide variety of substances, because substrates are often transported bound to albumin. A diminished serum albumin concentration can be an indicator of protein malnutrition, a protein-losing disease such as nephrotic syndrome, or a severe reduction in the synthetic capacity of the liver.

Serologic and Genetic Testing

Antigen and antibody detection is the cornerstone in elucidating the differential diagnosis of viral and/or autoimmune hepatitis. Similarly, abnormal levels of protein markers are diagnostic in α_1- antitrypsin deficiency, Wilson's disease, and hepatocellular carcinoma, and genetic testing can be a valuable adjunct for confirmation of the suspected diagnosis of certain heritable liver diseases.

HYPERBILIRUBINEMIA

Gilbert's Syndrome

The most common example of a hereditary hyperbilirubinemia (present in varying degrees in about 10% of the general population) is Gilbert's syndrome, inherited as an autosomal dominant trait with variable penetrance. The primary defect is a mutation in the glucuronosyl transferase enzyme, but usually about one third of normal enzyme activity is present. Plasma bilirubin concentrations seldom exceed 5 mg/dL but will increase twofold to threefold with fasting or illness or stress.

Crigler-Najjar Syndrome

Crigler-Najjar syndrome is a rare hereditary form of severe unconjugated hyperbilirubinemia that results from a mutation in the glucuronosyl transferase enzyme. Typically glucuronosyl transferase activity is reduced to less than 10% of normal. Children who lack effective enzyme function are jaundiced in the perinatal period. Kernicterus can develop. Optimal treatment for a neurologically intact child includes exchange transfusion in the neonatal period, daily phototherapy throughout childhood, and early liver transplantation before brain damage develops. Long-term phenobarbital therapy may decrease jaundice by stimulating the activity of glucuronosyl transferase.

Bilirubin phototherapy lights should be available for management of anesthesia in children with this syndrome. Fasting should be minimized because this stress is known to increase plasma bilirubin concentration. Morphine is metabolized by a glucuronosyl transferase enzyme system different from that deficient in Crigler-Najjar syndrome. Therefore, morphine can be safely administered to these patients. Barbiturates, inhaled anesthetics, and muscle relaxants are acceptable choices in these patients.

Dubin-Johnson Syndrome

Dubin-Johnson syndrome is caused by decreased ability to transport organic ions from hepatocytes into the biliary system, which results in conjugated hyperbilirubinemia. Despite the conjugated hyperbilirubinemia, these patients are not cholestatic. Inheritance of this syndrome is autosomal recessive. The disorder is benign.

Benign Postoperative Intrahepatic Cholestasis

Benign postoperative intrahepatic cholestasis may occur when surgery is prolonged, especially if it is complicated by hypotension, hypoxemia, and the need for blood transfusion. The hyperbilirubinemia may be caused by an increase in bilirubin production (breakdown of transfused red blood cells or resorption of a hematoma) and/or decreased hepatic clearance of bilirubin. Jaundice with conjugated hyperbilirubinemia is usually apparent within 24 to 48 hours. Results of liver function tests other than those for bilirubin and alkaline phosphatase are usually normal or only mildly abnormal. This condition typically resolves in tandem with improvement in the underlying surgical or medical condition.

Progressive Familial Intrahepatic Cholestasis

Progressive familial intrahepatic cholestasis is a rare hereditary metabolic disease presenting as cholestasis in infancy and end-stage cirrhosis before adulthood. Pruritus may be severe. The precise metabolic defect responsible for this disease has not been identified. Liver transplantation is the only curative treatment. Management of anesthesia in patients with progressive familial intrahepatic cholestasis or cirrhosis is influenced by the presence of malnutrition, portal hypertension, coagulation abnormalities, hypoalbuminemia, and chronic hypoxemia.

DISEASES OF THE BILIARY TRACT

Cholelithiasis and inflammatory biliary tract disease constitute major health problems in the United States. Approximately 30 million Americans have gallstones. The prevalence of gallstones is significantly higher in women than in men. The prevalence rises with increasing age, obesity, rapid weight loss, and pregnancy. Gallstone formation is most likely related to abnormalities in the physicochemical characteristics of the various components of bile. Approximately 90% of gallstones in countries consuming a Western diet high in protein and fat are radiolucent, composed primarily of cholesterol. The remaining gallstones are usually radiopaque and are typically composed of calcium bilirubinate. These gallstones develop most often in patients with cirrhosis or hemolytic anemia.

Acute Cholecystitis

Patients who have gallbladder or biliary tract stones can exhibit no symptoms (silent disease), acute symptomatic disease, or chronic intermittently symptomatic disease. Obstruction of the cystic duct or common bile duct by a gallstone causes acute inflammation. Cholelithiasis is present in 95% of patients with acute cholecystitis. Obstruction of the cystic duct, which is nearly always due to a gallstone, produces acute inflammation of the gallbladder.

Signs and symptoms of acute cholecystitis include nausea, vomiting, fever, abdominal pain, and right upper quadrant tenderness. Severe pain that begins in the mid-epigastrium, moves to the right upper quadrant, and may radiate to the back, and is caused by a stone lodged in a duct is designated *biliary colic*. This pain is extraordinarily intense and usually begins abruptly and subsides gradually. Patients may notice dark urine and scleral icterus. Most jaundiced patients have stones in the common bile duct at the time of surgery. Laboratory testing commonly demonstrates leukocytosis.

Patients with a clinical diagnosis of acute cholecystitis are treated with intravenous fluids and opioids to manage the pain. Febrile patients with leukocytosis are given antibiotics. Surgery is typically considered when the patient's condition has stabilized. Laparoscopic cholecystectomy is the procedure of choice. In approximately 5% of patients, laparoscopic cholecystectomy must be converted to open cholecystectomy because inflammation obscures the anatomy. Patients with septic shock, peritonitis, pancreatitis, or coagulopathy may undergo open cholecystectomy or ultrasonographically guided percutaneous cholecystostomy. Cholangiography can be performed during surgery, and common duct stones can be removed concurrently or subsequently by endoscopic retrograde cholangiopancreatography (ERCP).

Anesthetic considerations for laparoscopic cholecystectomy are similar to those for other laparoscopic procedures. Insufflation of the abdominal cavity (pneumoperitoneum) results in increased intraabdominal pressure that may interfere with the adequacy of ventilation and venous return. Changes in cardiovascular function resulting from insufflation include an immediate decrease in venous return and cardiac output and an increase in mean arterial pressure and systemic vascular resistance. During the next several minutes, there is partial restoration of cardiac output, but blood pressure and heart rate typically remain unchanged. This pattern of cardiovascular responses is most likely the result of interactions caused by increased abdominal pressure, neurohumoral responses, and absorbed carbon dioxide. Placement of the patient in reverse Trendelenburg's position favors movement of abdominal contents away from the operative site and may improve ventilation.

The use of opioids during anesthesia for this operation is controversial because these drugs can cause spasm of the sphincter of Oddi. However, opioids have often been used without any adverse effects, which emphasizes that not all patients respond to opioids with sphincter of Oddi spasm. It has been suggested that the incidence of opioid-induced sphincter spasm is quite low (<3%). It is possible to antagonize this spasm by intravenous administration of glucagon, or naloxone or nitroglycerin.

Choledocholithiasis

The term *choledocholithiasis* indicates that gallstones are present in the common bile duct. Stones typically lodge at the point of insertion of the common bile duct into the ampulla of Vater. Patients with choledocholithiasis may present with signs of cholangitis (fever, shaking chills, jaundice, right upper quadrant pain) or jaundice alone and a history of pain suggestive of cholecystitis. Not all stones obstruct the common duct. Some pass into the duodenum or into a pancreatic duct, which results in acute pancreatitis. Serum bilirubin and alkaline phosphatase concentrations typically increase markedly and abruptly when a stone obstructs the common bile duct. Aminotransferase concentrations are only modestly increased.

Acute obstruction of the common bile duct by a stone may mimic ureterolithiasis because of the similarities in location and severity of the pain, but liver function tests distinguish between these two conditions. Acute inflammation of the head of the pancreas may produce obstruction of the common bile duct. Computed tomography or ERCP helps distinguish pancreatitis from choledocholithiasis. Symptoms of an acute myocardial infarction or viral hepatitis may produce abdominal pain that is similar to that of biliary tract disease. The epigastric pain may be similar to that in patients with pancreatic carcinoma. Acute intermittent porphyria can also cause severe abdominal pain, but alkaline phosphatase and bilirubin concentrations are normal in this condition.

Endoscopic sphincterotomy is the initial treatment for patients with choledocholithiasis. ERCP can be used to identify the cause of common bile duct obstruction and can also be used to remove a stone or place a stent. Sphincterotomy is also the recommended treatment for patients with retained bile duct stones after gallbladder or biliary tract surgery. Operative exploration of the common bile duct is reserved for the few patients in whom endoscopic sphincterotomy is unsuccessful.

HEPATITIS

Hepatitis is an inflammatory disease of the liver parenchyma. It is often due to viral infection but can also be caused by autoimmune mechanisms or by ingestion of chemicals, such as drugs, alcohol, or solvents that are toxic.

Hepatitis may occur with minimal symptoms but is frequently complicated by at least malaise and jaundice. Acute hepatitis may be a self-limiting illness, but it can also progress to chronic hepatitis, cirrhosis, hepatocellular carcinoma, or liver failure.

Viral Hepatitis

The vast majority of cases of acute viral hepatitis in the United States are caused by one of four viruses: hepatitis A virus, hepatitis B virus, hepatitis C virus, or hepatitis D virus. However, there are other viruses such as herpes simplex virus, cytomegalovirus, and Epstein-Barr virus that can also cause acute hepatitis. Hepatitis A virus is the most common cause of acute viral hepatitis (50%), followed in incidence by hepatitis B virus (35%) and hepatitis C virus (15%). Hepatitis D virus occurs only in patients with hepatitis B and is present as a co-infection. Differentiating the various kinds of viral hepatitis is difficult based solely on the clinical presentation and routine laboratory testing of liver function (bilirubin, AST, ALT, and alkaline phosphatase levels). A definitive diagnosis requires serologic testing (Table 13-2) and, occasionally, liver biopsy.

Treatment of acute viral hepatitis is symptomatic. Avoidance of alcohol consumption, restriction of excessive physical exertion, and good nutrition are essential. In addition, it is necessary to monitor for signs of progression to either fulminant liver failure or chronic hepatitis.

Viral hepatitis can be prevented by avoidance of exposure to activities with a high risk of viral exposure and active

TABLE 13-2 ■ **Characteristic features of viral hepatitis**

Parameter	Type A	Type B	Type C	Type D
Mode of transmission	Fecal-oral Sewage-contaminated shellfish	Percutaneous Sexual	Percutaneous	Percutaneous
Incubation period	20-37 days	60-110 days	35-70 days	60-110 days
Results of serum antigen and antibody tests	IgM early, IgG appears during convalescence	HBsAg and anti-HBcAg early and persist in carriers	Anti-HCV in 6 wk to 9 mo	Anti-HDV late, may be short-lived
Immunity	Antibodies in 45%	Antibodies in 5%-15%	Unknown	Protected if immune to type B
Course	Does not progress to chronic liver disease	Chronic liver disease develops in 1%-5% of adults and 80%-90% of children	Chronic liver disease develops in up to 75%	Coinfection with type B
Prevention after exposure	Pooled gamma globulin Hepatitis A vaccine	Hepatitis B immunoglobulin Hepatitis B vaccine	Interferon plus ribavirin	Unknown
Mortality	<0.2%	0.3%-1.5%	Unknown	Acute icteric hepatitis: 2%-20%

Adapted from Keefe EB. Acute hepatitis. *Sci Am Med.* 1999:1-9.

HBcAg, Hepatitis B core antigen; *HBsAg,* hepatitis B surface antigen; *HCV,* hepatitis C virus; *HDV,* hepatitis D virus; *IgG,* immunoglobulin G; *IgM,* immunoglobulin M.

immunization with virus-specific vaccine. After successful vaccination, regular serum antibody titer monitoring is prudent. If needed, a booster immunization can ensure effective protection. In cases of acute viral exposure, passive immunization with pooled gamma globulin is recommended.

The development of cirrhosis and primary hepatocellular carcinoma are risks of chronic hepatitis B and C infection, although decades may pass before the adverse effects occur.

Drug-Induced Hepatitis

A large variety of medications (analgesics, anticonvulsants, antibiotics, antihypertensives, and many others) can cause hepatic inflammation resulting from idiosyncratic reaction or dose-related toxicity. The onset of clinical signs is usually 2 to 6 weeks after exposure but can be delayed for as long as 6 months after starting the medication. Because the clinical symptoms and signs and the histologic appearance of the liver can be identical to those of acute viral hepatitis, prompt and accurate diagnosis is imperative. Failure to identify and discontinue the offending drug may have dire consequences.

Acetaminophen overdose is a well-known cause of hepatocellular toxicity and liver necrosis. High concentrations of toxic metabolites of this compound overwhelm the conjugative capacity of the liver by exhausting glutathione stores. Oral N-acetylcysteine administration within the first 8 hours after acetaminophen ingestion can dramatically reduce the extent of parenchymal injury (see Chapter 25).

Autoimmune Hepatitis

By definition, autoimmune hepatitis is an inflammatory condition of the liver that is caused by a cellular immune response against self-antigens in the native liver. This illness has a prevalence of 10 to 20 per 100,000 and is much more common in women (70%) than in men. A concurrent autoimmune illness is often present. The diagnosis is confirmed by the combination of clinical findings, laboratory test results (for bilirubin, liver enzymes, serum autoantibodies, immunoglobulin G concentration), and histologic evaluation.

There is no curative intervention to treat autoimmune hepatitis, so the goal of treatment is to induce a long-lasting remission with the use of corticosteroids and/or other immunosuppressive drugs. In case of progression to end-stage liver disease, liver transplantation may be considered.

Halothane Hepatitis

For anesthesiologists, halothane hepatitis is an especially relevant and unique form of hepatitis. In genetically susceptible individuals, certain volatile anesthetics (halothane, enflurane, isoflurane, desflurane) can elicit an immune-mediated hepatotoxic reaction. The most compelling evidence for this is the presence of circulating immunoglobulin G antibodies in the majority of patients with a diagnosis of halothane hepatitis. These antibodies are directed against microsomal proteins on the surface of hepatocytes that have been covalently modified by the reactive oxidative trifluoroacetyl halide metabolite of halothane to form neoantigens. This acetylation of liver proteins, in effect, changes these proteins from "self" to "nonself" (neoantigens), which results in the formation of antibodies against this new protein and a form of autoimmune hepatitis. Antitrifluoroacetyl antibody testing is specific to this condition. Because of its relatively high degree of drug metabolism, halothane is the most common volatile anesthetic to cause hepatitis, with an estimated incidence of about 1 in 20,000 administrations in adult patients. Sensitized individuals may show cross-reactivity with other fluorinated volatile anesthetic agents. Sevoflurane is an exception, however, because it has a different chemical structure and does not produce trifluoro-acetylated metabolites.

Postoperative Hepatic Dysfunction

New-onset postoperative jaundice is best evaluated via a systematic approach. First, the prospect of benign post-operative intrahepatic cholestasis—a relatively common occurrence—should be considered; the prevalence of this condition increases with prolonged surgery, hypotension, hypoxemia, and massive blood transfusion. Next, the presence of a large occult hematoma, hemolysis, or sepsis should be considered. Finally, drug-induced or immune-mediated hepatotoxicity can be considered. Discontinuation of all possible contributing drugs and supportive therapy (intra-vascular volume restoration, oxygen supplementation, drainage of pathologic fluid collections, intravenous antibi-otics, etc.) are essential while the reason for the jaundice is being established.

Chronic Hepatitis

Chronic hepatitis is defined as any hepatic inflammation that lasts longer than 6 months. This diagnosis is corroborated by elevated serum concentrations of liver enzymes and/or bilirubin and histologic evidence of ongoing inflammation. In the United States alcoholic liver disease is the most com-mon cause of chronic liver disease and cirrhosis. Chronic hepatitis C infection is the second most prevalent cause of chronic hepatitis. There can be a wide range of disease sever-ity in chronic hepatitis, so the prognosis can be quite vari-able. Mild forms of chronic hepatitis may not significantly impact quality of life. However, advanced and progressive hepatitis does interfere with daily activities. Severe chronic hepatitis evolves into cirrhosis with compromise of multiple organ systems.

CIRRHOSIS

Progressive parenchymal liver damage and co-existent tissue regeneration disrupt normal hepatic architecture and lead to nodular transformation. This altered morphology is observ-able with computed tomography, magnetic resonance imag-ing, and ultrasonography. Histologic examination may help to differentiate the cause of cirrhosis (alcoholic cirrhosis, postne-crotic cirrhosis, primary or secondary biliary cirrhosis, non-alcoholic steatohepatitis, hemochromatosis, Wilson's disease, α_1-antitrypsin deficiency, or other disorders.)

Fatigue, malaise, and jaundice are typically present, and later the symptoms and signs of advanced liver disease such as spider angiomata, gynecomastia, testicular atrophy, and asci-tes appear.

Laboratory findings include elevated bilirubin, aminotrans-ferase, and alkaline phosphatase concentrations; an increased INR; thrombocytopenia; and a decreased serum albumin

concentration. Hypoglycemia is common due to inadequate gluconeogenesis.

Portal Hypertension

In tandem with the fibrotic degeneration of the liver in cir-rhosis and the resultant increase in resistance to intrahepatic blood flow, portal vein blood flow decreases and portal hyper-tension develops. Ascites, hepatomegaly, splenomegaly, and peripheral edema are typically present.

Ascites and Spontaneous Bacterial Peritonitis

Ascites and cirrhosis frequently co-exist. Contributory factors for the development of ascites include portal hypertension, hypoal-buminemia, and sodium and water retention (Figure 13-1).

When ascites formation is significant, medical therapy is directed at correcting the underlying hypoalbuminemia and the sodium and water retention. Adherence to a low-sodium diet and administration of an aldosterone antagonist, such as spironolactone, can promote a gradual diuresis and a reduc-tion in the volume of ascites. Diuresis should not exceed 1 L of fluid per day to prevent hypovolemia and azotemia. For ascites that is resistant to medical therapy, paracentesis or insertion of a transjugular intrahepatic portosystemic shunt can be con-sidered. Less commonly the ascitic fluid can be returned to the intravascular space by a LeVeen shunt, which is a subcuta-neous one-way conduit between the peritoneal cavity and the internal jugular vein.

If the clinical condition of a patient with ascites deteriorates suddenly, the ascitic fluid must be analyzed for turbidity, leu-kocytosis, and bacterial growth. *Spontaneous bacterial perito-nitis* has a very high morbidity and mortality even with timely initiation of antibiotic therapy.

Gastroesophageal Varices

Because portal hypertension interferes with splanchnic venous blood flow, submucosal veins at the gastroesophageal junc-tion become dilated to allow for increased collateral flow via the azygous and hemiazygous veins. Not all cirrhotic patients develop varices, and not all patients with varices develop bleeding. However, if variceal bleeding occurs, it is usually hemodynamically significant. Patients with massive bleeding or co-existent hepatic encephalopathy may require endotra-cheal intubation to protect the airway and prevent pulmonary aspiration.

Variceal bleeding can be controlled by endoscopic therapy, including variceal banding and sclerotherapy. To prevent recurrent bleeding, a transjugular intrahepatic portosystemic shunt (TIPS) can be inserted or a surgical portosystemic shunt created in selected patients. These shunts may not prolong overall survival, but they are effective in preventing recurrent bleeding. Medical treatment of esophageal varices includes administration of propranolol or nadolol, which reduces por-tal hypertension and reduces the risk of rebleeding.

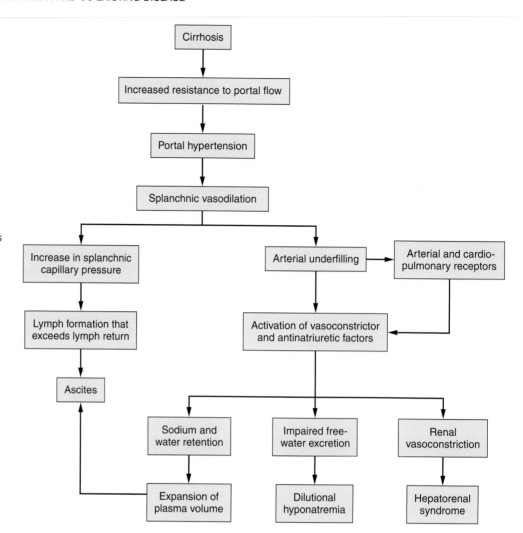

FIGURE 13-1 Pathogenesis of ascites. *(From Gines P, Cardenas A, Arroyo V, et al. Management of cirrhosis and ascites.* N Engl J Med. *2004;350:1646-1654. Copyright 2004 Massachusetts Medical Society. All rights reserved.)*

Hepatic Encephalopathy

Neuropsychiatric changes often appear with declining liver function. Affected areas may include cognition, motor function, personality, and consciousness. Asterixis and slow or flattened waves on the electroencephalogram are pathognomonic signs of advanced liver disease with encephalopathy. Portosystemic shunting may exacerbate hepatic encephalopathy by allowing ammonia and other metabolic byproducts to bypass hepatic clearance.

The treatment of hepatic encephalopathy includes restriction of protein intake to reduce ammonia production, enteral administration of nonabsorbable disaccharides (lactulose) or antibiotics (neomycin) to decrease ammonia absorption, correction of electrolyte imbalances, and avoidance of all forms of opioids, sedative-hypnotic drugs, and anesthetic drugs if possible.

Hyperdynamic Circulation

Hepatic cirrhosis is frequently accompanied by a hyperdynamic circulation, which is characterized by diminished systemic vascular resistance and a compensatory increase in cardiac output. It is presumed that accumulation of vasodilatory compounds such as prostaglandins or interleukins is at least partially responsible for the increased cardiac output and the arteriovenous shunting seen in cirrhosis. Reduced blood viscosity resulting from hypoalbuminemia and anemia may also play a role.

Cirrhosis may also be associated with cardiomyopathy or diastolic dysfunction, so intraoperative management of hemodynamics can be challenging.

Hepatopulmonary Syndrome

In addition to the peripheral vasodilation seen with hepatic cirrhosis, significant intrapulmonary shunting and ventilation/perfusion mismatch occurs in up to one quarter of these patients. Signs and symptoms include dyspnea and hypoxemia, which may worsen in the upright position. Differentiation between intrapulmonary shunting and right-to-left intracardiac shunting can be achieved using contrast echocardiography.

The only definitive treatment for severe hepatopulmonary syndrome is liver transplantation. Administration of somatostatin and supplemental oxygen is used as supportive therapy until a donor organ becomes available.

Portopulmonary Hypertension

Co-existent portal vein and pulmonary artery hypertension has a prevalence of less than 4% in cirrhotic patients. Portopulmonary hypertension typically presents years after the diagnosis of cirrhosis, and symptoms can include dyspnea, fatigue, and syncope. Right-sided heart dysfunction is common. The severity of portopulmonary hypertension is independent of the severity of the cirrhosis.

Cirrhotic patients with portopulmonary hypertension have a very limited life expectancy. Liver transplantation is the only known curative therapy, but it can be recommended only if pulmonary vascular resistance is not severely increased. Patients with end-stage liver disease who have a mean pulmonary artery pressure of more than 45 mm Hg are poor candidates for liver transplantation. The 1-year mortality in this subset of patients is more than 80% with or without surgery. In rare cases, if severe pulmonary hypertension is responsive to medical therapy, such as treatment with prostaglandins or nitric oxide, then liver transplantation might be attempted. Perioperative monitoring and treatment of such a patient should be carried out in concert with an experienced pulmonologist.

Hepatorenal Syndrome

Functional renal failure that is associated with severe liver disease is called *hepatorenal syndrome*. The prognosis of this disorder is very poor even though there is no intrinsic renal abnormality. The exact pathophysiology of hepatorenal syndrome is unknown, but it appears that dehydration and diminished renal blood flow often precede the decrease in glomerular filtration rate and development of azotemia.

Renal replacement therapy is the mainstay of supportive treatment until the underlying liver dysfunction can be normalized or a donor organ becomes available for transplantation.

Hepatorenal syndrome can be categorized into type 1 and type 2 forms based on rapidity of onset, that is, how fast the serum creatinine level rises and creatinine clearance declines. Short-term mortality is very high in both varieties of hepatorenal syndrome.

Coagulopathy

The liver synthesizes most of the coagulation factors of the coagulation cascade. In addition, hepatocytes produce a number of anticoagulant proteins (protein S, protein C, protein Z, antithrombin III) and the antifibrinolytic plasminogen activator inhibitor. The liver is also essential for clearance of activated coagulation factors from the circulation. End-stage liver disease can be accompanied by numerous disturbances in this intricate system of clot formation and clot dissolution.

In patients with end-stage liver disease evaluation of coagulation function requires insight into the complex hemostatic abnormalities that can be present and interpretation of the results of a number of both quantitative and qualitative tests of coagulation function.

ACUTE LIVER FAILURE

Definition

Acute liver failure is defined as the rapid development of severe liver damage with impaired synthetic function and encephalopathy in someone who previously had normal liver function or well-compensated liver disease. By definition, acute liver failure develops in less than 4 weeks (measured from the first appearance of physical signs such as jaundice to the loss of 80% to 90% of hepatic function). Acute liver failure includes *fulminant hepatic failure,* that is, liver failure that occurs within 8 days of the onset of symptoms. Acute liver failure often affects young people and carries a very high mortality. The underlying cause and the grade of encephalopathy on presentation are important determinants of outcome.

Impaired synthetic function and encephalopathy are critical events in this disorder. In most cases of acute liver failure there is widespread hepatocellular necrosis and a variable amount of hepatic parenchymal inflammation. Patients with acute liver failure are at increased risk of progressing from mild encephalopathy to cerebral edema, increased intracranial pressure, and coma.

Etiology

Common causes of acute liver failure are acetaminophen overdose, idiosyncratic drug reaction, acute viral hepatitis, alcoholic hepatitis, and acute fatty liver of pregnancy. Less common causes include Wilson's disease and Reye's syndrome.

Treatment

Coagulopathy, renal failure, cardiorespiratory complications, and severe metabolic derangements are frequent. Intensive care unit admission and close observation are essential; supportive therapy must include restoring intravascular fluid volume, normalizing electrolyte concentrations, and providing mechanical ventilation if needed. "Liver dialysis" (using an extracorporeal system somewhat like a kidney dialysis machine that pumps blood through a series of filters to remove unwanted materials) is evolving as a therapeutic option and is available as an experimental treatment at some medical centers.

Intracranial pressure monitoring is controversial. Information about intracranial pressure could be very helpful in controlling this pressure, but placement of an intracranial pressure sensor in the presence of severe coagulopathy carries a significant risk of intracranial hemorrhage.

Outcome

Mortality from acute liver failure is high, in excess of 80%, despite the accessibility of sophisticated multidisciplinary intensive care. Survival is strongly dependent on what caused the liver failure and whether a known antidote for the specific underlying cause exists, such as *N*-acetylcysteine for acetaminophen poisoning. Liver transplantation is an option if a donor organ is available, but the short-term mortality is still higher than 65% even with transplantation.

ANESTHESIA FOR PATIENTS WITH DECREASED LIVER FUNCTION

Identifying the population of patients with liver disease can be challenging, because clinical manifestation of liver dysfunction occur only after a substantial decline in liver function has occurred. However, routine preoperative liver function testing in *all* preoperative patients is not a practical way to find the occasional person with liver dysfunction. Currently, with the prevalence of alcoholic and hepatitis C–related cirrhosis increasing, the number of patients with compromised liver function requiring surgery is on the rise. An estimated 1 in 700 patients undergoing elective surgery has abnormal liver enzyme levels and is at increased risk for perioperative morbidity and mortality related to hepatic dysfunction.

Risk Assessment

Patients with liver disease have a diminished physiologic reserve with which to respond to surgical stress and, as a result, are at increased risk for bleeding, infection, hepatic decompensation, and death. The extent of liver damage and the type of surgery are the two main determinants of perioperative risk.

Child-Pugh Score

The Child-Pugh score was developed specifically to predict surgical mortality in patients with cirrhosis. It assigns points for five variables (total bilirubin level, serum albumin level, INR, ascites, and hepatic encephalopathy) that are combined into a single score to categorize patients into Child-Pugh class A, B, or C (Tables 13-3 and 13-4). The predicted perioperative mortality for intraabdominal surgery in these patient groups is 10%, 30%, and 80%, respectively.

In general, patients in Child-Pugh classes A and B are suitable candidates for surgery when preoperative optimization and attentive perioperative care are provided. Patients in

Child-Pugh class C are usually treated medically if the disease process permits. Surgery, if necessary, should be delayed until liver function improves (Figure 13-2).

Optimal preoperative management may decrease the incidence of perioperative complications and death. In addition to the standard history taking, physical examination, medication review, and laboratory assessment, evaluation for acute or ongoing hepatic deterioration is critically important.

Perioperative Care

NUTRITION, METABOLISM, AND ELECTROLYTE LEVELS
Malnutrition and malabsorption are common in patients with advanced liver disease. Vitamin deficiencies and hypoalbuminemia have consequences for a number of organ functions and for pharmacokinetics as well. Improvement in diet, especially caloric enhancement, protein enrichment as tolerated, and vitamin supplementation, are desirable.

TABLE 13-3 ■ Child-Pugh scoring system to assess severity of liver disease

Sign of hepatic dysfunction	1 Point	2 Points	3 Points
Encephalopathy (grade)	None	Grade I-II	Grade III-IV
Ascites	Absent	Mild	Severe
Bilirubin (mg/dL)	<2	2-3	>3
Albumin (g/dL)	>3.5	2.8-3.5	<2.8
International normalized ratio	<1.7	1.7-2.2	>2.2

TABLE 13-4 ■ Survival statistics according to Child-Pugh class

Points	Class	One-year survival	Two-year survival
5-6	A	100%	85%
7-9	B	81%	57%
10-15	C	45%	35%

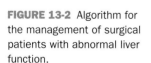

FIGURE 13-2 Algorithm for the management of surgical patients with abnormal liver function.

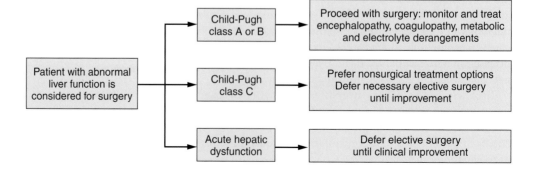

Patient with abnormal liver function is considered for surgery

Child-Pugh class A or B → Proceed with surgery: monitor and treat encephalopathy, coagulopathy, metabolic and electrolyte derangements

Child-Pugh class C → Prefer nonsurgical treatment options Defer necessary elective surgery until improvement

Acute hepatic dysfunction → Defer elective surgery until clinical improvement

As a consequence of diminished hepatic gluconeogenesis, hypoglycemia is likely. Blood glucose monitoring is warranted, and a glucose infusion may be required during surgery.

Hyponatremia despite an increased total body sodium content is common, because the degree of free water retention exceeds the degree of sodium retention. Administration of an aldosterone antagonist combined with consumption of a low-sodium diet help to correct this abnormality. In patients receiving diuretic therapy creatinine and electrolyte levels should be monitored.

ENCEPHALOPATHY

The degree of preoperative hepatic encephalopathy may or may not parallel the extent of liver dysfunction. Encephalopathy is exaggerated by infection, gastrointestinal bleeding, and the presence of a transjugular intrahepatic portosystemic shunt. New onset of neurologic symptoms and signs requires investigation for the potential cause. Lethargic or unconscious patients may require endotracheal intubation for airway protection. The presence of preoperative encephalopathy is associated with a greatly increased perioperative mortality rate in patients undergoing nonhepatic surgery.

PULMONARY COMORBIDITIES AND AIRWAY MANAGEMENT

In addition to evaluation for the possible presence of hepatopulmonary syndrome and/or portopulmonary hypertension, preoperative assessment of liver function must include an evaluation of the risk of aspiration and measurement of oxygen saturation with the patient breathing room air, pulmonary function testing, and measurement of pulmonary artery pressure if appropriate.

Patients with chronic liver disease, especially those with ascites, frequently have increased gastric volumes and delayed gastric emptying. Therefore, rapid-sequence induction of general anesthesia with cricoid pressure is prudent to facilitate endotracheal intubation and airway protection.

RENAL FUNCTION

Patients with cirrhosis are at increased risk of developing renal dysfunction. Gastrointestinal bleeding, hypotension, hypoperfusion, large-volume paracentesis, and administration of potentially nephrotoxic medications all increase the likelihood of acute renal deterioration. An increasing serum creatinine concentration and a decreasing creatinine clearance are ominous signs in patients with marginal liver function. Hepatorenal syndrome has no specific remedy. However, maintenance of euvolemia and renal replacement therapy are essential while the patient tries to recover from the underlying hepatic dysfunction.

Patients benefit from monitoring for the presence of metabolic acidosis, particularly lactic acidosis, and correction of acid-base and electrolyte imbalances.

CIRCULATION

A hyperdynamic circulation is a prominent feature of hepatic insufficiency. The decreased systemic vascular resistance is, to some extent, compensated for by an increased cardiac output. However, hypoalbuminemia and the resulting decrease in plasma oncotic pressure can cause fluid to shift to the interstitial space, so edema is common.

In hypotensive patients, invasive monitoring (arterial line, cardiac output measurement), intravascular volume replacement, and vasopressor therapy may be necessary. In euvolemic, vasodilated patients, vasopressor administration can help restore blood pressure without compromising tissue perfusion. Phenylephrine, norepinephrine, and vasopressin are commonly used for this purpose during liver transplantation.

COAGULATION

Coagulopathy is very common. The combination of reduced procoagulant factor production and simultaneous decreases in anticoagulant modulator concentrations typically result in excessive bleeding. Laboratory testing of clotting factor concentrations, fibrinogen levels, platelet counts, and other parameters, combined with clinical observation of bleeding and thromboelastography may be particularly helpful in diagnosing the cause of the bleeding diathesis and devising an optimal treatment plan.

If malnutrition is present, vitamin K administration is helpful to enhance hemostasis via production of vitamin K–dependent clotting factors. Transfusion of fresh frozen plasma, cryoprecipitate, platelets, or a combination of these products may be indicated. Transfusion therapy is best guided by laboratory analysis of the underlying problem rather than simply use of an empiric formula for infusion of the various blood products. A dysfunctional liver has a diminished capacity to metabolize citrate, a component of blood products and cell saver infusates, so monitoring of ionized calcium concentration is necessary. Intravenous calcium administration is often indicated.

PHARMACOKINETICS

Pharmacokinetics in patients with hepatic dysfunction can be altered by impaired hepatic synthetic function, increased volume of distribution, decreased plasma protein binding of medications, and decreased clearance of drugs. For example, a larger initial dose of nondepolarizing muscle relaxant is necessary to achieve an effective plasma concentration resulting from the increase in volume of distribution, but subsequent doses of these drugs should be reduced to reflect decreased hepatic drug clearance. Cisatracurium may be particularly useful in patients with liver disease because its elimination is independent of liver function.

Postsurgical Recovery

Liver failure is the most common cause of postoperative death in patients with cirrhosis. For optimal postoperative observation and care, admission to an intensive care unit is prudent, especially if the patient's condition was unstable during surgery. In addition to monitoring postoperative liver function, critical care will also include maintaining hemodynamics, ensuring satisfactory oxygenation and ventilation, frequently assessing neurologic function, controlling electrolyte disturbances and coagulation disorders, and monitoring renal function.

Early enteral feeding has been shown to improve outcome and should be considered.

LIVER TRANSPLANTATION

Approximately 7000 liver transplantation surgeries are performed annually in the United States. The 1-year survival is more than 85%, the 3-year survival is currently more than 80%, and the 5-year survival is more than 70%. Liver transplantation, once considered an experimental surgical procedure, has become the treatment of choice for various forms of severe or irreversible liver dysfunction.

More than 90% of livers for transplantation are cadaveric organs. Live donor liver transplantation, which usually involves removal of an entire lobe of the liver, produces excellent results in children. However, adult-to-adult live donor liver transplantation is often problematic because of size mismatching. The small-for-size syndrome is not uncommon and manifests as liver dysfunction within the first week after surgery. It appears that cirrhotic patients do better with a donor liver at least as large as their native liver.

Indications

Alcoholism, chronic progressive hepatitis (especially that caused by hepatitis C virus), and hepatocellular carcinoma were all considered contraindications to liver transplantation in the past, but now these entities have become the most frequent indications for this surgery. Less common indications include primary sclerosing cholangitis, α_1-antitrypsin deficiency, nonalcoholic steatohepatitis, hemochromatosis, Wilson's disease, and acute liver failure.

Organ Allocation

To facilitate fair distribution of the limited number of allografts among the 17,000 patients or so on the national liver transplantation waiting lists, the United Network for Organ Sharing and Eurotransplant International Foundation use the Model for End-Stage Liver Disease (MELD) scoring system. This replaced the Child-Pugh system for liver transplant purposes. The MELD score is used to predict the chance of 90-day mortality *without* liver transplantation and is calculated based on three laboratory test results:

$$3.8 \times \log_e (\text{bilirubin in mg} / \text{dL}) + 11.2 \times \log_e (\text{INR}) + 9.6 \times \log_e (\text{creatinine in mg} / \text{dL}) + 0.643$$

MELD scores can range from 6 to 40, and patients are ranked on the waiting list according to their scores. The patients with the highest scores are at the top of the list. Patients' MELD scores are recalculated regularly to reflect the frequently changing conditions in potential transplant recipients. When MELD score does not reflect the severity of the underlying liver disease and its prognosis, as in patients with hepatocellular carcinoma, a MELD score is assigned based on the staging of the cancer, often according to the Milan criteria, which classify a single liver tumor of 5 cm or less or a total of not more than three tumors with none larger than 3 cm as potentially suitable for treatment by liver transplantation.

Surgical Procedure

Surgery for removal of the native liver and implantation of the donor liver has three phases: the dissection phase, the anhepatic phase, and the reperfusion or neohepatic phase.

The *dissection phase* involves mobilizing the vascular structures around the liver (hepatic artery, portal vein, suprahepatic and infrahepatic vena cava), isolating the common bile duct, and removing the native liver. Cardiovascular instability resulting from hemorrhage, venous pooling as a result of decreases in intraabdominal pressure, and impaired venous return resulting from surgical retraction are not uncommon during this phase.

The *anhepatic stage* begins when the blood supply to the native liver is interrupted by clamping of the hepatic artery and portal vein. To avoid a marked decrease in venous return and cardiac output as well as splanchnic venous congestion during occlusion of the inferior vena cava, a venovenous bypass system is often used. Placement of the donor liver may require vigorous retraction near the diaphragm, leading to compromise of ventilation and oxygenation. Because of the lack of liver metabolic function during the anhepatic phase, metabolic acidosis, decreased drug metabolism, and citrate intoxication are likely. A calcium infusion may be needed to treat hypocalcemia.

The *reperfusion* or *neohepatic phase* begins after surgical anastomosis of the major vascular structures to the donor liver. Before the vascular clamps are removed, the allograft is flushed to remove air, debris, and preservative solutions. Despite this step, subsequent unclamping can cause significant hemodynamic instability, dysrhythmias, severe bradycardia, hypotension, and hyperkalemia. Once the allograft begins to function, hemodynamic and metabolic stability are gradually restored and urine output increases. Recovery of the capacity to metabolize drugs occurs soon after reperfusion of the graft. Clotting parameters usually normalize with administration of clotting factors. Postoperative support of ventilation and oxygenation may be required.

Liver function test results return to normal following successful liver transplantation. Liver transplantation also results in reversal of the hyperdynamic circulation that characterizes liver failure. Oxygenation improves, although intrapulmonary shunts may persist and contribute to ventilation/perfusion abnormalities. Normal physiologic mechanisms that protect hepatic blood flow are blunted after liver transplantation. The liver is normally an important source of autotransfusion of blood volume in shock states via a vasoconstrictive response, and this mechanism may be impaired after liver transplantation.

Recent Advances in Liver Transplantation

The most recent developments in liver transplantation include blood-sparing transfusion strategies and early extubation after surgery.

BLOOD TRANSFUSION

Current understanding of the complexities of hemostatic mechanisms and the widespread use of advanced diagnostic tests of coagulation function have resulted in a dramatic reduction in the amount of blood transfusion per case. This reduction in blood transfusion has also reduced the incidence of citrate toxicity and hypervolemia and has positively affected postoperative outcome. Intensive care unit and hospital lengths of stay have become shorter.

EARLY POSTOPERATIVE EXTUBATION

When the duration of surgery is shorter and the intraoperative course is uneventful, shortening the usual period of postoperative mechanical ventilation may be considered in some patients. Transplantation centers are becoming increasingly interested in *fast-tracking* appropriate patients, to optimize both patient care and perioperative resource utilization.

KEY POINTS

- Diseases of the liver and biliary tract can be categorized as parenchymal liver disease (hepatitis and cirrhosis) and cholestasis with or without obstruction of the extrahepatic biliary pathway.
- Bilirubin is the degradation product of hemoglobin and myoglobin. Unconjugated bilirubin is transported to the liver, where it is conjugated by glucuronosyl transferase. Unconjugated hyperbilirubinemia occurs with an increase in bilirubin production, decreased hepatic uptake of bilirubin, or decreased conjugation of bilirubin. Conjugated hyperbilirubinemia occurs with decreased canalicular transport of bilirubin, acute or chronic hepatocellular dysfunction, or obstruction of the bile ducts.
- The use of opioids during anesthesia for gallbladder or common bile duct surgery is controversial because these drugs can cause spasm of the sphincter of Oddi. However, it is possible to antagonize this spasm with intravenous administration of glucagon, nitroglycerin, or naloxone.
- Acute hepatitis is most often a result of viral infection but can also be caused by drugs and toxins. In the United States, approximately 50% of acute viral hepatitis in adults is due to infection with hepatitis A virus, 35% to infection with hepatitis B virus, and 15% to infection with hepatitis C virus.
- Major complications of hepatitis B and C infection include the development of chronic hepatitis, cirrhosis, and hepatocellular carcinoma.
- Drugs (analgesics, volatile anesthetics, antibiotics, antihypertensives, anticonvulsants, tranquilizers) can cause hepatitis indistinguishable histologically from acute viral hepatitis. Many of these drug reactions are idiosyncratic; that is, they are rare, unpredictable, and not dose dependent. Failure to discontinue the offending drug may result in progressive hepatitis and even death.

- Halothane hepatitis, a rare form of hepatic dysfunction, can follow administration of volatile anesthetics, especially halothane, in genetically susceptible individuals. Microsomal proteins on the surface of hepatocytes that have been modified by the trifluoroacetyl halide metabolite of halothane form neoantigens. Formation of antibodies against these proteins produces a form of autoimmune hepatitis.
- Enflurane, isoflurane, and desflurane can form trifluoroacetyl metabolites, which results in cross-sensitivity with halothane. However, the incidence of hepatitis after use of these anesthetics is very much lower than after halothane administration because they undergo a much lower degree of metabolism. Sevoflurane does not undergo metabolism to trifluoroacetylated metabolites. Therefore, unlike the other fluorinated volatile anesthetics, sevoflurane does not produce immune-mediated hepatotoxicity.
- Chronic hepatitis is characterized by long-term abnormalities in levels of liver function markers and evidence of inflammation on liver biopsy specimens. Chronic hepatitis is defined as disease that lasts 6 months or longer. The most common diseases that cause chronic hepatitis are autoimmune hepatitis and chronic viral hepatitis (infection with hepatitis B or C virus).
- Portal hypertension is the result of an increase in resistance to blood flow through the portal venous system as a result of the fibrotic cirrhotic process. Portal hypertension combined with hypoalbuminemia and increased secretion of vasoconstrictor and antinatriuretic factors and antidiuretic hormone causes development of ascites.
- Surgery for liver transplantation is characterized by three phases: the dissection phase, the anhepatic phase, and the reperfusion or neohepatic phase. The dissection phase involves mobilizing the vascular structures around the liver (hepatic artery, portal vein, suprahepatic and infrahepatic vena cava), isolating the common bile duct, and removing the native liver. The anhepatic stage begins when the blood supply to the native liver is interrupted by clamping of the hepatic artery and portal vein. The reperfusion or neohepatic phase begins after surgical anastomosis of the major vascular structures to the donor liver.

RESOURCES

Child CG, Turcotte JG. Surgery and portal hypertension. *Major Probl Clin Surg.* 1964;1:1-85.

del Olmo JA, Flor-Lorente B, Flor-Civera B, et al. Risk factors for nonhepatic surgery in patients with cirrhosis. *World J Surg.* Jun 2003;27(6):647-652.

Faust TW, Reddy KR. Postoperative jaundice. *Clin Liver Dis.* 2004;8:151-166.

Friedman LS. The risk of surgery in patients with liver disease. *Hepatology.* Jun 1999;29(6):1617-1623.

Gines P, Cardenas A, Arroyo V, et al. Management of cirrhosis and ascites. *N Engl J Med.* 2004;350:1646-1654.

Hannaman MJ, Hevesi ZG. Anesthesia care for liver transplantation. *Transplant Rev.* 2011 Jan;25(1):36-43.

Keegan MT, Plevak DJ. Preoperative assessment of the patient with liver disease. *Am J Gastroenterol.* Sep 2005;100(9):2116-2127.

Mandell MS, Lockrem J, Kelley SD. Immediate tracheal extubation after liver transplantation: experience of two transplant centers. *Anesth Analg.* 1997;84:249-253.

Millwala F, Nguyen GC, Thuluvath PJ. Outcomes of patients with cirrhosis undergoing non-hepatic surgery: risk assessment and management. *World J Gastroenterol.* Aug 14, 2007;13(30):4056-4063.

O'Leary JG, Friedman LS. Predicting surgical risk in patients with cirrhosis: from art to science. *Gastroenterology.* Apr 2007;132(4):1609-1611.

Rizvon MK, Chou CL. Surgery in the patient with liver disease. *Med Clin North Am.* Jan 2003;87(1):211-227.

Teh SH, Nagorney DM, Stevens SR, et al. Risk factors for mortality after surgery in patients with cirrhosis. *Gastroenterology.* Apr 2007;132(4):1261-1269.

Diseases of the Gastrointestinal System

HOSSAM TANTAWY ■
TORI MYSLAJEK ■

The principal function of the gastrointestinal (GI) tract is to provide the body with a supply of water, nutrients, and electrolytes. Each division of the GI tract—esophagus, stomach, and small and large intestines—is adapted for specific functions, such as passage, storage, digestion, and absorption of food. Impairment of any part of the GI tract may have significant effects on a patient coming for surgery.

ESOPHAGEAL DISEASES

Dysphagia is the classic symptom of all disorders of the esophagus. To evaluate dysphagia, a barium contrast study is recommended, followed by esophagoscopy, which permits direct viewing of esophageal abnormalities as well as collection of biopsy and cytology specimens.

Diffuse Esophageal Spasm

Diffuse esophageal spasm typically occurs in elderly patients and is most likely due to autonomic nervous system dysfunction. Pain produced by esophageal spasm may mimic angina pectoris and frequently responds favorably to treatment with nitroglycerin, which further confuses the clinical picture. Nifedipine and isosorbide, which decrease lower esophageal sphincter (LES) pressure, may also relieve pain produced by esophageal spasm.

Achalasia

Achalasia is classified as a neuromuscular disorder of the esophagus. It is defined as dysfunction of both the esophageal muscles and the LES. The incidence of achalasia is 6 per 100,000 persons per year. The current theory of the etiology of achalasia is that the primary pathologic process is destruction of the nerves to the LES followed by degeneration of the function of the esophageal body. The result is hypertension of the LES, failure of the LES to relax when swallowing, reduced peristalsis, and esophageal dilation. Symptoms consist of the triad of dysphagia, weight loss, and regurgitation. Long-term disease is associated with an increased risk of esophageal cancer. Aspiration is common with resultant pneumonia, lung abscess, and/or bronchiectasis. The diagnosis can be made by esophagram, which reveals the classic "bird's beak" appearance. However, manometry is the definitive test for the diagnosis of achalasia.

TREATMENT

All treatments for achalasia are palliative, because they can relieve the obstruction caused by the LES but cannot correct the decreased motility of the esophagus. Medications, including nitrates, nitroglycerin, and calcium channel blockers, can be used to attempt to relax the LES. Endoscopic interventions include dilations and/or injections of botulinum toxin. Surgical esophagomyotomy offers better results than endoscopic dilation. Surgery now is typically a modified laparoscopic Heller myotomy. Esophagectomy can be considered in very advanced disease and would eliminate the risk of cancer as well as mitigate symptoms. Patients with achalasia are at increased risk of perioperative aspiration and must be treated using full-stomach precautions.

Esophagectomy

Esophagectomy can be a curative or palliative option for malignant esophageal lesions (10% to 50% cure rate). It may also be considered when benign conditions, such as obstructive lesions, are not responsive to conservative management. There are several surgical approaches to esophagectomy, including transthoracic, transhiatal, and minimally invasive (laparoscopic, thoracoscopic, or robotically assisted) techniques.

MORBIDITY AND MORTALITY

The morbidity and mortality of esophagectomy is quite high, with rates of 10% to 15% reported. Most major postoperative complications are respiratory complications, and these contribute to poor outcomes. Acute lung injury and/or acute respiratory distress syndrome (ARDS) may occur up to 10% to 20% of esophagectomies. The mortality approaches 50% if ARDS occurs. The cause of ARDS in the setting of esophagectomy is not completely understood, but it is thought that inflammatory mediators and gut-related endotoxins may be triggers. Other contributing factors may include the use of prolonged one-lung ventilation resulting in ischemia-reperfusion injury of the lung. A history of smoking, low body mass index, long duration of surgery, cardiopulmonary instability, and the occurrence of a postoperative anastomotic leak may also increase the risk of ARDS. Other common postoperative complications include anastomotic leaks (11% to 21% incidence), dumping syndrome, and esophageal stricture.

ANESTHETIC IMPLICATIONS

Patients may be malnourished (protein-calorie malnutrition) before esophagectomy and for many months afterward. However, over the past decade regular surveillance of patients with Barrett's esophagus has lead to the diagnosis of esophageal cancer in very early stages. Such patients typically arrive for surgery in good nutritional balance. Some patients coming for esophagectomy have had chemotherapy and/or radiation therapy before the procedure, so pancytopenia, dehydration, and lung injury can be present.

In the early postoperative period patients may need to return to the operating room, and they may have any of the conditions noted earlier, including acute lung injury. Patients with anastomotic leak may have sepsis and/or shock. There is a very significant risk of aspiration in all patients who have had an esophagectomy. This risk persists for life.

Gastroesophageal Reflux Disease

PHYSIOLOGY AND PATHOPHYSIOLOGY

Currently, *gastroesophageal reflux disease* (GERD) is described as reflux of gastric contents into the esophagus associated with symptoms. Natural antireflux mechanisms consist of the LES, the crural diaphragm, and the anatomic location of the

TABLE 14-1 ▪ Effect of drugs on lower esophageal sphincter tone

Increase	Decrease	No Change
Metoclopramide	Atropine	Propranolol
Domperidone	Glycopyrrolate	Oxprenolol
Prochlorperazine	Dopamine	Cimetidine
Cyclizine	Sodium nitroprusside	Ranitidine
Edrophonium	Ganglion blockers	Atracurium
Neostigmine	Thiopental	?Nitrous
Succinylcholine	Tricyclic antidepressants	oxide
Pancuronium	β-Adrenergic stimulants	
Metoprolol	Halothane	
α-Adrenergic	Enflurane	
stimulants	Opioids	
Antacids	?Nitrous oxide	
	Propofol	

gastroesophageal junction below the diaphragmatic hiatus. The LES opens with swallowing and closes afterward to prevent gastric acid in the stomach from refluxing into the esophagus. At rest, the LES typically exerts a pressure high enough to prevent reflux. With inappropriate relaxation or weakness of the LES, gastric acid reenters the esophagus, causing irritation (Table 14-1).

The primary defect causing GERD seems to be a decrease in the resting tone of the LES (average of 13 mm Hg in patients with GERD vs. 29 mm Hg in patients without GERD). Chronic peptic esophagitis is caused by reflux of acidic gastric fluid into the esophagus, producing retrosternal discomfort ("heartburn"). Reflux into the pharynx, larynx, and tracheobronchial tree can result in chronic cough, bronchoconstriction, pharyngitis, laryngitis, bronchitis, or pneumonia. Morning hoarseness may also be noted. Recurrent pulmonary aspiration can also result in aspiration pneumonia, pulmonary fibrosis, or asthma.

INCIDENCE OF ASPIRATION

Reflux esophagitis is a common clinical problem. More than one third of healthy adults experience symptoms of heartburn at least once a month. In terms of anesthetic management, GERD represents an aspiration risk. Factors that contribute to the likelihood of intraoperative aspiration include urgent or emergent surgery, a difficult airway, inadequate anesthetic depth, use of the lithotomy position, autonomic neuropathy, insulin-dependent diabetes mellitus, pregnancy, increased intraabdominal pressure, depressed consciousness, severe illness, and obesity.

By extrapolation from early studies in rhesus monkeys subjected to direct instillation of gastric contents into the lungs, it is believed that patients are at risk of aspiration pneumonitis if there is at least 0.4 mL/kg of gastric volume and the pH of the gastric contents is less than 2.5.

COMPLICATIONS

In addition to being at increased risk of aspiration, patients with GERD may develop other complications that can affect anesthetic management. These include (1) *mucosal* complications, such as esophagitis or esophageal stricture (the stricture causes esophageal dilation and compounds the risk for aspiration); and (2) *extraesophageal* or *respiratory complications*, such as laryngitis, bronchitis, bronchospasm, recurrent pneumonia, and progressive pulmonary fibrosis. Up to 50% of patients with asthma have either endoscopic evidence of esophagitis or an increased esophageal acid exposure on 24-hour ambulatory pH monitoring.

PROPHYLAXIS AND TREATMENT

The decision to include anticholinergic drugs in preoperative medication must be balanced against the known ability of these drugs to decrease LES tone. Theoretically, anticholinergic drugs, by decreasing LES pressure, can increase the likelihood of silent regurgitation and the possibility of pulmonary aspiration. However, occurrence of this potential adverse effect has not been documented. Succinylcholine increases LES pressure and intragastric pressure, but the barrier pressure (LES pressure minus intragastric pressure) is unchanged.

Depending on the planned surgery and anesthetic, medications to treat GERD may be given preoperatively. Cimetidine and ranitidine decrease gastric acid secretion and increase gastric pH. Cimetidine's effect begins in 1 to 1.5 hours and lasts for 3 hours. Ranitidine is four to six times more potent than cimetidine and has fewer side effects. Famotidine and nizatidine can also be given intravenously and are similar in effect to ranitidine but have a longer duration of action. Proton pump inhibitors are generally given orally the night before surgery and again on the morning of surgery. Very recent evidence indicates that proton pump inhibitors inhibit the antiplatelet effects of clopidogrel and possibly aspirin. This may be of particular concern in patients with coronary or other vascular stents. There may be an increased risk of stent thrombosis or occlusion.

Sodium citrate is an oral nonparticulate antacid that increases gastric pH. It should be given with a gastrokinetic agent such as metoclopramide, and its use should be restricted to those who are diabetic, severely clinically obese, or pregnant.

Cricoid pressure compresses the lumen of the pharynx between the cricoid cartilage and the cervical vertebrae. It is usually applied by an assistant under the direction of the anesthesia provider and maintained until successful endotracheal intubation is verified. The force applied should be sufficient to prevent aspiration but not so great as to cause airway obstruction or esophageal rupture in the event of vomiting.

Endotracheal intubation is essential for protecting the airway from aspiration in anesthetized patients with GERD. The endotracheal tube is superior to all other airway devices in reducing aspiration risk.

Hiatal Hernia

A *hiatal hernia* is a herniation of part of the stomach into the thoracic cavity through the esophageal hiatus in the diaphragm. A *sliding hiatal hernia* is one in which the gastroesophageal junction and fundus of the stomach slide upward.

This type of hernia is seen in approximately 30% of patients undergoing upper GI tract radiographic examination. Many of these patients are asymptomatic, that is, have no clinical symptoms of reflux. This hernia may result from weakening of the anchors of the gastroesophageal junction to the diaphragm, from longitudinal contraction of the esophagus, or from increased intraabdominal pressure. A *paraesophageal hernia* is one in which the esophagogastric junction remains in its normal location and a pouch of stomach is herniated next to the gastroesophageal junction through the esophageal hiatus. Hiatal hernias are only infrequently repaired. Most patients with hiatal hernias do not have symptoms of reflux esophagitis, which emphasizes the importance of the integrity of the LES.

Esophageal Diverticula

Diverticula are outpouchings of the wall of the esophagus. The most common sites are pharyngoesophageal (Zenker's diverticulum), (midesophageal), and epiphrenic (supradiaphragmatic diverticulum).

Zenker's diverticulum appears in a natural zone of weakness in the posterior hypopharyngeal wall (Killian's triangle) and can cause significant bad breath from food particles consumed up to several days previously. This food can also be regurgitated. If such a diverticulum becomes large and filled with food, it can compress the esophagus and cause dysphagia or aspiration pneumonia. Nasogastric tube and echocardiography probe insertion should be performed with utmost care in these patients to prevent perforation of the diverticulum.

A midesophageal diverticulum may be caused by traction from old adhesions or inflamed lymph nodes or by propulsion associated with esophageal motility abnormalities. An epiphrenic diverticulum may be associated with achalasia. Small or medium-sized Zenker's diverticula and midesophageal and epiphrenic diverticula are usually asymptomatic.

TREATMENT

Symptomatic Zenker's diverticulum is treated by cricopharyngeal myotomy with or without diverticulectomy. Large symptomatic esophageal diverticula are removed surgically.

Mucosal Tear (Mallory-Weiss Syndrome)

A mucosal tear is usually caused by vomiting, retching, or vigorous coughing. The tear typically involves the gastric mucosa near the squamocolumnar mucosal junction. Patients have upper GI tract bleeding. In most patients, bleeding ceases spontaneously, but continued bleeding may require vasopressin therapy or angiographic embolization.

PEPTIC ULCER DISEASE

Burning epigastric pain exacerbated by fasting and improved with meal consumption is the symptom complex associated with *peptic ulcer disease.* The lifetime prevalence of peptic ulcer disease in the United States is approximately 12% in men and 10% in women. Interestingly, an estimated 15,000 deaths per year occur as a consequence of complicated peptic ulcer disease. Bleeding, peritonitis, dehydration, perforation, and sepsis, especially in elderly debilitated and malnourished patients, are risk factors for death caused by peptic ulcer disease. Such patients pose significant anesthetic challenges.

Protective Function of the Gastric Lining

The *mucus-bicarbonate layer* serves as a physicochemical barrier to multiple chemicals, including hydrogen ions. Gastroduodenal surface epithelial cells secrete mucus. The mucous gel impedes diffusion of ions and molecules such as pepsin. Bicarbonate, secreted by surface epithelial cells of the gastroduodenal mucosa into the mucous gel, forms a pH gradient ranging from 1 to 2 at the gastric luminal surface and reaching 6 to 7 along the epithelial cell surface. Bicarbonate secretion is stimulated by calcium, prostaglandins, cholinergic input, and luminal acidification.

Surface epithelial cells provide the next line of defense by several mechanisms, including mucus production, epithelial cell ionic transporters that maintain intracellular pH and bicarbonate production, and intracellular tight junctions. If the preepithelial barrier is breached, gastric epithelial cells bordering the site of injury can migrate to the area and restore the damaged region.

Prostaglandins play a central role in gastric epithelial cell defenses and repair. These metabolites of arachidonic acid are formed by cyclooxygenase. Cyclooxygenase-1 present in the stomach, platelets, kidneys, and endothelial cells regulates the release of mucosal bicarbonate and mucus and inhibits parietal cell secretion. These functions are important in maintaining mucosal blood flow and epithelial cell structure.

Causes of Injury

Hydrochloric acid and pepsinogen are the two principal gastric secretory products capable of inducing mucosal injury. Acid secretion occurs under basal and stimulated conditions. Basal acid production occurs in a circadian pattern, with the highest levels occurring during the night and the lowest levels during the morning hours. Cholinergic input via the vagus nerve and histaminergic input from local gastric sources are the principal contributors to basal acid secretion. Stimulated gastric acid secretion occurs primarily in three phases based on the site at which the signal originates (cephalic, gastric, or intestinal). The sight, smell, and taste of food are the components of the cephalic phase of gastric acid secretion, which stimulates gastric secretion via the vagus nerve. The gastric phase is activated once food enters the stomach. Distention of the stomach wall also leads to gastrin release and acid production. The last phase of gastric acid secretion is initiated as food enters the intestine and is mediated by luminal distention. This fact explains why blocking one receptor type (histamine 2, or H_2) decreases acid secretion stimulated by agents that activate different parts of the pathway (gastrin, acetylcholine).

HELICOBACTER PYLORI

Many lines of evidence have established that *Helicobacter pylori* is a factor in the pathogenesis of duodenal ulceration. *H. pylori* infection is virtually always associated with chronic active gastritis, but only 10% to 15% of infected individuals develop actual peptic ulceration. Ironically, the earliest stages of *H. pylori* infection are accompanied by a marked *decrease* in gastric acid secretion. Then it induces increased acid secretion through both direct and indirect actions of the organism and proinflammatory cytokines (interleukin-1 [IL-1] and IL-8 and tumor necrosis factor) on G, D, and parietal cells. *H. pylori* also decreases duodenal mucosal bicarbonate production.

Complications

BLEEDING

Hemorrhage is the leading cause of death associated with peptic ulcer disease, and the incidence of this complication has not changed since the introduction of H_2-receptor antagonists. The lifetime risk of hemorrhage in patients with duodenal ulcer who have not had surgery and do not receive continuing maintenance drug therapy is approximately 35%. The current risk of mortality from bleeding is 10% to 20%.

PERFORATION

The lifetime risk of perforation in patients with duodenal ulceration who do not receive therapy is approximately 10%. Perforation is usually accompanied by sudden and severe epigastric pain caused by the spillage of highly acidic gastric secretions into the peritoneum. The mortality of emergent ulcer operations is correlated with the presence of preoperative shock, significant co-existing medical illnesses, and perforation longer than 48 hours before surgery.

OBSTRUCTION

Gastric outlet obstruction can occur acutely or chronically. Hence, patients with gastric outlet obstruction should be considered to have a full stomach when they come for surgery. Acute obstruction is caused by edema and inflammation in the pyloric channel and the first portion of the duodenum. Pyloric obstruction is suggested by recurrent vomiting, dehydration, and hypochloremic alkalosis resulting from loss of acidic gastric secretions. Treatment consists of nasogastric suction, rehydration, and intravenous administration of antisecretory drugs. In most instances, acute obstruction resolves within 72 hours with these supportive measures. However, repeated episodes of ulceration and healing can lead to pyloric scarring and a subsequent fixed stenosis and chronic gastric outlet obstruction.

Gastric Ulcer

Benign gastric ulcers are a form of peptic ulcer disease occurring with one third the frequency of benign duodenal ulcers (Table 14-2).

TABLE 14-2 ■ Classification of gastric ulcers

Type of gastric ulcer	Location
Type I	Along the lesser curvature close to incisura; no acid hypersecretion
Type II	Two ulcers, first on gastric body, second duodenal; usually acid hypersecretion
Type III	Prepyloric with acid hypersecretion
Type IV	At lesser curvature near gastroesophageal junction; no acid hypersecretion
Type V	Anywhere in stomach, usually seen with use of nonsteroidal antiinflammatory drugs

Stress Gastritis

Major trauma accompanied by shock, sepsis, respiratory failure, hemorrhage, massive transfusion, or multiorgan injury is often associated with the development of *acute stress gastritis*. Acute stress gastritis is particularly prevalent after thermal injury involving more than 35% of body surface area, central nervous system injury, or intracranial hypertension. The major complication of stress gastritis is gastric hemorrhage. The incidence of gastric bleeding is significantly associated with coagulopathy, thrombocytopenia, an international normalized ratio of more than 1.5, and a partial thromboplastin time of more than twice the normal value.

Treatment

ANTACIDS

Antacids are rarely, if ever, used by clinicians as the primary therapeutic agents for gastritis. However, patients often use them for symptomatic relief of dyspepsia. The most commonly used antacids are mixtures of aluminum hydroxide and magnesium hydroxide. Many of the frequently used antacids (e.g., Maalox, Mylanta) contain a combination of both aluminum and magnesium hydroxide to avoid the side effects of constipation or diarrhea. Neither magnesium- nor aluminum-containing preparations should be used in patients with chronic renal failure. The former can cause hypermagnesemia and the latter can cause neurotoxicity. Other potent antacids include calcium carbonate (Tums) and sodium bicarbonate. Long-term use of calcium carbonate can lead to milk-alkali syndrome (hypercalcemia and hyperphosphatemia) with possible development of renal stones and progression to renal insufficiency. Sodium bicarbonate use may induce systemic alkalosis.

H_2-RECEPTOR ANTAGONISTS

Four H_2-receptor antagonists—cimetidine, ranitidine, famotidine, and nizatidine—are currently available, and their structures share homology with histamine. All will significantly inhibit basal and stimulated gastric acid secretion. This class of drugs is effective for the treatment of active ulcer disease (4 to 6 weeks of treatment) and as an adjuvant (with antibiotics) for the management of *H. pylori* infection. Cimetidine was the first H_2-receptor antagonist used for the treatment of acid peptic disorders, with healing rates approaching 80% at 1 month. Ranitidine, famotidine, and nizatidine are more potent H_2-receptor antagonists than cimetidine. Cimetidine and ranitidine, but not famotidine and nizatidine, bind to hepatic cytochrome P-450. Therefore, careful monitoring of treatment with drugs such as warfarin, phenytoin, and theophylline that use cytochrome P-450 for metabolism is indicated.

PROTON PUMP INHIBITORS

Omeprazole, esomeprazole, lansoprazole, rabeprazole, and pantoprazole are substituted benzimidazole derivatives that covalently bind and irreversibly inhibit hydrogen–potassium–adenosine triphosphatase (H^+,K^+-ATPase). These are the most potent acid-inhibitory drugs available. Proton pump inhibitors inhibit all phases of gastric acid secretion. Onset of action is rapid, with a maximum effect achieved between 2 and 6 hours and a duration of gastric acid inhibition lasting up to 72 hours. As with any agent that leads to significant hypochlorhydria, proton pump inhibitors may interfere with absorption of drugs such as ketoconazole, ampicillin, iron, and digoxin. Hepatic cytochrome P-450 may also be inhibited by some proton pump inhibitors (omeprazole, lansoprazole). Patients receiving clopidogrel as maintenance therapy after placement of coronary or other vascular stents should avoid proton pump inhibitors because of the decreased antiplatelet effect of clopidogrel when used in conjunction with a proton pump inhibitor.

PROSTAGLANDIN ANALOGUES

Because of their central role in maintaining mucosal integrity and repair, prostaglandin analogues were developed for the treatment of peptic ulcer disease. At present, the prostaglandin E_1 derivative misoprostol is the only drug in this class approved by the U.S. Food and Drug Administration for clinical use in the prevention of gastroduodenal mucosal injury induced by nonsteroidal antiinflammatory drugs. Prostaglandin analogues enhance mucosal bicarbonate secretion, stimulate mucosal blood flow, and decrease mucosal cell turnover. The most common side effect is diarrhea. Other toxicities include uterine contractions and uterine bleeding. Therefore, misoprostol is contraindicated in women who may be pregnant, and women of child-bearing age must be made aware of this potential drug effect.

CYTOPROTECTIVE AGENTS

Sucralfate is a complex sucrose salt in which the hydroxyl groups have been substituted by aluminum hydroxide and sulfate. It can act by several mechanisms. In the gastric environment, aluminum hydroxide dissociates, leaving the polar sulfate anion, which can then bind to positively charged tissue proteins found within the ulcer bed. This process provides a physicochemical barrier impeding further tissue injury by

acid and pepsin. Sucralfate may also induce a trophic effect by binding growth factors such as endothelial growth factor, enhance prostaglandin synthesis, stimulate mucus and bicarbonate secretion, and enhance mucosal defense and repair. Toxicity from sucralfate is rare, and constipation is the most common side effect. Sucralfate should be avoided in patients with chronic renal insufficiency to prevent aluminum-induced neurotoxicity.

Colloidal bismuth subcitrate and bismuth subsalicylate (Pepto-Bismol) are the most widely used bismuth-containing antacids or antiulcer drugs. The mechanism by which these agents induce ulcer healing is unclear. Potential mechanisms include ulcer coating, prevention of further pepsin and hydrochloric acid–induced damage, binding of pepsin, and stimulation of prostaglandins, bicarbonate, and mucus secretion. Long-term use of high dosages, especially of colloidal bismuth subcitrate, may lead to neurotoxicity.

MISCELLANEOUS DRUGS

Anticholinergic drugs, designed to inhibit activation of the muscarinic receptor in parietal cells, have limited success in ulcer healing because of their relatively weak acid-inhibiting effect and significant side effects (dry eyes, dry mouth, urinary retention).

TREATMENT OF *HELICOBACTER PYLORI* INFECTION

The National Institutes of Health, American Digestive Health Foundation, and European Maastricht and Asia Pacific consensus conferences recommend that *H. pylori* be eradicated in patients with peptic ulcer disease. Eradication of this organism is associated with a dramatic decrease in ulcer recurrence. No single agent is effective in eradicating this organism. Combination therapy for 14 days provides the greatest efficacy. The antibiotics used with the greatest frequency are amoxicillin, metronidazole, tetracycline, clarithromycin, and bismuth compounds. Treatment protocols combine a proton pump inhibitor with two antibiotics, clarithromycin and either metronidazole or amoxicillin. The most feared complication with amoxicillin is pseudomembranous colitis, but this occurs in fewer than 1% to 2% of patients.

SURGICAL TREATMENT

Operative intervention is reserved for the treatment of complicated ulcer disease. The most common complications requiring surgery are hemorrhage, perforation, and obstruction as well as failure of a recurrent ulcer to respond to medical therapy and/or the inability to exclude malignant disease. The first goal of any surgical treatment should be removal of the ulcer diathesis so that ulcer healing is achieved and recurrence is minimized. The second goal is treatment of co-existing anatomic complications, such as pyloric stenosis or perforation. The third major goal should be preventing undesirable long-term side effects from the surgery.

Three procedures—truncal vagotomy and drainage, truncal vagotomy and antrectomy, and proximal gastric vagotomy—have been widely used for the operative treatment of peptic ulcer disease. Surgical treatment now, however, is often directed exclusively at correcting the immediate problem (e.g., closure of a duodenal perforation) *without* gastric denervation. Division of both vagal trunks at the esophageal hiatus (truncal vagotomy) denervates the acid-producing fundic mucosa as well as the remainder of the vagally supplied viscera. Because denervation results in impairment of gastric emptying, truncal vagotomy must be combined with a procedure to eliminate pyloric sphincter function, usually a pyloroplasty. Truncal vagotomy can also be combined with resection of the gastric antrum, which results in even further reduction in acid secretion, presumably by removing the antral source of gastrin. Restoration of GI continuity is achieved by gastroduodenostomy. Proximal gastric vagotomy (or parietal cell vagotomy) differs from truncal vagotomy in that only the nerve fibers to the acid-secreting fundic mucosa are divided. Vagotomy also diminishes parietal cell responsiveness to gastrin and histamine. Basal acid secretion is reduced by approximately 80% in the period immediately after surgery.

ZOLLINGER-ELLISON SYNDROME

In 1955 Zollinger and Ellison described two patients with gastroduodenal and intestinal ulceration together with gastrin hypersecretion and a non–beta islet cell tumor of the pancreas (gastrinoma). The incidence of *Zollinger-Ellison syndrome* varies from 0.1% to 1% of individuals with peptic ulcer disease. Men are affected more often than women, and in the majority of cases the disorder is identified when the patient is between the ages of 30 and 50.

Pathophysiology

Gastrin stimulates acid secretion through gastrin receptors on parietal cells and through induction of histamine release. It also exerts a trophic effect on gastric epithelial cells. Longstanding hypergastrinemia leads to markedly increased gastric acid secretion by both parietal cell stimulation and increased parietal cell mass. This increased gastric acid output leads to peptic ulcer disease, erosive esophagitis, and diarrhea.

Signs and Symptoms

Abdominal pain and peptic ulceration are seen in up to 90% of patients with Zollinger-Ellison syndrome; diarrhea is seen in 50%, with 10% having diarrhea as their only symptom. Gastroesophageal reflux is seen in about half of patients. Initial presentation and ulcer location in the duodenal bulb may be indistinguishable from those in ordinary peptic ulcer disease. Ulcers in unusual locations (second part of the duodenum and beyond), ulcers refractory to standard medical therapy, and ulcer recurrence after acid-reducing surgery or ulcers presenting with complications (bleeding, obstruction, and perforation) create suspicion of a gastrinoma. Gastrinomas can develop in the presence of multiple endocrine neoplasia type I (MEN I) syndrome, a disorder involving primarily three organ

TABLE 14-3   Causes of increased fasting serum gastrin level

Hypochlorhydria and achlorhydria (± pernicious anemia)	*Helicobacter pylori* infection
	Retained gastric antrum
	Gastric outlet obstruction
G-cell hyperplasia	Massive small bowel obstruction
Renal insufficiency	Vitiligo
Rheumatoid arthritis	Diabetes mellitus
Pheochromocytomas	Use of antisecretory drugs

sites: the parathyroid glands (80% to 90%), pancreas (40% to 80%), and pituitary gland (30% to 60%). In view of the stimulatory effect of calcium on gastric secretion, the hyperparathyroidism and hypercalcemia seen in MEN I patients may have a direct effect on ulcer disease. Resolution of hypercalcemia by parathyroidectomy reduces gastrin and gastric acid output in gastrinoma patients.

Diagnosis

The first step in the evaluation of a patient with suspected Zollinger-Ellison syndrome is obtaining a fasting gastrin level (Table 14-3). Gastric acid induces feedback inhibition of gastrin release. Such feedback is absent in Zollinger-Ellison syndrome. Up to 50% of patients with gastrinomas have metastatic disease at the time of diagnosis.

Treatment

Patients with duodenal ulcers as part of Zollinger-Ellison syndrome are treated initially with proton pump inhibitors at doses higher than those used to treat GERD and peptic ulcer disease, and then these drugs are continued at dosages guided by gastric acid measurements. Curative surgical resection of a gastrinoma is indicated in the absence of evidence of MEN I syndrome and metastatic disease.

Management of Anesthesia

Management of anesthesia for gastrinoma excision must consider the presence of gastric hypersecretion as well as the likely presence of large gastric fluid volumes. Esophageal reflux is common in these patients despite the ability of gastrin to increase LES tone. Depletion of intravascular fluid volume and electrolyte imbalances (hypokalemia, metabolic alkalosis) may accompany profuse watery diarrhea. The associated endocrine abnormalities (MEN I syndrome) can also influence the management of anesthesia. Antacid prophylaxis with proton pump inhibitors and H_2-receptor antagonists is maintained up to the time of surgery. A preoperative coagulation screen and liver function tests may be recommended, since alterations in fat absorption can influence production of clotting factors. Intravenous administration of ranitidine is useful for preventing gastric acid hypersecretion during surgery.

POSTGASTRECTOMY SYNDROMES

A number of syndromes have been described following gastric operations performed for peptic ulcer disease or gastric neoplasm. The overall occurrence of severe postoperative symptoms is low, perhaps 1% to 3% of cases, but the disturbances can be rather disabling. The two most common postgastrectomy syndromes are dumping and alkaline reflux gastritis.

Dumping

Dumping syndrome consists of a series of vasomotor and GI signs and symptoms. There are two phases of dumping: early and late. Dumping is caused by the entry of hyperosmolar gastric contents into the proximal small bowel, which results in a shift of fluid into the gut lumen, plasma volume contraction, and acute intestinal distention. Release of vasoactive GI hormones may also play a role. Early dumping symptoms occur 15 to 30 minutes after a meal and include nausea, diarrhea, epigastric discomfort, diaphoresis, crampy abdominal pain, tachycardia, palpitations, and, in extreme cases, dizziness or even syncope. Late dumping symptoms follow a meal by 1 to 3 hours and can include vasomotor symptoms that are thought to be secondary to hypoglycemia, which occurs as a result of excessive insulin release. Dietary modifications—consumption of frequent small meals, intake of few simple sugars, and a reduction in the amount of fluid ingested with a meal—can be very helpful. Octreotide therapy has been reported to improve dumping symptoms in diet-refractory cases. The drug is administered subcutaneously before a meal. Somatostatin analogues have beneficial effects on the vasomotor symptoms of dumping that are postulated to occur as a result of the pressor effects of these compounds on splanchnic blood vessels. In addition, somatostatin analogues inhibit the release of vasoactive peptides from the gut, decrease peak plasma insulin levels, and slow intestinal transit. Acarbose, an α-glucosidase inhibitor that delays the digestion of ingested carbohydrates, is often beneficial in late dumping.

Alkaline Reflux Gastritis

Alkaline reflux gastritis is identified by the occurrence of the clinical triad of (1) postprandial epigastric pain often associated with nausea and vomiting, (2) evidence of reflux of bile into the stomach, and (3) associated histologic evidence of gastritis. There is no pharmacologic treatment for alkaline reflux gastritis. The only proven treatment is operative diversion of intestinal contents from contact with the gastric mucosa. The most common surgical procedure for this purpose is a Roux-en-Y gastrojejunostomy.

IRRITABLE BOWEL SYNDROME

Patients with *irritable bowel syndrome* (spastic or mucous colitis) often complain of generalized abdominal discomfort. Commonly, the frequency of stools is increased, and the stool is covered with mucus. Many patients have associated symptoms of vasomotor instability, including tachycardia, hyperventilation, fatigue, diaphoresis, and headaches. Air trapped in the splenic flexure may produce pain in the left shoulder that radiates down the left arm (*splenic flexure syndrome*). Despite the frequent occurrence of irritable bowel syndrome, there is no known specific etiologic agent or structural or biochemical defect.

INFLAMMATORY BOWEL DISEASE

Inflammatory bowel diseases are the most common chronic inflammatory disorders after rheumatoid arthritis. The diagnosis of ulcerative colitis and Crohn's disease, and the differentiation between these disorders, is based on nonspecific clinical and histologic patterns that are often obscured by intercurrent infection, iatrogenic events, medication, or surgery. The incidence of inflammatory bowel disease in the United States is approximately 18 per 100,000 people.

Ulcerative Colitis

Ulcerative colitis is a mucosal disease involving the rectum and extending proximally to involve all or part of the colon. Approximately 40% to 50% of patients have disease limited to the rectum and rectosigmoid, 30% to 40% have disease extending beyond the sigmoid but not involving the entire colon, and 20% have a total colitis. Proximal spread occurs in continuity without areas of spared mucosa. In more severe disease, the mucosa is hemorrhagic, edematous, and ulcerated. In long-standing disease, inflammatory polyps (pseudopolyps) may be present. After many years of disease, the mucosa may appear atrophic and featureless, and the entire colon narrows and shortens. The major symptoms of ulcerative colitis are diarrhea, rectal bleeding, tenesmus, passage of mucus, and crampy abdominal pain. Symptoms in moderate to severe disease may also include anorexia, nausea, vomiting, fever, and weight loss. Active disease can be associated with an increase in levels of acute phase reactants, platelet count, and erythrocyte sedimentation rate, and a decrease in hematocrit. In severely ill patients, the serum albumin level is low and leukocytosis may be present.

COMPLICATIONS

Catastrophic illness is an initial presentation in only 15% of patients with ulcerative colitis. In 1% of patients, a severe episode may be accompanied by massive hemorrhage, which usually stops with treatment of the underlying disease. However, if the patient requires 6 to 8 units of blood within 24 to 48 hours, colectomy is frequently performed. *Toxic megacolon* is defined as a dilated transverse colon with loss of haustrations. It occurs in approximately 5% of episodes and can be triggered by electrolyte abnormalities or narcotics. About half of the time, toxic megacolon will resolve with medical therapy, but urgent colectomy may be required in those who do not experience improvement with conservative treatment. Perforation of the colon is the most dangerous complication of ulcerative colitis, and the physical signs of peritonitis may not be obvious, especially if the patient is receiving glucocorticoids. The mortality rate associated with this complication is approximately 15%. Some patients can develop toxic colitis and such severe ulcerations that the bowel may perforate without dilating. Obstructions caused by benign stricture formation occur in 10% of patients.

Crohn's Disease

Although Crohn's disease usually presents as acute or chronic bowel inflammation, the inflammatory process typically evolves into one of two patterns of disease, a penetrating-fistulous pattern or an obstructing pattern, each with different treatments and prognoses.

The most common site of inflammation is the terminal ileum. Therefore, the usual presentation of ileocolitis is a history of recurrent episodes of right lower quadrant pain and diarrhea. Sometimes the initial presentation mimics that of acute appendicitis with pronounced right lower quadrant pain, a palpable mass, fever, and leukocytosis. A spiking fever suggests intraabdominal abscess formation. Weight loss, typically 10% to 20% of body weight, is common and is a consequence of diarrhea, anorexia, and fear of eating. An inflammatory mass may be palpated in the right lower quadrant of the abdomen. Local extension of the mass can cause obstruction of the right ureter or inflammation of the bladder, manifested as dysuria and fever. Bowel obstruction may take several forms. In the early stages, bowel wall edema and spasm produce intermittent obstruction and increasing postprandial pain. Over several years, persistent inflammation gradually progresses to fibrostenotic narrowing and stricture. Diarrhea decreases and is replaced by chronic bowel obstruction. Severe inflammation of the ileocecal region may lead to localized wall thinning, with microperforation and formation of fistulas to the adjacent bowel, the skin, the urinary bladder, or an abscess cavity in the mesentery.

Extensive inflammatory disease is associated with a loss of digestive and absorptive surfaces, which results in malabsorption and steatorrhea. Nutritional deficiencies can also result from poor intake and enteric losses of protein and other nutrients, causing hypoalbuminemia, hypocalcemia, hypomagnesemia, coagulopathy, and hyperoxaluria with nephrolithiasis. Vertebral fractures are caused by a combination of vitamin D deficiency, hypocalcemia, and prolonged glucocorticoid use. Pellagra from niacin deficiency can occur in extensive small bowel disease, and malabsorption of vitamin B_{12} can lead to a megaloblastic anemia and neurologic symptoms.

Diarrhea is a sign of active disease caused by bacterial overgrowth in obstructed areas, fistulization, bile acid malabsorption resulting from a diseased or resected terminal ileum, and intestinal inflammation with decreased water absorption and increased secretion of electrolytes.

Patients with colitis have low-grade fever, malaise, diarrhea, crampy abdominal pain, and sometimes hematochezia. Gross bleeding is not as common as in ulcerative colitis and appears in about half of patients with Crohn's disease involving only the colon. Only 1% to 2% bleed massively. Pain is caused by passage of fecal material through narrowed and inflamed segments of large bowel. Toxic megacolon is rare but may be seen with severe inflammation. Stricture formation can produce symptoms of bowel obstruction. Colonic disease may fistulize into the stomach or duodenum, causing feculent vomitus, or into the proximal or middle small bowel, causing malabsorption by "short-circuiting" bacterial overgrowth.

Symptoms and signs of upper GI tract disease include nausea, vomiting, and epigastric pain. Patients usually have an *H. pylori*–negative gastritis. The second portion of the duodenum is more commonly involved than the duodenal bulb. Patients with advanced gastroduodenal Crohn's disease may develop chronic gastric outlet obstruction.

Up to one third of patients with Crohn's disease have at least one extraintestinal manifestation of the disease. Patients with perianal Crohn's disease are at higher risk of developing extraintestinal manifestations (Table 14-4).

Treatment of Inflammatory Bowel Disease

SURGICAL TREATMENT

Crohn's disease is a recurring disorder that cannot be cured by surgical resection. Surgery can only provide palliation. Current surgical procedures for treatment of obstructing

TABLE 14-4	Extraintestinal manifestation of inflammatory bowel disease (IBD)
Dermatologic	Erythema nodosum in 10%-15% of IBD cases; pyoderma gangrenosum in 1%-12%
Rheumatologic	Peripheral arthritis in 15%-20% of IBD cases
Ocular	1%-10% of IBD cases; conjunctivitis, anterior uveitis/iritis, episcleritis
Hepatobiliary	Approximately 50% of IBD cases; hepatomegaly; fatty liver due to chronic debilitating illness, malnutrition, and glucocorticoid therapy; cholelithiasis caused by malabsorption of bile acids; primary sclerosing cholangitis leading to biliary cirrhosis and hepatic failure
Urologic	Calculi in 10%-20% of IBD cases; ureteral obstruction
Other	Thromboembolic disease (pulmonary embolism, cerebrovascular accidents, arterial emboli) due to thrombocytosis; increased levels of fibrinopeptide A, factor V, factor VIII, and fibrinogen; accelerated thromboplastin generation; antithrombin III deficiency due to increased gut losses or increased catabolism; free protein S deficiency
	Endocarditis, myocarditis, and pleuropericarditis
	Interstitial lung disease
	Secondary/reactive amyloidosis

TABLE 14-5 ■ **Indications for surgery in inflammatory bowel disease**

ULCERATIVE COLITIS

Massive hemorrhage, perforation, toxic megacolon obstruction, intractable and fulminant disease, cancer

CROHN'S DISEASE

Stricture, obstruction, hemorrhage, abscess, fistulas, intractable and fulminant disease, cancer, unresponsive perianal disease

Crohn's disease include resection of the diseased segment and strictureplasty. A diverting colostomy may help heal severe perianal disease or a rectovaginal fistula, but disease almost always recurs after takedown of the colostomy. Often, patients require a total proctocolectomy and ileostomy. Resection of one half to two thirds of the small bowel represents the upper limit of resection, because removal of more than two thirds of the small intestine results in *short bowel syndrome* and the need for total parenteral nutrition.

Nearly half of patients with extensive chronic ulcerative colitis undergo surgery within the first 10 years of their illness. The indications for surgery are listed in Table 14-5. The complication rate is approximately 20% in elective, 30% in urgent, and 40% in emergent proctocolectomy. The complications are primarily hemorrhage, sepsis, and neural injury. Although single-stage total proctocolectomy with ileostomy has traditionally been the operation of choice, newer operations maintain continence while surgically removing the involved rectal mucosa.

MEDICAL TREATMENT

Sulfasalazine is the mainstay of therapy for mild to moderate inflammatory bowel disease. It was originally developed to deliver both antibacterial (sulfapyridine) and antiinflammatory (5-acetylsalicylic acid) therapy into the connective tissues of joints and the colonic mucosa. It is effective in inducing remission in both ulcerative colitis and Crohn's disease and in maintaining remission in ulcerative colitis. Up to 30% of patients experience allergic reactions or significant side effects such as headache, anorexia, nausea, and vomiting that are attributable to the sulfapyridine moiety. Hypersensitivity reactions can include rash, fever, hepatitis, agranulocytosis, hypersensitivity pneumonitis, pancreatitis, worsening of colitis, and impairment of folate absorption. Newer sulfa-free aminosalicylate preparations deliver increased amounts of the pharmacologically active ingredients of sulfasalazine (5-acetylsalicylic acid, mesalamine) to the site of active bowel disease while limiting systemic toxicity. The most commonly used of these newer drugs are Asacol and Pentasa, both of which contain mesalamine. Asacol is an enteric-coated form of mesalamine, but it has a slightly different release pattern, with 5-acetylsalicylic acid liberated at a pH higher than 7.0.

The majority of patients with moderate to severe ulcerative colitis benefit from oral or parenteral glucocorticoids.

Prednisone is usually started at dosages of 40 to 60 mg/day for active ulcerative colitis that is unresponsive to sulfa therapy. Parenteral glucocorticoids or corticotropin is occasionally preferred for glucocorticoid-naive patients despite a risk of adrenal hemorrhage. Topically applied glucocorticoids are also beneficial for distal colitis and may serve as an adjunct in those who have rectal involvement. These glucocorticoids are absorbed from the rectum in significant amounts and can lead to adrenal suppression after prolonged administration.

Glucocorticoids are also effective for treatment of moderate to severe Crohn's disease. Controlled ileal-release budesonide is nearly equipotent to prednisone in treating ileocolonic Crohn's disease and has fewer glucocorticoid side effects. Steroids play no role in maintenance therapy in either ulcerative colitis or Crohn's disease. Once clinical remission has been induced, corticosteroids should be tapered and discontinued.

Antibiotics have no role in the treatment of active or quiescent ulcerative colitis. However, "pouchitis," which occurs in approximately one third of ulcerative colitis patients after colectomy, usually responds to treatment with metronidazole or ciprofloxacin. These two antibiotics should be used as first-line drugs in perianal and fistulous Crohn's disease and as second-line therapy in active Crohn's disease after 5-acetylsalicylic acid agents become ineffective.

Azathioprine and 6-mercaptopurine (6-Mp) are purine analogues commonly used in the management of glucocorticoid-dependent inflammatory bowel syndromes. Azothioprine is readily absorbed and then converted to 6-Mp, which is then metabolized to an active end product. Efficacy is typically seen within 3 to 4 weeks. Pancreatitis occurs in 3% to 4% of patients, generally within the first few weeks of therapy, and is completely reversible when the drug is discontinued. Other side effects include nausea, fever, rash, and hepatitis. Bone marrow suppression (particularly leukopenia) is dose related and often delayed.

Methotrexate inhibits dihydrofolate reductase, which results in impaired DNA synthesis. Additional antiinflammatory properties may be related to a decrease in IL-1 production. Potential toxicities include leukopenia, hypersensitivity reactions, hepatic fibrosis, and pneumonitis.

Cyclosporine alters the immune response by acting as a potent inhibitor of T cell–mediated responses. Although cyclosporine acts primarily via inhibition of IL-2 production by helper T cells, it also decreases recruitment of cytotoxic T cells and blocks other cytokines, interferon-γ, and tumor necrosis factor. It has a more rapid onset of action than 6-mercaptopurine and azathioprine. Renal function should be monitored frequently. Hypertension, gingival hyperplasia, hypertrichosis, paresthesias, tremors, headaches, and electrolyte abnormalities are common side effects of cyclosporine. Creatinine elevation requires a dosage reduction or discontinuation of the drug.

PSEUDOMEMBRANOUS ENTEROCOLITIS

The cause of pseudomembranous enterocolitis is unknown. It is often associated with antibiotic therapy, bowel obstruction, uremia, congestive heart failure, and intestinal ischemia.

TABLE 14-6 ■ Secretory characteristics of carcinoid tumors in various sites

	Foregut	Midgut	Hindgut
Serotonin secretion	Low	High	Rare
Other substances secreted	ACTH, 5-HTP, GRF	Tachykinins; rarely 5-HTP, ACTH	Rarely 5-HTP, ACTH; other numerous peptides
Carcinoid syndrome	Atypical	Typical	Rare

ACTH, Corticotropin; *GRF,* growth hormone–releasing factor; *5-HT,* 5-hydroxytryptamine; *5-HTP,* 5-hydroxy-L-tryptophan.

TABLE 14-7 ■ Location and presentation of carcinoid tumors

Carcinoid location	Presentation
Small intestine	Abdominal pain (51%), intestinal obstruction (31%), tumor (17%), gastrointestinal bleeding (11%)
Rectum	Bleeding (39%), constipation (17%), diarrhea (17%)
Bronchus	Asymptomatic (31%)
Thymus	Anterior mediastinal mass
Ovary and testicle	Mass discovered on physical examination or ultrasonography
Metastases	In the liver; frequently presents as hepatomegaly

Clinical manifestations include fever, watery diarrhea, dehydration, hypotension, cardiac dysrhythmias, skeletal muscle weakness, ileus, and metabolic acidosis.

CARCINOID TUMORS

The incidence of clinically significant carcinoid tumors is 7 to 13 cases per million people per year. Carcinoid tumors can occur in almost any GI tissue. However, most (70%) originate from one of three sites: a bronchus, the jejunoileum, or the colon-rectum. These tumors typically secrete GI peptides and/or vasoactive substances (Table 14-6).

Carcinoid Tumors without Carcinoid Syndrome

Carcinoid tumors (Table 14-7) are often found incidentally during surgery for suspected appendicitis. Symptoms are often vague, and so the diagnosis is usually delayed by about 2 years from the onset of the symptoms.

Carcinoid Tumors with Systemic Symptoms due to Secreted Products

Carcinoid tumors can contain GI peptides, including gastrin, insulin, somatostatin, motilin, neurotensin, tachykinins (substance K, substance P, neuropeptide K), glucagon, gastrin-releasing peptide, vasoactive intestinal peptide, pancreatic peptide, other biologically active peptides (corticotropin, calcitonin, growth hormone), prostaglandins, and bioactive amines (serotonin). These substances may or may not be released in sufficient amounts to cause symptoms. Foregut carcinoids are more likely to produce various peptides than midgut carcinoids.

Carcinoid Syndrome

Carcinoid syndrome occurs in approximately 20% of patients with carcinoid tumors as a result of the large amounts of serotonin and vasoactive substances reaching the systemic circulation. The two most common signs are flushing and diarrhea.

The characteristic flush is of sudden onset. Physically it appears as a deep red blush, especially in the neck and face, often associated with a feeling of warmth and occasionally associated with pruritus, tearing, diarrhea, or facial edema. Flushes may be precipitated by stress, alcohol, exercise, certain foods, and drugs such as catecholamines, pentagastrin, and serotonin reuptake inhibitors. Cardiac tumors may have cardiac manifestations resulting from fibrosis involving the endocardium, primarily on the right side of the heart. Left-sided lesions can occur with pulmonary involvement or via a right-to-left intracardiac shunt (atrial septal defect, ventricular septal defect, patent foramen ovale). Pulmonic stenosis and tricuspid regurgitation are the typical valvular lesions. The carcinoid triad is (1) cardiac involvement, (2) flushing, and (3) diarrhea. Other clinical manifestations include wheezing or asthma-like symptoms and pellagra-like skin lesions. Retroperitoneal fibrosis can cause ureteral obstruction.

In most of patients with carcinoid syndrome, serotonin is overproduced and is responsible for the diarrhea through its effects on gut motility and intestinal secretion. Serotonin receptor antagonists (especially 5-hydroxytryptamine 3, [5-HT$_3$] antagonists) relieve the diarrhea in most patients. Serotonin does not appear to be involved in the flushing. In patients with gastric carcinoid tumors, the red, patchy pruritic flush is likely due to histamine release and can be prevented by H$_1$- and H$_2$-receptor blockers. Both histamine and serotonin may be responsible for bronchoconstriction.

A potentially life-threatening complication of carcinoid syndrome is development of a *carcinoid crisis.* Clinically, this manifests as intense flushing, diarrhea, abdominal pain, and cardiovascular signs, including tachycardia, hypertension, or hypotension. If not adequately treated, it can be fatal. The crises may occur spontaneously or may be provoked by stress, chemotherapy, or biopsy. Anesthetic drugs that can precipitate a carcinoid crisis are noted in Table 14-8.

The diagnosis of carcinoid syndrome relies on measurement of urinary or plasma serotonin concentrations or measurement of serotonin metabolites in the urine. The measurement

TABLE 14-8 ▪ Pharmacologic agents associated with carcinoid crisis

DRUGS THAT MAY PROVOKE MEDIATOR RELEASE

Succinylcholine, mivacurium, atracurium, D-tubocurarine
Epinephrine, norepinephrine, dopamine, isoproterenol,
   thiopental

DRUGS NOT KNOWN TO RELEASE MEDIATORS

Propofol, etomidate, vecuronium, cisatracurium, rocuronium,
   sufentanil, alfentanil, fentanyl, remifentanil
All inhalation agents; desflurane may be the better choice in
   patients with liver metastasis because of its low rate of
   metabolism

of 5-hydroxyindoleacetic acid (5-HIAA) is performed most frequently. False-positive test results may occur if the patient is eating serotonin-rich foods.

TREATMENT

Therapy for carcinoid tumors includes avoiding conditions that precipitate flushing, treating heart failure and/or wheezing, providing dietary supplementation with nicotinamide, and controlling diarrhea. If the patient continues to have symptoms, serotonin receptor antagonists or somatostatin analogues are useful. Many of these drugs have very short half-lives and must be given as continuous infusions. The 5-HT$_1$ and 5-HT$_2$ receptor antagonists methysergide, cyproheptadine, and ketanserin have all been used to control diarrhea but usually do not decrease flushing. The use of methysergide is limited because it can cause or exacerbate retroperitoneal fibrosis. The 5-HT$_3$ receptor antagonists ondansetron, tropisetron, and alosetron can control diarrhea and nausea in the majority of patients and even occasionally ameliorate the flushing. A combination of H$_1$- and H$_2$-receptor antagonists (i.e., diphenhydramine and cimetidine or ranitidine) may be useful in controlling the flushing in patients with foregut carcinoid tumors.

Synthetic analogues of somatostatin, such as octreotide, control symptoms in more than 80% of patients. Lanreotide is now the most widely used drug to control the symptoms of carcinoid syndrome. It is given in a sustained release form by subcutaneous injection and can last up to 2 weeks. Somatostatin analogues are effective in relieving symptoms and decreasing urinary 5-HIAA levels. In patients with carcinoid crises, somatostatin analogues are effective in treating the condition as well as preventing its development during known precipitating events such as surgery, anesthesia, chemotherapy, and stress. Octreotide should be administered 24 to 48 hours before surgery and then continued throughout the procedure. Short-term side effects occur in 40% to 60% of patients receiving subcutaneous somatostatin analogues. These include pain at the injection site, abdominal discomfort, and nausea. Important long-term side effects include gallstone formation, steatorrhea, and glucose intolerance.

Surgery is the only potentially curative therapy for nonmetastatic carcinoid tumors.

Invasive arterial blood pressure monitoring is necessary during the intraoperative management of patients with carcinoid syndrome because of the potential for rapid changes in hemodynamic variables. Administration of octreotide preoperatively and before manipulation of the tumor will attenuate most adverse hemodynamic responses. General anesthesia is typically used for this surgery, and any combination of drugs is suitable for the anesthetic. However, increased levels of serotonin have been associated with delayed awakening. Ondansetron, a serotonin antagonist, is a useful and logical antiemetic choice.

Use of epidural analgesia in patients who have been adequately treated with octreotide is a safe technique provided the local anesthetic is administered in a gradual manner accompanied by careful hemodynamic monitoring.

ACUTE PANCREATITIS

Acute pancreatitis is an acute inflammatory disorder of the pancreas. The incidence of acute pancreatitis has increased 10-fold since the 1960s, which perhaps reflects increased alcohol abuse and/or improved diagnostic techniques.

Pathogenesis

The pancreas contains numerous digestive enzymes (proteases). Autodigestion of the pancreas is prevented by packaging of the proteases in precursor form, synthesis of protease inhibitors, and the low intrapancreatic concentration of calcium, which decreases trypsin activity. Loss of any of these protective mechanisms leads to enzyme activation, autodigestion, and acute pancreatitis.

Gallstones and alcohol abuse are the causative factors in 60% to 80% of patients with acute pancreatitis. Gallstones are believed to cause pancreatitis by transiently obstructing the ampulla of Vater, which leads to pancreatic ductal hypertension. Acute pancreatitis is common in patients with acquired immunodeficiency syndrome and those with hyperparathyroidism and its associated hypercalcemia. Trauma-induced acute pancreatitis is generally associated with blunt trauma rather than penetrating injury. This blunt trauma may compress the pancreas against the spine. Postoperative pancreatitis occurs after abdominal and noncardiac or cardiac thoracic surgery, especially procedures that require cardiopulmonary bypass. Clinical pancreatitis develops in 1% to 2% of patients following endoscopic retrograde cholangiopancreatography (ERCP).

Signs and Symptoms

Excruciating, unrelenting midepigastric abdominal pain that radiates to the back occurs in almost every patient with acute pancreatitis. Sitting and leaning forward may decrease the pain. Nausea and vomiting can occur at the peak of the pain. Abdominal distention with ileus often develops. Dyspnea may reflect the presence of pleural effusions or ascites. Low-grade fever, tachycardia, and hypotension are fairly common. Shock may occur as a result of (1) hypovolemia from the exudation of blood and plasma into the retroperitoneal space, (2) release of kinins that cause vasodilation and increased capillary permeability, and (3) systemic effects of pancreatic enzymes released into the general circulation.

Obtundation and psychosis may reflect alcohol withdrawal. Development of tetany may occur as a result of hypocalcemia (calcium binds to free fatty acids and forms soaps).

Diagnosis

The hallmark of acute pancreatitis is an increase in serum amylase concentration. Serum lipase concentration is also elevated. Contrast-enhanced computed tomography is the best noninvasive test for documenting the morphologic changes associated with acute pancreatitis. ERCP can be useful for both evaluating and treating certain forms of pancreatitis, such as traumatic pancreatitis (localization of injury) and severe gallstone pancreatitis (papillotomy, stone removal, and drainage).

The differential diagnosis of acute pancreatitis includes a perforated duodenal ulcer, acute cholecystitis, mesenteric ischemia, and bowel obstruction. Acute myocardial infarction may cause severe abdominal pain, but serum amylase concentration is not increased. Patients with pneumonia may also have significant epigastric pain and fever.

It is important to identify patients with acute pancreatitis who are at significant risk of dying from the disease. Multifactor scoring systems have been devised to help identify these high-risk patients. One such system is the Ranson criteria. These criteria are (1) age older than 55 years, (2) white blood cell count of more than 16,000 cells/mm^3, (3) blood urea nitrogen concentration of more than 16 mmol/L, (4) aspartate transaminase level of more than 250 units/L, (5) arterial Pao$_2$ of less than 60 mm Hg, (6) fluid deficit of more than 6 L, (7) blood glucose level of more than 200 mg/dL in a person without a history of diabetes mellitus, (8) lactate dehydrogenase level of more than 350 IU/L, (9) corrected calcium concentration of less than 8 mg/dL, (10) a decrease in hematocrit of more than 10, and (11) metabolic acidosis with a base deficit of more than 4 mmol/L. It is noteworthy that the serum amylase concentration is not one of the criteria.

In the Ranson scoring system, mortality is related to the number of criteria met. Patients fulfilling zero to two criteria have a mortality of less than 5%. Patients meeting three or four criteria have a 20% mortality; those fulfilling five or six criteria have a 40% mortality. The presence of seven or eight criteria is associated with 100% mortality.

Complications

Nearly 25% of patients who develop acute pancreatitis experience significant complications. Shock can develop early in the course of severe acute pancreatitis and is a major risk factor for death. Sequestration of large volumes of fluid in the peripancreatic space, hemorrhage, and systemic vasodilation contribute to hypotension. Arterial hypoxemia is often present early in the course of the disease. ARDS is seen in 20% of patients. Renal failure occurs in 25% of patients and is associated with a poor prognosis. GI hemorrhage and coagulation defects from disseminated intravascular coagulation may occur. Infection of necrotic pancreatic material or abscess formation is a serious complication associated with a mortality rate of more than 50%.

Treatment

Aggressive intravenous fluid administration is necessary to treat the significant hypovolemia that occurs in all patients, even those with mild pancreatitis. Colloid replacement may be necessary if there is significant bleeding or albumin loss. Traditionally, oral intake is stopped to rest the pancreas and prevent aggravation of the accompanying ileus. There are data to suggest that feeding patients via a postpyloric route such as a nasojejunal tube or feeding jejunostomy may be helpful, especially in patients who are intubated and mechanically ventilated as a result of ARDS or renal failure. Parenteral feeding is indicated if patients do not tolerate enteral feeding. Nasogastric suction may be needed to treat persistent vomiting or ileus. Opioids are typically administered to manage the severe pain. Endoscopic removal of obstructing gallstones is indicated within the first 24 to 72 hours of the onset of symptoms to decrease the risk of cholangitis. Drainage of intraabdominal collections of fluids or necrotic material can be done without surgery. Interventions via ERCP include drainage through tubes of various sizes that can be changed (upsized) if needed.

CHRONIC PANCREATITIS

The incidence of chronic pancreatitis is difficult to determine, since the disease may be asymptomatic or abdominal pain may be attributed to other causes. The persistent inflammation characteristic of chronic pancreatitis leads to irreversible damage to the pancreas. There is loss of both exocrine and endocrine function.

Pathogenesis

Chronic pancreatitis is most often due to chronic alcohol abuse. Alcohol may have a direct toxic effect on the pancreas. Diets high in protein seem to predispose alcoholic patients to the development of chronic pancreatitis. *Idiopathic* chronic pancreatitis is seen in up to 25% of adults in the United States with chronic pancreatitis. It is suggested that a significant number of "idiopathic" cases are related to genetic defects. Chronic pancreatitis also occurs in association with cystic fibrosis and hyperparathyroidism (hypercalcemia).

Signs and Symptoms

Chronic pancreatitis is often characterized by epigastric pain that radiates to the back and is frequently postprandial. However, 10% to 30% of patients have painless chronic pancreatitis.

Steatorrhea is present when at least 90% of pancreatic exocrine function is last. Diabetes mellitus is the end result of loss of endocrine function. Pancreatic calcifications develop in most patients with alcohol-induced chronic pancreatitis.

Diagnosis

The diagnosis of chronic pancreatitis may be based on a history of chronic alcohol abuse and demonstration of pancreatic calcifications. Patients who have chronic pancreatitis are often thin and even emaciated. This is due to the maldigestion of proteins and fats seen when the amount of pancreatic enzymes entering the duodenum is reduced to 10% to 20% of normal. Serum amylase concentrations are usually normal. An abdominal radiograph may reveal pancreatic calcifications. Ultrasonography is useful for documenting the presence of an enlarged pancreas or identifying a pseudocyst. Computed tomography in patients with chronic pancreatitis demonstrates dilated pancreatic ducts and changes in the size of the pancreas. ERCP is the most sensitive imaging test for detecting *early* changes in the pancreatic ducts caused by chronic pancreatitis.

Treatment

Treatment of chronic pancreatitis includes management of pain, malabsorption, and diabetes mellitus. Opioids are often required for adequate pain control, and in some patients, celiac plexus blockade may be considered. An internal surgical drainage procedure (pancreaticojejunostomy) or endoscopic placement of stents and/or extraction of stones may be helpful in patients whose pain is resistant to medical management. Enzyme supplements are administered to facilitate fat and protein absorption. Insulin is administered as needed.

MALABSORPTION AND MALDIGESTION

Malabsorption of nutrients usually involves impaired absorption of fat (steatorrhea), although other substances (iron, calcium, bile salts, specific amino acids, saccharides) may be selectively poorly absorbed in the absence of steatorrhea. Steatorrhea is most frequently caused by small bowel, liver, or biliary tract disease or pancreatic exocrine insufficiency. Patients with small bowel disease may develop hypoalbuminemia as a result of leakage of protein through diseased intestinal mucosa. Deficiencies of fat-soluble vitamins (vitamins A, D, E, K), hypocalcemia, and hypomagnesemia may be present in patients with liver and biliary tract disease.

Gluten-Sensitive Enteropathy

Gluten-sensitive enteropathy (previously termed *celiac disease* in children and *nontropical sprue* in adults) is a disease of the small intestine resulting in malabsorption (steatorrhea), weight loss, abdominal pain, and fatigue. Treatment is removal of gluten-containing foods, such as wheat, rye, and barley, from the diet.

Extensive Small Bowel Resection

Extensive small bowel resection for mesenteric ischemia, volvulus, or Crohn's disease may result in malabsorption if the remaining small intestinal surface area for absorption of nutrients is decreased below a critical level. Clinical manifestations of the resulting *short bowel syndrome* include diarrhea, steatorrhea, trace element deficiencies, and electrolyte imbalances, especially hyponatremia and hypokalemia. Total parenteral nutrition may be needed if frequent small feedings are not effective in maintaining nutritional balance.

GASTROINTESTINAL BLEEDING

GI bleeding (Table 14-9) most often originates in the upper GI tract (from peptic ulcer disease). Bleeding in the lower GI tract from diverticulosis or tumor accounts for 10% to 20% of all cases of GI bleeding and primarily affects older patients.

Upper Gastrointestinal Tract Bleeding

Patients with acute upper GI tract bleeding may experience hypotension and tachycardia if blood loss exceeds 25% of total blood volume. Patients with orthostatic hypotension characterized by a positional decrease in systolic blood pressure of 10 to 20 mm Hg and a corresponding increase in heart rate generally have a hematocrit of less than 30%. The hematocrit may be normal early in the course of acute hemorrhage because of insufficient time for equilibration of plasma volume. After fluid resuscitation, anemia becomes more overt. Melena indicates that bleeding has occurred at a site above the cecum.

TABLE 14-9 ■ Common causes of upper and lower gastrointestinal tract bleeding

Cause	Incidence (%)
UPPER GASTROINTESTINAL TRACT BLEEDING	
Peptic ulcer	
Duodenal ulcer	36
Gastric ulcer	24
Mucosal erosive disease	
Gastritis	6
Esophagitis	6
Esophageal varices	6
Mallory-Weiss tear	3
Malignancy	2
LOWER GASTROINTESTINAL TRACT BLEEDING	
Colonic diverticulosis	42
Colorectal malignancy	9
Ischemic colitis	9
Acute colitis of unknown cause	5
Hemorrhoids	5

Adapted from Young HS. Gastrointestinal bleeding. *Sci Am Med.* 1998:1-10.

Blood urea nitrogen levels are typically more than 40 mg/dL because of the absorbed nitrogen load from the blood in the small intestine. Elderly individuals, those with esophageal variceal bleeding, those with malignancy, and those who develop bleeding during hospitalization for other medical conditions have an acute mortality rate of more than 30%. Multiple organ system failure, rather than hemorrhage, is the usual cause of death in these patients. Upper endoscopy after hemodynamic stabilization is the diagnostic-therapeutic procedure of choice in patients with acute upper GI tract bleeding.

For patients with bleeding peptic ulcers, endoscopic coagulation (thermotherapy, or injection with epinephrine or a sclerosing material) is indicated when active bleeding is visible. Even patients receiving anticoagulants can be safely treated with endoscopic coagulation of a peptic ulcer. Perforation occurs in approximately 0.5% of patients undergoing endoscopic coagulation. In patients with bleeding esophageal varices, endoscopic ligation of the bleeding varices is as effective as sclerotherapy. A transjugular intrahepatic portosystemic shunt may be used in patients with esophageal variceal bleeding resistant to control by endoscopic coagulation or sclerotherapy. However, insertion of such a shunt can lead to worsening encephalopathy. Mechanical tamponade of bleeding varices can be accomplished with a Sengstaken-Blakemore tube or a Minnesota tube. These devices have balloons to mechanically tamponade the bleeding varices. Such devices are rarely used now that endoscopic therapy for bleeding varices is so successful. Surgical treatment of nonvariceal upper GI tract bleeding may be undertaken to oversew an ulcer or to perform gastrectomy for diffuse hemorrhagic gastritis in patients who continue to bleed despite optimal supportive therapy and in whom endoscopic coagulation is unsuccessful.

Lower Gastrointestinal Tract Bleeding

Lower GI tract (colonic) bleeding usually occurs in older patients and typically presents as abrupt passage of bright red blood and clots via the rectum. Causes include diverticulosis, tumors, ischemic colitis, and certain forms of infectious colitis. Sigmoidoscopy to exclude anorectal lesions is indicated as soon as patients are in hemodynamically stable condition. Colonoscopy can be performed after the bowel has been cleansed. If bleeding is persistent and brisk, angiography and embolic therapy may be attempted. Up to 15% of patients with lower GI tract bleeding require surgical intervention to control it.

Occult Gastrointestinal Bleeding

Occult GI bleeding may present as unexplained iron deficiency anemia or as intermittently positive results on tests for occult blood in the stool. Peptic ulcer disease and colonic neoplasm are the most common causes of occult GI bleeding. The site of occult bleeding is determined by upper GI tract endoscopy and colonoscopy. Occasionally other tests such as a radioactive tagged red blood cell scan or angiography are needed to define the bleeding site.

DIVERTICULOSIS AND DIVERTICULITIS

Colonic diverticula are herniations of the mucosa and submucosa through the muscularis propria layer. These occur most often in individuals who consume low-fiber diets. Diverticulitis is inflammation of one or more diverticula, mostly in the sigmoid or descending colon. Mild diverticulitis typically manifests with fever and lower abdominal pain and tenderness. Nausea, vomiting, constipation, diarrhea, dysuria, tachycardia, and leukocytosis may be noted. Right colon diverticulitis is often indistinguishable from appendicitis. Severe diverticulitis is characterized by the development of a diverticular abscess that may rupture and produce purulent peritonitis. Fistula formation can occur and most commonly is a connection between the sigmoid colon and the bladder. Abdominal computed tomography is the most useful study for evaluation of suspected diverticulitis.

Treatment for mild distress in patients tolerating oral hydration should include 7 to 10 days of oral broad-spectrum antimicrobial therapy (including coverage for anaerobic organisms). Patients with diverticulitis severe enough to require hospitalization are treated with intravenous fluids, bowel rest, broad-spectrum antibiotics, and parenteral analgesics. If, despite adequate supportive therapy, the patient's condition does not improve within 48 hours, complications of diverticulitis likely exist. Further therapy is necessary and may include surgery. Surgical treatment of acute diverticulitis consists of resection of the diseased segment of colon.

APPENDICITIS

Incidence and Epidemiology

The peak incidence of acute appendicitis is in the second and third decades of life. It is relatively rare at the extremes of age, but perforation and increased mortality are more common in infants and the elderly. Among infants younger than 2 years of age there is a 70% to 80% incidence of perforation and generalized peritonitis. In the elderly, pain and tenderness are often blunted, and thus the diagnosis is frequently delayed, so there is a 30% incidence of perforation in patients older than 70 years. The mortality rate has decreased steadily in Europe and the United States from 8.1 per 100,000 people in 1941 to fewer than 1 per 100,000 in 1970 and subsequently. Interestingly, the overall incidence of appendicitis is much *lower* in underdeveloped countries and in lower socioeconomic groups.

Pathogenesis

Luminal obstruction can be identified in only 30% to 40% of cases, and ulceration of the mucosa is the initial event in the majority of cases. Obstruction, if present, is most commonly caused by a fecalith. Enlarged lymphoid follicles associated with viral infections (e.g., measles), inspissated barium, worms (e.g., pinworms, ascaris), and tumors (e.g., carcinoid) may also obstruct the lumen. Luminal bacteria multiply and invade the appendiceal wall. Venous engorgement and subsequent arterial compromise result from high intraluminal pressures. Perforation and/or gangrene may eventually occur. If the appendiceal inflammatory process evolves slowly, adjacent organs such as the terminal ileum, cecum, and omentum may wall off the appendiceal area so that a localized abscess develops. Rapid progression of appendicitis and vascular impairment causes perforation into the peritoneal cavity.

Signs and Symptoms

History and symptoms are important diagnostic features of appendicitis. The initial symptom is almost invariably mild crampy abdominal pain resulting from appendiceal contractions or distention of the appendiceal lumen. It is initially poorly localized in the periumbilical or epigastric region and accompanied by the urge to defecate or pass flatus, neither of which relieves the pain. As inflammation spreads to the parietal peritoneal surfaces, the pain becomes steady and more severe, aggravated by motion or cough, and by then is usually located in the right lower quadrant. Anorexia is very common. Nausea and vomiting occur in 50% to 60% of cases. Urinary frequency and dysuria can occur if the appendix lies adjacent to the bladder. Body temperature is usually normal or slightly elevated. A temperature of more than 38.3° C suggests perforation. Early perforation is rare, but the perforation rate may approach 80% after 48 hours. Moderate leukocytosis of 10,000 to 18,000 cells/mm^3 is frequent, but the absence of leukocytosis does not rule out acute appendicitis. Leukocytosis of more than 20,000 cells/mm^3 suggests perforation. Appendicitis occurs in about 1 in every 1000 pregnancies and is the most common extrauterine condition requiring abdominal surgery during pregnancy. The differential diagnosis of acute appendicitis is presented in Table 14-10.

Treatment

Appendectomy should be performed as soon as the patient can be prepared. The only circumstance in which operation is *not* indicated is the presence of a palpable mass 3 to 5 days after the onset of symptoms. Such patients have a periappendiceal abscess. Surgery at this time is frequently associated with complications, so medical therapy is typically used instead. This includes broad-spectrum antibiotics, fluids, and rest. Resolution of the mass and symptoms often occurs within a week. Appendectomy can be done safely a few months later.

PERITONITIS

Peritonitis is an inflammation of the peritoneum. It may be localized or diffuse, acute or chronic, and infectious or aseptic. Acute peritonitis is most often infectious and is usually related to a perforated viscus (*secondary peritonitis*). When no bacterial source is identified, infectious peritonitis is called *primary* or *spontaneous.*

Pathogenesis

Infectious agents gain access to the peritoneal cavity through a perforated viscus, a penetrating wound of the abdominal wall, or external introduction of a foreign object that is or becomes infected, such as a peritoneal dialysis catheter. In the absence of immune compromise, host defenses are capable of eradicating small contaminations. The conditions that most commonly result in the introduction of bacteria into the peritoneum are noted in Table 14-11. Bacterial peritonitis can also occur in the apparent absence of an intraperitoneal source of bacteria (primary or spontaneous bacterial peritonitis). This condition typically occurs in the setting of ascites and cirrhosis, especially in patients with ascites with a low protein concentration (<1 g/L). It is postulated that spontaneous bacterial peritonitis actually develops due to translocation of bacteria from the intestinal lumen to regional lymph nodes with subsequent bacteremia and infection of the ascitic fluid.

Aseptic peritonitis may be due to irritation of the peritoneum by the presence of normal physiologic fluids (e.g., gastric juice, bile, pancreatic enzymes, blood, urine) in an abnormal location (the peritoneum) or the presence of sterile foreign bodies, such as surgical sponges or instruments or starch from surgical gloves, in the peritoneal cavity. It can also be a complication of certain systemic diseases such as lupus erythematosus, porphyria, or familial Mediterranean fever.

TABLE 14-10 ▪ Differential diagnosis of appendicitis		
Mesenteric lymphadenitis	Ureteral calculus	Pelvic inflammatory disease
Ruptured graafian follicle	Acute cholecystitis	Corpus luteum cyst
Acute pancreatitis	Acute gastroenteritis	Strangulating intestinal obstruction
Perforated ulcer	Acute diverticulitis	No organic disease

TABLE 14-11 ▪ Causes of peritonitis
BOWEL PERFORATION
Trauma, iatrogenic causes (endoscopic perforation, ischemia, anastomotic leak, catheter perforation) ingested foreign body, inflammatory bowel disease, vascular causes, (embolus, ischemia), strangulated hernia, volvulus, intussusception
OTHER ORGAN LEAK
Pancreatitis, cholecystitis, salpingitis, bile leak after biopsy, urinary bladder rupture
PERITONEAL DISRUPTION
Peritoneal dialysis, intraperitoneal chemotherapy, retained postoperative foreign body, penetrating fistulous pattern, trauma

Signs and Symptoms

The cardinal manifestations of peritonitis are acute abdominal pain and tenderness, usually with fever. Generalized peritonitis is associated with widespread inflammation and diffuse abdominal tenderness, including rebound tenderness. Rigidity of the abdominal wall is common. Bowel sounds are usually absent. Tachycardia, hypotension, and signs of dehydration are common as are leukocytosis and acidosis. If ascites is present, diagnostic paracentesis with cell counts, measurement of protein and lactate dehydrogenase levels, and culture is essential for diagnosis. In the elderly and immunosuppressed, signs of peritoneal irritation may be muted and therefore more difficult to detect.

Treatment and Prognosis

Treatment of peritonitis consists of hydration, correction of electrolyte abnormalities, administration of antibiotics, and, if needed, surgical correction of the underlying problem. Mortality rates are less than 10% for uncomplicated peritonitis in otherwise healthy persons. Mortality rates of 40% or more have been reported in the elderly, those with underlying illnesses, and those in whom peritonitis has been present for longer than 48 hours.

ACUTE COLONIC PSEUDO-OBSTRUCTION

Acute colonic pseudo-obstruction is a form of colonic ileus characterized by massive dilation of the colon in the absence of mechanical obstruction. The disorder is characterized by loss of effective colonic peristalsis and subsequent distention of the colon. This syndrome generally develops in seriously ill patients hospitalized for significant medical problems. Typically such patients have electrolyte disorders, are immobile, or have received narcotic or anticholinergic medications. The disorder can also be observed in surgical patients after a variety of non-GI operations. If left untreated, the massive colonic dilation can result in ischemia of the right colon and cecum, and perforation. One current hypothesis as to the etiology of colonic pseudo-obstruction invokes an imbalance in neural input to the colon distal to the splenic flexure. It suggests an excess of sympathetic stimulation and a paucity of parasympathetic input, therefore resulting in spastic contraction of the distal colon and functional obstruction. Plain radiographs of the abdomen reveal dilation of the proximal colon and a decompressed distal colon with some air in the rectosigmoid region. For patients in whom the cecal diameter is less than 12 cm (the risk of perforation is much greater if the cecal diameter exceeds 12 cm), an initial trial of conservative therapy is indicated that includes correction of electrolyte disorders, avoidance of narcotic and anticholinergic agents, hydration, mobilization, tap water enemas, and nasogastric suction. The 70% of cases that will resolve with conservative therapy do so within 2 days, which suggests that a 48-hour trial of conservative management is warranted in patients in stable condition.

However, patients for whom conservative therapy fails should be considered for active intervention. This could include intravenous administration of neostigmine. Intravenous neostigmine at a dose of 2 to 2.5 mg given over 3 to 5 minutes results in immediate colonic decompression in 80% to 90% of patients. Because symptomatic bradycardia is a serious side effect of neostigmine administration, all patients being treated with this drug require cardiac monitoring. Decompressive colonoscopy or placement of a cecostomy are other active interventions that may be needed.

KEY POINTS

- Natural antireflux mechanisms consist of the lower esophageal sphincter, the crural diaphragm, and the anatomic location of the gastroesophageal junction below the diaphragmatic hiatus.
- Factors that contribute to the likelihood of aspiration include urgency of surgery, a difficult airway, inadequate anesthetic depth, lithotomy position, increased intraabdominal pressure, insulin-dependent diabetes mellitus, autonomic neuropathy, pregnancy, depressed consciousness, severe illness, and obesity.
- Patients with silent aspiration may present with symptoms and signs of bronchial asthma.
- All patients who have undergone esophagectomy have a very significant risk of aspiration.
- Major trauma accompanied by shock, sepsis, respiratory failure, hemorrhage, massive transfusion, or multiorgan injury is often associated with the development of acute stress gastritis.
- Cimetidine and ranitidine bind to hepatic cytochrome P-450. Therefore, monitoring of drugs that also use this enzyme system, such as warfarin, phenytoin, and theophylline, is indicated.
- Following gastric surgery for peptic ulcer disease or gastric neoplasm, patients may develop dumping syndrome or alkaline reflux gastritis.
- Inflammatory bowel diseases are the most common chronic inflammatory diseases after rheumatoid arthritis. Ulcerative colitis and Crohn's disease can be associated with abdominal pain, fluid and electrolyte disturbances, bleeding bowel perforation, peritonitis, fistula formation, GI tract obstruction, cancer, and numerous extraintestinal inflammatory conditions.
- Carcinoid tumors may be associated with carcinoid syndrome due to release of large amounts of serotonin and other vasoactive substances into the systemic circulation causing flushing, diarrhea, tachycardia, and hypertension or hypotension.
- Gallstones and alcohol abuse cause the majority of cases of acute pancreatitis. Chronic pancreatitis is usually caused by chronic alcohol abuse, but up to 25% of cases are labeled as idiopathic in origin.
- Gastrointestinal bleeding most often originates in the upper GI tract due to peptic ulcer disease. About 20% of GI

bleeding originates in the lower GI tract and can be due to diverticulosis, tumors, ischemic colitis, or certain forms of infectious colitis.

■ Peritonitis is an inflammation of the peritoneum that may be localized or diffuse, acute or chronic, and infectious or aseptic. Acute peritonitis is most often infectious and is a result of a perforated viscus.

RESOURCES

Aitkenhead AR. Anaesthesia and bowel surgery. *Br J Anaesth*. 1984;56:95-101.

Cortinez FLI. Refractory hypotension during carcinoid resection surgery. *Anaesthesia*. 2000;55:505-506.

Dierdorf SF. Carcinoid tumor and carcinoid syndrome. *Curr Opin Anaesthesiol*. 2003;16:343-347.

Hunter AR. Colorectal surgery for cancer: the anaesthetist's contribution? *Br J Anaesth*. 1986;58:825-826.

Kasper DL, Fauci AS, Longo DL, eds. Part 13. Disorders of the alimentary track. In *Harrison's Principles of Internal Medicine*. 16th ed. New York, NY: McGraw-Hill; 2005.

Mulholland MW, Lillemoe KD, Doherty GM. *Greenfield's Surgery: Scientific Principles and Practice.*. Philadelphia, PA: Lippincott Williams & Wilkins; 2006.

Ng A, Smith G. Gastroesophageal reflux and aspiration of gastric contents in anesthetic practice. *Anesth Analg*. 2001;93:494-513.

Redmond MC. Perianesthesia care of the patient with gastroesophageal reflux disease. *J Perianesthesia Nurs*. 2003;18:535-544:quiz 345–347.

Sontag SJ, O'Connell S, Khandewal S, et al. Most asthmatics have gastroesophageal reflux with or without bronchodilator therapy. *Gastroenterology*. 1990;99:613-620.

Steinberg W, Tenner S. Acute pancreatitis. *N Engl J Med*. 1994;330:1198-1210.

Young HS. Diseases of the pancreas. *Sci Am Med*. 1997:1-16.

Young HS. Gastrointestinal bleeding. *Sci Am Med*. 1998:1-10.

CHAPTER 15

Inborn Errors of Metabolism

HOSSAM TANTAWY ■
TORI MYSLAJEK ■

The presence of nutritional disturbances or inborn errors of metabolism will significantly influence the management of anesthesia (Table 15-1). The pathophysiology and the associated anesthetic implications of the most frequently encountered of these diseases are highlighted in this chapter. Inborn errors of metabolism manifest as a variety of metabolic defects that may complicate the management of anesthesia. In some instances, these defects are clinically asymptomatic and manifest only in response to specific triggering events, such as ingestion of certain drugs or foods.

PORPHYRIAS

Porphyrias are a group of metabolic disorders each of which results from the deficiency of a specific enzyme in the heme synthetic pathway. Therefore, this category of inborn errors of metabolism is characterized by overproduction of porphyrins. Porphyrins are essential for many vital physiologic functions, including oxygen transport and storage. The synthetic pathway involved in the production of porphyrins is determined by a sequence of enzymes. A defect in any of these enzymes results in accumulation of the preceding intermediate form of porphyrin and produces a form of porphyria (Figure 15-1). In human physiology, heme is the most important porphyrin and is bound to proteins to form hemoproteins that include hemoglobin and cytochrome P-450 isoenzymes. Production of heme is regulated by the activity of aminolevulinic acid (ALA) synthetase, which is present in mitochondria. The formation of ALA synthetase is controlled by the endogenous concentration of heme, which ensures that the level of heme production parallels requirements. ALA synthetase is readily inducible, and therefore supply can respond rapidly to increased heme requirements such as those resulting from administration of drugs that need cytochrome P-450 isoenzymes for their metabolism. In the presence of porphyria, any increase in heme requirements results in accumulation of pathway intermediates, that is, those chemicals compounds immediately preceding the site of enzyme block.

TABLE 15-1 ■ Inborn errors of metabolism

Porphyria
Purine metabolism disorders
Hyperlipidemia
Carbohydrate metabolism disorders
Amino acid metabolism disorders
Mucopolysaccharidoses
Gangliosidoses

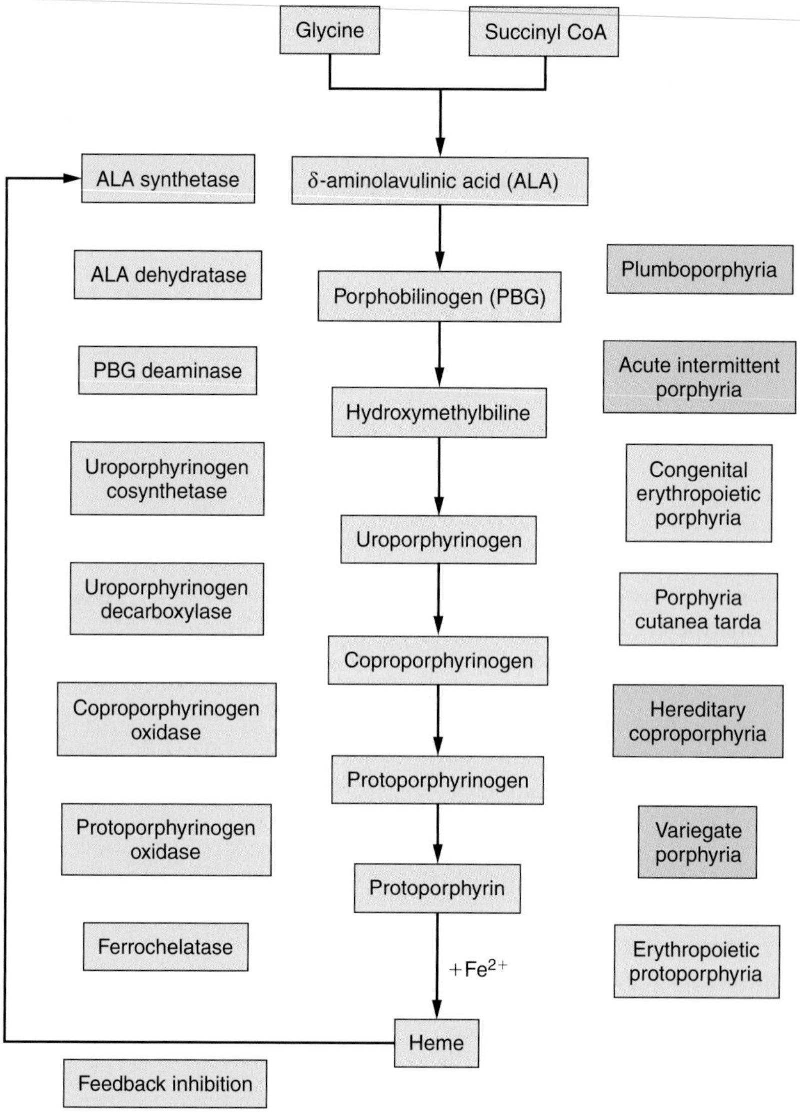

FIGURE 15-1 Metabolic pathways for heme synthesis. Enzymes are noted on the feedback inhibition loop of the sequence, and the type of porphyria associated with the enzyme deficiency is designated on the right. Examples of acute porphyrias are indicated by the dark boxes. *CoA,* Coenzyme A. *(Adapted from James MF, Hift RJ. Porphyrias. Br J Anaesth. 2000;85:143-153.)*

Classification

Porphyrias are classified as either hepatic or erythropoietic depending on the primary site of overproduction or accumulation of the precursors or porphyrins (Table 15-2). Only acute forms of porphyria are relevant to the management of anesthesia, because they are the only forms of porphyria that may result in life-threatening reactions in response to certain drugs.

Acute Porphyria

Acute porphyrias are inherited autosomal dominant disorders with variable expression. The enzyme defects in porphyria are deficiencies rather than absolute deficits. Although there is no direct influence of gender on the pattern of inheritance, attacks occur more frequently in women and are most frequent during the third and fourth decades of life. Attacks are rare before puberty or following the onset of menopause. Acute attacks of porphyria are most commonly precipitated by events that

TABLE 15-2   Classification of porphyrias

HEPATIC

Acute intermittent porphyria
Variegate porphyria
Hereditary coproporphyria
Aminolevulinic acid dehydratase porphyria
Porphyria cutanea tarda

ERYTHROPOIETIC

Congenital erythropoietic porphyria
Erythropoietic protoporphyria

decrease heme concentrations and thus increase the activity of ALA synthetase and stimulate the production of porphyrinogens. Enzyme-inducing drugs are the most important triggering factors in the development of acute porphyria. These acute attacks may also be precipitated by physiologic hormonal fluctuations such as those that accompany menstruation, fasting (such as before elective surgery), dehydration, stress (such as that associated with anesthesia and surgery), and infection. Pregnancy in these patients is often associated with spontaneous abortion. Furthermore, pregnancy may be complicated by systemic hypertension and an increased incidence of low-birth-weight infants.

SIGNS AND SYMPTOMS

Acute attacks of porphyria are characterized by severe abdominal pain, autonomic nervous system instability, electrolyte disturbances, and neuropsychiatric manifestations ranging from mild to life-threatening events. Skeletal muscle weakness that may progress to quadriparesis and respiratory failure is the most potentially lethal neurologic manifestation of an acute attack of porphyria. Central nervous system involvement with upper motor neuron lesions, cranial nerve palsies, and abnormalities of the cerebellum and basal ganglia are seen less frequently. However, these lesions in combination with autonomic neuropathy and hypovolemia can cause significant cardiovascular instability. Seizures may occur during an attack of acute porphyria. Psychiatric disturbances may develop but, despite classic tales of werewolf behavior and other bizarre psychiatric problems, mental disorders are not very common. Gastrointestinal symptoms include abdominal pain, vomiting and diarrhea. However, notwithstanding severe abdominal pain that may mimic acute appendicitis, acute cholecystitis, or renal colic, clinical examination of the abdomen typically yields normal findings. Abdominal pain is thought to be related to autonomic neuropathy. Dehydration and electrolyte disturbances involving sodium, potassium, and magnesium may be prominent. Tachycardia and hypertension or, less commonly, hypotension are manifestations of cardiovascular instability.

Complete and prolonged remissions are likely between episodes, and many individuals with the genetic defect never develop symptoms. It is important to note, however, that patients at known risk of porphyria but previously asymptomatic (silent or latent porphyria) may experience their first symptoms in response to administration of triggering drugs during the perioperative period. ALA synthetase concentrations are increased during all acute attacks of porphyria.

TRIGGERING DRUGS

Drugs may trigger an acute attack of porphyria by inducing the activity of ALA synthetase or interfering with its negative feedback control at the final common pathway of heme synthesis (see Figure 15-1). It is not possible to predict which drugs will be porphyrinogenic, although chemical groupings such as the allyl groups present on barbiturates and certain steroid structures have been incriminated in the induction of porphyria. Only the acute forms of porphyria are affected by drug-induced enzyme induction. It is not clear why the manifestations of nonacute porphyrias are apparently unaffected by enzyme-inducing drugs. For example, potent enzyme inducers of ALA synthetase, including the anticonvulsants, do not exacerbate or precipitate porphyria cutanea tarda or

the erythropoietic porphyrias. The labeling of drugs as safe or unsafe for patients with porphyria is often based on anecdotal experience with the use of particular agents in porphyric patients and reports of the induction of acute attacks. Drugs may be tested in cell culture models for their ability to induce ALA synthetase activity or for their effects on porphyrin synthesis. Alternatively, the action of drugs on the porphyrin synthetic pathway can be investigated in animal models. Both cell culture and animal models tend to *overestimate* the porphyrinogenicity of drugs.

It is difficult to assess the porphyrinogenic potential of anesthetic drugs, since other factors such as sepsis or stress may also precipitate a porphyric crisis in the perioperative period. Any classification of anesthetic drugs with regard to their ability to precipitate a porphyric crisis is likely to be imperfect (Table 15-3). Particular care is needed when selecting drugs for patients with acute intermittent porphyria or clinically active forms of porphyria and when prescribing drugs in combination, because exacerbation of porphyria is more likely under these circumstances.

Acute Intermittent Porphyria

Of all the acute porphyrias, acute intermittent porphyria affecting the central and peripheral nervous system produces the most serious symptoms (systemic hypertension, renal dysfunction) and is the one most likely to be life threatening. The defective enzyme is porphobilinogen deaminase, and the gene encoding this enzyme is located on chromosome 11.

Variegate Porphyria

Variegate porphyria is characterized by neurotoxicity and cutaneous photosensitivity in which bullous skin eruptions occur on exposure to sunlight as a result of the conversion of porphyrinogens to porphyrins. The enzyme defect is at the level of protoporphyrinogen oxidase, and the gene encoding this enzyme is on chromosome 1. The incidence of variegate porphyria is highest in South Africa.

Hereditary Coproporphyria

Acute attacks of hereditary coproporphyria are less common and less severe than attacks of acute intermittent porphyria or variegate porphyria. These patients typically experience neurotoxicity and cutaneous hypersensitivity, although these signs tend to be less severe than is seen in variegate porphyria. The defective enzyme is coproporphyrinogen oxidase, encoded by a gene on chromosome 9.

Porphyria Cutanea Tarda

Porphyria cutanea tarda is due to an enzymatic defect (decreased hepatic activity of uroporphyrinogen decarboxylase) transmitted as an autosomal dominant trait. ALA synthetase activity is unimportant in this form of porphyria,

TABLE 15-3 ■ Recommendations regarding the use of anesthetic drugs in the presence of acute porphyrias

Drug	Recommendation	Drug	Recommendation
INHALED ANESTHETICS		**ANTICHOLINERGICS**	
Nitrous oxide	Safe	Atropine	Safe
Isoflurane	Probably safe*	Glycopyrrolate	Safe
Sevoflurane	Probably safe*		
Desflurane	Probably safe*	**ANTICHOLINESTERASE**	
		Neostigmine	Safe
INTRAVENOUS ANESTHETICS			
Propofol	Safe	**LOCAL ANESTHETICS**	
Ketamine	Probably safe*	Lidocaine	Safe
Thiopental	Avoid	Tetracaine	Safe
Thiamylal	Avoid	Bupivacaine	Safe
Methohexital	Avoid	Mepivacaine	Safe
Etomidate	Avoid	Ropivacaine	No data
ANALGESICS		**SEDATIVES AND ANTIEMETICS**	
Acetaminophen	Safe	Droperidol	Safe
Aspirin	Safe	Midazolam	Probably safe†
Codeine	Safe	Lorazepam	Probably safe†
Morphine	Safe	Cimetidine	Probably safe†
Fentanyl	Safe	Ranitidine	Probably safe†
Sufentanil	Safe	Metoclopramide	Probably safe†
Ketorolac	Probably avoid†	Ondansetron	Probably safe†
Phenacetin	Probably avoid†		
Pentazocine	Avoid	**CARDIOVASCULAR DRUGS**	
		Epinephrine	Safe
NEUROMUSCULAR BLOCKING DRUGS		α-Agonists	Safe
Succinylcholine	Safe	β-Agonists	Safe
Pancuronium	Safe	β-Antagonists	Safe
Atracurium	Probably safe*	Diltiazem	Probably safe*
Cisatracurium	Probably safe*	Nitroprusside	Probably safe*
Vecuronium	Probably safe*	Nifedipine	Probably avoid†
Rocuronium	Probably safe*		
Mivacurium	Probably safe*		
OPIOID ANTAGONIST			
Naloxone	Safe		

Adapted from James MFM, Hift RJ. Porphyrias. *Br J Anaesth*. 2000;85:143-153.
*Although safety is not conclusively established, the drug is unlikely to provoke acute porphyria.
†Use only if expected benefits outweigh the risks.

and drugs capable of precipitating attacks in other forms of porphyria do not provoke attacks of porphyria cutanea tarda. Likewise, neurotoxicity does not accompany this form of porphyria. Signs and symptoms of porphyria cutanea tarda most often appear as photosensitivity reactions, especially in men older than 35 years of age. Porphyrin accumulation in the liver can be associated with hepatocellular necrosis. Anesthetic drugs are not hazardous in affected patients, although the choice of drugs should take into consideration the likely presence of liver disease.

Erythropoietic Uroporphyria

Erythropoietic uroporphyria is a rare form of porphyria transmitted as an autosomal recessive trait. In contrast to porphyrin synthesis in the liver, porphyrin synthesis in the erythropoietic system is responsive to changes in hematocrit and tissue oxygenation. Hemolytic anemia, bone marrow hyperplasia, and splenomegaly are often present. Infections are common, and photosensitivity can be severe. Of note, the urine of affected patients turns red when exposed to light. Neurotoxicity and abdominal pain do not occur, and administration of barbiturates does *not* adversely alter the course of the disease. Death usually occurs during early childhood.

Erythropoietic Protoporphyria

Erythropoietic protoporphyria is a more common, but less debilitating, form of erythropoietic porphyria. Signs and symptoms include photosensitivity, vesicular cutaneous eruptions, urticaria, and edema. In occasional patients cholelithiasis develops secondary to increased excretion of protoporphyrin. Administration of barbiturates does *not* adversely affect the course of the disease, and survival to adulthood is common.

Preoperative Evaluation

The principles of safe anesthetic management of patients with porphyria include the identification of susceptible individuals and the determination of potentially porphyrinogenic drugs. Laboratory identification of porphyric individuals is not easy since many show only subtle or even no biochemical abnormalities during an asymptomatic phase. In the presence of a suggestive family history, determination of erythrocyte porphobilinogen activity is the most appropriate screening test for patients with suspected acute intermittent porphyria. A careful family history should be obtained and a thorough physical examination performed (although there is often no clinical evidence or only subtle skin lesions), and the presence or absence of peripheral neuropathy and autonomic nervous system instability should be noted.

Guidelines for drug selection include the following: (1) There is evidence that a single exposure to a potent inducer can be well tolerated, but not during an acute attack. (2) Exposure to multiple potential inducers is more dangerous than exposure to any single agent. (3) Lists of "safe" and "unsafe" anesthetic drugs and adjuncts may be based on animal or cell culture experiments, so the actual clinical effects of these agents may be unknown. Note that the American Porphyria Foundation maintains up-to-date information on all aspects of these diseases, and a drug database with information about drugs and acute porphyria can be found at http://www.drugs-porphyria.com.

If an acute exacerbation of porphyria is suspected during the perioperative period, particular attention must be given to skeletal muscle strength and cranial nerve function, since these symptoms and signs may predict impending respiratory failure and an increased risk of pulmonary aspiration. Cardiovascular examination may reveal systemic hypertension and tachycardia, which necessitate treatment before induction of anesthesia. Postoperative mechanical ventilation may be required during an acute porphyric crisis. During an acute exacerbation, severe abdominal pain may mimic a surgical abdomen. Patients experiencing an acute porphyric crisis must be assessed carefully for fluid balance and electrolyte status, especially the presence of hyponatremia.

Preoperative starvation should be minimized, but if a prolonged fast is unavoidable, administration of a glucose-saline infusion should be considered, since caloric restriction has been linked to the precipitation of attacks of acute porphyria.

PREOPERATIVE PREMEDICATION

Benzodiazepines are commonly selected for preoperative anxiolysis. Aspiration prophylaxis that includes antacids and/or histamine-2 receptor antagonists is acceptable. Interestingly, cimetidine has been recommended for treatment of acute porphyric crises since this drug may decrease heme consumption and inhibit ALA synthetase activity. Cimetidine cannot, however, prevent an acute attack of porphyria.

PROPHYLACTIC THERAPY

No specific prophylactic therapy has shown proven benefit. However, because carbohydrate administration can suppress porphyrin synthesis, administration of oral carbohydrate supplements (20 g/hr) preoperatively may be recommended. If oral feedings are not possible, then infusion of 10% glucose in saline is an option.

Management of Anesthesia

Anesthesia has been implicated in triggering acute attacks of porphyria. However, most patients with porphyria can be safely anesthetized if appropriate precautions are taken. Patients with evidence of active porphyria or a history of acute porphyric crises are at increased risk. Short-acting anesthetic drugs are presumed to be safe because their rapid elimination limits the time of exposure for enzyme induction. However, repeated or prolonged use of these drugs, such as by continuous intravenous infusion, could result in a different clinical outcome. A number of case reports have described the successful use of intermittent propofol administration in patients with porphyria, but there are not enough data to validate propofol administration by continuous infusion in porphyria patients. It is likely that exposure to several potential enzyme-inducing drugs may be more dangerous than exposure to any one drug, so the anesthetic plan must take this into account.

REGIONAL ANESTHESIA

There is no absolute contraindication to the use of regional anesthesia in patients with porphyria. However, if a regional anesthetic is being considered, it is essential to perform a neurologic examination before initiating the blockade to minimize the likelihood that worsening of any preexisting neuropathy would be erroneously attributed to the regional anesthetic. Autonomic nervous system blockade induced by the regional anesthetic could unmask cardiovascular instability, especially in the presence of autonomic neuropathy, hypovolemia, or both. There is no evidence that any local anesthetic has ever induced an acute attack of porphyria or neurologic damage in porphyric individuals. Regional anesthesia has been safely used in parturient women with acute intermittent porphyria. Regional anesthesia is used very infrequently, however, in patients experiencing an attack of acute intermittent porphyria because of concerns about hemodynamic instability, mental confusion, and porphyria-related neuropathy.

GENERAL ANESTHESIA

The total dose of drugs administered and the length of exposure to anesthetic drugs may influence the risk of triggering a porphyric crisis in vulnerable patients (see Table 15-3). The availability of relatively short-acting anesthetic drugs has likely contributed to the safety of anesthesia in the presence of porphyria. Perioperative monitoring should consider the frequent presence of autonomic dysfunction and the possibility of blood pressure lability.

Induction of Anesthesia

Propofol has been used safely for induction of anesthesia in patients with porphyria, although the use of prolonged continuous infusions of this drug is of unproven safety. Ketamine has been used safely in the presence of quiescent acute intermittent porphyria. The use of etomidate is controversial. *All barbiturates must be considered unsafe for anesthetic use even if the porphyria is in a quiescent phase.*

Maintenance of Anesthesia

Nitrous oxide is well established as a safe inhaled anesthetic in patients with porphyria. Safe use of isoflurane has also been described. The relatively short duration of action of sevoflurane and desflurane are desirable characteristics for drugs in this patient population. However, experience is too limited to make firm recommendations about their use. Opioids have been administered safely to these patients. Neuromuscular blocking drugs do not seem to introduce any predictable risk when administered to these patients.

Cardiopulmonary Bypass. In theory, cardiopulmonary bypass is a potential risk factor for patients with porphyria because of the additional stresses introduced by hypothermia, pump-induced hemolysis, blood loss and the consequent increase in heme demand by the bone marrow, and the large number of drugs that are typically administered. Interestingly, clinical experience does not support an increased incidence of porphyric crises in patients undergoing cardiopulmonary bypass.

TREATMENT OF A PORPHYRIC CRISIS

The first step in treating an acute porphyric crisis is removal of any known triggering factors. Adequate hydration and carbohydrate loading are necessary, via either an enteral or a parenteral route. Sedation using a phenothiazine can be useful. Pain often necessitates administration of opioids. Nausea and vomiting are treated with conventional antiemetics. β-Blockers can be administered to control tachycardia and hypertension. Since traditional anticonvulsants are regarded as *unsafe*, seizures may be treated with a benzodiazepine or propofol. Electrolyte disturbances, including hypomagnesemia, must be treated aggressively.

Administration of heme (3 to 4 mg/kg IV daily for 4 days) is indicated after a day or two of the crisis if the patient is no better after receiving conservative therapy. Heme may be administered as hematin, heme albumin, or heme arginine. It is presumed that heme supplements the intracellular pool of heme and thus suppresses ALA synthetase activity. Heme arginine is more stable than hematin and lacks the potential adverse effects associated with hematin (renal failure, coagulopathy, thrombophlebitis). Somatostatin decreases the rate of formation of ALA synthetase and, in combination with plasmapheresis, may effectively decrease pain and induce remission.

DISORDERS OF PURINE METABOLISM

Gout

Gout is a disorder of purine metabolism and may be classified as primary or secondary. Primary gout is due to an inherited metabolic defect that leads to overproduction of uric acid. Secondary gout is hyperuricemia resulting from an identifiable cause, such as administration of chemotherapeutic drugs leading to the rapid lysis of purine-containing cells. Gout is characterized by hyperuricemia with recurrent episodes of acute arthritis caused by deposition of urate crystals in joints. Deposition of urate crystals typically initiates an inflammatory response that causes pain and limited motion of the joint. At least half of the initial attacks of gout are confined to the first metatarsophalangeal joint, that is, the joint at the base of the great toe. Persistent hyperuricemia also results in deposition of urate crystals in extraarticular locations, manifested most often as nephrolithiasis. Urate crystal deposition can also occur in the myocardium, aortic valve, and extradural spinal regions. The incidence of systemic hypertension, ischemic heart disease, and diabetes mellitus is increased in patients with gout.

TREATMENT

Treatment of gout is designed to decrease the plasma concentrations of uric acid by administration of uricosuric drugs (such as probenecid) or drugs that inhibit the conversion of purines to uric acid by xanthine oxidase (allopurinol). Colchicine, which lacks any effect on purine metabolism, is considered the drug of choice for management of acute gouty arthritis. It relieves joint pain presumably by modifying leukocyte migration and phagocytosis. Side effects of colchicine include vomiting and diarrhea. Large doses of colchicine can also produce hepatorenal dysfunction and agranulocytosis.

MANAGEMENT OF ANESTHESIA

Management of anesthesia in the presence of gout focuses on prehydration to facilitate continued renal elimination of uric acid. Administration of sodium bicarbonate to alkalinize the urine also facilitates excretion of uric acid. Even with appropriate precautions, acute attacks of gout often follow surgical procedures in patients with a history of gout.

Extraarticular manifestations of gout and side effects of drugs used to control the disease deserve consideration when formulating the plan for anesthesia management. Renal function is evaluated, since clinical manifestations of gout usually increase with deteriorating renal function. Abnormalities detected on the electrocardiogram could reflect urate deposits in the myocardium. The increased incidence of systemic hypertension, ischemic heart disease, and diabetes mellitus in patients with gout must be considered. Although rare, adverse renal and hepatic effects may be associated with the use of probenecid and colchicine. Limited temporomandibular joint motion from gouty arthritis, if present, can make direct laryngoscopy difficult.

Lesch-Nyhan Syndrome

Lesch-Nyhan syndrome is a genetically determined disorder of purine metabolism that occurs exclusively in males. Biochemically, the defect is characterized by decreased or absent activity of hypoxanthine-guanine phosphoribosyltransferase, which leads to excessive purine production and increased uric acid concentrations throughout the body. Clinically, patients are often mentally retarded and exhibit characteristic spasticity and self-mutilation. Self-mutilation usually involves trauma to perioral tissues, and subsequent scarification may caused difficulties with direct laryngoscopy for tracheal intubation. Seizure disorders associated with this syndrome are often treated with benzodiazepines. Athetoid dysphagia may increase the likelihood of aspiration if vomiting occurs. Malnutrition is often present. Hyperuricemia is associated with nephropathy, urinary tract calculi, and arthritis. Death is often due to renal failure.

Management of anesthesia is influenced by co-existing renal dysfunction and possible impaired metabolism of drugs administered during anesthesia. The presence of a spastic skeletal muscle disorder suggests caution in using succinylcholine. The sympathetic nervous system response to stress is enhanced, which requires caution in the administration of exogenous catecholamines to these patients.

DISORDERS OF CARBOHYDRATE METABOLISM

Disorders of carbohydrate metabolism typically reflect genetically determined enzyme defects (Table 15-4). The defect can result in a deficiency or an excess of a precursor or end product of metabolism that is normally involved in the production of glycogen from glucose. In some instances, an alternate metabolic pathway is used. Ultimately, the signs and symptoms of a specific disorder of carbohydrate metabolism are a reflection of the effects produced by alterations in the amount of precursors or end products of metabolism that result from the enzyme defects.

Glycogen Storage Disease Type 1a

Glycogen storage disease type 1a (von Gierke's disease) is due to absent or insufficient amounts of the enzyme glucose-6-phosphatase. As a result, glycogen cannot be hydrolyzed in hepatocytes, neutrophils, and possibly other cells, which leads to its intracellular accumulation. Hypoglycemia can be severe, and oral feedings are required every 2 to 3 hours to maintain acceptable blood glucose concentrations. Chronic metabolic acidosis is present and may lead to osteoporosis. Mental retardation, growth retardation, and seizures resulting from hypoglycemia are likely. Hepatomegaly results from accumulation of glycogen in the liver. Renal enlargement, also caused by accumulation of glycogen, can manifest as chronic pyelonephritis. A hemorrhagic diathesis may be due to platelet dysfunction, and recurrent epistaxis and bleeding after minor trauma and surgery may occur. Facial and truncal obesity is present. Survival beyond 2 years of age is unusual, although surgical creation of a portocaval shunt may benefit some patients.

Management of anesthesia must include provision of exogenous glucose to prevent intraoperative hypoglycemia.

TABLE 15-4 ■ **Disorders of carbohydrate metabolism**

Glycogen storage disease type 1a (von Gierke's disease)
Glycogen storage disease type 1b
Pompe's disease
McArdle's disease
Galactosemia
Fructose 1,6-diphosphate deficiency
Pyruvate dehydrogenase deficiency

Monitoring of the arterial pH and blood glucose concentration is helpful, because these patients often become acidotic because of an inability to convert lactic acid to glycogen. Lactate-containing solutions for intravenous infusion are also avoided to minimize the theoretical possibility of metabolic acidosis because of lactate administration during the perioperative period.

Glycogen Storage Disease Type 1b

Glycogen storage disease type 1b is a rare autosomal recessive disease in which glucose-6-phosphate, a product of metabolic cleavage of glycogen, cannot be transported to the inner surface of microsomes because of a deficiency in its transport system. Thus, this disease is a variant of glycogen storage disease type 1a. In glycogen storage disease type 1b, glycogen accumulates in the liver, kidneys, and intestinal mucosa, and glucose availability to tissues is impaired. Hypoglycemia and lactic acidosis ensue. Clinical signs and symptoms resemble those described for glycogen storage disease type 1a. In addition, patients with type 1b experience recurrent infections resulting from impaired neutrophil activity.

If surgery is planned, preoperative fasting is minimized, and glucose-containing infusions are administered intravenously throughout the perioperative period. Strict asepsis is important. Preoperative normalization of the blood glucose concentration may improve platelet function and decrease the likelihood of intraoperative bleeding. Intraoperative monitoring of blood glucose concentration is recommended, since hypoglycemia may be profound and difficult to recognize during general anesthesia. Lactic acidosis develops as a result of the incomplete conversion of glycogen. For this reason, monitoring of arterial pH is helpful. Administration of lactate-containing solutions is not recommended. Iatrogenic hyperventilation and its associated respiratory alkalosis may stimulate the release of lactate from skeletal muscles and aggravate metabolic acidosis. Treatment of significant metabolic acidosis might include administration of sodium bicarbonate.

DISORDERS OF AMINO ACID METABOLISM

Although there are more than 70 known disorders of amino acid metabolism, most are extremely rare. Classic manifestations include mental retardation, seizures, and aminoaciduria (Table 15-5). In addition, metabolic acidosis,

TABLE 15-5 ▪ Disorders of amino acid metabolism

Disorder	Mental retardation	Seizures	Metabolic acidosis	Hyperammonemia	Hepatic failure	Thromboembolism	Other
Phenylketonuria	Yes	Yes	No	No	No	No	Friable skin
Homocystinuria	Yes/no	Yes	No	No	No	Yes	
Hypervalinemia	Yes	Yes	Yes	No	No	No	Hypoglycemia
Citrullinemia	Yes	Yes	No	Yes	Yes	No	
Branched-chain aciduria (maple syrup urine disease)	Yes	Yes	Yes	No		Yes	Hypoglycemia Neurologic deterioration during perioperative period
Methylmalonyl-coenzyme A mutase deficiency			Yes	Yes			Acidosis intraoperatively Avoid nitrous oxide?
Isoleucinemia	Yes	Yes	Yes	Yes	Yes	No	Hypovolemia
Methioninemia	Yes	No	No	No	No	No	Thermal instability
Histidinuria	Yes	Yes/no	No	No	No	No	Erythrocyte fragility
Neutral aminoaciduria (Hartnup's disease)	Yes/no		Yes	No	No	No	Dermatitis
Argininemia	Yes		No	Yes	Yes	No	

hyperammonemia, hepatic failure, and thromboembolism can occur.

Management of anesthesia in patients with disorders of amino acid metabolism is directed toward maintenance of intravascular fluid volume and acid-base homeostasis. Use of anesthetics that could evoke seizure activity should be avoided, since these patients are likely to have seizure disorders.

Phenylketonuria

Phenylketonuria is the prototype of disorders attributable to abnormal amino acid metabolism. Phenylalanine accumulates as a result of an enzymatic deficiency of phenylalanine hydroxylase. Clinical features include mental retardation and seizures. The skin may be friable and vulnerable to damage from pressure or friction created by adhesive materials. Also, these patients are likely to have associated vitamin B_{12} deficiency, especially with their strict die. If this is the case and the patient has B_{12} deficiency resulting from a lack of supplementary vitamin treatment, nitrous oxide should probably be avoided. These patients may also be more sensitive to narcotics.

Homocystinuria

Homocystinuria is due to failure of transsulfuration of precursors of cystine, an important constituent of cross-linkages in collagen. Manifestations of the disease caused by increased blood and urine concentrations of homocystine reflect weakened collagen and include dislocation of the lens, osteoporosis, a marfanoid habitus, kyphoscoliosis, brittle light-colored hair, malar flush, and vascular disease in the coronary, cerebral, and renal arteries. Complications arising from this vascular disease are the most common causes of morbidity and mortality early in life. Mental retardation may also be a prominent finding. The diagnosis of homocystinuria is confirmed by demonstrating homocystine in the urine. Plasma homocystine acts as an atherogenic and thrombophilic agent. Thromboembolism can be life threatening and is presumed to reflect activation of Hageman factor by homocystine, which results in increased platelet adhesiveness. Measures to minimize the risk of thromboembolism during the perioperative period should include administration of pyridoxine or betaine, both of which decrease homocystine concentrations and thus platelet adhesiveness. Preoperative hydration, infusion of dextran, and early ambulation may also help prevent deep vein thrombosis.

Maple Syrup Urine Disease

Maple syrup urine disease is a rare inborn error of metabolism that results from defective carboxylation of branched-chain amino acids. In the absence of adequate enzyme activity, consumption of foods containing branched-chain amino acids results in the accumulation of these amino acids as well as ketoacids in tissues and blood. Excess concentrations of leucine are usually higher than those of isoleucine or valine since leucine is the predominant amino acid in most proteins. The presence of these amino acids in the urine gives it a maple syrup odor.

Growth retardation and delayed psychomotor development are often a consequence of this chronic metabolic imbalance. Infection or fasting commonly results in acute metabolic decompensation, with increased plasma levels of branched-chain amino acids and ketoacids resulting from the breakdown of endogenous proteins. Increased plasma levels of ketoacids contributes to the production of metabolic acidosis. Hypoglycemia is a possibility and presumably reflects the ability of increased plasma leucine concentrations to stimulate release of insulin. A potentially fatal encephalopathy may accompany this disease.

Treatment is directed at decreasing the plasma levels of branched-chain amino acids and ketoacids with peritoneal dialysis or hemodialysis. Parenteral nutrition using preparations devoid of branched-chain amino acids may also be effective.

Surgery and anesthesia introduce a number of hazards in the perioperative management of patients with maple syrup urine disease. For example, catabolism of body proteins produced by surgery or infection can result in increased blood concentrations of branched-chain amino acids. Even blood in the gastrointestinal tract, as can occur following tonsillectomy, produces an added metabolic load in patients with maple syrup urine disease. Accumulation of branched-chain amino acids in the circulation can produce neurologic deterioration during the perioperative period. The danger of hypoglycemia in affected patients is exacerbated by the period of fasting that precedes elective surgery. Therefore, it is useful to initiate an intravenous infusion of glucose-containing solution intraoperatively. Measurement of arterial pH is helpful for detecting metabolic acidosis caused by accumulation of ketoacids.

Methylmalonyl-Coenzyme A Mutase Deficiency

Methylmalonyl-coenzyme A mutase deficiency is an inborn error of metabolism that can result in methylmalonicacidemia. Acute treatment includes intravenous administration of crystalloid solution containing bicarbonate. Events during the perioperative period that increase protein catabolism (fasting, bleeding into the gastrointestinal tract, stress, tissue destruction) may predispose to acidosis.

Experience with anesthesia in patients with this disorder is limited, and recommendations are based more on theory than on clinical experience. For example, nitrous oxide may be avoided based on the theoretic concern that this inhaled anesthetic could predispose to methylmalonicacidemia in susceptible patients, because of nitrous oxide–induced inhibition of cobalamin coenzymes. The impact of preoperative fasting on amino acid metabolism and intravascular fluid volume is lessened by permitting ingestion of clear fluid up to 2 hours before surgery. Generous administration of intravenous fluids and glucose is also helpful in minimizing hypovolemia and protein catabolism.

KEY POINTS

■ Acute attacks of porphyria are characterized by severe abdominal pain, autonomic nervous system instability, electrolyte disturbances, and neuropsychiatric manifestations. These can range from mild disturbances to life-threatening events.

■ Skeletal muscle weakness that may progress to quadriparesis and respiratory failure is the potentially most lethal neurologic manifestation of an acute attack of porphyria. Seizures may also occur.

■ Because carbohydrate administration can suppress porphyrin synthesis, carbohydrate supplementation preoperatively may be recommended to reduce the risk of an attack of acute porphyria.

■ In a patient with phenylketonuria and vitamin B_{12} deficiency, nitrous oxide should probably be avoided.

RESOURCES

American Porphyria Foundation. http://www.porphyriafoundation.com.

Diaz JH, Belani KG. Perioperative management of children with mucopolysaccharidoses. *Anesth Analg.* 1993;77:1261-1270.

Gorchein A. Drug treatment in acute porphyria. *Br J Clin Pharmacol.* 1997;44:427-434.

Herrick IA, Rhine EJ. The mucopolysaccharidoses and anaesthesia: a report of clinical experience. *Can J Anaesth.* 1988;35:67-73.

James MF, Hift RJ. Porphyrias. *Br J Anaesth.* 2000;85:143-153.

Jensen NF, Fiddler DS, Striepe V. Anesthetic considerations in porphyrias. *Anesth Analg.* 1995;80:591-599.

CHAPTER **16**

Nutritional Diseases: Obesity and Malnutrition

BROOKE E. ALBRIGHT ■
WANDA M. POPESCU ■

Nutritional diseases are caused by either an underconsumption of essential nutrients or an overconsumption of poor nutrients. Both result in forms of *malnutrition*. Currently, the most prevalent nutritional disease worldwide is obesity. Because of its detrimental impact on overall health and functional status, obesity is now considered one of the leading preventable causes of medical illness in the world. The U.S. Surgeon General considers obesity a "national epidemic" and "a serious public health threat." Most evidence suggests that obesity is due to a combination of elements, including genetic, environmental, psychologic, and socioeconomic factors. Controlling the obesity epidemic will depend on a better understanding of its causes as well as a systems-based team approach to its medical management.

OBESITY

Definition

Obesity is defined as an abnormally high amount of adipose tissue compared with lean muscle mass (20% or more over ideal body weight). It is associated with increased morbidity

and mortality due to a wide spectrum of medical and surgical diseases (Table 16-1). Body mass index (BMI) is the most commonly used quantifier of obesity despite the fact that it does not measure adipose tissue directly. BMI is calculated as weight in kilograms divided by the square of the height in meters (BMI = kg/m^2). This BMI ratio is used because of its simplicity. However, there are flaws in the formula that should be taken into consideration when using the BMI clinically. For example, those persons with an unusually high percentage of lean muscle mass, such as body builders, may have a high BMI that does not correlate with a high ratio of adipose tissue. In general, calculation of BMI provides a useful predictive indicator of weight categories that may lead to health problems (Table 16-2). It should be noted that the weight category term *morbid obesity* has been replaced with the term *clinically severe obesity*.

Epidemiology

Over the past 20 years, obesity has increased dramatically, and it is now recognized as a national public health threat. In the United States in 2007 and 2008, it was estimated that approximately two thirds of adults (73 million people) were overweight or obese. Obesity prevalence has steadily increased, and in 2007 and 2008, it affected approximately 32% of men and 35% of women. Over the last few years, the prevalence of childhood obesity has nearly tripled and is currently estimated at about 25%. As the prevalence of obesity increases, so do its associated health care costs. On average, the annual health care costs for an obese patient are approximately 42% more than for a normal-weight patient. In 2008, $147 billion was spent on obesity-related medical problems.

Currently, obesity is the sixth most important risk factor for disease worldwide. In addition to being associated with major comorbid conditions, including diabetes, hypertension, and cardiovascular disease, obesity is also associated with a

TABLE 16-1 ■ **Medical and surgical conditions associated with obesity**

Organ system	Comorbid conditions
Respiratory system	Obstructive sleep apnea Obesity hypoventilation syndrome Restrictive lung disease
Cardiovascular system	Systemic hypertension Coronary artery disease Congestive heart failure Cerebrovascular disease, stroke Peripheral vascular disease Pulmonary hypertension Hypercoagulable syndromes Hypercholesterolemia Hypertriglyceridemia Sudden death
Endocrine system	Metabolic syndrome Diabetes mellitus Cushing's syndrome Hypothyroidism
Gastrointestinal system	Nonalcoholic steatohepatitis Hiatal hernia Gallstones Fatty liver infiltration Gastroesophageal reflux disease, delayed gastric emptying
Musculoskeletal system	Osteoarthritis of weight-bearing joints Back pain Inguinal hernia Joint pain
Malignancy	Pancreatic Kidney Breast Prostate Cervical, uterine, endometrial Colorectal
Other	Kidney failure Depression Overall shorter life expectancy

Modified from Adams JP, Murphy PG. Obesity in anaesthesia and intensive care. *Br J Anaesth.* 2000;85:91-108.

TABLE 16-2 ■ **Body mass index (BMI) weight categories**

Category	BMI range (kg/m^2)
ADULTS	
Underweight	<18.5
Normal	18.5-24.9
Overweight	25-29.9
Obese class I	30-34.9
Obese class II	35-39.9
Obese class III (severe, morbid)	≥40
CHILDREN (2-18 YR)	
Overweight	85th-94th percentile
Obese	95th percentile or ≥30
Severely obese	99th percentile

decrease in life expectancy. The risk of premature death is doubled in the obese population and the risk of death resulting from cardiovascular disease is increased fivefold in the obese compared with the nonobese.

Pathophysiology

Weight gain results when caloric intake exceeds energy expenditure. Energy expenditure is primarily determined by basal metabolic rate, which is responsible for maintaining homeostasis of bodily functions. Most metabolic activity occurs within lean tissue and involves small sources of energy expenditure, including the thermal effect of physical activity and the heat produced by food digestion, absorption, and storage. Exercise can increase energy consumption not only during exercise but for up to 18 hours afterward. It does so by increasing the thermal effects of physical activity, and with regular exercise over time, the body's basal metabolic rate increases. Caloric restriction (i.e., fasting) *without exercise,* on the other hand, leads to a reduction in basal metabolic rate due to promotion of the body's efforts to conserve energy. This reduction in basal metabolic rate leads to slow weight loss during the dieting phase but rapid weight gain when normal caloric intake is resumed.

FAT STORAGE

A positive caloric balance is stored by the body as fat in adipocytes. This fat is primarily in the form of triglycerides. Triglycerides serve as an efficient form of energy storage because of their high caloric density and hydrophobic nature. Adipocytes are able to increase to a maximum size, and then they begin dividing. It is believed that at BMIs of up to 40 kg/m^2, adipocytes are only increased in size, whereas in clinically severe obesity, there exists an absolute increase in the total number of fat cells. The storage of triglycerides is regulated by lipoprotein lipase. This enzyme's activity varies in different parts of the body, and it is more active in abdominal fat than in hip fat. The increase in metabolic activity of abdominal fat may contribute to the higher incidence of metabolic disturbances associated with central obesity. Abdominal obesity is more common in men and is therefore known as *android* fat distribution. Peripheral fat around the hips and buttocks is more common in women and is known as *gynecoid* fat distribution. It is currently accepted that a *waist-to-hip ratio* of more than 1.0 in men and more than 0.8 in women is a strong predictor of ischemic heart disease, stroke, diabetes, and death independent of the total amount of body fat. Environmental factors such as stress and cigarette smoking stimulate cortisol production, which may facilitate deposition of extra calories as abdominal fat.

CELLULAR DISTURBANCES

Obesity leads to severe metabolic derangements, mainly because of disturbances in insulin regulation. At a cellular level, fatty infiltration of the pancreas leads to decreased secretion of insulin while, at the same time, engorgement of adipocytes promotes insulin resistance. In addition, the engorged adipocytes are capable of secreting various cytokines, including interleukin-1 (IL-1) and IL-6 and tumor necrosis factor-α. These cytokines worsen glucose intolerance by decreasing the secretion of adiponectin, a powerful insulin sensitizer. Leptin, another hormone secreted by adipose tissue, travels centrally to the ventromedial hypothalamus and modulates the secretion of neuropeptides that regulate energy expenditure and food intake. Leptin induces satiety when present in high concentrations. Leptin secretion accelerates inflammatory changes by activating monocytes and decreasing the capacity of neutrophils to migrate and activate. Acting in opposition to leptin, the hormone ghrelin increases appetite. Ghrelin appears to modulate appetite both peripherally and centrally by affecting the mechanosensitivity of gastric vagal afferents, making them less sensitive to distention and thus facilitating overeating. An antiobesity vaccine directed against the hormone ghrelin is currently under development. The developers are hoping to produce a vaccine that induces an autoimmune response against ghrelin, preventing it from reaching the central nervous system so that its effects on appetite are suppressed. With abdominal obesity, the high level of fatty infiltration of omental adipocytes (usually devoid of fat) leads to an increased influx of fatty acids, hormones, and cytokines. All of these substances eventually stimulate the liver to produce increased levels of very low-density lipoproteins and apolipoprotein B. As a result the pancreas is stimulated to secrete more insulin and more pancreatic polypeptides. The end result is diffuse intracellular inflammatory changes.

GENETIC FACTORS

From a Darwinian perspective, the ability of the body to conserve and store energy probably conferred a survival advantage. However, in affluent societies where food is very calorie dense and serving sizes are abnormally large, this ability to conserve and store energy may actually prove deleterious to survival. For this reason, scientists are looking for specific genes that may favor energy storage and diminish energy expenditure as possible explanations for the current obesity epidemic. The discovery of the various hormones responsible for signaling satiety in the brain and thus maintaining a normal body weight has lead scientists to believe that overeating resulting in obesity may be due to genetic mutations. In fact, research suggests that many forms of severe obesity may be related to a combination of inherited gene mutations. Genetic factors have been shown to influence the degree of weight gain and to predict which individuals are most likely to gain weight. Statistical analyses suggest that more than half of the variations in individual BMIs are genetically influenced. For example, mutations in the gene that controls the hypothalamic melanocortin receptor, which is involved in appetite suppression, explains about 5% of severe early childhood obesity. Homozygous mutations in genes responsible for leptin and ghrelin secretion and receptor activity are also associated with extreme

childhood obesity. However, it is clear that the metabolic consequences from inheritance of maladaptive genes are not entirely responsible for the current obesity epidemic.

ENVIRONMENT FACTORS

Environmental factors, including the consumption of high-calorie foods in combination with decreased physical activity and aging, are also important considerations in the development of obesity. The technologic developments of the past 50 years have contributed significantly to a decline in physical activity. From the automobile and the TV remote control to electronic gaming systems, our modern environment is designed to promote a sedentary lifestyle. There has also been a change in our food habits with the development of "fast food" and intense food marketing and industry competition. These new food habits only amplify the obesity problem.

Some people try to solve their weight problem by following popular fad diets that claim to aid in weight loss. Although these "lose-weight-quick" diets appear to work initially, it is unlikely that they contribute to sustained weight loss. Both proteins and carbohydrates can be metabolically converted into fat. Evidence is lacking to prove that changing the relative proportions of protein, carbohydrates, and fat in the diet without reducing overall caloric intake will promote weight loss. The bottom line is quite simple: if an individual is to lose weight and keep the weight off, daily energy expenditure must exceed daily caloric intake. If daily caloric (energy) intake exceeds energy expenditure by only 2%, the cumulative effect after 1 year is approximately a 2.3-kg (5-lb) increase in body weight. The critical elements of weight loss are both diet and exercise. Even slight exertion has been shown to provide some benefit to a highly sedentary adult, and the benefit is not exclusively related to weight loss. Exercise has a positive impact on cardiovascular health and glucose control. It limits the progressive decline in lean body tissue with age, decreases the risk of developing osteoporosis, and improves overall psychologic well-being.

PSYCHOLOGIC AND SOCIOECONOMIC FACTORS

In many societies obesity historically was viewed as a sign of wealth and elite socioeconomic status. Today, however, much more emphasis is placed on appearing slim and fit. Media and marketing pressures are leading overweight individuals, particularly women, to experiment with quick weight-loss schemes and to develop obsessive, unhealthy eating disorders to avoid discrimination. Nearly 37% of women in the United States are at risk of developing major depression related to obesity. Eating disorders linked with both depression and obesity include binge eating disorder and night eating syndrome (Table 16-3). These eating disorders are seen in a large proportion of patients attending obesity clinics. It is important to recognize the characteristics of eating disorders, as well as signs of depression and anxiety, because psychologic assessment and counseling are essential for treatment of these conditions. Use of antidepressants to

TABLE 16-3 ▪ Criteria for common eating disorders

BINGE EATING DISORDER

Consumption of large meals rapidly and without control

Three or more of the following: rapid eating, solitary or secretive eating, eating despite fullness, eating without hunger, self-disgust, guilt, depression

Striking distress while eating

No compensatory features, that is, no excess exercise, purging, or fasting

Persistence for >2 days/wk for 6 mo

If vomiting is part of the disorder, it is classified as bulimia

NIGHT EATING SYNDROME

Evening hyperphagia (>50% of daily intake occurs after the evening meal)

Guilt, tension, and anxiety while eating

Frequent waking with more eating

Morning anorexia

Consumption of sugars and other carbohydrates at inappropriate times

Persistence for >2 mo

Adapted from Stunkard AJ. Binge-eating disorder and the night-eating syndrome. In: Wadden TA, Stunkard AJ, eds. *Handbook of Obesity Treatment*. New York, NY: Guilford Press; 2002:107-121.

TABLE 16-4 ▪ Drugs causing weight gain

Anticonvulsants: phenytoin, sodium valproate

Antidepressants: tricyclics, selective serotonin reuptake inhibitors, monoamine oxidase inhibitors, mirtazapine, lithium

Antihistamines

Antipsychotics, especially olanzapine

Corticosteroids

Insulin

Oral contraceptive and progestogenic compounds and blockers

Oral hypoglycemic agents: glitazones (peripheral rather than visceral gain), sulfonylureas

Adapted from Haslam DW, James WPT. Obesity. *Lancet*. 2005;366:1197-1209.

treat depression related to obesity can be risky, because many of these drugs are associated with weight gain themselves (Table 16-4).

Lack of U.S. Food and Drug Administration (FDA) regulation of the labeling of the nutritional content of food has allowed the food industry to sell foods rich in potentially harmful chemicals that prolong the shelf life of the food and to add ingredients that increase the caloric density of the food without increasing its macronutrient content. Fast food restaurants have made huge profits by attracting consumers with sugary and salty foods rich in fats, extracted sugars, and refined starches. All of these may taste good but, when eaten in large quantities, are toxic to the body. Clever marketing trends to "supersize" meal portions to fool consumers into believing they are getting more value for their dollar has also led to an unhealthy and unnecessary increase in calorie consumption.

Diseases Associated with Obesity

Obesity can have detrimental effects on many organ systems. The most profound effects are on the endocrine, cardiovascular, respiratory, gastrointestinal, immune, musculoskeletal, and nervous systems. Clinically severely obese individuals have limited mobility and may therefore appear to be asymptomatic even in the presence of significant respiratory and cardiovascular impairment.

ENDOCRINE DISORDERS

Many of the comorbid conditions caused by obesity are related to the *metabolic syndrome,* also known as *syndrome X.* This syndrome has been defined in a number of ways. The most accepted definition requires the presence of at least three of the following signs: large waist circumference, high triglyceride levels, low levels of high-density lipoprotein cholesterol, glucose intolerance, and hypertension.

Glucose Intolerance and Diabetes Mellitus Type 2

Excess weight is an important risk factor for the development of non–insulin-dependent (type 2) diabetes mellitus. Increased adipose tissue leads to increased resistance of peripheral tissues to the effects of insulin, which ultimately results in glucose intolerance and diabetes mellitus. Events that increase stress levels in these patients, such as surgery, may necessitate the use of exogenous insulin. Resolution of type 2 diabetes can be achieved in more than three quarters of obese patients by weight loss.

Endocrinopathies Causing Obesity

Certain diseases of the endocrine system may promote the development of obesity. Examples are hypothyroidism and Cushing's disease. It is important to consider the possibility of an endocrine disorder when evaluating obese patients.

CARDIOVASCULAR DISORDERS

Cardiovascular disease is a major cause of morbidity and mortality in obese individuals and may manifest as systemic hypertension, coronary artery diseases, and heart failure. In patients with clinically severe obesity, cardiac function is best at rest and exercise is poorly tolerated. Physical activity may cause exertional dyspnea and/or angina pectoris. Any increase in cardiac output is achieved by an increase in heart rate without an increase in stroke volume or ejection fraction. Changing position from sitting to supine is associated with an increase in pulmonary capillary wedge pressure and mean pulmonary artery pressure as well as a decrease in heart rate and systemic vascular resistance. Obese individuals with cardiac dysfunction may choose to sleep sitting up in a chair to avoid symptoms of orthopnea and paroxysmal nocturnal dyspnea. A history of such a sleep pattern should raise concern about the patient's cardiovascular status.

Systemic Hypertension

Mild to moderate systemic hypertension is three to six times more frequent in obese than in lean patients and is seen in approximately 50% to 60% of obese patients. The

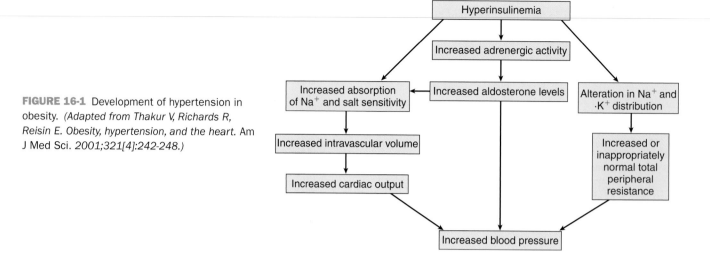

FIGURE 16-1 Development of hypertension in obesity. *(Adapted from Thakur V, Richards R, Reisin E. Obesity, hypertension, and the heart. Am J Med Sci. 2001;321[4]:242-248.)*

mechanism of hypertension in obesity is multifactorial (Figure 16-1). Obesity-induced hypertension is related to insulin effects on the sympathetic nervous system and extracellular fluid volume. Hyperinsulinemia appears to increase circulating levels of norepinephrine; norepinephrine has direct pressor activity and increases renal tubular reabsorption of sodium and calcium, which results in hypervolemia. Cardiac output increases by an estimated 100 mL/min for each kilogram of adipose tissue weight gain. At the cellular level, insulin activates adipocytes to release angiotensinogen, which activates the renin-angiotensin-aldosterone pathway; this in turn leads to sodium retention and development of hypertension. An increase in circulating cytokines is seen in obesity, and this may cause damage to and fibrosis of the arterial wall, thereby increasing arterial stiffness. If hypertension is not well controlled, a mixed eccentric and concentric left ventricular hypertrophy can develop that eventually leads to heart failure and pulmonary hypertension. Weight loss can significantly improve or even completely resolve hypertension. In general, a decrease of 1% in body weight can decrease systolic blood pressure by 1 mm Hg and diastolic blood pressure by 2 mm Hg.

Cardiac Disease

Coronary Artery Disease. Obesity seems to be an independent risk factor for the development of ischemic heart disease, and this coronary artery disease is more common in obese individuals with central (abdominal) fat distribution. This risk is compounded by the presence of dyslipidemia, a chronic inflammatory state, hypertension, and diabetes mellitus. Insulin resistance and abnormal glucose tolerance are associated with progression of atherosclerosis. Young obese patients are showing a significant incidence of single-vessel coronary artery disease, particularly in the right coronary artery. Obese men seem to be affected 10 to 20 years before women, which may reflect a protective effect from estrogen that dissipates after menopause.

Heart Failure. Obesity is an independent risk factor for heart failure. Possible mechanisms for the development of this heart failure are structural and functional modifications of the heart resulting from volume overload and vascular stiffness. These changes in obese patients cause pressure overload that leads to concentric left ventricular hypertrophy, a progressively less compliant left ventricle, left ventricular diastolic dysfunction, and, finally, left ventricular systolic dysfunction. Increased metabolic demands and a larger circulating blood volume result in a hyperdynamic circulation. Right ventricular afterload may be increased because of associated sleep-disordered breathing and changes in left ventricular function (Figure 16-2). Insulin resistance also appears to play a significant role in the development of heart failure. Cardiac steatosis, lipoapoptosis, and activation of specific cardiac genes that promote left ventricular remodeling and cardiomyopathy may contribute to obesity-related cardiomyopathy. The increased demands placed on the cardiovascular system by obesity decrease cardiovascular reserve and limit exercise tolerance. Cardiac dysrhythmias in obese individuals may be precipitated by arterial hypoxemia, hypercarbia, ischemic heart disease, obesity hypoventilation syndrome, and fatty infiltration of the cardiac conduction system. It is important to note that ventricular hypertrophy and dysfunction worsen with the duration of obesity. However, some of these structural and functional changes are reversible with significant weight loss.

RESPIRATORY DISORDERS

Respiratory derangements associated with obesity are related to the presence of redundant tissue in the upper airway, thorax, and abdomen that affects lung volumes, gas exchange, lung compliance, and work of breathing.

Lung Volumes

Obesity can produce an extrinsic restrictive pattern of ventilation resulting from the added weight of the thoracic cage or chest wall and abdomen. The added weight impedes motion of the diaphragm, especially in the supine position, which

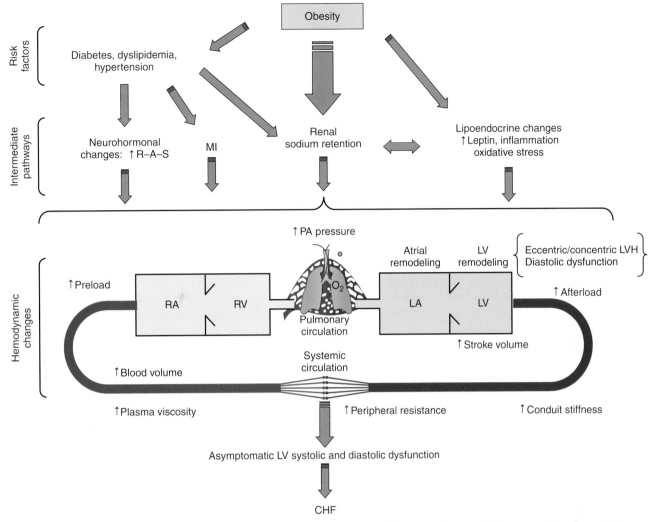

FIGURE 16-2 Cardiac changes in obesity leading to heart failure. ↑, Increased; *CHF*, congestive heart failure; *LA*, left atrium; *LV*, left ventricle; *LVH*, left ventricular hypertrophy; *MI*, myocardial infarction; *PA*, pulmonary artery; *RA*, right atrium; *RAS*, renin-angiotensin system; *RV*, right ventricle. *(Adapted from Vasan RS. Editorial: cardiac function and obesity. Heart. 2003;89:1127-1129.)*

results in an overall decrease in functional residual capacity (FRC), expiratory reserve volume, and total lung capacity. FRC declines exponentially with increasing BMI. FRC may decrease to the point that small airway closure occurs, that is, closing volume becomes greater than FRC. This results in ventilation/perfusion mismatching, right-to-left intrapulmonary shunting, and arterial hypoxemia. General anesthesia accentuates these changes. A 50% decrease in FRC occurs in obese anesthetized patients compared with a 20% decrease in nonobese individuals. Application of positive end-expiratory pressure (PEEP) can improve FRC and arterial oxygenation but at the potential expense of cardiac output and oxygen delivery.

The decrease in FRC impairs the ability of obese patients to tolerate periods of apnea, such as during direct laryngoscopy for endotracheal intubation. Obese individuals are likely to experience oxygen desaturation following induction of anesthesia despite adequate preoxygenation. This phenomenon reflects a decreased oxygen reserve secondary to the reduced FRC and an increase in oxygen consumption

resulting from the increased metabolic activity of excess adipose tissue.

Gas Exchange and Work of Breathing

Because of the obese patient's increased body mass, oxygen consumption and carbon dioxide production are increased. To maintain normocapnia, obese patients must increase minute ventilation, which also increases the work of breathing. Obese patients will typically increase their minute ventilation by rapid shallow breathing, because this breathing pattern utilizes the least amount of energy and may prevent fatigue from the increased work of breathing. Clinically severely obese individuals may exhibit only modest decreases in arterial oxygenation and modest increases in the alveolar-arterial oxygen difference. The Paco₂ and ventilatory response to carbon dioxide remain within the normal range in obese patients, which reflects the high diffusing capacity and favorable characteristics of the carbon dioxide dissociation curve. However, arterial oxygenation may deteriorate markedly on induction of anesthesia (increased oxygen consumption and decreased oxygen reserves) so that a high fraction of inspired oxygen (FIO_2) is required to maintain an acceptable level of PaO_2 and oxygen saturation as measured by pulse oximetry.

Lung Compliance and Airway Resistance

Increased BMI is associated with decreased lung compliance and increased airway resistance. The decrease in lung compliance is caused by accumulation of fat tissue in and around the chest wall and abdomen and the added effects of increased pulmonary blood volume. Decreased lung compliance is associated with decreases in FRC and impaired gas exchange. These changes in lung compliance and resistance are most marked when obese individuals assume the supine position.

Obstructive Sleep Apnea

Obstructive sleep apnea (OSA) is defined as cessation of breathing for longer than 10 seconds during sleep. There may be frequent episodes of apnea and hypopnea during sleep. *Hypopnea* is a reduction in the size or number of breaths compared with normal ventilation and is associated with some degree of arterial desaturation. Apnea occurs when the pharyngeal airways collapse. Pharyngeal patency depends on the action of dilator muscles that prevent upper airway collapse. The pharyngeal muscle tone is decreased during sleep, and in many individuals, this reduced tone leads to a significant narrowing of the upper airway, resulting in turbulent airflow and snoring. In susceptible individuals this may progress to severe snoring and, ultimately, to sleep apnea. Sleep fragmentation is the most likely explanation for the daytime somnolence, which is associated with impaired concentration, memory problems, and even motor vehicle accidents in patients with sleep apnea. Airway obstruction may induce physiologic changes that include arterial hypoxemia, arterial hypercarbia, polycythemia, systemic hypertension, pulmonary hypertension, and right ventricular failure. In addition, patients may complain of morning headaches caused by nocturnal carbon dioxide retention and cerebral vasodilation. OSA is diagnosed using polysomnography in a sleep laboratory, where episodes of apnea during sleep can be observed and quantified. The severity of OSA is measured by the average number of incidents per hour. More than five incidents per hour is considered sleep apnea syndrome. The main predisposing factors for the development of OSA are male gender, middle age, and obesity (BMI > 30 kg/m^2). Other factors such as evening alcohol consumption or use of pharmacologic sleep aids can worsen the problem. Treatment of OSA is aimed at applying enough positive airway pressure through a nasal mask to sustain patency of the upper airway during sleep. Patients treated with positive airway pressure demonstrate improved neuropsychiatric function and a lessening of daytime somnolence. Patients with mild OSA who do not tolerate positive airway pressure may benefit from nighttime application of oral appliances designed to enlarge the airway by keeping the tongue in an anterior position or by displacing the mandible forward. The use of drugs such as protriptyline and fluoxetine to treat OSA has not been shown to be reliably

effective. Nocturnal oxygen therapy is another possibility for individuals who experience significant oxygen desaturation. In severe cases of sleep apnea surgical treatment, including uvulopalatopharyngoplasty, tracheostomy, or maxillofacial surgery (i.e., genioglossal advancement), may be performed. In many instances, weight loss results in a significant improvement in or even complete resolution of OSA symptoms.

Obesity Hypoventilation Syndrome

Obesity hypoventilation syndrome (OHS) is the long-term consequence of OSA. It is characterized by nocturnal episodes of central apnea (apnea without respiratory efforts) reflecting progressive desensitization of the respiratory center to nocturnal hypercarbia. At its extreme, OHS culminates in pickwickian syndrome, which is characterized by obesity, daytime hypersomnolence, arterial hypoxemia, polycythemia, hypercarbia, respiratory acidosis, pulmonary hypertension, and right ventricular failure. In patients with OHS, even light sedation can cause complete airway collapse and/or respiratory arrest. All patients with a history of OSA or OHS must be thoroughly evaluated preoperatively.

GASTROINTESTINAL DISORDERS

Hepatobiliary Disease

The risk of developing gallbladder and biliary tract disease is increased threefold in obese people, which perhaps reflects abnormal cholesterol metabolism. Abnormal liver function test results and fatty infiltration of the liver are frequent findings. Therefore, caution should be used when selecting medications known to cause liver dysfunction. Interestingly, the increased metabolism of volatile anesthetics (defluorination) seen in obese patients has not been shown to result in hepatic dysfunction.

Nonalcoholic Fatty Liver Disease/Nonalcoholic Steatohepatitis

Obesity is the most important risk factor associated with *nonalcoholic fatty liver disease* (NAFLD), also known as *nonalcoholic steatohepatitis*. Obesity causes an excess of intrahepatic triglycerides, impaired insulin activity, and additional release of inflammatory cytokines. These factors can lead to destruction of hepatocytes and disruption of hepatic physiology and architecture. Because of the increasing prevalence of obesity, NAFLD has become one of the most common causes of end-stage liver disease in the United States. Approximately one third of *overweight* children, adolescents, and adults have nonalcoholic steatohepatitis. About 85% of *severely obese* adults have NAFLD. In most cases, this form of hepatitis follows a benign course. However, in severe cases it may progress to cirrhosis, portal hypertension, and/or hepatocellular carcinoma requiring liver transplantation. Most patients are asymptomatic, but some may experience fatigue and abdominal discomfort. Liver function test results may be abnormal. Among patients with NAFLD, 22% also develop diabetes mellitus, 22% develop systemic hypertension, and 25% die of coronary heart disease within 5 to 7 years. Weight reduction, especially bariatric surgery–induced weight loss, has been shown to significantly improve the metabolic abnormalities associated with fatty liver disease or even cure this form of hepatic inflammation.

Gallbladder Disease

Gallbladder disease is closely associated with obesity. Most commonly, obese patients have cholelithiasis resulting from supersaturation of bile with cholesterol resulting from abnormal cholesterol metabolism. Women with a BMI of more than 32 kg/m^2 have a three times higher risk of developing gallstones and those with a BMI of more than 45 kg/m^2 have a seven times higher risk of gallstones than lean people. Paradoxically, rapid weight loss, especially after bariatric surgery, *increases* the risk of gallstones.

Gastric Emptying and Gastroesophageal Reflux Disease

Obesity per se is not a risk factor for delayed gastric emptying or gastroesophageal reflux disease (GERD). Indeed, most obese patients may actually have increased gastric emptying, although obese patients have greater gastric fluid volumes. Not all obese patients require routine administration of prophylactic proton pump inhibitors, antacids, or rapid-sequence induction for general anesthesia.

INFLAMMATORY SYNDROME OF OBESITY

A higher rate of perioperative infection is seen in the obese population. This phenomenon may be due to the inability of neutrophils to activate, migrate, and adhere at sites of inflammation as a result of adipose tissue secretion of various proinflammatory cytokines or "adipokines." Markers of inflammation, such as C-reactive protein, interleukins (IL-6, IL-18), and tumor necrosis factor, are released by adipocytes. The elevated concentrations of these inflammatory markers consistently decrease after weight-loss surgery. In addition, adiponectin, an adipose tissue–derived cytokine that is associated with insulin sensitivity, decreases in obese states and increases with weight loss.

CANCER

The depressed immune function of the obese patient significantly increases the risk of development of certain cancers. The World Health Organization International Agency for Research on Cancer estimates that obesity and lack of physical activity are responsible for 25% to 33% of breast, colon, endometrial, renal, and esophageal cancers. Prostate and uterine cancer are also seen in a higher percentage of overweight patients. Peripheral conversion of sex hormones in adipose tissue by aromatase, together with decreased concentrations of plasma sex steroid–binding globulin, may be responsible for the increased incidence of some of these cancers.

THROMBOEMBOLIC DISORDERS

The risk of deep vein thrombosis in obese patients undergoing surgery is approximately double that of nonobese individuals. This increased risk of thromboembolic disease presumably reflects the compounded effects of polycythemia, increased intraabdominal pressure, increased fibrinogen levels associated with a chronic inflammatory state, and immobilization leading to venostasis. At a cellular level, adipocytes produce excessive plasminogen activator inhibitor and tissues have a decreased capacity for synthesis of tissue plasminogen activator. As a result there is a decrease in fibrinolysis that renders the obese patient susceptible to development of deep vein thrombosis or fatal pulmonary embolism. This phenomenon is worsened in the perioperative period. The use of low-molecular-weight heparin has been advocated to decrease thromboembolic complications during this period. In calculating the dosing for heparin, some suggest that the dose be based on total body weight, since this correlates with drug clearance. Perioperative use of sequential compression stockings is also indicated.

The risk of stroke is increased in obese patients. Studies report an association between stroke and an increased BMI and waist/hip ratio. For every 1 unit increase in above normal BMI, there is a 4% increase in the risk of ischemic stroke and a 6% increase in the risk of hemorrhagic stroke. This increased stroke risk may be related to the prothrombotic and chronic inflammatory state that accompanies excess adipose tissue accumulation.

MUSCULOSKELETAL DISORDERS

Degenerative Joint Disease

Osteoarthritis and degenerative joint disease are being seen more frequently in men and women 40 to 60 years of age, a trend that closely parallels the obesity epidemic. Obesity leads to joint pain and arthritis of the hips, knees, and carpometacarpal joints of the hands, not only because of mechanical loading of weight-bearing joints, but also because of the accompanying inflammatory and metabolic effects of increased adipose tissue. Co-existing disorders of glucose intolerance, lipid metabolism, hyperuricemia, gout, and vitamin D deficiency may further contribute to the problem of osteoarthritis in obese patients. Extra care must be taken in the positioning of patients with arthritis or degenerative joint disease in the operating room.

NERVOUS SYSTEM

Obese patients, especially those affected by diabetes, may have symptoms of autonomic nervous system dysfunction and peripheral neuropathy. Deficiencies of essential micronutrients such as Vitamin B_{12}, thiamine, folate, trace minerals, iron, and calcium, in combination with hyperglycemia, can lead to autonomic nervous system dysfunction. Weight loss in severely obese patients is associated with significant improvement in autonomic cardiac modulation. Because pressure sores and nerve injuries are more common in the superobese and diabetic populations, particular attention must be given to padding the extremities and protecting pressure-prone areas during surgery.

Treatment of Obesity

Successful treatment of obesity relies on a significant degree of patient motivation. It is estimated that fewer than 20% of obese patients are sufficiently motivated to accept treatment. Only after patients have acknowledged their weight problem and shown themselves capable of complying with a weight-loss program (even if unsuccessful) should pharmacologic or surgical treatment be considered. Genuine patient motivation is required to achieve sustained positive results because, ultimately, the treatment of obesity requires a lifelong commitment to lifestyle alterations in the form of increased physical activity and decreased caloric intake. The benefits of weight loss in obesity are well documented. Medical and surgical weight-loss plans should be aimed at decreasing the morbidity of obesity rather than meeting a cosmetic standard of thinness. A weight loss of only 5 to 20 kg can be associated with a decrease in systemic blood pressure and plasma lipid concentrations and better control of diabetes mellitus.

NONPHARMACOLOGIC THERAPY

The first step in any weight-loss program is dieting. Caloric restriction to 500 to 1000 kcal/day less than a regular diet promotes weight loss. Restricting caloric intake beyond this amount may initially help the patient lose weight faster. However, the likelihood of long-term adherence to such a restricted diet is very low. Behavior modification therapy may be required to help patients remain motivated and adhere to lifestyle alterations. The addition of exercise programs to dieting programs helps in maintaining successful long-term weight loss. Unfortunately, in most patients with severe obesity, weight loss is not maintained over time without pharmacologic or surgical intervention.

MEDICAL THERAPY

Current recommendations of the National Institutes of Health and the European Union suggest adding pharmacotherapy to weight-management programs in patients with a BMI of 27 kg/m^2 or higher and a persistent comorbid condition such as hypertension or glucose intolerance and in patients with a BMI of more than 30 kg/m^2 with no comorbidities. When used properly, weight-loss drugs increase by threefold to fourfold the proportion of patients achieving at least a 5% weight loss at 1 year.

Drugs designed to control caloric intake include serotonin reuptake inhibitors (phentermine) and mixed serotonin/norepinephrine/dopamine reuptake inhibitors. Caution must be used when prescribing these drugs, since they may increase blood pressure and heart rate, and have led to pulmonary hypertension in some patients. Fenfluramine/phentermine ("fen-phen") and dexfenfluramine, selective serotonin reuptake inhibitors, were taken off the market in 2009 by the FDA because of evidence linking the drugs with cardiac valvular disease. Sibutramine, a mixed serotonin/norepinephrine/dopamine reuptake inhibitor, was taken off the market in October 2010 because of evidence of a significant increase in risk of major cardiovascular events including heart attack and stroke. Currently, only phentermine (an appetite suppressant related to amphetamine) is FDA approved to treat obesity.

Another class of drugs used to treat obesity includes drugs that bind gastric and pancreatic lipases in the gut and prevent the hydrolysis of dietary fat into absorbable free fatty acids.

This promotes weight loss via malabsorption of fats. The only FDA-approved lipase inhibitor is orlistat. Another category of weight-loss medications includes those drugs that increase energy expenditure and may contain ephedrine or ephedra alkaloids. Ephedra was often found in over-the-counter diet drugs and herbal supplements. These medications can cause unexpected cardiovascular events, including severe hypertension, cardiac dysrhythmias, myocardial infarction, stroke, and even death. The FDA banned the sale of these drugs in 2004.

SURGICAL THERAPY

Adult bariatric surgery results in significant sustained weight loss in patients who are severely obese. Bariatric surgery also improves obesity-related comorbid conditions, especially hypertension and diabetes. Such surgery is the most cost-effective treatment for patients with a BMI of more than 40 kg/m^2 or patients with a BMI of 35 kg/m^2 or more and significant comorbid conditions. With the recognition of the long-term benefits of this surgery for clinically severely obese patients, bariatric surgery is performed much more often now than a decade ago. In the United States bariatric surgery is performed as frequently as cholecystectomy. It appears that the mean percentage of excess weight loss after Roux-en-Y gastric bypass is 68%. It is 62% for gastric banding. Patients have a 77% likelihood of resolution of diabetes and a 62% likelihood of resolution of hypertension.

Current strategies for surgically assisted weight loss fall into one of three categories: gastric restriction, intestinal malabsorption, or combined restrictive-malabsorptive bariatric surgery (Table 16-5). Most often these surgeries are performed laparoscopically. Laparoscopic techniques have the advantages of decreased pain, decreased rates of complication (i.e., pulmonary complications, thromboembolism, wound infection, hernia development), and shorter recovery times, and their efficacy is comparable to that of open procedures.

Types of Bariatric Surgery

Restrictive Bariatric Procedures. Laparoscopic adjustable gastric banding, sleeve gastrectomy, and vertical banded gastroplasty are examples of restrictive procedures, in which a small gastric pouch with a small outlet (10 to 12 mm in diameter) is created. The mechanism of weight loss with this operation may be related to appetite suppression and early satiety or possibly to vagal nerve compression or reduced secretion of gastric hormones, such as ghrelin. Gastroplasty is rarely performed now because of its poor weight-loss results. Adjustable gastric banding is the most commonly performed bariatric procedure in Europe, Latin America, and Australia. It has been used in the United States since 2001 and is gaining in popularity. The surgery entails placement of an adjustable silicone band around the upper end of the stomach, which creates a small pouch and restrictive stoma that slows the passage of food into the small intestine. This procedure requires no cutting of, or entry into, the stomach or small intestine and should therefore be associated with a low complication rate. The gastric band is adjusted after surgery by injection of saline into

TABLE 16-5 Most common bariatric surgeries

	Combined restrictive-malabsorptive	Restrictive	Malabsorptive
Name	Roux-en-Y gastric bypass	Adjustable gastric banding (Lap-Band surgery) Laparoscopic sleeve gastrectomy	Jejunoileal bypass or biliopancreatic diversion
How stomach is made smaller	Upper portion of stomach is stapled to lower part of intestines leaving only a small gastric pouch	Gastric banding: silicone band is placed around top portion of stomach and adjusted until desired size of stomach is achieved Sleeve gastrectomy: greater curvature of stomach is resected, with ~25% of stomach remaining	80% of stomach is removed along with a significant portion of small intestine, which leaves behind a smaller absorptive area
Hospital stay	2-3 days	Overnight	1-2 days
Operating time	2 hr	1 hr	1.5 hr
Advantages	Greatest weight loss of all types of surgery with improvement in obesity-related health issues	Lower mortality and morbidity with banding because band is adjustable and placement does not require cutting, stapling, or rerouting stomach Nutritional deficiencies usually not an issue since intestines left intact	Significant weight loss
Disadvantages	Need for continuous lifelong nutritional surveillance and supplementation	Need for more frequent outpatient visits and longest time to achieve weight loss	Malabsorption of essential vitamins and nutrients like B_{12}, folic acid, and iron, as well as protein-caloric malnutrition

a subcutaneous port (placed at the time of surgery) to adjust the stoma size. Sleeve gastrectomy involves resection of the greater curvature of the stomach, which compromises about 75% of the stomach. The smaller gastric reservoir produces early satiety, and the remnant stomach secretes decreased levels of gastric hormones. The normal absorptive physiology of the entire small intestine is left intact in all of these restrictive procedures, so specific nutrient deficiencies are rare unless there is a significant change in eating habits or complications such as stomal stenosis occur.

Malabsorptive Bariatric Procedures. Malabsorptive procedures include (1) distal gastric or jejunoileal bypass, (2) biliopancreatic diversion (BPD), and (3) duodenal switch. These operations typically combine gastric volume reduction with a bypass of various lengths of small intestine. After creation of a gastric pouch (200 to 250 mL in volume), the small bowel is divided proximal to the ileocecal valve and connected directly to the gastric pouch, which produces a *gastroileostomy*. The remaining proximal limb of small intestine (biliopancreatic conduit) is anastomosed end to side to the distal ileum, proximal to the ileocecal valve. This provides a common channel that allows for mixture of nutrients with digestive enzymes in the ileum. The length of the common channel determines the degree of malabsorption. Because these procedures induce weight loss by extensively bypassing the small intestine and promoting malabsorption, they are associated with a high incidence of anemia, deficiency of fat-soluble vitamins, and protein-calorie malnutrition in the first year after surgery.

Because of these increased risks of nutritional and metabolic complications, these operations are not performed as frequently as the restrictive procedures.

Combined Bariatric Procedure. The combined bariatric procedure, called *Roux-en-Y gastric bypass* (RYGB), includes both gastric restriction and some degree of malabsorption. It is the preferred surgical approach for clinically severe obesity. In the RYGB procedure, the surgeon creates a very small (15- to 50-mL) proximal gastric pouch that is connected to a Roux limb via an enteroenterostomy to the jejunum near the ligament of Treitz. The procedure bypasses the distal stomach, duodenum, and proximal jejunum, so there is a marked loss of absorptive surface area for nutrients, electrolytes, and bile salts. The RYGB procedure requires the longest operating time and postoperative hospital stay compared with other forms of bariatric surgery. However, it results in the greatest weight loss and improvement in obesity-related health issues.

Surgical Complications

Complications and mortality rates for bariatric surgery depend on several factors: patient age, gender, BMI, existing comorbid conditions, procedure type and complexity, and the experience of the surgeon and surgical center. Higher mortality rates have been associated with abdominal obesity, male gender, BMI of 50 kg/m² or more, diabetes mellitus, sleep apnea, older age, and performance of the surgery at a lower-volume bariatric surgery center. Recent improvements in mortality rates are likely due to the use of laparoscopic techniques and better anesthesia, monitoring, and perioperative care. Overall 30-day mortality for bariatric surgery ranges from 0.1% to 2%. Gastric banding has the lowest mortality rate. Mortality for gastric bypass and sleeve gastrectomy is 0.5%. Malabsorptive operations are associated with a higher mortality rate. The mortality of RYGB ranges from 0.5% to 1.5%. The most severe complications of bariatric surgery include anastomotic leaks, stricture formation, pulmonary embolism, sepsis, gastric prolapse, and bleeding. Less common complications are wound dehiscence, hernia or seroma formation, lymphocele, lymphorrhea, and suture extrusion.

Nutritional complications are seen after malabsorptive and combined bariatric procedures. These complications are a result of the marked reduction in vitamin and mineral uptake. The majority of patients can maintain a relatively normal nutritional status after RYGB, but deficiencies of iron, vitamin B_{12}, vitamin K, and folate are common. Some patients develop subclinical micronutrient deficiency. Taking multivitamins with mineral supplements reduces, but does not totally prevent, the development of vitamin or mineral deficiencies. Chronic vitamin K deficiency can lead to an abnormal prothrombin time with a normal partial thromboplastin time. Patients who come for elective surgery with vitamin K deficiency and coagulopathy respond to administration of a vitamin K analogue such as phytonadione within 6 to 24 hours. Fresh frozen plasma may be required for prothrombin time correction for emergency surgery or active bleeding.

Additional complications of bariatric surgery include occurrence of an undesirable *dumping syndrome* in some patients. Other patients experience major nutritional complications. Three of the most clinically significant nutritional complications are (1) protein-calorie malnutrition, (2) Wernicke's encephalopathy, and (3) peripheral neuropathy. In the long term, patients are also at risk of metabolic bone disease. Pregnant women and adolescents are at higher risk of nutritional complications after RYGB because of their higher physiologic nutritional needs. Long-term nutritional follow-up is essential to promote a healthy life after weight-loss surgery. Even when surgery-related mortality is taken into account, several studies have shown a significant survival benefit in patients who underwent bariatric surgery compared with those who did not. The survival benefit is specifically due to a decrease in the rate of myocardial infarction, resolution of diabetes mellitus, and fewer cancer-related deaths.

Protein-Calorie Malnutrition. Severe malnutrition is the most serious metabolic complication of bariatric surgery. Red meat is poorly tolerated after bariatric surgery because it is much harder to break down and pass through the small stomach outlet. If the outlet becomes plugged, vomiting will result. If the patient does not consume enough alternative protein sources, such as milk, yogurt, eggs, fish, and poultry, protein malnutrition can develop. Protein-calorie malnutrition is generally more common with BPD and is very rare with vertical banded gastroplasty. Protein-calorie malnutrition has a reported incidence of 7% to 12% in patients who have

undergone BPD. Hypoalbuminemia has been reported as early as 1 year after BPD. Revision of the common channel from 50 to 200 cm in length has been shown to correct the hypoalbuminemia associated with excessive weight loss. In cases of severe malnutrition, enteral or parenteral nutrition therapy may be necessary. Mild to moderate cases usually respond to dietary counseling. More frequent monitoring may be necessary for patients prone to protein-calorie malnutrition.

Fat Malabsorption. Fat-soluble vitamin malabsorption and fat malabsorption (evidenced by steatorrhea) are common with RYGB and BPD. Indeed, this phenomenon is the principal means by which BPD promotes weight loss. The length of the common channel in BPD regulates the degree of fat absorption and determines the severity of malabsorption. Evidence has shown that a 100-cm common channel is better tolerated than a 50-cm channel and is associated with less diarrhea and steatorrhea and improved protein metabolism. Problems with fat-soluble vitamin imbalances and fat malabsorption are rarely seen with vertical banded gastroplasty.

Consideration of Bariatric Surgery in Pediatric and Adolescent Patients

With over 10% of children now classified as overweight or obese, the appropriateness of bariatric surgery in adolescents is being considered. In 2005, a National Institutes of Health consensus statement indicated that bariatric surgery in adolescents is safe and effective for long-term sustained weight loss and resolution of comorbid conditions. The American Society for Bariatric Surgery has expanded the patient population suitable for bariatric surgery to include adolescents and possibly individuals with a BMI of 30 to 34.9 kg/m^2 who have associated comorbid conditions. Although these updated guidelines suggest that bariatric surgery be considered for adolescents, the risks and benefits of this aggressive intervention must be weighed by an interdisciplinary team at an experienced bariatric surgery center.

Management of Anesthesia in Obese Patients

PREOPERATIVE EVALUATION

A thorough preoperative evaluation is necessary for all patients with clinically severe obesity coming for surgery. The focus of the history taking and physical examination should be on the cardiovascular and respiratory systems and airway evaluation. Many of these patients lead sedentary lifestyles, so eliciting symptoms associated with cardiorespiratory disease may be difficult. Even a thorough history and physical examination with electrocardiography (ECG) may underestimate the extent of cardiovascular disease in these patients. In some cases, more extensive preoperative diagnostic testing including standard blood work, chest radiography, sleep studies, cardiac stress testing, transthoracic echocardiography, and room air arterial blood gas sampling may be necessary to fully evaluate the health status of an obese patient.

The anesthesiologist should inquire about the presence of chest pain, shortness of breath at rest or with minimal exertion, and palpitations, and the position in which the patient sleeps. The most common symptoms of pulmonary hypertension are exertional dyspnea, fatigue, and syncope, which reflect an inability to increase cardiac output during activity. If pulmonary hypertension is suspected, then avoidance of hypoxemia, nitrous oxide, and other drugs that may further worsen pulmonary vasoconstriction is warranted. Intraoperatively, inhaled anesthetics may be beneficial because they cause bronchodilation and decrease hypoxic pulmonary vasoconstriction.

Symptoms of OSA, such as snoring, apneic episodes during sleep, daytime somnolence, morning headaches, and frequent sleep arousals, should be sought. If a diagnosis of severe OSA or OHS is suspected, further evaluation may be required. Symptoms of acid reflux, coughing, inability to lie flat without coughing, or heartburn may indicate GERD or delayed gastric emptying. If these symptoms are not already controlled with antacids or proton pump inhibitors, it may be necessary to start these medications preoperatively. Prolonging the period of preoperative fasting from the standard 8 hours to 12 hours and prohibiting the intake of clear liquids starting at 8 hours preoperatively may be prudent. In patients with a history of hypertension, eliciting symptoms such as frequent headaches and changes in vision can indicate whether the blood pressure is well controlled. In those with uncontrolled hypertension, referral to the primary care doctor for optimization should be considered. In diabetic patients, symptoms of claudication, peripheral neuropathy, renal dysfunction, or retinopathy, or an elevated hemoglobin A_{1c} level should signal the possibility of advanced diabetes, poorly controlled glucose levels, and microvascular and macrovascular disease.

Obese patients have unique issues that may contribute to cardiovascular, pulmonary, and thromboembolic complications. High-risk patients should be identified early to ensure optimal management of co-existing diseases before surgery. A look at prior anesthetic and surgical records, with special attention to induction and intubation, may help identify problems with airway management and indicate the weight of the patient at the time of the previous surgery.

Physical Examination and Airway Examination

The physical examination should attempt to identify signs suggestive of cardiac and respiratory disease. Signs of left or right ventricular failure such as increased jugular venous pressure, extra heart sounds, rales, hepatomegaly, and peripheral edema may be very difficult to elicit in the morbidly obese patient because of body habitus. Pedal edema is a very common finding in obese patients and may be due to right-sided heart failure, varicose veins, or extravasation of intravascular fluid associated with decreased mobility.

A detailed assessment of the upper airway must be performed to look for the following anatomic features: fat face and cheeks, short neck, large tongue, large tonsillar size, excessive palatal and pharyngeal soft tissue, restricted mouth opening, limited cervical and/or mandibular mobility, large breasts, increased neck circumference at the level of the thyroid cartilage, or a Mallampati score of 3 or higher.

A history of sleep apnea should raise the possibility of upper airway abnormalities that may predispose to difficulties with mask ventilation and exposure of the glottic opening during direct laryngoscopy, such as decreased anatomic space to accommodate anterior displacement of the tongue. When awake, these patients may compensate for their compromised airway anatomy by increasing the craniocervical angulation, which increases the space between the mandible and cervical spine and elongates the tongue and soft tissues of the neck. This compensation is lost when these patients become unconscious.

Studies have not shown a statistically significant link between obesity per se and the likelihood of difficult intubation. Rather, physical examination findings such as a very thick neck or a Mallampati score higher than 3 more reliably predict the possibility of a difficult intubation. In selected patients, awake endotracheal intubation using fiberoptic laryngoscopy may be the most appropriate method for securing the airway, but it is important to remember that neither clinically severe obesity nor a high BMI is an absolute indication for an awake intubation. In fact, with the recent advent of the videolaryngoscope, awake fiberoptic intubation is being performed much less frequently.

The obese patient should also be evaluated for ease of peripheral intravenous catheter placement. If severe difficulty with intravenous access is anticipated, then the patient should be informed of the possibility of placement of a central intravenous catheter before induction. If a patient is found to be at very high risk of intraoperative or postoperative deep vein thrombosis, then placement of an inferior vena cava filter before surgery should be considered.

Preoperative Diagnostic Tests

ECG examination may demonstrate findings suggestive of right ventricular hypertrophy, left ventricular hypertrophy, cardiac dysrhythmias, or myocardial ischemia or infarction. It is important to keep in mind that the ECG may not always be reliable in the clinically severely obese patient because of morphologic features such as (1) displacement of the heart by an elevated diaphragm, (2) increased cardiac workload with associated cardiac hypertrophy, (3) increased distance between the heart and the recording electrodes caused by excess adipose tissue in the chest wall and possibly increased epicardial fat, and (4) the potential for associated chronic lung disease to alter the ECG. Chest radiographic examination may show signs of heart failure, increased vascular markings, pulmonary congestion, pulmonary hypertension, hyperinflated lungs, or other pulmonary disease. Transthoracic echocardiography is useful to evaluate left and right ventricular systolic and diastolic function as well as to identify pulmonary hypertension. In cases of severe OSA, results of arterial blood gas analysis on a sample drawn with the patient breathing room air may be helpful in guiding intraoperative and postoperative ventilatory management.

Home Medications

Most home medications should be continued preoperatively, with the exception of oral hypoglycemics, angiotensin-converting enzyme inhibitors, angiotensin receptor blockers, anticoagulants (warfarin, aspirin, clopidogrel [Plavix]), and nonsteroidal antiinflammatory drugs. Patients taking histamine-2 receptor blockers such as famotidine, nonparticulate antacids, or proton pump inhibitors should be counseled to take these medications on the morning of surgery. Obese patients are at high risk of acute postoperative pulmonary embolism because of their chronic inflammatory state, so perioperative deep vein thrombosis prophylaxis with either unfractionated or low-molecular-weight heparin is indicated.

If continuous positive airway pressure (CPAP) or bilevel positive airway pressure (BIPAP) is used at home, the patient should be advised to bring the mask on the day of surgery so that this therapy can be continued in the postoperative period. Currently, no data exist to support the preoperative initiation of CPAP or BIPAP to improve postoperative outcomes in patients with sleep apnea.

INTRAOPERATIVE MANAGEMENT

Positioning

Specially designed operating tables (or two regular tables joined together) may be required for bariatric surgery. Regular operating room tables have a maximum weight limit of approximately 205 kg, but operating tables capable of holding up to 455 kg, with a little extra width to accommodate the extra girth, are now available. To transfer the patient from the stretcher to the operating table, an air transfer mattress device (e.g., Hover-Matt) can be used to laterally transfer and reposition patients and minimize injury to staff. Some severely obese patients will require "ramping," which is a means of positioning the patient using a ramp that extends from behind the low back to the neck and allows the head to be positioned above the chest in a horizontal plane formed between the sternal notch and the external auditory meatus. This position allows better ventilatory mechanics and facilitates intubation (Figure 16-3). Particular care should be paid to protecting pressure areas (elbows, heels), because pressure sores and nerve injuries are more common in the superobese and obese patients with diabetes. Brachial plexus, sciatic, and ulnar nerve palsies have been reported in patients with increased BMI. Upper and lower limbs, because of their increased weight, have a higher likelihood of sliding off the operating table, which produces peripheral nerve injuries. It is desirable to keep the arms in neutral position on the arm boards so that their position can be monitored and excess pressure from tight tucking and draping can be avoided.

Laparoscopic Surgery

The degree of intraabdominal pressure determines the effects of pneumoperitoneum on venous return, myocardial performance, and ventilatory status. There is a biphasic cardiovascular response to increases in intraabdominal pressure. At an intraabdominal pressure of approximately 10 mm Hg, there is an *increase* in venous return, probably from a reduction in splanchnic sequestration of blood. This is associated with an increase in cardiac output and arterial pressure. Hypovolemia, however, blunts this response. Compression of the inferior vena cava occurs at intraabdominal pressures of approximately 20 mm Hg, and this results in *decreased* venous return from the lower body, increased renal vascular resistance, decreased renal blood flow, and decreased glomerular filtration. Concomitantly, obese patients manifest a disproportionate increase in systemic vascular resistance caused not only by aortic compression but also by increased secretion of vasopressin. These patients have higher left ventricular end-systolic wall stress *before* pneumoperitoneum (caused by increased end-systolic left ventricular dimensions) and *during* pneumoperitoneum. Since higher left ventricular end-systolic wall stress is a determinant of myocardial oxygen demand, more aggressive control of blood pressure (ventricular afterload) may be needed in clinically severely obese patients to optimize myocardial oxygen supply and demand. Femoral venous blood flow can be reduced by both pneumoperitoneum and Trendelenburg positioning, with an associated increased risk of lower extremity thrombosis. High intraabdominal pressure in conjunction with placement in Trendelenburg's position increases intrathoracic pressure and may impede adequate ventilation. Moreover, absorption of carbon dioxide can worsen hypercarbia and induce acidosis, thereby increasing pulmonary hypertension.

Choice of Anesthesia

According to the American Society of Anesthesiologists (ASA) Practice Guidelines, local or regional anesthesia should be the primary anesthetic choice for obese patients undergoing surgery, with general anesthesia used only when necessary.

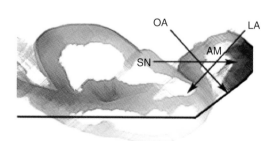 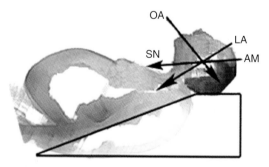

FIGURE 16-3 "Ramping" to achieve proper positioning for airway management. AM, Auditory meatus; LA, [laryngeal axis]; OA, [oral axis]; SN, sternal notch. *(Illustration by Brooke E. Albright, MD.)*

Placement of an epidural or peripheral nerve block can significantly aid in managing postoperative pain and reduce the need for narcotics, which decreases the incidence of postoperative respiratory depression.

Regional Anesthesia

Regional anesthesia, including spinal anesthesia, epidural anesthesia, and peripheral nerve block, may be technically difficult in obese patients, since landmarks are obscured by excess adipose tissue. It is estimated that the risk of a failed block is about 1.5 times higher in patients with a BMI of more than 30 kg/m^2 than in patients with a low BMI. There is also a higher likelihood of block-related complications. The success rate for blocks is significantly higher when ultrasonographic guidance is used to assist in needle placement. A distinct advantage of regional anesthesia in the obese patient is the ability to limit the amount of intraoperative and postoperative opioid use, which thereby limits the risk of respiratory depression and improves patient safety and satisfaction. Interestingly, obese patients require as much as 20% *less* local anesthetic for spinal or epidural anesthesia than nonobese patients, presumably because of fatty infiltration and vascular engorgement from increased intraabdominal pressure, which decreases the volume of the epidural space. It is difficult to reliably predict the sensory level of anesthesia that will be achieved by neuraxial blockade in these patients.

General Anesthesia

Induction of general anesthesia in the obese patient is not without risks. The anesthetic plan, including all risks, benefits, and alternatives to general anesthesia, should be discussed thoroughly with the patient and surgeon before the operation. The possible need for postoperative respiratory support via CPAP, BIPAP, or mechanical ventilation should also be discussed.

Premedication

Use of anxiolytic premedications such as benzodiazepines in the obese population is controversial, and the decision to premedicate should be made on a case-by-case basis depending on the risk of upper airway obstruction.

Airway Management

Management of the airway is one of the greatest challenges associated with general anesthesia in the obese patient. An emergency airway cart that provides access to rescue intubating devices such as supraglottic devices, a flexible bronchoscope, a light wand, and resuscitation drugs should be immediately available. The use of an intubating laryngeal mask airway has been shown to be successful for tracheal *intubation* in 96% of obese patients and for successful *ventilation* in less than 1 minute in 100% of obese patients. Use of a videolaryngoscope may facilitate tracheal intubation. Since the introduction of videolaryngoscopy, awake fiberoptic tracheal intubation is used much less frequently, but it remains an option for airway management in certain patients. For very high-risk patients with extremely limited pulmonary reserve or abnormal airway anatomy, an ear, nose, and throat surgeon should be immediately available to perform an emergency tracheostomy if needed.

Before intubation there must be adequate time for positioning and preoxygenation. Proper patient positioning is essential to successful intubation of the trachea. Often the large body habitus, particularly a large chest, short neck, or excess neck soft tissue, limits placement of the laryngoscope and glottic exposure. Successful intubation is contingent upon adequate alignment of the oral, pharyngeal, and laryngeal axes, also known as the *sniffing* position. To achieve this position, the obese patient may require ramping, in which a wedge-shaped device is placed behind the torso and a pillow is placed behind the head to slightly extend the neck so that the sternal notch is in line horizontally with the auditory meatus (see Figure 16-3). Adequate preoxygenation is critically important in obese patients, since these patients have a decreased FRC and higher oxygen consumption. Therefore they experience desaturation much faster than nonobese patients when they are apneic. Studies have shown that when patients undergo 5 minutes of preoxygenation with an Fio$_2$ of 100% via CPAP at a pressure of 10 cm H$_2$O, then the time that apnea can be tolerated without desaturation increases by 50%, which allows more time for direct laryngoscopy and tracheal intubation.

The decision to perform a rapid-sequence induction should be made on a case-by-case basis. Multiple risk factors for pulmonary aspiration may be present in the obese population: higher gastric residual volume, lower pH of gastric contents, higher intraabdominal pressure, and higher incidence of GERD and diabetes. However, no studies have documented an increased incidence of pulmonary aspiration solely related to an increased BMI.

Management of Ventilation

In the obese population, several factors make controlled mechanical ventilation problematic in the operating room. Obese patients already have a decreased FRC and decreased lung oxygen reserves, and experience desaturation faster during periods of hypoventilation or apnea than do normal-weight individuals. Positioning for adequate surgical exposure (prone or Trendelenburg's position) can worsen ventilation problems by decreasing chest wall compliance. If pneumoperitoneum is required for surgical exposure (laparoscopic or robotic surgery), ventilation may be impaired by the increased abdominal pressure, which worsens lung compliance. Recruitment maneuvers, such as Valsalva's maneuver, can be used to prevent atelectasis. There are no data to indicate which mode of ventilation is best for obese patients. PEEP improves ventilation/perfusion matching and arterial oxygenation in obese patients, but at high levels (PEEP of 15 to 20 cm H$_2$O) adverse effects on cardiac output and oxygen delivery offset these benefits. Using pressure-controlled ventilation and changing the inspiration/exhalation ratio can help limit peak airway pressure. When spontaneous ventilation is resumed at the conclusion of surgery, it is best to maintain the patient in a semi-upright position and apply pressure-support ventilation with PEEP to help reduce the risk of atelectasis. In a spontaneously breathing obese patient, the supine position is often associated with hypoxia.

INDUCTION AND MAINTENANCE OF ANESTHESIA

Any combination of drugs can be used for the induction and maintenance of general anesthesia in clinically severely obese patients. However, some drugs appear to have a better pharmacokinetic profile for obese patients.

Pharmacokinetics of Anesthetic Drugs

The physiologic changes associated with obesity may lead to alterations in the distribution, binding, and elimination of many drugs. The volume of distribution in obese individuals may be influenced by a variety of factors, including increased blood volume and cardiac output, decreased total body water (fat contains less water than other tissues), altered protein binding of drugs, and the lipid solubility of the drug being administered. The effect of obesity on protein binding is variable. Despite the occasional presence of liver dysfunction, hepatic clearance of drugs is usually not altered. Heart failure and decreased hepatic blood flow could slow elimination of drugs that are highly dependent on liver clearance. Renal clearance of drugs may increase in obese individuals because of increased renal blood flow and glomerular filtration rate.

The impact of obesity on dosing of injected drugs is difficult to predict. Total blood volume is likely to be increased, which would tend to decrease the plasma concentration achieved following intravenous injection of a drug. However, fat has a relatively low blood flow, so an increased dose of drug calculated based on *total body weight* could result in an excessive plasma concentration. Cardiac output is increased in the obese patient, which affects drug distribution and dilution in the first minute after administration. Because both cardiac output and plasma volume are increased, an initially higher dose of drug may be required for loading to attain peak plasma concentration. The most clinically useful approach is to calculate the initial dose of drug to be injected into an obese patient based on *lean body weight* rather than total body weight. Lean body weight is total body weight minus fat weight (Figure 16-4). In clinically severe obesity, lean body weight is increased and accounts for 20% to 40% of excess body weight. *Ideal body weight* does not take into account the increase in lean body weight in severely obese patients. Therefore, lean body weight is more highly correlated with cardiac output and drug clearance and should be used for initial dosing. Subsequent doses of drugs should be based on the pharmacologic response to the initial dose. Repeated injections of a drug, however, can result in cumulative drug effects and prolonged responses, reflecting storage of drugs in fat and subsequent release from this inactive depot into the systemic circulation as the plasma concentration of drug declines. It is important to note that *oral absorption* of drugs is *not* influenced by obesity.

An increased incidence of fatty liver infiltration in obese patients warrants caution when selecting drugs that have been associated with postoperative liver dysfunction. Increased

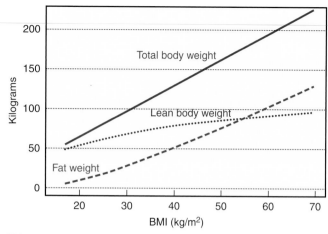

FIGURE 16-4 Comparison of total body weight, lean body weight, and fat weight with increasing body mass index (BMI) in a male of standard height. *(Adapted from Lemmens H. Perioperative pharmacology in morbid obesity. Curr Opin Anaesthesiol. 2010;23:485-491.)*

defluorination of volatile anesthetics in obese patients has not been shown to result in hepatic or renal dysfunction. This increased defluorination observed after the administration of certain volatile anesthetics to obese patients does not occur with administration of sevoflurane. Awakening of obese patients is more prompt after exposure to desflurane or sevoflurane than after administration of either isoflurane or propofol. The rapid elimination of nitrous oxide is useful, but the frequent need for increased supplemental oxygen limits the usefulness of nitrous oxide in obese patients.

Maintenance of anesthesia is best managed with drugs with minimal potential for accumulation in adipose tissue. Propofol, benzodiazepines, barbiturates, atracurium, cisatracurium, and narcotics such as sufentanil and fentanyl are highly lipophilic and accumulate in fatty tissue when administered by infusion over a long period. Usually, highly lipophilic drugs show a significant increase in volume of distribution in obese patients, and it would seem that dosing should be based on total body weight. However, because the majority of these drugs have the potential to accumulate in adipose tissue over time, a prolonged effect can be seen. An exception is remifentanil. This drug is also highly lipophilic; however, because it is rapidly metabolized by plasma esterases, it has limited potential for accumulation in fat tissue and is therefore favored over other narcotics for intraoperative analgesia. Ketamine and dexmedetomidine may also be useful anesthetic adjuncts in patients who are susceptible to narcotic-induced respiratory depression. For common anesthetic drug dosing recommendations, refer to Table 16-6.

Administration of hydrophilic substances, such as muscle relaxants, should be based on lean body weight, because their peak plasma concentrations are independent of the volume of distribution, which is greatly increased in obese patients. The large volume of distribution is due to the high ratio of extracellular to intracellular fluid, since the water content of adipose tissue is almost completely extracellular. Because the effect of

TABLE 16-6 ■ Recommended weight basis for dosing of common anesthetic drugs in obese patients

Total body weight	Lean body weight
Propofol: loading	Propofol: maintenance
Midazolam	Thiopental
Succinylcholine	Vecuronium
Cisatracurium and	Cisatracurium and
atracurium: loading	atracurium: maintenance
Pancuronium*	Rocuronium
	Remifentanil
	Fentanyl
	Sufentanil

*Pancuronium requires higher dosing to maintain 90% depression of twitch height in obese patients, but will also have a longer duration of action at higher dosages.

this increased extracellular fluid on neuromuscular blockade is unclear, it is recommended that neuromuscular blockers be dosed based on *lean body weight* and that the degree of blockade be carefully monitored.

The pharmacokinetics of succinylcholine are unique. Because the level of plasma pseudocholinesterase and the volume of distribution is increased, clinically severely obese patients have larger absolute succinylcholine dose requirements than normal-weight patients. Therefore, to achieve profound neuromuscular blockade and facilitate intubation, administration of succinylcholine should be based on *total body weight* rather than lean body weight.

Monitoring

The extent of surgery and concomitant comorbid conditions should be the primary factors that determine the need for and extent of monitoring beyond routine monitoring. For surgery performed under local or regional anesthesia with moderate sedation, the ASA Practice Guidelines recommend continuous capnography to decrease the risk of undetected airway obstruction, which is especially prevalent in the obese population. For surgery performed under general anesthesia, hemodynamic monitoring may be needed in selected patients. The technical difficulty of placing invasive hemodynamic monitors may be increased in this patient population. If noninvasive blood pressure cuffs are used, it is important to fit a correctly sized cuff. If the cuff is too small, then blood pressure measurements may be falsely elevated. Alternative to standard blood pressure cuffs include noninvasive blood pressure monitoring systems that detect blood pressure in the radial artery or in the finger. An intraarterial catheter should be inserted if noninvasive monitoring is inadequate or if the obese patient has severe cardiopulmonary disease. When intravenous access is problematic, use of ultrasonography to guide the placement of peripheral and/or central lines may increase the success rate and decrease the complication rate associated with these procedures. Transesophageal echocardiography (TEE) and pulmonary artery catheterization can be

performed intraoperatively in patients with heart failure, pulmonary hypertension, or other medical conditions that make continuous assessment of volume status or cardiac function necessary. Continuous TEE monitoring allows immediate detection of alterations in cardiac function as well as accurate assessment of volume status to guide fluid management. However, TEE monitoring requires expensive equipment and trained personnel and may not be readily available in all hospital settings.

Fluid Management

Calculation of fluid requirements in the obese patient should be based on lean body weight with a goal of euvolemia. Achieving this goal in the obese population may be very difficult, however, especially since there is a high association between severe obesity and diastolic dysfunction. In patients with preexisting cardiac disease, large fluid loads may not be tolerated well, and development of pulmonary edema is more likely. During laparoscopic surgery, decreased urinary output does not necessarily reflect hypovolemia, and liberal fluid administration may have a negative impact on overall outcome.

POSTOPERATIVE MANAGEMENT

Although episodic arterial hypoxemia may occur any time from the immediate postoperative period to as late as 2 to 5 days after surgery, no data support routine intensive care unit admission to decrease morbidity and mortality. Early episodic arterial hypoxemia may be due to perioperative opioid use. The patients at highest risk for developing postoperative hypoxemia are those with a history of OSA. The sitting position is a useful posture to improve arterial oxygenation. Routine administration of oxygen during the postoperative period is controversial, because oxygen administration can increase the duration of apnea by delaying the arousal effect produced by arterial hypoxemia. Therefore, it is preferable to provide supplemental oxygen only if arterial oxygen desaturation occurs. Once the patient's saturation can be maintained at baseline levels or higher than 90% on room air with good pain control, then pulse oximetry may be discontinued.

Transport

Before transport from the operating room to the recovery room, the obese patient should be fully awake and alert, sitting in a semi-upright position, receiving supplemental oxygen, and monitored by pulse oximetry. Verbal contact should be maintained throughout transport to assess wakefulness and adequacy of respiratory effort.

Emergence

Tracheal extubation is considered when obese patients are fully awake and alert, and have recovered from the depressant effects of the anesthetics. Although there are no specific studies to guide the practice of tracheal extubation in obese patients, certain maneuvers can facilitate better respiratory mechanics before extubation. These include placement in the semi-upright position (30 degrees or more head up), provision of pressure-support ventilation with PEEP or CPAP until extubation, oxygen supplementation, and placement of a nasopharyngeal airway to help maintain airway patency. A history of OSA or OHS mandates intense postoperative respiratory monitoring to ensure a patent upper airway and acceptable oxygenation and ventilation. In certain high-risk patients, placement of a tube exchanger before extubation may be prudent and is usually well tolerated even if left in place for several hours.

The notion that slow emergence of clinically severely obese patients from the effects of general anesthesia reflects delayed release of volatile anesthetics from fat stores is not accurate. Poor total fat blood flow limits the delivery of volatile anesthetics for storage. Overall, recovery times are often comparable in obese and lean individuals undergoing surgery that requires anesthesia for less than 4 hours.

Postoperative Analgesia

Because opioid-induced ventilatory depression is a concern, a multimodal approach to postoperative pain control is usually employed. This includes use of techniques that decrease narcotic requirements. Peripheral and central nerve block with continuous infusion of local anesthetic with or without small doses of opioids is an effective method for postoperative analgesia in obese patients. Supplementation with nonsteroidal antiinflammatory drugs (NSAIDs), α_2-receptor agonists, N-methyl-d-aspartate (NMDA) receptor antagonists, sodium channel blockers, or other nonopioid analgesics is highly recommended, since these drugs do not contribute to postoperative respiratory depression. Ketorolac is an NSAID that has been used successfully to reduce pain in the postoperative period. The principal side effects are gastrointestinal discomfort and the potential for increased operative site bleeding. Ketorolac is not suitable for use in patients who have undergone bariatric surgery because these patients are at especially high risk for development of gastrointestinal bleeding. An intravenous preparation of acetaminophen was recently approved by the FDA. Dosing of intravenous acetaminophen for patients who weigh more than 50 kg should be 1 g IV every 6 hours as needed, not to exceed 4 g in 24 hours. Because acetaminophen is metabolized by the liver and excreted in the urine, dosage should be decreased in patients with liver or kidney disease. Both dexmedetomidine, a selective α_2-receptor agonist, and clonidine, a less selective α_2-receptor agonist, have been shown to reduce opioid requirements if administered by continuous infusion in the perioperative period. Ketamine has been shown to enhance the analgesic effects of morphine by inhibiting opioid activation of NMDA receptors. Given in small doses postoperatively, ketamine can decrease pain and increase wakefulness and oxygen saturation. If opioids are eventually required to control postoperative pain, then patient-controlled analgesia is a good option. Dosages of opioids are best based on lean body weight.

Respiratory and Cardiovascular Monitoring and Management

The adequacy of ventilation should be assessed and monitored for at least 24 to 48 hours postoperatively. If the patient was on CPAP or BIPAP ventilation at home, this ventilation mode should be resumed postoperatively. If the patient had not been diagnosed with sleep apnea preoperatively but experiences frequent airway obstruction and hypoxemic episodes in the recovery room, then CPAP or BIPAP can be considered. These noninvasive ventilatory modes should be used very cautiously in the period immediately after gastric bypass surgery, however, because some risk of stomal dehiscence is associated with their use. Respiratory monitoring in the first few postoperative hours should be intensive. Any sign suggestive of respiratory fatigue or cardiovascular instability should be evaluated and treated immediately. If obese patients require reintubation, it is best performed in a controlled fashion rather than in an emergent situation.

Discharge to an unmonitored Setting

The decision about when to discharge patients to a regular hospital room or to home can be difficult in obese patients. It is considered safe to discharge a patient to an unmonitored setting (regular hospital bed or home) when pain is adequately controlled and the patient is no longer at significant risk of postoperative respiratory depression.

Postoperative Complications

Postoperative morbidity and mortality rates are higher in obese patients than in nonobese patients. This is due primarily to the presence of preexisting medical illnesses and the risk of aspiration during endotracheal intubation. Wound infection is twice as common in obese patients. Postoperative mechanical ventilation is often needed in obese patients who have a history of carbon dioxide retention and have undergone prolonged surgery. The hazards of OSA and OHS may extend several days into the postoperative period. The maximum decrease in Pao_2 typically occurs 2 to 3 days postoperatively. Weaning from mechanical ventilation may be difficult because of increased work of breathing, decreased lung volumes, and ventilation/perfusion mismatching. The likelihood of deep vein thrombosis and pulmonary embolism is increased, which emphasizes the importance of early postoperative ambulation and the potential need for prophylactic anticoagulation. Obese patients tend not to be able to mobilize their fat stores during critical illness and need to rely on carbohydrates for energy. This increased carbohydrate metabolism raises the respiratory quotient and accelerates protein catabolism. If these patients take nothing by mouth for a prolonged period, a protein malnutrition syndrome may develop.

The incidence of obesity is increasing worldwide and with it comes adverse health consequences and increased health care costs. Continued efforts in research, education, and public awareness will help us better identify and understand the causes of obesity, improve management, discover new treatment modalities, and ultimately decrease the adverse impact of the obesity epidemic. Anesthetic management of patients with clinically severe obesity presents numerous challenges.

MALNUTRITION AND VITAMIN DEFICIENCIES

Malnutrition

Nutrients are essential for the maintenance of biochemical pathways that control systems such as cardiac function, respiration, immune responses, and cognition. Proteins are especially important for muscle and tissue synthesis, and their component amino acids have a wide range of biologic roles. Malnutrition results from an imbalance in nutritional intake or inadequate caloric support. It can be due to loss of appetite, overconsumption or underconsumption of nutrients in the diet, or malabsorption. Estimates suggest that malnourished patients have hospital stays 50% longer than well-nourished patients and are at higher risk of wound infection, immunosuppression, renal dysfunction, and other complications. Anemia and vitamin B_{12} deficiency further impair recovery. To minimize the risk of malnutrition, it is recommended that *all* patients admitted to a hospital be screened and monitored for signs of malnutrition. Biologic markers suggestive of malnutrition include serum albumin concentration of less than 3 g/dL, transferrin level of less than 200 mg/dL, and prealbumin level of less than 15 mg/dL. Cholesterol, zinc, iron, vitamin B_{12}, and folic acid levels may also be significantly reduced in malnourished patients. Of all these markers, prealbumin may be the most useful, because its half-life is only 2 days and changes in nutritional status can be detected quite early. However, prealbumin levels should always be measured in conjunction with C-reactive protein levels, since inflammation can raise the level of prealbumin and affect interpretation of results. In the presence of low levels of both prealbumin and C-reactive protein, it is likely that the patient is malnourished. Treatment of malnutrition is aimed at balancing nutritional intake with energy needs, depending on the level of activity or stress of the patient. If nutritional therapy is necessary, then enteral feeding or parenteral nutrition can be initiated.

ENTERAL NUTRITION

When the gastrointestinal tract is functioning, enteral nutrition can be provided by means of nasogastric or gastrostomy tube feedings or by postpyloric methods, such as nasojejunal tubes or feeding jejunostomy tubes. Continuous infusion is the usual method for administering enteral feedings. The rate, composition, and volume of the feeding solution will be individualized based on laboratory data. The question of when to stop postpyloric feedings in patients requiring surgery is still unclear. However, nasogastric and orogastric feedings should be stopped 8 hours before surgery and the stomach should be suctioned before the patient is taken to the operating room. Complications of enteral feedings are infrequent but include

TABLE 16-7 ■ Complications of total and peripheral parenteral nutrition

Hypokalemia
Hypophosphatemia
Bacterial translocation from the gastrointestinal tract
Renal dysfunction
Nonketotic hyperosmolar hyperglycemic coma
Hypomagnesemia
Venous thrombosis
Osteopenia
Hyperchloremic metabolic acidosis
Hypocalcemia
Infection, sepsis
Elevated liver enzyme levels
Fluid overload
Refeeding syndrome

hyperglycemia causing osmotic diuresis and hypovolemia. Exogenous insulin administration may be a consideration if blood glucose concentrations are elevated. The osmolarity of elemental diets (i.e., tube feedings) is high at 550 to 850 mOsm/L, and this often causes diarrhea.

PARENTERAL NUTRITION

Parenteral nutrition is indicated when the gastrointestinal tract is not functioning. *Peripheral parenteral nutrition* using an isotonic solution delivered through a peripheral vein is limited by osmolality and volume constraints. It may be useful as a supplement to oral intake or when the anticipated need for nutritional support is less than 14 days. *Total parenteral nutrition* (TPN) is used when the daily caloric requirements exceed 2000 kcal or prolonged nutritional support is required. In such cases a catheter is inserted into a central vein to permit infusion of hypertonic solutions in a daily volume of approximately 40 mL/kg.

Potential complications of TPN are numerous (Table 16-7). Blood glucose concentrations must be monitored, because hyperglycemia is very common and may require treatment with *exogenous* insulin. Hypoglycemia may occur if the TPN infusion is abruptly discontinued, since the increased circulating *endogenous* concentrations of insulin will persist. Hyperchloremic metabolic acidosis may occur because of the liberation of hydrochloric acid during the metabolism of amino acids present in most parenteral nutrition solutions. Parenteral feeding of patients with compromised cardiac function is associated with the risk of congestive heart failure from fluid overload. Increased production of carbon dioxide resulting from metabolism of large amounts of glucose may result in the need to initiate mechanical ventilation or failure to wean intubated patients.

Vitamin Deficiencies

Table 16-8 lists the more common vitamin deficiencies.

TABLE 16-8 ◼ Vitamin deficiencies

Vitamin deficiency	Causes of deficiency	Signs of deficiency
Thiamine (B_1) (beriberi)	Chronic alcoholism, which results in decreased intake of thiamine	Low systemic vascular resistance; high cardiac output; polyneuropathy (demyelination, sensory deficit, paresthesia); exaggerated blood pressure response to hemorrhage, change in body position, positive pressure ventilation
Riboflavin (B_2)	Almost always caused by dietary deficiency, photodegradation of milk or other dairy products	Magenta tongue, angular stomatitis, seborrhea, cheilosis
Niacin (B_3) (pellagra)	Carcinoid tumor; niacin (nicotinic acid) is synthesized from tryptophan; in carcinoid tumor, tryptophan is used to form serotonin instead of niacin, which makes patients with these tumors more susceptible to deficiency	Mental confusion, irritability, peripheral neuropathy, achlorhydria, diarrhea, vesicular dermatitis, stomatitis, glossitis, urethritis, excessive salivation
Pyridoxine (B_6)	Alcoholism, isoniazid therapy	Seborrhea, glossitis, convulsions, neuropathy, depression, confusion, microcytic anemia
Folate (B_9)	Alcoholism; therapy with sulfasalazine, pyrimethamine, or triamterene	Megaloblastic anemia, atrophic glossitis, depression, increased homocysteine level
Cyanocobalamin (B_{12})	Gastric atrophy (pernicious anemia), terminal ileal disease, strict vegetarianism	Megaloblastic anemia, loss of vibratory and positional sense, abnormal gait, dementia, impotence, loss of bladder and bowel control, increased levels of homocysteine and methylmalonic acid
Biotin	Ingestion of *raw* egg whites; contain the protein avidin, which strongly binds the vitamin and reduces its bioavailability	Mental changes (depression, hallucinations); paresthesias; a scaling rash around the eyes, nose, and mouth; alopecia
Ascorbic acid (C) (scurvy)	Smoking, alcoholism	Capillary fragility, petechial hemorrhage, joint and skeletal muscle hemorrhage, poor wound healing, catabolic state, loosened teeth and gangrenous alveolar margins, low potassium and iron levels
A	Dietary lack of leafy vegetables and animal liver, malabsorption	Loss of night vision, conjunctival drying, corneal destruction, anemia
D (rickets)	Limited sun exposure, inflammatory bowel disease and other fat malabsorption syndromes	Thoracic kyphosis, which can lead to hypoventilation; alkaline to less calcium absorption; parathyroid hormone activity, which leads to increased osteoclastic activity and bone resorption
E	Occurs only with fat malabsorption or genetic abnormalities of vitamin E metabolism or transport	Peripheral neuropathy, spinocerebellar ataxia, skeletal muscle atrophy, retinopathy
K	Prolonged antibiotic therapy that eliminates the intestinal bacteria that form the vitamin; failure of fat absorption	Bleeding

KEY POINTS

◼ Obesity is the most prevalent nutritional disease and is considered one of the most preventable causes of illness worldwide.

◼ Obesity leads to an increased incidence of glucose intolerance, diabetes mellitus, systemic hypertension, coronary artery diseases, heart failure, cancer, and thromboembolic events. A waist/hip ratio higher than 1.0 in men and 0.8 in women is a strong predictor of ischemic heart disease, stroke, diabetes, and death independent of total body fat.

◼ Compared with the normal-weight population, the risk of premature death is doubled and the risk of death resulting from cardiovascular disease is increased fivefold in the obese population.

◼ Bariatric surgery results in significant and sustained weight loss, as well as a diminution in obesity-related comorbid conditions. It is associated with a survival benefit.

◼ Regional anesthesia is the preferred method of primary anesthesia in the severely obese patient. Use of ultrasonography in clinical practice has significantly increased the success rate of regional anesthesia.

◼ Airway management is one of the greatest challenges associated with general anesthesia in obese patients. Mask ventilation is difficult due to the presence of increased soft tissues in the head, neck, and chest. The videolaryngoscope has improved the safety of tracheal intubation after induction of anesthesia. Therefore, awake intubations are now required less often.

- In the obese population, pneumoperitoneum during laparoscopic surgery may have a significant deleterious impact on cardiopulmonary performance as indicated by decreased cardiac output and stroke volume, increased systemic vascular resistance, and decreased FRC.
- The impact of obesity on appropriate dosing of intravenous anesthetic drugs is difficult to predict. A useful clinical approach is to calculate the initial dose of injected drug based on lean body weight rather than total body weight.
- A multimodal approach to postoperative pain control is usually employed to decrease the risk of opioid-induced respiratory depression in the obese patient.
- Current guidelines recommend screening and monitoring for signs of malnutrition in all patients admitted to the hospital. In situations in which oral intake is prohibited and treatment of malnutrition is needed, supplementation can be provided by initiating enteral or parenteral nutrition.

RESOURCES

Adams KF, Schatzkin A, Harris TB, et al. Overweight, obesity, and mortality in a large prospective cohort of persons 50 to 71 years old. *N Engl J Med.* 2006;355(8):763-778.

Bergland A, Gislason H, Raeder J. Fast-track surgery for bariatric laparoscopic gastric bypass with focus on anaesthesia and peri-operative care. Experience with 500 cases. *Acta Anaesthesiol Scand.* 2008;52:1394-1399.

Flegal KM, Carroll MD, Ogden CL, et al. Prevalence and trends in obesity among US adults, 1999-2008. *JAMA.* 2010;303:235-241.

Gonzalez H, Minville V, Delanoue K, et al. The importance of increased neck circumference to intubation difficulties in obese patients. *Anesth Analg.* 2008;106:1132-1136.

Haslam DW, James WPT. Obesity. *Lancet.* 2005;366:1197-1209.

Lemmens H. Perioperative pharmacology in morbid obesity. *Curr Opin Anaesthesiol.* 2010;23:485-491.

Levi D, Goodman ER, Patel M, et al. Critical care of the obese and bariatric surgical patient. *Crit Care Clin.* 2003;19:11-32.

McCullough PA, Gallagher MJ, Dejong AT, et al. Cardiorespiratory fitness and short-term complications after bariatric surgery. *Chest.* 2006;130:517-525.

Mears E. Outcomes of continuous process improvement of a nutritional care program incorporating serum prealbumin measurements. *Nutrition.* 1996;12:479-484.

Poirier P, Cornier MA, Mazzone T, et al. on behalf of the American Heart Association Obesity Committee of the Council on Nutrition and Physical Activity, and Metabolism. Bariatric surgery and cardiovascular risk factors: a scientific statement from the American Heart Association. *Circulation.* 2011;123:1683-1701.

Vasan RS. Editorial: cardiac function and obesity. *Heart.* 2003;89:1127-1129.

Renal Disease

NATALIE F. HOLT ■

The kidneys are responsible for, or contribute to, a number of essential functions, including water conservation, electrolyte homeostasis, acid-base balance, and several neurohumoral and hormonal functions. Knowing how the kidneys perform these important functions aids in understanding the clinical presentation, signs and symptoms, and treatment of renal diseases.

The kidneys are the most highly perfused organs in the body, receiving 20% to 25% of the cardiac output. Each kidney consists of approximately a million nephrons, each of which has distinct anatomic parts: Bowman's capsule, proximal tubule, loop of Henle, distal tubule, and collecting duct. Renal blood flow is autoregulated between mean arterial pressures of 50 and 150 mm Hg. A glomerulus, which is a tuft of capillaries, is surrounded by Bowman's capsule and is supplied by an afferent arteriole and drained by a slightly smaller efferent arteriole. The juxtaglomerular apparatus is a specialized structure between the afferent arteriole and distal tubule that contributes to the control of renal perfusion and extrarenal hemodynamics. The glomeruli filter the plasma at a rate of 180 L/day, allowing all but protein and polysaccharides to pass into the nephron. As the plasma flows along the nephron, virtually all the fluid and solutes are reabsorbed by a number of active and passive transport systems. The main function of the kidneys is water and sodium homeostasis, which are intimately linked and regulated by a number of feedback loops and hormonal controls.

TABLE 17-1 ■ Tests used to evaluate renal function

Test	Reference Value
GLOMERULAR FILTRATION RATE	
Blood urea nitrogen concentration	10-20 mg/dL
Serum creatinine concentration	0.6-1.3 mg/dL
Creatinine clearance	110-140 mL/min
Urine protein (albumin) excretion	<150 mg/day
RENAL TUBULAR FUNCTION AND/OR INTEGRITY	
Urine specific gravity	1.003-1.030
Urine osmolality	50-1400 mOsm/L
Urine sodium excretion	<40 mEq/L
Glucosuria	
Enzymuria	
N-Acetyl-β-glucosaminidase	
α-Glutathione S-transferase	
FACTORS THAT INFLUENCE INTERPRETATION	
Dehydration	
Variable protein intake	
Gastrointestinal bleeding	
Catabolism	
Advanced age	
Skeletal muscle mass	
Accurate timing of urine volume measurement	

TABLE 17-2 ■ Calculations used to measure or estimate glomerular filtration rate

CREATININE CLEARANCE

$$\text{Creatinine clearance (mL/min)} = (U_{Cr} \times U_{Volume}) / [P_{Cr} \times \text{time (min)}]$$

COCKCROFT-GAULT EQUATION

$$\text{GFR (mL/min)} = \{[(140 - \text{age}) \times \text{Lean body weight (kg)}] / (P_{Cr} \times 72)\} \times 0.85 \text{ (for women)}$$

MODIFICATION OF DIET IN RENAL DISEASE (MDRD) EQUATION

$$\text{GFR (mL/min/1.73m}^2) = 170 \times (P_{Cr})^{-0.999} \times (\text{Age})^{-0.176} \times (P_{BUN})^{-0.170} \times (P_{Albumin})^{0.318} \times 0.762 \text{ (for women)} \times 1.180 \text{ [for blacks]}$$

Adapted from Cockcroft DW, Gault MH. Prediction of creatinine clearance from serum creatinine. *Nephron*. 1976;16:31-41; and Levey AS, Bosch JP, Lewis JB, et al. A more accurate method to estimate glomerular filtration equation from serum creatinine: a new prediction equation. *Ann Intern Med*. 1999;130(6):461-470.

Urine and plasma concentrations of creatinine and BUN are measured in mg/dL. Plasma albumin concentration is measured in g/dL. Urine volume is measured in mL.

GFR, Glomerular filtration rate, $P_{Albumin}$, plasma albumin concentration; P_{BUN}, plasma urea nitrogen concentration; P_{Cr}, plasma creatinine concentration; U_{Cr}, urine creatinine concentration; U_{Volume}, urine volume.

CLINICAL ASSESSMENT OF RENAL FUNCTION

There are a number of tests that are useful in evaluating renal function and diagnosing disease (Table 17-1).

Glomerular Filtration Rate

The glomerular filtration rate (GFR) is considered the best measure of renal function, because it parallels the various functions of the nephrons. The GFR may be calculated from timed urine volumes plus urinary and plasma creatinine concentrations (creatinine clearance), or from direct measurements of the clearance of either endogenous or exogenous substances (creatinine and inulin, respectively). Alternatively, a number of formulas exist that estimate the GFR from various serum and urinary indices (Table 17-2). Normal values for GFR are 125 mL/min to 140 mL/min and vary with gender, body weight, and age. GFR decreases by approximately 1% per year after the age of 20.

Clinical manifestations of uremia generally appear when the GFR falls below 15 mL/min/1.73 m² (normal level is ≥90 mL/min/1.73 m²). Alterations in the GFR are also associated with predictable changes in erythropoietic activity.

Creatinine Clearance

Creatinine, an endogenous marker of renal filtration, is produced at a relatively constant rate by hepatic conversion of skeletal muscle creatinine. Creatinine is freely filtered by the kidney and is not reabsorbed. As a result, creatinine clearance is the most reliable measure of GFR (see Table 17-1).

Creatinine clearance does not depend on corrections for age or the presence of a steady state.

Serum Creatinine

Serum creatinine levels can be used as an estimate of the GFR. Normal serum creatinine concentrations range from 0.6 to 1.0 mg/dL in women and 0.8 to 1.3 mg/dL in men, which reflects differences in skeletal muscle mass. A number of factors (accelerated creatinine production, decreased tubular secretion of creatinine, presence of chromogens in the blood) can increase serum creatinine concentrations in the absence of a concomitant decrease in GFR. Conversely, small reductions in serum creatinine level can reflect large decreases in GFR. For example, the maintenance of normal serum creatinine concentrations in elderly patients with known decreases in the GFR reflects decreased creatinine production owing to the decreased skeletal muscle mass that accompanies aging. Serum creatinine values are also slow to reflect acute changes in renal function. For example, if acute renal failure occurs and the GFR decreases from 100 mL/min to 10 mL/min, serum creatinine values do not increase correspondingly for approximately 7 days.

Blood Urea Nitrogen

Blood urea nitrogen (BUN) concentrations vary with the GFR. Nevertheless, the influences of dietary intake, co-existing disease, and intravascular fluid volume on BUN concentrations make it potentially misleading as a test of renal function. For example, production of urea is increased by consumption of a high-protein diet or gastrointestinal bleeding, which results in increased BUN concentrations despite a normal GFR. Other causes of increased BUN concentrations despite a normal GFR include dehydration and increased catabolism, as occurs during a febrile illness. Increased BUN concentrations in the presence of dehydration most likely reflect increased urea absorption owing to slow movement of fluid through the renal tubules. When the latter is responsible for increased BUN concentrations, the serum creatinine levels remain normal. BUN concentrations can also remain normal with consumption of a low-protein diet (as in hemodialysis patients) despite decreases in the GFR. Even with these extraneous influences, however, BUN concentrations higher than 50 mg/dL usually reflect a decreased GFR.

Renal Tubular Function and Integrity

Renal tubular function is most often assessed by measuring the urine concentrating ability. The presence of proteinuria may reflect renal tubular damage. Enzymes present in the renal tubular cells (N-acetyl-β-D-glucosaminidase, α-glutathione S-transferase) may be detectable in the urine following sevoflurane anesthesia, which presumably reflects transient drug-induced tubular dysfunction that is not accompanied by changes in the BUN or serum creatinine concentrations.

URINE CONCENTRATING ABILITY

The diagnosis of renal tubular dysfunction is established by demonstrating that the kidneys do not produce appropriately concentrated urine in the presence of a physiologic stimulus for the release of antidiuretic hormone. In the absence of diuretic therapy or glucosuria, a urine-specific gravity higher than 1.018 suggests that the ability of renal tubules to concentrate urine is adequate. Treatment with diuretics or the presence of hypokalemia or hypercalcemia may interfere with the ability of renal tubules to concentrate urine. The inorganic fluoride resulting from metabolism of sevoflurane is theoretically capable of interfering with the urine concentrating ability of the renal tubules; however, the clinical significance of this observation has yet to be established.

PROTEINURIA

Proteinuria is relatively common and is present in 5% to 10% of tested adults during screening examinations. Transient proteinuria may be associated with fever, congestive heart failure, seizure activity, pancreatitis, and exercise. This form of proteinuria resolves with treatment of the underlying condition. Orthostatic proteinuria occurs in up to 5% of adolescents while in the upright position and disappears with recumbency. Generally, orthostatic proteinuria resolves spontaneously and is not associated with any deterioration in renal function. Persistent proteinuria generally connotes significant renal disease. Microalbuminuria is the earliest sign of diabetic nephropathy. Severe proteinuria may result in hypoalbuminemia, with associated decreases in plasma oncotic pressures and increases in unbound drug concentrations.

TABLE 17-3 ■ Calculation of fractional excretion of sodium (Fe_Na)

$$Fe_{Na}(\%) = [(P_{Cr} \times U_{Na}) / (P_{Na} \times U_{Cr})] \times 100$$

Urine and plasma concentrations of creatinine and sodium are measured in mg/dL.
P_{Cr}, Plasma creatinine concentration; P_{Na}, plasma sodium concentration; U_{Cr}, urine creatinine concentration; U_{Na}, urine sodium concentration.

FRACTIONAL EXCRETION OF SODIUM

The fractional excretion of sodium (Fe_Na) is a measure of the percentage of filtered sodium that is excreted in the urine (Table 17-3). It is most useful in differentiating between prerenal and renal causes of azotemia. An Fe_Na higher than 2% (or urinary sodium concentration of >40 mEq/L) reflects decreased ability of the renal tubules to conserve sodium and is consistent with tubular dysfunction. An Fe_Na of less than 1% (or urinary sodium excretion of <20 mEq/L) occurs when normally functioning renal tubules are conserving sodium and is suggestive of prerenal azotemia.

URINALYSIS

Examination of the urine is useful for diagnosing renal and urinary tract disease. Urinalysis is intended to detect the presence of protein, glucose, acetoacetate, blood, and leukocytes. The urine pH and solute concentrations (specific gravity) are determined, and sediment microscopy is used to identify the presence of cells, casts, microorganisms, and crystals. Hematuria may be caused by bleeding anywhere between the glomerulus and urethra. Microhematuria may be benign (focal nephritis) or may reflect glomerulonephritis, renal calculi, or cancer of the genitourinary tract. Joggers may experience transient hematuria, presumably as a result of trauma to the urinary tract. Sickle cell disease is a consideration in African Americans who exhibit hematuria. In the absence of protein or red blood cell casts in the urine, glomerular disease as a cause of hematuria is unlikely. Red blood cell casts are pathognomonic of acute glomerulonephritis. White blood cell casts are most commonly seen with pyelonephritis.

NOVEL BIOMARKERS OF RENAL FUNCTION

Cystatin C is a protein produced by all nucleated cells and freely filtered but not resorbed by the kidneys. Its serum concentration is independent of age, gender, or muscle mass, and for this reason it may turn out to be a better marker of GFR than serum creatinine concentration. Neutrophil gelatinase–associated lipocalin is a protein produced by renal tubular cells in response to injury and has shown promise as an early indicator of acute kidney injury.

ACUTE KIDNEY INJURY

Acute kidney injury (AKI) is characterized by deterioration of renal function over a period of hours to days, resulting in failure of the kidneys to excrete nitrogenous waste products and to maintain fluid and electrolyte homeostasis. Commonly used definitions of AKI include an increase in serum creatinine concentration of more than 0.5 mg/dL compared with the baseline value, a 50% decrease in the calculated creatinine clearance, or a change in serum creatinine concentration of greater than 0.3 mg/dL within 48 hours of an acute insult. AKI may be oliguric (urinary output < 400 mL/day) or nonoliguric (urinary output > 400 mL/day). Despite major advances in dialysis therapy and critical care, the mortality rate among patients with severe AKI requiring dialysis remains high. When AKI occurs in the setting of multiorgan failure, the mortality rate often exceeds 50%. The most common causes of death are sepsis, cardiovascular dysfunction, and pulmonary complications.

Etiology

The incidence of AKI depends on the definition used and the patient population studied. Some degree of AKI is thought to affect 5% to 7% of all hospitalized patients. AKI is associated with a number of other systemic diseases, acute clinical conditions, drug treatments, and interventional therapies. It almost invariably accompanies multiorgan failure syndromes in the critically ill patient population.

The causes of AKI are classically divided into prerenal, intrarenal (or intrinsic), and postrenal (Table 17-4). Azotemia is a condition marked by abnormally high serum concentrations of nitrogen-containing compounds such as BUN and creatinine, and is a hallmark of AKI, regardless of cause.

PRERENAL AZOTEMIA

Prerenal azotemia accounts for nearly half of hospital-acquired cases of AKI. Prerenal azotemia is rapidly reversible if the underlying cause is corrected. If left untreated, sustained prerenal azotemia is the most common factor that predisposes patients to ischemia-induced acute tubular necrosis. Elderly patients are uniquely susceptible to prerenal azotemia because of their predisposition to hypovolemia (poor fluid intake) and high incidence of renovascular disease. Among hospitalized patients, prerenal azotemia is often due to congestive heart failure, liver dysfunction, or septic shock. Reduced renal blood flow may be a result of anesthetic drug–induced decreases in perfusion pressure, particularly in the presence of hypovolemia and surgical blood loss.

Assessment of volume status, hemodynamics, and drug therapy is required to identify prerenal causes of acute oliguria. Invasive monitoring (central venous catheter, pulmonary artery catheter) may be necessary to assess intravascular volume status. Urinary indices are often helpful in distinguishing prerenal from intrinsic AKI (Table 17-5). The use of urinary indices is based on the assumption that the ability of renal tubules to reabsorb sodium and water is maintained in the presence of prerenal causes of AKI, whereas these functions are impaired in the presence of tubulointerstitial disease or acute tubular necrosis. Blood and urine specimens for determination of urinary indices must be obtained before

TABLE 17-4 ■ **Causes of acute kidney injury**

PRERENAL AZOTEMIA

Hemorrhage
Gastrointestinal fluid loss
Trauma
Surgery
Burns
Cardiogenic shock
Sepsis
Hepatic failure
Aortic or renal artery clamping
Thromboembolism

RENAL AZOTEMIA

Acute glomerulonephritis
Vasculitis
Interstitial nephritis (drug allergy, infiltrative diseases)
Acute tubular necrosis
    Ischemia
    Nephrotoxic drugs (aminoglycosides, nonsteroidal antiinflammatory drugs)
    Solvents (carbon tetrachloride, ethylene glycol)
    Heavy metals (mercury, cisplatin)
    Radiographic contrast dyes
    Myoglobinuria
    Intratubular crystals (uric acid, oxalate)

POSTRENAL AZOTEMIA

Nephrolithiasis
Benign prostatic hyperplasia
Clot retention
Bladder carcinoma

Adapted from Klahr S, Miller SB. Acute oliguria. *N Engl J Med.* 1998;338:671-675; and Thadhani R, Pascual M, Bonventre JV. Acute renal failure. *N Engl J Med.* 1996;334(22):1148-1169.

the administration of fluids, dopamine, mannitol, or other diuretic drugs.

RENAL AZOTEMIA

Intrinsic renal diseases that result in AKI are categorized according to the primary site of injury (glomerulus, renal tubules, interstitium, renal vasculature). Injury to the renal tubules is most often due to ischemia or nephrotoxins (aminoglycosides, radiographic contrast agents). Prerenal azotemia and ischemic tubular necrosis are a continuum, with the initial decreases in renal blood flow leading to ischemia of the renal tubular cells. Although some cases of ischemic AKI are reversible if the underlying cause is corrected, irreversible cortical necrosis occurs if the ischemia is severe or prolonged. Injury may also occur during reperfusion because of an influx of inflammatory cells, cytokines, and oxygen-free radicals.

Ischemia and toxins often combine to cause AKI in severely ill patients with conditions such as sepsis or acquired immunodeficiency syndrome (AIDS). AKI resulting from acute interstitial nephritis is most often caused by allergic reactions to drugs. Other causes of renal azotemia include glomerulonephritis, pyelonephritis, renal artery emboli, renal vein thrombosis, and vasculitis.

TABLE 17-5   Characteristic urinary indices in patients with acute oliguria resulting from prerenal or renal causes

Index	Prerenal causes	Renal causes
Urinary sodium concentration (mEq/L)	<20	>40
Urine osmolality (mOsm/kg)	>500	<400
Fractional excretion of sodium (%)	<1	>1
Ratio of blood urea nitrogen to creatinine concentration	>20	10-20
Ratio of urine to plasma creatinine concentration	>40	<20
Ratio of urine to plasma osmolarity	>1.5	<1.1
Sediment	Normal, occasional hyaline casts	Renal tubular epithelial cells, granular casts

Adapted from Klahr S, Miller SB. Acute oliguria. *N Engl J Med*. 1998;338(10):671-675; and Schrier RW, Wang W, Poole B, et al. Acute renal failure: definition, diagnosis, pathogenesis, and therapy. *J Clin Invest*. 2004;114(1):5-14.

POSTRENAL AZOTEMIA

AKI occurs when urinary outflow tracts are obstructed, as with prostatic hyperplasia or cancer of the prostate or cervix. It is important to diagnose postrenal causes of AKI promptly, because the potential for recovery is inversely related to the duration of the obstruction. Renal ultrasonography is often useful for determining the presence of obstructive nephropathy. Percutaneous nephrostomy can relieve obstruction and improve outcomes.

Risk Factors

Risk factors for the development of AKI include preexisting renal disease, advanced age, congestive heart failure, peripheral vascular disease, diabetes, emergency surgery, and major operative procedures such as coronary revascularization and aortic aneurysm repair (Table 17-6). Sepsis and multiple organ system dysfunction resulting from trauma introduce the risk of AKI. Iatrogenic components that predispose to AKI include inadequate fluid replacement, hypotension, delayed treatment of sepsis, and administration of nephrotoxic drugs or dyes.

Appropriate hydration and optimal preservation of the intravascular fluid volume are essential to maintain renal perfusion. It is also important to maintain adequate systemic blood pressure and cardiac output and to prevent peripheral vasoconstriction. Hypotension may result in inadequate renal perfusion and loss of renal autoregulation. Potentially nephrotoxic substances (nonsteroidal antiinflammatory drugs, aminoglycosides, radiographic contrast dyes) are logically avoided in patients with prerenal oliguria, and diuretic therapy is contraindicated.

TABLE 17-6   Risk factors for perioperative renal failure

Advanced age	High-risk surgical procedures
Preexisting renal insufficiency	Renal vascularization
Congestive heart failure	Aortic cross-clamping
Diabetic nephropathy	Cardiopulmonary bypass
Hypertensive nephropathy	Urologic surgery
Liver failure	Transplantation
Pregnancy-induced hypertension	Trauma
Sepsis	Nephrotoxins
Shock	Aminoglycoside antibiotics
	Radiocontrast dyes
	Nonsteroidal antiinflammatory drugs

Adapted from Sladen RN. Oliguria in the ICU: systemic approach to diagnosis and treatment. *Anesthesiol Clin North Am*. 2000;18(4):739-752.

Diagnosis

Signs and symptoms of AKI are often absent in the early stages, and a high degree of suspicion is required to identify subtle changes that accompany the development of AKI. Patients may show generalized malaise or demonstrate evidence of fluid overload such as dyspnea, edema, and hypertension. As protein and amino acid metabolites accumulate, patients become lethargic, nauseated, and confused. Hyperkalemia and acidosis may affect cardiac rhythm and contractility. Encephalopathy, coma, seizures, and death may ensue. Other signs and symptoms of AKI are associated with its specific cause, such as hypotension, jaundice, hematuria, or urinary retention.

The diagnosis of AKI is usually made based on laboratory data demonstrating an acute increase in serum creatinine concentration. Urinary output may or may not fall, and depending on this, the term *oliguric* or *nonoliguric* is used to qualify AKI. There are a number of definitions of oliguria, the most common of which is less than 0.5 mL/kg/hr or less than 400 mL/day. Anuria is defined as less than 100 mL/day, with complete anuria being very unusual.

Urinalysis is often helpful in diagnosing whether the cause of AKI is prerenal, intrarenal, or postrenal (see Table 17-4).

Complications

Complications of AKI manifest in the central nervous, cardiovascular, hematologic, and gastrointestinal systems. Metabolic derangements are also common. In addition, infections occur frequently in patients who develop AKI and are leading causes of morbidity and mortality.

Neurologic complications of AKI include confusion, asterixis, somnolence, seizures, and polyneuropathy. These changes appear to be related to the build-up of protein and amino acids in the blood, and symptoms may be ameliorated by dialysis.

Cardiovascular complications include systemic hypertension, congestive heart failure, and pulmonary edema, principally as reflections of sodium and water retention. The presence of congestive heart failure or pulmonary edema suggests the need to decrease the intravascular fluid volume. Cardiac dysrhythmias may develop; peaked T waves and widened QRS complexes are indicative of hyperkalemia. Uremic pericarditis may also occur.

Hematologic complications include anemia and coagulopathy. Hematocrit values between 20% and 30% are common as a result of hemodilution and decreased erythropoietin production. Patients with renal insufficiency are also at increased risk of bleeding complications caused by uremia-induced platelet dysfunction. Preoperative dialysis may be indicated in high-risk patients. Alternatively, 1-desamino-8-D-arginine vasopressin (desmopressin [DDAVP]) can be administered preoperatively to temporarily increase concentrations of von Willebrand factor (vWF) and factor VIII and improve coagulation.

Metabolic derangements include hyperkalemia and metabolic acidosis. Sodium and water retention result in hypertension and edema. Frequent monitoring of arterial blood gas concentrations and electrolyte levels is indicated.

Gastrointestinal complications include anorexia, nausea, vomiting, and ileus. Gastrointestinal bleeding occurs in as many as one third of patients who develop AKI and may contribute to anemia. Gastroparesis may occur as a result of uremia. Administration of histamine-2 (H_2) receptor antagonists and/or proton pump inhibitors may decrease the risk of gastrointestinal bleeding.

Infection commonly affects the respiratory and urinary tracts and sites where breaks in normal anatomic barriers have occurred because of indwelling catheters. Impaired immune responses resulting from uremia may contribute to the increased likelihood of infections in patients with AKI.

Treatment

There are no specific treatment modalities for AKI. Management is aimed at limiting further renal injury and correcting fluid, electrolyte, and acid-base derangements. Underlying causes should be sought and terminated or reversed, if possible. Specifically, hypovolemia, hypotension, and low cardiac output should be corrected and sepsis treated. A mean arterial pressure of 65 mm Hg should be attained, but there is no evidence supporting a better outcome with supraphysiologic values of either systemic pressure or cardiac output.

Fluid resuscitation and vasopressor therapy are universally emphasized in the prevention and treatment of AKI. There is no evidence to support the use of colloid over crystalloid. In fact, administration of hydroxyethyl starch has been shown in some studies to exacerbate renal injury. Traditionally, 0.9% saline was the preferred crystalloid for use in patients with renal dysfunction because it lacks potassium. However, recent research suggests that it may cause hyperchloremic metabolic acidosis and secondarily lead to hyperkalemia. Therefore, lactated Ringer's or other bicarbonate-containing balanced salt solutions may be a better choice.

With regard to the use of vasopressors in the treatment of AKI associated with sepsis, concern has been expressed that renal vasoconstriction may exacerbate tubular injury. It is true that α_1-agonists such as norepinephrine reduce renal blood flow in healthy volunteers. However, in patients with sepsis-related AKI, their effects depend on the balance of a variety of factors. In general, it appears that improved systemic pressure is accompanied by reduced renal sympathetic tone and vasodilation, and in this context, direct α_1-agonist–mediated renal vasoconstriction is of minor importance. Therefore, the overall effect of using norepinephrine in septic patients is to increase the GFR and urinary output. Arginine vasopressin is an alternative to traditional vasopressors in the treatment of septic shock and may be effective when other agents have failed. This drug appears to selectively constrict renal efferent arterioles; therefore, it may help preserve the GFR and urinary output better than α_1-agonists. However, its superiority in the management of septic shock has yet to be demonstrated.

The use of dopamine either to treat or to prevent AKI is not supported by the literature; in fact, dopamine use has been associated with a number of undesirable side effects. Fenoldopam is a dopamine analogue with exclusively dopamine-1 agonist activity. At low dosages, fenoldopam causes renal vasodilation, whereas at higher dosages, peripheral vasodilation occurs. Preliminary evidence suggests that fenoldopam provides renal protection in patients at high risk who are undergoing cardiac, vascular, and transplant surgery.

The practice of trying to convert oliguric to nonoliguric AKI by using diuretics is not advised and may actually increase mortality risk and permanent renal injury. However, the incidence of posttransplantation acute tubular necrosis may be lower in patients treated with mannitol plus hydration than in those treated with hydration alone. The mechanism of action presumably relates to mannitol's ability to cause renal vasodilation through the production of renal prostaglandins. Mannitol is also commonly used in the treatment of pigment-induced nephropathies; however, clinical evidence of its benefits in this context is weak.

Prophylactic administration of *N*-acetylcysteine, a thio-containing antioxidant that acts as a free radical scavenger, may provide protection against radiographic dye–induced nephropathy. However, because of conflicting data and the risk of complications such as anaphylactoid reactions, it is not universally recommended.

Alkalinization of urine with sodium bicarbonate is helpful in the treatment of pigment-induced nephropathy such as that caused by rhabdomyolysis, because it increases the solubility of myoglobin and prevents the formation of tubular precipitates. Prophylactic administration of sodium bicarbonate also appears to reduce the incidence of contrast-induced nephropathy by decreasing the formation of damaging free radicals.

In severe sepsis, administration of activated protein C and steroid replacement (in those patients who demonstrate adrenal insufficiency) may reduce mortality.

TABLE 17-7 ■ Analgesic dosage adjustments in patients with renal insufficiency

Drug	Adjustment method	GFR > 50 mL/min	GFR 10-50 mL/min	GFR < 10 mL/min
Acetaminophen	↑ Interval	q4h	q6h	q8h
Acetylsalicylic acid	↑ Interval	q4h	q4-6h	Avoid
Alfentanil	↔ Dose	100%	100%	100%
Codeine	↓ Dose	100%	75%	50%
Fentanyl	↓ Dose	100%	75%	50%
Ketorolac	↓ Dose	100%	50%	25%-50%
Meperidine	↓ Dose	100%	75%	50%
Methadone	↓ Dose	100%	100%	50%–75%
Morphine	↓ Dose	100%	75%	50%
Remifentanil	↔ Dose	100%	100%	100%
Sufentanil	↔ Dose	100%	100%	100%

Adapted from Schrier RW, ed. *Manual of Nephrology.* 7th ed. Philadelphia, PA: Lippincott Williams & Wilkins; 2009.
↑, Increase; ↓, decrease; ↔, no change; *GFR*, glomerular filtration rate.

Dialysis (also known as *hemofiltration* or *renal replacement therapy*) is still the mainstay of treatment for severe AKI. There are five main indications for its use: volume overload, hyperkalemia, severe metabolic acidosis, symptomatic uremia, and overdose with a dialyzable drug. Two dialysis methods exist: hemodialysis and peritoneal dialysis. The purpose of both is to remove excess fluid and solutes from the blood and optimize electrolyte balance. Dialysis may be performed as a continuous or intermittent therapy, and controversy exists as to whether one or the other method is superior.

Prognosis

The overall prognosis for hospital-acquired AKI is poor. Many AKI study series report mortality rates of more than 20%, and once dialysis is required, mortality rates are invariably in excess of 50%. Those who succumb usually die of failure of other organ systems after prolonged and complex hospital courses. Only about 15% of patients developing AKI will fully recover renal function. Five percent of AKI patients will retain a degree of renal insufficiency that remains stable, and another 5% will experience continued deterioration of renal function throughout the remainder of their lives. Fifteen percent will be left with stable renal insufficiency for a period but remain at high risk of developing chronic renal failure later in life.

Drug Dosing in Patients with Renal Impairment

Renal impairment affects most of the organ systems of the body and, consequently, the pharmacology of many drugs. Selecting drugs that do not rely on the kidneys for excretion is ideal but not always possible.

The first step in tailoring drug dosing for patients with renal impairment is to estimate the creatinine clearance, since the rate of elimination of drugs excreted by the kidneys is proportional to the GFR. If the patient is oliguric, the creatinine clearance can be approximated by a value of 5 mL/min. If the normal drug regimen starts with a loading dose to rapidly achieve therapeutic levels, the following guidelines may be used: If after clinical examination, the extracellular fluid volume appears to be normal, use the loading dose suggested for patients with normal renal function. If the extracellular fluid is contracted, reduce the loading dose. If the extracellular fluid is expanded, use a higher loading dose. There are also formulas to calculate loading and maintenance doses based on renal function, depending on either the fraction of drug excreted in the urine or the difference in drug half-life in patients with normal renal function and those with impaired function.

For medications with wide therapeutic ranges or long plasma half-lives, the interval between doses is generally increased. For medications with narrow therapeutic ranges or short plasma half-lives, reduced doses at normal intervals are advised. In reality, a combination of the two methods of dosage adjustment is frequently used (Table 17-7).

Management of Anesthesia

Because of the high morbidity and mortality, only lifesaving surgery should be undertaken in patients with AKI. The principles that guide the management of anesthesia are the same as those that guide supportive treatment of AKI, namely, maintenance of an adequate systemic blood pressure and cardiac output and the avoidance of further renal insults, including hypovolemia, hypoxia, and exposure to nephrotoxins. Invasive hemodynamic monitoring is mandatory, as are frequent blood gas analyses and electrolyte measurements.

In general, the administration of diuretics to maintain urine output in those patients who are not oliguric has not been shown to improve either renal outcome or patient survival. However, when a dilutional anemia has been caused by overzealous hydration, use of diuretics may minimize the risk of fluid overload caused by the administration of blood or

TABLE 17-8 ■ **Causes of chronic kidney disease**

Glomerulopathies
   Primary glomerular disease
   Focal glomerulosclerosis
   Membranoproliferative glomerulonephritis
   Membranous nephropathy
   Immunoglobulin A nephropathy
   Diabetes mellitus
   Amyloidosis
   Postinfective glomerulonephritis
   Systemic lupus erythematosus
   Wegener's granulomatosis
Tubulointerstitial diseases
   Analgesic nephropathy
   Reflux nephropathy with pyelonephritis
   Myeloma kidney
   Sarcoidosis
Heredity diseases
   Polycystic kidney disease
   Alport's syndrome
   Medullary cystic disease
Systemic hypertension
Renal vascular disease
Obstructive uropathy
Human immunodeficiency virus infection

Adapted from Tolkoff-Rubin NE, Pascual M. Chronic renal failure. *Sci Am Med.* 1998:1-12.

TABLE 17-9 ■ **Stages of chronic kidney disease**

Stage	Description	GFR (mL/min/1.73 m^2)
1	Kidney damage with normal or increased GFR	≥90
2	Kidney damage with mildly decreased GFR	60-89
3	Moderately decreased GFR	30-59
4	Severely decreased GFR	15-29
5	Kidney failure	<15 or dialysis

Adapted from National Kidney Foundation. KDOQI clinical practice guidelines for chronic kidney disease: evaluation, classification, and stratification. Available at: http://www.kidney.org/professionals/kdoqi/guidelines_ckd/toc.htm. Accessed August 5, 2011.
Chronic kidney disease is defined as either the presence of kidney damage or a GFR of <60 mL/min/1.73 m^2 for ≥3 mo. Kidney damage may be diagnosed based on evidence of a pathologic abnormality, laboratory biomarkers, or imaging studies.
GFR, Glomerular filtration rate.

blood products. For patients who meet the criteria, postoperative dialysis should be initiated as soon as the patient is in hemodynamically stable condition.

CHRONIC KIDNEY DISEASE

Chronic kidney disease (CKD) is the progressive, irreversible deterioration of renal function that results from a wide variety of diseases (Table 17-8). In the United States, diabetes mellitus is the leading cause of end-stage renal disease (ESRD), followed closely by systemic hypertension. The clinical manifestations of CKD are typically independent of the initial insult and instead reflect the overall inability of the kidneys to excrete nitrogenous waste products, regulate fluid and electrolyte balance, and secrete hormones. In most patients, regardless of the cause, a decrease in the GFR to less than 25 mL/min eventually progresses to ESRD requiring dialysis or transplantation (Table 17-9).

The best source of data on the incidence and etiology of CKD and ESRD is the U.S. Renal Data System of the National Institutes of Health. According to these data, in 2008 the prevalence of ESRD reached 1699 per million, or approximately half a million individuals. Prevalence continues to increase, partly due to aging of the population and partly because patients with ESRD are surviving longer. However, the incidence of ESRD has flattened and is quoted as 351 per million in 2008, or more than 112,000 individuals.

There are striking racial and ethnic variations in the incidence and prevalence of ESRD. Based on data from 2008, the incidence of ESRD among African American and Native American populations is 3.6 and 1.8 times greater, respectively, than the rate among whites. The rate of ESRD among Hispanics is 1.5 times higher than among non-Hispanics. Furthermore, African Americans and Hispanics tend to reach ESRD at a younger age than whites. Hypertensive nephropathy accounts for a relatively higher proportion of ESRD cases among African Americans compared with other racial or ethnic groups. A combination of genetic variables and disparities in health care access are likely to underlie these differences.

Diagnosis

Signs of CKD are often undetectable (Table 17-10). When symptoms do appear, complaints are nonspecific, such as fatigue, malaise, and anorexia. In most patients the diagnosis is made during routine testing. In addition to serum creatinine level, urinary sediment analysis is helpful in establishing the diagnosis and possible cause of renal dysfunction.

Progression of Chronic Kidney Disease

Intrarenal hemodynamic changes (glomerular hypertension, glomerular hyperfiltration and permeability changes, glomerulosclerosis) are likely responsible for progression of renal disease. Decreases in both systemic and glomerular hypertension can be achieved by the administration of angiotensin-converting enzyme (ACE) inhibitors and/or angiotensin receptor blockers (ARBs). In addition to having beneficial effects on intraglomerular hemodynamics and systemic pressures, ACE inhibitors and ARBs have renoprotective effects that manifest as reductions in proteinuria and slowing of the progression of glomerulosclerosis in patients with diabetic and nondiabetic nephropathy. Other antihypertensive drugs that lower the systemic pressure to similar degrees do not provide comparable renoprotective effects.

TABLE 17-10   Manifestations of chronic kidney disease

Electrolyte imbalances
  Hyperkalemia
  Hypermagnesemia
  Hyperphosphatemia
  Hypocalcemia
Metabolic acidosis
Unpredictable intravascular fluid volume status
Anemia
  Increased cardiac output
  Rightward shift of oxyhemoglobin dissociation curve
Uremic coagulopathy
  Increased bleeding time
  Platelet dysfunction
Neurologic changes
  Autonomic dysfunction
  Encephalopathy
  Peripheral neuropathy
Cardiovascular changes
  Congestive heart failure
  Dyslipidemia
  Systemic hypertension
Renal osteodystrophy
Pruritus

In animal models, protein intake can influence the progression of renal disease, and consequently, moderate protein restriction is recommended for all patients with renal insufficiency. In patients who are diabetic, strict control of blood glucose concentrations can delay the onset of proteinuria and slow the progression of nephropathy, neuropathy, and retinopathy. There is no evidence in humans that restricting dietary phosphate or lipid intake slows the progression of renal disease.

Adaptation to Chronic Kidney Disease

Normally functioning kidneys precisely regulate the concentrations of solutes and water in the extracellular fluid despite large variations in daily dietary intake. Because of substantial renal reserve function, patients with CKD often remain relatively asymptomatic until renal function is less than 10% of normal.

The kidneys demonstrate three stages of adaptation to progressive impairment of renal function. The first stage involves substances such as creatinine and urea, which are dependent largely on glomerular filtration for urinary excretion. As the GFR decreases, the plasma concentrations of these substances begin to rise, but the increase is not directly proportional to the degree of GFR impairment. For example, serum creatinine concentrations frequently remain within normal limits despite a 50% decrease in GFR. Beyond a certain point, however, when the renal reserve has been exhausted, even minimal further decreases in the GFR can result in significant increases in the serum creatinine and urea concentrations.

The second stage of adaptation to progressive renal impairment is seen with solutes such as potassium. Serum potassium concentrations are maintained within normal limits until GFR approaches 10% of normal, at which point hyperkalemia manifests. As nephrons are lost, the remaining nephrons increase their secretion of potassium through increased blood flow and increased sodium delivery to the collecting tubules. In addition, because aldosterone secretion increases in patients with renal failure, there is a greater loss of potassium through the gastrointestinal tract. This system of enhanced gastrointestinal secretion is an effective compensatory mechanism in the presence of normal dietary intake of potassium but can be easily overwhelmed by an acute exogenous potassium load (e.g., administration of potassium, such as during the perioperative period) or acute endogenous potassium load (e.g., hemolysis, tissue trauma such as that associated with surgery).

The third stage of adaptation involves sodium homeostasis and regulation of the extracellular fluid compartment volume. In contrast to the levels of other solutes, sodium balance remains intact despite progressive deterioration in renal function and variations in dietary intake. Nevertheless, the system can be overwhelmed by abruptly increased sodium intake (resulting in volume overload) or decreased sodium intake (resulting in volume depletion).

Complications

UREMIC SYNDROME

Uremic syndrome is a constellation of signs and symptoms (anorexia, nausea, vomiting, pruritus, anemia, fatigue, coagulopathy) that reflect the kidney's progressive inability to perform its excretory, secretory, and regulatory functions. Although it is questionable whether urea itself produces the signs and symptoms (except at high concentrations), the BUN concentration is a useful clinical indicator of the severity of the uremic syndrome and the patient's response to therapy. This is in contrast to the serum creatinine concentration, which correlates poorly with uremic symptoms. Traditional treatment of uremic syndrome is dietary protein restriction to decrease protein catabolism and urea production.

RENAL OSTEODYSTROPHY

Changes in bone structure and mineralization are common in patients with progressive CKD. The most important factors are secondary hyperparathyroidism and decreased vitamin D production by the kidneys. Decreased vitamin D production by the kidneys impairs intestinal absorption of calcium. Hypocalcemia stimulates parathyroid hormone (PTH) secretion, which leads to bone resorption to restore serum calcium concentrations. As the GFR decreases, there is a parallel decrease in phosphate clearance and an increase in serum phosphate concentrations. This results in reciprocal decreases in serum calcium concentrations. Radiographs demonstrate evidence of bone demineralization. Further evidence of bone resorption is the presence of increased serum alkaline phosphatase concentrations. Treatment of renal osteodystrophy is intended to prevent skeletal complications and includes restriction of dietary phosphate intake and oral calcium and vitamin D supplementation. Antacids may be administered to bind phosphorus in the gastrointestinal tract; however, magnesium-containing antacids introduce the risk of hypermagnesemia, and aluminum-containing antacids are equally undesirable. If medical therapies fail to control hypocalcemia resulting from secondary hyperparathyroidism, subtotal parathyroidectomy is often recommended.

Accumulation of aluminum in patients undergoing long-term renal dialysis, although decreasing in frequency, may result in bone pain, fractures, and weakness. Hyperparathyroidism seems to protect against aluminum-induced bone disease. If aluminum toxicity is present, deferoxamine chelation therapy is helpful.

ANEMIA

Anemia frequently accompanies CKD and is presumed to be responsible for many of the symptoms (fatigue, weakness, decreased exercise tolerance) characteristic of uremic syndrome. This anemia is normochromic and normocytic, and is due primarily to decreased erythropoietin production by the kidneys. Excess PTH appears also to contribute to anemia by replacing bone marrow with fibrous tissue.

The anemia of CKD is treated with recombinant human erythropoietin or darbepoetin. Blood transfusions are avoided if possible, because the resultant sensitization to antigens of the human leukocyte antigen (HLA) complex makes future kidney transplantation less successful. Intermittent injections of parenteral iron are recommended to maximize the response to erythropoietin. The development or exacerbation of systemic hypertension is a risk of erythropoietin administration.

UREMIC BLEEDING

Patients with CKD have an increased tendency to bleed despite the presence of a normal platelet count, prothrombin time, and plasma thromboplastin time. The bleeding time is the screening test that best correlates with the tendency to bleed. Hemorrhagic episodes (gastrointestinal bleeding, epistaxis, hemorrhagic pericarditis, subdural hematoma) are significant sources of morbidity in patients with CKD and contribute to persistent anemia.

Treatment of uremic bleeding may include the administration of cryoprecipitate to provide factor VIII–vWF complex or the use of desmopressin. A significant deterrent to the use of cryoprecipitate is the risk of viral disease transmission. Desmopressin, an analogue of antidiuretic hormone, increases circulating levels of factor VIII–vWF complex and thereby improves coagulation. In patients with uremia, the intravenous infusion or subcutaneous injection of desmopressin is particularly useful for preventing clinical hemorrhage when invasive procedures such as surgery are planned. Desmopressin is fast acting and short-lived. The maximal effect is present within 2 to 4 hours and lasts for about 6 to 8 hours. Tachyphylaxis appears to develop with repeat doses and may be related to depletion of endothelial stores of vWF (Table 17-11).

TABLE 17-11 ◼ **Treatment of uremic bleeding**

Drug	Dosage	Onset of effect	Peak effect	Duration of effect
Cryoprecipitate	10 units IV over 30 min	<1 hr	4-12 hr	12-18 hr
Desmopressin (DDAVP)	0.3 mcg/kg IV or SC	<1 hr	2-4 hr	6-8 hr
Conjugated estrogen	0.6 mg/kg/day IV for 5 days	6 hr	5-7 days	14 days

Adapted from Tolkoff-Rubin NE, Pascual M. Chronic renal failure. *Sci Am Med.* 1998:1-12.
IV, Intravenous; *SC,* subcutaneous.

Conjugated estrogens have also been shown to improve bleeding times in patients with uremia. The time to onset of action is about 6 hours, but the effects last for 14 to 21 days. It has also been observed that erythropoietin shortens bleeding times by enhancing platelet aggregation and increasing platelet counts.

NEUROLOGIC CHANGES

Neurologic changes may be early manifestations of progressive renal insufficiency. Initially, symptoms may be mild (impaired abstract thinking, insomnia, irritability), but as renal disease progresses, more significant changes (seizures, obtundation, uremic encephalopathy, coma) may develop. A disabling complication of advanced renal failure is the development of a distal, symmetrical mixed motor and sensory polyneuropathy, marked by paresthesias or hyperesthesias or distal weakness of the lower extremities. The arms may also be affected, but the incidence is less than in the legs. Diabetic neuropathy may be superimposed on uremic neuropathy. Hemodialysis may improve some aspects of uremic encephalopathy and reduce the severity of peripheral neurologic symptoms.

CARDIOVASCULAR CHANGES

Systemic hypertension is the most significant risk factor accompanying CKD and contributes to the congestive heart failure, coronary artery disease, and cerebrovascular disease that occur in these patients. Uncontrolled systemic hypertension also speeds the progression of renal dysfunction. The pathogenesis of systemic hypertension in these patients involves intravascular volume expansion resulting from retention of sodium and water and activation of the renin-angiotensin-aldosterone system.

Dyslipidemias are common at all stages of CKD and increase the risk of cardiovascular morbidity and mortality. Along with lifestyle and dietary modifications, therapy is advised when fasting triglyceride levels are 500 mg/dL or higher and/or low-density lipoprotein levels are 100 mg/dL or more.

Silent myocardial ischemia is probably common due to peripheral neuropathy. Chemical stress testing may be preferred to exercise stress testing, because patients in renal failure are often unable to exercise adequately. However, dipyridamole thallium testing may be less accurate in patients with uremia, probably as a result of decreased sensitivity of the microvasculature to dipyridamole. The baseline electrocardiogram may be altered by metabolic derangements. For unknown reasons, baseline plasma creatine kinase concentrations are commonly increased in patients with CKD. Because this increase is accounted for principally by the MM isoenzyme, the value of the MB fraction for diagnosis of an acute myocardial infarction remains intact.

Dialysis is the indicated treatment for patients who are hypertensive because of hypervolemia (volume is removed to attain "dry weight") and those who develop uremic pericarditis. Dialysis is less likely to control systemic hypertension because of activation of the renin-angiotensin-aldosterone system. Increasing dosages of antihypertensive drugs are recommended for these patients. ACE inhibitors are used cautiously in patients in whom GFR is dependent on increased efferent arteriolar vasoconstriction (bilateral renal artery stenosis, transplanted kidney with unilateral stenosis), which is mediated by angiotensin II. Administration of ACE inhibitors to these patients can result in efferent arteriolar dilation and decreased GFR, leading to a sudden deterioration in renal function.

Cardiac tamponade and hemodynamic instability associated with uremic pericarditis is an indication for prompt drainage of the effusion, often via placement of a percutaneous pericardial catheter. In occasional patients, surgical drainage with creation of a pericardial window or pericardiectomy is necessary. The development of hypotension unresponsive to intravascular fluid volume replacement may be an important clue that cardiac tamponade is present.

Treatment

Management of patients with CKD includes aggressive treatment of the underlying cause, pharmacologic therapy to delay disease progression and prevent complications, and preparation for renal replacement therapy as ESRD ensues.

BLOOD PRESSURE

Since hypertension is both a cause and a consequence of CKD and is directly correlated with deterioration of renal function, blood pressure control is imperative. Hypertension in CKD is difficult to treat, and most patients require therapy with three or more antihypertensive agents to achieve target blood pressure (<130/80 mm Hg). Considering that a driving force in the pathophysiology of CKD is the renin-angiotensin-aldosterone system, most guidelines recommend treatment with either ACE inhibitors or ARBs, whether or not hypertension is present. Treatment with these agents has been shown in many clinical trials to decrease proteinuria, slow the progression of renal dysfunction, and reduce mortality and cardiac events.

β-Blockers (specifically carvedilol) and diuretics are also commonly used.

NUTRITION

A number of studies involving both diabetic and nondiabetic patients with CKD have demonstrated that modest protein restriction reduces the progression of renal disease. However, an overly restrictive diet places patients at risk for malnutrition and its associated complications. A daily protein intake of 0.6 to 0.8 mg/kg is currently advised.

Dietary phosphorus should be restricted to 800 to 1000 mg/day when serum phosphorus or PTH levels are elevated. Phosphate binders are used when dietary restriction alone is ineffective. Vitamin D supplementation is also sometimes used to help normalize phosphorus and calcium levels. In patients with advanced disease and chronic metabolic acidosis, administration of alkali salts is advised. Sodium intake should be restricted to less than 2.4 g/day to prevent hypertension and fluid overload.

Long-term follow-up of diabetic patients with CKD has shown that euglycemia is associated with reversal of the typical lesions seen in diabetic nephropathy and a reduction in proteinuria. However, this is a long-term change, and the benefits may not manifest for 5 to 10 years. Current guidelines recommend a glycosylated hemoglobin level of less than 7%. Metformin is recommended for most patients with type 2 diabetes and stable stage 1, 2, or 3 CKD. However, owing to the risk of lactic acid accumulation, metformin should be discontinued if there are acute changes in renal function or the patient is at risk of such changes, such as during illness or in the perioperative period.

ANEMIA

Anemia often accompanies CKD and is associated with a decreased health-related quality of life. The decision to initiate treatment should be individualized, with consideration of the potential benefits and risks of therapy. Anemia is responsive to treatment with erythropoietin in all stages of CKD. In general, the target hemoglobin level should be in the range of 11 to 12 mg/dL.

RENAL REPLACEMENT THERAPY

Dialysis is usually advised when the GFR reaches 15 mL/min/1.73 m^2 or less. There is clear evidence that the dialysis dose is significantly correlated with survival. Since clinical signs and symptoms are not reliable indicators of dialysis adequacy, the delivered dose should be measured and monitored routinely (Table 17-12). Dialysis dose can be calculated from a number of different formulas or models. All of them essentially measure the clearance of urea by estimating the difference in predialysis and postdialysis plasma BUN levels. Urea is used to calculate dialysis dose because it is a small, readily dialyzed solute that accounts for 90% of the waste nitrogen that accumulates between hemodialysis treatments. Furthermore, the fractional clearance of urea has been shown to correlate with morbidity and mortality in dialysis patients.

TABLE 17-12	Findings suggestive of inadequate hemodialysis

CLINICAL

Anorexia, nausea, vomiting
Poor nutritional status
Depressed sensorium
Pericarditis
Ascites
Minimal weight gain or weight loss between treatments
Fluid retention and systemic hypertension

CHEMICAL

Decrease in blood urea nitrogen concentration during hemodialysis of <65%
Albumin concentration of <4 g/dL
Predialysis blood urea concentration of <50 mg/dL (a sign of malnutrition)
Predialysis serum creatinine concentration of <5 mg/dL (a sign of malnutrition)
Persistent anemia (hematocrit <30%) despite erythropoietin therapy

Adapted from Ifudu O. Care of patients undergoing hemodialysis. *N Engl J Med.* 1998;339(15):1054-1062.

Hemodialysis and Associated Clinical Challenges

Hemodialysis involves the diffusion of solutes across a semipermeable membrane between the blood and a dialysis solution. This results in the removal of metabolic waste products and excess fluid volume, as well as the replenishment of body buffers. During the procedure, blood is heparinized and passed through a plastic dialyzer. The dose of dialysis, type of dialysis membrane, and solute clearance are the most important modifiable factors. A typical dialysis session lasts for 3 or 4 hours and results in a 65% to 70% reduction in BUN. The annual mortality for patients receiving hemodialysis is nearly 25% and is most often attributed to cardiovascular causes or infection.

Vascular Access. A surgically created vascular access site is necessary for effective hemodialysis. Native arteriovenous fistulas (cephalic vein anastomosed to the radial artery) are superior to polytetrafluoroethylene grafts as sites of vascular access because of their longer life span and lower incidence of thrombosis and infection. The most common access-related complication is intimal hyperplasia, which results in stenosis proximal to the venous anastomosis. Other complications related to access include thrombosis, infection, aneurysm formation, and limb ischemia. When dialysis is urgently required, vascular access is obtained with a double-lumen dialysis catheter, most often using the jugular or femoral vein.

Complications

INTRADIALYTIC COMPLICATIONS. Hypotension is the most common adverse event during hemodialysis and most likely reflects osmolar shifts and ultrafiltration-induced volume depletion. Hypotensive episodes may also be due to myocardial ischemia, cardiac dysrhythmias, or pericardial effusion with cardiac tamponade. Arrhythmias may be due to rapid changes in potassium concentration. Most hypotensive episodes are successfully treated by slowing the rate of ultrafiltration and/or administering intravenous saline.

Hypersensitivity reactions to the ethylene oxide used to sterilize dialysis machines, as well as adverse reactions to the specific hemodialysis membrane material polyacrylonitrile, may occur. Reactions to polyacrylonitrile are seen most commonly in patients receiving ACE inhibitors. When blood comes in contact with the polyacrylonitrile membrane, the membrane's high negative surface charge stabilizes enzymes, which generate bradykinins. Normally, bradykinin is degraded by kinases, but ACE inhibitors block this response, and profound peripheral vasodilation and hypotension occurs.

Dialysis disequilibrium syndrome is marked by nausea, headaches, and fatigue, but may progress to seizures or coma. The condition is thought to result from rapid changes in pH and solute concentrations in the central nervous system. Management includes reducing the rate of dialysate and blood flow and using dialyzers with smaller surface area.

Muscle cramps are a frequent complaint and most likely reflect changes in potassium concentrations.

NUTRITION AND FLUID BALANCE. During progressive renal failure, catabolism and anorexia lead to loss of lean body mass, but concomitant fluid retention masks weight loss and may even lead to weight gain. Protein-calorie malnutrition is extremely common. Decreased oral intake, hemodialysis-induced catabolism, and hormonal imbalances are common factors. Amino acids as well as water-soluble vitamins are removed by dialysis, which contributes to malnutrition. Routine assessment of nutritional status using plasma biomarkers (albumin, prealbumin) is advised, and many patients benefit from oral or parenteral nutritional supplements.

There is no justification for stringent restriction of dietary potassium in patients undergoing hemodialysis. Patients with ESRD have decreased total body potassium stores and an inexplicable tolerance of hyperkalemia. The expected cardiac and neuromuscular responses to hyperkalemia are less pronounced in patients receiving hemodialysis than in those with normal renal function. Clearance of potassium by hemodialysis is efficient, and because most potassium is intracellular, it is likely that hypokalemia will be suggested by a blood sample obtained soon after completion of hemodialysis and before transcellular equilibration has occurred.

Patients should receive counseling with regard to regulation of sodium and fluid intake. Normal weight gain between dialysis treatments is 3% to 4% of total body mass.

Decreased catabolism of insulin in many patients receiving hemodialysis may result in decreased insulin requirements compared with needs before the initiation of hemodialysis. The presentation of diabetic ketoacidosis may be atypical, with respiratory acidosis and alkalosis but without metabolic acidosis and hypovolemia.

INFECTION. Infection is the second leading cause of death in patients with ESRD. Contributing factors include impaired phagocytosis and neutrophil chemotaxis, and malnutrition.

It is recommended that all patients receiving hemodialysis be immunized against pneumococcus, hepatitis B virus, and influenza virus. Malnutrition or inadequate dialysis may impair antibody response to vaccines, however, and the diagnosis of infection may be difficult because many patients do not show typical symptoms such as fever.

Tuberculosis in patients receiving hemodialysis is usually extrapulmonary and often presents with atypical symptoms that mimic those of inadequate dialysis. Because anergy in response to skin testing is common, unexplained weight loss and anorexia, with or without persistent fever, should prompt further testing to rule out tuberculosis.

Hepatitis B or C virus infection in patients receiving hemodialysis is often asymptomatic, and liver aminotransferase concentrations may not be increased. A substantial proportion of patients undergoing hemodialysis have antibodies to hepatitis C. Of note, dosage adjustments of drugs used to treat human immunodeficiency virus (HIV) infection are not required during hemodialysis.

Peritoneal Dialysis

Peritoneal dialysis requires placing an anchored plastic catheter in the peritoneal cavity for infusion of a dialysate that remains in place for several hours. During that time, diffusive solute transport occurs across the peritoneal membrane until fresh fluid is exchanged for the old fluid. Automated peritoneal dialysis, in which a mechanized cycler infuses and drains peritoneal dialysate at night, is used in many patients.

Peritoneal dialysis may be desirable for patients with congestive heart failure or unstable angina who may not tolerate the rapid fluid shifts or fluctuations in systemic blood pressure that often accompany hemodialysis. Peritoneal dialysis is also indicated for patients with extensive vascular disease that prevents the creation of a vascular access site for hemodialysis.

In patients with diabetes, insulin can be infused with the dialysate to provide precise regulation of blood glucose concentrations.

The presence of abdominal hernias or adhesions may interfere with the ability to use peritoneal dialysis effectively. Peritonitis presenting as abdominal pain and fever is the most common serious complication of peritoneal dialysis. Treatment is with antibiotics, which may include cephalosporins, aminoglycosides, and vancomycin. Survival rates and annual costs are similar with peritoneal dialysis and hemodialysis, but hospitalization rates are higher among patients treated with peritoneal dialysis.

Drug Clearance in Patients Undergoing Dialysis

Patients who are undergoing dialysis require special consideration with respect to drug dosing intervals. Supplemental dosing may be needed for drugs that are cleared by dialysis. When possible, drug doses are best scheduled for administration after completion of a dialysis session.

Drug properties that influence clearance by dialysis include protein binding, water solubility, and molecular weight.

Low-molecular-weight (<500 Da), water-soluble, nonprotein-bound drugs are readily cleared by dialysis. Continuous renal replacement therapies, such as continuous venovenous hemofiltration and continuous arteriovenous hemofiltration, efficiently remove drugs unless they are bound to protein.

Perioperative Hemodialysis

Patients should undergo adequate dialysis within 24 hours of elective surgery to minimize the likelihood of volume overload, hyperkalemia, and uremic bleeding. Depending on the planned surgery, the use of heparin may be avoided or minimized during preoperative hemodialysis. Patients receiving peritoneal dialysis who are undergoing abdominal surgery are generally switched to hemodialysis in the immediately postoperative period.

Urgent hemodialysis is not required after radiocontrast dye studies in those who are undergoing regular hemodialysis. Although these dyes can be removed by hemodialysis, the volume administered in most studies does not result in pulmonary edema in patients maintained on an adequate dialysis regimen, and nephrotoxicity is not a concern in patients with ESRD.

Management of Anesthesia

Management of anesthesia in patients with CKD requires an understanding of the pathologic changes that accompany renal disease, co-existing medical conditions, and the impact of reduced renal function on drug pharmacokinetics (Table 17-13). Optimal management of modifiable risk factors and the development of an anesthetic management plan aimed at minimizing further kidney injury are imperative.

PREOPERATIVE EVALUATION

Preoperative evaluation of patients with CKD includes consideration of renal function, underlying pathologic processes, and comorbid conditions. In addition to identifying patients with preexisting renal dysfunction, it is important to recognize those who are at high risk of developing perioperative renal failure.

Evaluation of the trend in serum creatinine concentration is useful to determine whether renal function is stable. Blood volume status may be estimated by comparing body weight before and after hemodialysis, monitoring vital signs (orthostatic hypotension, tachycardia), and measuring atrial filling pressures. Because diabetes is often present in these patients, glucose management is of concern. Blood pressure should be well controlled before elective surgery. Antihypertensive therapy is frequently continued; however, ACE inhibitors and ARBs are often withheld on the day of surgery to reduce the risk of intraoperative hypotension. Preoperative medication must be individualized, with recognition that these patients may exhibit unexpected sensitivity to central nervous system depressant drugs.

A common recommendation is that the serum potassium concentration should not exceed 5.5 mEq/L on the day of surgery. The patient should be evaluated preoperatively for

TABLE 17-13 ■ **Drugs used in anesthesia practice that depend significantly on renal elimination**

Class	Drugs
Induction agents	Phenobarbital
	Thiopental
Muscle relaxants	Gallamine
	Metocurine
	Pancuronium
	Vecuronium
Cholinesterase inhibitors	Edrophonium
	Neostigmine
Cardiovascular drugs	Atropine
	Digoxin
	Glycopyrrolate
	Hydralazine
	Milrinone
Antimicrobials	Aminoglycosides
	Cephalosporins
	Penicillins
	Sulfonamides
	Vancomycin
Analgesics	Codeine
	Meperidine
	Morphine

Adapted from Malhotra V, Sudheendra V, O'Hara J, et al. Anesthesia and the renal and genitourinary systems. In: Miller RD, Eriksson LI, Fleisher LA, et al, eds. *Miller's Anesthesia.* 7th ed. Philadelphia, PA: Churchill Livingstone; 2009.

the presence of anemia, but the introduction of recombinant human erythropoietin therapy has decreased the number of patients with renal failure who come for elective surgery with a hematocrit of less than 30%. The preoperative presence of a coagulopathy may be addressed with the administration of desmopressin. Gastric aspiration prophylaxis should be considered, especially in diabetic patients. However, all H_2-receptor blockers are excreted renally; therefore dosage adjustment is required. Patients maintained on dialysis should undergo dialysis within the 24 hours preceding elective surgery.

INDUCTION OF ANESTHESIA

Induction of anesthesia and tracheal intubation can be safely accomplished with most of the intravenous drugs (propofol, etomidate, thiopental). Thiopental has an increased volume of distribution and reduced protein binding in patients with CKD; therefore, a dose reduction is advised. Many patients with ESRD respond to induction of anesthesia as if they were hypovolemic. The likelihood of hypotension is increased by uremia as well as by the administration of antihypertensives. Exaggerated central nervous system effects of anesthetic induction drugs may also reflect uremia-induced disruption of the blood–brain barrier.

If indicated, rapid-sequence induction with succinylcholine may be performed if the potassium concentration is less than 5.5 mg/dL. Potassium release following administration of succinylcholine is not exaggerated in patients with CKD.

Alternatively, a nondepolarizing muscle relaxant with a short onset of action, such as rocuronium, may be selected.

Attenuated sympathetic nervous system activity impairs compensatory peripheral vasoconstriction; thus, small decreases in blood volume, institution of positive pressure ventilation, abrupt changes in body position, or drug-induced myocardial depression can result in an exaggerated decrease in systemic blood pressure. Patients being treated with ACE inhibitors or ARBs may be at increased risk of experiencing intraoperative hypotension, especially in the setting of acute surgical blood loss or neuraxial anesthesia.

MAINTENANCE OF ANESTHESIA

A balanced anesthetic technique using a volatile agent, muscle relaxant, and opioids is most often employed. Elimination of volatile anesthetics is not dependent on renal function. Sevoflurane may be avoided because of concerns related to fluoride nephrotoxicity or production of compound A, although there is no evidence that patients with co-existing renal disease are at increased risk of renal dysfunction after administration of sevoflurane. Total intravenous anesthesia is also an option.

Potent volatile anesthetics are useful for controlling intraoperative systemic hypertension and decreasing the doses of muscle relaxants needed for adequate surgical relaxation. Excessive depression of cardiac output is a potential hazard of volatile anesthetics. Decreases in blood flow must be minimized to avoid jeopardizing oxygen delivery to the tissues.

Selection of nondepolarizing muscle relaxants for maintenance of skeletal muscle paralysis during surgery is influenced by the known clearance mechanisms of these drugs. Renal disease may slow excretion of vecuronium and rocuronium, whereas clearance of mivacurium, atracurium, and cisatracurium from plasma is independent of renal function. Renal failure may delay clearance of laudanosine, the principal metabolite of atracurium and cisatracurium. Laudanosine lacks effects at the neuromuscular junction, but at high plasma concentrations, it may stimulate the central nervous system. Regardless of the drug selected, it is prudent to decrease the initial dose and administer subsequent doses based on the responses observed using a peripheral nerve stimulator.

Opioids are useful because they lack cardiodepressant effects and may help minimize the need for volatile anesthetics. Both morphine and meperidine undergo metabolism to potentially neurotoxic compounds (morphine-3-glucoronide and normeperidine, respectively) that rely on renal clearance. Morphine-6-glucoronide, a morphine metabolite more potent that its parent compound, may also accumulate in patients with CKD and result in profound respiratory depression. Hydromorphone also has an active metabolite, hydromorphone-3-glucoronide, that may accumulate in patients with CKD; however, hydromorphone may be used safely with proper monitoring and dose adjustment. Alfentanil, fentanyl, remifentanil, and sufentanil lack active metabolites. However, the elimination half-life of fentanyl may be prolonged in patients with CKD.

Renal excretion accounts for approximately 50% of the clearance of neostigmine and approximately 75% of the elimination of edrophonium and pyridostigmine. Therefore, the risk of recurarization following reversal of muscle relaxant is low, because the half-lives of these agents are likely to be prolonged to a greater extent than the half-lives of the nondepolarizing muscle relaxants.

Fluid Management and Urine Output

Patients with severe renal dysfunction who do not require hemodialysis and those without renal disease undergoing operations associated with a high incidence of postoperative renal failure may benefit from preoperative hydration with balanced salt solutions. Indeed, most patients come to the operating room with a contracted extracellular fluid volume. A bolus of balanced salt solution to restore circulating volume (500 mL IV) should increase urine output in the presence of hypovolemia. Lactated Ringer's solution (potassium 4 mEq/L) or other potassium-containing fluids should be used with caution. Maintaining a urine output of at least 0.5 mL/kg/hr is generally considered reasonable.

Stimulation of urine output with osmotic (mannitol) or tubular (furosemide) diuretics in the absence of adequate intravascular fluid volume replacement is not advised. Intraoperative urine output has not been shown to be predictive of postoperative renal insufficiency. Indeed, the most likely cause of oliguria is an inadequate circulating fluid volume, and administration of diuretics in this setting may further compromise renal function. Preliminary results suggest that fenoldopam, a dopamine-1 agonist, may provide renal protection in patients at high risk who are undergoing cardiac, vascular, or transplant surgery. A dose of 0.1 mcg/kg/min initiated at the induction of surgery may therefore be considered.

Patients dependent on hemodialysis require special attention with respect to perioperative fluid management. An absence of renal function narrows the margin of safety between insufficient and excessive fluid administration. Noninvasive operations require replacement of only insensible water losses. The small amount of urine output can be replaced with 0.45% sodium chloride. Thoracic or abdominal surgery can be associated with loss of significant intravascular fluid volume to the interstitial spaces. This loss is often replaced with balanced salt solutions or colloid. Blood transfusions are considered if the oxygen-carrying capacity must be increased or if blood loss is excessive. Measuring the central venous pressure is often useful for guiding fluid replacement.

Monitoring

To preserve blood vessels for future dialysis access, venipuncture should be avoided entirely in the nondominant arm, as well as in the upper part of the dominant arm. Similarly, it is recommended that radial and ulnar artery cannulation be avoided in case these vessels are needed for an arteriovenous fistula in the future. The same may be said of the brachial and even the axillary arteries. Use of the femoral arteries carries the risk of line infection, particularly since these patients may already be immunocompromised. Remaining options include the dorsalis pedis or posterior tibial arteries, which may be inconvenient because of positioning or difficult to access because of edema and tissue induration. Whichever site is chosen, it is important to note that neither the arterial pressure nor the arterial blood gas concentrations will be accurate if the cannula is placed in the same extremity as a functioning or partially patent fistula.

Venous pressure monitoring is often extremely helpful, if not necessary, since a volume load is not well tolerated by patients with even modest decreases in renal function. The choice of right atrial or pulmonary artery pressure monitoring is guided by the presence of underlying cardiopulmonary disease. Strict asepsis must be maintained when placing these lines, because patients with CKD are extremely prone to infection. Central venous access may be difficult in patients who have a tunneled venous access device or temporary dialysis catheter in situ or who have had many such catheters previously placed with subsequent stenosis of the veins. Transesophageal echocardiography is an additional option for monitoring hemodynamic status.

Although their use is discouraged, temporary dialysis catheters may be employed if intravenous access proves difficult. However, it must be remembered that (1) the catheter must be accessed aseptically, just as it is at the time of dialysis; (2) heparin must be aspirated before connecting to an intravenous line or pressure transducer; and (3) heparin must be reintroduced and the line aseptically sealed at the discontinuation of its use.

Associated Concerns

Attention to patient positioning on the operating room table is important. Poor nutritional status renders the skin particularly prone to bruising and sloughing, and extra padding is required to protect vulnerable nerves around the elbows, knees, and ankles. Fistulas must be protected at all costs and be well padded to prevent pressure injury. Blood pressure cuffs should not be applied to the arm with the fistula. If at all possible, the arm with the fistula should not be tucked but should be positioned so that the fistula thrill can be checked periodically throughout surgery.

Regional Anesthesia

Neuraxial anesthesia may be considered in patients with CKD. A sympathetic blockade of T4 to T10 levels may theoretically improve renal perfusion by attenuating catecholamine-induced renal vasoconstriction and suppressing the surgical stress response. However, platelet dysfunction and the effects of residual heparin in patients receiving hemodialysis must also be considered. In addition, adequate intravascular fluid volume must be maintained to minimize hypotension.

Brachial plexus blockade is useful for placing the vascular shunts necessary for long-term hemodialysis. In addition to providing analgesia, this form of regional anesthesia abolishes vasospasm and produces vasodilation that facilitates the surgical procedure. The suggestion that the duration of brachial plexus anesthesia is shortened in patients with CKD has not been confirmed in controlled studies. The presence of uremic neuropathies should be excluded before induction of regional anesthesia. Co-existing metabolic acidosis may decrease the threshold for seizures in response to local anesthetics.

Postoperative Management

Although residual neuromuscular blockade after apparent reversal of nondepolarizing neuromuscular blockade with anticholinesterase drugs is rare, this diagnosis should be considered in anephric patients who manifest signs of skeletal muscle weakness during the early postoperative period. Other explanations (antibiotics, acidosis, electrolyte imbalance) should also be considered when muscle weakness persists or reappears in patients with renal dysfunction.

Caution should be exercised in the use of parenteral opioids for postoperative analgesia in view of the potential in these patients for exaggerated central nervous system depression and hypoventilation after administration of even small doses of opioids. Administration of naloxone may be necessary if depression of ventilation is severe. Selection of opioids that do not have active metabolites and do not rely on the kidneys for excretion is appropriate. Nonsteroidal antiinflammatory agents are best avoided, because they may exacerbate hypertension, precipitate edema, and increase the risk of cardiovascular complications.

Continuous monitoring of the electrocardiogram is helpful for detecting cardiac dysrhythmias, such as those related to hyperkalemia. Continuation of supplemental oxygen into the postoperative period is a consideration, especially if anemia is present. It is prudent to check levels of electrolytes, BUN, and creatinine as well as hematocrit postoperatively. A chest radiograph may be useful if pulmonary edema is a concern. Uremic coagulopathy should be considered in the workup of postoperative bleeding. Controversy exists over the preferred maintenance fluid for patients with CKD. Although 0.9% saline was traditionally favored because it lacks potassium, it may exacerbate preexisting acidosis.

RENAL TRANSPLANTATION

Candidates for renal transplantation are selected from among patients with ESRD who are being maintained on established programs of long-term renal replacement therapy. In adults, the most common causes of ESRD are diabetes mellitus, systemic hypertension, and glomerulonephritis. Despite concerns regarding recurrence of disease in the donor kidney, such disease generally progresses slowly. A kidney from a cadaver donor can be preserved by perfusion at low temperatures for up to 48 hours, which makes its transplantation a semi-elective surgical procedure. Attempts are made to match HLA antigens and ABO blood groups between donor and recipient. Paradoxically, the presence of certain common shared HLA antigens in the blood administered to a potential transplant recipient has been observed to induce tolerance to donor antigens and thus improve graft survival. The donor kidney is placed in the lower abdomen and receives its vascular supply from the iliac vessels. The ureter is anastomosed directly to the bladder. Immunosuppressive therapy is instituted during the perioperative period.

Management of Anesthesia

GENERAL ANESTHESIA

Although both regional and general anesthesia have been successfully used for renal transplantation, general anesthesia is more common. General anesthesia offers the advantage of allowing controlled ventilation, because respiratory mechanics may be compromised by surgical retraction in the area of the diaphragm. Renal function after kidney transplantation is not predictably influenced by choice of volatile anesthetic. Decreased cardiac output resulting from negative inotropic effects of volatile anesthetics is minimized to avoid jeopardizing the adequacy of tissue oxygen delivery (especially if anemia is present) and to promote renal perfusion. A high-normal systemic blood pressure is required in the presence of euvolemia to maintain adequate urine flow. The selection of muscle relaxants is influenced by their dependence on renal clearance. In this regard, atracurium and cisatracurium are attractive selections, because their clearance from the plasma is organ independent. A newly transplanted kidney is able to clear neuromuscular blockers and the anticholinesterase drugs used for their reversal at the same rate as healthy native kidneys.

Central venous pressure monitoring is useful for guiding the rate and volume of crystalloid infusions. Optimal hydration during the intraoperative period is intended to maximize renal blood flow and improve early function of the transplanted kidney. Mannitol is often administered to facilitate urine formation by the newly transplanted kidney and to reduce the risk of acute tubular necrosis. Mannitol is an osmotic diuretic that facilitates urine output by decreasing excess tissue and intravascular fluid. In addition, mannitol increases renal blood flow through the local release of prostaglandins. Albumin may also be helpful when a cadaveric kidney is transplanted to expand intravascular volume and promote urine production.

When the vascular clamps are released, renal preservative solution from the transplanted kidney and venous drainage from the legs are released into the circulation. Cardiac arrest has been described after completion of the arterial anastomosis to the transplanted kidney and release of the vascular clamp. This event is most likely due to sudden hyperkalemia caused by washout of the potassium-containing preservative solutions from the newly perfused kidney. Unclamping may also be followed by hypotension resulting from the abrupt addition of up to 300 mL to the capacity of the intravascular fluid space and the release of vasodilating chemicals from previously ischemic tissues.

REGIONAL ANESTHESIA

The advantage of regional anesthesia compared with general anesthesia is avoidance of the need for tracheal intubation and administration of neuromuscular blocking drugs. This advantage is negated, however, if regional anesthesia must be extensively supplemented with injected or inhaled agents. Furthermore, blockade of the peripheral sympathetic nervous system, as produced by regional anesthesia, can complicate control of systemic blood pressure, especially considering the unpredictable intravascular fluid volume status of many of these patients. The use of regional anesthesia, particularly epidural anesthesia, is controversial in the presence of abnormal coagulation.

Postoperative Complications

The newly transplanted kidney may undergo acute immunologic rejection, which manifests in the vasculature of the transplanted kidney. It can be so rapid that inadequate circulation is evident almost immediately after the blood supply to the kidney is established. The only treatment for this acute rejection reaction is removal of the transplanted kidney, especially if the rejection process is accompanied by disseminated intravascular coagulation. A hematoma also may arise in the graft postoperatively, causing vascular or ureteral obstruction.

Delayed signs of graft rejection include fever, local tenderness, and deterioration of urine output. Treatment with high doses of corticosteroids and antilymphocyte globulin may be helpful. The acute tubular necrosis that occurs in the transplanted kidney secondary to prolonged ischemia usually responds to hemodialysis. Cyclosporine toxicity may also cause AKI. Ultrasonography and needle biopsy are performed to differentiate between the possible causes of kidney malfunction.

Opportunistic infections resulting from long-term immunosuppression are common after renal transplantation. Long-term survival is unsatisfactory in renal transplant recipients who are immunosuppressed and who also carry hepatitis B surface antigen. The frequency of cancer is 30 to 100 times higher in transplant recipients than in the general population, which presumably reflects the loss of protective effects resulting from immunosuppression. Large cell lymphoma is a well-recognized complication of transplantation; it occurs almost exclusively in patients with evidence of Epstein-Barr virus infection.

Anesthetic Considerations in Renal Transplant Recipients Undergoing Surgery

Renal transplant recipients are often elderly individuals with co-existing cardiovascular disease and diabetes mellitus. The side effects of immunosuppressant drugs (systemic hypertension, lowered seizure thresholds, anemia, thrombocytopenia) must be considered when planning the management of anesthesia in these patients. Serum creatinine concentrations are likely to be normal in the presence of normally functioning renal grafts. Nevertheless, the GFR and renal blood flow are likely to be lower than those in healthy individuals, and the activity of drugs excreted by the kidneys may be prolonged. The presence of azotemia, proteinuria, and systemic hypertension may indicate chronic rejection of the kidney transplant.

Drugs that are potentially nephrotoxic or dependent on renal clearance should be avoided, and diuretics should be administered only after careful evaluation of the patient's intravascular volume status. Decreases in renal blood flow resulting from hypovolemia or other causes should be minimized.

PRIMARY DISEASES OF THE KIDNEYS

A number of pathologic processes can primarily involve the kidneys or occur in association with dysfunction of other organ systems. Knowledge of the associated pathologic features and other characteristics of these diseases is important when managing these patients during the perioperative period.

Glomerulonephritis

Acute glomerulonephritis is usually due to deposition of antigen-antibody complexes in the glomeruli. The source of antigens may be exogenous (after streptococcal infection) or endogenous (collagen vascular diseases). Clinical manifestations of glomerular disease include hematuria, proteinuria, hypertension, edema, and increased serum creatinine concentration. The presence of urinary red blood cell casts is also highly suggestive of renal dysfunction resulting from a glomerular process. Proteinuria reflects an increase in glomerular permeability. Prompt diagnosis is important, because treatment with immunosuppressive drugs may help prevent permanent kidney injury.

Two general patterns of glomerular disease exist. A nephritic pattern is associated with inflammation and an active urine sediment containing red and white blood cells, and a variable amount of proteinuria. A nephrotic pattern is characterized by marked proteinuria and a relatively inactive urine sediment.

Nephrotic Syndrome

Nephrotic syndrome is defined as daily urinary protein excretion exceeding 3.5 g associated with sodium retention, hyperlipoproteinemia, and thromboembolic and infectious complications. Diabetic nephropathy is the most frequent cause of nephrotic proteinuria. In the absence of diabetes, the most common cause of nephrotic syndrome in adults is membranous glomerulonephritis, which is frequently associated with neoplasia (carcinoma, sarcoma, lymphoma, leukemia). HIV infection may cause nephrotic proteinuria and renal insufficiency; in some patients, this is the first clinical manifestation of AIDS. Pregnancy-induced hypertension is also often associated with nephrotic syndrome.

SIGNS AND SYMPTOMS

Sodium retention and edema formation in patients with nephrotic syndrome have been presumed to reflect decreased plasma oncotic pressure with resultant hypovolemia. Increased tubular reabsorption of sodium was assumed to be a homeostatic response to hypovolemia. More recent evidence suggests that sodium retention is a primary event that precedes the development of proteinuria. Increased sodium reabsorption by the distal renal tubules may be due to an inappropriately low natriuretic response to atrial natriuretic peptide. Patients with nephrotic syndrome may experience hypovolemia with associated orthostatic hypotension, tachycardia, peripheral vasoconstriction, and occasionally even AKI in response to the administration of diuretics. The risk of AKI is increased in elderly patients and those who receive nonsteroidal antiinflammatory drugs. Infusion of albumin corrects the clinical signs of hypovolemia. Hyperlipidemia accompanies nephrotic syndrome and may be associated with an increased risk of vascular disease.

THROMBOEMBOLIC COMPLICATIONS

Thromboembolic complications such as renal vein thrombosis, pulmonary embolism, and deep vein thrombosis are major risks in patients with nephrotic syndrome, particularly those who have membranous glomerulonephritis. Arterial thromboses are less common than venous thromboses, although the risk of acute myocardial infarction in these patients may be increased. Prophylactic administration of heparin or oral anticoagulants may be considered in patients at high risk.

Infection

Pneumococcal peritonitis has been responsible for fatalities in children with nephrotic syndrome. Viral infections may be more likely in immunosuppressed patients, whereas susceptibility to bacterial infections seems to be related to decreased levels of immunoglobulin G.

Protein Binding

Plasma levels of vitamins and hormones may be decreased in patients with nephrotic syndrome as a result of proteinuria. Hypoalbuminemia decreases the available binding sites for many drugs and increases the circulating levels of unbound drug. In this regard, when plasma drug levels are monitored, low levels of highly protein-bound drugs do not necessarily indicate low therapeutic concentrations.

Nephrotic Edema

Generalized edema is a function of an increase in total body sodium content. Potent loop diuretics such as furosemide are needed to offset the kidney's propensity to retain sodium. In addition, thiazide or potassium-sparing diuretics may be added to decrease sodium reabsorption in the distal nephrons. The goal is to decrease edema slowly, because abrupt natriuresis may cause hypovolemia and even AKI; it may also produce hemoconcentration, which increases the risk of thromboembolic complications. Albumin solutions are administered to expand the plasma volume only if symptomatic hypovolemia is present. In particularly severe cases, plasma ultrafiltration may be considered.

Goodpasture's Syndrome

Goodpasture's syndrome is a rare autoimmune disease that manifests as rapidly progressing glomerulonephritis in combination with pulmonary hemorrhage. It occurs most often in young males. Anti–glomerular basement membrane antibodies account for renal dysfunction and apparently also react with similar antigens in the lungs, producing alveolitis and subsequent hemoptysis. Typically, hemoptysis precedes clinical evidence of renal disease. Plasmapheresis is sometimes used to remove the disease-causing antibodies. Corticosteroids are also employed to reduce inflammatory damage. The prognosis is poor, and most patients develop renal failure within a year of diagnosis.

Interstitial Nephritis

Interstitial nephritis has been observed as an allergic reaction to drugs, including sulfonamides, allopurinol, phenytoin, and diuretics. Other less common causes include autoimmune diseases (systemic lupus erythematosus) and infiltrative diseases (sarcoidosis). Patients exhibit decreased urine concentrating ability, proteinuria, and systemic hypertension. Renal failure caused by acute interstitial nephritis is often reversible after withdrawal of the offending agent or treatment of the underlying disease. Corticosteroid therapy may be beneficial.

Hereditary Nephritis

Hereditary nephritis (Alport's syndrome) is often accompanied by hearing loss and ocular abnormalities. The disorder is more common in males than in females. In women, the disease is usually mild, but in men, the symptoms are more severe and progressive. Drug therapy has not proven successful, although lowering the intraglomerular pressure with ACE inhibitors may slow the progression of renal disease. ESRD is likely before the age of 50.

Polycystic Kidney Disease

Polycystic kidney disease is a genetic disorder most commonly inherited as an autosomal dominant trait. The condition is marked by the development of cysts in the kidney, as well as in other organs such as the liver and pancreas. Intracranial aneurysms and cardiac valve abnormalities may also be present. Mild systemic hypertension, hematuria, kidney stones, and urinary tract infections are common. The disease typically progresses slowly until renal failure occurs during middle age. Hemodialysis or renal transplantation is eventually necessary in most patients.

Fanconi's Syndrome

Fanconi's syndrome results from inherited or acquired disturbances of proximal renal tubular function. There is renal loss of substances normally conserved by the proximal renal tubules, including potassium, bicarbonate, phosphate, amino acids, glucose, and water. Symptoms include polyuria, polydipsia, metabolic acidosis, and skeletal muscle weakness. Dwarfism and osteomalacia, reflecting loss of phosphate, are also common, and patients may have vitamin D–resistant rickets. Management of anesthesia includes attention to fluid and electrolyte abnormalities and the recognition that left ventricular cardiac failure secondary to uremia is often present in advanced stages of the disease.

Bartter's and Gitelman's Syndromes

Bartter's syndrome and Gitelman's syndrome are inherited renal salt-wasting disorders caused by defects in sodium, chloride, and potassium channels in the thick ascending limb of the distal convoluted tubule. Juxtaglomerular hyperplasia, hyperaldosteronism, and hypokalemic acidosis are pathognomic of these disorders. Treatment relies on ACE inhibitors, spironolactone, and sodium and potassium supplementation. These syndromes alone do not lead to renal failure. However, if patients develop ESRD for other reasons, transplantation of a kidney from a healthy donor results in normal renal solute handling.

Renal Tubular Acidosis

Renal tubular acidosis (RTA) is a syndrome that causes metabolic acidosis resulting from inappropriate acidification of the urine. Several subtypes of the disorder are recognized. Type 1 RTA is caused by impaired bicarbonate reabsorption in the proximal renal tubule. Type 2 RTA is due to impaired secretion of hydrogen ions in the distal tubule. The result of either defect is a hypokalemic, hyperchloremic metabolic acidosis and inappropriately basic urine. These conditions may be hereditary or secondary to an underlying systemic illness. Type 4 RTA also causes a metabolic acidosis, but is distinct from the other types in that it is associated with hyperkalemia rather than hypokalemia. Type 4 RTA occurs when plasma aldosterone levels are inappropriately low or the kidney fails to respond to aldosterone normally. Type 4 RTA is often seen in patients with CKD.

Nephrolithiasis

Although the pathogenesis of nephrolithiasis is poorly understood, several predisposing factors are recognized for the five major types of renal stones that occur (Table 17-14). Most stones are composed of calcium oxalate and result from excess calcium excretion by the kidneys. In these patients, causes of hypercalcemia (hyperparathyroidism, sarcoidosis, cancer) must be considered. Urinary tract infections with ureasplitting organisms that produce ammonia favor the formation of magnesium ammonium phosphate stones. Formation of uric acid stones is favored by a persistently acidic urine (pH < 6.0), which decreases the solubility of uric acid. Approximately 50% of patients with uric acid stones have gout.

Stones in the renal pelvis are typically painless unless their presence is complicated by infection or obstruction. By contrast, renal stones passing down the ureter can produce intense flank pain, often radiating to the groin, associated with nausea and vomiting, and mimicking an acute surgical abdomen. Hematuria is common during ureteral passage of stones, whereas ureteral obstruction may precipitate renal failure.

TREATMENT

Treatment of a renal stone depends on identifying the composition of the stone and correcting predisposing factors, such as hyperparathyroidism, urinary tract infection, or gout. High fluid intake sufficient to maintain a daily urine output of 2 to 3 L is often part of the therapy. Extracorporeal shock wave lithotripsy is a noninvasive treatment for renal stones that uses focused, high-intensity acoustic impulses to break up stones into pieces that may be excreted in the urine. The advantages of this approach, as an alternative to percutaneous nephrolithotomy, are that it is associated with low morbidity and can be performed on an outpatient basis. Cardiac dysrhythmias may occur during extracorporeal shock wave lithotripsy, presumably as a result of premature stimulation of the atria by the electrical discharge that precedes each shock wave. Lithotripsy devices are equipped with electrocardiogram gating that helps limit the risk of ventricular fibrillation caused by the "R-on-T" phenomenon.

Renal Hypertension

Renal disease is the most common cause of secondary systemic hypertension. Accelerated or malignant hypertension is likely to be associated with renal disease. Furthermore, the

TABLE 17-14 ■ Composition and characteristics of renal stones			
Type of stone	Incidence (%)	Radiographic appearance	Cause
Calcium oxalate	70	Opaque	Primary hyperparathyroidism Idiopathic hypercalciuria Hyperoxaluria
Magnesium ammonium phosphate (struvite)	15	Opaque	Alkaline urine (usually resulting from chronic bacterial infection)
Calcium phosphate	8	Opaque	Renal tubular acidosis
Uric acid	5	Translucent	Acid urine Gout Hyperuricosuria
Cystine	2	Opaque	Cystinuria

appearance of systemic hypertension in young patients suggests the diagnosis of renal rather than essential hypertension. Hypertension due to renal dysfunction reflects parenchymal disease of the kidneys or renovascular disease.

Chronic pyelonephritis and glomerulonephritis are parenchymal diseases often associated with systemic hypertension, particularly in younger patients. Less common forms of renal parenchymal disease that can cause systemic hypertension include diabetic nephropathy, cystic disease of the kidneys, and renal amyloidosis.

Renovascular disease is caused by narrowing of the renal arteries resulting from either fibromuscular dysplasia or atheroma. The sudden onset of a marked increase in systemic blood pressure or the presence of hypertension before the age of 30 years should arouse suspicion of renovascular disease. A bruit may be audible on auscultation of the abdomen over the kidneys. Systemic hypertension due to renovascular disease does not respond well to treatment with antihypertensive drugs.

The mechanism that produces systemic hypertension in the presence of renal parenchymal or renovascular disease has not been established. Stimulation of the renin-angiotensin-aldosterone system is a possible, but unproven, mechanism. Regardless of the mechanism, treatment of systemic hypertension due to renal parenchymal disease is usually with antihypertensive drugs, including β-adrenergic antagonists, which inhibit the release of renin from the kidneys. Treatment of renovascular hypertension is with renal artery endarterectomy or nephrectomy.

Uric Acid Nephropathy

Acute uric acid nephropathy occurs when uric acid crystals precipitate in the renal collecting tubules or ureters, producing acute oliguric renal failure. This precipitation occurs when uric acid concentrations reach a saturation point in acidic urine. The condition is particularly likely to occur when uric acid production is greatly increased, as in patients with myeloproliferative disorders being treated with chemotherapeutic drugs. These patients are particularly vulnerable to uric acid nephropathy when they become dehydrated or acidotic because of decreased caloric intake.

Hepatorenal Syndrome

Acute oliguria manifesting in patients with decompensated cirrhosis of the liver is called *hepatorenal syndrome*. Indeed, cirrhosis of the liver is associated with decreased GFR and renal blood flow that precede overt renal dysfunction by several weeks. The typical patient is deeply jaundiced and moribund; ascites, hypoalbuminemia, and hypoprothrombinemia are present. Renal failure in these patients reflects reduction in effective circulating volume, partly as a result of diuretic treatment and partly as a result of splanchnic arteriolar dilatation. Treatment is directed at restoring intravascular fluid volume. Administration of normal saline may aggravate

ascites. Therefore, whole blood or packed red blood cells may be a more appropriate form of volume replacement. Vasopressin analogues such as orniptressin and terlipressin cause splanchnic vasoconstriction, and may help to increase renal perfusion and GFR. A peritoneal-venous shunt for the treatment of ascites may also be associated with improved renal function.

There is an increased incidence of postoperative AKI in patients with obstructive jaundice who undergo surgery. The cause of renal failure in these patients is unclear, but preoperative administration of mannitol may be recommended in the hope of providing some renoprotective effect.

Benign Prostatic Hyperplasia

Benign prostatic hyperplasia (BPH) is a nonmalignant enlargement of the prostate caused by excessive growth of both the glandular and stromal elements of the gland. Symptoms occur as a result of compression of the urethral canal and disruption of the normal flow of urine. BPH is common worldwide in men older than 40 years of age.

MEDICAL THERAPY

Prostatic tissue growth is androgen sensitive, so that androgen deprivation decreases the size of the prostate and thereby the resistance to outflow through the prostatic urethra. Finasteride, an inhibitor of the 5α-reductase enzyme, is moderately effective for symptomatic treatment of BPH. Side effects of 5α-reductase inhibitors are minimal. α-Adrenergic antagonists (terazosin, doxazosin, tamsulosin) are administered to block adrenergic receptors in hyperplastic prostatic tissue, the prostatic capsule, and the bladder neck, and thereby decrease smooth muscle tone and resistance to urinary flow. These drugs also have antihypertensive effects and may cause orthostatic hypotension in some patients.

INVASIVE TREATMENTS

The most commonly used minimally invasive treatments of BPH are transurethral microwave thermotherapy (TUMT) and transurethral needle ablation (TUNA). These procedures rely on the generation of heat to cause tissue necrosis and shrinkage of the prostate.

Surgical treatments include transurethral incision of the prostate (TUIP) and transurethral resection of the prostate (TURP). TUIP is usually effective in patients whose prostates weigh 30 g or less and in whom the primary urinary outlet obstruction is located at the bladder neck. As the incisions are deepened, the bladder neck and prostatic urethra spring open, and the bladder outlet obstruction is relieved. TURP involves resection of prostatic tissue using electrocautery or sharp excision. The procedure is associated with a fair amount of bleeding; patients are admitted postoperatively for continuous bladder irrigation to prevent the formation of obstructing blood clots.

Newer procedures using laser therapy to destroy prostate tissue have also been developed. Advantages of laser ablation

TABLE 17-15   Signs and symptoms of transurethral resection of the prostate (TURP) syndrome

System	Signs and Symptoms	Cause
Cardiovascular	Hypertension, reflex bradycardia, pulmonary edema, cardiovascular collapse, ECG changes (wide QRS, elevated ST segment, ventricular arrhythmias)	Rapid fluid absorption, reflex bradycardia (secondary to hypertension or increased ICP), third-spacing secondary to hyponatremia and hypo-osmolality
Respiratory	Tachypnea, hypoxemia, Cheyne-Stokes breathing	Pulmonary edema
Neurologic	Nausea, restlessness, visual disturbances, confusion, somnolence, seizure, coma, death	Hyponatremia and hypo-osmolality causing cerebral edema and increased ICP, hyperglycinemia (glycine is an inhibitory neurotransmitter that potentiates NMDA receptor activity), hyperammonemia
Hematologic	Disseminated intravascular coagulation, hemolysis	Hyponatremia and hypo-osmolality
Renal	Renal failure	Hypotension, hyperoxaluria (oxalate is a metabolite of glycine)
Metabolic	Acidosis	Deamination of glycine to glyoxylic acid and ammonia

ECG, Electrocardiogram; *ICP,* intracranial pressure; *NMDA,* N-methyl-D-aminotransferase.

of the prostate are brief operating time (≤20 minutes) and the absence of perioperative hemorrhage.

Transurethral Resection of the Prostate (TURP) Syndrome

During TURP, an irrigation solution (glycine, sorbitol, mannitol) is used to provide surgical visualization and remove blood and resected tissue. The procedure is accompanied by absorption of irrigating fluid via direct intravascular access through the prostatic venous plexus or more slowly through absorption from the retroperitoneal and perivesical spaces. TURP syndrome is characterized by intravascular fluid volume shifts and the effects of plasma solute absorption (Table 17-15). Solute changes may alter neurologic function independent of volume-related effects. Although monitoring of serum sodium concentrations during TURP is effective for assessing intravascular fluid absorption, there may be benefit in monitoring serum osmolality as well. Hypo-osmolality appears to be the principal factor contributing to the neurologic and hypovolemic changes considered to reflect TURP syndrome. Supportive care remains the most important therapeutic approach for managing cardiovascular, central nervous system, and renal complications of TURP syndrome.

Neuraxial anesthesia has conventionally been the anesthetic technique of choice for TURP because it allows for monitoring of TURP syndrome symptoms during the procedure.

Intravascular Volume Expansion. Rapid intravascular fluid volume expansion due to systemic absorption of irrigating fluids (absorption rates may reach 200 mL/min) can cause systemic hypertension and reflex bradycardia. Patients with poor left ventricular function may develop pulmonary edema due to acute circulatory volume overload. Factors that influence the amount of irrigating solution absorbed include the intravesicular pressure, which is determined by the height of the irrigation bag above the prostatic sinuses (height should be limited to 40 cm above the prostate) and the number of prostatic sinuses opened (resection time should be limited to 1

hour and a rim of tissue should be left on the capsule). If intravesical pressures are maintained below 15 cm H_2O, absorption of irrigating fluids is minimal.

The most widely used indicator of intravascular fluid volume gain is hyponatremia. Before treating TURP syndrome with hypertonic saline, it is important to exclude the presence of hypervolemia with near-normal plasma sodium concentrations. Cardiovascular compromise and impaired arterial oxygenation due to pulmonary edema require aggressive intervention, which may include administration of inotropic drugs or diuretics.

Intravascular Volume Loss. Perioperative hypotension during TURP is sometimes preceded by systemic hypertension. It is conceivable that hyponatremia in association with systemic hypertension can result in water flux along osmotic and hydrostatic pressure gradients out of the intravascular space and into the lungs with resultant pulmonary edema and hypovolemic shock. Sympathetic nervous system blockade produced by regional anesthesia may compound the hypotension, as may intraoperative endotoxemia, which is common during TURP.

Hyponatremia. Acute hyponatremia due to intravascular absorption of sodium-free irrigating fluids may cause confusion, agitation, visual disturbances, pulmonary edema, cardiovascular collapse, and seizures. Changes on the electrocardiogram may accompany progressive decreases in serum sodium concentrations. Spinal anesthesia associated with hypotension may cause nausea and vomiting indistinguishable from that caused by acute hyponatremia. Furthermore, some hyponatremic patients show no signs of water intoxication.

Hypo-osmolality. Hypo-osmolality rather than hyponatremia appears to be the crucial physiologic derangement leading to central nervous system dysfunction in TURP syndrome. This is predictable, because the blood–brain barrier is essentially impermeable to sodium but freely permeable to water. Cerebral edema caused by acute hypo-osmolality can result in increased intracranial pressure with resultant bradycardia and hypertension.

Diuretics administered to treat hypervolemia during TURP may accentuate hyponatremia and hypo-osmolality. A patient's serum sodium concentration and osmolality may continue to decrease following TURP because of continued absorption of irrigating solutions from the perivesicular and retroperitoneal spaces. If the serum osmolality is near normal, no interventions to correct serum sodium concentrations are recommended for asymptomatic patients even in the presence of hyponatremia. Instituting treatment in the absence of symptoms risks too rapid a correction, because the correction rate is difficult to control. The most feared complication of correction of hyponatremia is central pontine myelinolysis (osmotic demyelination syndrome), which has been observed after both rapid and slow correction of serum sodium concentrations in patients undergoing TURP.

Hyperammonemia. Hyperammonemia is a result of the use of glycine-containing irrigation solutions with subsequent systemic absorption of glycine and its oxidative deamination to glyoxylic acid and ammonia. Alterations in central nervous system function may accompany hyperammonemia, but its role in TURP syndrome remains unclear. Endogenous arginine in the liver prevents hepatic release of ammonia and facilitates conversion of ammonia to urea. The time necessary to deplete endogenous arginine stores may be as brief as 12 hours, which approximates the preoperative fasting time. Prophylactic administration of intravenous arginine blunts the increase in serum ammonia concentrations associated with the presence of glycine in the systemic circulation.

Hyperglycinemia. Glycine is an inhibitory neurotransmitter similar to γ-aminobutyric acid in the spinal cord and brain. The use of glycine-containing irrigation solutions may cause visual disturbances, including transient blindness during TURP syndrome, which reflects the role of glycine as an inhibitory neurotransmitter in the retina. Therefore, glycine likely affects retinal physiology independent of the cerebral edema caused by hyponatremia and hypo-osmolality. Vision returns to normal within 24 hours as serum glycine concentrations approach baseline values. Reassurance that unimpaired vision will return is probably the best treatment.

Glycine may also lead to encephalopathy and seizures through its ability to potentiate the effects of N-methyl-d-aspartate (NMDA), an excitatory neurotransmitter. Magnesium exerts a negative control on the NMDA receptor, and hypomagnesemia caused by dilution (resulting from systemic absorption of irrigating solutions during TURP or administration of loop diuretics) may increase the susceptibility to seizures. For this reason, a trial of magnesium therapy may be indicated in patients who develop seizures and in whom glycine-containing irrigating solutions have been used.

Glycine may also exert toxic effects on the kidneys. Hyperoxaluria due to metabolism of glycine to oxalate and glyoxylic acid may compromise renal function in patients with preexisting renal disease.

KEY POINTS

- The kidneys are involved in water conservation, electrolyte homeostasis, acid-base balance, and several neurohumoral and hormonal functions. Some or all of these functions are affected by renal disease.
- Patient risk factors for perioperative AKI include advanced age, preexisting renal dysfunction, diabetes, hypertension, and peripheral vascular disease. High-risk surgical procedures include those requiring aortic cross-clamping and cardiopulmonary bypass. Prevention of AKI hinges on maintaining adequate renal perfusion and avoiding nephrotoxins. Fenoldopam, a dopamine-1 agonist, may also be helpful in patients at high risk.
- Treatment of AKI is supportive, aimed at limiting further injury by maintaining hemodynamic stability and adequate intravascular fluid volume. Mannitol and sodium bicarbonate may be useful in treating pigment- or contrast-induced nephropathies.
- Preoperative evaluation of patients with CKD should take into consideration not only baseline renal function, but also the high prevalence of comorbid conditions, including cardiovascular disease and diabetes.
- National guidelines advise that patients with CKD should have their blood pressure maintained below 130/80 mm Hg. ACE inhibitors and/or ARBs are first-line therapies, but most patients require treatment with multiple antihypertensive drugs.
- Provision of anesthesia for patients with CKD focuses on meticulous fluid and electrolyte management, acid-base maintenance, and attention to drug disposition in renal failure. Vessels of the nondominant forearm should be preserved in anticipation of vascular access requirements for hemodialysis.
- During renal transplantation, hypotension and cardiac dysrhythmias may develop when the vascular clamps are released. This event is likely due to washout of potassium-containing preservative fluid from the newly perfused kidney, abrupt addition of fluid to the intravascular space, and the release of vasodilating chemicals from previously ischemic tissues.

RESOURCES

Graven stein D. Transurethral resection of the prostate (TURP) syndrome: a review of the pathophysiology and management. *Anesth Analg.* 1997;84(2):438-446.

Josephs SA, Thakar CV. Perioperative risk assessment, prevention, and treatment of acute kidney injury. *Int Anesthesiol Clin.* 2009;47(4):89-105.

Kelly AM, Dwamena B, Cronin P, et al. Meta-analysis: effectiveness of drugs for preventing contrast-induced nephropathy. *Ann Intern Med.* 2008;148(4):284-294.

Kheterpal S, Tremper KK, Heung M, et al. Development and validation of an acute kidney injury risk index for patients undergoing general surgery: results from a national data set. *Anesthesiology.* 2009;110(3):505-515.

Prowle JR, Bellomo R. Fluid administration and the kidney. *Curr Opin Crit Care.* 2010;16(4):332-336.

Sear JW. Kidney dysfunction in the postoperative period. *Br J Anaesth.* 2005;95(1):20-32.

Singri N, Ahya SN, Levin ML. Acute renal failure. *JAMA.* 2003;289(6):747-751.

Sladen RN. Oliguria in the ICU: systemic approach to diagnosis and treatment. *Anesthesiol Clin North Am.* 2000;18(4):739-752.

Sprung J, Kapural L, Bourke DL, et al. Anesthesia for kidney transplant surgery. *Anesthesiol Clin North America.* 2000;18(4):919-951.

Wagener G, Brentjens TE. Anesthetic concerns in patients presenting with renal failure. *Anesthesiol Clin.* 2010;28(1):39-54.

Zacharias M, Conlin NP, Herbison GP, et al. Interventions for protecting renal function in the perioperative period. *Cochrane Database Syst Rev.* 2008(4):CD003590.

CHAPTER 18

Fluid, Electrolyte, and Acid-Base Disorders

ROBERT B. SCHONBERGER ■

Alterations of water, osmolal, and electrolyte content and distribution as well as acid-base disturbances are common in the perioperative period and rarely happen in isolation, because they are inherently interrelated. They both affect and are affected by the function and stability of disparate organ systems. Central nervous system impairment, cardiac dysfunction, and neuromuscular changes are especially common in the presence of water, osmolal, electrolyte, and acid-base disturbances. Several perioperative events can exacerbate such alterations (Table 18-1). Management of patients with these disturbances is based on an assessment of the cause and severity of the condition, an understanding of the interrelationships among these disturbances, and an awareness of the patient's comorbid conditions.

ABNORMALITIES OF WATER, OSMOLALITY, AND ELECTROLYTES

Water and Osmolal Homeostasis

In the nonobese adult, total body water comprises approximately 60% of body weight (adiposity decreases this proportion). Body water is divided into intracellular fluid (ICF) and extracellular fluid (ECF) compartments according to the location of the water relative to cell membranes (Figure 18-1). ECF consists primarily of an interstitial compartment (three fourths of ECF) and an intravascular plasma compartment (one fourth of ECF). Water shifts between compartments according to the balance of hydrostatic and oncotic pressure across membranes, and thus water homeostasis relies on the maintenance of osmolality within a narrow physiologic range. The integrity of living cells depends on the preservation of water homeostasis, as well as on the energy-intensive maintenance of intracellular and extracellular concentrations of ions, also termed *electrolytes*. These electrolytes, in addition to being a major determinant of both osmolality and acid-base balance, are responsible for electrical potentials across cell membranes. Changes in electrolyte homeostasis may especially impact excitable cells in the central nervous system and musculature that rely on action potentials for the rapid and organized transfer of information.

Water and osmolal homeostasis are predominantly mediated by osmolality sensors, neurons located in the anterior hypothalamus. In response to osmolal elevations, these neurons stimulate thirst and cause pituitary release of vasopressin (antidiuretic hormone). Vasopressin is stored as granules in the posterior pituitary and acts through G protein–coupled receptors in the collecting ducts of the kidney to cause water retention, which in turn decreases serum osmolality. As a

TABLE 18-1 ■ Common causes of water, osmolal, electrolyte, and acid-base disturbances during the perioperative period

Disease states
  Endocrinopathies
  Nephropathies
  Gastroenteropathies
Drug therapy
  Diuretics
  Corticosteroids
Nasogastric suction
Surgery
  Transurethral resection of the prostate
  Translocation of body water due to tissue trauma
  Resection of portions of the gastrointestinal tract
Management of anesthesia
  Intravenous fluid administration
  Alveolar ventilation
  Hypothermia

TABLE 18-2 ■ Factors and drugs affecting vasopressin secretion

Stimulation of vasopressin release	Inhibition of vasopressin release	Drugs that stimulate vasopressin release and/or potentiate the renal action of vasopressin
Contracted ECF volume	Expanded ECF volume	Amitriptyline
Hypernatremia	Hyponatremia	Barbiturates
Hypotension	Hypertension	Carbamazepine
Nausea and vomiting		Chlorpropamide
Congestive heart failure		Clofibrate
Cirrhosis		Morphine
Hypothyroidism		Nicotine
Angiotensin II		Phenothiazines
Catecholamines		Selective serotonin reuptake inhibitors
Histamine		
Bradykinin		

ECF, Extracellular fluid.

TOTAL BODY WATER = 0.6 × BODY WEIGHT

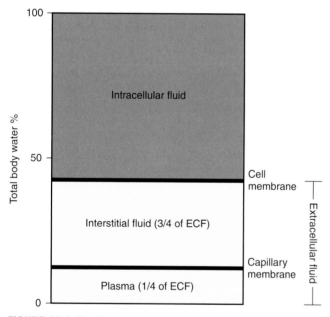

FIGURE 18-1 Total body water (approximately 60% of total body weight) is designated as intracellular fluid (ICF) or extracellular fluid (ECF) depending on the location of the water relative to cell membranes. ECF is further divided into interstitial and plasma compartments depending on its location relative to vascular walls. Of total body water, two thirds is ICF. Of ECF, 75% is interstitial and 25% is intravascular.

The osmolality of serum represents the total number of osmotically active particles (i.e., solutes) per kilogram of solvent. When osmolality is assessed, a shorthand indirect measurement of serum osmolality can easily be calculated as 2[Na] + [Glucose]/18 + [BUN]/2.8, and this calculated value should always be compared with direct, laboratory-measured osmolality. A significant difference in these values—an "osmolal gap"—should alert the clinician to the presence of unmeasured, osmotically active particles. Increases in serum osmolality may be encountered as a result of free water depletion (e.g., dehydration or diabetes insipidus) or the presence of additional solutes (most commonly from the ingestion of ethanol or other toxins, hyperglycemia, or the iatrogenic administration of osmolal loads such as mannitol or glycine). Perioperative attempts to induce fluid shifts by deliberate administration of osmolal loads should take into consideration the patient's preexisting serum osmolality to avoid extreme increases in serum osmolality (>320 mOsm/kg). Mannitol should not be administered to an intoxicated patient with elevated intracranial pressure, for example, without prior consideration of the preexisting effects of ethanol molecules and water diuresis on the osmolal state of the patient.

Although vasopressin is predominantly secreted in response to increased osmolality, release is also stimulated by large iso-osmolar decreases in effective circulating volume. In addition, the pain and stress of the perioperative period are upregulators of vasopressin release, and the stress response to critical illness can include water retention, oliguria, and dilutional hyponatremia (Table 18-2).

In contrast to osmolal homeostasis, the homeostatic response to isotonic changes in total body water relies on juxtaglomerular sensation of changes in effective circulating volume and consequent changes in kidney renin excretion. Renin converts angiotensinogen into angiotensin I,

major site of vasopressin effects, the kidney is responsible for maintaining water homeostasis by excreting urine with large variations in total osmolality. Under normal circumstances, serum osmolality is tightly regulated by thirst and renal control of water excretion. The normal range of serum osmolality is 280 to 290 mOsm/kg.

which is converted to angiotensin II in the lung. Angiotensin II induces adrenal release of aldosterone, which promotes sodium reabsorption and potassium loss in the distal tubules and also leads to increases in water resorption. Elevations in circulating volume also cause increased release of natriuretic peptides that promote a return to water homeostasis.

Fluid resuscitation in patients with hypovolemia necessitates consideration of cause, severity, and patient comorbid conditions. Crystalloid administration should take into consideration a patient's electrolyte and acid-base balance as well as concerns regarding the acute cardiovascular effects of additional volume and the neurologic effects of changes in volume, osmolality, and glucose levels.

Infusion of colloids, including blood products, should be done in the context of appropriate goals for hemoglobin, platelets, and coagulation factors, which must take into consideration the course of any ongoing blood loss and the health status of the patient. Artificial volume expanders may offer the advantage of reduced tissue edema compared with crystalloids.

DISORDERS OF SODIUM

As the ion with the highest concentration in the ECF, sodium contributes most of the effective osmoles to serum. This underlying connection between serum sodium concentration and osmolality is critical for understanding disorders of sodium homeostasis. Under normal circumstances, serum sodium concentration is maintained between 136 and 145 mmol/L primarily by the action of vasopressin on water and osmolal homeostasis. Variations in measured sodium concentration frequently occur along with derangements in total body water.

Assessment and treatment of changes in sodium concentration must therefore consider osmolality as well as the total body water of the patient. Total body water can be increased, normal, or decreased in the context of derangements in sodium concentration, and the cause and treatment of serum sodium disorders depend on the osmolality and volume status of the patient.

Hyponatremia

Hyponatremia commonly exists in concert with hypo-osmolality when water retention or water intake exceeds the renal excretion of dilute urine. Hyponatremia exists in approximately 15% of hospitalized patients, most commonly as a dilutional effect in the setting of increased vasopressin release. In the outpatient setting, hyponatremia is more likely to be a result of chronic disease.

SIGNS AND SYMPTOMS

The signs and symptoms of hyponatremia depend on the rate at which the hyponatremia has developed and are less pronounced in chronic cases. In addition, younger patients

TABLE 18-3 ■ **Symptoms and signs of hyponatremia**

Symptoms	Signs
Anorexia	Abnormal sensorium
Nausea	Disorientation, agitation
Lethargy	Cheyne-Stokes breathing
Apathy	Hypothermia
Muscle cramps	Pathologic reflexes
	Pseudobulbar palsy
	Seizures
	Coma
	Death

appear to tolerate a decrease in serum sodium better than elderly patients.

Anorexia, nausea, and general malaise may occur early, but central nervous system signs and symptoms predominate later in the course and in acutely deteriorating cases of hyponatremia (Table 18-3). As mentioned earlier, hyponatremia usually occurs along with extracellular hypotonicity. The associated osmolal gradient allows water to move into brain cells, which results in cerebral edema and increased intracranial pressure. Brain cells may compensate over time by lowering intracellular osmolality through the movement of potassium and organic solutes out of brain cells. This reduces water movement into the intracellular space. However, when adaptive mechanisms fail or hyponatremia progresses, central nervous system manifestations of hyponatremia can present as a change in sensorium, seizures, brain herniation, and death.

DIAGNOSIS

Although hyponatremia usually co-exists with hypo-osmolality, osmolality should be measured in all cases of hyponatremia, particularly to avoid overlooking a pathologic hyperosmolar state caused by dangerous concentrations of glucose or exogenous toxins, or iatrogenic infusions of osmolal loads.

In such hyperosmolal situations, plasma volume expands as interstitial and intracellular water migrates into the intravascular space, causing a relative dilution of the serum sodium concentration without reduction in the amount of total body sodium. Total body water may be increased, unchanged, or decreased depending on the competing effects of water coadministered with the osmolal load and the likely presence of osmotic diuresis.

In patients with normal osmolality, a pseudohyponatremia can be seen as a laboratory artifact in cases of severe hyperlipidemia or hyperproteinemia when plasma volume is increased in the presence of normal serum sodium concentrations. Measuring sodium concentrations in *serum* rather than in plasma avoids the misinterpretation of this nonelectrolyte problem.

Once the two situations of hyperosmolality and normal osmolality have been excluded, the approach to the diagnosis of hypo-osmolal hyponatremia should be to evaluate the severity of the electrolyte derangement and the underlying volume status of the patient. Hypervolemic hyponatremia suggests the possibility of renal failure, congestive heart failure, or a hypo-albuminemic state such as cirrhosis or nephrotic syndrome. Normovolemic hyponatremia is commonly seen in the syndrome of inappropriate secretion of antidiuretic hormone or in situations of habitual ingestion of hypotonic substances as seen in psychogenic polydipsia. Hypovolemic hyponatremia should prompt an investigation into the source of free water loss—either renal losses (e.g., from diuretics, mineralocorticoid deficiency, or other salt-wasting nephropathy) or extrarenal losses (e.g., gastrointestinal losses or third spacing).

Sometimes the clinical context offers the answer. For example, massive absorption of irrigating solutions that do not contain sodium, such as during transurethral resection of the prostate, is a relatively common cause of intraoperative hyponatremia. When the clinical context does not lead to a diagnosis, urinary sodium concentration measured from a spot urine sample can further differentiate among the various causes of hyponatremia (Figure 18-2).

TREATMENT

Treatment of hypotonic hyponatremia will depend on the volume status of the patient. In hypovolemic hyponatremia, appropriate volume resuscitation should be pursued, usually with normal saline. If renal sodium losses are suspected, mineralocorticoid deficiency and the possibility of adrenal insufficiency should not be overlooked. Cases of massive third spacing such as can accompany pancreatitis or burns requires tailored resuscitation based on the totality of electrolyte and hematologic derangements.

In euvolemic or hypervolemic patients, treatment involves withholding free water and encouraging free water excretion with a loop diuretic. Administration of saline is necessary only if significant symptoms are present. In these as in all cases of hyponatremia, the rate of correction depends on whether the development of hyponatremia was acute (i.e., occurred in <48 hours) or was chronic.

Acute *symptomatic* hyponatremia must be treated promptly. Solute-free fluids are withheld and hypertonic saline (3% NaCl) and furosemide are administered to enhance renal excretion of free water. Serum electrolyte levels should be checked frequently and this treatment continued until symptoms disappear, which will likely occur before the serum sodium concentration returns to normal.

Chronic *symptomatic* hyponatremia should be corrected slowly to avoid the risk of osmotic demyelination. During the development of chronic hyponatremia, brain cells retain their

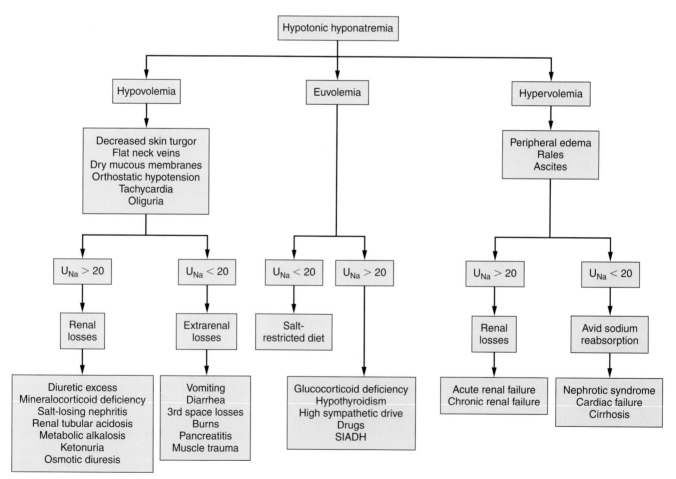

FIGURE 18-2 Diagnostic algorithm for hypotonic hyponatremia. *SIADH,* Syndrome of inappropriate secretion of antidiuretic hormone; U_{Na}, urinary sodium concentration (mEq/L) in a spot urine sample. *(Adapted from Schrier RW. Manual of Nephrology. 6th ed. Philadelphia, PA: Lippincott Williams & Wilkins; 2006.)*

normal intracellular volume as the serum sodium decreases by exporting "effective osmoles." Approximately half of these effective osmoles are potassium ions and anions, and the remainder are small organic compounds. While hyponatremia is being corrected, brain cells must reaccumulate these effective osmoles or water will move out of the cells into the now relatively hypertonic ECF, causing cell shrinkage. Such shrinkage can trigger central pontine myelinolysis, which can result in quadriplegia, seizures, coma, and death. The risk of osmotic demyelination is higher in patients who are malnourished or potassium depleted. Guidelines for correction of chronic symptomatic hyponatremia call for an initial correction in serum sodium concentration of approximately 10 mEq/L. Thereafter, correction should not exceed 1 to 1.5 mEq/L/hr or a daily maximum increase of 12 mEq/L.

Treatment of chronic *asymptomatic* hyponatremia should consider the underlying cause of the electrolyte disturbance. Appropriate sodium intake and volume restriction are often the cornerstones of treatment. Patients with hypervolemic hyponatremia secondary to congestive heart failure respond very well to the combination of an angiotensin-converting enzyme inhibitor and a loop diuretic.

MANAGEMENT OF ANESTHESIA

If at all possible, significant hyponatremia, especially if symptomatic, should be corrected before surgery. If the surgery is urgent, then appropriate corrective treatment should continue throughout the surgery and into the postoperative period. Frequent measurement of serum sodium concentration is necessary to avoid overly rapid correction of hyponatremia with resultant osmotic demyelination or overcorrection resulting in hypernatremia. If the treatment of hyponatremia includes hypertonic sodium infusion during surgery, it should be infused via a pump while losses caused by the surgery are replaced with standard crystalloid or colloid solutions as required. Treatment of the underlying cause of the hyponatremia should also continue throughout the perioperative period.

Induction and maintenance of anesthesia in patients with hypovolemic hyponatremia are fraught with the risk of hypotension. In addition to fluid therapy, vasopressors and/or inotropes may be required to treat the hypotension and should be made available before the start of induction. Hypervolemic hyponatremic patients, particularly those with heart failure, may benefit from invasive hemodynamic monitoring to assess cardiac function and guide fluid therapy.

Transurethral Resection of the Prostate (TURP) Syndrome

Benign prostatic hyperplasia is often treated surgically by transurethral resection of the prostate (TURP). This procedure involves resection via a cystoscope with continuous irrigation of the bladder to aid in visualization and removal of blood and resected material. The irrigating fluid is usually a nearly isotonic, nonelectrolyte fluid containing glycine or a mixture of sorbitol and mannitol. This irrigating fluid may be absorbed rapidly via open venous sinuses in the prostate gland, which causes volume overload and hyponatremia. The use of hypotonic irrigating solutions has mostly fallen out of favor but would also lead to hypo-osmolality. The constellation of findings associated with absorption of bladder irrigation solution is known as *TURP syndrome.* This syndrome is more likely to occur when resection is prolonged (>1 hour), when the irrigating fluid is suspended more than 40 cm above the operative field, when hypotonic irrigation fluid is used, and when the pressure in the bladder is allowed to increase above 15 cm H_2O. TURP syndrome (Table 18-4) manifests principally with cardiovascular signs of fluid overload and neurologic signs and symptoms of hyponatremia. Use of hypotonic irrigating solutions can

TABLE 18-4   Signs and symptoms of transurethral resection of the prostate (TURP) syndrome

System	Signs and symptoms	Cause
Cardiovascular	Hypertension, reflex bradycardia, pulmonary edema, cardiovascular collapse	Rapid fluid absorption (reflex bradycardia may be secondary to hypertension or increased ICP)
	Hypotension	Third spacing secondary to hyponatremia and hypo-osmolality; cardiovascular collapse
	ECG changes (wide QRS, elevated ST segments, ventricular arrhythmias)	Hyponatremia
Respiratory	Tachypnea, oxygen desaturation, Cheyne-Stokes breathing	Pulmonary edema
Neurologic	Nausea, restlessness, visual disturbances, confusion, somnolence, seizures, coma, death	Hyponatremia and hypo-osmolality causing cerebral edema and increased ICP, hyperglycinemia (glycine is an inhibitory neurotransmitter that potentiates NMDA receptor activity), hyperammonemia
Hematologic	Disseminated intravascular hemolysis	Hyponatremia and hypo-osmolality
Renal	Renal failure	Hypotension, hyperoxaluria (oxalate is a metabolite of glycine)
Metabolic	Acidosis	Deamination of glycine to glyoxylic acid and ammonia

ECG, Electrocardiogram; *ICP,* intracranial pressure; *NMDA,* N-methyl-D-aminotransferase; *TURP,* transurethral resection of the prostate.

also induce hemolysis, because red blood cells encounter a significant influx of free water from hypotonic ECF. Hypertension and pulmonary edema are common. If a glycine irrigant is used, transient blindness can occur that is thought to result from the inhibitory neurotransmitter effects of glycine. Glycine breaks down into glyoxylic acid and ammonia, and excessive ammonia levels themselves are known to cause encephalopathy.

Monitoring for the development of TURP syndrome includes direct neurologic assessment in patients under regional anesthesia and measurement of hemodynamics, serum sodium concentration, and osmolality in patients under general anesthesia. Treatment consists of terminating the surgical procedure so that no more fluid is absorbed, administration of loop diuretics if needed for relief of cardiovascular symptoms, and administration of hypertonic saline if severe neurologic symptoms are present or the serum sodium concentration is less than 120 mEq/L.

Hypernatremia

Hypernatremia, defined as a serum sodium concentration of more than 145 mEq/L, is much less common than hyponatremia because the vasopressin-driven thirst mechanism is very effective in responding to the hypertonic state of hypernatremia. Even in patients with renal disorders of sodium retention or severe water loss, patients will regulate their serum sodium concentration close to or within the normal range if they have access to water. Therefore, hypernatremia is much more likely to be seen in the very young, the elderly, and people who are debilitated, have altered mental status, or are unconscious.

In the perioperative setting, hypernatremia is most likely a result of iatrogenic overcorrection of hyponatremia or treatment of acidemia with sodium bicarbonate. Free water losses from diabetes insipidus and extrarenal gastrointestinal losses will also lead to hypernatremia. Because sodium is the major contributor to ECF osmolality, hypernatremia induces the movement of water across cell membranes into the ECF. Hypernatremia and the associated hyperosmolality will always lead to cellular dehydration and shrinkage.

SIGNS AND SYMPTOMS

Signs and symptoms of hypernatremia can vary from mild to life threatening (Table 18-5). The earliest signs and symptoms are restlessness, irritability, and lethargy. As hypernatremia progresses, muscular twitching, hyperreflexia, tremors, and ataxia may develop. The signs and symptoms progress as the osmolality increases above 325 mOsm/kg. Muscle spasticity, seizures, and death may ensue. The very young and the very old and those with preexisting central nervous system disease exhibit more severe symptoms at any given serum sodium concentration or degree of hyperosmolality.

The most prominent abnormalities in hypernatremia are neurologic. Dehydration of brain cells occurs as water shifts out of the cells into the hypertonic interstitium. Capillary and

TABLE 18-5	Symptoms and signs of hypernatremia
Symptoms	**Signs**
Polyuria	Muscle twitching
Polydipsia	Hyperreflexia
Orthostasis	Tremor
Restlessness	Ataxia
Irritability	Muscle spasticity
Lethargy	Focal and generalized seizures
	Death

venous congestion as well as venous sinus thrombosis have all been reported. As the brain cells shrink, cerebral blood vessels may stretch and tear, which results in intracranial hemorrhage.

Usually the signs and symptoms are more severe when hypernatremia is acute rather than chronic and when excessive elevations in serum sodium levels are present. Mortality rates of up to 75% have been reported in adults with severe acute hypernatremia (serum sodium concentration > 160 mEq/L), and survivors of severe acute hypernatremia often have permanent neurologic sequelae. During the development of chronic hypernatremia, brain cells generate "idiogenic osmoles" that restore intracellular water in spite of the ongoing hypernatremia and protect against brain cell dehydration. If chronic hypernatremia is corrected too rapidly, these idiogenic osmoles predispose to the development of cerebral edema.

DIAGNOSIS

The diagnosis and treatment of hypernatremia should focus on assessing the severity of the derangement and on ascertaining the volume status of the patient. The presence of hypervolemia, euvolemia, or hypovolemia dictates the appropriate diagnostic and treatment modalities (Figure 18-3).

In hypovolemic hypernatremia, the patient has lost more water than sodium via renal or extrarenal routes. This may occur as a result of excessive hypotonic diuresis, gastrointestinal losses, or insensible fluid losses from burns or sweating.

Patients with hypervolemic hypernatremia will show signs of ECF volume expansion, such as jugular venous distention, peripheral edema, and pulmonary congestion. The differential diagnosis includes a history of hypertonic fluid administration, oral intake of salt tablets, and endocrine abnormalities marked by excessive aldosterone secretion.

Euvolemic and hypovolemic hypernatremia occur secondary to water loss without concomitant salt loss and may be seen with either extrarenal pathologic conditions (e.g., gastrointestinal tract losses or insensible losses from burns or sweating) or from renal losses (e.g., diabetes insipidus, loop diuretics, or osmotic diuresis).

As with hyponatremia, testing of a spot urine sample for sodium concentration and osmolality can help distinguish among the causes of hypernatremia (see Figure 18-3).

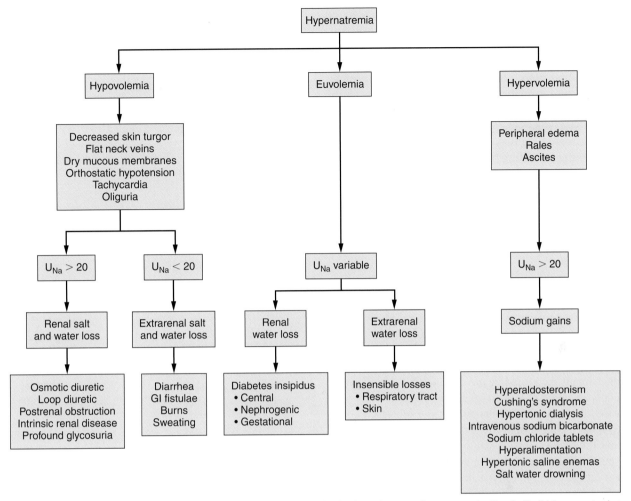

FIGURE 18-3 Diagnostic algorithm for hypernatremia. *GI,* Gastrointestinal; U_{Na}, urinary sodium concentration (mEq/L) in a spot urine sample. *(Adapted from Schrier RW. Manual of Nephrology. 6th ed. Philadelphia, PA: Lippincott Williams & Wilkins; 2006.)*

TREATMENT

Treatment is determined by how severe the hypernatremia is and how rapidly it developed and whether the ECF volume is increased or decreased.

In hypovolemic hypernatremia, the water deficit is replenished with normal saline or a balanced electrolyte solution until the patient is euvolemic and then the plasma osmolality is corrected with hypotonic saline or 5% dextrose solution.

In patients with hypervolemic hypernatremia, the primary treatment is diuresis with a loop diuretic, but if the cause of the hypervolemic hypernatremia is renal failure, then hemofiltration or hemodialysis may be needed.

Patients with euvolemic hypernatremia require water replacement either orally or with 5% dextrose intravenously. Treatment of diabetes insipidus is covered in Chapter 19 and depends on whether there is a central deficit of vasopressin release or a renal insensitivity to vasopressin's actions.

Acute hypernatremia should be corrected over several hours. However, to avoid cerebral edema, chronic hypernatremia should be corrected more slowly, over 2 to 3 days. Ongoing sodium and water losses should also be calculated and replaced.

MANAGEMENT OF ANESTHESIA

If at all possible, surgery should be delayed until the hypernatremia has been corrected and the associated symptoms have abated. Frequent serum sodium measurements and urine output monitoring will be required perioperatively, and invasive hemodynamic monitoring may be useful to assess volume status. Hypovolemia will be exacerbated by induction and maintenance of anesthesia, and prompt correction of hypotension with fluids, vasopressors, and/or inotropes may be required. The volume of distribution of hydrophilic drugs will be altered in hypovolemia and hypervolemia. An accentuated hemodynamic response to anesthetic drug administration, however, is more likely a consequence of vasodilatory and cardiodepressant responses in a hypovolemic patient than a result of changes in the volume of distribution.

DISORDERS OF POTASSIUM

Potassium is the major intracellular cation. The normal total body potassium content depends on muscle mass; it is maximal in young adults and decreases progressively with age. Less than 1.5% of total body potassium is found in the extracellular space. Therefore, serum potassium concentration is often a reflection more of factors that regulate transcellular potassium distribution than of total body potassium. Total body potassium is regulated over longer periods of time, principally by the distal nephron in the kidneys; the distal nephron secretes potassium in response to aldosterone, which leads to an increase in urine volume and nonresorbable anions, and metabolic alkalosis. More than 90% of the potassium taken in by diet is excreted in the urine, and most of the remainder is eliminated in the feces. As the glomerular filtration rate decreases in renal failure, the amount of potassium excreted by the gastrointestinal route increases.

Hypokalemia

SIGNS AND SYMPTOMS

Signs and symptoms of hypokalemia are generally restricted to the cardiac and neuromuscular systems and include dysrhythmias, muscle weakness, cramps, paralysis, and ileus.

DIAGNOSIS

Hypokalemia is diagnosed by the presence of a serum potassium concentration of less than 3.5 mmol/L and results from decreased net intake, intracellular shifts, or increased potassium losses. Differential diagnosis requires determining whether the hypokalemia is acute and secondary to intracellular potassium shifts, such as might be seen with hyperventilation or alkalosis, or whether the hypokalemia is chronic and associated with depletion of total body potassium stores (Table 18-6). If the hypokalemia is the result of potassium losses, a spot urinary potassium reading will guide the diagnosis toward either renal or extrarenal causes. Renal potassium losses are associated with a spot urinary potassium value of more than 15 to 20 mEq/L despite the presence of hypokalemia. Appropriately low urine potassium concentrations in the setting of hypokalemia point to a normally functioning kidney in the setting of inadequate potassium intake or gastrointestinal losses. In cases of renal loss, assessment of the transtubular potassium concentration gradient, hemodynamics, and acid-base status will further guide diagnosis. Hypertension with hypokalemia is usually the result of a hyperaldosterone state. Renal losses in the setting of acidemia point to a diagnosis of renal tubular acidosis or diabetic ketoacidosis. Renal losses in the setting of alkalemia can indicate a response to diuretics or can be seen in genetic disorders such as Liddle's syndrome (associated with hypertension) or Bartter's syndrome (which has tubular effects similar to those of loop diuretics). Hypomagnesemia can also exacerbate renal potassium losses. Hypokalemia without a change in total body potassium stores can be caused by familial hypokalemic periodic paralysis. Unusual causes of hypokalemia from ICF shifts include conditions causing rapid cell growth, such as after initiation of treatment for pernicious anemia or other anabolic states.

TABLE 18-6 ■ Causes of hypokalemia
HYPOKALEMIA DUE TO INCREASED RENAL POTASSIUM LOSS
Thiazide diuretics
Loop diuretics
Mineralocorticoids
High-dose glucocorticoids
Antibiotics (penicillin, nafcillin, ampicillin)
Drugs associated with magnesium depletion (aminoglycosides)
Surgical trauma
Hyperglycemia
Hyperaldosteronism
HYPOKALEMIA DUE TO EXCESSIVE GASTROINTESTINAL LOSS OF POTASSIUM
Vomiting and diarrhea
Zollinger-Ellison syndrome
Jejunoileal bypass
Malabsorption
Chemotherapy
Nasogastric suction
HYPOKALEMIA DUE TO TRANSCELLULAR POTASSIUM SHIFT
β-Adrenergic agonists
Tocolytic drugs (ritodrine)
Insulin
Respiratory or metabolic alkalosis
Familial periodic paralysis
Hypercalcemia
Hypomagnesemia

Adapted from Gennari JF. Hypokalemia. *N Engl J Med*. 1998;339:451-458.

TREATMENT

Treatment of hypokalemia depends on the degree of potassium depletion and the underlying cause. If the hypokalemia is profound or is associated with life-threatening signs, potassium must be administered intravenously. In the presence of paralysis or malignant dysrhythmias, the rate of potassium repletion can be as high as 20 mEq over 30 to 45 minutes, repeated as needed. If a malignant dysrhythmia appears after potassium repletion is initiated, the differential diagnosis may implicate the potassium administration as the cause. Therefore electrocardiographic (ECG) monitoring is required whenever rapid potassium repletion is undertaken. In the setting of urgent repletion, delivering potassium solutions in a dextrose carrier is suboptimal, because the resultant insulin secretion will further induce intracellular potassium transfer.

Largely because of the risks of intravenous potassium administration, in cases of nonemergent potassium repletion the enteral route is preferred. If intravenous repletion is chosen in a nonemergency situation, it should proceed at a rate of less than 20 mmol/hr. Peripheral infusion may result in pain or venous damage at the intravenous site, and central administration is preferred.

MANAGEMENT OF ANESTHESIA

Whether or not to treat hypokalemia before surgery is an ongoing subject of debate and depends on the chronicity and severity of the deficit. Because of the limitations on rate of repletion and the large total body potassium deficits that accompany chronic hypokalemia, the safe repletion of total body potassium stores often requires days. Although total body depletion is variable in its relationship to serum potassium concentrations, chronic hypokalemia with serum concentrations of less than 3.0 mmol/L may require delivery of 600 mmol or more of potassium to achieve full normalization. It is therefore unlikely that the administration of small aliquots of potassium immediately before surgery will make any significant difference in potassium balance. Moreover, such interventions carry the risk of inadvertent serum hyperkalemia that may exacerbate susceptibility to dysrhythmias in the perioperative period. However, it has also been suggested that even small improvements in potassium balance may help normalize transmembrane potentials and reduce the incidence of perioperative dysrhythmias. Recommendations on this controversial issue are based more on expert opinion, clinical judgement, and local practice patterns than on evidence from peer-reviewed studies.

It may be prudent to correct significant hypokalemia in patients with other risk factors for dysrhythmias such as those with congestive heart failure, those taking digoxin, and those with ECG evidence of hypokalemia. ECG abnormalities associated with potassium derangement are illustrated in (Figure 18-4). Classically, U waves are seen in the presence of hypokalemia. Anesthetic management of patients with significant hypokalemia should also prevent further decreases in serum potassium concentration by avoiding the administration of insulin, glucose, β-adrenergic agonists, bicarbonate, and diuretics, as well as by avoiding hyperventilation and respiratory alkalosis.

Because of the effect of hypokalemia on skeletal muscle, there is the theoretical possibility of prolonged action of muscle relaxants. Doses of neuromuscular blockers should be guided by nerve stimulator testing.

Potassium levels should be measured frequently if repletion is ongoing or changes resulting from drug administration, surgical progress, or ventilation are expected.

Hyperkalemia

Hyperkalemia is defined as a serum potassium concentration of more than 5.5 mEq/L. As with hypokalemia, hyperkalemia can result from transcellular movement of potassium out of cells or from alterations in potassium intake or excretion. In hospitalized patients, hyperkalemia is frequently the result of iatrogenic potassium loads (Table 18-7).

SIGNS AND SYMPTOMS

Signs and symptoms of hyperkalemia depend on the acuity of the increase. Chronic hyperkalemia is often asymptomatic, and dialysis-dependent patients can withstand considerable

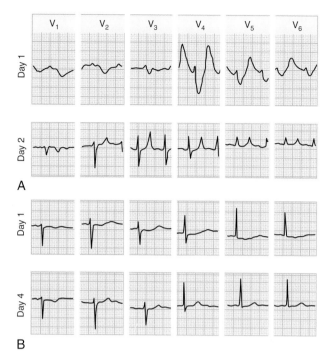

FIGURE 18-4 Electrocardiographic changes in hyperkalemia (**A**) and hypokalemia (**B**). **A,** On day 1, at a K+ level of 8.6 mEq/L, the P wave is no longer recognizable and the QRS complex is diffusely prolonged. Initial and terminal QRS delays are characteristic of K+-induced intraventricular conduction slowing and are best illustrated in leads V$_2$ and V$_6$. On day 2, at a K+ level of 5.8 mEq/L, the P wave is recognizable, with a PR interval of 0.24 seconds; the duration of the QRS complex is approximately 0.10 seconds, and the T waves are characteristically "tented." **B,** On day 1, at a K+ level of 1.5 mEq/L, the T and U waves are merged. The U wave is prominent and the QU interval is prolonged. On day 4, at a K+ level of 3.7 mEq/L, the tracing is normal. *(From Bonow R, Mann D, Zipes D, et al, eds.* Braunwald's Heart Disease: A Textbook of Cardiovascular Medicine. *9th ed. Philadelphia, PA: Saunders; 2011. Courtesy Dr. C. Fisch.)*

variations in serum potassium concentration between dialysis sessions (usually 2 to 3 days) with remarkably few symptoms. Chronic hyperkalemia may be associated with nonspecific symptoms such as general malaise and mild gastrointestinal disturbances. More acute or significant increases in potassium manifest as membrane depolarization and associated cardiac and neuromuscular changes, including weakness, paralysis, nausea, vomiting, and bradycardia or asystole.

DIAGNOSIS

The first step in the diagnosis of hyperkalemia is to rule out a spuriously high potassium level secondary to hemolysis of the specimen. A spuriously high potassium level may also occur with thrombocytosis and leukocytosis resulting from leakage of potassium from the cells in vitro. True hyperkalemia can be identified on ECG tracings first as a peaked T wave, followed in more severe cases by disappearance of the P wave and prolongation of the QRS complex, which progresses to sine waves and then eventually to asystole (see Figure 18-4).

TABLE 18-7   Causes of hyperkalemia

INCREASED TOTAL BODY POTASSIUM CONTENT

Acute oliguric renal failure

Chronic renal disease

Hypoaldosteronism

Drugs that impair potassium excretion

  Triamterene

  Spironolactone

  Nonsteroidal antiinflammatory drugs

Drugs that inhibit the renin-angiotensin-aldosterone system

ALTERED TRANSCELLULAR POTASSIUM SHIFT

Succinylcholine

Respiratory or metabolic acidosis

Lysis of cells resulting from chemotherapy

Iatrogenic bolus

PSEUDOHYPERKALEMIA

Hemolysis of blood specimen

Thrombocytosis/leukocytosis

Common causes of hyperkalemia in the perioperative period include acidosis, rhabdomyolysis, and succinylcholine administration. If the increase in serum potassium level is thought to be associated with increased total body potassium, then decreased renal excretion or increased potassium intake is likely. Measurement of the urinary potassium excretion rate can aid in the differential diagnosis between cellular potassium shifts and problems with potassium excretion.

TREATMENT

Immediate treatment of hyperkalemia is required if life-threatening dysrhythmias or ECG signs of severe hyperkalemia are present. This treatment is aimed at antagonizing the effects of a high potassium level on the transmembrane potential and redistributing the potassium intracellularly. Calcium chloride or calcium gluconate is administered intravenously to stabilize cellular membranes. The onset of action is immediate. Potassium can be driven intracellularly by the action of insulin with or without glucose. This measure will be effective within 10 to 20 minutes. Other adjuvant therapies include sodium bicarbonate administration and hyperventilation to promote alkalosis and movement of potassium intracellularly. Potassium driven intracellularly may eventually move out of the cells again, so therapy may need to continue beyond acute correction of the derangement.

When hyperkalemia is secondary to increased total body stores of potassium, then potassium must be eliminated from the body. This can be achieved by administration of a loop diuretic such as furosemide, infusion of saline to encourage diuresis, or use of an ion exchange resin. The primary potassium exchange resin used is sodium polystyrene sulfonate (Kayexalate) given either orally or by enema. Dialysis may be required to remove potassium in cases of emergent hyperkalemia or in patients with poor renal function.

MANAGEMENT OF ANESTHESIA

It is recommended that the serum potassium concentration be below 5.5 mEq/L for elective surgery. Correction of hyperkalemia before surgery is preferable, but if this is not feasible, steps should be taken to lower the potassium level immediately before induction of anesthesia by the methods indicated previously. Potassium levels may influence the selection of drugs for induction and maintenance of anesthesia, because preoperative medications that induce hypocapnia and acidosis may cause further transcellular potassium shifts. Also, succinylcholine increases serum potassium concentration by approximately 0.5 mEq/L in healthy patients and is best avoided in the absence of an urgent need for it. The effects of muscle relaxants may be exaggerated if there is muscle weakness from the hyperkalemia. Respiratory and metabolic acidosis must be avoided, since either will exacerbate the hyperkalemia and its effects. Potassium-containing intravenous fluids such as lactated Ringer's solution (which contains 4 mEq/L of potassium) and Normosol (which contains 5 mEq/L of potassium) should be avoided. Dialysis patients who are scheduled for surgery in which intraoperative potassium loads can be anticipated may be managed preoperatively by decreasing the potassium content of the dialysate to reduce serum potassium levels in anticipation of surgery.

DISORDERS OF CALCIUM

Only 1% of total body calcium is present in the ECF. The remainder is stored in bone. Of the calcium in the ECF, 60% is free or coupled with anions and thus filterable, and the remaining 40% is bound to proteins, mainly albumin. Only the ionized calcium in the extracellular space is physiologically active. Ionized calcium concentrations are affected by both albumin concentration and the pH of plasma. Net calcium balance occurs when absorption from the diet equals losses of calcium in feces and urine. Several hormones regulate calcium metabolism: parathyroid hormone, which increases bone resorption and renal tubular reabsorption of calcium; calcitonin, which inhibits bone resorption; and vitamin D, which augments intestinal absorption of calcium. The activity of these hormones is altered in response to changes in plasma ionized calcium concentration. Other hormones, including thyroid hormone, growth hormone, and adrenal and gonadal steroids, also affect calcium homeostasis, but their secretion is determined by factors other than plasma calcium concentration.

Hypocalcemia

Hypocalcemia is defined as a reduction in serum ionized calcium concentration. It is important to note that many blood chemistry analysis systems measure total calcium rather than ionized calcium. Several formulas exist to convert total calcium to ionized calcium, but none of these is totally reliable.

Binding of calcium to albumin is pH dependent, and acid-base disturbances can change the fraction and therefore the concentration of ionized calcium without changing total body

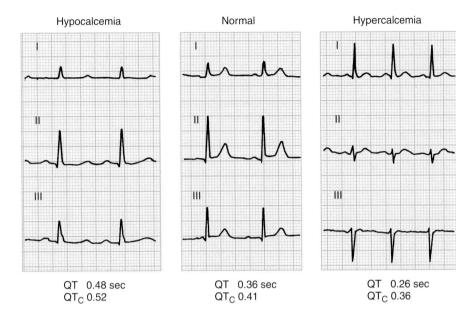

Hypocalcemia	Normal	Hypercalcemia

QT 0.48 sec
QT_C 0.52

QT 0.36 sec
QT_C 0.41

QT 0.26 sec
QT_C 0.36

FIGURE 18-5 Electrocardiographic changes in calcium disorders. Prolongation of the QT interval (ST-segment portion) is typical of hypocalcemia. Hypercalcemia may cause abbreviation of the ST segment and shortening of the QT interval. *(Data from Goldberger AL. Clinical Electrocardiography: A Simplified Approach. 6th ed. St Louis, MO: Mosby; 1999.)*

calcium. Alkalosis reduces the ionized calcium concentration, so ionized calcium may be significantly reduced after bicarbonate administration or in the setting of hyperventilation. Many hospitalized patients are also hypoalbuminemic, and the reduction in bound calcium will reduce the measured serum calcium level. When serum calcium concentration is interpreted in the setting of a low albumin level, corrected calcium concentration can be calculated as follows: measured calcium (mg/dL) + 0.8 [4 – albumin (mg/dL)].

SIGNS AND SYMPTOMS

The signs and symptoms of hypocalcemia depend on the rapidity and the degree of reduction in ionized calcium. Most of these signs and symptoms are evident in the cardiovascular and neuromuscular systems and include paresthesias, irritability, seizures, hypotension, and myocardial depression. ECG changes associated with hypocalcemia are marked by prolongation of the QT interval (Figure 18-5). In the postoperative period after parathyroid resection, hypocalcemia-induced laryngospasm can be life threatening.

DIAGNOSIS

Hypocalcemia is often caused by decreased parathyroid hormone secretion, end-organ resistance to parathyroid hormone, or disorders of vitamin D metabolism. These are usually seen clinically as complications of thyroid or parathyroid surgery, magnesium deficiency, and renal failure. In the operative theater, acute hypocalcemia is often encountered as a result of calcium binding to citrate preservative during massive transfusion.

TREATMENT

Acute symptomatic hypocalcemia with seizures, tetany, and/or cardiovascular depression must be treated immediately with intravenous calcium. The duration of treatment will be dependent on serial calcium measurements. Treatment of hypocalcemia in the presence of hypomagnesemia is ineffective unless

magnesium is also replenished. Metabolic or respiratory *alkalosis* should be corrected. If metabolic or respiratory *acidosis* is present with hypocalcemia, then the calcium level should be corrected before the acidosis is treated, because correcting an acidosis with bicarbonate or hyperventilation will only exacerbate the hypocalcemia.

Less acute and asymptomatic hypocalcemia may be treated with oral calcium and vitamin D supplementation.

MANAGEMENT OF ANESTHESIA

Symptomatic hypocalcemia must be treated before surgery, and every effort must be made to minimize any further decrease in serum calcium level intraoperatively. This might occur with hyperventilation or administration of bicarbonate. Ionized calcium levels should always be considered during massive transfusion of blood containing citrate. Hypothermia, liver disease, and renal failure impair citrate clearance and further increase the likelihood of significant hypocalcemia in transfusion recipients.

Sudden decreases in ionized calcium levels may be seen in the early postoperative period after thyroidectomy or parathyroidectomy and may precipitate laryngospasm.

Hypercalcemia

Hypercalcemia results from increased calcium absorption from the gastrointestinal tract (milk-alkali syndrome, vitamin D intoxication, granulomatous diseases such as sarcoidosis), decreased renal calcium excretion in renal insufficiency, and increased bone resorption of calcium (primary or secondary hyperparathyroidism, malignancy, hyperthyroidism, and immobilization).

SIGNS AND SYMPTOMS

Hypercalcemia is associated with neurologic and gastrointestinal signs and symptoms such as confusion, hypotonia, depressed deep tendon reflexes, lethargy, abdominal pain, and nausea and vomiting, especially if the increase in serum calcium level is relatively acute. A shortened ST segment and QT interval are seen (Figure 18-5). Chronic hypercalcemia is often associated with polyuria, hypercalciuria, and nephrolithiasis.

DIAGNOSIS

Almost all patients with hypercalcemia have either hyperparathyroidism or cancer. Primary hyperparathyroidism is usually associated with a serum calcium concentration of less than 11 mEq/L and no symptoms, whereas malignancy often presents with acute symptoms and a serum calcium level higher than 13 mEq/L.

TREATMENT

Treatment of hypercalcemia is directed toward increasing urinary calcium excretion and inhibiting bone resorption and further gastrointestinal absorption of calcium.

Since hypercalcemia is frequently associated with hypovolemia secondary to polyuria, volume expansion with saline not only corrects the fluid deficit but also increases urinary excretion of calcium along with administered sodium. Loop diuretics also enhance urinary excretion of both sodium and calcium but should be used only after appropriate volume resuscitation.

Calcitonin, bisphosphonates, or mithramycin may be required in disorders associated with osteoclastic bone resorption. Hydrocortisone may reduce gastrointestinal absorption of calcium in granulomatous disease, vitamin D intoxication, lymphoma, and myeloma. Oral phosphate may also be given to reduce gastrointestinal uptake of calcium if renal function is normal. Dialysis may be required for life-threatening hypercalcemia. Surgical removal of the parathyroid glands may be required to treat primary or secondary hyperparathyroidism.

MANAGEMENT OF ANESTHESIA

Management of anesthesia for emergency surgery in a patient with hypercalcemia is aimed at restoring intravascular volume before induction and increasing urinary excretion of calcium with loop diuretics (thiazide diuretics should be avoided, because they *increase* renal tubular reabsorption of calcium). Ideally, surgery should be postponed until calcium levels have normalized.

Central venous pressure or pulmonary artery pressure monitoring may be advisable in some patients requiring fluid resuscitation and diuresis as part of the perioperative treatment of hypercalcemia. Dosing of muscle relaxants must be guided by neuromuscular monitoring if muscle weakness, hypotonia, or loss of deep tendon reflexes is present.

DISORDERS OF MAGNESIUM

Magnesium is predominantly found intracellularly and in mineralized bone. Between 60% and 70% of serum magnesium is ionized, with 10% complexed to citrate, bicarbonate, or phosphate and approximately 30% bound to protein, mostly albumin. There is little difference between extracellular and intracellular ionized magnesium concentrations, so there is only a small transmembrane gradient for ionized magnesium. It is the ionized fraction of magnesium that is associated with clinical effects.

Magnesium is absorbed from and secreted into the gastrointestinal tract and filtered, reabsorbed, and excreted by the kidneys. Renal reabsorption and excretion are passive, following sodium and water.

Hypomagnesemia

Some degree of hypomagnesemia occurs in up to 10% of hospitalized patients. An even higher percentage of patients in intensive care units, especially those receiving parenteral nutrition or dialysis, have hypomagnesemia. Coronary care unit patients with hypomagnesemia have a higher mortality rate that those with normal serum levels of magnesium.

SIGNS AND SYMPTOMS

Signs and symptoms of hypomagnesemia are similar to those of hypocalcemia and involve mostly the cardiac and neuromuscular systems. Dysrhythmias, weakness, muscle twitching, tetany, apathy, and seizures can be seen. Hypokalemia and/or hypocalcemia that had been refractory to supplementation will respond after correction of hypomagnesemia.

DIAGNOSIS

Hypomagnesemia is most commonly due to reduced gastrointestinal uptake (reduced dietary intake or reduced absorption from the gastrointestinal tract) or to renal wasting of magnesium. These entities can be differentiated by measuring the urinary magnesium excretion rate. Much less frequently, hypomagnesemia is due to intracellular shifts of magnesium with no overall change in total body magnesium, to hungry bone syndrome after parathyroidectomy, or to exudative cutaneous losses after burn injury.

TREATMENT

Treatment of hypomagnesemia depends on the severity of the deficiency and the signs and symptoms that are present. If cardiac dysrhythmias or seizures are present, magnesium is administered intravenously as a bolus (2 g of magnesium sulfate equals 8 mEq of magnesium), and the dose is repeated until symptoms abate. After life-threatening signs have resolved, a slower infusion of magnesium sulfate can be continued for several days to allow for equilibration of intracellular and total body magnesium stores. If renal wasting is present, supplementation must be increased to account for the magnesium lost in the urine.

Hypermagnesemia is a potential side effect of the treatment of hypomagnesemia, so the patient should be monitored for signs of hypotension, facial flushing, and loss of deep tendon reflexes.

MANAGEMENT OF ANESTHESIA

Management of anesthesia in patients with hypomagnesemia includes attention to the signs of magnesium deficiency, magnesium supplementation, and treatment of refractory hypokalemia or hypocalcemia if needed. If the hypomagnesemia is secondary to malnutrition or alcoholism, the anesthetic implications of these diseases must be considered.

Ventricular dysrhythmias should be anticipated and treated as necessary. Muscle relaxation should be guided by the results of peripheral nerve stimulation, since hypomagnesemia can be associated with both muscle weakness and muscle excitation. Fluid loading (particularly with sodium-containing solutions) and the use of diuretics should be avoided, because the renal excretion of magnesium passively follows sodium excretion.

Hypermagnesemia

Hypermagnesemia (i.e., a serum magnesium concentration of >2.5 mEq/L) is much less common than hypomagnesemia because a magnesium load can be briskly excreted if renal function is normal. Even patients with renal failure rarely have symptomatic hypermagnesemia unless there is a significantly increased dietary or intravenous intake. However, milder elevations in serum magnesium levels are frequently found in intensive care unit and dialysis patient populations. Hypermagnesemia may be a complication of magnesium sulfate administration to treat preeclampsia/eclampsia or to provide perinatal neurologic protection in premature delivery. Magnesium infusion during pheochromocytoma surgery is popular in some centers but may also result in hypermagnesemia.

SIGNS AND SYMPTOMS

Signs and symptoms of hypermagnesemia begin to occur at serum levels of 4 to 5 mEq/L and include lethargy, nausea and vomiting and facial flushing. At levels above 6 mEq/L, a loss of deep tendon reflexes and hypotension occur. Paralysis, apnea, heart block, and/or cardiac arrest are likely if the magnesium level exceeds 10 mEq/L.

DIAGNOSIS

Evaluation of hypermagnesemia involves assessing renal function (creatinine clearance) and detecting any source of excess magnesium intake, such as parenteral infusion, oral ingestion of antacids, and administration of magnesium-based enemas or cathartics. Once these have been excluded, less common causes of hypermagnesemia, including hypothyroidism, hyperparathyroidism, Addison's disease, and lithium therapy, can be considered.

TREATMENT

Life-threatening signs of hypermagnesemia may be temporarily ameliorated with intravenous calcium administration, but hemodialysis may be required. Lesser degrees of hypermagnesemia can be treated with forced diuresis with saline and loop diuretics to increase renal excretion of magnesium.

MANAGEMENT OF ANESTHESIA

Invasive cardiovascular monitoring may be necessary perioperatively to measure and treat the hypotension and vasodilation associated with hypermagnesemia and to guide fluid resuscitation and ongoing replacement of fluids during forced diuresis. Acidosis exacerbates hypermagnesemia, so careful attention must be paid to ventilation and arterial pH. Initial and subsequent doses of muscle relaxant should be reduced in the presence of muscle weakness and guided by results of peripheral nerve stimulation. Hypermagnesemia and skeletal muscle weakness are not uncommon causes of failure to wean from mechanical ventilation in the intensive care setting, especially in patients with renal failure.

ACID-BASE DISORDERS

Arterial acid-base balance is normally tightly regulated within the pH range of 7.35 to 7.45 to ensure optimal conditions for cellular enzyme function. Values of arterial blood pH less than 7.35 are termed *acidemia,* and values higher than 7.45 are termed *alkalemia.* The related terms *acidosis* and *alkalosis* refer to acid-base derangements that produce either excess H^+ or excess OH^-, respectively, but that may be present regardless of arterial pH. Intracellular pH is lower than extracellular pH and is maintained at a closely regulated level of 7.0 to 7.3. Acid-base regulation in the setting of normal metabolism requires handling of the continuous production of acidic metabolites totalling approximately 1 mEq/kg body weight per day.

Stability of pH is accomplished by a system of intracellular and extracellular buffers, most importantly the HCO_3/CO_2 buffer pair. Carbon dioxide can enter or leave the body via the lungs, and bicarbonate can enter or leave the body via the kidneys. Maintenance of a normal bicarbonate concentration relative to carbon dioxide tension results in an optimal ratio of approximately 20:1. Maintenance of this ratio of 20:1 allows for a relatively normal pH despite deviations from normal of either bicarbonate concentration or carbon dioxide tension. Other buffers include proteins, bone apatite, and phosphate ions.

The relationship of the CO_2/HCO_3 buffer system to pH is expressed by the Henderson-Hasselbalch equation: $pH = 6.1 + log$ (serum bicarbonate concentration/$0.03 \times Paco_2$).

Changes in respiration regulate carbon dioxide tension, whereas renal regulation modifies bicarbonate concentration. These changes may be the cause of a primary acid-base disorder or can occur as a compensatory mechanism in response to another underlying disorder. In non–mechanically ventilated and nonsedated patients, compensatory respiratory or renal responses can normalize an altered pH but will not overcompensate and alter the pH to the point of reversing the primary disorder. This is not always true in the operating room, where the potential for overcompensation for acid-base disorders makes familiarity with the clinical history a key part of understanding the patient's primary acid-base abnormality.

Renal compensation for acid-base derangements may include increases in resorption or secretion of filtered bicarbonate in the proximal tubule. In addition, protons (i.e., hydrogen ions) can be reabsorbed in the distal tubule and collecting duct or excreted into the urine. Hydrogen ion excretion in the urine regenerates the bicarbonate originally consumed by buffering a hydrogen ion in the ECF. The excreted hydrogen

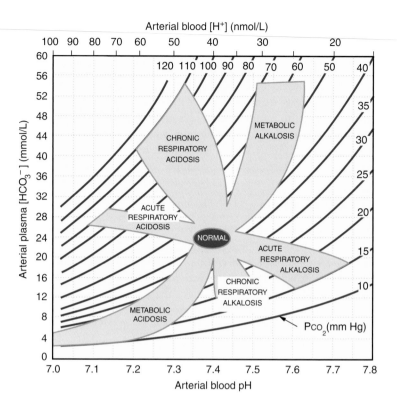

FIGURE 18-6 Acid-base nomogram (map). Shaded areas represent the 95% confidence limits of the normal respiratory and metabolic compensations for primary acid-base disturbances. Data falling outside the shaded areas denote a mixed disorder if a laboratory error is not present. *(Data from Brenner B, Clarkson M, Oparil S, et al, eds. Brenner and Rector's The Kidney. 8th ed. Philadelphia, PA: Saunders; 2007.)*

ions are themselves buffered by titratable renal buffers (mainly ammonia) and lost in the urine.

Evaluation of acid-base disturbances begins with a determination of the primary pH derangement by measurement of arterial pH, $Paco_2$, and HCO_3. A high or low pH will demonstrate the primary acid-base disorder and allow evaluation of whether there is appropriate compensation. In cases of normal pH, there may still be chronic compensated acidosis or alkalosis that can offer insight into the patient's comorbid condition.

Identification of acid-base disturbance follows a series of steps:

1. Identify whether the pH is increased or decreased. An increase defines alkalemia and a decrease defines acidemia.
2. Identify the change in $Paco_2$ and bicarbonate from their normal levels of 40 mm Hg and 24 mEq/L, respectively.
3. If both $Paco_2$ and bicarbonate change in the same direction (i.e., both are increased or both are decreased), then there is a primary acid-base disorder with a compensatory secondary disorder that brings the ratio of bicarbonate to carbon dioxide tension back toward 20:1.
4. If bicarbonate and $Paco_2$ change in opposite directions, then there is a mixed acid-base disorder.
5. Determine the primary acid-base disorder by comparing the fractional change of the measured bicarbonate or carbon dioxide tension to the normal value.
6. There are equations and nomograms that calculate the expected change in one of the three parameters involved in acid-base determination (pH, bicarbonate, or carbon dioxide tension) for a given change in one of the other two parameters (Figure 18-6). If the actual change is markedly

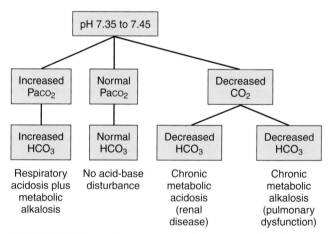

FIGURE 18-7 Diagnostic approach to the interpretation of a normal arterial pH based on $Paco_2$ and bicarbonate concentration.

different from the expected change, then there is a mixed acid-base disorder.

7. Finally, calculate the anion gap to determine whether there is an anion gap metabolic acidosis. Elevation in the anion gap requires subsequent identification of the unmeasured anion.

Figures 18-7, 18-8, and 18-9 provide an overview of the diagnostic approaches to simple acid-base disorders with a normal, low, or high pH.

SIGNS AND SYMPTOMS

Major adverse consequences of severe systemic acidosis (pH < 7.2) can occur independently of whether the acidosis

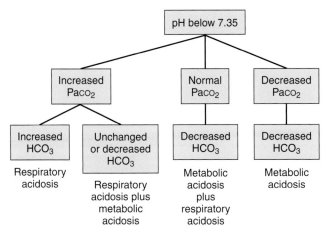

FIGURE 18-8 Diagnostic approach to interpretation of an arterial pH of less than 7.35 based on $Paco_2$ and bicarbonate concentration.

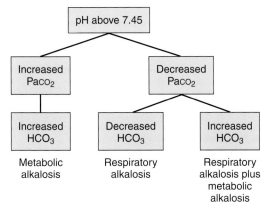

FIGURE 18-9 Diagnostic approach to interpretation of an arterial pH of more than 7.45 based on $Paco_2$ and bicarbonate concentration.

is of respiratory, metabolic, or mixed origin (Table 18-8). The effects of acidosis are particularly detrimental to the cardiovascular system. Acidosis decreases myocardial contractility, although clinical effects are minimal until the pH decreases to less than 7.2, which perhaps reflects the effects of catecholamine release in response to the acidosis. When the pH is less than 7.1, cardiac responsiveness to catecholamines decreases and compensatory inotropic effects are diminished. The detrimental effects of acidosis may be accentuated in those with underlying left ventricular dysfunction or myocardial ischemia and in those in whom sympathetic nervous system activity is impaired, such as by β-adrenergic blockade or general anesthesia.

Major adverse consequences of severe systemic alkalosis (pH > 7.60) reflect impairment of cerebral and coronary blood flow caused by arteriolar vasoconstriction (Table 18-9). Associated decreases in serum ionized calcium concentration probably contribute to the neurologic abnormalities associated with systemic alkalosis. Alkalosis predisposes patients, especially those with co-existing heart disease, to refractory

TABLE 18-8 ■ Adverse consequences of severe acidosis

NERVOUS SYSTEM
Obtundation
Coma

CARDIOVASCULAR SYSTEM
Impaired myocardial contractility
Decreased cardiac output
Decreased arterial blood pressure
Sensitization to reentrant cardiac dysrhythmias
Decreased threshold for ventricular fibrillation
Decreased responsiveness to catecholamines

VENTILATION
Hyperventilation
Dyspnea
Fatigue of respiratory muscles

METABOLISM
Hyperkalemia
Insulin resistance
Inhibition of anaerobic glycolysis

Adapted from Adrogué HJ, Madias NE. Management of life-threatening acid-base disorders. *N Engl J Med.* 1998;338:26-34.

TABLE 18-9 ■ Adverse consequences of alkalosis

NERVOUS SYSTEM
Decreased cerebral blood flow
Seizures
Lethargy
Delirium
Tetany

CARDIOVASCULAR SYSTEM
Arteriolar vasoconstriction
Decreased coronary blood flow
Decreased threshold for angina pectoris
Predisposition to refractory dysrhythmias

VENTILATION
Hypoventilation
Hypercarbia
Arterial hypoxemia

METABOLISM
Hypokalemia
Hypocalcemia
Hypomagnesemia
Hypophosphatemia
Stimulation of anaerobic glycolysis

Adapted from Adrogué JH, Madias NE. Management of life-threatening acid-base disorders. *N Engl J Med.* 1998;338:107-111.

TABLE 18-10 ■ Causes of respiratory acidosis
Drug-induced ventilatory depression
Permissive hypercapnia
Upper airway obstruction
Status asthmaticus
Restriction of ventilation (rib fractures/flail chest)
Disorders of neuromuscular function
Malignant hyperthermia
Hyperalimentation

TABLE 18-11 ■ Causes of respiratory alkalosis
Iatrogenic (mechanical hyperventilation)
Decreased barometric pressure
Arterial hypoxemia
Central nervous system injury
Hepatic disease
Pregnancy
Salicylate overdose

ventricular dysrhythmias. Alkalosis depresses ventilation and can frustrate efforts to wean patients from mechanical ventilation. Hypokalemia accompanies both metabolic and respiratory alkalosis but is more prominent in the presence of metabolic alkalosis. Alkalosis stimulates anaerobic glycolysis and increases the production of lactic acid and ketoacids. Although alkalosis can decrease the release of oxygen to the tissues by tightening the binding of oxygen to hemoglobin, chronic alkalosis negates this effect by increasing the concentration of 2,3-diphosphoglycerate in erythrocytes.

Respiratory Acidosis

Respiratory acidemia is present when a decrease in alveolar ventilation results in an increase in the $Paco_2$ sufficient to decrease arterial pH to less than 7.35 (Table 18-10). The most likely cause of respiratory acidosis during the perioperative period is drug-induced depression of ventilation by opioids, general anesthetics, or paralytics. Respiratory acidosis may be complicated by metabolic acidosis when renal perfusion is decreased to the extent that reabsorption mechanisms in the renal tubules are impaired. For example, cardiac output and renal blood flow may be so decreased in patients with chronic obstructive pulmonary disease and cor pulmonale as to lead to metabolic acidosis.

Respiratory acidosis is treated by correcting the disorder responsible for hypoventilation. Mechanical ventilation is necessary when the increase in $Paco_2$ is marked, and carbon dioxide narcosis may create a self-reinforcing disorder. It must be remembered that rapid lowering of chronically increased $Paco_2$ levels by mechanical ventilation decreases body stores of carbon dioxide much more rapidly than the kidneys can produce a corresponding decrease in serum bicarbonate concentration. The resulting metabolic alkalosis can cause neuromuscular irritability and excitation of the central nervous system manifesting as seizures. It is best to decrease the $Paco_2$ slowly to permit sufficient time for renal tubular elimination of bicarbonate.

Metabolic alkalosis may accompany respiratory acidosis when the body stores of chloride and potassium are decreased. For example, decreased serum chloride concentrations facilitate renal tubular reabsorption of bicarbonate, which leads to metabolic alkalosis. Hypokalemia stimulates renal tubules to excrete hydrogen, which may produce metabolic alkalosis or aggravate a co-existing alkalosis caused by chloride deficiency.

Treatment of metabolic alkalosis associated with these electrolyte disturbances requires administration of potassium chloride.

Respiratory Alkalosis

Respiratory alkalosis is present when an increase in alveolar ventilation results in a decrease in $Paco_2$ sufficient to increase the pH to greater than 7.45 (Table 18-11). The most likely cause of acute respiratory alkalosis during the perioperative period is iatrogenic hyperventilation as may occur during general anesthesia. Respiratory alkalosis occurs normally during pregnancy and is an important adaptive response to high altitude.

Treatment of respiratory alkalosis is directed at correcting the underlying disorder responsible for alveolar hyperventilation. During anesthesia, this is most often accomplished by adjusting the ventilator to decrease alveolar ventilation. The hypokalemia and hypochloremia that may co-exist with respiratory alkalosis may also require treatment.

Metabolic Acidosis

Metabolic acidosis lowers blood pH, which stimulates the respiratory center to hyperventilate and lower carbon dioxide tension. Respiratory compensation does not in general fully counterbalance the increased acid production, but the pH will return *toward* normal.

Acidoses of metabolic origin are typically divided into those with a normal anion gap and those with a high anion gap.

A high anion gap occurs when a fixed acid is added to the extracellular space. The acid dissociates, the hydrogen ion combines with bicarbonate forming carbonic acid, and the decreased bicarbonate concentration produces an increased anion gap. Lactic acidosis, ketoacidosis, renal failure, and the acidoses associated with many poisonings are examples of high anion gap metabolic acidoses.

Non–anion gap metabolic acidosis is the result of a net increase in chloride concentration. Bicarbonate loss is counterbalanced by a net gain of chloride ions to maintain electrical neutrality. Therefore, a normal anion gap acidosis is often called a *hyperchloremic* metabolic acidosis. The most common causes of a normal anion gap acidosis are intravenous infusion of sodium chloride and gastrointestinal and renal losses of bicarbonate (diarrhea, renal tubular acidosis, early renal failure).

TABLE 18-12 ■ Causes of metabolic acidosis

Lactic acidosis
Diabetic ketoacidosis
Renal failure
Hepatic failure
Methanol and ethylene glycol intoxication
Aspirin intoxication
Increased skeletal muscle activity
Cyanide poisoning
Carbon monoxide poisoning

TABLE 18-13 ■ Causes of metabolic alkalosis

Hypovolemia
Vomiting
Nasogastric suction
Diuretic therapy
Bicarbonate administration
Hyperaldosteronism
Chloride-wasting diarrhea

SIGNS AND SYMPTOMS

Since acidosis is secondary to an underlying disorder, the presentation of acidosis is complicated by the signs and symptoms of the causative disorder. Derangements of pH have wide-ranging effects on tissue, organ, and enzyme function, and the signs and symptoms attributable to an acidosis relate to these effects. The clinical features of metabolic acidosis depend also on the rate of development of the acidosis and are likely to be more dramatic in rapidly developing acidosis in which compensatory respiratory or renal changes are not able to limit the fall in pH.

DIAGNOSIS

Diagnosis depends on a high index of suspicion and laboratory testing. Most commonly, arterial blood is analyzed for pH, carbon dioxide tension, bicarbonate concentration, and anion gap. Common causes of metabolic acidosis are listed in Table 18-12.

Metabolic acidosis can be of renal or nonrenal origin. Metabolic acidosis of renal origin involves a primary disorder of renal acidification. This occurs when the kidneys are unable to regenerate sufficient bicarbonate to replace that lost by the buffering of normal endogenous acid production (distal renal tubular acidosis) or when an abnormally high fraction of filtered bicarbonate is not reabsorbed in the proximal tubule and is subsequently lost in the urine (proximal renal tubular acidosis or acetazolamide use). Combined defects occur in renal failure. The most common causes of extrarenal sources of a metabolic acidosis are gastrointestinal bicarbonate losses, ketoacidosis, and lactic acidosis.

TREATMENT

Treatment of metabolic acidosis includes treatment of the cause of the acidosis, for example, insulin and fluids for diabetic ketoacidosis and improvement in tissue perfusion for lactic acidosis. Administration of sodium bicarbonate for acute treatment of metabolic acidosis is very controversial. Many recommend that bicarbonate be given only if the pH is less than 7.1 or the bicarbonate concentration is less than 10 mEq/L. It is thought that the bicarbonate reacts with hydrogen ions, generating carbon dioxide, which diffuses into cells and lowers intracellular pH even more than before the bicarbonate treatment. It is also postulated that administration of bicarbonate to patients with chronic metabolic acidosis may result in transient tissue hypoxia. Acute changes in pH toward normal (or alkalosis) may negate the rightward shift of the oxyhemoglobin dissociation curve caused by acidemia (Bohr effect) and result in increased hemoglobin affinity for oxygen, which reduces oxygen delivery at the tissue level.

The 2005 American Heart Association Guidelines for Cardiopulmonary Resuscitation and Emergency Cardiovascular Care do not recommend administering sodium bicarbonate routinely during cardiac arrest and cardiopulmonary resuscitation. However, sodium bicarbonate may be considered for life-threatening hyperkalemia or cardiac arrest associated with hyperkalemia, or for cardiac arrest associated with a preexisting metabolic acidosis.

MANAGEMENT OF ANESTHESIA

Elective surgery should be postponed until an acidosis has been treated. For urgent surgery in a patient with metabolic acidosis, invasive hemodynamic monitoring should be considered to guide fluid resuscitation and to monitor cardiac function in marked acidosis. Laboratory measurement of acid-base parameters should be performed frequently throughout the perioperative period, because pH can change rapidly and significantly in response to changes in ventilation, volume status, circulation, and drug administration.

Acidosis affects the proportion of drug in the ionized and un-ionized states. Volume of distribution may also be affected in patients who have uncorrected hypovolemia.

Metabolic Alkalosis

Metabolic alkalosis is marked by an increase in plasma bicarbonate concentration and is usually compensated for by an increase in carbon dioxide tension. Common causes of metabolic alkalosis are listed in Table 18-13.

Metabolic alkalosis can be of renal or extrarenal origin and can be caused by either a net loss of hydrogen ions (such as loss of hydrochloric acid with vomiting) or a net gain of bicarbonate (such as being caused by tubular defects of bicarbonate reabsorption). Abnormal losses of chloride with or without hydrogen ion (e.g., in cystic fibrosis, villous adenoma) also induce increased renal bicarbonate reabsorption in an attempt to maintain electroneutrality. Therefore, metabolic alkaloses can be characterized as chloride responsive or chloride resistant. Another classification of metabolic alkalosis is volume-depletion alkalosis (resulting from vomiting, diarrhea, or chloride losses) and volume-overload alkalosis (resulting from primary or secondary mineralocorticoid excess).

Metabolic alkalosis can also occur secondary to renal compensation for chronic respiratory disease with hypercarbia. In these patients, bicarbonate levels may be quite high and associated with urinary losses of chloride along with obligatory losses of sodium and potassium. If the respiratory disorder is treated with mechanical ventilation and the carbon dioxide tension is reduced rapidly, a profound metabolic alkalosis may result.

SIGNS AND SYMPTOMS

Progressively more binding of calcium to albumin occurs as an alkalosis develops, so the signs and symptoms of alkalosis, especially those related to the neuromuscular and central nervous systems, may be very similar to those of hypocalcemia. Metabolic alkalosis may be accompanied by volume contraction, hypochloremia and hypokalemia, or volume overload and sodium retention, depending on the cause.

DIAGNOSIS

As with metabolic acidosis, the diagnosis of metabolic alkalosis is dependent on a high index of suspicion and laboratory testing. Metabolic alkaloses secondary to chloride losses are associated with low urinary chloride levels (typically <10 mEq/L) and volume contraction. In contrast, metabolic alkaloses associated with mineralocorticoid excess are typically associated with volume overload and spot urine chloride values of more than 20 mEq/L.

TREATMENT

Volume-depletion metabolic alkalosis is treated by chloride replacement along with fluid resuscitation using saline, which is itself weakly acidic. If the alkalosis has been caused by gastric losses of hydrochloric acid, then proton pump inhibitors can be given to stop the perpetuation of the alkalosis. Metabolic alkalosis associated with loop diuretics can be improved by adding or substituting potassium-sparing diuretics. In the case of volume-overload metabolic alkalosis, when excess mineralocorticoid is present, administration of spironolactone plus potassium chloride may be useful if the source of mineralocorticoid secretion cannot be eliminated.

MANAGEMENT OF ANESTHESIA

Management of anesthesia includes judicious volume replacement and adequate supplementation with chloride, potassium, and magnesium as needed. Invasive monitoring may be helpful in some patients. Care must be taken not to eliminate a compensatory metabolic alkalosis in patients with chronic lung disease and significant carbon dioxide retention, because successful weaning from mechanical ventilation will likely necessitate a return to the chronic respiratory acidosis and metabolic alkalosis the patient had at presentation.

KEY POINTS

- Total body water content is categorized as ICF and ECF, according to the location of the water relative to cell membranes. The distribution and concentration of electrolytes differ greatly between fluid compartments. The electrophysiology of excitable cells is dependent on the intracellular and extracellular concentrations of sodium, potassium, and calcium.

- Water balance is predominantly mediated by osmolality sensors, neurons located in the anterior hypothalamus that stimulate thirst and cause pituitary release of vasopressin (antidiuretic hormone). Vasopressin is stored as granules in the posterior pituitary and acts through G protein–coupled receptors in the collecting ducts of the kidney, causing water retention that in turn corrects serum osmolality.

- As hyponatremia develops, it is usually associated with extracellular hypotonicity, which results in water movement into cells and can manifest as cerebral edema and increased intracranial pressure. Initial compensation is afforded by the movement of ECF into the cerebrospinal fluid. Later compensation includes the lowering of intracellular osmolality by the movement of potassium and organic solutes out of brain cells. This reduces water movement into the intracellular space. However, when these adaptive mechanisms fail or hyponatremia progresses, central nervous system manifestations of hyponatremia occur.

- The volume overload, hyponatremia, and hypo-osmolality that may accompany transurethral resection of the prostate is known as *TURP syndrome*. This syndrome is more likely to occur when resection is prolonged (>1 hour), when the irrigating fluid is suspended more than 40 cm above the operative field, and when the pressure in the bladder is allowed to increase above 15 cm H_2O. TURP syndrome manifests principally with cardiovascular signs of volume overload and neurologic signs of hyponatremia.

- Hypokalemia is diagnosed by testing the serum potassium concentration. The differential diagnosis requires determining whether the hypokalemia is acute and secondary to intracellular potassium shifts such as might be seen with hyperventilation or alkalosis, or is chronic and associated with depletion of total body potassium stores.

- Immediate treatment of hyperkalemia is required if life-threatening dysrhythmias or ECG signs of severe hyperkalemia are present. This treatment is aimed at antagonizing the effects of a high potassium on the transmembrane potential and redistributing the potassium intracellularly. Calcium chloride or calcium gluconate is administered to stabilize cellular membranes. Hyperventilation, sodium bicarbonate administration, and insulin administration promote movement of potassium intracellularly.

- Binding of calcium to albumin is pH dependent, and acid-base disturbances can change the fraction and therefore the concentration of ionized calcium without changing total body calcium. Alkalosis reduces the ionized calcium concentration, so ionized calcium may be significantly reduced after bicarbonate administration or with hyperventilation.

■ Signs and symptoms of hypermagnesemia begin to occur at serum levels of 4 to 5 mEq/L and include lethargy, nausea and vomiting, and facial flushing. At levels above 6 mEq/L, a loss of deep tendon reflexes and hypotension occur. Paralysis, apnea, and/or cardiac arrest are likely if the magnesium level exceeds 10 mEq/L.

■ Major adverse consequences of severe systemic acidosis (pH < 7.2) can occur independently of whether the acidosis is of respiratory, metabolic, or mixed origin. Acidosis decreases myocardial contractility, although clinical effects are minimal until the pH decreases below 7.2, which perhaps reflects the effects of catecholamine release in response to the acidosis. When the pH is less than 7.1, cardiac responsiveness to catecholamines decreases and compensatory inotropic effects are diminished. The detrimental effects of acidosis may be accentuated in those with underlying left ventricular dysfunction or myocardial ischemia and in those in whom sympathetic nervous system activity is impaired, such as by β-adrenergic blockade or general anesthesia.

■ Major adverse consequences of severe systemic alkalosis (pH > 7.60) reflect impairment of cerebral and coronary blood flow due to arteriolar vasoconstriction. Associated decreases in serum ionized calcium concentration contribute to the neurologic abnormalities associated with systemic alkalosis. Alkalosis predisposes patients, especially those with co-existing heart disease, to refractory ventricular dysrhythmias. Alkalosis also depresses ventilation.

RESOURCES

Adrogué HJ, Madias NE. Hyponatremia. *N Engl J Med.* 2000;342:1581-1589.

Adrogué HJ, Madias NE. Management of life-threatening acid-base disorders. *N Engl J Med.* 1998;338:26-34:107-111.

Bonow R, Mann D, Zipes D, et al. eds. *Braunwald's Heart Disease: A Textbook of Cardiovascular Medicine.* 9th ed. Philadelphia, PA: Saunders; 2011.

Brenner B, Clarkson M, Oparil S, et al. eds. *Brenner and Rector's The Kidney.* 8th ed. Philadelphia, PA: Saunders; 2007.

Fauci AS, Braunwald E, Hauser SL, et al. eds. *Harrison's Principles of Internal Medicine.* 17th ed. New York, NY: McGraw Hill; 2007.

Gennari FJ. Hypokalemia. *N Engl J Med.* 1998;339:451-458.

2010 American Heart Association guidelines for cardiopulmonary resuscitation and emergency cardiovascular care science. *Circulation.* 2010;122:S729-S767.

Wahr JA, Parks R, Boisvert D, et al. Preoperative serum potassium levels and perioperative outcomes in cardiac surgical patients. *JAMA.* 1999;281:2203-2210.

CHAPTER 19

Endocrine Disease

RUSSELL T. WALL, III ■

DIABETES MELLITUS

Normal glucose physiology is marked by a balance between glucose utilization and endogenous production or dietary delivery (Figure 19-1). The liver is the primary source of endogenous glucose production via glycogenolysis and gluconeogenesis. Following a meal, plasma glucose level increases, which stimulates an increase in plasma insulin secretion that promotes glucose utilization. Late in the postprandial period (2 to 4 hours after eating) when glucose utilization exceeds glucose production, a transition from exogenous glucose delivery to endogenous production becomes necessary to maintain a normal plasma glucose level. Approximately 70% to 80% of glucose released by the liver is metabolized by insulin-insensitive tissues such as the brain, gastrointestinal tract, and red blood cells. During this time, diminished insulin secretion is fundamental to the maintenance of a normal plasma glucose concentration. Hyperglycemia-producing hormones (glucagon, epinephrine, growth hormone, cortisol) comprise the glucose counterregulatory system and support glucose production. Glucagon plays a primary role by stimulating glycogenolysis and gluconeogenesis, and inhibiting glycolysis. Epinephrine predominates when glucagon secretion is deficient.

Diabetes mellitus results from an inadequate supply of insulin and/or an inadequate tissue response to insulin. This leads to increased circulating glucose levels with eventual microvascular and macrovascular complications. Type 1a diabetes is caused by autoimmune destruction of beta cells within pancreatic islets resulting in complete absence or minimal circulating levels of insulin. Type 1b diabetes is a rare disease of absolute insulin deficiency that is not immune mediated. Type 2 diabetes also is not immune mediated and results from defects in insulin receptors and postreceptor intracellular signaling pathways.

Signs and Symptoms

TYPE 1 DIABETES

Between 5% and 10% of all cases of diabetes are type 1. There are 1.4 million individuals with type 1 diabetes in the United States and 10 to 20 million globally. Currently, the incidence is increasing by 3% to 5% per year. The disorder is usually diagnosed before the age of 40 and is one of the most common chronic childhood illnesses.

Type 1 diabetes is caused by a T cell–mediated autoimmune destruction of beta cells in the pancreas. The exact cause is unknown, although environmental triggers such as

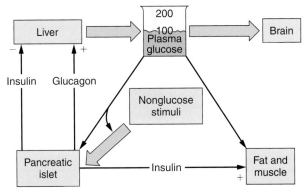

FIGURE 19-1 The pancreatic islets act as glucose sensors to balance hepatic glucose release to insulin-insensitive tissues (brain) and insulin-sensitive tissues (fat, muscle). Insulin inhibits glucose release by the liver and stimulates glucose utilization by insulin-sensitive tissues. With hyperglycemia, insulin secretion increases. With hypoglycemia, the reverse occurs. *(Adapted from Porte D Jr. Beta-cells in type II diabetes mellitus. Diabetes. 1991;40:166-180.)*

viruses (especially enteroviruses), dietary proteins, or drugs or chemicals may initiate the autoimmune process in genetically susceptible hosts. A long preclinical period (9 to 13 years) characterized by production of antibodies to beta cell antigens with loss of beta cell function precedes the onset of clinical diabetes in the majority of patients. At least 80% to 90% of beta cell function must be lost before hyperglycemia occurs. The autoimmune attack initially presents as islet inflammation (insulitis), with immune cells infiltrating the pancreatic islets. Circulating antibodies signify islet cell injury.

The presentation of clinical disease is often sudden and severe secondary to loss of a critical mass of beta cells. Patients demonstrate hyperglycemia over several days to weeks associated with fatigue, weight loss, polyuria, polydipsia, blurring of vision, and signs of intravascular volume depletion. The diagnosis is based on the presence of a random blood glucose level of more than 200 mg/dL and a hemoglobin A_{1c} (Hb A_{1c}) level of more than 7.0%. The presence of ketoacidosis indicates severe insulin deficiency and unrestrained lipolysis. Beta cell destruction is complete within 3 years of diagnosis in most children, with the process being slower in adults.

TYPE 2 DIABETES

Type 2 diabetes is responsible for 90% of all cases of diabetes mellitus in the world. In 2000, there were approximately 150 million individuals with type 2 diabetes globally, and the number is expected to double by 2025. Patients with type 2 diabetics are typically in the middle to older age group and are overweight, although there has been a significant increase in younger patients and even children with type 2 diabetes over the past decade. Type 2 diabetes continues to be underrecognized and underdiagnosed because of its subtle presentation. It is estimated that most individuals with type 2 diabetes had the disease for approximately 4 to 7 years before the disorder was diagnosed.

Type 2 diabetes is characterized by relative beta cell insufficiency and insulin resistance. In the initial stages of the disease, an insensitivity to insulin on the part of peripheral tissues leads to an increase in pancreatic insulin secretion to maintain normal plasma glucose levels. As the disease progresses and pancreatic cell function decreases, insulin levels are unable to compensate and hyperglycemia occurs. Three important defects are seen in type 2 diabetes: (1) an increased rate of hepatic glucose release, (2) impaired basal and stimulated insulin secretion, and (3) inefficient use of glucose by peripheral tissues (i.e., insulin resistance) (Figure 19-2). The increase in hepatic glucose release is caused by the reduction of insulin's normal inhibitory effects on the liver, as well as abnormalities in regulation of glucagon secretion. Although relative beta cell insufficiency is significant, type 2 diabetes is characterized by insulin resistance in skeletal muscle, adipose tissue, and the liver. Causes of insulin resistance include an abnormal insulin molecule; circulating insulin antagonists, including counter-regulatory hormones, free fatty acids, antiinsulin and insulin receptor antibodies, and cytokines; and target tissue defects at insulin receptors and/or postreceptor sites. It appears that insulin resistance is an inherited component of type 2 diabetes, with obesity and a sedentary lifestyle being acquired and contributing factors. Impaired glucose tolerance is associated with an increase in body weight, a decrease in insulin secretion, and a reduction in peripheral insulin action. The transition to clinical diabetes is characterized by these same factors plus an increase in hepatic glucose production.

The increasing prevalence of type 2 diabetes among children and adolescents appears related to obesity, since 85% of affected children are overweight or obese at the time of diagnosis. Obese patients exhibit a compensatory hyperinsulinemia to maintain normoglycemia. These increased insulin levels may desensitize target tissues, causing a reduced response to insulin. The mechanisms for hyperinsulinemia and insulin resistance from weight gain remain elusive.

Metabolic syndrome, or insulin-resistance syndrome, is a constellation of clinical and biochemical characteristics frequently seen in patients who have, or are at risk of developing, type 2 diabetes (Table 19-1). This syndrome combines insulin resistance with hypertension, dyslipidemia, a procoagulant state, and obesity, and is associated with premature atherosclerosis and subsequent cardiovascular disease. This syndrome affects at least 25% of people in the United States.

Diagnosis

The American Diabetes Association has established diagnostic criteria for diabetes mellitus (Table 19-2). Measurement of fasting plasma glucose level is the recommended screening test for diabetes mellitus. The upper limit for normal fasting glucose level is 100 mg/dL. Hyperglycemia not sufficient to meet the diagnostic criteria for diabetes is classified as either impaired fasting glucose or impaired glucose tolerance, depending on whether it is identified through measurement of fasting plasma glucose level or an oral glucose tolerance test.

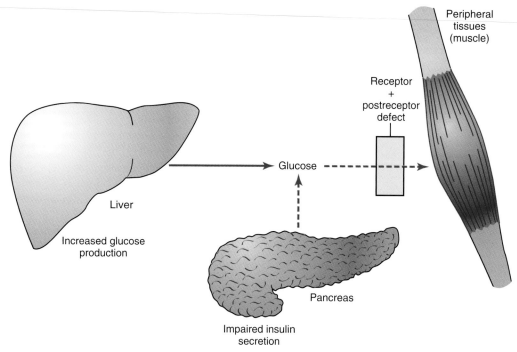

FIGURE 19-2 Abnormalities in type 2 diabetes. *(Adapted from Inzucchi S, ed.* The Diabetes Mellitus Manual: A Primary Care Companion to Ellenberg and Rifkin's Sixth Edition. *New York, NY: McGraw-Hill; 2005:79.)*

TABLE 19-1 ■ Diagnostic features of metabolic syndrome

At least three of the following:
    Fasting plasma glucose level ≥ 110 mg/dL
    Abdominal obesity (waist girth > 40 inches in men,
       35 inches in women)
    Serum triglyceride level ≥ 150 mg/dL
    Serum high-density lipoprotein cholesterol level < 40 mg/dL
      in men, < 50 mg/dL in women
    Blood pressure ≥ 130/85 mm Hg

Adapted from Expert Panel on Detection, Evaluation, and Treatment of High Blood Cholesterol in Adults: Executive summary of the Third Report of the National Cholesterol Education Program (NCEP) Expert Panel on Detection, Evaluation, and Treatment of High Blood Cholesterol in Adults (Adult Treatment Panel III). *JAMA.* 2001;285:2486-2497.

TABLE 19-2 ■ Diagnostic criteria for diabetes mellitus

Symptoms of diabetes (polyuria, polydipsia, unexplained
    weight loss) plus a random plasma glucose concentration
    ≥ 200 mg/dL

or

Fasting (no caloric intake for ≥ 8 hr) plasma glucose level
    ≥ 126 mg/dL

or

2-hr plasma glucose level > 200 mg/dL during an oral glucose
    tolerance test

Adapted from Diagnosis and classification of diabetes mellitus. American Diabetes Association. *Diabetes Care.* 2010;33(suppl 1):S62.

Any fasting glucose level between 101 and 125 mg/dL is categorized as impaired fasting glucose. Glucose levels, especially in type 2 diabetics, usually increase over years to decades, progressing from the normal range to the impaired glucose tolerance range and finally to clinical diabetes. Although rarely used in routine practice, the oral glucose tolerance test is recommended for diagnosis when glucose values are equivocal.

The Hb A_{1c} test provides a valuable measure of long-term glycemic control. Hemoglobin is nonenzymatically glycosylated by glucose, which freely crosses red blood cell membranes. The percentage of hemoglobin molecules participating in this reaction is proportional to the average plasma glucose concentration during the preceding 60 to 90 days. The normal range for Hb A_{1c} is 4% to 6%. Increased risk of microvascular and macrovascular disease begins when the Hb A_{1c} proportion is 6.5% or higher.

Treatment

The cornerstones of treatment for type 2 diabetes are dietary adjustments along with weight loss, exercise therapy, and oral antidiabetic drugs. Reduction of body weight through diet and exercise is the first therapeutic measure to control type 2 diabetes. The decrease in adiposity improves hepatic and peripheral tissue insulin sensitivity, enhances postreceptor insulin action, and may possibly increase insulin secretion. Nutritional guidelines of the American Diabetes Association emphasize maintenance of optimal plasma glucose and lipid levels.

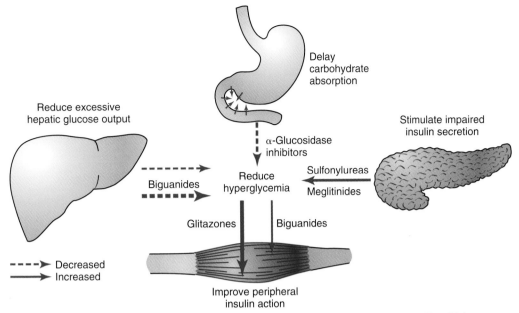

FIGURE 19-3 Sites of action of oral antidiabetic agents. *(Adapted from Inzucchi S, ed. The Diabetes Mellitus Manual: A Primary Care Companion to Ellenberg and Rifkin's Sixth Edition. New York, NY: McGraw-Hill; 2005:168.)*

ORAL ANTIDIABETIC DRUGS

The four major classes of oral antidiabetic medications are (1) the secretagogues (sulfonylureas, meglitinides), which increase insulin availability; (2) the biguanides (metformin), which suppress excessive hepatic glucose release; (3) the thiazolidinediones or glitazones (rosiglitazone, pioglitazone), which improve insulin sensitivity; and (4) the α-glucosidase inhibitors (acarbose, miglitol), which delay gastrointestinal glucose absorption (Figure 19-3). These agents are used to maintain glucose control, which is defined as a fasting glucose level of 90 to 130 mg/dL, peak postprandial glucose level of less than 180 mg/dL, and HbA$_{1c}$ level of less than 7% in the initial stages of the disease.

The sulfonylureas are usually the initial pharmacologic treatment for type 2 diabetes mellitus. They act by stimulating insulin secretion from pancreatic beta cells; they can also enhance insulin-stimulated peripheral tissue utilization of glucose. The second-generation agents (glyburide, glipizide, glimepiride) are more potent and have fewer side effects than their predecessors. Unfortunately, because of the natural history of type 2 diabetes characterized by decreasing beta cell function, these drugs are not effective indefinitely. Hypoglycemia is the most common side effect. Whether or not harmful cardiac effects from sulfonylureas have been demonstrated is controversial. Potassium adenosine triphosphate (ATP) channels in the myocardium mediate ischemic preconditioning, which appears critical for myocardial protection and limitation of infarction size. Sulfonylureas may inhibit this protective response and potentially delay contractile recovery, which results in larger myocardial infarction areas.

The biguanides decrease hepatic gluconeogenesis and, to a lesser degree, enhance utilization of glucose by skeletal muscle and adipose tissue by increasing glucose transport across cell membranes. In addition to lowering glucose levels, they decrease plasma levels of triglycerides and low-density lipoprotein cholesterol and reduce postprandial hyperlipidemia and plasma-free fatty acids. The risk of hypoglycemia is less than that with the sulfonylureas. Lactic acidosis is a rare but serious side effect of the biguanides; the risk is particularly high in patients with renal insufficiency. It is much less common with metformin than with its predecessor phenformin.

The thiazolidinediones or glitazones are insulin sensitizers that decrease insulin resistance by binding to peroxisome proliferator–activated receptors located in skeletal muscle, liver, and adipose tissue. These drugs influence the expression of genes encoding proteins for glucose and lipid metabolism, endothelial function, and atherogenesis and, as a result, may influence diabetic dyslipidemia in addition to hyperglycemia.

The α-glucosidase inhibitors inhibit α-glucosidase enzymes in the brush border of enterocytes in the proximal small intestine, which results in a delay in the intraluminal production and subsequent absorption of glucose. They are administered before a main meal to ensure their presence at the site of action.

In most patients, therapy is initiated with a sulfonylurea or biguanide and titrated to achieve fasting and peak postprandial glucose levels recommended by the American Diabetes Association (Figure 19-4). Combination therapy with oral agents directed at more than one mechanism is often effective. If combination oral therapy is unsuccessful, a bedtime dose of intermediate-acting insulin is added, since hepatic glucose overproduction is typically highest at night. If oral agents plus single-dose insulin therapy is ineffective, type 2 diabetic patients are switched to insulin therapy alone.

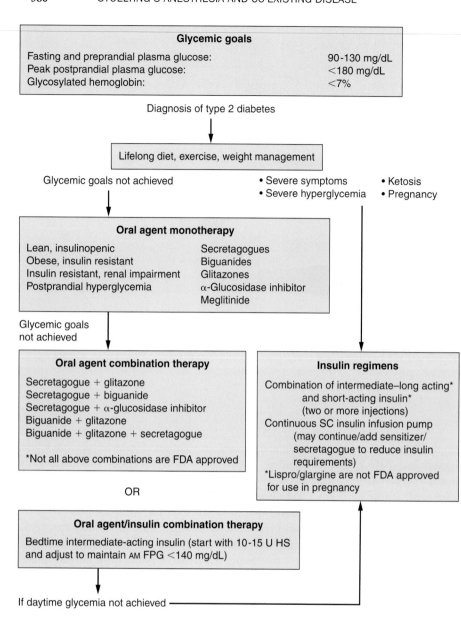

FIGURE 19-4 Algorithm for treatment of type 2 diabetes. *FDA,* U.S. Food and Drug Administration; *FPG,* fasting plasma glucose level; *HS,* at bedtime; *SC,* subcutaneous. *(Adapted from Inzucchi S, ed.* The Diabetes Mellitus Manual: A Primary Care Companion to Ellenberg and Rifkin's Sixth Edition. *New York, NY: McGraw-Hill; 2005:193.)*

TABLE 19-3 ■ Insulin preparations

Insulin	Onset	Peak	Duration
SHORT ACTING			
Human regular	30 min	2-4 hr	5-8 hr
Lispro (Humalog)	10-15 min	1-2 hr	3-6 hr
Aspart (NovoLog)	10-15 min	1-2 hr	3-6 hr
INTERMEDIATE			
Human NPH	1-2 hr	6-10 hr	10-20 hr
Lente	1-2 hr	6-10 hr	10-20 hr
LONG ACTING			
Ultralente	4-6 hr	8-20 hr	24-48 hr
Glargine (Lantus)	1-2 hr	—	24 hr

Tight control of type 2 diabetes provides significant benefits in preventing and slowing the progression of microvascular disease and possibly macrovascular disease. Not only must hyperglycemia be treated but all abnormalities of insulin resistance (metabolic syndrome) must be managed, with the goals of therapy including an Hb A_{1c} level of less than 7%, a low-density lipoprotein level of less than 100 mg/dL, a high-density lipoprotein level of more than 40 mg/dL in men and more than 50 mg/dL in women, a triglycerides level of less than 200 mg/dL, and a blood pressure of less than 130/80 mm Hg.

INSULIN

Insulin is necessary to manage all cases of type 1 diabetes and many cases of type 2 diabetes (Table 19-3). In the United States, 30% of patients with type 2 diabetes are treated with insulin. Conventional insulin therapy uses twice-daily injections. Intensive insulin therapy requires three or more daily injections or a continuous infusion (Figures 19-5 through 19-9).

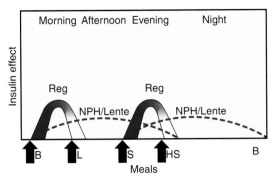

FIGURE 19-5 Insulin effect of two daily doses of NPH/Lente plus regular insulin. ↑, Time of insulin injection; *B*, breakfast; *L*, lunch; *S*, supper; *HS*, bedtime. *(Adapted from Hirsch IB, Farkas-Hirsch R, Skyler JS. Intensive insulin therapy for treatment of type I diabetes.* Diabetes Care. *1990;13:1265-1283.)*

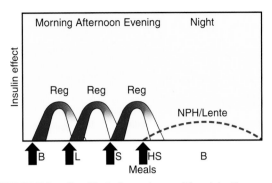

FIGURE 19-7 Insulin effect of a regimen of four injections per day: short-acting insulin before each meal and NPH/Lente at bedtime. ↑, Time of insulin injection; *B*, breakfast; *HS*, bedtime; *L*, lunch; *S*, supper.

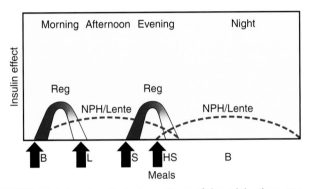

FIGURE 19-6 Insulin effect of a regimen of three injections per day: NPH/Lente plus regular insulin in morning, regular insulin before supper, NPH/Lente at bedtime. ↑, Time of insulin injection; *B*, breakfast; *HS*, bedtime; *L*, lunch; *S*, supper.

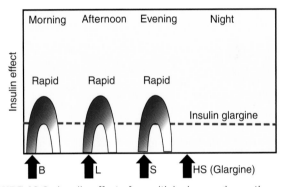

FIGURE 19-8 Insulin effect of a multiple-dose regimen: three premeal doses of rapid-acting insulin (lispro/aspart) plus basal insulin (glargine). ↑, Time of insulin injection; *B*, breakfast; *HS*, bedtime; *L*, lunch; *S*, supper.

The various forms of insulin include *basal insulins,* which are intermediate acting (NPH, Lente, lispro protamine, aspart protamine) administered twice daily or long-acting (Ultralente, glargine) administered once daily; and insulins that are *short acting* (regular) or *rapid acting* (lispro, aspart), which provide glycemic control at mealtimes. Conventional insulin therapy usually requires twice-daily injections of combinations of intermediate-acting and short- or rapid-acting insulins. A typical total daily basal dose of insulin equals weight (in kilograms) × 0.3, with the hourly rate obtained by dividing by 24.

Hypoglycemia is the most frequent and dangerous complication of insulin therapy. The hypoglycemic effect can be exacerbated by simultaneous administration of alcohol, sulfonylureas, biguanides, thiazolidinediones, angiotensin-converting enzyme (ACE) inhibitors, monoamine oxidase inhibitors, and nonselective β-blockers. β-Blockers may exacerbate hypoglycemia by inhibiting lipolysis of adipose tissue, which serves as an alternate fuel when patients become hypoglycemic. Defective counterregulatory responses by glucagon and epinephrine to reduced plasma glucose levels contribute to this complication.

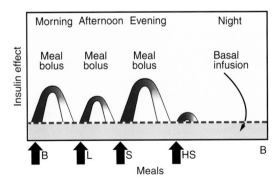

FIGURE 19-9 Insulin effect of continuous subcutaneous infusion of short- or rapid-acting insulin before meals and snacks. ↑, Time of insulin injection; *B*, breakfast; *HS*, bedtime; *L*, lunch; *S*, supper.

Repetitive episodes of hypoglycemia, especially at night, can result in *hypoglycemia unawareness,* a condition in which the patient does not respond with the appropriate autonomic warning symptoms before neuroglycopenia. The diagnosis in adults requires a plasma glucose level of

TABLE 19-4 ◾ Diagnostic features of diabetic ketoacidosis	
Serum glucose level (mg/dL)	≥300
pH	≤7.3
HCO_3^- (mEq/L)	≤18
Serum osmolarity (mOsm/L)	<320
Serum and urine ketone levels	Moderate to high

TABLE 19-5 ◾ Diagnostic features of hyperglycemic hyperosmolar syndrome	
Glucose level (mg/dL)	≥600
pH	≥7.3
HCO_3^- (mEq/L)	≥15
Serum osmolarity (mOsm/L)	≥350

less than 50 mg/dL. Symptoms are adrenergic (sweating, tachycardia, palpitations, restlessness, pallor) and neuroglycopenic (fatigue, confusion, headache, somnolence, convulsions, coma). Treatment includes the administration of sugar in the form of sugar cubes, glucose tablets, or soft drinks if the patient is conscious, and glucose 0.5 g/kg IV or glucagon 0.5 to 1.0 mg IV, IM, or SC if the patient is unconscious.

Complications

DIABETIC KETOACIDOSIS

Diabetic ketoacidosis (DKA) is a complication of decompensated diabetes mellitus. The signs and symptoms of DKA are primarily the result of abnormalities in carbohydrate and fat metabolism. Episodes of DKA occur more commonly in patients with type 1 diabetes and are precipitated by infection or acute illness. High glucose levels exceed the threshold for renal tubular absorption, which creates a significant osmotic diuresis with marked hypovolemia. A tight metabolic coupling between hepatic gluconeogenesis and ketogenesis leads to an overproduction of ketoacids by the liver. DKA results in an excess of glucose counterregulatory hormones, with glucagon activating lipolysis and free fatty acids providing the substrate for ketogenesis. An increase in production of ketoacids (β-hydroxybutyrate, acetoacetate, acetone) creates an anion gap metabolic acidosis (Table 19-4). Substantial deficits of water, potassium, and phosphorus exist, although laboratory values of these electrolytes may be normal or increased. Hyponatremia results from the effect of hyperglycemia and hyperosmolarity on water distribution. The deficit of potassium is usually substantial (3 to 5 mEq/kg), and the deficit of phosphorus can lead to diaphragmatic and skeletal muscle dysfunction and impaired myocardial contractility.

The treatment of DKA consists of administration of large amounts of normal saline and effective doses of insulin, and electrolyte supplementation. An intravenous loading dose of 0.1 unit/kg of regular insulin plus a low-dose insulin infusion of 0.1 unit/kg/hr is initiated. Insulin administration must be continued until a normal acid-base status is achieved. The insulin rate is reduced when hyperglycemia is controlled, the blood pH is higher than 7.3, and bicarbonate level is more than 18 mEq/L. Potassium and phosphate are replaced with KCl and K_2PO_4. Magnesium is replaced as needed. Sodium

bicarbonate is administered if the blood pH is less than 7.1. The infrequent but devastating development of cerebral edema can result from correction of hyperglycemia without simultaneous correction of serum sodium level. The overall mortality rate from DKA is 5% to 10%, but it is significantly higher in patients older than 65 years of age and in those who are comatose at presentation.

HYPERGLYCEMIC HYPEROSMOLAR SYNDROME

Hyperglycemic hyperosmolar syndrome is characterized by severe hyperglycemia, hyperosmolarity, and dehydration. It usually occurs in patients with type 2 diabetes who are older than 60 years of age in the context of an acute illness. The syndrome evolves over days to weeks with a persistent glycosuric diuresis. When the glucose load exceeds the renal tubular maximum for glucose reabsorption, a massive solute diuresis occurs with total body water depletion. The patient experiences polyuria, polydipsia, hypovolemia, hypotension, tachycardia, and organ hypoperfusion. Hyperosmolarity (>340 mOsm/L) is responsible for mental obtundation or coma (Table 19-5). Patients may have some degree of metabolic acidosis but do not demonstrate ketoacidosis. Vascular occlusions secondary to low-flow states and diffuse intravascular coagulation are important complications of hyperglycemic hyperosmolar syndrome.

Treatment includes significant fluid resuscitation, insulin administration, and electrolyte supplementation. If the plasma osmolarity is greater than 320 mOsm/L, large volumes of hypotonic saline (1000 to 1500 mL/hr) should be administered until the osmolarity is less than 320 mOsm/L, at which time large volumes of isotonic saline (1000 to 1500 mL/hr) can be given. Insulin therapy is initiated with an intravenous bolus of 15 units of regular insulin followed by a 0.1 unit/kg/hr infusion. The insulin infusion is decreased to 2 to 3 units/hr when the glucose level decreases to approximately 250 to 300 mg/dL. Electrolyte deficits are significant but usually less severe than in DKA. The mortality rate of hyperglycemic hyperosmolar syndrome is 10% to 15%.

MICROVASCULAR COMPLICATIONS

Microvascular dysfunction is unique to diabetes and is characterized by nonocclusive, microcirculatory disease and impaired autoregulation of blood flow and vascular tone. Hyperglycemia is essential for the development of these changes, and intensive glycemic control delays the onset and slows the progression of microvascular effects.

Nephropathy

Approximately 30% to 40% of individuals with type 1 diabetes and 5% to 10% of those with type 2 diabetes develop end-stage renal disease. The kidneys demonstrate glomerulosclerosis with glomerular basement membrane thickening, arteriosclerosis, and tubulointerstitial disease. The clinical course is characterized by hypertension, albuminuria, peripheral edema, and a progressive decrease in glomerular filtration rate. When the glomerular filtration rate decreases to less than 15 to 20 mL/min, the ability of the kidneys to excrete potassium and acids is impaired and patients develop hyperkalemia and metabolic acidosis. Hypertension, hyperglycemia, hypercholesterolemia, and microalbuminuria accelerate the decrease in the glomerular filtration rate. Treatment of hypertension can markedly slow the progression of renal dysfunction. ACE inhibitors are particularly beneficial in diabetic patients because they retard the progression of proteinuria and the decrease in glomerular filtration rate. If end-stage renal disease develops, there are four options: hemodialysis, peritoneal dialysis, continuous ambulatory peritoneal dialysis, and transplantation. Patients who receive a kidney transplant, especially if the organ is from a living human HLA-identical donor, demonstrate a longer survival than those who undergo dialysis. Combined kidney-pancreas transplantation results in lower mortality than dialysis or renal transplantation alone and may prevent recurrence of diabetic nephropathy in the transplanted kidney.

Peripheral Neuropathy

More than 50% of patients who have had diabetes for longer than 25 years develop a peripheral neuropathy. A distal symmetric diffuse sensorimotor polyneuropathy is the most common form. Sensory deficits usually overshadow motor abnormalities and appear in the toes or feet and progress proximally toward the chest in a "stocking and glove" distribution. Loss of large sensory and motor fibers produces loss of light touch and proprioception as well as muscle weakness. Loss of small fibers decreases the perception of pain and temperature and produces dysesthesia, paresthesia, and neuropathic pain. Foot ulcers develop from mechanical and traumatic injury as a result of loss of cutaneous sensitivity to pain and temperature and impaired perfusion. Significant morbidity results from recurrent infection, foot fractures (Charcot's joint), and subsequent amputations. The treatment of peripheral neuropathy includes optimal glucose control, as well as the use of nonsteroidal antiinflammatory drugs, antidepressants, and anticonvulsants for pain control.

Retinopathy

Diabetic retinopathy results from a variety of microvascular changes, including blood vessel occlusion, dilation, increased permeability, and microaneurysm formation resulting in hemorrhage, exudation, and growth of abnormal blood vessels and fibrous tissue. Visual impairment can range from minor changes in color vision to total blindness. Strict glycemic control and blood pressure control can reduce the risk of development and progression of retinopathy.

Autonomic Neuropathy

Diabetic autonomic neuropathy can affect any part of the autonomic nervous system and is the result of damaged vasoconstrictor fibers, impaired baroreceptor function, and ineffective cardiovascular reactivity. Symptomatic autonomic neuropathy is rare and is present in fewer than 5% of diabetics. The pathogenesis is not completely understood, but may involve metabolic, microvascular, and/or autonomic abnormalities. Cardiovascular signs of autonomic neuropathy include abnormalities in heart rate control as well as central and peripheral vascular dynamics. Resting tachycardia and loss of heart rate variability during deep breathing are early signs. A heart rate that fails to respond to exercise is indicative of significant cardiac denervation and is likely to result in substantially reduced exercise tolerance. The heart may demonstrate systolic and diastolic dysfunction with a reduced ejection fraction. Dysrhythmias may be responsible for sudden death. In advanced stages, severe orthostatic hypotension is present. The presence of cardiovascular autonomic neuropathy can be demonstrated by measuring orthostatic changes in heart rate and blood pressure and the hemodynamic response to exercise.

Diabetic autonomic neuropathy may also impair gastric secretion and gastric motility, eventually causing gastroparesis diabeticorum in approximately 25% of diabetic patients. Although it is often clinically silent, symptomatic patients will have nausea, vomiting, early satiety, bloating, and epigastric pain. Treatment of gastroparesis includes strict blood glucose control, consumption of multiple small meals, reduction of the fat content of meals, and use of prokinetic agents such as metoclopramide. Diarrhea and constipation are also common among diabetic patients and may be related to diabetic autonomic neuropathy. In addition, patients with diabetic autonomic neuropathy may demonstrate altered respiratory reflexes and impaired ventilatory responses to hypoxia and hypercapnia.

MACROVASCULAR COMPLICATIONS

Cardiovascular disease is a major cause of morbidity and the leading cause of mortality in diabetic individuals. Between 20% and 30% of patients coming to the hospital with a myocardial infarction have diabetes. Patients with poorly controlled diabetes demonstrate elevated triglyceride levels, low levels of high-density lipoprotein cholesterol, and an abnormally small, dense, more atherogenic low-density lipoprotein cholesterol. This dyslipidemia is caused by lack of appropriate insulin signaling and is exacerbated by poor glucose control. Measures to prevent coronary artery disease include maintaining lipid levels, glucose level, and blood pressure within normal limits. Aspirin and statin therapy should be considered for all diabetic patients.

Management of Anesthesia

PREOPERATIVE EVALUATION

The preoperative evaluation should emphasize the cardiovascular, renal, neurologic, and musculoskeletal systems. The index of suspicion should be high for myocardial ischemia and infarction. Silent ischemia is possible if autonomic neuropathy is present, and stress testing should be considered in patients with multiple cardiac risk factors and poor or indeterminate exercise tolerance. For renal disease, control of hypertension is important. Meticulous attention to hydration status, avoidance of nephrotoxins, and preservation of renal blood flow are also essential. The presence of autonomic neuropathy predisposes the patient to perioperative dysrhythmias and intraoperative hypotension. In addition, loss of compensatory sympathetic responses interferes with the detection and treatment of hemodynamic insults. Preoperative evaluation of the musculoskeletal system should look for limited joint mobility caused by nonenzymatic glycosylation of proteins and abnormal cross-linking of collagen. Firm, woody, nonpitting edema of the posterior neck and upper back (scleredema of diabetes) coupled with impaired joint mobility may limit range of motion of the neck and render endotracheal intubation difficult. Gastroparesis may increase the risk of aspiration, regardless of nothing-by-mouth status.

Management of insulin in the preoperative period depends on the type of insulin that the patient takes and the timing of dosing. If a patient takes subcutaneous insulin each night at bedtime, two thirds of this dose (NPH and regular) should be administered the night before surgery, and one half of the usual morning NPH dose should be given on the day of surgery. The daily morning dose of regular insulin should be held. If the patient uses an insulin pump, the overnight rate should be decreased by 30%. On the morning of surgery, the pump can be kept infusing at the basal rate or discontinued and replaced with a continuous insulin infusion at the same rate; alternatively, the patient can be given subcutaneous glargine and the pump discontinued 60 to 90 minutes after administration. If the patient uses glargine and lispro or aspart for daily glycemic control, the patient should take two thirds of the glargine dose and the entire lispro or aspart dose the night before surgery and hold all morning dosing. Oral hypoglycemics should be discontinued 24 to 48 hours preoperatively. It is advised that sulfonylureas be avoided during the entire perioperative period, because they block the myocardial potassium ATP channels that are responsible for ischemia- and anesthetic-induced preconditioning.

INTRAOPERATIVE MANAGEMENT

Aggressive glycemic control is important intraoperatively (Table 19-6). Ideally, a continuous infusion of insulin should be initiated at least 2 hours before surgery. Intraoperative serum glucose levels should be maintained between 120 and 180 mg/dL. Levels above 200 mg/dL are likely to cause glycosuria and dehydration and to inhibit phagocyte function and wound healing. Typically, 1 unit of insulin lowers glucose approximately 25 to 30 mg/dL. The initial hourly rate for a continuous insulin infusion is determined by dividing the total daily insulin requirement by 24. A typical rate is 0.02 unit/kg/hr, or 1.4 units/hr in a 70-kg patient. An insulin infusion can be prepared by mixing 100 units of regular insulin in 100 mL of normal saline (1 unit/mL). Insulin infusion requirements are higher

for patients undergoing coronary artery bypass graft surgery, patients receiving steroids, patients with severe infection, and patients receiving hyperalimentation or vasopressor infusions. An insulin infusion should be accompanied by an infusion of 5% dextrose in half-normal saline with 20 mEq KCl at 100 to 150 mL/hr to provide enough carbohydrate (at least 150 g/day) to inhibit hepatic glucose production and protein catabolism. Serum glucose level should be monitored at least every hour and even every 30 minutes in patients undergoing coronary artery bypass surgery or patients with high insulin requirements. Glucose determination is preferentially made using venous plasma or serum samples; arterial and capillary blood yields glucose values approximately 7% higher than those for venous blood, and whole-blood determinations are usually 15% lower than plasma or serum values. Urine glucose monitoring is not reliable.

Avoidance of hypoglycemia is especially critical, since recognition of hypoglycemia may be delayed in patients receiving anesthetics, sedatives, analgesics, β-blockers, or sympatholytics and in those with autonomic neuropathy. If hypoglycemia does occur, treatment consists of administration of 50 mL of 50% dextrose in water, which typically increases the glucose level 100 mg/dL or 2 mg/dL/mL.

POSTOPERATIVE CARE

The postoperative management of diabetic patients requires meticulous monitoring of insulin requirements. Hyperglycemia has been associated with poor outcomes in postoperative and critically ill patients. However, the optimal target for blood glucose level in the perioperative period has not yet been defined. In addition, this target may be different for patients with newly diagnosed hyperglycemia than for those with preexisting diabetes. The risks of hypoglycemia must also be considered. Currently, the American Diabetes Association recommends that glucose levels be maintained between 140 and 180 mg/dL in critically ill patients and that insulin treatment be initiated if serum glucose levels exceed 180 mg/dL.

INSULINOMA

Insulinomas are rare, benign insulin-secreting pancreatic islet cell tumors. They usually occur as an isolated finding but may present as part of multiple endocrine neoplasia syndrome type I (insulinoma, hyperparathyroidism, and a pituitary tumor). They occur in women twice as often as in men and usually in the fifth or sixth decade of life. The diagnosis is made by demonstrating Whipple's triad: (1) symptoms of hypoglycemia with fasting, (2) a glucose level of less than 50 mg/dL with symptoms, and (3) relief of symptoms by administration of glucose. An inappropriately high insulin level (>5 to 10 microunits/mL) during a 48- to 72-hour fast confirms the diagnosis. Preoperative localization of these often small lesions is challenging, and several studies (computed tomography [CT], magnetic resonance imaging [MRI], endoscopic or transabdominal ultrasonography, transhepatic portal vein sampling, and/or intraarterial calcium stimulation) are commonly utilized in combination to improve tumor localization.

TABLE 19-6 ▪ Inpatient insulin algorithm

Goal BG: _____ mg/dL
Standard drip: Regular insulin 100 units/100 mL 0.9% NaCl via infusion device
Initiation of infusion:
  Bolus dose: Regular insulin 0.1 unit/kg = _____ units
  Algorithm 1: Start here for most patients.
  Algorithm 2: Start here if patient has undergone CABG, solid organ transplant, or islet cell transplant; is receiving glucocorticoids or vasopressors; or is diabetic and receiving >80 units/day of insulin as an outpatient.

ALGORITHM 1		ALGORITHM 2		ALGORITHM 3		ALGORITHM 4	
BG	Units/hr	BG	Units/hr	BG	Units/hr	BG	Units/hr
<60 = Hypoglycemia (See below for treatment)							
<70	Off	<70	Off	<70	Off	<70	Off
70-109	0.2	70-109	0.5	70-109	1	70-109	1.5
110-119	0.5	110-119	1	110-119	2	110-119	3
120-149	1	120-149	1.5	120-149	3	120-149	5
150-179	1.5	150-179	2	150-179	4	150-179	7
180-209	2	180-209	3	180-209	5	180-209	9
210-239	2	210-239	4	210-239	6	210-239	12
240-269	3	240-269	5	240-269	8	240-269	16
270-299	3	270-299	6	270-299	10	270-299	20
300-329	4	300-329	7	300-329	12	300-329	24
330-359	4	330-359	8	330-359	14	>330	28
>360	6	>360	12	>360	16		

MOVING FROM ALGORITHM TO ALGORITHM

Moving up: Move to higher algorithm when current algorithm fails, defined as BG outside goal range for 2 hr (see above goal) and failure of level to change by at least 60 mg/dL within 1 hr.

Moving down: Move to lower algorithm when BG is <70 mg/dL for two checks OR BG decreases by >100 mg/dL in 1 hr.

Tube feeds or TPN: Decrease infusion by 50% if nutrition (tube feeds or TPN) is discontinued or significantly reduced. Reinstitute hourly BG checks every 4 hr.

Patient monitoring: Check capillary BG every hour until it is within goal range for 4 hr, then decrease to every 2 hr for 4 hr, and if it remains at goal, may decrease to every 4 hr.

TREATMENT OF HYPOGLYCEMIA (BG <60 MG/DL)

Discontinue insulin drip.

  and

Give $D_{50}W$ IV
  Patient conscious: 25 mL (½ amp)
  Patient unconscious: 50 mL (1 amp)
  Recheck BG every 20 min and repeat 25 min of $D_{50}W$ IV if <60 mg/dL. Restart drip once BG is >70 mg/dL for two checks. Restart drip with lower algorithm (see Moving Down).

INTRAVENOUS FLUIDS

Most patients will need 5-10 g of glucose per hour (D_5W or D_5 ½ NS at 100-200 mL/hr or equivalent [TPN, enteral feeds]).

amp, Ampule; *BG*, blood glucose level; *CABG*, coronary artery bypass graft; *D₅W*, 5% dextrose in water; *D₅ ½ NS*, 5% dextrose in half-normal saline; *D₅₀W*, 50% dextrose in water; *IV*, intravenously; *TPN*, total parenteral nutrition.

Preoperatively, patients are often managed with diazoxide, an agent that directly inhibits insulin release from beta cells. Other medical therapies include verapamil, phenytoin, propranolol, glucocorticoids, and the somatostatin analogues octreotide and lanreotide. Surgical treatment is curative. Ninety percent of insulinomas are benign, and tumor enucleation is the procedure of choice. Laparoscopic resection is used in selected cases.

Profound hypoglycemia can occur intraoperatively, particularly during manipulation of the tumor; however, marked hyperglycemia can follow removal of the tumor. In a few medical centers, an artificial pancreas that continuously analyzes the blood glucose concentration and automatically infuses insulin or glucose has been used for intraoperative management of these patients. In most cases, serial blood glucose measurements (every 15 minutes) are taken using a standard glucometer. Since evidence

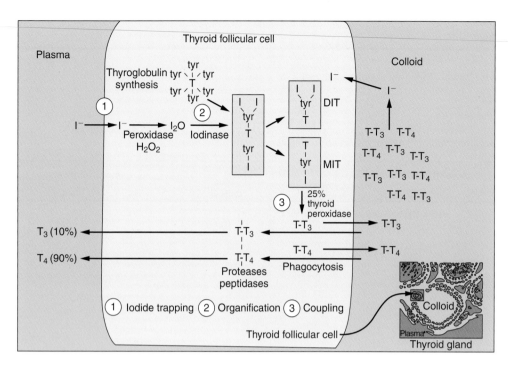

FIGURE 19-10 Thyroid follicular cell. *DIT,* Diiodotyrosine; *MIT,* monoiodotyrosine; *T,* thyroglobulin; T_3, 3,5,3'-triiodothyronine (triiodothyronine); T_4, 3,5,3',5'-tetraiodothyronine (thyroxine); tyr, tyrosine.

of hypoglycemia may be masked under anesthesia, it is probably wise to include glucose in intravenously administered fluids.

THYROID DISEASE

The thyroid gland weighs approximately 20 g and is composed of two lobes joined by an isthmus. The gland is closely affixed to the anterior and lateral aspects of the trachea, with the upper border of the isthmus located just below the cricoid cartilage. A pair of parathyroid glands is located on the posterior aspect of each lobe. A rich capillary network permeates the entire gland. The gland is innervated by the adrenergic and cholinergic nervous systems. The recurrent laryngeal nerve and external motor branch of the superior laryngeal nerve are in intimate proximity to the gland. Histologically, the thyroid is composed of numerous follicles filled with proteinaceous colloid. The major constituent of colloid is thyroglobulin, an iodinated glycoprotein that serves as the substrate for thyroid hormone synthesis. The thyroid gland also contains parafollicular C cells, which produce calcitonin.

Production of normal quantities of thyroid hormones depends on the availability of exogenous iodine. The diet is the primary source of iodine. Iodine is reduced to iodide in the gastrointestinal tract, rapidly absorbed into the blood, then actively transported from the plasma into thyroid follicular cells (Figure 19-10). Binding of iodine to thyroglobulin (i.e., organification) is catalyzed by an iodinase enzyme and yields inactive monoiodotyrosine and diiodotyrosine. Approximately 25% of the monoiodotyrosine and diiodotyrosine undergo coupling via thyroid peroxidase to form the active compounds triiodothyronine (T_3) and thyroxine (T_4). The remaining 75% never becomes hormones, and eventually the iodine is cleaved and recycled. T_3 and T_4 remain attached to thyroglobulin and are stored as colloid until they are released

into the circulation. Since the thyroid contains a large store of hormones and has a low turnover rate, there is protection against depletion if synthesis is impaired or discontinued.

The T_4/T_3 ratio of secreted hormones is 10:1. Upon entering the blood, T_4 and T_3 bind reversibly to three major proteins: thyroxine-binding globulin (80% of binding), prealbumin (10% to 15%), and albumin (5% to 10%). Only the small amount of free fraction of hormone, however, is biologically active. Although only 10% of thyroid hormone secretion is T_3, T_3 is three to four times more active than T_4 per unit of weight and may be the only active thyroid hormone in peripheral tissues. In the periphery, T_3 traverses cell membranes and binds to receptors in the cell nucleus, stimulating messenger RNA synthesis, which in turn controls protein synthesis. Also, binding with mitochondria stimulates oxidative phosphorylation and ATP formation. At the plasma membrane level, T_3 influences transcellular flux of substrates and cations. Thyroid hormones stimulate virtually all metabolic processes. They influence growth and maturation of tissues, enhance tissue function, and stimulate protein synthesis and carbohydrate and lipid metabolism.

Thyroid hormone acts directly on cardiac myocytes and vascular smooth muscle cells. In the heart, T_3 is transported via specific proteins across the myocyte cell membrane and enters the nucleus, binding to nuclear receptors that in turn bind to specific target genes. T_3-responsive genes code for structural and regulatory proteins in the heart (myosin, β-adrenergic receptors, Ca^{2+}-activated ATPase, phospholamban, and Ca^{2+}, Na^+, and K^+ channels) that are important for systolic contractile function and diastolic relaxation. Thyroid hormone increases myocardial contractility directly, decreases systemic vascular resistance via direct vasodilation, and increases intravascular volume. Most recent studies emphasize the direct effects of T_3 on the heart and vascular smooth muscle as responsible for the exaggerated hemodynamic effects of hyperthyroidism. Even though hyperthyroid patients appear to have increased numbers of β-adrenergic receptors, these receptors demonstrate little or no increased sensitivity to adrenergic stimulation, and surprisingly, these patients have normal or low serum concentrations of catecholamines.

Regulation of thyroid function is controlled by the hypothalamus, pituitary, and thyroid glands, which participate in a classic feedback control system. Thyrotropin-releasing hormone (TRH) is secreted from the hypothalamus, traverses the pituitary stalk, and promotes release of thyrotropin-stimulating hormone (TSH) from the anterior pituitary. TSH binds to specific receptors on the thyroid cell membrane and enhances all processes of synthesis and secretion of T_4 and T_3. A decrease in TSH causes a reduction in synthesis and secretion of T_4 and T_3, a decrease in follicular cell size, and a decrease in the gland's vascularity. An increase in TSH yields an increase in hormone production and release and an increase in gland cellularity and vascularity. TSH secretion is also influenced by plasma levels of T_4 and T_3 via a negative feedback loop. In addition to the feedback system, the thyroid gland has an autoregulatory mechanism that maintains a consistent level of hormone stores.

Diagnosis

The third generation of the TSH assay is now the single best test of thyroid hormone action at the cellular level. Small changes in thyroid function cause significant changes in TSH secretion. The normal level of TSH is 0.4 to 5.0 milliunits/L. A TSH level of 0.1 to 0.4 milliunits/L with normal levels of free T_3 (FT_3) and free T_4 (FT_4) is diagnostic of subclinical hyperthyroidism. A TSH level of less than 0.03 milliunits/L with elevated T_3 and T_4 is diagnostic of overt hyperthyroidism. A TSH level of 5.0 to 10 milliunits/L with normal levels of FT_3 and FT_4 is diagnostic of subclinical hypothyroidism. A TSH level of more than 20 milliunits/L (may be as high as 200 or even 400 milliunits/L) with reduced levels of T_3 and T_4 is diagnostic of overt hypothyroidism.

The TRH stimulation test assesses the functional state of the TSH-secreting mechanism in response to TRH and is used to test pituitary function. Other tests that may be helpful in detecting thyroid dysfunction include measurement of serum antimicrosomal antibodies, antithyroglobulin antibodies, and thyroid-stimulating immunoglobulins. Thyroid scans using iodine 123 (^{123}I) or technetium 99m evaluate thyroid nodules as "warm" (normally functioning), "hot" (hyperfunctioning), or "cold" (hypofunctioning). Ultrasonography is 90% to 95% accurate in determining whether a lesion is cystic, solid, or mixed.

Hyperthyroidism

SIGNS AND SYMPTOMS

Hyperthyroidism refers to hyperfunctioning of the thyroid gland with excessive secretion of active thyroid hormones. The majority of cases of hyperthyroidism result from one of three pathologic processes: Graves' disease, toxic multinodular goiter, or a toxic adenoma. Regardless of the cause, the signs and symptoms of hyperthyroidism are those of a hypermetabolic state. The patient is anxious, restless, and hyperkinetic and may be emotionally unstable. The skin is warm and moist, the face is flushed, the hair is fine, and the nails are soft and fragile. The patient may demonstrate increased sweating and complain of heat intolerance. The eyes exhibit a wide-eyed stare with retraction of the upper eyelids (exophthalmos or proptosis) resulting from an infiltrative process that involves retrobulbar fat and the eyelids. Wasting, weakness, and fatigue of the proximal limb muscles are common. The patient usually complains of extreme fatigue but an inability to sleep. Increased bone turnover and osteoporosis may occur. A fine tremor of the hands and hyperactive tendon reflexes are common. Weight loss despite an increased appetite occurs secondary to increased calorigenesis. Bowel movements are frequent and diarrhea is not uncommon.

The cardiovascular system is most threatened by hypermetabolism of peripheral tissues, increased cardiac work with tachycardia, arrhythmias (commonly atrial) and palpitations, a hyperdynamic circulation, increased myocardial contractility and cardiac output, and cardiomegaly. The cardiac responses are due to the direct effects of T_3 on the myocardium and the peripheral vasculature. Although cardiac failure rarely occurs, a thyrotoxic cardiomyopathy has been described characterized by a lymphocytic and eosinophilic infiltration of the myocardium with fibrotic and fatty changes. Elderly patients with unexplained cardiac failure or rhythm disturbances—especially atrial in origin—should be evaluated for thyrotoxicosis.

Graves' disease or toxic diffuse goiter occurs in 0.4% of the U.S. population and is the leading cause of hyperthyroidism. The disease typically occurs in females (female/male ratio is 7:1) between the ages of 20 and 40 years. Although the etiology is unknown, Graves' disease appears to be a systemic autoimmune disease caused by thyroid-stimulating antibodies that bind to TSH receptors in the thyroid, activating adenyl cyclase and stimulating thyroid growth, vascularity, and hypersecretion of T_4 and T_3. The thyroid is usually diffusely enlarged, becoming two to three times its normal size. An ophthalmopathy occurs in 30% of cases and may include upper lid retraction, a wide-eyed stare, muscle weakness, proptosis, and an increase in intraocular pressure. When severe, the condition is termed *malignant exophthalmos*. Steroid therapy, bilateral tarsorrhaphy, external radiation therapy, or surgical decompression may be necessary in these cases. Fortunately, most cases are mild, follow a benign course, and remit spontaneously. The diagnosis of Graves' disease is confirmed by the presence of thyroid-stimulating antibodies in the context of low TSH level and elevated T_4 and T_3 levels.

Toxic multinodular goiter usually arises from long-standing simple goiter and occurs mostly in patients older than 50 years of age. It may present with extreme thyroid enlargement that can cause dysphagia, globus sensation, and possibly inspiratory stridor from tracheal compression. The latter is especially common when the mass extends into the thoracic inlet behind the sternum. In severe cases, superior vena cava obstruction syndrome may also be present. The diagnosis is confirmed by a thyroid scan demonstrating "hot" patchy foci throughout the gland or one or two "hot" nodules. Radioactive iodine uptake and serum T_4 and T_3 levels may only be slightly elevated. The goiter must be differentiated from a neoplasm, and a CT scan and biopsy may be necessary.

TREATMENT

The first line of treatment for hyperthyroidism is an antithyroid drug, either methimazole or propylthiouracil (PTU). These agents interfere with the synthesis of thyroid hormones by inhibiting organification and coupling. PTU has the added advantage of inhibiting the peripheral conversion of T_4 to T_3. A euthyroid state can almost always be achieved in 6 to 8 weeks with either drug if a sufficient dosage is used. Side effects occur in 3% to 12% of patients, with agranulocytosis being the most serious.

Iodide in high concentrations inhibits release of hormones from the hyperfunctioning gland. High concentrations of iodide decrease all phases of thyroid synthesis and release, and result in reduced gland size and possibly a decrease in vascularity. Its effects occur immediately but are short-lived. Therefore, iodide is usually reserved for preparing hyperthyroid patients for surgery, managing patients with actual or impending thyroid storm, and treating patients with severe thyrocardiac disease. There is no need to delay surgery in a patient with otherwise well-controlled thyrotoxicosis in order to initiate iodide therapy.

Iodide is administered orally as a saturated solution of potassium iodide (SSKI), 3 drops PO every 8 hours for 10 to 14 days. The radiographic contrast dye ipodate or iopanoic acid (0.5 to 3.0 g every day) contains iodide and demonstrates beneficial effects similar to those of inorganic iodide. In addition, ipodate inhibits the peripheral conversion of T_4 to T_3 and may also antagonize thyroid hormone binding to receptors. Antithyroid drug therapy should precede the initiation of iodide treatment, because administration of iodide alone will increase thyroid hormone stores and exacerbate the thyrotoxic state. Lithium carbonate 300 mg PO every 6 hours may be given in place of potassium iodide or ipodate to patients who are allergic to iodide.

β-Adrenergic antagonists do not affect the underlying thyroid abnormality but may relieve signs and symptoms of increased adrenergic activity such as anxiety, sweating, heat intolerance, tremors, and tachycardia. Propranolol offers the added features of impairing the peripheral conversion of T_4 to T_3.

Ablative therapy with radioactive iodine 131 (^{131}I) or surgery is recommended for patients with Graves' disease for whom medical management has failed, as well as for patients with toxic multinodular goiter or a toxic adenoma. Standard doses of ^{131}I deliver approximately 8500 rad to the thyroid and destroy the follicular cells. The remission rate is 80% to 98%. A major disadvantage of therapy is that 40% to 70% of treated patients become hypothyroid within 10 years.

Surgery (i.e., subtotal thyroidectomy or possibly total thyroidectomy) results in prompt control of disease and is associated with a lower incidence of hypothyroidism (10% to 30%) than radioactive iodine therapy. Subtotal thyroidectomy corrects thyrotoxicosis in more than 95% of patients; mortality rate for the procedure is less than 0.1%. Complications from surgery include hypothyroidism, hemorrhage with tracheal compression, unilateral or bilateral damage to the recurrent laryngeal nerve(s), damage to the motor branch of the superior laryngeal nerve, and damage to or inadvertent removal of the parathyroid glands.

Hyperthyroidism during pregnancy is treated with low dosages of antithyroid drugs. However, these drugs do cross the placenta and can cause fetal hypothyroidism. If the mother remains euthyroid while taking small dosages of an antithyroid drug, the occurrence of fetal hypothyroidism is rare. Radioactive iodine treatment is contraindicated during pregnancy, as is oral iodide therapy, because it can cause fetal goiter and hypothyroidism. The long-term use of propranolol during pregnancy is controversial since intrauterine growth retardation has been attributed to its use. Fortunately, pregnancy appears to attenuate the severity of hyperthyroidism, and dosages of antithyroid drugs can usually be kept low (i.e., PTU < 200 mg/day). If dosages higher than 300 mg/day of PTU are needed during the first trimester, a subtotal thyroidectomy should be performed in the second trimester. Thyroid storm occurring in pregnancy is managed in the same way as in nonpregnant patients.

MANAGEMENT OF ANESTHESIA

In hyperthyroid patients undergoing surgery, euthyroidism should definitely be established preoperatively. In elective cases, this may mean waiting a substantial time (6 to 8 weeks) for antithyroid drugs to become effective. In emergency cases, the use of an intravenous β-blocker, ipodate, glucocorticoids, and PTU is usually necessary. No intravenous preparation of PTU is available, so the drug must be taken orally, via a nasogastric tube, or rectally. Glucocorticoids (dexamethasone 2 mg IV every 6 hours) should be administered to decrease hormone release and reduce the peripheral conversion of T_4 to T_3. The anesthesiologist should be prepared to manage thyroid storm, especially in patients with uncontrolled or poorly controlled disease.

Evaluation of the upper airway for evidence of tracheal compression or deviation caused by a goiter is an important part of the preoperative evaluation. Examination of chest radiographs and CT scans is often helpful in this regard. Intraoperatively, the need for invasive monitoring is determined on an individual basis and depends on the type of surgery to be performed and the medical condition of the patient. Controlled studies in hyperthyroid animals demonstrate no clinically significant increase in anesthetic requirements (i.e., minimum alveolar concentration). Establishment of adequate anesthetic depth is extremely important to avoid exaggerated sympathetic nervous system responses. Drugs that stimulate the sympathetic nervous system (i.e., ketamine, pancuronium, atropine, ephedrine, epinephrine) should be avoided. Thiopental, because of its thioureylene nucleus, decreases the peripheral conversion of T_4 to T_3 and may have a slight advantage over other agents for anesthesia induction. Eye protection (eyedrops, lubricant, eye pads) is critical, especially for patients with proptosis.

For maintenance of anesthesia, any of the potent inhalation agents may be used. A concern in hyperthyroid patients is organ toxicity secondary to an increase in drug metabolism. Although animal studies demonstrate an increase in hepatotoxicity in hyperthyroid rats following exposure to isoflurane, these results have not been substantiated in humans. Nitrous oxide and opioids are safe and effective in hyperthyroid patients. Hyperthyroid patients may have co-existing muscle disease (e.g., myasthenia gravis) with reduced requirements for the nondepolarizing muscle relaxants; therefore, careful titration is required. For the treatment of intraoperative hypotension, a direct-acting vasopressor (phenylephrine) is preferred. Ephedrine, epinephrine, norepinephrine, and dopamine should be avoided or administered in extremely low doses to prevent exaggerated hemodynamic responses. Regional anesthesia can be safely performed and in fact may be a preferred technique. Epinephrine-containing local anesthetic solutions should be avoided.

Removal of the thyrotoxic gland does not mean immediate resolution of thyrotoxicosis. The half-life of T_4 is 7 to 8 days; therefore, β-blocker therapy may need to be continued in the postoperative period.

THYROID STORM

Thyroid storm is a life-threatening exacerbation of hyperthyroidism precipitated by trauma, infection, medical illness, or surgery. Thyroid storm and malignant hyperthermia can present with similar intraoperative and postoperative signs and symptoms (i.e., hyperpyrexia, tachycardia, hypermetabolism); therefore, differentiation between the two may be extremely difficult. Surprisingly, thyroid hormone levels in thyroid storm may not be significantly higher than during uncomplicated hyperthyroidism. Thyroid function tests therefore may not be useful in making the diagnosis. The cause is probably a shift from protein-bound thyroid hormone to free hormone as a result of the presence of circulating inhibitors to binding.

Thyroid storm most often occurs in the postoperative period in untreated or inadequately treated hyperthyroid patients after emergency surgery. Patients manifest extreme anxiety, fever, tachycardia, cardiovascular instability, and altered consciousness. Treatment includes rapid alleviation of thyrotoxicosis and general supportive care. Dehydration is managed with intravenous administration of glucose-containing crystalloid solutions, and cooling measures (e.g., cooling blanket, ice packs, administration of cool humidified oxygen) are used to counter the fever. β-Blockers should be titrated to decrease heart rate to less than 90 beats per minute. Dexamethasone 2 mg every 6 hours or cortisol 100 to 200 mg every 8 hours can be used to decrease hormone release and conversion of T_4 to T_3. Antithyroid drugs (PTU 200 to 400 mg every 8 hours) may be administered through a nasogastric tube, orally, or rectally. If circulatory shock is present, intravenous administration of a direct vasopressor (phenylephrine) is indicated. A β-adrenergic blocker or digitalis is recommended for atrial fibrillation accompanied by a fast ventricular response. Serum thyroid hormone levels generally return to normal within 24 to 48 hours and recovery occurs within 1 week. The mortality rate for thyroid storm remains surprisingly high at approximately 20%.

Hypothyroidism

SIGNS AND SYMPTOMS

Hypothyroidism or myxedema is a relatively common disease affecting 0.5% to 0.8% of the adult population. Primary hypothyroidism results in decreased production of thyroid hormones despite adequate or increased levels of TSH and accounts for 95% of all cases of hypothyroidism. The most common cause in the United States is ablation of the gland by radioactive iodine or surgery. The second most common type of hypothyroidism is idiopathic and probably autoimmune in origin, with autoantibodies blocking TSH receptors in the thyroid. Unlike Graves' disease, this immune response destroys receptors instead of stimulating them. Hashimoto's thyroiditis is an autoimmune disorder characterized by goitrous enlargement and hypothyroidism that usually affects middle-aged women.

In adults, hypothyroidism has a slow, insidious, progressive course. There is gradual slowing of mental and physical activity. In mild cases, patients tire easily and experience weight gain. In moderate to severe cases, patients develop fatigue, lethargy, apathy, and listlessness. The speech becomes slow and the intellect becomes dull. With time, patients experience cold intolerance, decreased sweating, constipation, menorrhagia, and slowing of motor function secondary to muscle stiffness and cramping. They gain weight despite a decrease in appetite. Physically, they demonstrate dry thickened skin, coarse facial features, dry brittle hair, a large tongue, a deep hoarse voice, and periorbital and peripheral edema. Accumulation of hydrophilic mucopolysaccharides in the dermis and other tissues is responsible for the immobile, nonpitting edema.

Physiologically, cardiac output is decreased secondary to reductions in stroke volume and heart rate. Baroreceptor function is also impaired. The electrocardiogram (ECG) in patients with overt hypothyroidism shows flattened or inverted T waves, low-amplitude P waves and QRS complexes, and sinus bradycardia; ventricular dysrhythmias may also be present. Peripheral vascular resistance is increased and blood volume is reduced, which results in pale, cool skin. In advanced cases, myocardial contractility becomes reduced secondary to systolic and diastolic dysfunction, and the heart becomes enlarged and dilated (hypothyroid cardiomyopathy). Pericardial effusions are common. Hypothyroid patients usually have hypercholesterolemia and hypertriglyceridemia and may have coronary artery disease. Hyponatremia and impairment of free water excretion are also common, related to inappropriate secretion of antidiuretic hormone (ADH). Maximum breathing capacity and diffusion capacity are decreased, and ventilatory responsiveness to hypoxia and hypercarbia is depressed. Pleural effusions may result in dyspnea. Gastrointestinal function is slow, and an adynamic ileus may occur. Deep tendon reflexes demonstrate a prolonged relaxation phase.

Twenty percent of women older than 60 years of age have subclinical hypothyroidism. Subclinical disease is associated with an increased risk of coronary heart disease in patients with a TSH level of more than 10 milliunits/L. Although most patients have few if any signs or symptoms, changes in myocardial structure and contractibility can occur secondary to systolic and diastolic dysfunction. Even though these changes are reversible with L-thyroxine therapy, use of thyroid replacement for subclinical disease remains controversial.

Secondary hypothyroidism is diagnosed by reduced levels of FT_4, T_4, and T_3, as well as a reduced TSH level. A TRH stimulation test can confirm pituitary abnormality as the cause. This test measures the responsiveness of the pituitary gland to intravenously administered TRH, the hypothalamic stimulator of TSH. In primary hypothyroidism, basal levels of TSH are elevated, and the elevation is exaggerated after TRH administration. With pituitary dysfunction, there is a blunted or absent response to TRH.

Euthyroid sick syndrome is the occurrence of abnormal results on thyroid function tests in critically ill patients with significant nonthyroidal illness. Characteristic findings include low levels of T_3 and T_4 and a normal TSH level. As illness increases in severity, the T_3 and T_4 levels decrease further. The etiology of this response is not understood. Euthyroid sick syndrome may be a physiologic response to stress, and it can be induced by surgery. No treatment for thyroid function is necessary. Differentiating hypothyroidism from euthyroid sick syndrome can be extremely difficult. A serum TSH level is the best aid. Levels higher than 10 milliunits/L indicate hypothyroidism, whereas levels lower than 5.0 milliunits/L indicate euthyroidism.

Changes in thyroid function test results have also been documented following uncomplicated acute myocardial infarctions, congestive heart failure, and cardiopulmonary bypass. Significant depression of T_3 levels occurs, but the administration of T_3 does not appear efficacious. In addition, the use of T_3 as an inotrope has not been show to result in any substantial improvement in cardiac performance.

TREATMENT

L-Thyroxine (levothyroxine sodium) is usually administered for the treatment of hypothyroidism. The first evidence of a therapeutic response to thyroid hormone is sodium and water diuresis and a reduction in the TSH level. In patients with hypothyroid cardiomyopathy, a measurable improvement in myocardial function is often achieved with therapy.

Although angina is uncommon in hypothyroidism, it can appear or worsen during treatment of the hypothyroid state with thyroid hormone. Medical management of such patients is particularly difficult. Therefore, patients who have both hypothyroidism and angina should undergo angiographic evaluation of the coronary arteries before hormone replacement is initiated. If surgically remediable disease is demonstrated, coronary artery bypass graft surgery can be successfully accomplished despite hypothyroidism. Coronary revascularization can permit the necessary thyroid hormone replacement and reinstitution of the euthyroid state.

MANAGEMENT OF ANESTHESIA

Hypothyroid patients may be at increased risk when undergoing either general or regional anesthesia for a number of reasons. Airway compromise secondary to a swollen oral cavity, edematous vocal cords, or goitrous enlargement may be present. Decreased gastric emptying increases the risk of regurgitation and aspiration. A hypodynamic cardiovascular system characterized by decreased cardiac output, stroke volume, heart rate, baroreceptor reflexes, and intravascular volume may be compromised by surgical stress and cardiac-depressant anesthetic agents. Decreased ventilatory responsiveness to hypoxia and hypercarbia is enhanced by anesthetic agents. Hypothermia occurs quickly and is difficult to treat. Hematologic abnormalities such as anemia (25% to 50% of patients) and dysfunction of platelets and coagulation factors (especially factor VIII), electrolyte imbalances (hyponatremia), and hypoglycemia are common and require close monitoring intraoperatively. Decreased neuromuscular excitability is exacerbated by anesthetic drugs.

These patients can be extremely sensitive to narcotics and sedatives and may even be lethargic secondary to their disease; therefore, preoperative sedation should be undertaken with caution. Hypothyroid patients also appear to have an increased sensitivity to anesthetic drugs, although the effect of thyroid activity on the minimum alveolar concentration of volatile anesthetics is negligible. Increased sensitivity is probably secondary to reduced cardiac output, decreased blood volume, abnormal baroreceptor function, decreased hepatic metabolism, and decreased renal excretion of drugs. In patients with a hypodynamic cardiovascular system invasive monitoring and/or transesophageal echocardiography may be needed to monitor intravascular volume and cardiac status.

General anesthetics should be administered through an endotracheal tube following either rapid-sequence induction or awake intubation if a difficult airway is present. Hypothyroid patients are very sensitive to the myocardial-depressant effects of the potent inhalational agents. Vasodilation in the presence of possible hypovolemia and impaired baroreceptor activity can produce significant hypotension. Pharmacologic support for intraoperative hypotension is best provided with ephedrine, dopamine, or epinephrine and not a pure α-adrenergic agonist (phenylephrine). Unresponsive hypotension may require supplemental steroid administration.

From a cardiovascular standpoint, pancuronium is a preferred muscle relaxant; however, reduced skeletal muscle activity in these patients coupled with a reduction in hepatic metabolism necessitates cautious dosing. Controlled ventilation is recommended in all cases, since these patients tend to hypoventilate if allowed to breathe spontaneously. Dextrose in normal saline is the recommended intravenous fluid to avoid hypoglycemia and minimize hyponatremia secondary to impaired free water clearance.

If emergency surgery is necessary, the potential for severe intraoperative cardiovascular instability and myxedema coma in the postoperative period is high. Intravenous thyroid replacement therapy should be initiated as soon as possible. Although intravenous L-thyroxine takes 10 to 12 days to yield a peak basal metabolic rate, intravenous triiodothyronine is effective in 6 hours with a peak basal metabolic rate seen in 36 to 72 hours. L-Thyroxine 300 to 500 mcg IV or L-triiodothyronine 25 to 50 mcg IV is an acceptable initial dose. Steroid coverage with hydrocortisone or dexamethasone is necessary, since decreased adrenal cortical function often accompanies hypothyroidism. Phosphodiesterase inhibitors such as milrinone may be effective in the treatment of reduced myocardial contractility because their mechanism of action does not depend on β-receptors, whose number and sensitivity may be reduced in hypothyroidism.

MYXEDEMA COMA

Myxedema coma is a rare severe form of hypothyroidism characterized by delirium or unconsciousness, hypoventilation, hypothermia (80% of patients), bradycardia, hypotension, and a severe dilutional hyponatremia. It occurs most commonly in elderly women with a long history of hypothyroidism. Infection, trauma, cold, and central nervous system depressants predispose hypothyroid patients to myxedema coma. Ironically, most patients are not comatose. Hypothermia (as low as 27° C) is a cardinal feature and results from impaired thermoregulation caused by defective function of the hypothalamus (a target tissue of thyroid hormone). Myxedema coma is a medical emergency with a mortality rate higher than 50%. Intravenous L-thyroxine or L-triiodothyronine is the treatment of choice. Intravenous hydration with glucose-containing saline solutions, temperature regulation, correction of electrolyte imbalances, and stabilization of the cardiac and pulmonary systems are necessary. Mechanical ventilation is frequently required. Heart rate, blood pressure, and temperature usually improve within 24 hours, and a relative euthyroid state is achieved in 3 to 5 days. Hydrocortisone 100 to 300 mg/day IV is also prescribed to treat possible adrenal insufficiency.

Goiter and Thyroid Tumors

A goiter is a swelling of the thyroid gland that results from compensatory hypertrophy and hyperplasia of follicular epithelium secondary to a reduction in thyroid hormone output. The cause may be a deficient intake of iodine, ingestion of a dietary (i.e., cassava) or pharmacologic (i.e., phenylbutazone, lithium) goitrogen, or a defect in the hormonal biosynthetic pathway. The size of the goiter is determined by the level and duration of hormone insufficiency. In most cases, a goiter is associated with a euthyroid state, with the increased mass and cellular activity eventually overcoming the impairment in hormone synthesis. However, hypothyroidism or hyperthyroidism occurs in some cases. Patients with simple, nontoxic goiter are euthyroid. Nevertheless, simple, nontoxic goiter is a forerunner of toxic multinodular goiter. In the United States, most cases of simple nontoxic goiter are of unknown cause and are treated with L-thyroxine. Surgery is indicated only if medical therapy is ineffective and the goiter is compromising the airway or is cosmetically unacceptable.

The anesthetic management of a patient undergoing surgical removal of a large goiter or thyroid mass that compromises the airway presents a major challenge. Examination of a CT scan of the neck will demonstrate anatomic abnormalities.

Sedatives and narcotics should be avoided or used with great caution before and during endotracheal tube placement. Awake intubation with an armored (anode) tube using fiberoptic bronchoscopy is probably the safest method to assess the degree of obstruction and establish the airway. Surgical removal of the mass may reveal underlying tracheomalacia and a collapsible airway. Tracheal extubation should be performed with as much caution and concern as intubation.

If the mass extends into the substernal regional (i.e., anterior mediastinal mass), superior vena cava obstruction, major airway obstruction, and/or cardiac compression may occur. The latter two may become apparent only upon induction of general anesthesia. Airway obstruction appears to result from changes in lung and chest wall mechanics that occur with changes in patient position or with the onset of muscle paralysis. During spontaneous respiration, the larger airways are supported by negative intrathoracic pressure, and the effects of extrinsic compression may be apparent in only the most severe cases. With cessation of spontaneous respiration, compensatory mechanisms are removed and airway obstruction occurs. In addition, positive pressure ventilation may demonstrate total airway occlusion. A preoperative history of dyspnea in the upright or supine position is predictive of possible airway obstruction during general anesthesia. A CT scan must be examined to assess the extent of the tumor. Flow-volume loops in the upright and supine positions will demonstrate the site of obstruction and the degree of obstruction to airflow in the upper airway and trachea. Limitations in the inspiratory limb of the loop indicate extrathoracic airway obstruction, and delayed flow in the expiratory limb indicates intrathoracic obstruction. Echocardiography with the patient in the upright and supine positions can indicate the degree of cardiac compression.

If practical, local anesthesia is recommended for patients requiring surgery. If general anesthesia is necessary, preoperative shrinkage of a thyroid tumor by radiation or chemotherapy is recommended unless the altered histologic appearance would prevent an accurate diagnosis, as when a biopsy specimen is required for diagnosis. Unfortunately, goiters are not sensitive to radiation therapy. In such patients, an awake intubation with fiberoptic bronchoscopy using an anode tube is recommended. The patient is placed in semi-Fowler's position, and volatile anesthetic with nitrous oxide and oxygen is administered using spontaneous ventilation. Muscle relaxants are avoided. It must be possible to change the patient's position.

Following tumor resection, the airway should be examined by fiberoptic bronchoscopy to detect tracheomalacia and determine whether and when tracheal extubation is appropriate. A rigid bronchoscope should be available to reestablish the airway if collapse occurs. Cardiopulmonary bypass equipment should be on standby during the case.

Complications of Thyroid Surgery

Morbidity from thyroid surgery approaches 13%. Recurrent laryngeal nerve injury may be unilateral or bilateral and temporary or permanent. The injury may result from excess trauma to the nerve(s) (abductor and/or adductor fibers of the recurrent laryngeal nerve), inadvertent ligation, or transection. When paralysis of the abductor muscles to the vocal cord occurs, the involved cord assumes a median or paramedian position. If trauma is unilateral, the patient experiences hoarseness but no airway obstruction, and function usually returns in 3 to 6 months. Ligation or transection of the nerve results in permanent hoarseness. Bilateral involvement is more serious, since the patient usually experiences airway obstruction and problems with coughing and respiratory toilet. Depending on the degree of damage, a temporary or permanent tracheostomy is usually necessary. Injury to the adductor fibers of the recurrent laryngeal nerve(s) results in paralysis of the adductor muscle(s) and increases the risk of pulmonary aspiration. Injury to the motor branch of the superior laryngeal nerve, which innervates the inferior pharyngeal constrictor and cricothyroid muscles, can also occur during thyroid dissection. This injury results in weakening of the voice and the inability to create high tones.

Hypoparathyroidism is also a complication of thyroid surgery. It usually results from damage to the blood supply of the parathyroid glands rather than inadvertent removal. One functioning parathyroid gland with an adequate blood supply is all that is necessary to avoid hypoparathyroidism. The signs and symptoms of hypocalcemia occur in the first 24 to 48 hours postoperatively. Anxiety, circumoral numbness, tingling of the fingertips, muscle cramping, and positive Chvostek's and Trousseau's signs are indicative of hypocalcemia. A positive Chvostek sign consists of facial muscle twitching produced by manual tapping over the area of the facial nerve at the angle of the mandible. A positive Trousseau sign is carpopedal spasm in response to 3 minutes of limb ischemia produced by a tourniquet. Stridor can occur and can proceed to laryngospasm. Immediate treatment with intravenous calcium gluconate (1 g, 10 mL of a 10% solution) or calcium chloride (1 g, 10 mL of a 10% solution) is necessary. A continuous infusion of calcium for several days is also recommended. For long-term management, oral calcium and vitamin D_3 are prescribed or autotransplantation of parathyroid tissue may be performed.

Tracheal compression from an expanding hematoma may cause rapid respiratory compromise in the period immediately after thyroid surgery. Immediate hematoma evacuation is the first line of treatment. If time permits, the patient should be returned to the operating room. If necessary, the wound should be opened at the bedside, clots evacuated, and bleeding vessels secured to relieve airway obstruction. A thyroid tray, including a tracheostomy set, should always be available at the bedside during the postoperative period so that sutures or clips can be removed and the wound opened emergently. Tracheostomy is not required if the wound is decompressed early.

PHEOCHROMOCYTOMA

Pheochromocytomas are catecholamine-secreting tumors that arise from chromaffin cells of the sympathoadrenal system. Although pheochromocytomas account for fewer than 0.1% of all cases of hypertension in adults, their detection is imperative, since they have lethal potential and are one of the few truly curable forms of hypertension. Uncontrolled catecholamine release can result in malignant hypertension, cerebrovascular accident, and myocardial infarction.

The precise cause of a pheochromocytoma is unknown. Pheochromocytomas are usually an isolated finding (90% of cases). Ten percent of pheochromocytomas are inherited (familial) as an autosomal dominant trait. Familial pheochromocytomas usually occur as bilateral adrenal tumors or as extraadrenal tumors that appear in the same anatomic site over successive generations. Both sexes are equally affected, and the peak incidence is in the third to fifth decades of life. Ten percent of pheochromocytomas occur in children, and in this population, multiple, extraadrenal, and bilateral tumors are relatively more common than in adults. Variability in clinical presentation leads to difficulties in diagnosis. Recent advances in genetic testing allow early identification of patients with a familial pheochromocytoma before signs and symptoms occur.

Familial pheochromocytomas can also be part of the multiple endocrine neoplastic syndromes and can occur in association with several neuroectodermal dysplasias (e.g., von Hippel–Lindau syndrome). Patients with multiple endocrine neoplasia syndrome type IIA have a pheochromocytoma, medullary carcinoma of the thyroid, and hyperparathyroidism. Patients with multiple endocrine neoplasia syndrome type IIB have a pheochromocytoma, medullary carcinoma of the thyroid, alimentary tract ganglioneuromatosis, thickened corneal nerves, and a marfanoid habitus. Almost 100% of patients with multiple endocrine neoplasia syndrome type II have or will develop bilateral benign adrenal medullary pheochromocytomas.

Eighty percent of pheochromocytomas are located in the adrenal medulla. The organ of Zuckerkandl near the aortic bifurcation is the most common extraadrenal site. Two percent of extraadrenal pheochromocytomas occur in the neck and thorax. Failure of involution of chromaffin tissue in childhood is the best explanation for the development of extraadrenal pheochromocytomas. Most extraadrenal pheochromocytomas follow a benign course. Malignant pheochromocytomas usually spread via venous and lymphatic channels with a predilection for liver and bone. The 5-year survival rate for patients with malignancy is 44%. Following resection of benign tumors, 5% to 10% of patients have a benign recurrence.

Most pheochromocytomas secrete norepinephrine, either alone or, more commonly, in combination with a smaller amount of epinephrine in a ratio of 85:15—the inverse of the secretion ratio in the normal adrenal gland. Approximately 15% of tumors secrete predominantly epinephrine. Some dopamine-secreting pheochromocytomas have also been described. Most pheochromocytomas are not under neurogenic control and secrete catecholamines autonomously.

Signs and Symptoms

The clinical presentation of pheochromocytoma is variable; attacks range from infrequent (i.e., once a month or fewer) to numerous (i.e., many times per day) and may last from less than a minute to several hours. They may occur spontaneously or be precipitated by physical injury, emotional stress, or medications. Hypertension, either continuous or paroxysmal, is the most frequent manifestation of pheochromocytoma. Headache, sweating, pallor, and palpitations are other classic signs and symptoms. Orthostatic hypotension is also a common finding and is considered to be secondary to hypovolemia and impaired vasoconstrictor reflex responses.

Hemodynamic signs depend on the predominant catecholamine secreted. With norepinephrine, α-adrenergic effects predominate, and patients usually have systolic and diastolic hypertension and a reflex bradycardia. With epinephrine, β-adrenergic effects predominate, and patients usually have systolic hypertension, diastolic hypotension, and tachycardia. Despite the 10-fold higher levels of circulating catecholamines, the hemodynamics are not greatly different in patients with pheochromocytomas and in patients with essential hypertension. Both groups have an increased systemic vascular resistance, usually a normal cardiac output, and a slightly decreased plasma volume. Long-term exposure to high levels of catecholamines does not appear to produce hemodynamic responses characteristic of acute administration. A desensitization of the cardiovascular system or a downregulation of adrenergic receptors may explain this finding.

Cardiomyopathy is a complication of pheochromocytoma. The cause appears multifactorial and includes catecholamine-induced permeability changes in the sarcolemmal membranes leading to excess calcium influx, toxicity from oxidized products of catecholamines, and myocardial damage by free radicals. In addition, high catecholamine levels result in coronary vasoconstriction through α-adrenergic pathways, which reduces coronary blood flow and potentially creates ischemia. Both dilated and hypertrophic cardiomyopathies, as well as left ventricular outflow tract obstruction, have been demonstrated echocardiographically. ECG abnormalities may include elevation or depression of the ST segment, flattening or inversion of T waves, prolongation of the QT interval, high or peaked P waves, left axis deviation, and arrhythmias. The cardiomyopathy appears reversible if catecholamine stimulation is removed early before fibrosis has occurred. Distinct from a cardiomyopathy, pheochromocytoma patients may develop cardiac hypertrophy with congestive heart failure secondary to sustained hypertension.

Although pheochromocytoma patients rarely have frank diabetes, most have an elevated blood glucose level secondary to catecholamine stimulation of glycogenolysis and inhibition of insulin release.

Diagnosis

When a pheochromocytoma is clinically suspected, excess catecholamine secretion must be demonstrated. For patients with a low probability of having a pheochromocytoma, a 24-hour urine collection for measurement of metanephrines and catecholamines is a useful screening test. However, the most sensitive test for patients at high risk (familial

pheochromocytoma or classic symptoms) is measurement of plasma-free metanephrines. Catecholamines are metabolized to free metanephrines within tumor cells, and these metabolites are continuously released into the circulation. A plasma-free normetanephrine level higher than 400 pg/mL and/or a metanephrine level higher than 220 pg/mL confirms the diagnosis of pheochromocytoma. A pheochromocytoma is excluded if normetanephrine level is less than 112 pg/mL and metanephrine level is less than 61 pg/mL.

Results are equivocal in 5% to 10% of patients, and in these cases, the clonidine suppression test may be used. Clonidine is an α$_2$-agonist that acts on the central nervous system to diminish efferent sympathetic outflow. In patients with a pheochromocytoma, increased plasma catecholamines result from tumor release, which bypasses normal storage and release mechanisms. Clonidine acts to lower plasma catecholamine levels in patients without a pheochromocytoma but has no effect on catecholamine levels in patients with a pheochromocytoma.

In the past, provocative testing with histamine or tyramine was used to elicit excess catecholamine release from the tumor. However, owing to the relatively high incidence of morbidity, these tests have been abandoned. A glucagon stimulation test is now considered to be the safest and most specific provocative test. Glucagon acts directly on the tumor to induce release of catecholamines. A positive response to the test yields a plasma catecholamine increase of at least three times the baseline values or more than 2000 pg/mL within 1 to 3 minutes of glucagon administration. This test should be performed only in patients with a diastolic blood pressure of less than 100 mm Hg.

Tumor location can be predicted by the pattern of catecholamine production (Table 19-7). CT detects more than 95% of adrenal masses larger than 1.0 cm in diameter. MRI offers advantages over CT, including better identification of small adrenal lesions, better differentiation of various types of adrenal lesions, no need for intravenous contrast, and lack of radiation exposure. In contrast to CT and MRI, which provide primarily anatomic information, testing with ^{131}I-metaiodobenzylguanidine (MIBG) and ^{123}I-MIBG provides functional information. MIBG is an analogue of guanethidine, similar in structure to norepinephrine. It is taken up by adrenergic neurons and concentrated in catecholamine-secreting tumors. MIBG is detected by

TABLE 19-7 **Pattern of catecholamine production by site of pheochromocytoma**

	Adrenal	Extraadrenal	Adrenal + extraadrenal
Norepinephrine	61%	31%	8%
Epinephrine	100%	—	—
Norepinephrine + epinephrine	95%	—	5%

Adapted from Kaser H. Clinical and diagnostic findings in patients with chromaffin tumors: pheochromocytomas, pheochromoblastomas. *Recent Results Cancer Res.* 1990;118:97-105.

scintigraphy. MIBG scintigraphy is especially useful in detecting extraadrenal pheochromocytomas and metastatic deposits. CT, MRI, and ^{131}I-MIBG scintigraphy are complementary studies in localizing pheochromocytomas. Positron emission scanning and selective venous catheterization with sampling of catecholamines from the adrenal veins and other sites are additional useful tests.

Management of Anesthesia

PREOPERATIVE MANAGEMENT

Since most pheochromocytomas secrete predominantly norepinephrine, medical therapy has depended on α-blockade to lower blood pressure, increase intravascular volume, prevent paroxysmal hypertensive episodes, allow resensitization of adrenergic receptors, and decrease myocardial dysfunction. Although a significantly reduced intravascular volume may accompany a pheochromocytoma, the majority of patients have a normal or only slightly decreased intravascular volume. α-Blockade appears to protect myocardial performance and tissue oxygenation from the adverse effects of catecholamines.

Phenoxybenzamine is the most frequently prescribed α-blocker for preoperative use. It is a noncompetitive $α_1$-antagonist with some $α_2$-blocking properties. Because it is a noncompetitive blocker, it is difficult for excess catecholamines to overcome the blockade. Its long duration of action permits oral dosing only twice daily. The goal of therapy is normotension, a resolution of symptoms, elimination of ST-segment and T-wave changes on the ECG, and elimination of arrhythmias. Overtreatment can result in severe orthostatic hypotension. The optimal duration of α-blockade therapy is undetermined and may range from 3 days to 2 weeks or longer. Because of the prolonged effect of phenoxybenzamine on α-receptors, the recommendation has been to discontinue its use 24 to 48 hours before surgery to avoid vascular unresponsiveness immediately following removal of the tumor. Some anesthesiologists administer only one half to two thirds of the morning dose preceding surgery to address similar concerns. Some surgeons request its discontinuation 48 hours preoperatively so that they can use hypertensive episodes intraoperatively as cues in localizing areas of metastasis. Prazosin and doxazosin, pure $α_1$-competitive blockers, are alternatives to phenoxybenzamine. They are shorter acting, cause less tachycardia, and are easier to titrate to a desired end point than phenoxybenzamine.

If tachycardia (i.e., heart rates > 120 beats per minute) or other arrhythmias result after α-blockade with phenoxybenzamine, a β-adrenergic blocker is prescribed. A nonselective β-blocker should never be administered before α-blockade, because blockade of vasodilatory $β_2$-receptors results in unopposed α-agonism, leading to vasoconstriction and hypertensive crises. Propranolol, a nonselective β-blocker with a half-life longer than 4 hours, is most frequently used. Atenolol, metoprolol, and labetalol have also been used successfully. The degree of α- and β-blockade provided by labetalol (i.e., β effects exceed α effects) may not be appropriate for certain

pheochromocytoma patients. In very rare circumstances, β-blockade may be initiated before α-blockade. A patient with a pheochromocytoma secreting solely epinephrine and with coronary artery disease may benefit greatly from the $β_1$-selective antagonist esmolol. Esmolol has a fast onset and short elimination half-life and can be administered intravenously in the period immediately before surgery.

α-Methylparatyrosine (metyrosine) inhibits the rate-limiting enzyme tyrosine hydroxylase of the catecholamine synthetic pathway and may decrease catecholamine production by 50% to 80%. In combination with phenoxybenzamine, it has been shown to facilitate intraoperative hemodynamic management. It is especially useful for malignant and inoperable tumors. Side effects, including extrapyramidal reactions and crystalluria, have limited its application.

Calcium channel blockers and ACE inhibitors may also be used to control hypertension. Calcium is a trigger for catecholamine release from the tumor, and excess calcium entry into myocardial cells contributes to a catecholamine-mediated cardiomyopathy. Nifedipine, diltiazem, and verapamil have all been used to control preoperative hypertension, as has captopril. An $α_1$-blocker plus a calcium channel blocker is an effective combination in treatment-resistant cases.

INTRAOPERATIVE MANAGEMENT

Optimal preparation for pheochromocytoma resection involves preoperative administration of an α-adrenergic blocker with or without a β-blocker with or without α-methylparatyrosine, as well as correction of possible hypovolemia. Intraoperative goals include avoidance of drugs or maneuvers that may provoke catecholamine release or potentiate catecholamine actions, and maintenance of cardiovascular stability, preferably with short-acting drugs. Hypertension frequently occurs during pneumoperitoneum as well as during tumor manipulation. On the other hand, significant hypotension may develop following ligation of the tumor's venous drainage. Intraoperative monitoring should include standard plus invasive monitoring methods. An arterial catheter enables monitoring of blood pressure on a beat-to-beat basis. A central venous pressure catheter is usually sufficient for patients without cardiac symptoms or other clinical evidence of cardiac involvement. A pulmonary artery catheter or transesophageal echocardiography may be necessary to manage the large fluid requirements, major volume shifts, and possible underlying myocardial dysfunction in patients with very active tumors. A large positive fluid balance is usually required to manage hypotension and keep intravascular volumes within a normal range.

Intraoperative ultrasonography can be used to localize small, functional tumors and to perform adrenal-sparing procedures or partial adrenalectomies. Adrenal-sparing procedures are particularly valuable when bilateral adrenal pheochromocytomas must be removed. Laparoscopy can be used for tumors smaller than 4 to 5 cm and is becoming the surgical approach of choice for many endocrine surgeons.

Factors that stimulate catecholamine release such as fear, stress, pain, shivering, hypoxia, and hypercarbia must be minimized in the perioperative period. Although all anesthetic drugs have been used with some degree of success, certain drugs should theoretically be avoided to prevent possible adverse hemodynamic responses. Morphine and atracurium can cause histamine release, which may provoke release of catecholamines from the tumor. Atropine, pancuronium, and succinylcholine are examples of vagolytic or sympathomimetic drugs that may stimulate the sympathetic nervous system.

Virtually all patients exhibit increases in systolic arterial pressure in excess of 200 mm Hg for periods of time intraoperatively irrespective of preoperative initiation of α-blockade. A number of antihypertensive drugs must be prepared and ready for immediate administration. Sodium nitroprusside, a direct vasodilator, is the agent of choice because of its potency, immediate onset of action, and short duration of action. Phentolamine, a competitive α-adrenergic blocker and a direct vasodilator, is effective, although tachyphylaxis and tachycardia are associated with its use. Nitroglycerin is effective, but large doses are often required and may cause tachycardia. Labetalol, with more β- than α-blocking properties, is preferred for predominantly epinephrine-secreting tumors. Magnesium sulfate inhibits release of catecholamines from the adrenal medulla and peripheral nerve terminals, reduces sensitivity of α-receptors to catecholamines, is a direct vasodilator, and is an antiarrhythmic. However, like all antihypertensive medications, it is suboptimal in controlling hypertension during tumor manipulation. Mixtures of antihypertensive drugs such as nitroprusside, esmolol, diltiazem, and phentolamine have been recommended to control refractory hypertension. Increasing the depth of anesthesia is also an option, although this approach may accentuate the hypotension accompanying tumor vein ligation.

Arrhythmias are usually ventricular in origin and are managed with either lidocaine or β-blockers. Lidocaine is short acting and has minimal negative inotropic action. Although propranolol has been widely used, esmolol, a selective β$_1$-blocker, offers several advantages. Esmolol has a rapid onset and is short acting (i.e., elimination half-life of 9 minutes), which allows adequate control of heart rate; it may also provide protection against catecholamine-induced ischemia and the development of postoperative hypoglycemia. Amiodarone, an antiarrhythmic agent that prolongs the duration of the action potential of atrial and ventricular muscle, has been used as an alternative to β-blockers to treat supraventricular tachycardia associated with hypercatecholaminemia.

Hypotension following tumor vein ligation is usually significant and occurs secondary to a combination of factors, including an immediate decrease in plasma catecholamine levels (half-lives of norepinephrine and epinephrine are approximately 1 to 2 minutes), vasodilation from residual α-blockade with phenoxybenzamine, intraoperative fluid and blood loss, and increased anesthetic depth. Hypotension with systolic pressures in the 70- to 79-mm Hg range is not infrequent. To prevent precipitous hypotension, volume expansion to a pulmonary capillary wedge pressure of 16 to 18 mm Hg should be attained before tumor vein ligation. Lactated Ringer's solution and physiologic saline are the recommended fluids for use before

tumor removal. Vasopressors and inotropes should be viewed as a secondary treatment modality. Residual α-adrenergic blockade and downregulation of receptors make patients relatively less responsive to vasopressors. Intraoperative administration of blood salvage products has resulted in postresection hypertension secondary to the catecholamine content of the blood. A decrease in anesthetic depth will also aid in controlling hypotension. With a decrease in plasma catecholamine levels immediately following resection, insulin levels increase and hypoglycemia may occur. Therefore, dextrose-containing solutions should be added after tumor removal. Glucocorticoid therapy should be administered if a bilateral adrenalectomy is performed or if hypoadrenalism is a possibility.

POSTOPERATIVE MANAGEMENT

The majority of patients become normotensive following complete tumor resection. However, plasma catecholamine levels do not return to normal until 7 to 10 days after surgery because of a slow release of stored catecholamines from peripheral nerves. Fifty percent of patients are hypertensive for several days after surgery, and 25% to 30% of patients remain hypertensive indefinitely. In these patients, hypertension is sustained rather than paroxysmal, lower than before surgery, and not accompanied by the classic features of hypercatecholaminemia. The differential diagnosis of persistent hypertension includes a missed pheochromocytoma, surgical complications with subsequent renal ischemia, and underlying essential hypertension.

Hypotension is the most frequent cause of death in the period immediately after surgery. Large volumes of fluid are necessary since the peripheral vasculature is poorly responsive to reduced levels of catecholamines. Vasopressors are a secondary consideration. Steroid supplementation may be necessary if hypoadrenalism is present. Dextrose-containing solutions should be included as part of the fluid therapy, and plasma glucose levels should be monitored for 24 hours.

ADRENAL GLAND DYSFUNCTION

Each adrenal gland consists of two components, the adrenal cortex and the adrenal medulla. The adrenal cortex is responsible for the synthesis of three groups of hormones classified as glucocorticoids, mineralocorticoids (aldosterone), and androgens. Corticotropin (ACTH) is secreted by the anterior pituitary gland in response to corticotropin-releasing hormone (CRH), which is synthesized in the hypothalamus and carried to the anterior pituitary in the portal blood. ACTH stimulates the adrenal cortex to produce cortisol. Maintenance of systemic blood pressure by cortisol reflects the importance of this hormone in facilitating conversion of norepinephrine to epinephrine in the adrenal medulla. Hyperglycemia in response to cortisol secretion reflects gluconeogenesis and inhibition of the peripheral use of glucose by cells. Retention of sodium and excretion of potassium are facilitated by cortisol. The antiinflammatory effects of cortisol and other glucocorticoids (cortisone, prednisone, methylprednisolone, dexamethasone, triamcinolone) are particularly apparent in the presence of high serum concentrations of these hormones. Aldosterone secretion is regulated by the renin-angiotensin system and the serum concentrations of potassium. Aldosterone regulates the extracellular fluid volume by promoting resorption of sodium by the renal tubules. In addition, aldosterone promotes renal tubular excretion of potassium.

The adrenal medulla is a specialized part of the sympathetic nervous system that is capable of synthesizing norepinephrine and epinephrine. The only important disease process associated with the adrenal medulla is pheochromocytoma. Adrenal medullary insufficiency is not known to occur.

Surgery is one of the most potent and best-studied activators of the hypothalamic-pituitary-adrenal (HPA) axis. The degree of activation of the axis depends on the magnitude and duration of surgery and the type and depth of anesthesia. In patients with an intact, normally functioning HPA axis, CRH, ACTH, and cortisol levels all increase significantly during surgery. Deep general anesthesia or regional anesthesia blunts but does not eliminate this response. Increases in ACTH begin with surgical incision and remain elevated during surgery, with the peak level occurring with pharmacologic reversal of muscle relaxants and extubation of the patient at the end of the procedure. Hormone levels remain elevated for several days postoperatively. During major surgery, cortisol release may increase from a preoperative level of 15 to 25 mg/day to 75 to 150 mg/day, which results in a plasma cortisol level of 30 to 50 mcg/dL. An uncomplicated cholecystectomy in an otherwise healthy patient will result in a plasma cortisol level of 27 to 34 mcg/dL 30 minutes after incision and 46 to 49 mcg/dL 5 hours after surgery. Patients in the intensive care unit (ICU) may have plasma cortisol levels of more than 60 mcg/dL.

Hypercortisolism (Cushing's Syndrome)

Cushing's syndrome is divided into two forms: ACTH dependent and ACTH independent. In ACTH-dependent Cushing's syndrome, inappropriately high plasma ACTH concentrations stimulate the adrenal cortex to produce excessive amounts of cortisol. The ACTH-independent variant is caused by excessive production of cortisol by abnormal adrenocortical tissue that is not regulated by secretion of CRH and ACTH. In this latter form of Cushing's syndrome, CRH and ACTH levels are actually suppressed. The term *Cushing's disease* is reserved for Cushing's syndrome caused by excessive secretion of ACTH by pituitary ACTH tumors (microadenomas). These microadenomas account for nearly 70% of cases of ACTH-dependent Cushing's syndrome. Acute ectopic ACTH syndrome is another form of ACTH-dependent Cushing's syndrome and is most often associated with small cell lung carcinoma. Benign or malignant adrenocortical tumors are the most common cause of ACTH-independent Cushing's syndrome.

DIAGNOSIS

There are no pathognomonic signs or symptoms that confirm the diagnosis of Cushing's syndrome. The most common symptom is the relatively sudden onset of weight gain, which is usually central and often accompanied by thickening of the facial fat, which rounds the facial contour (moon facies), and a florid complexion resulting from telangiectasias. Systemic hypertension, glucose intolerance, oligomenorrhea or amenorrhea in premenopausal women, decreased libido in men, and spontaneous ecchymoses are frequent concomitant findings. Skeletal muscle wasting and weakness manifest as difficulty climbing stairs. Depression and insomnia are often present. The diagnosis of Cushing's syndrome is confirmed by demonstrating cortisol hypersecretion based on 24-hour urinary secretion of cortisol. Determining whether a patient's hypercortisolism is ACTH dependent or ACTH independent requires reliable measurements of plasma ACTH using immunoradiometric assays. The high-dose dexamethasone suppression test distinguishes Cushing's disease from ectopic ACTH syndrome (presence of complete resistance). Imaging procedures provide no information about adrenal cortex function and are useful only for determining the location of a tumor.

TREATMENT

The treatment of choice for patients with Cushing's disease is transsphenoidal microadenomectomy if a clearly circumscribed microadenoma can be identified and is amenable to resection. Alternatively, patients may undergo 85% to 90% resection of the anterior pituitary. Pituitary irradiation and bilateral total adrenalectomy are necessary in some patients. Surgical removal of the adrenal gland is the treatment for adrenal adenoma or carcinoma.

MANAGEMENT OF ANESTHESIA

Management of anesthesia in patients with hypercortisolism must consider the physiologic effects of excessive cortisol secretion (Table 19-8). Preoperative evaluation of systemic blood pressure, electrolyte balance, and blood glucose concentration are especially important. Osteoporosis is a consideration when positioning patients for the operative procedure. The choice of drugs for preoperative medication, induction of anesthesia, and maintenance of anesthesia is not influenced by the presence of hypercortisolism. Etomidate may transiently decrease the synthesis and release of cortisol by the adrenal cortex. Doses of muscle relaxants should probably be decreased initially in view of the skeletal muscle weakness that frequently accompanies hypercortisolism. In addition, the presence of hypokalemia may influence responses to nondepolarizing muscle relaxants.

TABLE 19-8	Physiologic effects of excess cortisol secretion
Systemic hypertension	
Hyperglycemia	
Skeletal muscle weakness	
Osteoporosis	
Obesity	
Menstrual disturbances	
Poor wound healing	
Susceptibility to infection	

Mechanical ventilation of the patient's lungs during surgery is recommended, because skeletal muscle weakness, with or without co-existing hypokalemia, may decrease the strength of the muscles of breathing. Regional anesthesia is acceptable, but the likely presence of osteoporosis, with possible vertebral body collapse, is a consideration.

Plasma cortisol concentrations decrease promptly after micro-adenomectomy or bilateral adrenalectomy, and replacement therapy is recommended. In this regard, a continuous infusion of cortisol (100 mg/day IV) may be initiated intraoperatively. Likewise, patients with metastatic disease involving the adrenal glands may develop acute adrenal insufficiency, which requires the initiation of supplemental therapy. Transient diabetes insipidus and meningitis may also occur after microadenomectomy.

Primary Hyperaldosteronism (Conn's Syndrome)

Primary hyperaldosteronism (Conn's syndrome) is present when there is excess secretion of aldosterone from a functional tumor (aldosteronoma) that acts independently of a physiologic stimulus. Aldosteronomas occur more often in women than in men and only rarely in children. Occasionally, primary aldosteronism is associated with pheochromocytoma, primary hyperparathyroidism, or acromegaly. Secondary hyperaldosteronism is present when increased circulating serum concentrations of renin, as are associated with renovascular hypertension, stimulate the release of aldosterone. Aldosteronism associated with Bartter's syndrome (hyperplasia of the juxtaglomerular apparatus) is not accompanied by systemic hypertension. The prevalence of primary aldosteronism in patients with essential hypertension appears to be less than 1%.

SIGNS AND SYMPTOMS

Clinical signs and symptoms of primary aldosteronism are nonspecific, and some patients are completely asymptomatic. Symptoms may reflect systemic hypertension (headache) or hypokalemia (polyuria, nocturia, skeletal muscle cramps, skeletal muscle weakness). Systemic hypertension (diastolic blood pressure is often 100 to 125 mm Hg) is a function of aldosterone-induced sodium retention and increase in extracellular fluid volume. This hypertension may be resistant to treatment. Aldosterone promotes renal excretion of potassium, which results in hypokalemic metabolic alkalosis. Increased urinary excretion of potassium (more than 30 mEq/day) in the presence of hypokalemia suggests primary aldosteronism. Hypokalemic nephropathy can result in polyuria and loss of urine-concentrating ability. Skeletal muscle weakness is presumed to reflect hypokalemia. Hypomagnesemia and abnormal glucose tolerance may also be present.

DIAGNOSIS

Spontaneous hypokalemia in patients with systemic hypertension is highly suggestive of aldosteronism. Plasma renin activity is suppressed in almost all patients with untreated primary aldosteronism and in many with essential hypertension; with secondary aldosteronism, however, the plasma renin activity is high. A plasma aldosterone concentration of less than 9.5 ng/dL at the end of a saline infusion rules out primary aldosteronism. A syndrome exhibiting all the features of hyperaldosteronism (systemic hypertension, hypokalemia, suppression of the renin-angiotensin system) may result from long-term ingestion of licorice (glycyrrhizic acid).

TREATMENT

Initial treatment of hyperaldosteronism consists of potassium supplementation and administration of a competitive aldosterone antagonist such as spironolactone. Skeletal muscle weakness resulting from hypokalemia may require treatment with intravenous potassium. Systemic hypertension is treated with antihypertensive drugs. Accentuation of hypokalemia caused by drug-induced diuresis is decreased by use of a potassium-sparing diuretic such as triamterene. Definitive treatment for an aldosterone-secreting tumor is surgical excision. Bilateral adrenalectomy may be necessary if multiple aldosterone-secreting tumors are found.

MANAGEMENT OF ANESTHESIA

Management of anesthesia for the surgical treatment of hyperaldosteronism is facilitated by preoperative correction of hypokalemia and treatment of systemic hypertension. Persistence of hypokalemia may modify responses to nondepolarizing muscle relaxants. Intraoperative hyperventilation of the patient's lungs can decrease the plasma potassium concentration and should be avoided. Inhaled or injected drugs are acceptable for maintenance of anesthesia. The use of sevoflurane is questionable, however, if hypokalemic nephropathy and polyuria are present preoperatively.

Measurement of cardiac filling pressures via a right atrial or pulmonary artery catheter may be useful during surgery for adequate evaluation of the intravascular fluid volume and the response to intravenous infusion of fluids. Indeed, aggressive preoperative preparation can convert the excessive intravascular fluid volume status of these patients to unexpected hypovolemia, manifesting as hypotension in response to administration of vasodilating anesthetic drugs, positive pressure ventilation, changes in body position, or surgical blood loss. The detection of orthostatic hypotension during the preoperative evaluation is a clue to underlying hypovolemia. Acid-base status and plasma electrolyte concentrations should be measured frequently.

Supplementation with exogenous cortisol is probably unnecessary for surgical excision of a solitary adenoma in the adrenal cortex. Bilateral mobilization of the adrenal glands to excise multiple functional tumors, however, may introduce the need for exogenous cortisol administration. A continuous intravenous infusion of cortisol, 100 mg every 24 hours, may be initiated on an empirical basis if transient hypocortisolism resulting from surgical manipulation is a consideration.

Hypoaldosteronism

Hyperkalemia in the absence of renal insufficiency suggests the presence of hypoaldosteronism. Hyperkalemia is sometimes abruptly enhanced by hyperglycemia. Hyperchloremic metabolic acidosis is a predictable finding in the presence of hypoaldosteronism. Heart block secondary to hyperkalemia, orthostatic hypotension, and hyponatremia may also be present.

Isolated deficiency of aldosterone secretion may reflect congenital deficiency of aldosterone synthetase or hyporeninemia resulting from defects in the juxtaglomerular apparatus or treatment with ACE inhibitors leading to loss of angiotensin stimulation. Hyporeninemic hypoaldosteronism typically occurs in patients older than 45 years of age with chronic renal disease and/or diabetes mellitus. Indomethacin-induced prostaglandin deficiency is a reversible cause of this syndrome. Treatment of hypoaldosteronism includes liberal sodium intake and daily administration of fludrocortisone.

Adrenal Insufficiency

SIGNS AND SYMPTOMS

There are two types of adrenal insufficiency (AI): primary and secondary. In primary disease (Addison's disease), the adrenal glands are unable to elaborate sufficient quantities of glucocorticoid, mineralocorticoid, and androgen hormones. The most common cause of this rare endocrinopathy is bilateral adrenal destruction from autoimmune disease. More than 90% of the glands must be involved before signs of AI appear. The insidious onset of Addison's disease is characterized by fatigue, weakness, anorexia, nausea and vomiting, cutaneous and mucosal hyperpigmentation, hypovolemia, hyponatremia, and hyperkalemia. Secondary AI results from a failure in the production of CRH or ACTH caused by hypothalamic-pituitary disease or suppression of the hypothalamic-pituitary axis. Unlike in Addison's disease, there is only a glucocorticoid deficiency in secondary disease. In the majority of cases the cause is iatrogenic, such as pituitary surgery, pituitary irradiation, or most commonly the use of synthetic glucocorticoids. These patients lack cutaneous hyperpigmentation and may demonstrate only mild electrolyte abnormalities.

Cortisol is one of the few hormones essential for life. It participates in carbohydrate and protein metabolism, fatty acid mobilization, electrolyte and water balance, and the antiinflammatory response. It facilitates catecholamine synthesis and action; modulates β-receptor synthesis, regulation, coupling, and responsiveness; and contributes to normal vascular permeability, tone, and cardiac contractility. Cortisol accounts for 95% of the adrenal gland's glucocorticoid activity, with corticosterone and cortisone contributing some activity. Estimated daily cortisol secretion is the equivalent of 15 to 25 mg/day of hydrocortisone or 5 to 7 mg/day of prednisone.

DIAGNOSIS

The classic definition of AI includes a baseline plasma cortisol concentration of less than 20 mcg/dL and a cortisol level of less than 20 mcg/dL after ACTH stimulation. The short 250-mcg ACTH stimulation test is a reliable test of the integrity of the entire HPA axis. All steroids except dexamethasone must be discontinued for 24 hours before testing. Cortisol levels are measured at 30 and 60 minutes following the administration of ACTH. A normal ACTH stimulation test result is a plasma cortisol level greater than 25 mcg/dL. A positive test finding demonstrates a poor response to ACTH and indicates an impairment of the adrenal cortex. Absolute AI is characterized by a low baseline cortisol level and a positive result on the ACTH stimulation test. Relative AI is indicated when the baseline cortisol level is higher but the result on the ACTH stimulation test is positive.

TREATMENT

The most common cause of AI is exogenous steroids (Table 19-9). Patients are prescribed steroids to treat a number of illnesses, including arthritis, bronchial asthma, malignancies, allergies, collagen vascular diseases, and inflammatory conditions. Those who take steroids long term may exhibit signs and symptoms of AI during periods of stress, such as surgery or acute illness. For patients with a history of long-term steroid use, it may take 6 to 12 months from the time of discontinuation of the steroids for the adrenal glands to recover full function. Recovery from short courses of steroids may take several days. For example, prednisone 25 mg PO twice daily for 5 days results in a reduced response to exogenous ACTH for 5 days.

Preoperative glucocorticoid coverage should be provided for patients with a positive result on the ACTH stimulation test, Cushing's syndrome, or AI as well as for those at risk of HPA axis suppression or AI based on prior glucocorticoid therapy. Adrenal suppression is much more common than AI and is of concern because overt AI, although uncommon, may occur under the stressful conditions of surgery and anesthesia. Patients taking prednisone in dosages of less than 5 mg/day (morning dose) for any length of time, even years, do not demonstrate clinically significant HPA axis suppression and do not require perioperative supplementation, although they should receive their normal daily steroid dose. Any patient who received a glucocorticoid in dosages equivalent to more than 20 mg/day of prednisone for more than 3 weeks within the previous year is at risk of AI and should receive perioperative supplementation. Patients receiving dosages of steroids between these two extremes may have HPA axis suppression and should probably receive supplementation. Similarly, patients receiving more than 2 g/day of topical steroids or more than 0.8 mg/day of inhaled steroids on a long-term basis should probably receive supplementation.

Patients with known or suspected adrenal suppression or AI should receive their baseline steroid therapy plus supplementation in the perioperative period. Supplementation is individualized based on the surgery (Table 19-10). When more than 100 mg/day of hydrocortisone is administered, it may be wise to consider substituting methylprednisolone for hydrocortisone; given its lower mineralocorticoid activity, it is less likely to cause fluid retention, edema, and hypokalemia.

TABLE 19-9 ▪ **Glucocorticoid preparations**

Steroid	POTENCY		Equivalent dose (oral or IV, mg)
	Antiinflammatory (glucocorticoid)	Na⁺ retention (mineralocorticoid)	

Steroid	Antiinflammatory (glucocorticoid)	Na⁺ retention (mineralocorticoid)	Equivalent dose (oral or IV, mg)
SHORT ACTING			
Cortisol (hydrocortisone)	1	1	20
Cortisone	0.8	0.8	25
INTERMEDIATE ACTING			
Prednisone	4	0.8	5
Prednisolone	4	0.8	5
Methylprednisolone	5	0.5	4
Triamcinolone	5	0	4
LONG ACTING			
Dexamethasone	30-40	0	0.75

Adapted from Stoelting RK, Dierdorf SF. Endocrine disease. In: Stoelting RK, ed. *Anesthesia and Co-Existing Disease.* New York, NY: Churchill Livingstone; 1993:358.

IV, Intravenous.

TABLE 19-10 ▪ **Perioperative steroid (hydrocortisone) supplementation**

Superficial surgery (e.g., dental surgery, biopsy)	None
Minor surgery (e.g., inguinal hernia repair)	25 mg IV
Moderate surgery (e.g., cholecystectomy, colon resection)	50-75 mg IV, taper 1-2 days
Major surgery (e.g., cardiovascular surgery, Whipple's procedure)	100-150 mg IV, taper 1-2 days
Intensive care unit (e.g., sepsis, shock)	50-100 mg q6-8h for 2 days to 1 wk, followed by slow taper

IV, Intravenous.

MANAGEMENT OF ANESTHESIA

Acute AI should be considered in the differential diagnosis of hemodynamic instability, especially in patients unresponsive to the usual therapeutic interventions. Therapy includes treatment of the cause, repletion of circulating glucocorticoids, and replacement of water and sodium deficits. Glucocorticoid replacement may include intravenous hydrocortisone, methylprednisolone, or dexamethasone. If ACTH stimulation testing will be required to assist in establishing a diagnosis of primary or secondary disease, dexamethasone is preferred because it does not alter cortisol levels.

A bolus of 100 mg of hydrocortisone followed by a continuous infusion at 10 mg/hr is a recommended prescription. A 100-mg bolus of hydrocortisone every 6 hours is also an acceptable option. Continuous infusion has the advantage of maintaining the plasma cortisol concentration at stress levels greater than 830 nmol/L (30 mcg/dL). When the patient's condition stabilizes, the steroid dosage is reduced with eventual conversion to an oral preparation. Volume deficits may

be substantial (2 to 3 L), and 5% dextrose in normal saline is the fluid of choice. Hemodynamic support with vasopressors may be necessary. Metabolic acidosis and hyperkalemia usually resolve with fluid and steroid administration. In primary disease, administration of the mineralocorticoid fludrocortisone is not necessary acutely because isotonic saline replaces sodium loss.

No specific anesthetic agent(s) and/or technique(s) are recommended in managing patients with or at risk of AI. However, etomidate inhibits the synthesis of cortisol transiently and should be avoided in this patient population. Patients with untreated AI undergoing emergency surgery should be managed aggressively with invasive monitoring, intravenous corticosteroids, and fluid and electrolyte resuscitation. Minimal doses of anesthetic agents and drugs are recommended, since myocardial depression and skeletal muscle weakness are frequently part of the clinical presentation.

INTENSIVE CARE UNIT MANAGEMENT

AI is a common and underdiagnosed entity among critically ill patients. Patients at risk include those with infection and systemic inflammation from tuberculosis, meningococcemia, human immunodeficiency virus (HIV) infection, sepsis, and/or diffuse intravascular coagulation. The incidence of AI in high-risk, critically ill patients with hypotension, shock, and sepsis is approximately 30% to 40%. Approximately 33% of HIV–infected patients admitted to the ICU have AI, most likely caused by high levels of cytokines (interleukin-1, interleukin-6, interferon-α) and inflammatory peptides that impair the response of pituitary cells and inhibit the HPA axis. Cytokines also cause glucocorticoid resistance by impairing glucocorticoid receptor binding affinity. Hypotension is a common presentation, and hydrocortisone is required to maintain vascular tone, endothelial cell integrity, normal vascular permeability, β-receptor function, and catecholamine synthesis and action.

All patients suspected of having AI should be tested for serum cortisol concentration and undergo an ACTH stimulation test, especially if the stress level in uncertain. Free serum cortisol level, not total cortisol level, offers a better reflection of the HPA axis in critically ill patients with hypoproteinemia. With the exception of patients with vasopressor-dependent shock, significant doses of glucocorticoids should be reserved for patients with proven AI.

Administration of physiologic doses of glucocorticoids has been shown to confer survival advantage in patients with septic shock. Hydrocortisone dosages of 200 to 300 mg/day for a minimum of 5 to 7 days followed by a 5- to 7-day taper are commonly employed. Additional studies are needed to determine whether physiologic glucocorticoid dosages are beneficial to septic patients without shock or patients with shock but not vasopressor dependence.

PARATHYROID GLAND DYSFUNCTION

The four parathyroid glands are located behind the upper and lower poles of the thyroid gland and produce parathyroid hormone, a polypeptide hormone. Parathyroid hormone is released into the systemic circulation by a negative feedback mechanism that depends on the plasma calcium concentration. Hypocalcemia stimulates the release of parathyroid hormone, whereas hypercalcemia suppresses both hormonal synthesis and release. Parathyroid hormone maintains normal plasma calcium concentrations (4.5 to 5.5 mEq/L) by promoting the movement of calcium across three interfaces represented by the gastrointestinal tract, renal tubules, and bone.

Hyperparathyroidism

Hyperparathyroidism is present when the secretion of parathyroid hormone is increased. Serum calcium concentrations may be increased, decreased, or unchanged. Hyperparathyroidism is classified as primary, secondary, or ectopic.

PRIMARY HYPERPARATHYROIDISM

Primary hyperparathyroidism results from excessive secretion of parathyroid hormone due to a benign parathyroid adenoma, carcinoma of a parathyroid gland, or hyperplasia of one or more parathyroid glands. A benign parathyroid adenoma is responsible for primary hyperparathyroidism in approximately 90% of patients; carcinoma is responsible for fewer than 5% of cases. Hyperplasia usually involves all four parathyroid glands, although not all glands may be enlarged to the same degree. Hyperparathyroidism resulting from an adenoma or hyperplasia is the most common presenting symptom of multiple endocrine neoplasia syndrome type I.

Diagnosis

Hypercalcemia (serum calcium concentration >5.5 mEq/L and ionized calcium concentration >2.5 mEq/L) is the hallmark of primary hyperparathyroidism. Primary hyperparathyroidism is the most common cause of hypercalcemia in the general population, whereas cancer is the most common cause in hospitalized patients. Modest increases in plasma calcium concentrations discovered incidentally in otherwise asymptomatic patients are most likely due to parathyroid adenomas, whereas marked hypercalcemia (>7.5 mEq/L) is more likely due to cancer. Use of automated methods to measure serum calcium concentrations has detected primary hyperparathyroidism in a surprisingly large number of individuals, especially postmenopausal women. Patients in surgical ICUs for prolonged periods of time may develop hypercalcemia, which may reflect increased secretion of parathyroid hormone in response to repeated episodes of hypocalcemia resulting from sepsis, shock, and/or blood transfusions. Urinary excretion of cyclic adenosine monophosphate (cAMP) is increased in patients with primary hyperparathyroidism. Measurement of serum parathyroid hormone concentrations is not always sufficiently reliable to confirm the diagnosis.

Signs and Symptoms

Hypercalcemia is responsible for the broad spectrum of signs and symptoms that accompany primary hyperparathyroidism (Table 19-11). Symptoms due to hypercalcemia reflect changes in the ionized calcium concentration, which is the physiologically active form of calcium and represents approximately 45% of the total serum calcium concentration. The ionized serum calcium concentration is dependent on arterial pH and the plasma albumin concentration. For this reason, it is preferable to measure ionized calcium concentrations directly using an ion-specific electrode.

Early signs and symptoms of primary hyperparathyroidism and associated hypercalcemia include sedation and vomiting.

TABLE 19-11	Signs and symptoms of hypercalcemia due to hyperparathyroidism
Organ system	**Signs and symptoms**
Neuromuscular	Skeletal muscle weakness
Renal	Polyuria and polydipsia
	Decreased glomerular filtration rate
	Kidney stones
Hematopoietic	Anemia
Cardiac	Prolonged PR interval
	Shortened QT interval
	Systemic hypertension
Gastrointestinal	Vomiting
	Abdominal pain
	Peptic ulcer
	Pancreatitis
Skeletal	Skeletal demineralization
	Collapse of vertebral bodies
	Pathologic fractures
Nervous	Somnolence
	Decreased pain sensation
	Psychosis
Ocular	Calcifications (band keratopathy)
	Conjunctivitis

Skeletal muscle weakness and hypotonia are frequent complaints and may be so severe as to suggest the presence of myasthenia gravis. Loss of skeletal muscle strength and mass is most notable in the proximal musculature of the lower extremities. This skeletal muscle weakness is a neuropathy (muscle biopsy specimens resemble those in amyotrophic lateral sclerosis) and not a myopathy. Loss of sensation for pain and vibration may also be present. The cause of the neuropathy is unclear, but it is not related to hypercalcemia; it is reversible, because skeletal muscle strength often improves following surgical removal of excess parathyroid hormone–producing tissues.

Persistent increases in plasma calcium concentrations can interfere with urine concentrating ability, and polyuria results. Oliguric renal failure can occur in advanced cases of hypercalcemia. Renal stones, especially in the presence of polyuria and polydipsia, must arouse suspicion of primary hyperparathyroidism. Increased serum chloride concentration (>102 mEq/L) is most likely due to the influence of parathyroid hormone on renal excretion of bicarbonate, which produces a mild metabolic acidosis. Anemia, even in the absence of renal dysfunction, is a consequence of primary hyperparathyroidism. Peptic ulcer disease is frequent and may reflect potentiation of gastric acid secretion by calcium. Acute and chronic pancreatitis are associated with primary hyperparathyroidism. Even in the absence of peptic ulcer disease or pancreatitis, the abdominal pain that often accompanies hypercalcemia can mimic an acute surgical abdomen. Systemic hypertension is common, and the ECG may reveal a prolonged PR interval, whereas the QT interval is often shortened. When the serum calcium concentration exceeds 8 mEq/L, cardiac conduction disturbances are likely. The classic skeletal consequence of primary hyperparathyroidism is osteitis fibrosa cystica. Radiographic evidence of skeletal involvement includes generalized osteopenia, subcortical bone resorption in the phalanges and distal ends of the clavicles, and the appearance of bone cysts. Bone pain and pathologic fractures may be present.

In addition, patients may exhibit deficits of memory and cerebration, with or without personality changes or mood disturbances, including hallucinations.

Treatment

Primary hyperparathyroidism and the associated hypercalcemia are treated initially by medical means followed by definitive surgical removal of the diseased or abnormal portions of the parathyroid glands.

Medical Management. Saline infusion (150 mL/hr) is the basic treatment for all patients with symptomatic hypercalcemia. Intravascular fluid volume may be depleted by vomiting, polyuria, and urinary loss of sodium. The calcium-lowering effect of saline hydration alone is limited, and it is often necessary to add loop diuretics (furosemide 40 to 80 mg IV every 2 to 4 hours) to the therapeutic regimen. Loop diuretics inhibit sodium (and therefore calcium) reabsorption in the proximal loop of Henle. The goal is a daily urine output of 3 to 5 L. Addition of loop diuretics to saline hydration increases calcium excretion only if

the saline infusion is adequate to restore the intravascular fluid volume necessary for delivery of calcium to the renal tubules. Thiazide diuretics are not administered for treatment of hypercalcemia, because these drugs may enhance renal tubular reabsorption of calcium. Central venous pressure monitoring may be useful for guiding fluid replacement in these patients.

Bisphosphonates such as disodium etidronate administered intravenously are the drugs of choice for the treatment of life-threatening hypercalcemia. These drugs bind to hydroxyapatite in bone and act as potent inhibitors of osteoclastic bone resorption. Hemodialysis can also be used to lower serum calcium concentrations promptly, as can calcitonin, but the effects of this hormone are transient. Mithramycin inhibits the osteoclastic activity of parathyroid hormone, producing prompt lowering of serum calcium concentrations. The toxic effects of mithramycin (thrombocytopenia, hepatotoxicity, nephrotoxicity), however, limit its use.

Surgical Management. Definitive treatment of primary hyperparathyroidism is surgical removal of the diseased or abnormal portions of the parathyroid glands. Successful surgical treatment is reflected by normalization of serum calcium concentrations within 3 to 4 days and a decrease in the urinary excretion of cAMP. Postoperatively, the first potential complication is hypocalcemic tetany. The hypomagnesemia that occurs postoperatively aggravates the hypocalcemia and renders it refractory to treatment. Hyperchloremic metabolic acidosis, in association with deterioration of renal function, may occur transiently after parathyroidectomy. Acute arthritis may also occur following parathyroidectomy.

Management of Anesthesia

There is no evidence that any specific anesthetic drugs or techniques are necessary in patients with primary hyperparathyroidism undergoing elective surgical treatment. Maintenance of hydration and urine output is important in perioperative management of hypercalcemia. Careful positioning of hyperparathyroid patients is necessary because of the likely presence of osteoporosis and the associated vulnerability to pathologic fractures. The existence of somnolence before induction of anesthesia introduces the possibility that intraoperative anesthetic requirements could be decreased. Owing to its psychotropic effects, ketamine is an unlikely selection in patients with co-existing personality changes attributed to chronic hypercalcemia. The possibility of co-existing renal dysfunction is a consideration in the use of sevoflurane, because impaired urine concentrating ability associated with polyuria and hypercalcemia could be confused with anesthetic-induced fluoride nephrotoxicity. Co-existing skeletal muscle weakness suggests the possibility of decreased requirements for muscle relaxants, whereas hypercalcemia might be expected to antagonize the effects of nondepolarizing muscle relaxants. In view of the unpredictable response to muscle relaxants, it is advisable to decrease the initial dose of these drugs and titrate subsequent doses to effect.

The ECG should be monitored for manifestations of adverse cardiac effects of hypercalcemia, although there is evidence that the QT interval may not be a reliable index of changes in serum calcium concentrations during anesthesia. Theoretically, hyperventilation of the lungs is undesirable, because respiratory alkalosis lowers serum potassium concentrations and leaves the actions of calcium unopposed. Nevertheless, since it lowers levels of the ionized fractions of calcium, alkalosis could also be beneficial.

SECONDARY HYPERPARATHYROIDISM

Secondary hyperparathyroidism reflects an appropriate compensatory response of the parathyroid glands to counteract a disease process that produces hypocalcemia. For example, chronic renal disease impairs elimination of phosphorus and decreases hydroxylation of vitamin D, which results in hypocalcemia and compensatory hyperplasia of the parathyroid glands with increased release of parathyroid hormone. Because secondary hyperparathyroidism is adaptive rather than autonomous, it seldom produces hypercalcemia. Treatment of secondary hyperparathyroidism is directed at controlling the underlying disease, as is achieved by normalizing serum phosphate concentrations in patients with renal disease by administering an oral phosphate binder.

On occasion, transient hypercalcemia may follow otherwise successful renal transplantation. This response reflects the inability of previously hyperactive parathyroid glands to adapt quickly to normal renal excretion of calcium and phosphorus and to hydroxylation of vitamin D. The parathyroid glands usually return to normal size and function with time, although parathyroidectomy is occasionally necessary.

ECTOPIC HYPERPARATHYROIDISM

Ectopic hyperparathyroidism (humoral hypercalcemia of malignancy, pseudohyperparathyroidism) is due to secretion of parathyroid hormone (or a substance with similar endocrine effects) by tissues other than the parathyroid glands. Carcinoma of the lung, breast, pancreas, or kidney and lymphoproliferative disease are most commonly associated with ectopic parathyroid hormone secretion. Ectopic hyperparathyroidism is more likely than primary hyperparathyroidism to be associated with anemia and increased plasma alkaline phosphatase concentrations. A role for prostaglandins in the production of hypercalcemia in these patients is suggested by the calcium-lowering effects produced by indomethacin, which is an inhibitor of prostaglandin synthesis.

Hypoparathyroidism

Hypoparathyroidism is present when secretion of parathyroid hormone is absent or deficient or peripheral tissues are resistant to the effects of the hormone (Table 19-12). Absence or deficiency of parathyroid hormone is almost always iatrogenic, reflecting inadvertent removal of the parathyroid glands, as during thyroidectomy. Pseudohypoparathyroidism is a congenital disorder in which the release of parathyroid hormone is intact, but the kidneys are unable to respond to the hormone. Affected patients manifest mental retardation,

TABLE 19-12   Causes of hypoparathyroidism
DECREASED OR ABSENT PARATHYROID HORMONE
Accidental removal of parathyroid glands during thyroidectomy
Parathyroidectomy to treat hyperplasia
Idiopathic (DiGeorge's syndrome)
RESISTANCE OF PERIPHERAL TISSUES TO EFFECTS OF PARATHYROID HORMONE
Congenital
Pseudohypoparathyroidism
Acquired
Hypomagnesemia
Chronic renal failure
Malabsorption
Anticonvulsive therapy (phenytoin)
Osteoblastic metastases
Acute pancreatitis

calcification of the basal ganglia, obesity, short stature, and short metacarpals and metatarsals.

DIAGNOSIS

Measurements of serum calcium concentration and the ionized fraction of calcium are the most valuable diagnostic indicators for hypoparathyroidism. A serum calcium concentration of less than 4.5 mEq/L and an ionized calcium concentration of less than 2.0 mEq/L are indicative of hypoparathyroidism.

SIGNS AND SYMPTOMS

Signs and symptoms of hypoparathyroidism depend on the rapidity of the onset of hypocalcemia. Acute hypocalcemia can occur after accidental removal of the parathyroid glands during thyroidectomy and is likely to manifest as perioral paresthesias, restlessness, and neuromuscular irritability, as evidenced by a positive Chvostek sign or Trousseau sign. Inspiratory stridor reflects neuromuscular irritability of the intrinsic laryngeal musculature.

Chronic hypocalcemia is associated with complaints of fatigue and skeletal muscle cramps that may be associated with a prolonged QT interval on the ECG. The QRS complex, PR interval, and cardiac rhythm usually remain normal. Neurologic changes include lethargy, cerebration deficits, and personality changes reminiscent of those occurring in hyperparathyroidism. Chronic hypocalcemia is associated with formation of cataracts, calcification involving the subcutaneous tissues and basal ganglia, and thickening of the skull. Chronic renal failure is the most common cause of chronic hypocalcemia.

TREATMENT

Treatment of acute hypocalcemia consists of an infusion of calcium (10 mL of 10% calcium gluconate or 10 mL of 10% calcium chloride IV) until signs of neuromuscular irritability disappear. Correction of any co-existing respiratory or

TABLE 19-13   ◼   **Hypothalamic and related pituitary hormones**

Hypothalamic hormone	Action	Pituitary hormone or organ affected	Action
Corticotropin-releasing hormone	Stimulatory	Corticotropin	Stimulates secretion of cortisol and androgens
Thyrotropin-releasing hormone	Stimulatory	Thyrotropin	Stimulates secretion of thyroxine and triiodothyronine
Gonadotropin-releasing hormone	Stimulatory	Follicle-stimulating hormone, luteinizing hormone	Stimulate secretion of estradiol and progesterone,* stimulate ovulation,* stimulate secretion of testosterone,† stimulate spermatogenesis†
Growth hormone–releasing hormone	Stimulatory	Growth hormone	Stimulates production of insulin-like growth factor
Dopamine	Inhibitory	Prolactin	Stimulates lactation*
Somatostatin	Inhibitory	Pituitary, gastrointestinal tract, pancreas	Inhibits secretion of growth hormone and thyroid-stimulating hormone, suppresses release of gastrointestinal and pancreatic hormones
Vasopressin (antidiuretic hormone)	Stimulatory	Kidneys	Stimulates free water reabsorption
Oxytocin	Stimulatory	Uterus	Stimulates uterine contractions*
		Breasts	Stimulates milk ejection*

Adapted from Vance ML. Hypopituitarism. *N Engl J Med.* 1994;330:1651-1662.
*Actions in females.
†Actions in males.

metabolic alkalosis is indicated. For treatment of hypoparathyroidism not complicated by symptomatic hypocalcemia, the approach is oral administration of calcium and vitamin D. An exogenous parathyroid hormone replacement preparation practical for clinical use is not yet available. Thiazide diuretics may be useful, because these drugs cause sodium depletion without proportional potassium excretion and thereby tend to increase serum calcium concentrations.

MANAGEMENT OF ANESTHESIA

Management of anesthesia in the presence of hypocalcemia is designed to prevent any further decrease in the serum calcium concentration and to treat the adverse effects of hypocalcemia, particularly those involving the heart. In this regard, it is important to avoid iatrogenic hyperventilation, because it will further aggravate the clinical picture. Routine administration of whole blood containing citrate usually does not decrease serum calcium concentrations, because calcium is rapidly mobilized from body stores. Ionized calcium concentrations can be decreased, however, when infusions of blood are rapid (500 mL every 5 to 10 minutes, as during cardiopulmonary bypass or liver transplantation) or when metabolism or elimination of citrate is impaired by hypothermia, cirrhosis of the liver, or renal dysfunction.

PITUITARY GLAND DYSFUNCTION

The pituitary gland, located in the sella turcica at the base of the brain, consists of the anterior pituitary and posterior pituitary. The anterior pituitary secretes six hormones under the control of the hypothalamus (Table 19-13). The hypothalamus controls the function of the anterior pituitary by means of vascular connections (hormones travel via the hypophyseal portal veins to reach the anterior pituitary). The hypothalamic–anterior pituitary–target organ axis is composed of tightly coordinated systems in which hormonal signals from the hypothalamus stimulate or inhibit secretion of anterior pituitary hormones, which in turn act on target organs and modulate hypothalamic and anterior pituitary activity (closed-loop, negative feedback system). The posterior pituitary is composed of terminal neuron endings that originate in the hypothalamus. Vasopressin (ADH) and oxytocin are synthesized in the hypothalamus and are subsequently transported along the hypothalamic neuronal axons for storage in the posterior pituitary. The stimulus for the release of these hormones from the posterior pituitary arises from osmoreceptors in the hypothalamus that sense plasma osmolarity.

Overproduction of anterior pituitary hormones is most often associated with hypersecretion of ACTH (Cushing's syndrome) by anterior pituitary adenomas. Hypersecretion of other tropic hormones rarely occurs. Underproduction of a single anterior pituitary hormone is less common than generalized pituitary hypofunction (panhypopituitarism). The anterior pituitary gland is the only endocrine gland in which a tumor, most often a chromophobe adenoma, causes destruction by compressing the gland against the bony confines of the sella turcica. Metastatic tumor, most often from the breast or lung, also occasionally produces pituitary hypofunction. Endocrine features of panhypopituitarism are highly variable and depend on the rate at which the deficiency develops and the patient's age. Gonadotropin deficiency (amenorrhea, impotence) is typically the first manifestation of global pituitary dysfunction. Hypocortisolism occurs 4 to 14 days after hypophysectomy, whereas hypothyroidism is not likely to manifest before 4 weeks. CT and MRI are useful for radiographic assessment of the pituitary gland.

Acromegaly

Acromegaly is due to excessive secretion of growth hormone in adults, most often by an adenoma in the anterior pituitary gland. Failure of plasma growth hormone concentrations to decrease 1 to 2 hours after ingestion of 75 to 100 g of glucose is presumptive evidence of acromegaly, as are growth hormone concentrations higher than 3 ng/mL. A skull radiograph and CT are useful for detecting enlargement of the sella turcica, which is characteristic of anterior pituitary adenomas.

SIGNS AND SYMPTOMS

Manifestations of acromegaly reflect parasellar extension of the anterior pituitary adenoma and peripheral effects produced by the presence of excess growth hormone (Table 19-14). Headache and papilledema reflect increased intracranial pressure resulting from expansion of the anterior pituitary adenoma. Visual disturbances are due to compression of the optic chiasm by the expanding overgrowth of surrounding tissues.

Overgrowth of soft tissues of the upper airway (enlargement of the tongue and epiglottis) makes patients susceptible to upper airway obstruction. Hoarseness and abnormal movement of the vocal cords or paralysis of a recurrent laryngeal nerve may result from stretching caused by overgrowth of the surrounding cartilaginous structures. In addition, involvement of the cricoarytenoid joints can result in alterations in the patient's voice resulting from impaired movement of the vocal cords.

Peripheral neuropathy is common and likely reflects trapping of nerves by skeletal, connective, and soft tissue overgrowth. Flow through the ulnar artery may be compromised in patients exhibiting symptoms of carpal tunnel syndrome. Even in the absence of such symptoms, approximately one half of patients with acromegaly have inadequate collateral blood flow through the ulnar artery in one or both hands.

TABLE 19-14 ■ Manifestations of acromegaly

PARASELLAR TUMOR

Enlarged sella turcica

Headache

Visual field defects

Rhinorrhea

EXCESS GROWTH HORMONE

Skeletal overgrowth (prognathism)

Soft tissue overgrowth (lips, tongue, epiglottis, vocal cords)

Connective tissue overgrowth (recurrent laryngeal nerve paralysis)

Peripheral neuropathy (carpal tunnel syndrome)

Visceromegaly

Glucose intolerance

Osteoarthritis

Osteoporosis

Hyperhidrosis

Skeletal muscle weakness

Glucose intolerance and, on occasion, diabetes mellitus requiring treatment with insulin reflect the effects of growth hormone on carbohydrate metabolism. The incidence of systemic hypertension, ischemic heart disease, osteoarthritis, and osteoporosis seems to be increased in these patients. Lung volumes are increased, and ventilation/perfusion mismatching may be present. The patient's skin becomes thick and oily, skeletal muscle weakness may be prominent, and complaints of fatigue are common.

TREATMENT

Transsphenoidal surgical excision of pituitary adenomas is the preferred initial therapy. When adenomas have extended beyond the sella turcica, surgery or radiation therapy is no longer feasible; medical treatment with suppressant drugs (bromocriptine) may be an option in these cases.

MANAGEMENT OF ANESTHESIA

Management of anesthesia in patients with acromegaly is complicated by changes induced by excessive secretion of growth hormone. Particularly important are changes in the upper airway. Distorted facial anatomy may interfere with placement of an anesthesia face mask. Enlargement of the tongue and epiglottis predisposes to upper airway obstruction and interferes with visualization of the vocal cords by direct laryngoscopy. The distance between the lips and vocal cords is increased due to overgrowth of the mandible. The glottic opening may be narrowed, because of enlargement of the vocal cords. This, in addition to subglottic narrowing, may necessitate use of a tracheal tube with a smaller internal diameter than would be predicted based on the patient's age and size. Nasal turbinate enlargement may preclude the passage of nasopharyngeal or nasotracheal airways. A preoperative history of dyspnea on exertion or the presence of hoarseness or stridor suggests involvement of the larynx by acromegaly. In this instance, indirect laryngoscopy may be indicated to quantitate the extent of vocal cord dysfunction. When difficulty placing a tracheal tube is anticipated, it may be prudent to consider an awake fiberoptic tracheal intubation.

When a catheter is placed in the radial artery, it is important to consider the possibility of inadequate collateral circulation at the wrist. Monitoring blood glucose concentrations is useful if diabetes mellitus or glucose intolerance accompanies acromegaly. Peripheral nerve stimulation is used to guide dosing of nondepolarizing muscle relaxants, particularly if skeletal muscle weakness is present. The skeletal changes associated with acromegaly may make the use of regional anesthesia technically difficult or unreliable. There is no evidence that hemodynamic instability or alterations in pulmonary gas exchange accompany anesthesia in acromegalic patients.

Diabetes Insipidus

Diabetes insipidus reflects the absence of vasopressin (ADH) owing to destruction of the posterior pituitary (neurogenic diabetes insipidus) or failure of renal tubules to respond to

ADH (nephrogenic diabetes insipidus). Neurogenic and nephrogenic diabetes insipidus are differentiated based on the response to desmopressin (DDAVP), a vasopressin analogue that leads to concentration of the urine in the presence of neurogenic, but not nephrogenic, diabetes insipidus. Classic manifestations of diabetes insipidus are polydipsia and a high output of poorly concentrated urine despite increased serum osmolarity. Diabetes insipidus that develops during or immediately after pituitary gland surgery is generally due to reversible trauma to the posterior pituitary and is usually transient.

Initial treatment of diabetes insipidus consists of intravenous infusion of electrolyte solutions if oral intake cannot offset polyuria. Chlorpropamide, an oral hypoglycemic drug, potentiates the effects of ADH on renal tubules and may be useful for treating nephrogenic diabetes insipidus. Treatment of neurogenic diabetes insipidus is with ADH administered intramuscularly every 2 to 4 days or by intranasal administration of desmopressin.

Management of anesthesia for patients with diabetes insipidus includes monitoring the urine output and serum electrolyte concentrations during the perioperative period.

Inappropriate Secretion of Antidiuretic Hormone

Inappropriate secretion of ADH can occur in the presence of diverse pathologic processes, including intracranial tumors, hypothyroidism, porphyria, and carcinoma of the lung, particularly undifferentiated small cell carcinoma. Inappropriate secretion of ADH is alleged to occur in most patients following major surgery. Inappropriately increased urinary sodium concentrations and osmolarity in the presence of hyponatremia and decreased serum osmolarity are highly suggestive of inappropriate ADH secretion. Hyponatremia is due to dilution, reflecting expansion of the intravascular fluid volume secondary to hormone-induced resorption of water by the renal tubules. Abrupt decreases in serum sodium concentration, especially to less than 110 mEq/L, can result in cerebral edema and seizures.

Treatment of inappropriate secretion of ADH consists of restriction of oral fluid intake (to approximately 500 mL/day), antagonism of the effects of ADH on the renal tubules by administration of demeclocycline, and intravenous infusion of sodium chloride. Often fluid restriction is sufficient treatment for inappropriate secretion of ADH not associated with symptoms secondary to hyponatremia. However, restriction of oral fluid intake and administration of demeclocycline are not immediately effective in the management of patients manifesting acute neurologic symptoms resulting from hyponatremia. In these patients, intravenous infusions of hypertonic saline sufficient to increase serum sodium concentrations by 0.5 mEq/L/hr are recommended. Overly rapid correction of chronic hyponatremia has been associated with central pontine myelinolysis, a type of brain cell dysfunction caused by destruction of the myelin sheath of nerve cells in the brainstem.

KEY POINTS

- Diabetes mellitus results from an inadequate supply of and/or inadequate tissue response to insulin, which leads to increased circulating glucose levels.
- The effects of chronic hyperglycemia are many and include hypertension, coronary artery disease, congestive heart failure, peripheral vascular disease, cerebrovascular accident, chronic renal failure, and autonomic neuropathy.
- Aggressive perioperative glucose control has been shown to limit infection risk, improve wound healing, and result in overall reductions in morbidity and mortality.
- The direct effects of T_3 on the heart and vascular smooth muscle are responsible for the exaggerated hemodynamic effects of hyperthyroidism.
- The third-generation TSH assay is the single best test of thyroid hormone action at the cellular level.
- Every effort should be made to render patients euthyroid before surgery. When caring for surgical patients with hyperthyroidism or hypothyroidism, the clinician must be prepared to manage thyroid storm or myxedema coma during the perioperative period.
- Since most pheochromocytomas secrete predominantly norepinephrine, preoperative α-blockade is necessary to lower blood pressure, increase intravascular volume, prevent paroxysmal hypertensive episodes, allow resensitization of adrenergic receptors, and decrease myocardial dysfunction.
- During surgical excision of a pheochromocytoma, the patient often exhibits an exaggerated hypertensive response to anesthetic induction, intubation, surgical excision, and particularly tumor manipulation. Conversely, hypotension may occur following ligation of the tumor's venous drainage.
- The physiologic response to surgical stress is an increase in CRH, ACTH, and cortisol secretion that begins at surgical incision and continues into the postoperative period.
- The most common cause of AI is administration of exogenous steroids.
- Patients who received glucocorticoids in dosages equivalent to more than 20 mg/day of prednisone for longer than 3 weeks within the previous year are considered to have adrenal suppression and are at increased risk of AI. Such patients require perioperative corticosteroid supplementation.
- Hydrocortisone 200 to 300 mg/day for a minimum of 5 to 7 days followed by a tapering regimen over 5 to 7 days results in overall improvement in patients with vasopressor-dependent septic shock.
- Primary hyperparathyroidism is the most common cause of hypercalcemia in the general population and usually results from a benign parathyroid adenoma. Hypercalcemia can be treated medically by saline infusion, furosemide, and/or bisphosphonates before surgery.
- Overproduction of anterior pituitary hormones is most commonly manifested as Cushing's syndrome caused by ACTH hypersecretion by an adenoma in the anterior pituitary.
- Inappropriate secretion of ADH is common in the postoperative period and usually responds to fluid restriction.

RESOURCES

Akhtar S, Barash PG, Inzucchi SE. Scientific principles and clinical implications of perioperative glucose regulation and control. *Anesth Analg.* 2010;110:478-497.

Axelrod L. Perioperative management of patients treated with glucocorticoids. *Endocrinol Metab Clin North Am.* 2003;32:367-383.

Bravo EL. Evolving concepts in the pathophysiology, diagnosis, and treatment of pheochromocytoma. *Endocr Rev.* 1994;15:356-368.

Burch HB, Wartofsky L. Life-threatening thyrotoxicosis: thyroid storm. *Endocrinol Metab Clin North Am.* 1993;22:263-277.

Cooper MS, Stewart PM. Corticosteroid insufficiency in acutely ill patients. *N Engl J Med.* 2003;348:727-734.

DeWitt DE, Hirsch IB. Outpatient insulin therapy in type 1 and type 2 diabetes mellitus. *JAMA.* 2003;289:2254-2264.

Inzucchi S. *The Diabetes Mellitus Manual: A Primary Care Companion to Ellenberg and Rifkin's Sixth Edition.* New York, NY: McGraw-Hill; 2005.

Klein I, Ojamma K. Thyroid hormone and the cardiovascular system. *N Engl J Med.* 2001;344:501-509.

Mathur A, Gorden P, Libutti SK. Insulinoma. *Surg Clin North Am.* 2009;89(5):1105-1121.

Stathatos N, Wartofsky L. Perioperative management of patients with hypothyroidism. *Endocrinol Metab Clin North Am.* 2003;32:503-518.

Surks MI, Ortiz E, Daniels GH, et al. Subclinical thyroid disease: scientific review and guidelines for diagnosis and management. *JAMA.* 2004;291:228-238.

Hematologic Disorders

ADRIANA DANA OPREA ■

Disease states related to erythrocytes are anemia and polycythemia. *Anemia* is characterized by a decrease in the red cell mass, with the main adverse effect being a decrease in the oxygen-carrying capacity of blood. *Polycythemia* (*erythrocytosis*) represents an increase in hematocrit. Its consequences are primarily related to an expanded red cell mass and a resulting increase in blood viscosity.

PHYSIOLOGY OF ANEMIA

Anemia is a sign of disease manifesting clinically as a reduced absolute number of circulating red blood cells (RBCs). There is no single laboratory value that defines anemia. Although a decrease in hematocrit is most often used as an indicator, anemia has been defined as a reduction in one or more of the major RBC measures: hemoglobin (Hb) concentration, hematocrit, and RBC count. In adults, anemia is usually defined as an Hb concentration of less than 11.5 g/dL (hematocrit < 36%) for women and less than 12.5 g/dL (hematocrit < 40%) for men.

In acute blood loss the hematocrit may be unchanged initially. In parturient women, decreased hematocrit values reflect increases in plasma volume in relationship to the RBC mass (physiologic anemia). Decreases in hematocrit that exceed 1% every 24 hours can be explained only by acute blood loss or intravascular hemolysis.

The most important adverse effect of anemia is decreased tissue oxygen delivery due to associated decreases in arterial oxygen concentration (Cao_2). For example, decreases in Hb concentrations from 15 g/dL to 10 g/dL result in a 33% decrease in Cao_2. Initial compensation for decreased Cao_2 is accomplished by a rightward shift of the oxyhemoglobin dissociation curve, which facilitates release of oxygen from Hb to tissues. This is followed by tissue redistribution of blood to the myocardium, brain and muscles from the skin (which results in pallor) and kidneys (which subsequently stimulates erythroid precursors in the bone marrow to produce additional RBCs). Another compensatory mechanism is increased cardiac output as an indication of decreased blood viscosity. Fatigue and decreased exercise tolerance reflect the inability of cardiac output to increase further and maintain tissue oxygenation, especially in anemic patients who are physically active or patients with coronary artery disease. Orthopnea and dyspnea on exertion are followed by cardiomegaly, pulmonary congestion, ascites, and edema as a consequence of high-output heart failure in chronic, severe anemia.

There are many causes and forms of anemia. The most common causes of chronic anemia are iron deficiency, the presence of a chronic disease, thalassemia, and acute blood loss.

The Transfusion Trigger

The decision to perform transfusion before elective surgery is based on a combination of factors: the preoperative Hb level, the risks of anemia balanced against the risks of transfusion, the presence of co-existing diseases, and the magnitude of the anticipated blood loss. Transfusions of packed RBCs can be administered preoperatively to increase Hb concentrations, with recognition that a period of approximately 24 hours is needed to restore intravascular fluid volume. Compared with similar volumes of whole blood, packed RBCs produce about twice as high an increase in Hb concentration.

The most appropriate Hb level to serve as the trigger for perioperative blood transfusion is uncertain. Although the "10/30" rule (transfuse if the hemoglobin level is below 10 g/dL or the hematocrit is below 30%) used to be commonly cited as a reference point, there is no evidence that Hb values below this level mandate the need for perioperative RBC transfusion. There is clear evidence that patients with Hb levels of less than 6 g/dL should receive transfusions, whereas patients with compensated chronic anemia and hematocrit values between 6 and 10 g/dL can tolerate these levels without evidence of end-organ ischemia.

The strongest evidence regarding perioperative transfusion comes from the Transfusion Requirements in Critical Care trial, which found no significant differences in 30-day mortality rates between a group managed using a "restrictive" transfusion strategy (transfusions were administered as necessary to keep Hb values between 7 and 8 g/dL) and a group treated using a "liberal" strategy (Hb was kept between 10 and 12 g/dL). The restrictive regime did not cause a significant increase in mortality, cardiac morbidity, or duration of hospitalization.

RBC transfusions have been associated with direct transmission of infectious diseases, such as hepatitis B, hepatitis C, and human immunodeficiency virus (HIV) infection. In the critically ill and trauma patients, transfusions are independently associated with longer intensive care unit and hospital lengths of stay, higher mortality rates, increased incidence of ventilator-associated pneumonia, and increased mortality. The immunomodulatory effects of RBC transfusion can lead to cancer recurrence, postoperative bacterial infection, transfusion-related acute lung injury, and hemolytic transfusion reactions.

For surgery, an expected blood loss of 15% or less of total blood volume requires no replacement therapy. A loss of up to 30% can be replaced exclusively with crystalloid solutions. A loss of more than 30% to 40% generally requires RBC transfusion to restore oxygen-carrying capacity. The transfusion is given along with crystalloid and colloid solutions to restore intravascular volume and maintain tissue perfusion. In the case of massive transfusion (>50% of blood volume replaced within 24 hours), RBC transfusion should be accompanied by administration of fresh frozen plasma and platelets at a ratio of 1:1:1.

Patients with coronary artery disease merit special consideration. In vivo studies have found evidence of myocardial ischemia at Hb levels of 7 g/dL in the presence of coronary artery stenosis of 75% or more. The literature suggests that the transfusion trigger of a hematocrit of 28% to 30% should be used in patients with significant coronary artery disease, especially in those with unstable coronary syndromes.

Management of Anesthesia in Anemia

If elective surgery is performed in the presence of chronic anemia, it seems prudent to minimize the likelihood of significant changes that could further interfere with oxygen delivery to tissues. For example, drug-induced decreases in cardiac output or a leftward shift of the oxyhemoglobin dissociation curve due to respiratory alkalosis from iatrogenic hyperventilation could interfere with tissue oxygen delivery. Decreased body temperature also shifts the oxyhemoglobin dissociation curve to the left. Decreased tissue oxygen requirements may accompany the depressant effects of anesthetic drugs and hypothermia, offsetting the decrease in tissue oxygen delivery associated with anemia, although to unpredictable degrees. Signs and symptoms of inadequate tissue oxygen delivery due to anemia are difficult to appreciate during anesthesia. Efforts to offset the impact of surgical blood loss by such measures as normovolemic hemodilution and intraoperative blood salvage are considerations in selected patients. Effects of anesthesia on the sympathetic nervous system and cardiovascular responses may blunt the usual increase in cardiac output associated with acute normovolemic anemia.

Volatile anesthetics may be less soluble in the plasma of anemic patients, which reflects a decrease in the concentration of lipid-rich RBCs. As a result, uptake of volatile anesthetics in the plasma of anemic patients might be accelerated. However, the effect of decreased solubility of volatile anesthetics due to anemia is probably offset by the impact of an increased cardiac output. Therefore, it seems unlikely that clinically detectable differences in the rate of induction of anesthesia or vulnerability to an anesthetic overdose would be present in anemic patients compared with nonanemic patients.

HEMOLYTIC ANEMIA

Hemolytic anemia represents accelerated destruction (hemolysis) of erythrocytes caused most often by hemoglobinopathies and immune disorders. In hemolytic anemias either RBCs are removed from the circulation by the reticuloendothelial system (extravascular hemolysis) or the cells are lysed within the circulation (intravascular hemolysis). Therefore, RBC life span is shorter than the normal 120 days, and the resulting tissue hypoxia leads to hyperproduction of RBCs in the bone marrow.

Hemolytic anemia is characterized by reticulocytosis (>100,000 cells/mm^3) and increased mean corpuscular volume size, which reflect the presence of immature erythrocytes; unconjugated bilirubinemia; increased lactate dehydrogenase (LDH) level; and decreased serum level of haptoglobin. Confirmation of hemolytic anemia should be followed by performance of Coombs' test to rule out an immunologic cause, examination of a peripheral blood smear, and Hb electrophoresis.

Disorders of Red Cell Structure

The oxygen required by tissues for aerobic metabolism is supplied by the circulating mass of mature erythrocytes. The circulating RBC population is continually renewed by the erythroid precursor cells in the bone marrow under the control of both humoral and cellular growth factors. This cycle of normal erythropoiesis is a carefully regulated process. Oxygen sensors within the kidney detect minute changes in the amount of oxygen available to tissues and by releasing erythropoietin are able to adjust erythropoiesis to match tissue requirements.

The mature RBC has the shape of a biconcave disk. It lacks a nucleus and mitochondria, and one third of its contents is made up of a single protein, Hb. Intracellular energy requirements are largely supplied by glucose metabolism, which is targeted at maintaining Hb in a soluble, reduced state, providing appropriate amounts of 2,3-diphosphoglycerate (2,3-DPG), and generating adenosine triphosphate (ATP) to support membrane function. Without a nucleus or protein metabolic pathway, the cell has a limited life span of 100 to 120 days. However, the unique structure of the adult RBC provides maximum flexibility as the cell travels through the microvasculature.

HEREDITARY SPHEROCYTOSIS

Abnormalities in membrane protein composition can result in lifelong hemolytic anemia. *Hereditary spherocytosis* is inherited in an autosomal dominant pattern in most patients. It is the most common inherited hemolytic anemia in Europe and the United States, with a frequency of 1 in 5000 individuals. The principal defect is a deficiency in membrane skeletal proteins, usually spectrin and ankyrin. Affected cells show abnormal osmotic fragility and a shortened circulation half-life. Hereditary spherocytosis can be clinically silent, and about one third of patients have a very mild hemolytic anemia, with spherocytes rarely visible on peripheral blood smear. Some patients, however, have a more severe degree of hemolysis and anemia, and fewer than 5% of patients develop life-threatening anemia. Patients with hereditary spherocytosis often have splenomegaly and experience symptoms of easy fatigability in proportion to the degree of chronic anemia. These patients are at risk of episodes of hemolytic crisis, often precipitated by viral or bacterial infection. These crises worsen the chronic anemia and may be associated with jaundice. Infection with parvovirus B19 can produce a transient

(10 to 14 days) but profound aplastic crisis. The risk of pigment gallstones is high in patients with hereditary spherocytosis and should be considered in patients complaining of biliary colic.

Management of Anesthesia

Anesthetic risk in these patients is largely dictated by the severity of the anemia and whether the hemolysis is stable or in a period of exacerbation due to concurrent infection.

Episodic anemia, often triggered by viral or bacterial infection and cholelithiasis, must be considered in the preoperative evaluation. Patients undergoing cardiac surgery with cardiopulmonary bypass merit special consideration. The use of cardiopulmonary bypass may lead to excessive hemolysis, because spherocytes are more susceptible to mechanical and shear stress than normal erythrocytes. There are recommendations that mechanical heart valves be avoided, but short-term use of cardiopulmonary bypass may be safe.

HEREDITARY ELLIPTOCYTOSIS

Hereditary elliptocytosis is caused by an abnormality in one of the membrane proteins, spectrin or glycophorin, that makes the erythrocyte less pliable. Hereditary elliptocytosis is inherited as an autosomal dominant disorder and is prevalent in regions where malaria is endemic. In those areas the incidence may reach 3 in 100 people. Hereditary elliptocytosis is most often diagnosed as an incidental finding. The majority of cells demonstrate an elliptical or even rodlike appearance. Most patients with hereditary elliptocytosis are heterozygous and only rarely experience hemolysis. In contrast, those with homozygous or compound heterozygous defects may demonstrate greater degrees of hemolysis and more severe anemia.

ACANTHOCYTOSIS

Acanthocytosis is another defect in membrane structure found in patients with a congenital lack of β-lipoprotein (abetalipoproteinemia) and infrequently in patients with severe cirrhosis or pancreatitis. It results from cholesterol or sphingomyelin accumulation on the outer membrane of the erythrocyte. This accretion gives the membrane a spiculated appearance that signals the splenic macrophages of the reticuloendothelial system to remove it from the circulation, which produces hemolysis.

PAROXYSMAL NOCTURNAL HEMOGLOBINURIA

Paroxysmal nocturnal hemoglobinuria is a stem cell disorder that may arise in hematopoietic cells any time from the second to the eighth decade of life and result in complement-activated RBC hemolysis. A number of different associated mutations have been identified, but all result in abnormalities in or a reduction in amount of a membrane protein known as *glycosylphosphatidyl glycan*. Besides hemolytic anemia, patients are at risk for other complications such as venous thrombosis due to complement activation. The thromboses have an incidence of approximately 40% and can involve the hepatic and portal veins as well as other venous sites. In the absence of protectin, a critical glycosylphosphatidyl glycan–linked protein, patients can have a dysplastic or aplastic bone marrow suggestive of damage to all hematopoietic precursor cells. Paroxysmal nocturnal hemoglobinuria tends to be a chronic disorder, with hemolytic anemia and deficiencies in other marrow constituents. Median life expectancy after diagnosis is 8 to 10 years.

Management of Anesthesia

Nocturnal manifestation of the hemolysis is thought to be a result of carbon dioxide retention and subsequent acidosis. Therefore, during anesthesia, predisposing factors such as hypoxemia, hypoperfusion, and hypercarbia that can lead to acidosis and complement activation should be avoided. Inhalational agents and propofol may have a theoretical advantage over thiopental, which can be associated with complement-activated anaphylactoid reactions. Because of the risk of venous thrombosis, maintaining hydration is important.

Disorders of Red Cell Metabolism

Lacking a nucleus and having a limited life expectancy, the erythrocyte maintains only the very narrow spectrum of activities necessary to carry out its oxygen-transport function. The stability of the RBC membrane and the solubility of intracellular Hb depend on four glucose-supported metabolic pathways. These four pathways are illustrated in Figure 20-1. The most clinically relevant pathways are described in the following sections.

EMBDEN-MEYERHOF PATHWAY

The Embden-Meyerhof pathway (nonoxidative or anaerobic pathway) is responsible for generation of the ATP necessary for membrane function and the maintenance of cell shape and pliability. Defects in anaerobic glycolysis are associated with increased red cell rigidity and decreased survival, which produces a hemolytic anemia. Deficiencies of the glycolytic pathway are not associated with any typical morphologic red cell changes that herald their presence, nor do they lead to hemolytic crisis after exposure to oxidants. The severity of hemolysis is highly variable and largely unpredictable.

PHOSPHOGLUCONATE PATHWAY

The phosphogluconate pathway couples oxidative metabolism with nicotinamide adenine dinucleotide phosphate and glutathione reduction. It counteracts environmental oxidants and prevents globin denaturation. When patients lack either of the two key enzymes, glucose-6-phosphate dehydrogenase and glutathione reductase, denatured Hb precipitates on the inner surface of the RBC membrane, which results in membrane damage and hemolysis.

Glucose-6-Phosphate Dehydrogenase Deficiency

Glucose-6-phosphate dehydrogenase (G6PD) deficiency is an X-linked disorder and is the most common enzymatic disorder of RBCs, with more than 400 million people affected worldwide.

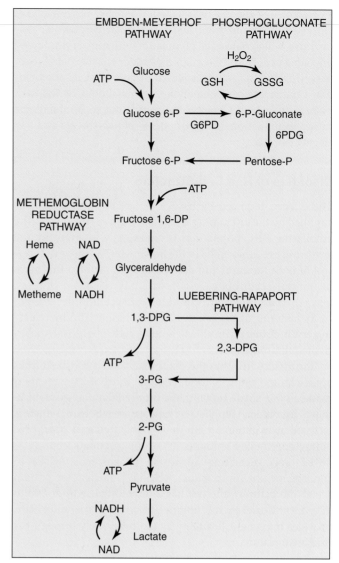

FIGURE 20-1 Diagrammatic representation of the four pathways involved in the most common disorders affecting red blood cell metabolism. *ATP,* Adenosine triphosphate; *1,6-DP,* 1,6-diphosphate; *1,3-DPG,* 1,3-diphosphoglycerate; *2,3,-DPG,* 2,3-diphosphoglycerate; *G6PD,* glucose-6-phosphate dehydrogenase; *GSH,* glutathione reductase; *GSSG,* oxidized glutathione; *NAD,* nicotinamide adenine dinucleotide; *NADH,* reduced form of nicotinamide adenine dinucleotide; *6-P,* 6-phosphate; *6PDG,* 6-phosphogluconate dehydrogenase; *2-PG,* 2-phosphoglycerate; *3-PG,* 3-phosphoglycerate; *6-P-Gluconate,* 6-phosphogluconate; *Pentose-P,* pentose phosphate.

G6PD activity is highest in young red cells and declines with age. The half-life of these erythrocytes is approximately 60 days. The clinical manifestations of the disorder depend of the level of the enzyme, with five classes described by the World Health Organization. Patients can have chronic hemolytic anemia (class I, <10% G6PD activity), intermittent hemolysis (class II, 10% G6PD activity), and hemolysis only with stressors (class III, 10% to 60% activity), or no hemolysis (classes IV and V).

The hemolysis is the result of the inability of the RBC to protect itself from oxidative stress. Acute insults that either precipitate new or aggravate preexisting hemolysis include infection, certain drugs, and ingestion of fava beans.

Management of Anesthesia. Anesthetic risk is largely a function of the severity and acuity of the anemia. The goal is to avoid the risk of hemolysis by not exposing the patient to oxidative drugs. In vitro studies show that codeine, midazolam, propofol, fentanyl, and ketamine are safe, but it might be wise to avoid isoflurane, sevoflurane, and diazepam, which depress G6PD activity in vitro. Methylene blue is a particular concern. If a patient with methemoglobinemia (with already compromised oxygen delivery) is also G6PD deficient, methylene blue administration may be life threatening. Drugs that can induce methemoglobinemia, such as lidocaine, prilocaine, and silver nitrate, should be avoided. Hypothermia, acidosis, hyperglycemia, and infection can precipitate hemolysis in the G6PD-deficient patient, and these conditions need to be aggressively treated in the perioperative period.

Pyruvate Kinase Deficiency

Pyruvate kinase deficiency, an autosomal recessive disorder, is the most common erythrocyte enzyme defect causing *congenital* hemolytic anemia. Pyruvate kinase deficiency is found worldwide, but shows a higher prevalence among people of northern European extraction and individuals from some regions of China. Although less prevalent than G6PD deficiency, pyruvate kinase deficiency is considerably more likely to produce a chronic hemolytic anemia. Accumulation of 2,3-DPG in the RBCs causes a shift of the oxyhemoglobin dissociation curve to the right to facilitate oxygen release to peripheral tissues. Splenectomy does not totally prevent hemolysis but does decrease the rate of RBC destruction. The severity of the clinical presentation ranges from a mild, fully compensated process without anemia to life-threatening, transfusion-requiring hemolytic anemia at birth. Severely affected individuals may have chronic jaundice, develop pigmented gallstones, and manifest splenomegaly. Splenectomy often improves the chronic hemolysis and may even eliminate the need for transfusion.

Management of Anesthesia. Anesthetic risk is largely a function of the severity and acuity of the anemia, as discussed previously.

The methemoglobin reductase pathway uses the pyridine nucleotide–reduced nicotinamide adenine dinucleotide generated from anaerobic glycolysis to maintain heme iron in its ferrous state. An inherited mutation of the methemoglobin reductase enzyme results in an inability to counteract oxidation of Hb to methemoglobin, the ferric form of Hb that will not transport oxygen. Patients with type I reduced nicotinamide adenine dinucleotide–diaphorase deficiency accumulate small amounts of methemoglobin in circulating red cells, whereas patients with type II disease have severe cyanosis and mental retardation.

The Luebering-Rapaport pathway is responsible for the production of 2,3-DPG. A single enzyme, 2,3 bisphosphoglycerate mutase, mediates both the synthase activity resulting in 2,3-DPG formation and the phosphatase activity that then converts 2,3-DPG to 3-phosphoglycerate, returning it to the glycolytic pathway. The balance of formation versus metabolism of 2,3-DPG is pH sensitive, with alkalosis favoring synthetase activity and acidosis favoring phosphatase activity. The 2,3-DPG response is also influenced by the supply of phosphate to the cell. Severe phosphate depletion in patients with diabetic ketoacidosis or nutritional deficiency can result in reduced 2,3-DPG production.

DISORDERS OF HEMOGLOBIN

The Hemoglobin Molecule

The RBC is basically a repository for Hb molecules, each containing active heme groups and representing 90% of the dry weight of the red cell. Each heme group is capable of binding to an oxygen molecule. The respiratory motion of Hb—that is, the uptake and release of oxygen to tissues—involves a specific change in molecular structure. As Hb shuttles from its deoxyhemoglobin to its oxyhemoglobin form, carbon dioxide and 2,3-DPG are expelled from their position between the β-globin chains, which opens the molecule to receive oxygen. Furthermore, oxygen binding by one of the heme groups increases the affinity of the other groups to load oxygen. This interaction is responsible for the sigmoid shape of the oxygen dissociation curve.

Inherited defects in Hb structure can interfere with this respiratory motion. Most defects are substitutions of a single amino acid in either the α- or β-globin chains. Some interfere with molecular movement, restricting the molecule to either a low- or high-affinity state, whereas others change the valency of heme iron from ferrous to ferric or reduce the solubility of the Hb molecule. Hb S (the abnormal Hb in sickle cell disease) is an example of an Hb with a single amino acid substitution that results in reduced solubility, which typically causes precipitation of the abnormal Hb.

Hemoglobin S and C

Sickle cell disease is a disorder caused by the substitution of valine for glutamic acid in the β-globin subunit. In the deoxygenated state, Hb S undergoes conformational changes exposing a hydrophobic region of the molecule. In extreme states of deoxygenation, the hydrophobic regions aggregate, and this results in distortion of the erythrocyte membrane, oxidative damage to the membrane, impaired deformability, and a shortened life span of 10 to 20 days.

Sickle cell anemia, the homozygous form of Hb S disease, presents early in life with severe hemolytic anemia and progresses to end-organ damage involving the bone marrow, spleen, kidneys, and central nervous system. Patients experience episodic painful crises (*vasoocclusive crises*) characterized by bone and joint pain that may or may not be associated with concurrent illness, stress, or dehydration. The severity and progression of the disease are remarkably varied. Organ damage can start early in childhood, with recurrent splenic infarction culminating in loss of splenic function in the first decade of life. The kidney is another prime target, with painless hematuria and loss of concentrating ability as an early feature progressing to chronic renal failure in the third or fourth decade of life. Pulmonary and neurologic complications are the leading causes of morbidity and mortality. Lung damage results from chronic persistent inflammation. *Acute chest syndrome,* a pneumonia-like complication, is characterized by the presence of a new pulmonary infiltrate involving at least one complete lung segment plus at least one of the following: chest pain, temperature higher than 38.5° C, tachypnea, wheezing, or cough. Neurologic complications include stroke, usually as a result of arterial disease rather than sickling. Adolescents present with cerebral infarction and adults develop hemorrhagic strokes.

Management of Anesthesia

Sickle cell trait does not cause an increase in perioperative morbidity or mortality. However, *sickle cell disease* is associated with a high incidence of perioperative complications. Risk factors for complications include advanced age; frequent and severe recent episodes of sickling; evidence of end-organ damage such as a low baseline oxygen saturation, elevated creatinine level, cardiac dysfunction, and history of stroke; and concurrent infection. Risks intrinsic to the type of surgery are also important considerations, with minor procedures such as inguinal hernia repair and extremity surgery considered to be low risk, intraabdominal operations such as cholecystectomy categorized as intermediate risk, and intracranial and intrathoracic procedures classified as high risk. Among orthopedic procedures, hip surgery and hip replacement, in particular, are associated with a considerable risk of complications, including excessive blood loss and sickle cell events.

The goals of preoperative transfusion management have changed in recent years. Studies examining the effects of aggressive transfusion strategies aimed at increasing the ratio of normal Hb to sickle Hb have found no benefit compared with the more conservative goal of achieving a preoperative hematocrit of 30%. Indeed, the aggressive strategy necessitated significantly more transfusion, and the complications of transfusion outweighed its benefits. Accordingly, patients undergoing low-risk procedures rarely require any preoperative transfusion, and patients undergoing moderate- to high-risk operations need only have preoperative anemia corrected to a target hematocrit of 30%. Choice of anesthetic technique does not appear to significantly affect the risk of complications stemming from sickle cell disease. Secondary goals of avoiding dehydration, acidosis, and hypothermia during anesthesia reduce the risk of perioperative sickling events. Use of occlusive orthopedic tourniquets is not contraindicated in sickle cell disease, although the incidence of perioperative complications is increased with their use. Postoperative pain requires aggressive management, since pain at the operative site and pain caused by vasoocclusive events can exacerbate complications of this disease. Patients often have a degree of tolerance to opioids, and a subset of patients may have opiate addiction, but these facts must not interfere with appropriate pain management.

Despite concerns that regional anesthesia might have detrimental effects in sickle cell patients, it is not contraindicated and may offer advantages in pain control.

Acute chest syndrome may develop 2 to 3 days into the postoperative period and demand treatment of hypoxemia, adequate analgesia, and, frequently, blood transfusion to correct anemia and improve oxygenation. Inhaled nitric oxide to reduce pulmonary hypertension and improve blood oxygenation has shown promise. In the postoperative period, patients also need to be monitored for pain crises, stroke, and infection.

SICKLE C HEMOGLOBIN

The prevalence of Hb C is about one fourth that of Hb S. Hb C causes the erythrocyte to lose water via enhanced activity of the potassium chloride cotransport system. This results in cellular dehydration that, in the homozygous state, may produce a mild to moderate hemolytic anemia. Ironically, the presence of both Hb S and Hb C *traits* (Hb SC) that in isolation cause no symptoms together produce a tendency to sickling and complications similar to those of Hb SS disease. It appears that the dehydration produced by Hb C increases the concentration of Hb S within the erythrocyte, exacerbating its insolubility and tendency to polymerize.

Management of Anesthesia

The anesthetic risks of Hb SC disease are not as well studied as those of Hb SS disease. However, one investigation suggested that perioperative transfusion considerably reduces the incidence of sickling complications in this subset of patients.

SICKLE HEMOGLOBIN–β-THALASSEMIA

Among African Americans, the frequency of the β-thalassemia gene is only one tenth that of the gene for Hb S. The clinical presentation of this compound heterozygous state is largely determined by whether it is associated with reduced amounts of Hb A (sickle cell–β⁺-thalassemia) or no Hb A whatsoever (sickle cell–β⁰-thalassemia). In the absence of any Hb A, patients experience acute vasoocclusive crises, acute chest syndrome, and other sickling complications at rates approaching those of patients with Hb SS.

Management of Anesthesia

Anesthetic considerations are the same as those for sickle cell disease.

UNSTABLE HEMOGLOBINS

Hbs are made unstable by structural changes that reduce their solubility or render them more susceptible to oxidation of amino acids within the globin chains. More than 100 unique unstable Hb variants have been documented, most associated with only minimal clinical manifestations. The mutations typically impair the globin folding or heme-globin binding that stabilizes the heme moiety within the hydrophobic globin pocket. Once freed from its cleft, the heme binds nonspecifically to other regions of the globin chains. This causes them to form a precipitate called the *Heinz body* that contains globin chains, chain fragments, and heme. Heinz bodies interact with the red cell membrane, reducing its deformability and favoring its removal by splenic macrophages. Unstable Hbs vary in their propensity to form Heinz bodies, and the severity of the associated anemia correspondingly varies. Hemolysis may be aggravated by the development of additional oxidative stresses, such as infection or ingestion of oxidizing agents. Patients with recurring bouts of severe hemolysis or morbidity because of chronic anemia may be considered candidates for splenectomy, which is usually effective in reducing or even eliminating symptoms.

Management of Anesthesia

Anesthetic management of patients with unstable hemoglobins is largely dictated by the degree of hemolysis. Transfusion during bouts of severe hemolysis and avoidance of oxidizing agents are important. These patients may have severe anemia and Hb-induced renal injury.

Thalassemias

Globin chains are assembled by cytoplasmic ribosomes under the control of two clusters of closely linked genes on chromosomes 11 and 16. The final globin molecule is a tetramer of two α-globin and two non–α-globin chains. In the adult, almost all Hb is made up of two α-globin and two β-globin chains (Hb A) with minor components of Hb F and Hb A_2.

An inherited defect in globin chain synthesis known as *thalassemia* is one of the leading causes of microcytic anemia in children and adults. This disorder shows a strong geographic influence, with β-thalassemia predominating in Africa and the Mediterranean area, and α-thalassemia and Hb E dominant in Southeast Asia.

THALASSEMIA MINOR

Most individuals with thalassemia have *thalassemia minor* and are heterozygous for either an α-globin (α-thalassemia trait) or β-globin (β-thalassemia trait) gene mutation. Although the mutation may decrease synthesis of the affected globin chain by up to 50% of normal, producing hypochromic and microcytic RBCs, the anemia is usually only modest with relatively little accumulation of the unaffected globin. Accordingly, morbidity associated with chronic hemolysis and ineffective erythropoiesis is rarely encountered.

THALASSEMIA INTERMEDIA

Patients with *thalassemia intermedia* show more severe anemia and prominent microcytosis and hypochromia. They have symptoms attributable both to anemia and to hepatosplenomegaly, cardiomegaly, and skeletal changes secondary to bone marrow expansion. These individuals may have a milder form of homozygous β-thalassemia, a combined α- and β-thalassemia defect, or β-thalassemia with high levels of Hb F.

THALASSEMIA MAJOR

Patients with *thalassemia major* develop severe, life-threatening anemia during their first few years of life. To survive childhood, they require repeated transfusion therapy to correct anemia and suppress the high level of ineffective erythropoiesis. The severity of thalassemia is remarkably variable, even among patients with seemingly identical genetic mutations. In its most severe forms, patients exhibit three defects that markedly depress their oxygen-carrying capacity: (1) ineffective erythropoiesis, (2) hemolytic anemia, and (3) hypochromia with microcytosis. The deficit in oxygen-carrying capacity produces maximum erythropoietin release, and marrow erythroblasts respond by increasing their unbalanced globin synthesis. The accumulating unpaired globins aggregate and precipitate, forming inclusion bodies that cause membrane damage to the RBCs. Some of these defective red cells are destroyed within the marrow, which results in ineffective erythropoiesis. Some abnormal erythrocytes escape into the circulation, where their altered morphology can cause accelerated clearance (hemolytic anemia) or, at best, reduced oxygen-carrying capacity resulting from the lowered Hb content (hypochromia with microcytosis). Other features of severe thalassemia include those attributable to bone marrow hyperplasia, including frontal bossing, maxillary overgrowth, stunted growth, and osteoporosis, as well as those caused by extramedullary hematopoiesis (hepatomegaly). Hemolytic anemia may produce splenomegaly together with dyspnea and orthopnea, which over time results in congestive heart failure and mental retardation. Transfusion therapy will ameliorate many of these changes, but complications resulting from iron overload such as cirrhosis, right-sided heart failure, and endocrinopathy frequently require chelation therapy. Some patients demonstrate reduced transfusion requirements after splenectomy. However, the risk of postsplenectomy sepsis in younger patients argues for deferment of surgery until after 5 years of age if possible. For patients receiving adequate transfusion and chelation therapy, splenectomy may not be indicated. Bone marrow transplantation was first performed for thalassemia major in 1982 and is a therapeutic option for younger patients with HLA-identical siblings.

MANAGEMENT OF ANESTHESIA

The severity of the thalassemia is a critical determinant of the degree of end-organ damage and the anesthetic risk. In its mildest forms, a chronic, compensated anemia is the major concern. With more severe forms of this disorder, the anemia is more significant, and associated features may include splenomegaly and hepatomegaly, skeletal malformations, congestive heart failure, mental retardation, and complications of iron overload such as cirrhosis, right-sided heart failure, and endocrinopathies. Skeletal malformations can make tracheal intubation and regional anesthesia difficult.

Disorders of Hemoglobin Resulting in Reduced or Ineffective Erythropoiesis

MACROCYTIC/MEGALOBLASTIC ANEMIA

Disruption of the erythroid precursor maturation sequence can result from deficiencies in vitamins such as folic acid and vitamin B_{12}, exposure to chemotherapeutic agents, or a preleukemic state. Since these are all defects in nuclear maturation, patients have *macrocytic anemia* and megaloblastic bone marrow morphology.

FOLATE AND VITAMIN B_{12} DEFICIENCY ANEMIA

Folic acid and vitamin B_{12} deficiency are primary causes of macrocytic anemia in adults. Both vitamins are essential for normal DNA synthesis, and high-turnover tissues such as bone marrow are the first to be affected when these vitamins are in short supply. In deficiency states, the marrow precursors appear much larger than normal and are unable to complete cell division. Accordingly, the marrow becomes megaloblastic, and macrocytic red cells are released into the circulation. The prevalence of deficiency of these vitamins varies considerably in different parts of the world. In developed countries, alcoholism is a frequent source of folate deficiency, both because of the poor dietary habits of alcoholic individuals and because of alcohol's interference with folate metabolism. In developing countries where tropical and nontropical sprue is more widespread, malabsorption may increase the frequency of vitamin B_{12} deficiency.

Sustained exposure to nitrous oxide can produce an impairment of vitamin B_{12} activity. Nitrous oxide can oxidize the cobalt atom of the vitamin, which reduces its cofactor activity and causes impairment in both methionine synthesis and S-adenosylmethionine synthesis. This action requires long exposure to high concentrations of nitrous oxide and pertains only to situations in which scavenging systems are inadequate, as might be found in dental offices or with recreational use of the gas.

A macrocytic anemia caused by folate or vitamin B_{12} deficiency may result in Hb levels of less than 8 to 10 g/dL, a mean red cell volume of 110 to 140 fL (normal = 90 fL), a normal reticulocyte count, and increased levels of LDH and bilirubin. In addition to causing megaloblastic anemia, vitamin B_{12} deficiency is associated with peripheral neuropathy due to degeneration of the lateral and posterior columns of the spinal cord. There are symmetrical paresthesias with loss of proprioceptive and vibratory sensations, especially in the lower extremities. Gait is unsteady, and deep tendon reflexes are diminished. Memory impairment and depression may be prominent. These neurologic deficits are progressive unless vitamin B_{12} is provided. Nonmedical abuse of nitrous oxide may be associated with neurologic findings similar to those that accompany vitamin B_{12} deficiency and pernicious anemia.

Folate and vitamin B_{12} deficiency can be corrected by vitamin administration. In cases of intestinal malabsorption the parenteral route is preferred. Emergency correction of life-threatening anemia or preparation for urgent surgery entails red cell transfusion.

Management of Anesthesia

Management of anesthesia in patients with megaloblastic anemia due to vitamin B_{12} deficiency is influenced by the need to maintain delivery of oxygenated arterial blood to peripheral tissues. The presence of neurologic changes may deter the selection of regional anesthetic techniques or peripheral nerve blockade. The use of nitrous oxide would not be prudent.

MICROCYTIC ANEMIA

Defects in hemoglobinization, such as those seen in severe iron deficiency, produce markedly ineffective erythropoiesis and microcytic, hypochromic anemia.

Iron Deficiency Anemia

Nutritional deficiency of iron as a cause of anemia is found only in infants and small children. In adults, iron deficiency anemia reflects depletion of iron stores caused by chronic blood loss. Typically this involves losses from the gastrointestinal tract or from the female genital tract (menstruation). Pregnant women are susceptible to development of iron deficiency anemia because of the increased RBC mass required during gestation and the needs of the fetus for iron.

Diagnosis. Patients experiencing chronic blood loss may not be able to absorb sufficient iron from the diet to form Hb as rapidly as RBCs are lost. As a result, RBCs are produced with too little Hb. Most cases of iron deficiency anemia in the United States are mild, exhibiting Hb concentrations of 9 to 12 g/dL. A decreased serum ferritin concentration (<30 ng/mL) is diagnostic of iron deficiency anemia. The absence of stainable iron in a bone marrow aspirate is also confirmatory evidence for iron deficiency anemia. Absence of reticulocytes, decreased serum iron level, and reduced transferrin saturation are also seen.

Treatment. Iron deficiency anemia is treated with ferrous iron salts administered orally. Iron stores are replenished slowly. Therapy should be continued for at least 1 year after the source of blood loss that caused the iron deficiency is corrected. A favorable response to iron therapy is evidenced by an increase in Hb concentration of approximately 2 g/dL in 3 weeks or return of Hb concentrations to normal in 6 weeks. Continued bleeding is reflected by reticulocytosis and failure of the Hb concentration to increase in response to iron therapy. It may be desirable to postpone elective surgery for up to 4 weeks and allow time for correction of anemia preoperatively.

Hemoglobins with Increased Oxygen Affinity

Hb mutations that increase the oxygen-binding avidity of the heme moiety cause the oxyhemoglobin dissociation curve to shift to the left, which reduces the P_{50} (i.e., the partial pressure of oxygen at which Hb is 50% saturated with oxygen). Many types of mutations can increase oxygen affinity. These Hbs bind oxygen more readily than normal and retain more oxygen at lower Po_2 levels. Accordingly, they deliver *less* oxygen to tissues at normal capillary Po_2, and blood returns to the lungs still saturated with oxygen. Since these variant Hbs cannot acquire excess oxygen in the lungs despite their higher oxygen affinity, the net result is a mild tissue hypoxia that triggers increased erythropoietin production leading to polycythemia.

MANAGEMENT OF ANESTHESIA

Tissue oxygen delivery at baseline may be barely adequate, so that even a modest decrease in hematocrit is potentially dangerous. Patients with only mild erythrocytosis do not require intervention. Patients with high hematocrits (>55% to 60%), whose blood viscosity may further compromise oxygen delivery, may require preoperative exchange transfusion, and careful avoidance of hemoconcentration is required in the perioperative period.

Hemoglobins with Decreased Oxygen Affinity

METHEMOGLOBINEMIA

Methemoglobin is formed when the iron moiety in Hb is oxidized from the ferrous (Fe^{2+}) state to the ferric (Fe^{3+}) state. Normal Hb, upon binding oxygen, partially transfers an electron from the iron to the oxygen, which moves the iron close to its ferric state, and the oxygen resembles a superoxide. Deoxygenation ordinarily returns the electron to the iron, but methemoglobin forms if the electron is not returned. The normal erythrocyte maintains methemoglobin levels at 1% or less by the methemoglobin reductase enzyme system. Methemoglobin moves the oxyhemoglobin dissociation curve markedly to the left and therefore delivers little oxygen to the tissues. Levels of methemoglobin below 30% of the total Hb content cause no compromise in tissue oxygenation. Levels between 30% and 50%, however, do initiate symptoms of oxygen deprivation, and levels higher than 50% can result in coma and death.

Methemoglobinemia of clinical importance can arise from three mechanisms: globin chain mutations favoring the formation of methemoglobin, mutations impairing the efficacy of the methemoglobin reductase system, and toxic exposure to substances that oxidize normal Hb iron at a rate that exceeds the capacity of the normal reducing mechanisms.

Hb M arises from mutations that stabilize heme iron in the ferric (Fe^{3+}) state, making it relatively resistant to reduction by the methemoglobin reductase system. The methemoglobin has a brownish blue color that does not change to red on exposure to oxygen, which gives patients a cyanotic appearance independent of their Pao_2. Patients with M-type Hbs are usually asymptomatic, since their methemoglobin levels rarely exceed 30% of total Hb.

Mutations impairing the methemoglobin reductase system rarely result in methemoglobinemia levels of more than 25%. Like their counterparts with Hb M, affected patients may exhibit a slate-gray *pseudocyanosis* despite normal Pao_2 levels. Exposure to chemical agents that directly oxidize Hb or produce reactive oxygen intermediates that oxidize Hb may produce an acquired methemoglobinemia in which life-threatening amounts of methemoglobin accumulate. Infants have lower levels of methemoglobin reductase in their erythrocytes and may manifest greater susceptibility to oxidizing agents.

Management of Anesthesia

Management of anesthesia in patients with methemoglobinemia focuses on avoiding tissue hypoxia. Pulse oximetry is unreliable in this setting and will typically give a value of 85% oxygen saturation. During surgery, an intraarterial catheter should be inserted for measurement of blood pressure, methemoglobin levels, and arterial blood gas concentrations. Acidosis should be corrected, and the electrocardiogram must be closely monitored for signs of ischemia. Patients with Hb M may be more sensitive to exposure to oxidizing agents. Therefore, local anesthetics, nitrates, and nitric oxide should be avoided.

In the setting of toxic methemoglobinemia, methylene blue should be available. The dosage is 1 to 2 mg/kg of a 1% solution in saline infused over 3 to 5 minutes. This treatment is usually effective, but may need to be repeated after 30 minutes. Methylene blue acts through the methemoglobin reductase system and requires the activity of G6PD. Patients who are G6PD deficient and patients severely affected by methemoglobin may require exchange transfusion.

DISORDERS OF RED CELL PRODUCTION

Hypoproliferation

Constitutional Aplastic Anemia (Fanconi's Anemia)
Fanconi's anemia is an autosomal recessive disorder that presents with severe pancytopenia in the first two decades of life and often progresses to acute leukemia. The gene frequency in Western societies is approximately 1 in 200 persons, whereas in white South Africans, it may be as high as 1 in 80. When fully expressed (as occurs in 1 per 100,000 live births), the disorder is associated with progressive bone marrow failure, multiple physical defects, chromosomal abnormalities, and a predisposition to cancer. Some patients may not have the classic physical defects, and the diagnosis should be considered in children and young adults with acute myelogenous leukemia.

ANEMIA DUE TO DRUG- AND RADIATION-ASSOCIATED MARROW DAMAGE

Anemia due to marrow damage is a predictable side effect of chemotherapy, and this anemia is usually mild except with the use of high-dose, multidrug chemotherapy that can produce pancytopenia. As long as the drugs do not irreversibly damage the bone marrow, recovery is usually complete. High-energy radiation can also produce anemia resulting from marrow damage, the degree of which is predictable from the type of radiation, the dose, and the extent of marrow exposure. Long-term exposure to low levels of external radiation or ingested radioisotopes can also produce aplastic anemia.

Several drugs have been associated with the development of severe, often irreversible, aplastic anemia. Table 20-1 lists classes of drugs that have been associated with marrow damage. Some, such as chloramphenicol, can produce severe, irreversible aplastic anemia after only a few doses of the drug, but most, such as phenylbutazone, propylthiouracil, and tricyclic antidepressants, are associated with a more gradual onset of pancytopenia, which is reversible if the drug is withdrawn.

TABLE 20-1	Classes of drugs associated with marrow damage

Antibiotics (chloramphenicol, penicillin, cephalosporins, sulfonamides, amphotericin B, streptomycin)
Antidepressants (lithium, tricyclics)
Antiepileptics (phenytoin, carbamazepine, valproic acid, phenobarbital)
Antiinflammatory drugs (phenylbutazone, nonsteroidals, salicylates, gold salts)
Antiarrhythmics (lidocaine, quinidine, procainamide)
Antithyroidal drugs (propylthiouracil)
Diuretics (thiazides, pyrimethamine, furosemide)
Antihypertensives (captopril)
Antiuricemics (allopurinol, colchicine)
Antimalarials (quinacrine, chloroquine)
Hypoglycemics (tolbutamide)
Platelet inhibitors (ticlopidine)
Tranquilizers (prochlorperazine, meprobamate)

ANEMIA DUE TO INFECTION-ASSOCIATED MARROW DAMAGE

Bone marrow damage can result from direct invasion of the marrow by an infectious agent. Miliary tuberculosis is perhaps the best example of this. Immunosuppression of stem cell growth can also produce anemia, even aplastic anemia. This can be seen following viral illnesses such as viral hepatitis, Epstein-Barr virus infection, HIV infection, and rubella. Parvovirus B19 infection can cause an acute, reversible pure red cell aplasia in patients with congenital hemolytic anemia. Although most of these anemias are reversible, some infections can produce fatal aplastic anemia.

ANEMIA DUE TO HEMATOLOGIC OR OTHER MARROW-INVOLVING MALIGNANCY

Anemia may be caused by any leukemia that reduces the number of erythroid precursors, whether by diverting the stem cells away from the erythroid pathway or by crowding them out of the marrow by their shear numbers. Solid tumors such as breast, lung, and prostate cancer may metastasize to the marrow, producing a similar hypoproliferative anemia. Myelodysplastic syndromes and myeloproliferative disorders are also capable of crowding out RBC precursors and thus leading to anemia.

MANAGEMENT OF ANESTHESIA.

Patients may come for surgery with anemia and thrombocytopenia severe enough so that transfusion is necessary preoperatively. The severity of the neutropenia will affect the need for and choice of antibiotic coverage. The use of granulocyte colony-stimulating factor preoperatively to increase neutrophil counts is controversial.

Polycythemia

Sustained hypoxia usually results in a compensatory increase in the RBC mass and hematocrit. Although this increases the oxygen-carrying capacity of the blood, it also increases blood viscosity. Tissue oxygen delivery is maximal at a hematocrit of 33% to 36% (Hb concentration of 11 to 12 g/dL), assuming no

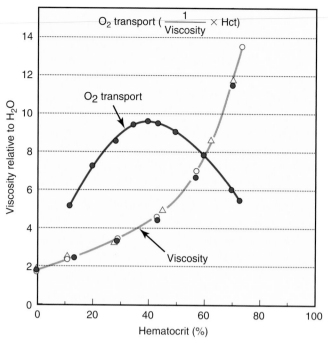

FIGURE 20-2 Viscosity of heparinized normal human blood as a function of hematocrit (Hct). Viscosity is measured with an Ostwald viscosimeter at 37° C and expressed in relation to the viscosity of saline solution. Oxygen transport is computed from hematocrit and oxygen flow (1/viscosity) and is recorded in arbitrary units. *(Data from Murray JF, Gold P, Johnson BL Jr, et al. Clinical manifestations and classification of erythrocyte disorders. In: Kaushansky K, Lichtman M, Beutler E, et al, eds. Williams Hematology. 8th ed. New York, NY: McGraw-Hill Medical; 2010.)*

changes occur in cardiac output or regional blood flow. Above this level, an increase in viscosity will tend to slow blood flow and decrease oxygen delivery. This effect is relatively minor until the hematocrit exceeds 55%, at which time blood flow to vital organs can be significantly reduced.

PHYSIOLOGY OF POLYCYTHEMIA

Polycythemia and *erythrocytosis* are terms that describe an abnormally high hematocrit. Even modest increases in the hematocrit can have a major impact on whole-blood viscosity. An increase in hematocrit can result from a reduction in plasma volume (*relative polycythemia*) without an actual increase in red cell mass. An acute decrease in plasma volume, as may be seen with preoperative fasting, can convert an asymptomatic polycythemia into one in which hyperviscosity threatens tissue perfusion. When the hematocrit rises to levels above 55% or 60%, whole-blood viscosity increases exponentially, especially in small blood vessels such as capillaries with low flow/shear rates. The cerebral circulation is particularly vulnerable to reductions in blood flow resulting from increased viscosity (Figures 20-2 and 20-3).

The clinical signs and symptoms of an elevated hematocrit vary depending on the underlying disease process and the rate of development. Patients with modest chronic polycythemia, such as that seen in chronic lung disease, will complain of few symptoms until the hematocrit exceeds 55% to 60%. Headaches and easy

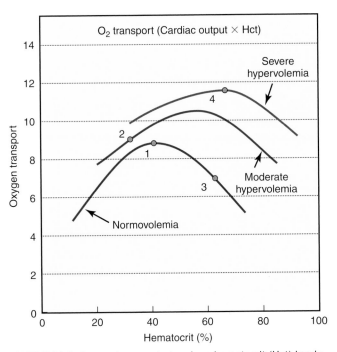

FIGURE 20-3 Oxygen transport at various hematocrit (Hct) levels in normovolemia, mild hypervolemia, and severe hypervolemia. Oxygen transport is estimated by multiplying hematocrit by cardiac output. *(Adapted from Murray JF, Gold P, Johnson BL Jr, et al. Clinical manifestations and classification of erythrocyte disorders. In: Kaushansky K, Lichtman M, Beutler E, et al, eds. Williams Hematology. 8th ed. New York, NY: McGraw-Hill Medical; 2010.)*

fatigability will then occur. Hematocrit levels above 60% can be life threatening because the increase in viscosity threatens organ perfusion. Patients with such high hematocrits are also at risk of venous and arterial thromboses. Forty percent of these patients experience at least one thrombotic event during their illness.

POLYCYTHEMIA VERA

Primary polycythemia, also known as *polycythemia vera* or PV, is a stem cell disorder characterized by proliferation of a clone of hematopoietic precursors, nearly all of which arise from a mutation in the *JAK2* (Janus kinase 2) gene. This clonal expansion most commonly produces an excess of erythrocytes, but numbers of platelets and leukocytes may also be increased. The criteria for a diagnosis of polycythemia vera include an elevated Hb level (>18.5 g/dL in men and >16.5 g/dL in women) and either the presence of the *JAK2* mutation or two of the following: hypercellularity of the bone marrow, a subnormal serum erythropoietin level, and endogenous erythroid colony formation. Polycythemia vera may appear at any age, but most patients develop the disease in their sixth or seventh decade. Patients can have a number of symptoms. Budd-Chiari syndrome is a common presentation, as is generalized pruritus and erythromelalgia. Coronary or cerebral thrombosis can often be the presenting symptom. Pulmonary hypertension occurs with increased frequency in this population. Patients generally require regular phlebotomy and may also require treatment with myelosuppressive drugs such as hydroxyurea to

control the hematocrit. Approximately 30% of patients will die of thrombotic complications and another 30% will succumb to cancer, most commonly, myelofibrosis and acute leukemia.

Patients with PV who are undergoing surgery are at increased risk of perioperative thrombosis and, paradoxically, hemorrhage. The increased risk of thrombosis is due to the predictable combination of baseline hypercoagulability augmented by the prothrombotic state of surgery. Hemorrhage is attributable to an acquired von Willebrand disease caused by abnormally low amounts of the ultralarge von Willebrand factor (vWF) multimers essential to normal platelet adhesion. The hyperviscosity associated with a high hematocrit favors a conformational change in vWF that renders it vulnerable to enzymatic cleavage. Therefore, the most hemostatically effective large multimers become depleted, which creates a risk of bleeding. Phlebotomy and avoidance of dehydration lower the risk of both thrombosis and hemorrhage during the perioperative period.

Management of Anesthesia.
Polycythemia vera patients are at risk for perioperative hypercoagulability and hemorrhage. Reduction of the hematocrit to 45% before surgery may reduce the risk of thrombohemorrhagic complications. Thrombocytosis should be decreased to 400,000 platelets/mm^3 or less. Aspirin therapy should be withheld for 7 days before surgery. Desmopressin and cryoprecipitate are beneficial in improving the levels of vWF and thus can reduce bleeding.

SECONDARY POLYCYTHEMIA DUE TO HYPOXIA

An increase in the RBC mass without evidence of change in other hematopoietic cell lines is a normal physiologic response to hypoxia, regardless of cause. Individuals living at high altitudes up to 7000 ft experience a compensatory polycythemia that is physiologically appropriate and not associated with clinical abnormalities. At higher altitudes, humans are at risk of both acute and chronic mountain sickness, manifested as severe headaches, nausea, vomiting, and disorientation resulting from cerebral edema.

Significant cardiopulmonary disease can also result in enough tissue hypoxia to induce polycythemia. Congenital heart disease with a significant right-to-left shunt and cyanosis is a good example. Extremely low cardiac output, whether congenital or acquired, may stimulate release of erythropoietin and be associated with an increased hematocrit. Pulmonary disease can result in hypoxic polycythemia. Extreme obesity with the development of hypoventilation (pickwickian syndrome) is a classic example. Inherited defects in Hb, such as high-affinity Hb and defects in the amount or function 2,3-DPG, may cause polycythemia resulting from reduced tissue oxygen delivery and a leftward shift in the oxyhemoglobin dissociation curve. Defects or drugs producing significant methemoglobinemia can also lead to a compensatory polycythemia. Individuals with disorders causing methemoglobinemia are distinguished by their *pseudocyanotic* appearance, which results from the brownish color of the ferric Hb because of its inability to reflect red light upon oxygenation.

SECONDARY POLYCYTHEMIA DUE TO INCREASED ERYTHROPOIETIN PRODUCTION

Renal disease and several erythropoietin-secreting tumors have been associated with secondary polycythemia. Hydronephrosis, polycystic kidney disease, renal cysts, and both benign and malignant renal tumors can result in increased erythropoietin production. Uterine myomas, hepatomas, and cerebellar hemangiomas have also been shown capable of secreting erythropoietin. After renal transplantation, patients can develop erythrocytosis that is unrelated to erythropoietin production. Angiotensin-converting enzyme inhibitors will reverse this polycythemia. Surreptitious use of recombinant erythropoietin by high-performance athletes also produces polycythemia.

Management of Anesthesia in Secondary Polycythemia

Management of patients with secondary polycythemia varies depending on the specific cause. Patients with mild hypoxic polycythemia require no specific treatment. In patients with a very high hematocrit, phlebotomy may be indicated to reduce the thrombotic and hemorrhagic complications of the disorder.

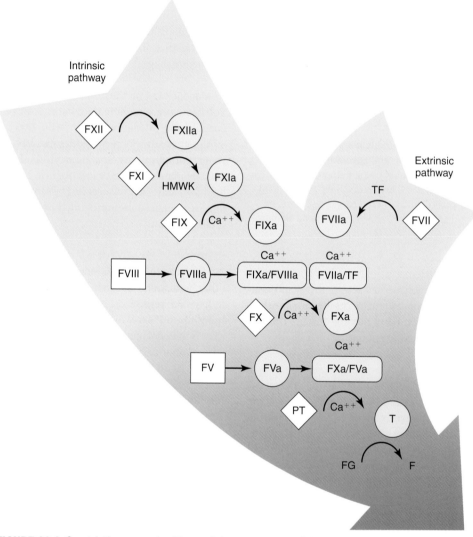

FIGURE 20-4 Coagulation cascade. Glycoprotein components of the intrinsic pathway include factors XII, XI, IX, VIII, X, and V; prothrombin; and fibrinogen. Glycoprotein components of the extrinsic pathway, initiated by the action of tissue factor located on cell surfaces, include factors VII, X, and V; prothrombin; and fibrinogen. Cascade reactions culminate in the conversion of fibrinogen to fibrin and the formation of a fibrin clot. Certain reactions, including activation of factor X and prothrombin, take place on membrane surfaces. Diamonds indicate proenzymes; squares indicate pro-cofactors; circles indicate enzymes and cofactors; shaded rectangles indicate macromolecular complexes on membrane surfaces. *F*, Fibrin; *FG*, fibrinogen; *HMWK*, high-molecular-weight kininogen; *PT*, prothrombin; *T*, thrombin; *TF*, tissue factor. *(From Furie B, Furie BC. Molecular basis of blood coagulation. In: Hoffman R, Benz EJ, Shattil SJ, et al, eds.* Hematology: Basic Principles and Practice. *5th ed. Philadelphia, PA: Churchill Livingstone; 2009:Fig 118-1.)*

DISORDERS OF HEMOSTASIS

Normal Hemostasis

Any disruption of vascular endothelium is a potent stimulus to clot formation. As a localized process, clotting acts to seal the break in vascular continuity, limit blood loss, and begin the process of wound healing. Prevention of an exuberant response that would result in pathologic thrombosis relies on several counterbalancing mechanisms, including the anticoagulant properties of intact endothelial cells, circulating inhibitors of activated coagulation factors, and localized fibrinolytic enzymes. Most abnormalities in hemostasis involve a defect in one or more of the steps in the coagulation process. It is important, therefore, to understand the physiology of hemostasis.

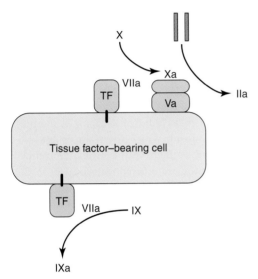

FIGURE 20-5 Initiation phase of the blood coagulation cascade. *TF,* Tissue factor. *(From Hoffmann M. Remodeling the blood coagulation cascade. J Thromb Thrombolysis. 2003;16[1-2]:17-20, Fig 2.)*

FIGURE 20-6 Amplification phase of the blood coagulation cascade. *TF,* Tissue factor; *TFPI,* tissue factor pathway inhibitor; *vWF,* von Willebrand factor. *(From Hoffmann M. Remodeling the blood coagulation cascade. J Thromb Thrombolysis. 2003;16[1-2]:17-20, Fig 3.)*

The cascade model of coagulation described 60 years ago consists of an extrinsic and an intrinsic pathway (Figure 20-4). The extrinsic system was represented by factor VIIa and tissue factor. By contrast, the intrinsic system was thought to be entirely intravascular. Both pathways could activate factor X, which, in complex with factor Va, could convert prothrombin to thrombin. The prothrombin time (PT) used to guide warfarin (Coumadin) therapy reflects the extrinsic pathway, whereas the activated partial thromboplastin time (aPTT) used to guide heparin therapy reflects the intrinsic pathway. Although this model correlates well with clotting assays, it does not accurately represent in vivo clotting.

In vivo coagulation follows exposure of blood to a source of tissue factor, typically from subendothelial cells, following damage to a blood vessel. The intrinsic, or contact, pathway of coagulation has no role in this earliest clotting event. Tissue factor–initiated coagulation has three phases: an *initiation* phase, an *amplification* phase, and a *propagation* phase.

The initiation phase begins as exposed tissue factor binds to factor VIIa (Figure 20-5). This factor VIIa–tissue factor complex catalyzes the conversion of small amounts of factor X to Xa, which in turn generates similarly small amounts of thrombin. During the amplification phase platelets, factor V, and factor XI are activated by the small amount of thrombin (Figure 20-6). The propagation phase is initiated by the activation of factor X by factors VIII and IX and calcium on the platelet surface (Figure 20-7). During this phase thrombin increases its own formation by activating platelets and factors V and VIII, which sets the stage for formation of the factor VIIIa-IXa complex. Formation of this complex allows factor Xa generation to switch from a reaction catalyzed by the factor VIIa–tissue factor complex to one produced by the intrinsic tenase (Xase) pathway. This switch is

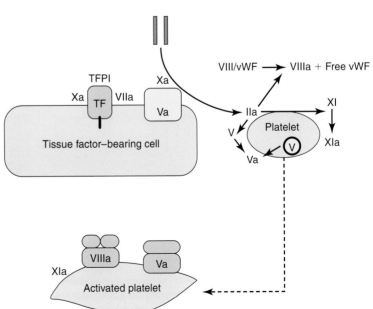
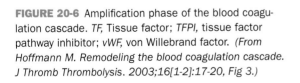

of enormous kinetic advantage, since the intrinsic Xase complex is 50 times more efficient at factor Xa generation. The bleeding diathesis associated with hemophilia, with its intact initiation phase and absent propagation phase, is evidence of the hemostatic importance of the propagation phase.

Commonly used laboratory tests of soluble coagulation factors measure only the kinetics of the initiation phase. The PT and aPTT both have as end points the first appearance of fibrin gel. This occurs after completion of less than 5% of the total reaction. These tests are sensitive in detecting severe deficiencies in clotting factors, such as hemophilia, and in guiding warfarin or heparin therapy. However, they do not model the sequence of events necessary for actual hemostasis and do not necessarily predict the risk of intraoperative bleeding.

In the venous circulation, the kinetic advantage of the coagulation cascade assembly on the platelet surface is readily apparent. However, relatively small numbers of platelets are needed to fulfill this function. To increase the risk of venous bleeding, the platelet count must decrease to very low levels, that is, fewer than 10,000/mm³. This contrasts sharply with the arterial circulation, in which the minimum platelet count needed to ensure hemostasis for surgery is at least five times that number.

Hemostatic Disorders Affecting Coagulation Factors of the Initiation Phase

Table 20-2 lists both inherited and acquired hemostatic disorders.

FACTOR VII DEFICIENCY
Hereditary deficiency of factor VII is a rare autosomal recessive disease with highly variable penetrance and clinical severity. Only patients with the homozygous deficiency have factor VII levels low enough (<15%) to have symptomatic bleeding.

These patients are easily recognized by their laboratory pattern of a prolonged PT but normal partial thromboplastin time (PTT).

Management of Anesthesia
The treatment of a single-factor deficiency depends on the severity of the deficiency. For surgery, factor levels of 20% to 25% provide adequate hemostasis. Several products are available to treat factor VII deficiency. Patients with factor VII levels of less than 1% generally require treatment with a concentrated source of factor VII. The preferred product for prophylaxis in patients with factor VII deficiency is Proplex T (factor IX complex) because it contains high levels of factor VII. Factor VII deficiency with active bleeding is treated with either Proplex T, factor VII concentrate, or the activated form of factor VII, recombinant factor VIIa. Patients with mild to moderate factor VII deficiency can be treated with infusion of fresh frozen plasma. Prothrombin complex concentrate can also be used, but it carries a high risk of thrombosis.

CONGENITAL DEFICIENCIES IN FACTOR X, FACTOR V, AND PROTHROMBIN (FACTOR II)
Congenital deficiencies in factor X, factor V, and prothrombin are inherited as autosomal recessive traits, and severe deficiencies are quite rare. Patients with a severe deficiency in any of these factors demonstrate prolongation of both the PT and PTT. Patients with factor V deficiency may also have a prolonged bleeding time because of the relationship between factor V and platelet function in supporting clot formation.

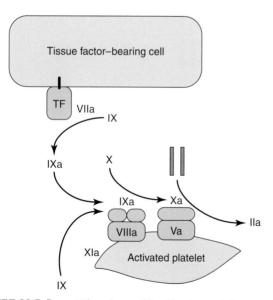

FIGURE 20-7 Propagation phase of the blood coagulation cascade. *TF,* Tissue factor. *(From Hoffmann M. Remodeling the blood coagulation cascade. J Thromb Thrombolysis. 2003;16[1-2]:17-20, Fig 4.)*

TABLE 20-2 ■ Categorization of coagulation disorders

HEREDITARY CAUSES

Hemophilia A
Hemophilia B
Von Willebrand's disease
Afibrinogenemia
Factor V deficiency
Factor VIII deficiency
Hereditary hemorrhagic telangiectasia
Protein C deficiency
Antithrombin III deficiency

ACQUIRED CAUSES

Disseminated intravascular coagulation
Perioperative anticoagulation
Intraoperative coagulopathies
Dilutional thrombocytopenia
Dilution of procoagulants
Massive blood transfusions
Certain types of surgery (cardiopulmonary bypass, brain surgery, orthopedic surgery, urologic surgery, obstetric delivery)
Drug-induced hemorrhage
Drug-induced platelet dysfunction
Idiopathic thrombocytopenic purpura
Thrombotic thrombocytopenic purpura
Catheter-induced thrombocytopenia
Vitamin K deficiency

Management of Anesthesia

Deficiencies in factor X, factor V, and prothrombin can be corrected with fresh frozen plasma. To obtain a significant increase in the level of any factor, a considerable volume of fresh frozen plasma must be infused. As a rule of thumb, 10 to 15 mL/kg of fresh frozen plasma is needed to obtain a 20% to 30% increase in the level of any missing factor. This represents a considerable volume of plasma and may present a significant cardiovascular challenge to some patients. The duration of effectiveness of this replacement therapy depends on the turnover time of each factor, which then dictates how often a repeat infusion of fresh frozen plasma will be needed. Factor V is stored in platelet granules, and in a bleeding patient platelet transfusion is an alternative way to deliver missing factor V to the site of bleeding.

For factor X, factor V, and prothrombin deficiency in patients facing surgery with a significant risk of blood loss, several prothrombin complex concentrates are available. The advantage of these products is that factor levels of 50% or more can be achieved without the risk of volume overload. The disadvantages of prothrombin complex concentrates are significant, however, and include the risk of inducing widespread thrombosis, thromboembolism, and disseminated intravascular coagulation. It is also important to recognize the variation in factor levels in the different products.

Hemostatic Disorders Affecting Coagulation Factors of the Propagation Phase

Defects in the propagation phase of coagulation are associated with a significant bleeding tendency. Some of these propagation phase defects are detected by an isolated prolongation of the aPTT. The X-linked recessive disorders hemophilia A and B are the principal examples of this type of abnormality. A marked reduction in either factor VIII or factor IX is associated with spontaneous and excessive hemorrhage, especially hemarthroses and muscle hematomas. A deficiency in factor XI also prolongs the aPTT but typically results in a less severe bleeding tendency.

Not all factor deficiencies causing prolongation of the aPTT are associated with bleeding. The initial activation stimulus for this laboratory test is surface contact activation of factor XII (Hageman's factor) to produce XIIa. This reaction is facilitated by the presence of high-molecular-weight kininogen and the conversion of prekallikrein to the active protease kallikrein. Deficiency in any of these three factors causes prolongation of the aPTT. However, these contact activation factors play no role in either the initiation phase or the propagation phase of clotting in vivo. Thus, deficiencies of factor XII, high-molecular-weight kininogen, and prekallikrein are *not* associated with clinical bleeding. Patients with deficiencies of these particular factors require no special management.

CONGENITAL FACTOR VIII DEFICIENCY: HEMOPHILIA A

The factor VIII gene is a very large gene on the X chromosome. Patients with the most severe hemophilia generally have an inversion or deletion of major portions of the X chromosome genome or a missense mutation resulting in factor VIII activity of less than 1% of normal. Other mutations, including point mutations and minor deletions, generally result in milder disease with factor VIII levels above 1%. In some patients, a functionally abnormal protein is produced, which causes a discrepancy between results on the immunologic assay of factor VIII antigen and results on the coagulation test of factor VIII activity.

The clinical severity of hemophilia A is best correlated with the factor VIII activity level. Patients with severe hemophilia have factor VIII activity levels that are less than 1% of normal and are usually diagnosed during childhood because of frequent, spontaneous hemorrhage into joints, muscles, and vital organs. They require frequent treatment with factor VIII replacement.

Factor VIII levels as low as 1% to 5% of normal are enough to reduce the severity of hemophilia, but these patients are still at increased risk of hemorrhage with surgery or trauma. They have much less difficulty with spontaneous hemarthroses or hematomas, however. Patients with factor levels of 6% to 30% have only mild disease that may go undiagnosed well into adult life. Nevertheless, they are at risk for excessive bleeding when undergoing a major surgical procedure. Female carriers of hemophilia A can also be at risk of excessive surgical bleeding. About 10% of female carriers have factor VIII activity of less than 30%.

Patients with severe hemophilia A have a significantly prolonged aPTT, whereas in those with milder disease, the aPTT may be only a few seconds longer than normal. The PT is normal.

Management of Anesthesia

Whenever major surgery is necessary in a patient with hemophilia A, the factor VIII level must be brought to near normal (100%) for the procedure. This requires an infusion of factor VIII concentrate. Since the half-life of factor VIII is approximately 12 hours in adults, repeated infusions every 8 to 12 hours will be needed to keep the factor VIII level above 50%. In children, the half-life of factor VIII may be as short as 6 hours, which requires more frequent infusions and laboratory assays to confirm efficacy. Peak and trough factor VIII levels should be measured to confirm the appropriate amount of factor VIII to be infused and the dosing interval. Therapy must be continued for up to 2 weeks to avoid postoperative bleeding that disrupts wound healing. Even longer periods of therapy may be required in patients who undergo bone or joint surgery. In this situation, 4 to 6 weeks of replacement therapy may be needed.

Up to 30% of patients with severe hemophilia A who are exposed to factor VIII concentrate or recombinant product will eventually develop inhibitor antibodies.

Fresh frozen plasma and cryoprecipitate can both be used to correct factor VIII levels. For patients with mild hemophilia desmopressin can also be administered either intravenously or intranasally. Fibrinolytic inhibitors, such as ε-aminocaproic acid (EACA) and tranexamic acid, can be given as adjunctive therapy for bleeding from mucous membranes and are particularly useful for dental procedures.

CONGENITAL FACTOR IX DEFICIENCY: HEMOPHILIA B

Patients with hemophilia B have a clinical spectrum of disease similar to that found in hemophilia A. Factor IX levels of less than 1% of normal are associated with severe bleeding, whereas more moderate disease is seen in patients with levels of 1% to 5%. Patients with factor IX levels of between 5% and 40% generally have very mild disease. Milder hemophilia (>5% factor IX activity) may not be detected until surgery is performed or the patient has a dental extraction. Similar to the laboratory findings in hemophilia A, patients with hemophilia B have a prolonged aPTT and a normal PT.

Management of Anesthesia

General guidelines for management of patients with hemophilia B do not differ significantly from those for management of hemophilia A patients. Recombinant or purified product or factor IX–prothrombin complex concentrates are used to treat mild bleeding episodes or administered as prophylaxis for minor surgery. Caution is needed when using factor IX–prothrombin complex concentrates. These agents can contain activated clotting factors. When given in amounts sufficient to increase factor IX levels to 50% or more, there is an increased risk of thromboembolic complications, especially in patients undergoing orthopedic procedures. Therefore, it is essential to use only recombinant factor IX to treat patients undergoing major orthopedic surgery and those with severe traumatic injuries or liver disease.

Purified factor IX concentrates or recombinant factor IX is used for several days to treat bleeding in patients with hemophilia B. Because of absorption into collagen sites in the vasculature, factor IX is less available than factor VIII, so that dosing is approximately double that for factor VIII concentrates. Factor IX has a half-life of 18 to 24 hours, so repeat infusion at 50% of the original dose every 12 to 24 hours is usually sufficient to keep the factor IX plasma level above 50%.

ACQUIRED FACTOR VIII OR IX INHIBITORS

Patients with hemophilia A are at significant risk of developing circulating inhibitors to factor VIII. This occurs in 30% to 40% of patients severely deficient in factor VIII. Patients with hemophilia B are less likely to develop inhibitors to factor IX. Only 3% to 5% of these patients develop inhibitors during their lifetime. A severe hemophilia-like syndrome can occur in genetically normal individuals because of the appearance of an acquired autoantibody to either factor VIII or factor IX. These patients are usually middle-aged or older with no personal or family history of abnormal bleeding who experience the sudden onset of severe, spontaneous hemorrhage.

A test known as a *mixing study* is required to detect the presence of an inhibitor. This study is performed by mixing *patient* plasma and *normal* plasma in a 1:1 ratio to determine whether the prolonged PTT shortens. The mixing study for a patient with classic hemophilia A who has a deficiency of factor VIII activity but no circulating factor VIII inhibitor will usually show a shortening of the PTT to within 4 seconds or less of the normal value. In contrast, in a patient with a factor VIII inhibitor, the PTT will not be corrected to that extent, if at all.

Management of Anesthesia

Management of a hemophilia A patient with circulating factor VIII inhibitors will vary according to whether the patient is a high or low responder. Low responders have low titers of inhibitors and do not show anamnestic responses to factor VIII concentrates. High responders have high titers of inhibitors and have dramatic anamnestic responses to therapy. Patients in the low-responder category can usually be managed with factor VIII concentrates. Larger initial and maintenance dosages of factor VIII are required, and frequent assays of factor VIII levels are essential to guide therapy. High responders cannot be treated with factor VIII concentrate. Major hemorrhage can be managed with "bypass" products such as activated prothrombin complex concentrates or recombinant factor VIIa. Recombinant factor VIIa is becoming the treatment of choice for patients with acquired inhibitors. Although the thrombin formed via factor VIIa is not as strong as that seen with factor VIII therapy, recombinant factor VIIa therapy is successful in controlling bleeding in more than 80% of patients with factor VIII inhibitors.

Hemophilia B patients with factor IX inhibitors can be managed in acute situations using recombinant VIIa or a prothrombin complex concentrate.

Patients who develop an autoantibody to factor VIII or IX without a history of hemophilia can experience life-threatening hemorrhage and may exhibit very high inhibitor levels. Treatment with recombinant factor VIIa or an activated prothrombin concentrate is required. Administration of factor VIII or IX alone will *not* be effective.

FACTOR XI DEFICIENCY

The only other coagulation factor defect causing an isolated prolongation of the PTT and a bleeding tendency is factor XI deficiency (Rosenthal's disease). It is inherited as an autosomal recessive trait. Factor XI deficiency is much rarer than either hemophilia A or B, but it affects up to 5% of Jews of Ashkenazi descent from Eastern Europe. Generally, the bleeding tendency is quite mild and may be apparent only following a surgical procedure. Hematomas and hemarthroses are very unusual, even in those patients with factor XI levels of less than 5%.

Management of Anesthesia

The treatment of factor XI deficiency depends on the severity of the deficiency and the bleeding history. Most patients can be treated with infusion of fresh frozen plasma. Treatment of patients with factor XI deficiency with active bleeding includes administration of prothrombin complex concentrates or recombinant factor VIIa with redosing according to PT results.

CONGENITAL ABNORMALITIES IN FIBRINOGEN

Hypofibrinogenemia and Afibrinogenemia. Congenital abnormalities in fibrinogen production interfere with the final step in the generation of a fibrin clot. Disorders with decreased fibrinogen levels, either *hypofibrinogenemia* or *afibrinogenemia,* are relatively rare conditions inherited as autosomal recessive traits. Patients with afibrinogenemia have a severe bleeding diathesis with both spontaneous and posttraumatic bleeding. The bleeding can begin during the first few days of life, and this condition may be initially confused with hemophilia. Hypofibrinogenemic patients usually do not have spontaneous bleeding but may have bleeding with surgery. Severe bleeding can be anticipated in patients with plasma fibrinogen levels of less than 50 to 100 mg/dL.

Dysfibrinogenemia

Production of an abnormal fibrinogen is a more common defect than very low levels of fibrinogen. Fibrinogen is synthesized in the liver under the control of three genes on chromosome 4. More than 300 different mutations producing dysfunctional and, at times, reduced amounts of fibrinogen have been reported. Many of these mutations are inherited as autosomal dominant traits. The clinical presentation of *dysfibrinogenemia* is highly variable. Patients who have both a reduced amount of fibrinogen and a dysfunctional fibrinogen (*hypodysfibrinogenemia*) usually have excessive bleeding. Most dysfibrinogenemic patients have abnormal results on coagulation tests but do not have a clinical bleeding tendency. Overall, approximately 60% of dysfibrinogenemias are clinically silent. The remainder can present with either a bleeding diathesis or, paradoxically, a thrombotic tendency. A small number of dysfibrinogenemias have been associated with spontaneous abortion and poor wound healing.

Laboratory evaluation of fibrinogen involves measurement of both concentration and function of fibrinogen. The most accurate quantitative measurement of total fibrinogen protein is provided by immunoassay or a protein precipitation technique. Other screening tests for fibrinogen dysfunction include the thrombin time and clotting time using a venom enzyme such as reptilase.

Management of Anesthesia

Most patients with dysfibrinogenemia have no clinical disease. Those who are symptomatic and at risk of bleeding during or after surgery require treatment with cryoprecipitate. To increase the fibrinogen level by at least 100 mg/dL in the average-size adult, 10 to 12 units of cryoprecipitate must be infused, followed by 2 to 3 units each day. Dysfibrinogenemia patients with a thrombotic tendency require long-term anticoagulant therapy.

FACTOR XIII DEFICIENCY

Stability of the fibrin clot is hemostatically important. Deficiency of factor XIII (fibrin-stabilizing factor) is a rare autosomal recessive disorder. Patients have persistent umbilical or circumcision bleeding at birth. Patients demonstrate a severe bleeding diathesis characterized by recurrent soft tissue bleeding, poor wound healing, and a high incidence of intracranial hemorrhage. Blood clots form but are weak and unable to maintain hemostasis. Fetal loss in women with factor XIII deficiency approaches 100%.

Factor XIII deficiency should be considered in a patient with a severe bleeding diathesis who has normal results on coagulation screening tests, including PT, PTT, fibrinogen level, platelet count, and bleeding time. Clot dissolution in urea can be used as a screening test. Patients at risk of severe hemorrhage have factor XIII levels of 1% of normal. Those with factor XIII levels of approximately 50% usually exhibit no bleeding tendency.

Management of Anesthesia

Factor XIII–deficient patients can be treated with fresh frozen plasma, cryoprecipitate, or a plasma-derived factor XIII concentrate. Factor XIII has a long circulating half-life of 7 to 12 days, and adequate hemostasis is achieved with even very low plasma concentrations (1% to 3%).

ARTERIAL COAGULATION

Disorders Affecting Platelet Number

The normal circulating platelet count is maintained within relatively narrow limits. Approximately one third of platelets are sequestered in the spleen at any given time. Since a platelet has a life span of approximately 9 to 10 days, some 15,000 to 45,000 platelets/mm^3 must be produced each day to maintain a steady state.

MANAGEMENT OF ANESTHESIA: GENERAL CONCEPTS FOR THROMBOCYTOPENIA

Regardless of the cause of thrombocytopenia, platelet transfusions are appropriate if the patient is experiencing a life-threatening hemorrhage, is bleeding into a closed space such as the cranium, or requires emergency surgery. Long-term management of thrombocytopenia requires other therapeutic maneuvers either to improve platelet production or to decrease platelet destruction.

Platelet transfusion therapy must be tailored to the severity of the thrombocytopenia, the presence of bleeding complications, and the patient's underlying disorder. For minor surgery the platelet count should be more than 20,000 to 30,000/mm^3. For major surgery the platelet count should be increased to 50,000/mm^3. However, for neurosurgical procedures platelets should be increased to 100,000/mm^3. Each unit of single-donor apheresis platelets or 6 units of random-donor platelets increases the platelet count in a normal-sized adult by approximately 50,000/mm^3. If there is alloimmunization or increased platelet consumption, measurement of platelet counts 1 hour after transfusion and at frequent intervals is important in planning further platelet transfusion needs.

One unit of single-donor apheresis platelets is equivalent to a random-donor pool of 4 to 8 units. For patients who become alloimmunized to random-donor platelets, blood banks can provide HLA-matched single-donor platelets. Random- and single-donor platelets do not need to be ABO compatible. However, sufficient RBCs are transfused in the platelet pool to increase the risk of sensitization in Rh-negative patients. Therefore, such patients, particularly women of childbearing age, should receive platelets from Rh-negative donors or be treated with Rh0(D) immune globulin (RhoGAM) following transfusion of Rh-positive product.

Patients with very low platelet counts, usually less than 15,000/mm³, can experience significant bleeding from multiple sites including the nose, mucous membranes, gastrointestinal tract, skin, and vessel puncture sites. One sign that strongly suggests thrombocytopenia is the appearance of a petechial rash involving the skin or mucous membranes. This condition is usually most pronounced over the lower extremities because of the increased hydrostatic pressure there. The differential diagnosis of thrombocytopenia is best organized according to the physiology of (1) platelet production, (2) distribution in the circulation, and (3) platelet destruction.

Disorders Resulting in Platelet Production Defects: Congenital

Platelet production disorders may be caused by megakaryocyte aplasia or hypoplasia in the bone marrow.

THROMBOCYTOPENIA–ABSENT RADIUS SYNDROME

Congenital hypoplastic thrombocytopenia with absent radii (*TAR syndrome*) is usually inherited in an autosomal recessive manner. Thrombocytopenia develops in the third trimester or soon after birth. The thrombocytopenia is initially severe (<30,000 platelets/mm³), but slowly improves over time, approaching the normal range by age 2. These patients often have bilateral radial anomalies, and abnormalities of other bones may also occur.

FANCONI'S ANEMIA

The hematologic manifestations of *Fanconi's anemia* do not usually appear until about 7 years of age. The bone marrow shows reduced cellularity and reduced numbers of megakaryocytes. Stem cell transplantation is curative in the majority of children once severe bone marrow failure has developed.

MAY-HEGGLIN ANOMALY

Patients with *May-Hegglin anomaly* typically have giant platelets in the circulation and Döhle's bodies (basophilic inclusions) in white blood cells. Platelet production is variably ineffective, with one third of patients having significant thrombocytopenia.

WISKOTT-ALDRICH SYNDROME

Wiskott-Aldrich syndrome is an X-linked disorder that presents with a combination of eczema, immunodeficiency, and thrombocytopenia. Circulating platelets are smaller than normal, function poorly because of granule defects, and have a reduced survival. Ineffective thrombopoiesis is the principal abnormality.

AUTOSOMAL DOMINANT THROMBOCYTOPENIA

Patients with *autosomal dominant thrombocytopenia* show an increased megakaryocyte mass but ineffective platelet production and release of macrocytic platelets into the circulation. Many of these patients also have nerve deafness and nephritis (*Alport's syndrome*).

Disorders Resulting in Platelet Production Defects: Acquired

A failure in platelet production can result from bone marrow damage. All aspects of normal hematopoiesis can be depressed, even to the point of bone marrow aplasia (aplastic anemia). Reductions in the marrow megakaryocyte mass are seen in response to radiation therapy or cancer chemotherapy, as a result of exposure to toxic chemicals (benzene, insecticides) or alcohol, and as a complication of viral hepatitis. Infiltration of the bone marrow by a malignant process can also disrupt thrombopoiesis. Hematopoietic malignancies, including multiple myeloma, acute leukemia, lymphoma, and myeloproliferative disorders, frequently produce platelet production defects.

Ineffective thrombopoiesis can also be seen in patients with vitamin B_{12} or folate deficiency (caused by alcoholism) and defective folate metabolism. Marrow megakaryocyte mass is increased, but effective platelet production is reduced. This failure of platelet production is rapidly reversed by appropriate vitamin therapy.

MANAGEMENT OF ANESTHESIA

Platelet transfusions are a mainstay in the management of patients with platelet production disorders. Patients with ineffective thrombopoiesis secondary to an intrinsic abnormality of megakaryocytes are treated similarly to those with a production disorder when there is need for urgent surgery. Ineffective thrombopoiesis associated with either vitamin B_{12} or folate deficiency should be treated with appropriate vitamin therapy. Recovery of the platelet count to normal occurs within days, which makes platelet transfusion unnecessary in all but the most acute situations.

Platelet Destruction Disorders: Nonimmune

Platelet consumption as a part of intravascular coagulation is seen in several clinical settings. If the entire coagulation pathway is activated, the process is referred to as *disseminated intravascular coagulation* (DIC). DIC can be dramatic, with severe thrombocytopenia and marked prolongation of results on coagulation factor assays, accompanied by bleeding, or it can be low grade, with little or no thrombocytopenia and less tendency for bleeding. Platelet consumption can also occur as an isolated process, so-called *platelet DIC*. Viral infection, bacteremia, malignancy, high-dose chemotherapy, and vasculitis can result in sufficient endothelial cell damage to dramatically increase the rate of platelet clearance without full activation of the coagulation pathway. Basically, this is an accentuation of the normal blood vessel repair process in which platelets adhere to exposed subendothelial surfaces and then aggregate with fibrinogen binding. With marked endothelial disruption, enough platelets can be consumed to result in thrombocytopenia. Blood vessel occlusion by formation of platelet thrombi is unusual but can occur with severe vasculitis. Patients with acquired immunodeficiency syndrome (AIDS) can develop a consumptive thrombocytopenia with end-organ damage secondary to arterial thrombosis.

Thrombotic thrombocytopenic purpura, hemolytic uremic syndrome, and HELLP syndrome (*h*emolysis, *e*levated
*l*iver enzymes, and *l*ow *p*latelet count) are the most important
examples of nonimmune platelet destruction. Although the
underlying pathophysiologies of these disorders are distinctly
different, these entities can lead to thrombus formation and
end-organ damage.

THROMBOTIC THROMBOCYTOPENIC PURPURA

Thrombotic thrombocytopenic purpura (TTP) is characterized by formation of platelet-rich thrombi in the arterial and
capillary microvasculature, leading to thrombocytopenia and
microangiopathic hemolytic anemia. Although this disease
was classically described as a complex of five symptoms and
signs—fever, renal failure, thrombocytopenia, microangiopathic hemolytic anemia, and neurologic symptoms—not all
of these are present in all patients with TTP. The presence of
thrombocytopenia and microangiopathic hemolytic anemia
(the latter documented by the findings of anemia, schistocy-
tosis, reticulocytosis, decreased haptoglobin level, increased
LDH level, and a negative result on Coombs' test) are considered sufficient for the diagnosis of TTP in the absence of other
possible explanations. TTP can occur as a familial disease, a
sporadic illness without apparent cause (idiopathic), a chronic
relapsing condition, or a complication of marrow transplantation or treatment with certain drugs (quinine, ticlopidine,
mitomycin C, interferon-α, pentostatin, gemcitabine, tacrolimus, and cyclosporine). Preeclampsia with HELLP syndrome
in pregnant women can evolve into TTP postpartum.

TTP is an excellent example of increased platelet destruction secondary to activation, aggregation, and thrombus
formation. The underlying mechanism in familial or cyclic
disease involves a deficiency of vWF-cleaving protease activity secondary to an inherited mutation of the gene that results
in persistent circulation of ultralarge vWF multimers. Plasma
exchange is effective in removing some of these multimers
and returning the vWF-cleaving protease activity to normal. Cases refractory to plasma exchange may respond to
immunosuppression.

HEMOLYTIC UREMIC SYNDROME

Hemolytic uremic syndrome (HUS) is a disorder similar to TTP
that is most often seen in children who come for treatment of
bloody diarrhea secondary to infection with a particular strain
of *Escherichia coli* or related bacteria that produce Shiga-like
toxin. Acute renal failure dominates the presentation. Thrombocytopenia and anemia are less pronounced than with TTP,
and neurologic signs are absent. These patients do not need
plasmapheresis or fresh frozen plasma therapy. Most children
recover spontaneously but may require hemodialysis for some
period. The mortality rate is less than 5%. Adults infected with
this strain of *E. coli* can have features of both HUS and TTP
but usually with less renal involvement. Since the mortality
rate in older children and adults is higher than that in young
children, they should be treated with plasma exchange and
hemodialysis, regardless of the pattern of their illness.

HELLP SYNDROME

Thrombocytopenia is a frequent complication of pregnancy.
Mild thrombocytopenia (platelet counts between 70,000 and
150,000/mm³) is seen in 6% to 7% of women nearing delivery
and represents a physiologic change similar to the dilutional
anemia of pregnancy. Thrombocytopenia associated with
hypertension is observed in 1% to 2% of pregnancies, and
as many as 50% of mothers with preeclampsia will develop
a DIC-like condition with severe thrombocytopenia (platelet
counts of 20,000 to 40,000/mm³) at the time of delivery. This
is referred to as *HELLP syndrome* when the combination of
red cell hemolysis (H), elevated liver enzyme levels (EL), and
low platelet count (LP) is present. Physiologically, HELLP syndrome resembles TTP. Control of the hypertension and completion of the delivery is usually enough to bring the process
to a halt. However, a few patients will go on to develop TTP–
HUS following delivery. Postpartum TTP is a life-threatening
illness with a poor prognosis. Treatment with both plasma
exchange and intravenous immunoglobulin has yielded variable results.

MANAGEMENT OF ANESTHESIA IN NONIMMUNE PLATELET DESTRUCTION DISORDERS

Proper management of patients with platelet destruction disorders depends on the diagnosis. In individuals who have
nonimmune destruction as a part of DIC, platelet and plasma
transfusions are supportive therapy. The only truly effective
therapy is treatment of the underlying cause of the DIC. If the
primary condition can be corrected, levels of coagulation factors and platelet counts will recover.

Patients with TTP or HUS should receive platelet transfusions only for life-threatening bleeding. With TTP or HUS
there is the potential for significant harm from platelet transfusion, since transfusion may lead to increased thrombosis
and end-organ damage secondary to marked platelet aggregation and activation. Surgery should be delayed whenever possible until the underlying disorder is controlled.

HUS and HELLP syndrome present a different therapeutic
challenge. HUS in children can usually be managed without
plasmapheresis, although dialysis may be necessary if renal
failure is severe. HELLP syndrome, like preeclampsia, usually
resolves with delivery of the fetus. However, a small number
of women will develop to a TTP-like syndrome postpartum.
These patients should be treated with plasma exchange. The
response to treatment is generally poor once end-organ damage has occurred.

Platelet Destruction Disorders: Autoimmune

Thrombocytopenia is a common manifestation of autoimmune disease. The severity of the thrombocytopenia is highly
variable. In some conditions, the platelet count falls to as
low as 1000 to 2000/mm³. In other patients, the ability of the
megakaryocytes to increase platelet production results in a
compensated state with platelet counts ranging from 20,000/
mm³ to near-normal levels.

The diagnosis of immune platelet destruction can usually be made from the clinical presentation, the findings of an increased number of reticulated (RNA-containing) platelets in blood, and demonstration of an increase in marrow megakaryocyte number and ploidy. Expansion of the megakaryocyte mass is evidence that platelet production is increasing markedly in an attempt to compensate for the shortened survival of the platelets in the circulation.

THROMBOCYTOPENIC PURPURA IN ADULTS

The differential diagnosis of autoimmune thrombocytopenia in adults begins with taking a thorough history to identify any exposure to potentially toxic drugs, receipt of blood products, or viral infection.

Posttransfusion Purpura

Adults can develop posttransfusion purpura following exposure to a blood product, most often RBCs or platelets. Although multiparous women negative for platelet antigen A1 are at greatest risk, posttransfusion purpura has been reported in both men and women. Usually, a potent alloantibody with platelet antigen A1 specificity is readily detected in the plasma.

Drug-Induced Autoimmune Thrombocytopenic Purpura

Several drugs can produce immune thrombocytopenia. Quinine, quinidine, and sedormid are the best known and have been studied extensively. Clinically, patients show severe thrombocytopenia, with platelet counts of less than 20,000/mm^3. These drugs act as haptens to trigger antibody formation and then serve as obligate molecules for antibody binding to the platelet surface. Thrombocytopenia can also occur within hours of the first exposure to a drug because of preformed antibodies. This has been reported with varying frequency (0% to 13%) with abciximab (ReoPro) and other glycoprotein IIb/IIIa inhibitors. Other drugs, such as α-methyldopa, sulfonamides, and gold salts, also stimulate autoantibodies.

Heparin-Induced Thrombocytopenia. The association of heparin with thrombocytopenia deserves special discussion. Heparin-induced thrombocytopenia (HIT) can take one of several forms. A modest decrease in the platelet count, HIT type 1 (*nonimmune HIT*) may be observed in a majority of patients within the first day of therapy with full-dose unfractionated heparin. This condition relates to passive heparin binding to platelets, which results in a modest shortening of the platelet life span. The effect is transient and clinically insignificant.

A second form of HIT, HIT type 2 (*immune-mediated HIT*), is more important. In this type of HIT, antibodies form to the heparin–platelet factor 4 complex, and these are capable of binding to platelet receptors and inducing platelet activation and aggregation. Platelet activation results in further release of heparin–platelet factor 4 and the appearance of platelet microparticles in the circulation. Both of these phenomena magnify the procoagulant state. In addition, heparin–platelet factor 4 complex binds to endothelial cells and stimulates thrombin production. This leads to both an increased clearance of platelets with resultant thrombocytopenia and venous and/or arterial thrombus formation, with the potential for severe end-organ damage and the potential for thromboses in unusual sites, such as the adrenal gland, the portal vein, and the skin.

The incidence of HIT type 2 varies with the type and dose of heparin and the duration of therapy. Between 10% and 15% of patients receiving *bovine* unfractionated heparin develop an antibody. Fewer than 6% of patients receiving *porcine* heparin develop antibodies. The risk of heparin-induced thrombosis is lower than the incidence of antibody formation. Fewer than 10% of those who develop an antibody to the heparin–platelet factor 4 complex will experience a thrombotic event. However, the risk varies considerably with the clinical situation and can reach 40% or higher in the period after orthopedic surgery. Some studies have suggested that the presence of the HIT antibody has a negative impact on clinical outcomes even in the absence of overt thrombosis. HIT antibody–positive patients undergoing coronary artery bypass surgery or receiving heparin therapy for unstable angina have been reported to have a significantly higher incidence of adverse events, including prolonged hospitalization, stroke, myocardial infarction, and death.

Immune-mediated HIT appears between days 5 and 10 of heparin use. There are two variants: an early-onset HIT that occurs in patients exposed to heparin within the previous 3 months and a delayed-onset HIT that appears after heparin is discontinued. The diagnosis is based on a scoring method called the *4Ts system* that considers the degree of *t*hrombocytopenia, the *t*iming of the platelet reduction, the presence of *t*hrombosis or other sequelae, and the presence of other causes of *t*hrombocytopenia (Table 20-3).

Patients who receive full-dose unfractionated heparin for longer than 5 days or who have previously received heparin should be routinely monitored with measurement of the platelet count every other day. A decrease in the platelet count of more than 50%, even if the absolute platelet count remains within the normal range, can signal the appearance of an HIT type 2 antibody. This mandates stopping administration of heparin and substituting a direct thrombin inhibitor for continued anticoagulation. If heparin is continued, even at low dosages, or low-molecular-weight heparin is substituted, there is still significant risk of a major thromboembolic event.

An acute form of HIT type 2 can occur when heparin therapy is restarted within 20 days of a previous exposure. If an HIT antibody is already present, a patient in whom heparin therapy is restarted can exhibit an acute drug reaction with sudden onset of severe dyspnea, rigors, diaphoresis, hypertension, and tachycardia. Such patients are at extreme risk of fatal thromboembolism if heparin administration is continued.

Management of Anesthesia. Platelet transfusions are appropriate if a patient with thrombocytopenia is experiencing life-threatening hemorrhage or is bleeding into a closed space. Platelet transfusion therapy must be tailored to the severity

TABLE 20-3 ◼ 4Ts scoring system for heparin-induced thrombocytopenia (HIT)

Category	2 Points	1 Point	0 Points
Thrombocytopenia	Platelet count decreased >50% from baseline *and* platelet nadir ≥20,000/mm³	Platelet count decreased 30%-50% from baseline *or* platelet nadir 10,000-19,000/mm³	Platelet count decreased <30% from baseline *or* platelet nadir <10,000/mm³
Timing of the platelet decrease	Clear onset between days 5 and 10 of heparin exposure *or* platelet decrease in less than a day with heparin exposure within the prior 30 days	Decrease in platelet counts consistent with onset between days 5 and 10 of heparin exposure but timing is not clear because of missing platelet counts *or* onset after day 10 of heparin exposure *or* decrease in platelet counts in less than a day with prior heparin exposure between 30 and 100 days earlier	Platelet count decrease within 4 days of heparin exposure
Thrombosis or other sequelae	New thrombosis, skin necrosis, or acute systemic reaction after unfractionated heparin exposure	Progressive/recurrent thrombosis or unconfirmed but clinically suspected thrombosis	No thrombosis or previous heparin exposure
Other causes of Thrombocytopenia	None apparent	Possible other causes present	Probable other causes present

Data from Crowther MA, Cook DJ, Albert M, et al. The 4Ts scoring system for heparin-induced thrombocytopenia in medical-surgical intensive care unit patients. *J Crit Care*. 2010;25:287-293.
The 4Ts score is assigned by summing the values for each of the four categories. A score of 1, 2, or 3 is considered to indicate low probability of HIT; 4 or 5 indicates intermediate probability of HIT; and 6, 7, or 8 indicates high probability of HIT.

of the thrombocytopenia, the presence of bleeding complications, and the patient's underlying disease. In patients with autoimmune thrombocytopenia secondary to drug ingestion, the most important management step is to discontinue the drug. Corticosteroid therapy may speed recovery in patients with an idiopathic thrombocytopenic purpura–like picture. The rate of recovery depends on both the clearance rate of the drug and the ability of marrow megakaryocytes to proliferate and increase platelet production. Even if the platelet count is very low, bleeding is unlikely and patients can be allowed to recover without platelet transfusion.

HIV-infected thrombocytopenic patients who require urgent surgery should be given platelet transfusions as appropriate. For elective surgery in patients who develop thrombocytopenia early in their HIV/AIDS disease, consideration may be given to treatment with zidovudine before scheduling surgery. About 60% of these patients will show a response, and up to 50% will have long-lasting improvement in platelet count. The effect, however, is not immediate. It can take up to 2 months before the platelet count improves. Among patients who do not respond to zidovudine, splenectomy can be helpful in more than 85% of cases if done early in the course of the thrombocytopenia. Corticosteroids, intravenous immunoglobulin, and intravenous Rh0(D) immune globulin have also been used in patients with AIDS. With disease progression, HIV-infected patients develop a platelet production defect that responds only to platelet transfusion therapy.

To prevent life-threatening thromboembolic events in patients with HIT, all forms of heparin must be stopped immediately. Any delay can put a patient at increased risk of thrombosis. Substitution of low-molecular-weight heparin for unfractionated heparin is not an option, because there is significant antibody cross-reactivity. If a thrombotic event occurs in HIT patients, treatment with a direct thrombin inhibitor should be initiated. Oral anticoagulants should never be started until there is continuous and successful coverage with a direct thrombin inhibitor. The immediate reduction in protein C levels that occurs with the initiation of warfarin therapy can lead to worsening thrombosis, including massive skin necrosis and limb gangrene. Since factor VII levels may mirror the decrease in protein C, limb gangrene can be associated with a rapid increase in the international normalized ratio after initiation of warfarin treatment. If this occurs, warfarin should be discontinued and vitamin K given to reverse its effect.

Cardiac surgery represents a challenge for patients with HIT, since heparin is the ideal anticoagulant for use during cardiopulmonary bypass. The procedure should be delayed until the HIT episode resolves or, if this is not possible, bivalirudin, a direct thrombin inhibitor, should be used for anticoagulation during cardiopulmonary bypass.

Idiopathic Thrombocytopenic Purpura

Thrombocytopenia unrelated to drug exposure, infection, or autoimmune disease is generally classified as *autoimmune idiopathic thrombocytopenic purpura* (ITP). This diagnosis can be made only by excluding all other causes of nonimmune and immune platelet destruction. Most adults with the disorder proceed to a chronic form of ITP in which a continued high level of marrow platelet production is required to maintain a chronically low to near-normal platelet count in the face of a shortened platelet life span. This condition is characterized by a high level of platelet destruction that is balanced by a high marrow production of platelets that have better than normal function. Severe bleeding does not occur until the platelet count is below 10,000/mm³. Patients with chronic ITP have platelet counts of 20,000 to 100,000/mm³.

Platelet survival in severely affected patients can be measured in hours rather than days, with destruction occurring mainly in the spleen. Transfused platelets also have a shortened life span. Some patients demonstrate only modest shortening of platelet survival, which suggests a subnormal rate of platelet production. Although most ITP patients receiving platelet transfusions rapidly destroy the infused platelets, up to 30% of patients demonstrate near-normal posttransfusion platelet survival.

Management of Anesthesia. Severe autoimmune ITP associated with bleeding in adults should be treated as a medical emergency with administration of high-dose corticosteroids for the first 3 days. If there is a need for emergency surgery or clinical evidence of intracranial hemorrhage, the patient should also be given intravenous immunoglobulin and platelet transfusions at least every 8 to 12 hours, regardless of the effect on the platelet count. Some patients who receive platelet transfusions will show a relatively normal posttransfusion platelet count and reasonable platelet survival. Even when there is no posttransfusion improvement in the platelet count, however, sufficient numbers of the transfused platelets may survive to improve hemostasis.

Some adults do not respond to corticosteroids and go on to develop chronic ITP. If ITP persists for longer than 3 to 4 months, it is extremely unlikely that the patient will spontaneously recover. In this case, splenectomy should be considered if the platelet count is less than 10,000 to 20,000/mm³. Approximately 50% of patients will achieve a permanent remission after splenectomy. If splenectomy is recommended for a patient with chronic ITP, it is important to immunize the patient with pneumococcal, meningococcal, and *Haemophilus influenza* vaccines before surgery to reduce the risk of postsplenectomy sepsis.

Management of chronic ITP in pregnancy deserves special attention. Most women with chronic ITP can be managed during their pregnancy with no medication, modest amounts of prednisone, or intermittent use of intravenous immunoglobulin. If the thrombocytopenia becomes severe, a higher daily dose of steroids together with weekly intravenous immunoglobulin, especially during the last 2 to 3 weeks of pregnancy, may be needed to prevent maternal bleeding. Even with severe ITP in the mother, most children are born with normal platelet counts. Platelet counts in neonates may decrease for 7 days or longer following delivery. Therefore, in children at risk, platelet counts should be checked every 2 to 3 days until the platelet count begins to increase.

Qualitative Platelet Disorders

Abnormalities in platelet function are often first noted as a complication of an acute illness or surgery. However, there may be several factors that could play a role in determining the severity of the bleeding tendency. Consequently, this is not a time when an accurate diagnosis is easily made, so treatment should address as many potential contributing factors as possible. Treatment should include discontinuing drugs that inhibit platelet function, empirically replacing vWF or treating with desmopressin, and even transfusing platelets. Although this approach lacks precision, it is effective.

CONGENITAL DISORDERS AFFECTING PLATELET FUNCTION
Von Willebrand's Disease
Von Willebrand's disease (vWD) is the most common inherited abnormality affecting platelet *function*. It is inherited as either an autosomal dominant or autosomal recessive trait with an estimated prevalence ranging from 1 in 100 to 3 in 100,000 individuals. Severe vWD with the occurrence of life-threatening bleeding is seen in fewer than 5 individuals per million in Western countries.

Patients with vWD usually experience mucocutaneous bleeding (especially epistaxis), easy bruising, menorrhagia, and gingival and gastrointestinal bleeding. The number of patients with slight to moderate reductions in vWF activity far exceeds the number with overt clinical bleeding, so there can be a marked overdiagnosis of vWD if measured vWF level is the sole criterion for diagnosis. The diagnosis of "clinically important" vWD should be limited to those cases in which abnormal bleeding occurs. If vWD is considered to be a contributing factor in a bleeding patient, it should be treated empirically, and laboratory evaluation should be postponed until the patient is in clinically stable condition and has not received either blood products or drugs for several weeks.

Screening laboratory evaluation for vWD should include measurement of the bleeding time, platelet count, PT, and aPTT. Patients with mild vWD generally have near-normal test results. In those with more severe disease, the bleeding time is markedly prolonged but the platelet count is normal. Patients with a severe deficiency of vWF or defective binding of factor VIII to vWF have a prolonged PTT secondary to low levels of factor VIII in plasma. Specific assays of vWF level and function are then necessary to confirm the diagnosis.

Full evaluation of patients with vWD requires measurements of factor VIII coagulant activity, vWF antigen, vWF activity, and vWF multimer distribution. These studies are of diagnostic importance in the classification of vWD, which, in turn, is essential in planning clinical management.

Type 1 Disease. Type 1 vWD (80% of cases) is the most common variant and represents a *quantitative* defect in plasma vWF levels. Clinical severity is quite variable, but generally correlates with the plasma levels of vWF and factor VIII. In patients and families with a history of repeated and severe bleeding episodes, vWF antigen and vWF activity are usually reduced to less than 15% to 25% of normal. These individuals should be treated for any bleeding episode and given prophylactic treatment for even minor surgical procedures.

Type 2 Disease. Type 2 vWD is characterized by a *qualitative* defect in plasma vWF. This can involve a reduction in the number of larger vWF multimers or variable changes in vWF antigen and factor VIII binding. The absence of larger multimers results in a disproportionate decrease in vWF activity.

Type 3 Disease. Type 3 vWD is characterized by the virtual absence of circulating vWF antigen and very low levels of both vWF activity and factor VIII (3% to 10% of normal). These patients experience severe bleeding with mucosal hemorrhage, hemarthroses, and muscle hematomas reminiscent of that in hemophilia A or B. However, unlike patients with hemophilia, these patients have a very prolonged bleeding time.

Management of Anesthesia. The type of vWD and its severity, as well as the nature, urgency, and location of the surgical procedure, all factor into the therapeutic management of a patient with vWD. Treatments for this disorder include desmopressin, a drug that optimizes plasma levels of endogenous vWF, and blood products that contain vWF in high concentrations.

Desmopressin is a synthetic analogue of the antidiuretic hormone vasopressin that, when given intravenously, stimulates release of vWF from endothelial cells to produce an immediate rise in plasma vWF and factor VIII activity. This enhances platelet function. It can be very effective in correcting the bleeding defect in vWD. Platelet function abnormalities resulting from aspirin, glycoprotein IIb/IIIa inhibitors, uremia, or liver disease can be partially corrected by desmopressin-stimulated release of very large vWF multimers.

Success in treating vWD patients with desmopressin depends on the disease type. Patients with type 1 vWD show the best response. The value of treatment with desmopressin in patients with type 2 disease is less certain. Patients with type 3 vWD do not respond to the drug since these patients lack endothelial stores of vWF. Both vWF and factor VIII must be provided to reliably treat bleeding in patients with type 3 vWD.

Desmopressin is available in both intravenous and intranasal preparations. Desmopressin is administered intravenously in a dose of 0.3 mcg/kg. A highly concentrated nasal spray can be self-administered by women with type 1 vWD for management of menorrhagia. This formulation can also be effective in controlling bleeding associated with tooth extraction or minor surgery.

Desmopressin therapy is most effective in treating mild bleeding episodes or in preventing bleeding during minor surgery. Patients with baseline vWF and factor VIII levels of more than 10 to 20 IU/dL seem to do best with this drug, demonstrating a threefold to fivefold increase in vWF levels. However, even if the response is suboptimal, bleeding may be partially contained, or, in the case of surgical prophylaxis, blood loss and the need for transfusion can be reduced. A disadvantage of desmopressin is its relatively short-lived effects. Improvement in the bleeding time and vWF level is limited to 12 to 24 hours. The response can decrease with repeated doses because of the development of tachyphylaxis. In situations in which control of bleeding is critical, such as following major surgery, desmopressin alone will be inadequate, and vWF replacement is necessary.

Replacement of vWF can be achieved by infusion of cryoprecipitate or purified concentrates containing the vWF–factor VIII complex. Cryoprecipitate is a readily available and effective blood product that contains concentrated amounts of fibrinogen, vWF, and factors VIII and XIII. Its administration results in an immediate shortening of the bleeding time, which reflects the infusion of larger vWF multimers. The dosing schedule for cryoprecipitate is empirical. Patients with severe type 1 or 3 disease are managed like patients with severe hemophilia A by increasing factor VIII levels to 50% to 70% of normal for major surgery and 30% to 50% of normal for minor surgery or less severe bleeding.

Because there is a risk of transfusion-transmitted infection with cryoprecipitate, purified commercial preparations of factor VIII–vWF concentrate are available and are recommended. A suitable concentrate must contain the larger vWF multimers to be effective. One preparation rich in vWF is Humate-P. Once bleeding is controlled, a single daily dose of concentrate is sufficient, since the half-life of the factor VIII–vWF complex in patients with vWD is about 24 hours.

ACQUIRED ABNORMALITIES OF PLATELET FUNCTION
Acquired platelet dysfunction is seen in association with hematopoietic disease, as part of a systemic illness, or as a result of drug therapy.

Myeloproliferative Disease
Patients with myeloproliferative disorders, such as polycythemia vera, myeloid metaplasia, idiopathic myelofibrosis, essential thrombocythemia, and chronic myelogenous leukemia, frequently exhibit abnormal platelet function. Some patients have very high platelet counts and demonstrate either abnormal bleeding or a tendency for arterial or venous thrombosis. In patients with polycythemia vera, expansion of the total blood volume and an increase in blood viscosity may contribute to the thrombotic risk. The most consistent laboratory abnormalities in patients with bleeding are defects in epinephrine-induced aggregation and in dense granule and α-granule function. Bleeding resulting from an acquired form of vWD may also be observed in these disorders, which results from a loss of higher-molecular-weight vWF multimers.

Dysproteinemia
Abnormal platelet function, including defects in adhesion, aggregation, and procoagulant activity, are observed in patients with dysproteinemia. Almost one third of patients with Waldenström's macroglobulinemia or immunoglobulin A myeloma have a demonstrable defect in platelet function. Multiple myeloma patients are less commonly affected. The concentration of the monoclonal protein spike appears to correlate with the abnormalities in platelet function.

Uremia

Uremic patients consistently show a defect in platelet function that correlates with the severity of the uremia and anemia. It appears that the uncleared metabolic product guanidinosuccinic acid acts as an inhibitor of platelet function by inducing endothelial cell nitric oxide release. Platelet adhesion, activation, and aggregation are abnormal and thromboxane A_2 generation is decreased.

Most patients with uremia have a prolonged bleeding time that is corrected by hemodialysis. Interestingly, the bleeding time also shortens with either RBC transfusion or erythropoietin therapy. For acute bleeding episodes, desmopressin therapy can improve platelet function transiently.

Liver Disease

In general, the most likely cause of hemorrhage in severe liver disease is a discrete defect, such as bleeding varices or a gastric or duodenal ulcer. However, if a cirrhotic patient has widespread bleeding, including ecchymoses and oozing from puncture sites, a coagulopathy should be considered. Such patients can have multiple defects in coagulation. Thrombocytopenia related to hypersplenism is common. Platelet dysfunction resulting from high levels of circulating fibrin degradation products increases the bleeding tendency. In addition, reduced production of factor VII and low-grade, chronic DIC with increased fibrinolysis add to the coagulopathy.

Inhibition by Drugs

Several classes of drugs can affect platelet function (Table 20-4). Aspirin and other nonsteroidal antiinflammatory drugs have a well-recognized impact on platelet function. Aspirin is a powerful inhibitor of platelet thromboxane A_2 synthesis because of its irreversible inhibition of cyclooxygenase function. Nonsteroidal antiinflammatory drugs such as indomethacin, ibuprofen, and sulfinpyrazone also inhibit platelet cyclooxygenase, but their effect is reversible and lasts only as long as the particular drug is in the circulation. Such agents are weak inhibitors of platelet function and are not usually associated with severe clinical bleeding. However, they can contribute to bleeding when other aggravating factors, such as treatment with other anticoagulants, a gastrointestinal disorder, or surgery, are present. Certain foods, food additives, vitamins, and herbal products—such as vitamins C and E, ω-3 fatty acids, and Chinese black tree fungus—can also reversibly inhibit platelet function through the cyclooxygenase pathway.

The impact of antibiotics on platelet function can be a major contributor to hemorrhage in critically ill patients. The penicillins, including carbenicillin, penicillin G, ticarcillin, ampicillin, nafcillin, and mezlocillin, can interfere with both platelet adhesion and platelet activation and aggregation. They bind to the platelet membrane and interfere with vWF binding and the response of platelets to agonists such as adenosine diphosphate and epinephrine. Significant clinical bleeding can occur if these antibiotics are administered in very high dosages. The presence of aggravating factors related to the critical illness must be important, since abnormal bleeding is rarely seen when these antibiotics are used in generally healthy patients. Platelet dysfunction has also been reported with some cephalosporins.

Volume expanders, such as dextran, can interfere with platelet aggregation and procoagulant activity when infused in large amounts. This can be a significant disadvantage in the trauma setting but can be useful in the vascular surgery setting to prevent platelet thrombosis. Hydroxyethyl starch is less likely to interfere with platelet function but can cause a detectable defect if given in amounts in excess of 2 L.

MANAGEMENT OF ANESTHESIA IN PATIENTS WITH QUALITATIVE PLATELET DISORDERS

The therapeutic goal in qualitative platelet disorders is less exact than in disorders resulting in thrombocytopenia. Because the platelets are dysfunctional, the absolute platelet number does not predict bleeding risk. Treatment with desmopressin may improve a mild to moderate platelet defect, especially if the risk of bleeding is relatively minor. If the bleeding risk is more substantial, platelet transfusions may be required. The bleeding time, results of platelet function analysis, or the thromboelastogram may be used to measure end points of coagulation but will not guarantee adequacy of platelet function for the challenge of surgery. As a general rule, sufficient platelet transfusions to increase the percentage of normal/functional platelets to the 10% to 20% range will be sufficient to correct drug-related platelet dysfunction.

Platelets become quite dysfunctional in the setting of hypothermia (temperature <35° C) and acidosis (pH <7.3), and platelets transfused into a patient with either or both of these conditions will rapidly become dysfunctional as well.

TABLE 20-4   Drugs that inhibit platelet function

STRONG ASSOCIATION

Aspirin (and aspirin-containing medications)

Clopidogrel, ticlopidine

Abciximab

Nonsteroidal antiinflammatory drugs: naproxen, ibuprofen, indomethacin, phenylbutazone, piroxicam, ketorolac

MILD TO MODERATE ASSOCIATION

Antibiotics, usually only in high dosages

  Penicillin, also carbenicillin, penicillin G, ampicillin, ticarcillin, nafcillin, mezlocillin

  Cephalosporins

  Nitrofurantoin

Volume expanders: dextran, hydroxyethyl starch

Heparin

Fibrinolytic agents: ε-aminocaproic acid, aprotinin

WEAK ASSOCIATION

Oncologic drugs: daunorubicin, mithramycin

Cardiovascular drugs: β-blockers, calcium channel blockers, nitroglycerin, nitroprusside, quinidine

Alcohol

HYPERCOAGULABLE DISORDERS

Sources of hypercoagulability can be divided into two major classes: a congenital predisposition caused by one or more genetic abnormalities, often referred to as *thrombophilia*, and acquired or environmental hypercoagulability.

Heritable Causes of Hypercoagulability

Hereditary conditions predisposing to venous thromboembolism (VTE) can conceptually be divided into conditions that either decrease endogenous antithrombotic proteins or increase prothrombotic proteins (Table 20-5).

THROMBOPHILIA DUE TO DECREASED ANTITHROMBOTIC PROTEINS

Hereditary Antithrombin Deficiency

Antithrombin III is the most important of the body's defenses against clot formation in healthy blood vessels or at the perimeter of a site of active bleeding. Antithrombin III deficiency is inherited as an autosomal dominant trait, with an estimated frequency of 1 per 1000 to 5000 individuals. Homozygous antithrombin deficiency is not compatible with life. Heterozygous patients have an antithrombin III level between 40% and 70% of normal. Individuals who are heterozygous for antithrombin III deficiency are roughly 20 times more likely than nondeficient individuals to develop VTE at some point in their lives. The thrombotic event usually occurs in association with some triggering event that further increases hypercoagulability.

In addition to anticoagulation, anesthetic management for these patients should include maintaining the antithrombin III level above 80% for 5 days after the procedure. This is done by administering antithrombin III concentrates.

Hereditary Protein C and Protein S Deficiency

Hereditary deficiency of protein C and protein S adversely affects thrombin regulation by restricting the activity of thrombin already formed and interfering with the ability to limit the rate of thrombin generation. The risk of VTE is about the same as with antithrombin III deficiency.

Synthesis of both protein C and protein S is vitamin K dependent, so individuals who are protein C deficient are at particular risk of thrombosis if warfarin therapy is initiated in the *absence of protective anticoagulation* with heparin. Specifically, during the first days of warfarin treatment, before inhibition of the vitamin K–dependent clotting factors is sufficient to provide the intended *anticoagulation,* modest suppression of protein C synthesis may compound the already subnormal protein C levels and result in heightened *hypercoagulability.* In addition to therapies to prevent or treat VTE, patients with protein C and S deficiency may require infusion of fresh frozen plasma and prothrombin complex concentrates to correct the levels of these proteins. In patients with protein C deficiency, purified protein C concentrate and activated protein C can be used.

THROMBOPHILIA DUE TO INCREASED PROTHROMBOTIC PROTEINS

Factor V Leiden

Factor V Leiden differs from normal factor V because of a genetic alteration that makes it very resistant to inactivation. Therefore, factor Va Leiden stays active in the circulation longer than normal, which promotes increased thrombin generation.

Factor V Leiden carries a low to intermediate procoagulant risk. Patients who are heterozygous for factor V Leiden have a fivefold to sevenfold increased risk of VTE, whereas the risk in homozygous individuals is increased up to 80-fold. The prevalence of factor V Leiden varies considerably in different ethnic populations. It is present in 5% of people of northern European descent but only rarely in those of African or Asian descent. Therefore, depending on the ethnic makeup of the community, up to 1 in 20 patients coming for routine surgery can be expected to have a degree of heightened risk of VTE attributable to factor V Leiden.

Prothrombin Gene Mutation

Another thrombophilia that operates via an increase in prothrombotic proteins is known as the *prothrombin gene mutation* (prothrombin 20210A), which causes levels of prothrombin to be considerably higher in affected individuals than in the general population. If this mutation is the only thrombophilic risk factor, the VTE risk is relatively low. The importance of this thrombophilia is similar to that of factor V Leiden and lies in the frequency of the gene rather than its potency. Also as with factor V Leiden, ethnicity plays a significant role in the prevalence of this gene. It occurs in about 4% of individuals of European descent but rarely in patients of African or Asian descent.

Acquired Causes of Hypercoagulability

MYELOPROLIFERATIVE DISORDERS

Myeloproliferative disorders, especially polycythemia vera, essential thrombocytosis, and paroxysmal nocturnal hemoglobinuria, are associated with an increased incidence

TABLE 20-5	**Major hereditary disorders linked to hypercoagulability***		
Disorder	**Prevalence in healthy controls(%)**	**Prevalence in patients with first DVT(%)**	**Likelihood of DVT by age 60 (%)**
Antithrombin deficiency	0.2	1.1	62
Protein C deficiency	0.8	3	48
Protein S deficiency	0.13	1.1	33
Factor V Leiden	3.5	20	6
Prothrombin 20210A	2.3	18	<5

DVT, Deep vein thrombosis.
*All values pertain to the heterozygous state of the given condition.

of thrombophlebitis, pulmonary embolism, and arterial occlusion. Patients with these conditions are also at risk of thrombosis of splenic, hepatic, portal, and mesenteric blood vessels. The pathogenesis of these thromboses is not clear, but increased activation and aggregation of platelets may be important for this hypercoagulable state.

MALIGNANCIES

Patients with certain malignancies demonstrate a marked thrombotic tendency. Adenocarcinoma of the pancreas, colon, stomach, and ovaries are the tumors most often associated with thromboembolic events. Indeed, these malignancies often present with an episode of deep vein thrombosis or migratory superficial thrombophlebitis. Of all patients who develop primary thrombophlebitis, 25% to 30% will have a recurrence, and 20% of these will turn out to have cancer. The pathogenesis of the thrombotic tendency appears to relate to a combination of release of one or more procoagulant factors by the tumor that can directly activate factor X, endothelial damage by tumor invasion, and blood stasis. Laboratory testing may show no abnormalities or some combination of thrombocytosis, elevation of the fibrinogen level, and low-grade DIC.

PREGNANCY AND ORAL CONTRACEPTIVE USE

Pregnancy and oral contraceptive use have been reported to increase the risk of thrombosis. The overall incidence of thrombosis is approximately 1 in 1500 pregnancies but is higher in women who have an inherited hypercoagulable state, a history of deep vein thrombosis or pulmonary embolism, or a family history of thromboembolic disease; who are obese; who are kept at bed rest for a prolonged period; or who require cesarean section. The risk of pulmonary embolism is highest during the third trimester and immediately postpartum and is a significant cause of maternal death. Antithrombin III–deficient women are at greatest risk and should receive anticoagulant therapy throughout pregnancy. Factor V Leiden and the prothrombin mutation are associated with much lower risk. Women with these inherited traits do not need to receive anticoagulant treatment.

The association of oral contraceptive use with thrombosis and thromboembolism appears to be multifactorial. Women who also smoke, have a history of migraine headaches, or have an inherited hypercoagulable defect are at increased risk (30-fold higher) of venous thrombosis, pulmonary embolism, and cerebrovascular thrombosis. There appears to be a weaker relationship between estrogen use at the time of menopause and the occurrence of thrombosis.

NEPHROTIC SYNDROME

Patients with nephrotic syndrome are at risk of thromboembolic disease including renal vein thrombosis. The reason is unclear but may be due to lower than normal levels of antithrombin III or protein C as a result of renal loss of coagulation proteins, factor XII deficiency, platelet hyperactivity, abnormal fibrinolytic activity, and higher than normal levels of other coagulation factors. Hyperlipidemia and hypoalbuminemia have also been proposed as possible etiologic factors.

ANTIPHOSPHOLIPID ANTIBODIES

The presence of antiphospholipid antibodies does not necessarily correlate with thrombosis. Patients with hepatitis C, mononucleosis, syphilis, Lyme disease, multiple sclerosis, or HIV infection can have circulating antiphospholipid antibodies but do not have a propensity for thrombosis.

The term *antiphospholipid antibody syndrome* is used when patients experience thromboses or pregnancy complications and have laboratory evidence of antiphospholipid antibodies in their blood. Antiphospholipid antibody syndrome can be primary, as the sole manifestation of autoimmune disease, or secondary in association with systemic lupus erythematosus (secondary antiphospholipid antibody syndrome). The diagnosis requires the following clinical findings: thrombosis or pregnancy-related morbidity, and the presence of one of the antiphospholipid antibodies (anticardiolipin, anti–β_2-glycoprotein I, or the lupus anticoagulant).

The antibodies are clinically defined by the method of detection. Lupus anticoagulant antibodies are detected by their prolongation of the PTT and the dilute Russell viper venom time, whereas anticardiolipin and anti–β_2-glycoprotein I antibodies are measured directly by immunoassay. The risk of thrombosis appears to be greater with lupus anticoagulants or antibodies with activity specifically directed at β_2-glycoprotein I.

The exact mechanism of the thrombotic action of these antibodies has yet to be defined. The antibodies might activate endothelial cells to increase the expression of vascular adhesion molecule 1 and E-selectin. This would increase the binding of white blood cells and platelets to the endothelial surface and lead to thrombus formation.

Patients with lupus anticoagulants have an increased propensity for thrombosis, with 30% to 60% of patients experiencing one or more thrombotic events during their lifetime. Isolated venous thrombosis or thromboembolism make up two thirds of the events and cerebral thrombosis accounts for the other third. Up to 20% of patients who have a VTE not associated with a disease, surgery, or trauma are found to have antiphospholipid antibodies. Along with factor V Leiden and the prothrombin gene mutation, the presence of an antiphospholipid antibody must be considered as a likely cause of thromboembolic disease in younger individuals. Patients can also develop *catastrophic antiphospholipid syndrome* characterized by multiorgan failure resulting from widespread small vessel thrombosis, thrombocytopenia, acute respiratory distress syndrome, DIC, and occasionally an autoimmune hemolytic anemia. This clinical picture is indistinguishable from that of TTP. Bacterial infection often appears to be a triggering event for this syndrome.

Management of Anesthesia in Venous Hypercoagulable Disorders

Current antithrombotic strategies range from simple management approaches such as early ambulation to a combination of elastic stockings and subcutaneous heparin therapy followed by conversion to outpatient warfarin therapy. Surgical patients may have a host of risk factors for VTE, all of which must be considered when balancing the degree of thrombotic risk and the costs (monetary expense and bleeding risk) of perioperative anticoagulation. A number of professional societies have espoused a four-tiered approach to risk stratification in surgical patients that permits the intensity of prophylaxis to be adjusted to the VTE risk (Table 20-6).

Prophylactic strategies may take pharmacologic and physical forms. Large trials suggest that subcutaneous administration of unfractionated or low-molecular-weight heparin confers a 60% to 70% reduction in risk of VTE. By contrast, aspirin provides relatively weak prophylactic effects. Physical methods of prophylaxis such as the use of graded elastic compression stockings are associated with a 40% to 45% risk reduction, whereas intermittent pneumatic compression stockings yield a risk reduction approaching that of heparin use.

A number of investigations published in the late 1970s and early 1980s presented evidence that regional anesthesia (usually neuraxial blockade) resulted in a decreased incidence of postoperative VTE. This was particularly true for lower extremity joint replacement surgery. As a result, regional anesthesia became the preferred anesthetic technique for this surgery and other procedures associated with a high risk of VTE. However, even when neuraxial anesthesia was combined with techniques such as early ambulation and intraoperative use of antiembolism stockings, the VTE risk was still unacceptably high. As a result, postoperative prophylactic anticoagulation with drugs such as warfarin or subcutaneous heparin became the standard of care for operations associated with a high risk of VTE (see Table 20-6).

Now that routine antithrombotic prophylaxis is utilized, the advantages of regional compared with general anesthesia are less clear in patients at high risk of VTE. Recent meta-analyses have found that regional and general anesthesia for hip surgery appear to produce comparable results in terms of most outcomes. Although there appears to be a slight reduction in VTE incidence with regional anesthesia and also a decreased need for transfusion, this does not translate into a significant difference in mortality. The U.S. Food and Drug Administration advisory prohibiting neuraxial anesthesia in patients receiving low-molecular-weight heparin resulting from an increased risk of epidural hematomas may further limit the use of regional anesthesia or its extension into the postoperative period. Postoperative pharmacologic prophylaxis for VTE is very effective, and so it may not be prudent to withhold these drugs to allow continued use of an epidural anesthetic postoperatively.

Patients with an absolute contraindication to anticoagulant therapy or those with a major bleeding complication may benefit from placement of a vena caval filter to prevent recurrent pulmonary emboli. The filters are effective and reduce the incidence of pulmonary embolism to less than 4%. In cancer patients for whom anticoagulant therapy has failed, a vena caval filter combined with continued anticoagulation may provide greater protection.

ANESTHETIC CONSIDERATIONS IN PATIENTS RECEIVING LONG-TERM ANTICOAGULANT THERAPY

Perioperative management of patients receiving anticoagulant therapy requires special attention. Certain operations such as some ophthalmic, dental, dermatologic, and gastrointestinal procedures can be carried out without interruption of oral anticoagulant therapy. The risk of perioperative thrombosis must be weighed against the risk of bleeding during and after surgery.

For most operations anticoagulation needs to be temporarily interrupted, and bridging therapy with unfractionated or low-molecular-weight heparin is instituted in patients at moderate and high risk of thrombosis. Bridging therapy reduces the risk of VTE by up to 80%. Warfarin should be stopped approximately 5 days before the procedure and heparin should be started 36 hours after the last dose of warfarin. In patients

---

TABLE 20-6 ☐ Levels of thromboembolism risk and recommended thromboprophylaxis in hospital patients

Level of risk	Approximate DVT risk without thromboprophylaxis (%)	Suggested thromboprophylaxis
LOW RISK		
Mobile patients undergoing minor surgery Medical patients who are fully mobile	<10	Early ambulation No specific thromboprophylaxis
MODERATE RISK		
Most general, open gynecologic, or urologic surgery patients Medical patients on bed rest Patients with moderate VTE risk plus high bleeding risk	10-40	LMWH Subcutaneous unfractionated heparin Fondaparinux Mechanical thromboprophylaxis
HIGH RISK		
Hip or knee arthroplasty patients Hip fracture surgery patients Patients with major trauma Spinal cord injury patients Patients with high VTE risk plus high bleeding risk	40-80	LMWH Fondaparinux Warfarin to INR of 2-3 Mechanical thromboprophylaxis

Data from Jaffer AK. Perioperative management of warfarin and antiplatelet therapy. *Cleve Clin J Med.* 2009;76(suppl 4):S37-S44.
DVT, Deep vein thrombosis; *INR,* international normalized ratio; *LMWH,* low-molecular-weight heparin; *VTE,* venous thromboembolism.

receiving heparin by continuous infusion, the infusion should be stopped 6 hours before surgery. Patients receiving low-molecular-weight heparin should receive the last dose no less than 18 hours preoperatively if they are on a twice-daily regimen and 30 hours preoperatively if they are on a once-daily regimen.

In cases in which neuraxial anesthesia is planned, the guidelines of the American Society of Regional Anesthesia and Pain Medicine recommend that needle placement for regional anesthesia take place 12 hours after the last dose of low-molecular-weight heparin if prophylactic dosing is used and 24 hours after the last dose of low-molecular-weight heparin if therapeutic dosing is used. Similarly, epidural catheter removal needs to be carefully coordinated with the heparin dosing (Table 20-7).

Resumption of anticoagulation postoperatively requires an evaluation of the risk of recurrent thrombosis and consideration of the degree to which surgery itself increases hypercoagulability. These factors must be weighed against the bleeding risk associated with resumption of anticoagulation. Since there is a delay of approximately 24 hours after warfarin administration before the international normalized ratio begins to increase, warfarin therapy should generally be resumed as soon as possible after surgery except in patients at high risk of bleeding. These patients can be managed with bridging therapy with heparin until the international normalized ratio reaches therapeutic levels.

Acquired Hypercoagulability of the Arterial Vasculature

HEART DISEASE

Patients with acute anterior wall myocardial infarction who, because of a wall motion abnormality, are likely to form a mural thrombus should receive warfarin for 2 to 3 months after the infarction. After that time there is little risk of embolism. Patients with atrial fibrillation, particularly atrial fibrillation associated with valvular disease, a dilated atrium, and evidence of heart failure or a prior embolus generally require moderate-dose warfarin therapy indefinitely. The need for anticoagulation in patients with atrial fibrillation is determined using the $CHADS_2$ scoring system, which takes into account the stroke risk factors of congestive heart failure, hypertension, age 75 years or older, diabetes mellitus, and prior stroke (Table 20-8). In patients with atrial fibrillation undergoing major surgery, oral anticoagulant therapy should be stopped and bridging therapy with heparin begun.

Dabigatran, an oral direct thrombin inhibitor recently approved for the prevention of stroke in patients with atrial fibrillation that is not associated with valvular heart disease, may pose a challenge. It is suggested that dabigatran be stopped 3 to 5 days before surgery in patients with impaired renal function (creatinine clearance <50 mL/min) and 2 to 3 days before surgery in others. If parenteral anticoagulant therapy is necessary, it should be initiated 12 to 24 hours after the last dose of dabigatran.

TABLE 20-7 ■ **Management of neuraxial anesthesia in patients receiving thromboprophylaxis**

Anticoagulant Drug	Recommendation
Subcutaneous unfractionated heparin	No contraindication with twice-daily dosing and total daily dose ≤ 10,000 units. Consider delaying heparin dose until after block if technical difficulty is anticipated.
Intravenous unfractionated heparin to be given during surgery	Heparinize 1 hr after neuraxial block. Remove catheter 24 hr after last heparin dose. No mandatory surgical delay if block placement is traumatic.
LMWH	*Twice-daily dosing:* Delay neuraxial block for at least 24 hr after last preoperative dose of heparin. First postoperative dose of LMWH should not be given sooner than 24 hr after surgery, regardless of anesthetic technique. Remove neuraxial catheter 2 hr before first postoperative LMWH dose. *Once-daily dosing:* Delay neuraxial block for at least 12 hr after last preoperative heparin dose. First postoperative LMWH dose can be given 6-8 hr after surgery and next dose 24 hr later. Indwelling neuraxial catheters can be maintained. Remove neuraxial catheter 12 hr after last LMWH dose.
Warfarin	INR should be normal before neuraxial anesthesia is induced. Remove catheter when INR < 1.5, that is, during initiation of warfarin therapy.
Fondaparinux	Use neuraxial blockade only if it can be accomplished with a single pass of an atraumatic needle and without an indwelling catheter.
Direct thrombin inhibitors	Avoid neuraxial techniques.

Adapted from Horlocker TT, Wedel DJ, Rowlingson JC, et al. Regional anesthesia in the patient receiving antithrombotic or thrombolytic therapy: American Society of Regional Anesthesia and Pain Medicine Evidence-Based Guidelines (third edition). *Reg Anesth Pain Med.* 2010;35(1):64-101. *INR,* International normalized ratio; *LMWH,* low-molecular-weight heparin.

TABLE 20-8 ■ **$CHADS_2$ scoring system for estimating the risk of stroke in nonrheumatic atrial fibrillation***

	Condition	Points
C	Congestive heart failure	1
H	Hypertension	1
A	Age ≥ 75 yr	1
D	Diabetes mellitus	1
S_2	Prior stroke or transient ischemic attack	2

*For risk stratification based on $CHADS_2$ score, see Table 20-9.

TABLE 20-9 ▪ Suggested risk stratification for perioperative thromboembolic events

Risk category	Mechanical heart valve	Atrial fibrillation	VTE
High	Any mitral valve prosthesis Caged-ball or tilting-disc aortic valve prosthesis Recent (within 6 mo) stroke or TIA	CHADS$_2$ score of 5 or 6 Recent (within 3 mo) stroke or TIA Rheumatic heart disease	Recent (within 3 mo) VTE Severe thrombophilia e.g., deficiency of protein C, protein S, or antithrombin III; presence of antiphospholipid antibodies; or multiple abnormalities
Moderate	Bileaflet aortic valve prosthesis and one of the following: atrial fibrillation, prior stroke or TIA, hypertension, diabetes, congestive heart failure, age >75 yr	CHADS$_2$ score of 3 or 4	VTE within the past 3 to 12 mo Mild to moderate thrombophilic condition Recurrent VTE Active cancer (treated within 6 mo or with palliative care)
Low	Bileaflet aortic valve prosthesis without atrial fibrillation and no other risk factors for stroke	CHADS$_2$ score of 0 to 2 No prior stroke or TIA	Single VTE occurring >12 mo earlier No other risk factors

Data from Douketis JD, Berger PB, Dunn AS, et al. The perioperative management of antithrombotic therapy: American College of Chest Physicians Evidence-Based Clinical Practice Guidelines (8th edition). *Chest.* 2008;133(6 suppl):299S-339S.
CHADS$_2$, System for predicting stroke likelihood based on the risk factors of congestive heart failure, hypertension, age ≥ 75 yr, diabetes mellitus, and prior stroke (see Table 20-8); *TIA,* transient ischemic attack; *VTE,* venous thromboembolism.

ANTIPHOSPHOLIPID ANTIBODIES

Patients with antiphospholipid antibodies (lupus anticoagulants) and a history of thromboembolic disease represent a major therapeutic challenge. These patients are at significant risk of both arterial and venous thromboses.

SUMMARY

In summary, hypercoagulability, a state of exaggerated activation of the coagulation system, plays a major role in the pathogenesis of VTE, a process that affects some 2 million Americans annually with an estimated annual mortality of 150,000 from pulmonary embolism. New heritable causes of hypercoagulability are being identified, and some genetic predisposition to thrombosis can be identified in more than half of patients with deep vein thrombosis. Anesthesiologists are being asked to care for an increasing number of patients carrying the diagnosis of hypercoagulability, many of whom are receiving long-term anticoagulation therapy. The perioperative period represents a time of high risk for VTE (Table 20-9). Some surgeries are associated with a more than 100-fold increase in the risk of thrombosis. Knowledge of the optimum operative management of these patients inevitably lags behind the identification of their pathophysiology, but it is incumbent upon the anesthesiologist to understand the mechanisms behind hypercoagulability and to make educated choices about the management of these patients. Hypercoagulability plays a less clearly defined role in the pathophysiology of arterial thrombotic events, but the high morbidity and mortality associated with arterial occlusion in the perioperative patient makes staying abreast of these developments an important part of patient care.

KEY POINTS

- The erythrocyte and its major protein constituent, Hb, are highly specialized so that oxygen delivery can be rapidly adjusted to meet local tissue needs. Disorders affecting the formation, structure, metabolism, and turnover of RBCs can impair their ability to perform this vital task in patients undergoing surgery.
- Preoperative management of patients with sickle cell disease no longer mandates exchange transfusion to decrease the ratio of sickle Hb to normal Hb; instead, transfusions are required only as needed to achieve a preoperative hematocrit of 30%.
- Recent advances in cell-based coagulation models have changed our fundamental understanding of in vivo clotting. This improved understanding has allowed a better appreciation of how specific defects in coagulation components affect the balance of hemostasis and what therapeutic interventions offer the best risk/benefit ratio.
- Sources of hypercoagulability can be divided into two major classes: a congenital predisposition that is usually lifelong and an acquired or environmental hypercoagulability such as occurs in surgery. In patients experiencing a first-time VTE, some congenital predisposition can be identified in up to 50% of cases. However, in almost all cases of VTE, some acquired or environmental hypercoagulability serves as a triggering event.
- Most disorders producing a state of venous hypercoagulability affect the generation or disposition of thrombin, whereas in the arterial circulation, platelet and endothelial function and regulation also critically affect the prothrombotic tendency.

RESOURCES

Crowther MA, Cook DJ, Albert M, et al. Canadian Critical Care Trials Group. The 4Ts scoring system for heparin-induced thrombocytopenia in medical-surgical intensive care unit patients. *J Crit Care*. 2010;25:287-293.

Douketis JD, Berger PB, Dunn AS, et al. The perioperative management of antithrombotic therapy: American College of Chest Physicians Evidence-Based Clinical Practice Guidelines (8th edition). *Chest*. 2008;133(suppl 6):299S-339S.

Firth PG, Head CA. Sickle cell disease and anesthesia. *Anesthesiology*. 2004;101:766-785.

Greinacher A, Farner B, Kroll H, et al. Clinical features of heparin-induced thrombocytopenia including risk factors for thrombosis. *Thromb Haemost*. 2005;94:132-135.

Gutt CN, Oniu T, Wolkener F, et al. Prophylaxis and treatment of deep vein thrombosis in general surgery. *Am J Surg*. 2004;189:14-22.

Hébert PC, Wells G, Blajchman MA, et al. A multicenter, randomized, controlled clinical trial of transfusion requirements in critical care. Transfusion Requirements in Critical Care Investigators, Canadian Critical Care Trials Group. *N Engl J Med*. 1999;340:409-417.

Hoffmann M. Remodeling the blood coagulation cascade. *J Thromb Thrombolysis*. 2003;16(1-2):17-20.

Horlocker TT, Wedel DJ, Rowlingson JC, et al. Regional anesthesia in the patient receiving antithrombotic or thrombolytic therapy: American Society of Regional Anesthesia and Pain Medicine Evidence-Based Guidelines (third edition). *Reg Anesth Pain Med*. 2010;35:64-101.

Jaffer AK. Perioperative management of warfarin and antiplatelet therapy. *Cleve Clin J Med*. 2009;76(suppl 4):S37-S44.

Levy JH, Key NS, Azran MS. Novel oral anticoagulants: implications in the perioperative setting. *Anesthesiology*. 2010;113(3):726-745.

Practice guidelines for perioperative blood transfusion and adjuvant therapies: an updated report by the American Society of Anesthesiologists Task Force on Perioperative Blood Transfusion and Adjuvant Therapies. *Anesthesiology*. 2006;105:198-208.

Schafer A, Levine M, Konkle B, et al. Thrombotic disorders: diagnosis and treatment. *Hematology Am Soc Hematol Educ Program*. 2003:520-539.

Tefferi A. Annual clinical updates in hematological malignancies: polycythemia vera and essential thrombocythemia: 2011 update on diagnosis, risk-stratification, and management. *Am J Hematol*. 2011;86(3):292-301.

Turpie AGG, Chin BSP, Lip GLH. Venous thromboembolism: pathophysiology, clinical features, and prevention. The ABCs of antithrombotic therapy. *BMJ*. 2002;325:887-890.

CHAPTER 21

Skin and Musculoskeletal Diseases

RAMACHANDRAN RAMANI ∎

Diseases of the skin and musculoskeletal system manifest with obvious clinical signs, since both are readily visible. However, less visible systemic effects of many of these disorders are also important.

SKIN AND CONNECTIVE TISSUE DISEASES

Epidermolysis Bullosa

Epidermolysis bullosa is a group of genetic diseases of mucous membranes and skin, particularly the oropharynx and esophagus. Epidermolysis bullosa can be categorized as simplex, junctional, and dystrophic. In the simplex type, epidermal cells are fragile because of mutations of genes encoding keratin intermediate filament proteins. In the dystrophic types the genetic mutation appears to be in the gene encoding the type of collagen that is the major component of anchoring fibrils.

SIGNS AND SYMPTOMS

Epidermolysis bullosa is characterized by bulla formation (blistering) resulting from intercellular separation within the epidermis followed by fluid accumulation. Bulla formation is typically initiated when lateral shearing forces are applied to the skin. Pressure applied perpendicular to the skin is not as great a hazard. Bullae can form after even minimal trauma and can even develop spontaneously.

The simplex form of epidermolysis bullosa has a benign course and development is normal. By contrast, patients with the junctional form of epidermolysis bullosa rarely survive beyond early childhood. Most die of sepsis. Features that distinguish junctional epidermolysis bullosa from other forms are generalized blistering beginning at birth, absence of scar formation, and generalized mucosal involvement (gastrointestinal, genitourinary, respiratory tracts). Manifestations of epidermolysis bullosa dystrophica include severe scarring with fusion of the digits (pseudosyndactyly), constriction of the oral aperture (microstomia), and esophageal stricture. The teeth are often dysplastic. Malnutrition, anemia, electrolyte derangements, and hypoalbuminemia are common, most likely reflecting chronic infection, debilitation, and renal dysfunction. Survival beyond the second decade is unusual. Diseases associated with epidermolysis bullosa include porphyria, amyloidosis, multiple myeloma, diabetes mellitus, and hypercoagulable states. Mitral valve prolapse may also accompany this disorder.

TREATMENT

Treatment of epidermolysis bullosa is symptomatic and supportive. Many of these patients are receiving corticosteroids. Infection of bullae with *Staphylococcus aureus* or β-hemolytic streptococci is common.

MANAGEMENT OF ANESTHESIA

Supplemental corticosteroids may be indicated during the perioperative period if patients have been receiving long-term treatment with these drugs. The main anesthetic concerns in patients with epidermolysis bullosa center on the serious complications that can occur if proper precautions are not taken during instrumentation. Avoidance of trauma to the skin and mucous membranes is crucial. Bulla formation can be caused by trauma from tape, blood pressure cuffs, tourniquets, adhesive electrodes, and rubbing of the skin with alcohol wipes. Blood pressure cuffs should be padded with a loose cotton dressing. Electrodes should have the adhesive portion removed. Petroleum jelly gauze can help hold the electrodes in place. Anything that touches a patient should be well padded. Intravenous and intraarterial catheters should be sutured or held in place with gauze wraps rather than tape. A nonadhesive pulse oximetry sensor should be used. A soft foam, sheepskin, or gel pad should be placed under the patient. All creases should be removed from the linen.

Trauma from the anesthetic face mask must be minimized by gentle application against the face. Lubrication of the face and mask with cortisol ointment or another lubricant can be helpful. Upper airway instrumentation should be minimized, because the squamous epithelium lining the oropharynx and esophagus is very susceptible to trauma. Frictional trauma to the oropharynx, such as that produced by an oral airway, can result in

formation of large intraoral bullae and/or extensive hemorrhage from denuded mucosa. Nasal airways are equally hazardous. Esophageal stethoscopes should be avoided. Hemorrhage from ruptured oral bullae has been treated successfully by application of epinephrine-soaked gauze directly to the bullae.

Interestingly, endotracheal intubation has not been associated with laryngeal or tracheal complications in patients with epidermolysis bullosa dystrophica. Indeed, laryngeal involvement is rare in this form of the disease, and tracheal bullae have not been reported. This finding is consistent with the greater resistance of columnar epithelium to disruption compared with fragile squamous epithelium. Generous lubrication of the laryngoscope blade with cortisol ointment and/or petroleum jelly and selection of a smaller-than-usual endotracheal tube are recommended. Chronic scarring of the oral cavity can result in a narrow oral aperture and immobility of the tongue, which makes tracheal intubation difficult. After intubation, the tube must be carefully immobilized with soft cloth bandages to prevent movement in the oropharynx, and the tube must be positioned so that it does not exert lateral forces at the corners of the mouth. Tape is not used to hold the endotracheal tube in place. Oropharyngeal suctioning can lead to life-threatening bulla formation. The risk of pulmonary aspiration may be increased in the presence of esophageal stricture.

Porphyria cutanea tarda has been reported to occur with increased frequency in patients with epidermolysis bullosa. This type of porphyria does not have the same implications for management of anesthesia as acute intermittent porphyria.

Propofol and ketamine are useful for avoiding airway manipulation when the operative procedure does not require controlled ventilation or skeletal muscle relaxation. Despite the presence of dystrophic skeletal muscle, there is no evidence that these patients are at increased risk of a hyperkalemic response when treated with succinylcholine. There are no known contraindications to the use of volatile anesthetics in these patients. As alternatives to general anesthesia, regional anesthetic techniques (spinal, epidural, brachial plexus block) have been recommended.

Pemphigus

Pemphigus refers to a group of chronic autoimmune blistering (vesiculobullous) diseases that may involve extensive areas of the skin and mucous membranes. Cutaneous pemphigus is characterized by bullae of the skin and mucous membranes (mouth, upper airway, genitalia). Two histopathologically and clinically different types of pemphigus have been recognized: pemphigus vulgaris and pemphigus foliaceus. Cutaneous pemphigus closely resembles the oral manifestations of epidermolysis bullosa dystrophica. Involvement of the oropharynx is present in approximately 50% of patients with pemphigus. Extensive oropharyngeal involvement makes eating painful, and patients may decrease oral intake to the point that severe malnutrition develops. Denuding of skin and bulla formation can result in significant fluid and protein losses. The risk of secondary infection is substantial.

Pemphigus is an autoimmune disorder in which circulating antibodies attack antigenic sites on the surface of epidermal cells, which results in destruction of these cells. Pemphigus may be associated with underlying malignancy, especially lymphoreticular cancer. As with epidermolysis bullosa, there may be an absence of intercellular bridges that normally prevent the separation of epidermal cells. Therefore, frictional trauma can result in bulla formation. Occasionally, infection or drug sensitivity is the inciting event for bulla formation. Pemphigus vulgaris is the most common form of pemphigus and is also the most significant because of its high incidence of oropharyngeal lesions.

TREATMENT

Treatment of pemphigus with corticosteroids has decreased the mortality associated with this disease from 70% to 5%. Biologic and immunosuppressive therapy with mycophenolate mofetil, rituximab, azathioprine, methotrexate, and cyclophosphamide has also been used successfully for early treatment of pemphigus. Immune globulin has replaced high-dose corticosteroids as a rescue therapy.

MANAGEMENT OF ANESTHESIA

Management of anesthesia in patients with pemphigus and epidermolysis bullosa is similar. Preoperative evaluation must consider current drug therapy. Supplementation with corticosteroids may be necessary. Electrolyte derangements may be present due to chronic fluid losses through bullous skin lesions. Dehydration and hypokalemia are not uncommon.

Airway management may be difficult because of bullae in the oropharynx. Airway manipulation, including direct laryngoscopy and endotracheal intubation, can result in acute bulla formation, upper airway obstruction, and bleeding. Regional anesthesia, although controversial, has been used successfully in these patients. Skin infection at the site selected for regional anesthesia is possible. Infiltration with a local anesthetic solution is usually avoided because of the risk of skin sloughing and bulla formation at the injection site. Propofol and ketamine are useful for general anesthesia in selected patients.

Psoriasis

Psoriasis is a common chronic dermatologic disorder affecting 1% to 3% of the world's population. It is characterized by accelerated epidermal growth resulting in inflammatory erythematous papules covered with loosely adherent scales (chronic plaque psoriasis). Skin lesions are remitting and relapsing. Onset may occur during adolescence and young adulthood or at an older age. Symmetrically distributed skin lesions typically involve the elbows, knees, hairline, and presacral region. An asymmetrical arthropathy occurs in about 5% to 8% of patients. This usually involves the small joints of the hands and feet, the large joints of the legs, or some combination of both. High-output heart failure has been observed. Generalized pustular psoriasis is a rare form of the disease

that may be complicated by hypoalbuminemia, sepsis, and renal failure.

TREATMENT

Treatment of psoriasis is directed at slowing the rapid proliferation of epidermal cells. Coal tar is effective because of its antimitotic action and its ability to inhibit enzymes. Although preparations containing coal tar can cause plaques to clear when used alone, they are generally used in combination with ultraviolet phototherapy. The use of coal tar is limited by its unpleasant odor and its potential to irritate normal skin. Coal tar is frequently used in shampoo preparations to prevent psoriatic scaling of the scalp. In rare cases, skin cancer has been associated with the therapeutic use of coal tar. Ointments containing salicylic acid are the most widely used keratolytic agents. They can be used alone or in combination with coal tar or topical corticosteroids. Topical corticosteroids are effective, but the disease promptly recurs when treatment is discontinued. Application of corticosteroids under occlusive dressings can result in significant systemic absorption and suppression of the pituitary-adrenal axis. Calcipotriene ointment (a vitamin D analogue) and tazarotene (a topical retinoid) can be used. Systemic therapy with methotrexate or cyclosporine and biologic therapy with etanercept (a tumor necrosis factor [TNF] inhibitor), infliximab (a monoclonal antibody to TNF), alefacept (an immunomodulatory fusion protein), or efalizumab (a monoclonal antibody to CD11a) may be required for severe cases. Toxic effects of these drugs include cirrhosis, renal failure, hypertension, and pneumonitis.

MANAGEMENT OF ANESTHESIA

Management of anesthesia must include evaluation of the drugs being used for the treatment of psoriasis, including topical corticosteroids and chemotherapeutic drugs. Skin trauma from venipuncture or the surgical incision can accentuate psoriasis in some patients. Patients with psoriasis often have a marked increase in skin blood flow that can contribute to altered thermoregulation.

Mastocytosis

Mastocytosis is a rare disorder of mast cell proliferation that can occur in a cutaneous form (urticaria pigmentosa) or in a systemic form. Urticaria pigmentosa is usually benign and asymptomatic. Children are most often affected. In nearly half of affected children, the small red-brown macules that are present on the trunk and extremities disappear by adulthood. In the systemic form of mastocytosis, mast cells proliferate in all organs (especially bone, liver, and spleen) but not in the central nervous system. Degranulation of mast cells with release of histamine, heparin, prostaglandins, and numerous enzymes (tryptases, hydrolases) may occur spontaneously or may be triggered by nonimmune factors, including physical or psychologic stimuli, alcohol, and drugs known to release histamine. A rare form of systemic mastocytosis, known as *malignant aggressive systemic mastocytosis,* is characterized by diffuse mast cell proliferation in parenchymal organs, thrombocytopenia, and hemorrhage. Patients with this form often require splenectomy.

SIGNS AND SYMPTOMS

Classic signs and symptoms of mastocytosis reflect degranulation of mast cells with anaphylactoid responses characterized by pruritus, urticaria, and flushing. These changes may be accompanied by hypotension and tachycardia. Hypotension may be so severe as to be life threatening. Although symptoms are usually attributed to histamine release from mast cells, histamine 1 and 2 (H_1 and H_2) receptor antagonists are not always protective. This suggests that vasoactive substances other than histamine (such as prostaglandins) may be involved. The incidence of bronchospasm is low. Bleeding is unusual in these patients, even though mast cells contain heparin.

MANAGEMENT OF ANESTHESIA

Management of anesthesia is influenced by the possibility of intraoperative mast cell degranulation and anaphylactoid reaction. Although the intraoperative period is usually uneventful, there are reports of life-threatening anaphylactoid reactions with even minor surgical procedures, which emphasizes the need to have resuscitation drugs such as epinephrine immediately available. Preoperative administration of H_1- and H_2-receptor antagonists may be considered to decrease the clinical response to histamine release. However, these drugs do not interfere with the actual release of histamine from mast cells. Cromolyn sodium does inhibit mast cell degranulation and may decrease the risk of bronchospasm.

Some recommend preoperative skin testing of anesthesia-related drugs to help define which anesthetics would provoke mast cell degranulation. Fentanyl, propofol, and vecuronium have been administered to these patients without causing mast cell degranulation as have succinylcholine and meperidine. Volatile anesthetics also appear to be acceptable in these patients. Monitoring serum tryptase concentration during the perioperative period may be useful for detecting the occurrence of mast cell degranulation.

Episodes of profound hypotension have been observed with administration of radiocontrast media to patients with mastocytosis. Therefore, it is prudent to pretreat these patients with H_1- and H_2-histamine receptor antagonists and a glucocorticoid before procedures involving contrast dye.

Atopic Dermatitis

Atopic dermatitis is the cutaneous manifestation of the atopic state. It is characterized by dry, scaly, eczematous, pruritic patches on the face, neck, and flexor surfaces of the arms and legs. Pruritus is the primary symptom. Systemic antihistamines are effective in decreasing pruritus, and corticosteroids may be indicated for short-term treatment of severe cases. Pulmonary manifestations of the atopic state, such as asthma, hay fever, otitis media, and sinusitis may influence anesthetic management.

Urticaria

Urticaria may be characterized as *acute urticaria, chronic urticaria,* or *physical urticaria.* Acute urticaria (hives) and angioedema affects 10% to 20% of the U.S. population at one time or another. In most people, the cause cannot be determined and the lesions resolve spontaneously or after administration of antihistamines. Only a minority of patients have lesions for a long period of time. With physical urticaria, physically stimulating the skin causes the formation of local wheals, itching, and, in some cases, angioedema. Cold urticaria accounts for 3% to 5% of all physical urticarias (Table 21-1). Urticarial

TABLE 21-1   Features of common types of chronic urticaria

Type of urticaria	Age range (yr)	Clinical features	Angioedema	Diagnostic test
Chronic idiopathic urticaria	20-50	Pink or pale edematous papules or wheals, wheals often annular, pruritus	Yes	
Symptomatic dermatographism	20-50	Linear wheals with a surrounding bright red flare at sites of stimulation, pruritus	No	Light stroking of skin causes wheal
Physical urticarias				
Cold	10-40	Pale or red swelling at sites of contact with cold surfaces or fluids, pruritus	Yes	Application of ice pack causes a wheal within 5 min of removing the ice (cold stimulation test)
Pressure	20-50	Swelling at sites of pressure (soles, palms, waist) lasting ≥2-24 hr, pain, pruritus	No	Application of pressure perpendicular to skin produces persistent red swelling after a latent period of 1-4 hr
Solar	20-50	Pale or red swelling at site of exposure to ultraviolet or visible light, pruritus	Yes	Radiation by a solar simulator for 30-120 sec causes wheals in 30 min
Cholinergic	10-50	Monomorphic pale or pink wheals on trunk, neck, and limbs, pruritus	Yes	Exercise or hot shower elicits wheals

Adapted from Greaves MW. Chronic urticaria. *N Engl J Med.* 1995;332:1767-1772.

vasculitis may be a presenting symptom of systemic lupus erythematosus and Sjögren's syndrome.

CHRONIC URTICARIA

Chronic urticaria is characterized by circumscribed wheals and localized areas of edema produced by extravasation of fluid through blood vessel walls. The wheals are smooth, pink to red, and surrounded by a bright red flare. They are usually intensely pruritic, can be found anywhere on hairless or hairy skin, and last less than 24 hours. Wheals lasting longer than 24 hours raise the possibility of other diagnoses, including urticarial vasculitis. Chronic urticaria affects approximately twice as many women as men and often follows a remitting and relapsing course, with symptoms typically increasing at night. Angioedema is urticaria involving the mucous membranes, particularly those of the mouth, pharynx, and larynx. Mast cells and basophils regulate urticarial reactions. When they are stimulated by certain nonimmunologic events or by immunologic factors (drugs, inhaled allergens), storage granules in these cells release histamine and other vasoactive substances such as bradykinin. These substances result in the localized vasodilation and transudation of fluid characteristic of urticarial lesions.

Except in patients with chronic urticaria for whom avoidable causes can be identified, treatment is symptomatic. A tepid shower temporarily alleviates pruritus. Antihistamines (H$_1$-receptor antagonists) are the principal treatment for mild cases of recurring chronic urticaria. Terfenadine has a low potential for sedation and is a common treatment for mild cases of chronic urticaria. High doses of this drug have been associated with cardiac dysrhythmias. Doxepin is a tricyclic antidepressant drug with significant H$_1$-antagonist actions that is particularly useful when severe urticaria is associated with depression. The combination of H$_1$- and H$_2$-receptor antagonists may be more efficacious than use of H$_1$-receptor antagonists alone. If antihistamines do not control chronic urticaria, a course of systemic corticosteroids may be considered. The period of treatment is usually limited to 21 days, because prolonged use of corticosteroids is invariably associated with a decrease in efficacy and an increase in side effects. A 2% topical spray of ephedrine is useful for treating oropharyngeal edema. Swelling involving the tongue may require urgent treatment with epinephrine.

All patients with chronic urticaria should be advised to avoid angiotensin-converting enzyme inhibitors, aspirin, and other nonsteroidal antiinflammatory drugs (NSAIDs).

COLD URTICARIA

Cold urticaria is characterized by development of urticaria and angioedema following exposure to cold. The most common triggering factors are cold air currents, rain, aquatic activities, snow, consumption of cold foods and beverages, and contact with cold objects. Severe cold urticaria may be life-threatening with laryngeal edema, bronchospasm, and hypotension. The diagnosis is based on skin stimulation at a temperature of 0° to 4° C for 1 to 5 minutes (cold stimulation test). Immunologic mechanisms may be associated with the development of cold urticaria. Immunoglobulin E concentrations may be increased. Cutaneous mast cells rather than basophils in the bloodstream are the target cells for degranulation, although basophil degranulation is possible with profound hypothermia. Tryptase is an important marker of mast cell degranulation.

The primary objective of treatment of cold urticaria is to prevent systemic reactions caused by known triggers. Antihistamines may decrease the incidence of recurrence and prolong the time that a cold stimulus is tolerated before a reaction occurs.

Management of Anesthesia

Management of anesthesia includes avoidance of drugs that are likely to evoke histamine release. Drugs requiring cold storage should be avoided or warmed before injection. Other prophylactic measures include warming intravenous fluids and increasing the ambient temperature of the operating room. Preoperative administration of H$_1$- and H$_2$-receptor antagonists and corticosteroids has been recommended, especially when intraoperative hypothermia is unavoidable, as may be the case during surgery requiring cardiopulmonary bypass.

Erythema Multiforme

Erythema multiforme is a recurrent disease of the skin and mucous membranes characterized by lesions ranging from edematous macules and papules to vesicular or bullous lesions that may ulcerate. Attacks are associated with viral infection (especially herpes simplex), infection with hemolytic streptococci, cancer, collagen vascular disease, and drug-induced hypersensitivity.

Stevens-Johnson syndrome (erythema multiforme major) is a severe manifestation associated with multisystem dysfunction. High fever, tachycardia, and tachypnea may occur. Drugs associated with the onset of this syndrome include antibiotics, analgesics, and certain over-the-counter medications. Corticosteroids are used in the management of severe cases.

MANAGEMENT OF ANESTHESIA

The hazards of administering anesthesia to patients with Stevens-Johnson syndrome are similar to those encountered in anesthetizing patients with epidermolysis bullosa. For example, involvement of the upper respiratory tract can make management of the airway and tracheal intubation difficult. The presence of pulmonary blebs makes these patients vulnerable to pneumothorax, particularly with positive pressure ventilation. Pulmonary blebs also prohibit the use of nitrous oxide. Patients with particularly severe Stevens-Johnson syndrome should be treated in a burn unit.

Scleroderma

Scleroderma (systemic sclerosis) is characterized by inflammation, vascular sclerosis, and fibrosis of the skin and viscera. Microvascular changes produce tissue fibrosis and organ sclerosis. Injury to vascular endothelial cells results in vascular obliteration and leakage of serum proteins into the interstitial space. These proteins produce tissue edema, lymphatic obstruction, and ultimately fibrosis. In some patients, the disease evolves into CREST syndrome (*c*alcinoses, *R*aynaud's phenomenon, *e*sophageal hypomotility, *s*clerodactyly, *t*elangiectasia). The prognosis is poor and is related to the extent of visceral involvement. No drugs or treatments have proved safe and effective in altering the underlying disease process.

The etiology of scleroderma is unknown, but the disease process has the characteristics of both a collagen vascular disease and an autoimmune disease. The typical age at onset is 20 to 40 years, and women are most often affected. Pregnancy accelerates the progression of scleroderma in approximately half of patients. The incidence of spontaneous abortion, premature labor, and perinatal mortality is high.

SIGNS AND SYMPTOMS

Manifestations of scleroderma occur in the skin and musculoskeletal system, nervous system, cardiovascular system, lungs, kidneys, and gastrointestinal tract.

Skin exhibits mild thickening and diffuse nonpitting edema. As scleroderma progresses, the skin becomes taut, which results in limited mobility and flexion contractures, especially of the fingers. Skeletal muscles may develop myopathy, manifested as weakness, particularly of proximal skeletal muscle groups. The plasma creatine kinase concentration is typically increased. Mild inflammatory arthritis can occur, but most limitation to joint movement is due to the thickened, taut skin. Avascular necrosis of the femoral head may occur.

Peripheral or cranial nerve neuropathy has been attributed to nerve compression by thickened connective tissue surrounding the nerve sheath. Facial pain suggestive of trigeminal neuralgia may occur as a result of this thickening. Keratoconjunctivitis sicca (dry eyes) exists in some patients and may predispose to corneal abrasions.

Changes in the myocardium reflect sclerosis of small coronary arteries and the conduction system, replacement of cardiac muscle with fibrous tissue, and the indirect effects of systemic and pulmonary hypertension. These changes result in cardiac dysrhythmias, cardiac conduction abnormalities, and congestive heart failure. Intimal fibrosis of pulmonary arteries is associated with a high incidence of pulmonary hypertension, which may progress to cor pulmonale. Pulmonary hypertension is often present, even in asymptomatic patients. Pericarditis and pericardial effusion with or without cardiac tamponade are not infrequent. Changes in the peripheral portion of the vascular tree are common and typically involve intermittent vasospasm in the small arteries of the digits. Raynaud's phenomenon occurs in most cases and may be the initial manifestation of scleroderma. Oral or nasal telangiectasias may be present.

The effects of scleroderma on the lungs are a major cause of morbidity and mortality. Diffuse interstitial pulmonary fibrosis may occur independent of the vascular changes that lead to pulmonary hypertension. Arterial hypoxemia resulting from decreased diffusion capacity is not unusual in these patients, even at rest. Although dermal sclerosis does not decrease chest wall compliance, pulmonary compliance is diminished by fibrosis.

Renal artery stenosis as a result of arteriolar intimal proliferation leads to decreased renal blood flow and systemic hypertension. Development of malignant hypertension and irreversible renal failure used to be the most common cause of death in patients with scleroderma, but now scleroderma renal crisis is relatively rare. Angiotensin-converting enzyme inhibitors are effective in controlling hypertension and in improving the impaired renal function that accompanies the hypertension. Corticosteroids can precipitate a renal crisis in patients with scleroderma.

Involvement of the gastrointestinal tract by scleroderma may manifest as dryness of the oral mucosa (xerostomia). Progressive fibrosis of the gastrointestinal tract causes hypomotility of the lower esophagus and small intestine. Dysphagia is a common complaint. Lower esophageal sphincter tone is decreased, and reflux of gastric fluid into the esophagus is common. Symptoms resulting from this esophagitis can be treated with antacids. Bacterial overgrowth resulting from intestinal hypomotility can produce a malabsorption syndrome. Coagulation disorders reflecting malabsorption of vitamin K may be present. Broad-spectrum antibiotics are effective in the treatment of this type of malabsorption syndrome. Intestinal hypomotility can also manifest as intestinal pseudo-obstruction. Somatostatin analogues such as octreotide may improve intestinal motility. Prokinetic drugs such as metoclopramide are not effective.

MANAGEMENT OF ANESTHESIA

Preoperative evaluation of patients with scleroderma must focus attention on the organ systems likely to be involved by this disease. Decreased mandibular motion and narrowing of the oral aperture resulting from taut skin must be appreciated before induction of anesthesia. Fiberoptic laryngoscopy may be necessary to facilitate endotracheal intubation through a small oral aperture. Oral or nasal telangiectasias may bleed profusely if traumatized during tracheal intubation. Intravenous access may be impeded by dermal thickening. Intraarterial catheterization for blood pressure monitoring introduces the same concerns as in patients with Raynaud's phenomenon. Cardiac evaluation may provide evidence of pulmonary hypertension. Because of chronic systemic hypertension and vasomotor instability, patients with scleroderma may have a contracted intravascular volume. This may produce hypotension during induction of anesthesia when anesthetic drugs with vasodilating properties exert their effects. Hypotonia of the lower esophageal sphincter puts patients at risk of regurgitation and pulmonary aspiration. Efforts to increase gastric fluid pH with antacids or H_2-receptor antagonists before induction of anesthesia are recommended.

Intraoperatively, decreased pulmonary compliance may require higher airway pressures to ensure adequate ventilation. Supplemental oxygen is indicated in view of the impaired diffusion capacity and vulnerability to the development of arterial hypoxemia. Events known to increase pulmonary vascular resistance, such as respiratory acidosis and arterial hypoxemia, must be prevented. These patients may be particularly sensitive to the respiratory depressant effects of opioids, and a period of postoperative ventilatory support may be required in patients with severe pulmonary disease.

The degree of renal dysfunction must be considered when selecting anesthetic drugs dependent on renal elimination. Regional anesthesia may be technically difficult because of the skin and joint changes that accompany scleroderma. Attractive features of regional anesthesia include peripheral vasodilation and postoperative analgesia. Measures to minimize peripheral vasoconstriction include maintenance of the operating room temperature above 21° C and administration of warmed intravenous fluids. The eyes should be protected to prevent corneal abrasions.

Pseudoxanthoma Elasticum

Pseudoxanthoma elasticum is a rare hereditary disorder of elastic tissue. Elastic fibers degenerate and calcify over time. The most striking feature of this condition, and often the basis for the diagnosis, is the appearance of angioid streaks in the retina. Substantial loss of visual acuity may result from these ocular changes. Additional visual impairment may occur when vascular changes predispose to vitreous hemorrhage. Skin changes, consisting of yellowish, rectangular, elevated xanthoma-like lesions, primarily in the neck, axilla, and inguinal regions, are among the earliest clinical features. Interestingly, some tissues rich in elastic fibers, such as the lungs, aorta, palms, and soles, are not affected by this disease process.

Gastrointestinal hemorrhage is a frequent occurrence. Degenerative changes in the arteries supplying the gastrointestinal tract are thought to prevent vasoconstriction of these blood vessels in response to mucosal injury. The incidence of hypertension and ischemic heart disease is increased in these patients. Endocardial calcification can involve the conduction system and predispose to cardiac dysrhythmias and sudden death. Involvement of cardiac valves is frequent. Calcification of peripheral arteries, particularly the radial and ulnar arteries, is common. Psychiatric disturbances often accompany this disease.

MANAGEMENT OF ANESTHESIA
Management of anesthesia in patients with pseudoxanthoma elasticum is based on an appreciation of the abnormalities associated with this disease. Cardiovascular derangements are probably the most important considerations. The increased incidence of ischemic heart disease is considered when establishing limits for acceptable changes in blood pressure and heart rate. Electrocardiographic monitoring is particularly important in view of the potential for cardiac dysrhythmias. Noninvasive blood pressure monitoring devices are usually selected. Trauma to the mucosa of the upper gastrointestinal tract, as may be produced by a gastric tube or esophageal

stethoscope, should be minimized. There are no specific recommendations regarding the choice of anesthetic drugs or techniques.

Ehlers-Danlos Syndrome

Ehlers-Danlos syndrome consists of a group of inherited connective tissue disorders caused by abnormal production of procollagen and collagen. It is estimated that 1 in 5000 people is affected by this syndrome. The only form of Ehlers-Danlos syndrome associated with an increased risk of death is the type IV (vascular) syndrome. This form may be complicated by rupture of large blood vessels or disruption of the bowel.

SIGNS AND SYMPTOMS
All forms of Ehlers-Danlos syndrome cause signs and symptoms of joint hypermobility, skin fragility or hyperelasticity, bruising and scarring, musculoskeletal discomfort, and susceptibility to osteoarthritis. The gastrointestinal tract, uterus, and vasculature are particularly well endowed with type III collagen, which accounts for complications such as spontaneous rupture of the bowel, uterus, or major arteries. Premature labor and excessive bleeding at the time of delivery are common obstetric problems. Dilation of the trachea is often present, and the incidence of pneumothorax is increased. Mitral regurgitation and cardiac conduction abnormalities are occasionally seen. Patients may exhibit extensive ecchymoses with even minimal trauma, although a specific coagulation defect has not been identified.

MANAGEMENT OF ANESTHESIA
Management of anesthesia in patients with Ehlers-Danlos syndrome must consider the cardiovascular manifestations of this disease and the propensity of these patients to bleed excessively. Avoidance of intramuscular injections or instrumentation of the nose or esophagus is important in view of the bleeding tendency. Trauma during direct laryngoscopy must be minimized. The decision regarding placement of an arterial or central venous catheter must consider the fact that hematoma formation may be extensive. Extravasation of intravenous fluids resulting from a displaced venous cannula may go unnoticed because of the extreme laxity of the skin. Maintenance of low airway pressure during assisted or controlled mechanical ventilation seems prudent in view of the increased incidence of pneumothorax. There are no specific recommendations for the selection of drugs to provide anesthesia. Regional anesthesia is not recommended because of the tendency of these patients to bleed and form extensive hematomas. Surgical complications may include hemorrhage and postoperative wound dehiscence.

Marfan's Syndrome

Marfan's syndrome, a connective tissue disorder, is inherited as an autosomal dominant trait. The incidence is 4 to 6 per 100,000 live births. Characteristically, these patients have long tubular bones, giving them a tall stature and an "Abe Lincoln" appearance. Additional skeletal abnormalities include a high-arched palate, pectus excavatum, kyphoscoliosis, and hyper-extensibility of the joints. Early development of emphysema is characteristic and may further accentuate the impact of lung disease related to kyphoscoliosis. There is a high incidence of spontaneous pneumothorax. Ocular changes such as lens dis-location, myopia, and retinal detachment occur in more than half of patients with Marfan's syndrome.

CARDIOVASCULAR SYSTEM

Cardiovascular abnormalities are responsible for nearly all premature deaths in patients with Marfan's syndrome. Defec-tive connective tissue in the aorta and heart valves can lead to aortic dilation, dissection, or rupture and to prolapse of cardiac valves, especially the mitral valve. Mitral regurgitation resulting from mitral valve prolapse is a common abnormality. The risk of bacterial endocarditis is increased in the presence of this valvular heart disease. Cardiac conduction abnormali-ties, especially bundle branch block, are common. Prophy-lactic β-blocker therapy is recommended for patients with a dilated thoracic aorta. Surgical replacement of the aortic valve and ascending aorta is indicated when the diameter of the ascending aorta exceeds 6 cm and substantial aortic regurgita-tion is present. Pregnancy poses a unique risk of rupture or dissection of the aorta in women with Marfan's syndrome.

MANAGEMENT OF ANESTHESIA

Preoperative evaluation of patients with Marfan's syndrome should focus on cardiopulmonary abnormalities. In most patients, skeletal abnormalities have little impact on the air-way. Care should be exercised, however, to avoid temporo-mandibular joint dislocation, to which these patients are susceptible. In view of the risk of aortic dissection, it is pru-dent to avoid any sustained increase in systemic blood pres-sure, as can occur during direct laryngoscopy or in response to painful surgical stimulation. Invasive monitoring including transesophageal echocardiography may be a consideration in selected patients. A high index of suspicion must be main-tained for the development of pneumothorax.

MUSCLE AND NEUROMUSCULAR DISEASES

Polymyositis and Dermatomyositis

Polymyositis and dermatomyositis are multisystem diseases of unknown etiology, manifesting as inflammatory myopathies. Dermatomyositis has characteristic skin changes in addi-tion to muscle weakness. These cutaneous changes include discoloration of the upper eyelids, periorbital edema, a scaly erythematous malar rash, and symmetrical erythematous atrophic changes over the extensor surfaces of joints. Abnor-mal immune responses may be responsible for the slowly progressive skeletal muscle damage of dermatomyositis and polymyositis. The concept that altered cellular immunity

causes polymyositis is supported by the fact that 10% to 20% of these patients have occult neoplasms.

SIGNS AND SYMPTOMS

Muscle weakness involves proximal skeletal muscle groups, especially the flexors of the neck, shoulders, and hips. Patients may have difficulty climbing stairs. Dysphagia, pulmonary aspiration, and pneumonia can result from paresis of pharyn-geal and respiratory muscles. Diaphragmatic and intercostal muscle weakness may contribute to ventilatory insufficiency. Increased serum creatine kinase concentrations parallel the extent and rapidity of skeletal muscle destruction. These dis-eases do *not* affect the neuromuscular junction.

Heart block secondary to myocardial fibrosis or atrophy of the conduction system, left ventricular dysfunction, and myo-carditis can occur. Polymyositis can also be associated with systemic lupus erythematosus, scleroderma, and rheumatoid arthritis. A widespread necrotizing vasculitis may be present in childhood forms of this disease.

DIAGNOSIS

The diagnosis of polymyositis or dermatomyositis is consid-ered when proximal skeletal muscle weakness, an increased serum creatine kinase concentration, and the characteristic skin rash are present. Electromyography may demonstrate the triad of spontaneous fibrillation potentials, decreased amplitude of voluntary contraction potentials, and repetitive potentials on needle insertion. Skeletal muscle biopsy findings support the clinical diagnosis. Muscular dystrophy and myas-thenia gravis can mimic polymyositis.

TREATMENT

Corticosteroids are the usual treatment for polymyositis. Immunosuppressive therapy with methotrexate, azathioprine, cyclophosphamide, mycophenolate, or cyclosporine may be effective when the response to corticosteroids is inadequate. Intravenous immunoglobulin may be useful in refractory cases.

MANAGEMENT OF ANESTHESIA

Management of anesthesia must consider the vulnerability of patients with polymyositis to pulmonary aspiration. In view of the skeletal muscle weakness, there has been concern that these patients could display abnormal responses to muscle relaxants. However, responses to nondepolarizing muscle relaxants and succinylcholine are *normal* in patients with polymyositis.

Muscular Dystrophy

Muscular dystrophy is a group of hereditary diseases char-acterized by painless degeneration and atrophy of skeletal muscles. There are progressive, symmetrical skeletal muscle weakness and wasting but no evidence of skeletal muscle denervation. Sensation and reflexes are intact. Increased permeability of skeletal muscle membranes precedes clinical evidence of muscular dystrophy. In order of decreasing frequency, muscular dystrophy can be categorized as pseudohypertrophic (Duchenne's muscular dystrophy), limb-girdle, facioscapulohumeral (Landouzy-Dejerine dystrophy), nemaline rod, or oculopharyngeal.

PSEUDOHYPERTROPHIC MUSCULAR DYSTROPHY (DUCHENNE'S MUSCULAR DYSTROPHY)

Pseudohypertrophic muscular dystrophy is the most common and most severe form of childhood progressive muscular dystrophy. The disease is caused by an X-linked recessive gene and becomes apparent in 2- to 5-year-old boys. Initial symptoms include a waddling gait, frequent falling, and difficulty climbing stairs, and these reflect involvement of the proximal skeletal muscle groups of the pelvic girdle. Affected muscles become larger as a result of fatty infiltration, and this accounts for the designation of this disorder as *pseudohypertrophic*. There is progressive deterioration in skeletal muscle strength, and typically these boys are confined to a wheelchair by age 8 to 10. Kyphoscoliosis can develop. Skeletal muscle atrophy can predispose to long bone fractures. Mental retardation is often present. Serum creatine kinase concentrations are 20 to 100 times normal, even early in the disease, reflecting increased permeability of skeletal muscle membranes and skeletal muscle necrosis. Approximately 70% of the female carriers of this disease also exhibit increased serum creatine kinase concentrations. Skeletal muscle biopsy specimens early in the course of the disease may demonstrate necrosis and phagocytosis of muscle fibers. Death usually occurs at 15 to 25 years of age as a result of congestive heart failure and/or pneumonia.

Degeneration of cardiac muscle invariably accompanies this muscular dystrophy. Characteristically, the electrocardiogram reveals tall R waves in V_1, deep Q waves in the limb leads, a short PR interval, and sinus tachycardia. Mitral regurgitation may occur as a result of papillary muscle dysfunction or decreased myocardial contractility.

Chronic weakness of the respiratory muscles and a weakened cough result in loss of pulmonary reserve and accumulation of secretions. These abnormalities predispose to recurrent pneumonia. Respiratory insufficiency often remains covert because overall activity is so limited. As the disease progresses, kyphoscoliosis contributes to further restrictive lung disease. Sleep apnea may occur and may contribute to development of pulmonary hypertension. Approximately 30% of deaths in individuals with pseudohypertrophic muscular dystrophy are due to respiratory causes.

Management of Anesthesia

Children with pseudohypertrophic muscular dystrophy may require anesthesia for muscle biopsy or correction of orthopedic deformities. Preparation for anesthesia must take into consideration the implications of increased skeletal muscle membrane permeability and decreased cardiopulmonary reserve. Hypomotility of the gastrointestinal tract may delay gastric emptying and, in the presence of weak laryngeal reflexes, can increase the risk of pulmonary aspiration.

Use of succinylcholine is contraindicated because of the risk of rhabdomyolysis, hyperkalemia, and/or cardiac arrest. Cardiac arrest may be due to hyperkalemia or to ventricular fibrillation. Indeed, ventricular fibrillation during induction of anesthesia that included succinylcholine administration has been observed in patients later discovered to have this form of muscular dystrophy. The response to nondepolarizing muscle relaxants is normal.

Rhabdomyolysis, with or without cardiac arrest, has been observed in association with administration of volatile anesthetics to these patients even in the absence of succinylcholine administration. Dantrolene should be available, because there is an increased incidence of malignant hyperthermia in these patients. Malignant hyperthermia has been observed after even brief periods of halothane administration, although most cases have been triggered by succinylcholine or prolonged inhalation of halothane. Regional anesthesia avoids the unique risks of general anesthesia in these patients. During the postoperative period, neuraxial analgesia may facilitate chest physiotherapy.

Monitoring is directed at early detection of malignant hyperthermia and cardiac depression. Postoperative pulmonary dysfunction should be anticipated and attempts made to facilitate clearance of secretions. Delayed pulmonary insufficiency may occur up to 36 hours postoperatively even though skeletal muscle strength has apparently returned to its preoperative levels.

LIMB-GIRDLE MUSCULAR DYSTROPHY

Limb-girdle muscular dystrophy is a slowly progressive but relatively benign disease. Onset occurs from the second to the fifth decade. Shoulder girdle or hip girdle muscles may be the only skeletal muscles involved.

FACIOSCAPULOHUMERAL MUSCULAR DYSTROPHY

Facioscapulohumeral muscular dystrophy is characterized by a slowly progressive wasting of facial, pectoral, and shoulder girdle muscles that begins during adolescence. Eventually the lower limbs are also involved. Early symptoms include difficulty raising the arms above the head and difficulty smiling. There is no involvement of cardiac muscle, and serum creatine kinase concentration is seldom increased. Recovery from atracurium-induced neuromuscular blockade may be faster than normal in these patients. The progression of this muscular dystrophy is slow and a long life is likely.

NEMALINE ROD MUSCULAR DYSTROPHY

Nemaline rod muscular dystrophy is an autosomal dominant disease characterized by slowly progressive or nonprogressive symmetrical dystrophy of skeletal and smooth muscle. The diagnosis is confirmed by skeletal muscle biopsy. Histologic examination demonstrates the presence of rods between normal myofibrils.

Affected individuals experience delayed motor development, generalized skeletal muscle weakness, a decrease in muscle mass, hypotonia, and loss of deep tendon reflexes. There are typical dysmorphic features and an abnormal gait, but intelligence is usually normal. Affected infants may present with hypotonia, dysphagia, respiratory distress, and cyanosis. Micrognathia and dental malocclusion are common. Other skeletal deformities include kyphoscoliosis and pectus excavatum. Restrictive lung disease may result from the myopathy and/or scoliosis. Cardiac failure resulting from dilated cardiomyopathy has been described.

Management of Anesthesia

Tracheal intubation may be difficult because of anatomic abnormalities such as micrognathia and a high-arched palate. Awake fiberoptic endotracheal intubation may be prudent. The respiratory depressant effects of drugs may be exaggerated in these patients due to respiratory muscle weakness and chest wall abnormalities. Ventilation/perfusion mismatching is increased, and the ventilatory response to carbon dioxide may be blunted. Bulbar palsy associated with regurgitation and aspiration may further complicate anesthetic management.

The response to succinylcholine and nondepolarizing neuromuscular blockers is *unpredictable.* There is no conclusive evidence that administration of succinylcholine evokes excessive potassium release. Indeed, resistance to succinylcholine has been described in some patients. Malignant hyperthermia has not been reported in patients with nemaline rod myopathy. Myocardial depression may accompany administration of volatile anesthetics if the disease process involves the myocardium. Plans for regional anesthesia must consider the possible respiratory compromise that could accompany a high motor block. In addition, the exaggerated lumbar lordosis and/or kyphoscoliosis may make neuraxial anesthesia technically difficult.

OCULOPHARYNGEAL DYSTROPHY

Oculopharyngeal dystrophy is a rare variant of muscular dystrophy characterized by progressive dysphagia and ptosis. Although experience is limited, these patients may be at risk of aspiration during the perioperative period, and their sensitivity to muscle relaxants may be increased.

EMERY-DREIFUSS MUSCULAR DYSTROPHY

Emery-Dreifuss muscular dystrophy is an X-linked recessive disorder characterized by development of skeletal muscle contractures that precede the onset of skeletal muscle weakness. These contractures are typically in a humeroperoneal distribution. Mental retardation is not present, and respiratory function is maintained. Cardiac involvement may be life-threatening and present as congestive heart failure, thromboembolism, or bradycardia. Unlike in other muscular dystrophies, female carriers of this disorder may experience cardiac impairment.

Myotonic Dystrophy

The term *myotonic dystrophy* designates a group of hereditary degenerative diseases of skeletal muscle characterized by persistent contracture (myotonia) after voluntary contraction of a

TABLE 21-2 ■ Classification of myotonic dystrophies
Myotonic dystrophy (myotonia atrophica, Steinert's disease)
Myotonia congenita (Thomsen's disease)
Paramyotonia congenita
Hyperkalemic periodic paralysis
Acid-maltase deficiency (Pompe's disease)
Schwartz-Jampel syndrome (chondrodystrophic myotonia)

muscle or following electrical stimulation (Table 21-2). Peripheral nerves and the neuromuscular junction are *not* affected. Electromyographic findings are diagnostic and are characterized by prolonged discharges of repetitive muscle action potentials. This inability of skeletal muscle to relax after voluntary contraction or stimulation results from abnormal calcium metabolism. Intracellular adenosine triphosphatase fails to return calcium to the sarcoplasmic reticulum, so unsequestered calcium remains available to produce sustained skeletal muscle contraction. Interestingly, general anesthesia, regional anesthesia, and neuromuscular blockade are *not* able to prevent or relieve this skeletal muscle contraction. Infiltration of contracted skeletal muscles with local anesthetic may induce relaxation. Quinine (300 to 600 mg IV) has also been reported to be effective in some cases. Increasing the ambient temperature of the operating room decreases the severity of myotonia and the incidence of postoperative shivering, which can precipitate skeletal muscle contraction. Most patients with myotonia survive to adulthood with little impairment, and it is common for them to conceal their symptoms, so they may come for surgery without the underlying myotonia being appreciated.

MYOTONIA DYSTROPHICA

Myotonia dystrophica is the most common and most serious form of myotonic dystrophy affecting adults. It is inherited as an autosomal dominant trait, with the onset of symptoms during the second or third decade. Unlike other myotonic syndromes, myotonia dystrophica is a multisystem disease, although skeletal muscles are affected most. Death from pneumonia or heart failure often occurs by the sixth decade of life. This reflects progressive involvement of skeletal muscle, cardiac muscle, and smooth muscle. Perioperative morbidity and mortality rates are high principally due to cardiopulmonary complications.

Treatment is symptomatic and may include use of phenytoin. Quinine and procainamide also have antimyotonic properties but can worsen cardiac conduction abnormalities. These three drugs depress sodium influx into skeletal muscle cells and delay the return of membrane excitability.

Signs and Symptoms

Myotonia dystrophica usually manifests as facial weakness (expressionless facies), wasting and weakness of the sternocleidomastoid muscles, ptosis, dysarthria, dysphagia, and inability to relax the hand grip (myotonia). Other characteristic features include the triad of mental retardation, frontal baldness, and cataracts. Endocrine gland involvement may be indicated by gonadal atrophy, diabetes mellitus, hypothyroidism, and adrenal insufficiency. Delayed gastric emptying and intestinal pseudo-obstruction may be present. Central sleep apnea may occur and may account for the frequent presence of hypersomnolence. There is an increased incidence of cholelithiasis, especially in men. Exacerbation of symptoms during pregnancy is common, and uterine atony and retained placenta often complicate vaginal delivery.

Cardiac dysrhythmias and conduction abnormalities presumably reflect myocardial involvement by the myotonic process. First-degree atrioventricular heart block is common and is often present before the clinical onset of the disease. Up to 20% of patients have asymptomatic mitral valve prolapse. Reports of sudden death may reflect development of complete heart block. Pharyngeal and thoracic muscle weakness makes these patients vulnerable to pulmonary aspiration.

Management of Anesthesia

Preoperative evaluation and management of anesthesia in patients with myotonia dystrophica must consider the likelihood of cardiomyopathy, respiratory muscle weakness, and the potential for abnormal responses to anesthetic drugs. Even asymptomatic patients have some degree of cardiomyopathy, so the myocardial depression produced by volatile anesthetics may be exaggerated. Cardiac dysrhythmias may need treatment. Anesthesia and surgery could aggravate cardiac conduction problems by increasing vagal tone.

Succinylcholine should not be administered because prolonged skeletal muscle contraction can result. However, the response to nondepolarizing neuromuscular blocking drugs is normal. Theoretically, reversal of neuromuscular blockade could precipitate skeletal muscle contraction, but adverse responses do not predictably occur with neostigmine use. Careful titration of neuromuscular blockers and administration of short-acting nondepolarizing muscle relaxants may obviate the need for reversal of neuromuscular blockade.

Patients with myotonia dystrophica are sensitive to the respiratory depressant effects of barbiturates, opioids, benzodiazepines, and propofol. This is most likely due to drug-induced central respiratory depression acting in tandem with weak and/or atrophic respiratory muscles. In addition, hypersomnolence and central sleep apnea contribute to the increased sensitivity to respiratory depressant drugs.

Myotonic contraction during surgical manipulation and/or the use of electrocautery may interfere with surgical access. Drugs such as phenytoin and procainamide, which stabilize skeletal muscle membranes, may be helpful in this situation. High concentrations of volatile anesthetics can also abolish myotonic contractions but at the expense of myocardial depression. Maintenance of normothermia and avoidance of shivering are very important since cold may induce myotonia.

MYOTONIA CONGENITA

Myotonia congenita is transmitted as an autosomal dominant trait and becomes manifest at birth or during early childhood. Skeletal muscle involvement is widespread, but other organ systems are not usually involved. Muscle hypertrophy and myotonia are present. The disease does not progress nor does it result in a decreased life expectancy. Patients with myotonia congenita respond to phenytoin, mexiletine, or quinine therapy. The response to succinylcholine administration is abnormal.

PARAMYOTONIA CONGENITA

Paramyotonia congenita is a rare autosomal dominant disorder characterized by generalized myotonia that is recognized during early childhood. Generalized muscle hypertrophy may occur. This myotonia is unusual because, in contrast to other myotonias, in paramyotonia the skeletal muscle stiffness is often exacerbated by exercise. In other myotonias, sustained exercise improves myotonia, the so-called warm-up phenomenon. Cold markedly aggravates the myotonia, and flaccid paralysis may be present after the muscles are warmed. Some patients develop muscle paralysis independent of myotonia. This could be related to the serum potassium concentration and may be the reason that there is some doubt whether paramyotonia congenita and hyperkalemic periodic paralysis are separate entities. The electromyogram may be normal when recorded at room temperature, but typical myotonic discharges become evident as muscles are cooled. Treatment is similar to that for myotonia congenita.

SCHWARTZ-JAMPEL SYNDROME

Schwartz-Jampel syndrome is a rare childhood disorder of progressive skeletal muscle stiffness, myotonia, and ocular, facial, and skeletal abnormalities including micrognathia. Tracheal intubation is predictably difficult. There is blepharospasm and tense puckering of the mouth. These children may be susceptible to malignant hyperthermia.

Periodic Paralysis

Periodic paralysis is a spectrum of diseases characterized by intermittent acute attacks of skeletal muscle weakness or paralysis (sparing only a few muscles such as the muscles of respiration) and associated with hypokalemia or hyperkalemia (Table 21-3). The hyperkalemic form is much rarer than the hypokalemic form. Attacks generally last for a few hours but may persist for days. Muscle strength is normal between attacks.

ETIOLOGY

The exact defect in familial periodic paralysis is unknown, although mutations in calcium and sodium channels are associated with hypokalemic and hyperkalemic periodic paralysis, respectively. It is recognized that the mechanism of this disease is not related to any abnormality at the neuromuscular junction but rather to loss of muscle membrane excitability. Skeletal muscle weakness provoked by a glucose-insulin infusion confirms the presence of *hypokalemic* familial periodic paralysis, and skeletal muscle weakness after oral administration of potassium confirms the presence of *hyperkalemic*

TABLE 21-3 ■ **Clinical features of familial periodic paralysis**

Type	Serum potassium concentration during symptoms (mEq/L)	Precipitating factors	Other features
Hypokalemic	<3.0	High-carbohydrate meal, strenuous exercise, glucose infusion, stress, menstruation, pregnancy, anesthesia, hypothermia	Cardiac dysrhythmias, electrocardiographic signs of hypokalemia
Hyperkalemic	>5.5	Exercise, potassium infusion, metabolic acidosis, hypothermia	Skeletal muscle weakness may be localized to tongue and eyelids

familial periodic paralysis. Acetazolamide is recommended for the treatment of both forms of familial periodic paralysis. Acetazolamide produces a non–anion gap acidosis, which protects against hypokalemia, and promotes renal potassium excretion, which protects against hyperkalemia as well.

A principal goal of anesthetic management is avoidance of any events that can precipitate skeletal muscle weakness. Hypothermia must be avoided in patients with periodic paralysis, regardless of the nature of the potassium sensitivity. In patients undergoing cardiac surgery, it may be necessary to maintain normothermia during cardiopulmonary bypass. Nondepolarizing muscle relaxants can be safely administered.

Hypokalemic Periodic Paralysis

Preoperative considerations include maintenance of carbohydrate balance, correction of electrolyte abnormalities, and avoidance of events known to trigger hypokalemic attacks (psychologic stress, cold, carbohydrate loads). High-carbohydrate meals can trigger hypokalemic episodes and should be avoided during the 24 hours preceding surgery. Glucose-containing solutions and drugs known to cause intracellular shifts of potassium, such as β-adrenergic agonists, must also be avoided. Mannitol can be administered in lieu of a potassium-wasting diuretic should the operative procedure require diuresis. Frequent perioperative monitoring of serum potassium concentration (every 30 to 60 minutes) is useful, and aggressive intervention to increase the serum potassium concentration (infusion of potassium chloride at a rate of up to 40 mEq/hr) may occasionally be needed. Hypokalemia may precede the onset of muscle weakness by several hours, so timely potassium supplementation may help to avoid muscle weakness. Short-acting neuromuscular blockers are preferable if skeletal muscle relaxation is required for the surgery. Succinylcholine with its ability to increase serum potassium concentration transiently is acceptable in these patients. Regional anesthesia has been safely used.

Hyperkalemic Periodic Paralysis

Management of anesthesia in patients with hyperkalemic periodic paralysis includes preoperative potassium depletion with diuretics, prevention of carbohydrate depletion by administration of glucose-containing solutions, and avoidance of potassium-containing solutions and potassium-releasing drugs such as succinylcholine. Frequent monitoring of serum potassium concentration is indicated, as is the ready availability of calcium for intravenous administration should signs of hyperkalemia appear on the electrocardiogram.

Myasthenia Gravis

Myasthenia gravis is a chronic autoimmune disorder caused by a decrease in functional acetylcholine receptors at the neuromuscular junction resulting from their destruction or inactivation by circulating antibodies (Figure 21-1). As many as 80% of functional acetylcholine receptors can be lost. This accounts for the weakness and easy fatigability of these patients and their marked sensitivity to nondepolarizing muscle relaxants. Indeed, the hallmarks of this disease are weakness and rapid exhaustion of voluntary muscles with repetitive use, followed by partial recovery with rest. Skeletal muscles innervated by cranial nerves (ocular, pharyngeal, and laryngeal muscles) are especially vulnerable, as indicated by the appearance of ptosis, diplopia, and dysphagia, which are often the initial symptoms of the disease. Myasthenia gravis is not a rare disease. It has a prevalence of 1 in 7500. Women 20 to 30 years of age are most often affected; men with myasthenia gravis are often older than 60 years of age when the disease presents. Receptor-binding antibodies are present in more than 80% of patients with myasthenia gravis. The origin of these antibodies is unknown, but a relationship to the thymus gland is suggested by the association of myasthenia gravis with thymus gland abnormalities. For example, thymic hyperplasia is present in two thirds of patients with myasthenia gravis, and 10% to 15% of these patients have thymomas. Other conditions that cause weakness of the cranial and somatic musculature must be considered in the differential diagnosis of myasthenia gravis (Table 21-4).

Myasthenia gravis is classified based on the skeletal muscles involved and the severity of symptoms. Type I is limited to involvement of the extraocular muscles. Approximately 10% of patients show signs and symptoms confined to the extraocular muscles and are considered to have ocular myasthenia gravis. Patients in whom the disease has been confined to the ocular

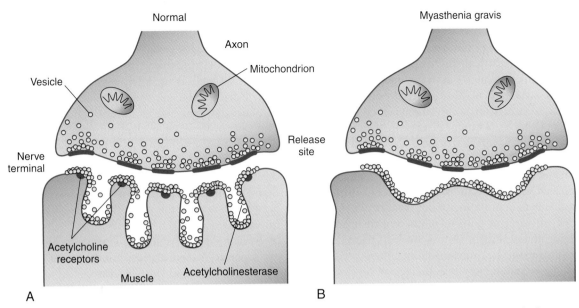

FIGURE 21-1 Normal (**A**) and myasthenic (**B**) neuromuscular junctions. Compared with normal neuromuscular junctions, myasthenic neuromuscular junctions have fewer acetylcholine receptors, simplified synaptic folds, and widened synaptic spaces. *(From Drachman DB. Myasthenia gravis. N Engl J Med. 1994;330:1797-1810. Copyright 1994 Massachusetts Medical Society. All rights reserved.)*

TABLE 21-4   Differential diagnosis of myasthenia gravis

Condition	Symptoms and characteristics	Comments
Congenital myasthenic syndromes	Rare, early onset, not autoimmune	Electrophysiologic and immunocytochemical tests required for diagnosis
Drug-induced myasthenia gravis Penicillamine Nondepolarizing muscle relaxants Aminoglycosides Procainamide	Triggers autoimmune myasthenia gravis Weakness in normal persons; exacerbation of myasthenia	Recovery within weeks of discontinuing the drug Recovery after drug discontinuation
Eaton-Lambert syndrome	Small cell lung cancer, fatigue	Incremental response on repetitive nerve stimulation, antibodies to calcium channels
Hyperthyroidism	Exacerbation of myasthenia gravis	Thyroid function abnormal
Graves' disease	Diplopia, exophthalmos	Thyroid-stimulating immunoglobulin present
Botulism	Generalized weakness, ophthalmoplegia	Incremental response on repetitive nerve stimulation, mydriasis
Progressive external ophthalmoplegia	Ptosis, diplopia, generalized weakness in some cases	Mitochondrial abnormalities
Intracranial mass compressing cranial nerves	Ophthalmoplegia, cranial nerve weakness	Abnormalities on computed tomography or magnetic resonance imaging

Adapted from Drachman DB. Myasthenia gravis. *N Engl J Med.* 1994;330:1797-1810. Copyright © 1994 Massachusetts Medical Society. All rights reserved.

muscles for longer than 3 years are unlikely to experience any progression in their disease. Type IIa is a slowly progressive, mild form of skeletal muscle weakness that spares the muscles of respiration. The response to anticholinesterase drugs and corticosteroids is good in these patients. Type IIb is a more rapidly progressive and more severe form of skeletal muscle weakness. The response to drug therapy is not as good, and the muscles of respiration may be involved. Type III is characterized by acute onset and rapid deterioration of skeletal muscle

strength within 6 months. It is associated with a high mortality rate. Type IV is a severe form of skeletal muscle weakness that results from progression of type I or type II myasthenia.

SIGNS AND SYMPTOMS
The clinical course of myasthenia gravis is marked by periods of exacerbation and remission. Muscle strength may be normal in well-rested patients, but weakness occurs promptly with exercise. Ptosis and diplopia resulting from extraocular

muscle weakness are the most common initial complaints. Weakness of pharyngeal and laryngeal muscles results in dysphagia, dysarthria, and difficulty handling saliva. Patients with myasthenia gravis are at high risk of pulmonary aspiration. Arm, leg, or trunk weakness can occur in any combination and is usually asymmetrical. Muscle atrophy does not occur. Myocarditis can result in atrial fibrillation, heart block, or cardiomyopathy. Other autoimmune diseases may occur in association with myasthenia gravis. For example, hyperthyroidism is present in approximately 10% of patients with myasthenia gravis. Rheumatoid arthritis, systemic lupus erythematosus, and pernicious anemia occur more commonly in patients with myasthenia than in those without myasthenia. Approximately 15% of neonates born to mothers with myasthenia gravis demonstrate transient (2 to 4 weeks) skeletal muscle weakness. Infection, electrolyte abnormalities, pregnancy, emotional stress, and surgery may precipitate or exacerbate muscle weakness. Antibiotics, especially the aminoglycosides, can aggravate the muscle weakness. Isolated respiratory failure may occasionally be the presenting manifestation of myasthenia gravis.

TREATMENT

Treatment modalities for myasthenia gravis include anticholinesterase drugs to enhance neuromuscular transmission, thymectomy, immunosuppression, and short-term immunotherapy, including plasmapheresis and administration of immunoglobulin.

Anticholinesterase drugs are the first line of treatment for myasthenia gravis. These drugs are effective because they inhibit the enzyme responsible for the hydrolysis of acetylcholine and thus increase the amount of neurotransmitter available at the neuromuscular junction. Pyridostigmine is the most widely used anticholinesterase drug for this purpose. The onset of effect occurs in 30 minutes, and peak effect is achieved in approximately 2 hours. Oral pyridostigmine lasts longer (3 to 6 hours) and produces fewer side effects than neostigmine. Pyridostigmine dosing is tailored to response, but the maximal dosage of pyridostigmine rarely exceeds 120 mg every 3 hours. Higher dosages may actually induce more muscle weakness, the so-called *cholinergic crisis.* The presence of significant muscarinic side effects (salivation, miosis, bradycardia) plus accentuated muscle weakness after administration of edrophonium (1 to 2 mg IV) confirms the diagnosis of a cholinergic crisis. Although anticholinesterase drugs benefit most patients, the improvements may be incomplete and may wane after weeks or months of treatment.

Thymectomy is intended to induce remission or at least allow the dosages of immunosuppressive medications to be reduced. Patients with generalized myasthenia gravis are candidates for thymectomy. Preoperative preparation should include optimizing strength and respiratory function. Immunosuppressive drugs should be avoided if possible, because they can increase the risk of perioperative infection. If the vital capacity is less than 2 L, plasmapheresis can be performed before surgery to improve the likelihood of adequate spontaneous respiration during the postoperative period. A surgical approach via median sternotomy optimizes visualization and removal of all thymic tissue. Mediastinoscopy through a cervical incision has been advocated as an alternative because it is associated with a smaller incision and less postoperative pain. The use of neuraxial analgesia minimizes postoperative pain and thus improves postoperative ventilation. The need for anticholinesterase medication may be decreased for a few days postoperatively, but the full benefit of thymectomy is often delayed for months after surgery. The mechanism by which thymectomy produces improvement is uncertain, although acetylcholine receptor antibody levels usually decrease following thymectomy.

Immunosuppressive therapy (corticosteroids, azathioprine, cyclosporine, mycophenolate) is indicated when skeletal muscle weakness is not adequately controlled by anticholinesterase drugs. Corticosteroids are the most commonly used and most consistently effective immunosuppressive drugs for the treatment of myasthenia gravis. They are also associated with the greatest likelihood of adverse effects.

Plasmapheresis removes antibodies from the circulation and produces short-term clinical improvement in patients with myasthenia gravis who are experiencing *myasthenic crises* or are being prepared for thymectomy. The beneficial effects of plasmapheresis are transient, and repeated treatment introduces the risk of infection, hypotension, and pulmonary embolism. The indications for administration of *immunoglobulin* are the same as for plasmapheresis. The effect is temporary, and this treatment has no effect on circulating concentrations of acetylcholine receptor antibodies.

MANAGEMENT OF ANESTHESIA

Patients with myasthenia gravis often require ventilatory support after surgery. Therefore, it is important to advise these patients during the preoperative interview that they may be intubated and ventilated when they awaken. Factors that correlate with the need for mechanical ventilation during the postoperative period following transsternal thymectomy include disease duration of longer than 6 years, the presence of chronic obstructive pulmonary disease unrelated to myasthenia gravis, a daily dose of pyridostigmine of more than 750 mg, and a vital capacity of less than 2.9 L. These factors are less predictive of the need for ventilatory support following transcervical thymectomy, which indicates that this less-invasive surgical approach produces less respiratory depression.

The acetylcholine receptor–binding antibodies of myasthenia gravis decrease the number of functional acetylcholine receptors, and this results in an increased sensitivity to nondepolarizing muscle relaxants. The balance between active and nonfunctional acetylcholine receptors modulates the sensitivity to nondepolarizing muscle relaxants. The initial muscle relaxant dose should be titrated according to response at the neuromuscular junction as monitored using a peripheral nerve stimulator. Monitoring these responses at the orbicularis oculi muscle may *overestimate* the degree of neuromuscular blockade but may help to avoid unrecognized persistent neuromuscular blockade in these patients.

It is possible that drugs used to treat myasthenia gravis can influence the response to muscle relaxants independent of the disease process. For example, anticholinesterase drugs inhibit not only true cholinesterase but also impair plasma pseudocholinesterase activity, which introduces the possibility of a prolonged response to succinylcholine. They could also antagonize the effects of nondepolarizing muscle relaxants. However, neither of these effects is seen clinically. Corticosteroid therapy does not alter the dose requirements for succinylcholine but has been reported to produce resistance to the neuromuscular blocking effects of steroidal muscle relaxants such as vecuronium.

Measurement of neuromuscular function in patients with myasthenia gravis treated with pyridostigmine demonstrates *resistance* to the effects of succinylcholine. The 95% effective dose (ED_{95}) is approximately 2.6 times higher than normal. Because the dose of succinylcholine commonly administered to patients without myasthenia gravis (1.0 to 1.5 mg/kg) represents three to five times the ED_{95}, it is likely that adequate intubating conditions can be achieved in patients with myasthenia gravis using these doses. The mechanism for the resistance to succinylcholine is unknown, but the decreased number of acetylcholine receptors at the postsynaptic neuromuscular junction may play a role.

In contrast to the resistance to succinylcholine, patients with myasthenia gravis exhibit marked sensitivity to nondepolarizing muscle relaxants. Even small doses of nondepolarizing muscle relaxant intended to block succinylcholine-induced fasciculations can produce profound skeletal muscle weakness in some patients. In patients with mild to moderate myasthenia gravis, the potency of atracurium and vecuronium is increased twofold compared with the response in patients without the disease. Despite the increase in potency, the duration of action of intermediate-acting muscle relaxants is short enough that skeletal muscle paralysis can be achieved and yet be predictably reversed at the conclusion of surgery.

Induction of anesthesia with a short-acting intravenous anesthetic is acceptable for patients with myasthenia gravis. However, the respiratory depressant effects of these drugs may be accentuated. Tracheal intubation can often be accomplished without neuromuscular blockers because of intrinsic muscle weakness and the relaxant effect of volatile anesthetics on skeletal muscle.

Maintenance of anesthesia is often provided with a volatile anesthetic with or without nitrous oxide. The use of volatile anesthetics can decrease the required dose of muscle relaxants or even eliminate the need for them. Should administration of a nondepolarizing neuromuscular blocker be necessary, the initial dose should be decreased by one half to two thirds and the response monitored using a peripheral nerve stimulator. The relatively short duration of action of intermediate-acting muscle relaxants is a desirable characteristic in this patient group. The respiratory effects of opioids, which can linger into the postoperative period, detract from their use for maintenance of anesthesia.

At the conclusion of surgery, it is important to postpone extubation until clear evidence of good respiratory function is present. Skeletal muscle strength often seems adequate during the early postoperative period but may deteriorate a few hours later. The need for mechanical ventilation during the postoperative period should be anticipated in those patients meeting the criteria known to correlate with inadequate ventilation after surgery.

Myasthenic Syndrome

Myasthenic syndrome (Eaton-Lambert syndrome) is a disorder of neuromuscular transmission that resembles myasthenia gravis (Table 21-5). This syndrome of skeletal muscle weakness, originally described in patients with small cell carcinoma of the lung, has subsequently been described in some patients without cancer. Myasthenic syndrome is an acquired autoimmune disease characterized by the presence of immunoglobulin G antibodies to voltage-sensitive calcium channels that causes a deficiency of these channels at the motor nerve terminal. This deficiency restricts calcium entry when the terminal is depolarized. Anticholinesterase drugs effective in the treatment of myasthenia gravis do *not* produce an improvement in patients with myasthenic syndrome. However, 3,4-diaminopyridine, which increases acetylcholine release at the neuromuscular junction, does improve muscle strength. Immunoglobulin also increases muscle strength temporarily (for 6 to 8 weeks).

TABLE 21-5	Comparison of myasthenic syndrome and myasthenia gravis	
Characteristic	**Myasthenic syndrome**	**Myasthenia gravis**
Manifestations	Proximal limb weakness (legs more than arms), exercise improves strength, muscle pain common, reflexes absent or decreased	Extraocular, bulbar, and facial muscle weakness; exercise causes fatigue; muscle pain uncommon; reflexes normal
Gender	Affects males more often than females	Affects females more often than males
Co-existing pathologic conditions	Small cell lung cancer	Thymoma
Response to muscle relaxants	Sensitive to succinylcholine and nondepolarizing muscle relaxants	Resistant to succinylcholine, sensitive to nondepolarizing muscle relaxants
	Poor response to anticholinesterases	Good response to anticholinesterases

Patients with myasthenic syndrome are sensitive to the effects of both depolarizing and nondepolarizing muscle relaxants. Antagonism of neuromuscular blockade with anticholinesterase drugs may be inadequate. The potential presence of myasthenic syndrome and the need to decrease doses of muscle relaxants should be considered in patients undergoing bronchoscopy, mediastinoscopy, or thoracoscopy for suspected lung cancer.

SKELETAL DISEASES

Osteoarthritis

Osteoarthritis is by far the most common joint disease in the United States, one of the leading chronic diseases of the elderly and a major cause of disability. Osteoarthritis is a degenerative process that affects articular cartilage. This process is different from rheumatoid arthritis because there is minimal inflammatory reaction in the joints. The pathogenesis is likely related to joint trauma from biomechanical stresses, joint injury, or abnormal joint loading resulting from neuropathy, ligamentous injury, or muscle atrophy. Pain is usually present on motion but is relieved by rest. Stiffness tends to disappear rapidly with joint motion, in contrast to the morning stiffness associated with rheumatoid arthritis, which can last for several hours.

One or several joints can be affected by osteoarthritis. The knees and hips are common sites of involvement. Bony enlargements, referred to as *Heberden's nodes,* are seen at the distal interphalangeal joints of the fingers. There may be degenerative disease of the vertebral bodies and intervertebral discs, which can be complicated by protrusion of the nucleus pulposus and compression of nerve roots. Degenerative changes are most significant in the middle to lower cervical spine and in the lower lumbar area. Radiographic findings include narrowing of the intervertebral disc spaces and osteophyte formation.

Although often overlooked, physical therapy and exercise programs can provide benefits for patients with osteoarthritis. Maintaining muscle function is important for both cartilage integrity and pain reduction. Pain can also be relieved by application of heat, use of simple analgesics such as acetaminophen, and treatment with antiinflammatory drugs. Symptomatic improvement with application of heat may be due to an increase in pain threshold in warm tissues compared with that in cold tissues. Transcutaneous nerve stimulation and acupuncture can be effective in some patients. Systemic corticosteroids have *no place* in the treatment of osteoarthritis. Joint replacement surgery may be recommended when pain caused by osteoarthritis is persistent and disabling or significant limitation of joint function is present.

Kyphoscoliosis

Kyphoscoliosis is a spinal deformity characterized by anterior flexion (*kyphosis*) and lateral curvature (*scoliosis*) of the vertebral column. Idiopathic kyphoscoliosis, which accounts for 80% of cases, commonly begins during late childhood and may progress in severity during periods of rapid skeletal growth. The incidence of idiopathic kyphoscoliosis is approximately 4 per 1000 population. There may be a familial predisposition to this disease, and females are affected four times more often than males. Diseases of the neuromuscular system, such as poliomyelitis, cerebral palsy, and muscular dystrophy, may also be associated with kyphoscoliosis.

Spinal curvature of more than 40 degrees is considered severe and is likely to be associated with physiologic derangements in cardiac and pulmonary function. Restrictive lung disease and pulmonary hypertension progressing to cor pulmonale are the principal causes of death in patients with kyphoscoliosis. As the scoliosis curve worsens, more lung tissue is compressed, which results in a decrease in vital capacity and dyspnea on exertion. The work of breathing is increased because of the abnormal mechanical properties of the distorted thorax and the increased airway resistance that results from small lung volumes. The alveolar-arterial oxygen difference is increased. Pulmonary hypertension is the result of increased pulmonary vascular resistance due to compression of lung vasculature and the response to arterial hypoxemia. The $PaCO_2$ is usually maintained at normal levels, but an insult such as bacterial or viral upper respiratory tract infection can result in hypercapnia and acute respiratory failure. A poor cough contributes to frequent pulmonary infection.

Preoperatively, it is important to assess the severity of the physiologic derangements produced by this skeletal deformity. Pulmonary function test results reflect the magnitude of restrictive lung disease. Arterial blood gas values are helpful for detecting unrecognized hypoxemia or acidosis that could be contributing to pulmonary hypertension. These patients may have preoperative pulmonary infection resulting from chronic aspiration. Certainly, any reversible component of pulmonary dysfunction, such as infection or bronchospasm, should be corrected before elective surgery.

Although no specific drug or drug combination can be recommended as optimal for patients with kyphoscoliosis, it should be remembered that nitrous oxide may increase pulmonary vascular resistance. This could be particularly problematic in patients with pulmonary hypertension. Monitoring central venous pressure may provide data suggesting an increase in pulmonary vascular resistance.

When the patient is undergoing surgery to correct the spinal curvature, special anesthetic considerations include the potential for blood loss and the risk of surgically induced spinal cord damage. Controlled hypotension as a way of decreasing the blood loss should be used with caution because of the risk of ischemic optic neuropathy and spinal cord ischemia. Prolonged surgery and a low transfusion threshold could increase the risk of ischemia. At the time that the spinal curvature is straightened or distracted, excessive traction on the spinal cord can result in spinal cord ischemia, which can produce paralysis. There are several maneuvers designed to detect spinal cord ischemia. One is the *wake-up test,* which entails determining that no significant neuromuscular blockade is present by discontinuing the anesthetic until the patient is sufficiently awake to move both legs on command and thus confirm that spinal cord motor pathways are intact. Anesthesia is then reestablished and the operation completed. Another method to confirm an intact spinal cord is to monitor somatosensory and motor evoked potentials. The advantage of this monitoring is that patients need not be awakened intraoperatively. However, many anesthetic drugs, especially volatile anesthetics and nitrous oxide, interfere with the monitoring of evoked potentials, and neuromuscular blockers cannot be used if motor evoked potentials are being monitored. Therefore, total intravenous anesthesia with an opioid and propofol or the combination of an opioid, propofol, and low-dose (0.33 MAC) volatile anesthetic is usually chosen to provide general anesthesia. These techniques make it easier to interpret changes in amplitude and latency resulting from spinal cord ischemia. A wake-up test may still be necessary if abnormalities persist. Measurement of evoked potentials is being used much more frequently than a wake-up test. At the conclusion of surgery, the principal concern is restoration of adequate ventilation. Postoperative mechanical ventilation may be necessary in some patients with severe kyphoscoliosis.

Back Pain

Low back pain is the most common musculoskeletal complaint requiring medical attention (Table 21-6). Risk factors for low back pain include male gender, frequent lifting of heavy objects, and smoking. In many patients, the cause of the back pain cannot be determined with certainty, and it is usually attributed to muscular or ligamentous strain, facet joint arthritis, or disc pressure on the annulus fibrosus, vertebral end plate, or nerve roots.

ACUTE LOW BACK PAIN

Back pain improves within 30 days in 90% of patients. Continuing ordinary activities within the limits permitted by the pain can lead to more rapid recovery than bed rest or back-mobilizing exercises. NSAIDs are often effective for analgesia for acute back pain. Pain arising from inflammation initiated by mechanical or chemical insult to a nerve root may be responsive to epidural administration of corticosteroids, but few patients experience symptomatic relief from epidural corticosteroids if radicular pain has been present for longer than 6 months or if laminectomy has been performed. A herniated disc should be considered in patients with radiculopathy that is suggested by pain radiating down a leg or by symptoms reproduced by straight leg raising. Most lumbar disc herniations producing sciatica occur at the L4-5 and L5-S1 levels. Magnetic resonance imaging can confirm a herniated disc, but findings should be interpreted with caution because many asymptomatic people also have disc abnormalities. Surgical

TABLE 21-6 ■ Causes of low back pain

MECHANICAL LOW BACK OR LEG PAIN (97%)
Idiopathic low back pain (lumbar sprain or strain) (70%)
Degenerative processes of discs and facets (age related) (10%)
Herniated disc (4%)
Spinal stenosis (3%)
Osteoporotic compression fractures (4%)
Spondylolisthesis (2%)
Traumatic fracture (<1%)
Congenital disease (<1%)
 Severe kyphosis
 Severe scoliosis
Spondylolysis

NONMECHANICAL SPINAL CONDITIONS (1%)
Cancer (0.7%)
 Multiple myeloma
 Metastatic cancer
 Lymphoma and leukemia
 Spinal cord tumors
 Retroperitoneal tumors
 Primary vertebral tumors
Infection (0.01%)
 Osteomyelitis
 Paraspinal abscess
 Epidural abscess
Inflammatory arthritis
 Ankylosing spondylitis
 Psoriatic spondylitis
 Reiter's syndrome
 Inflammatory bowel disease

VISCERAL DISEASE (2%)
Disease of pelvic organs
 Prostatitis
 Endometriosis
 Pelvic inflammatory disease
Renal disease
 Nephrolithiasis
 Pyelonephritis
 Perinephric abscess
Aortic aneurysm
Gastrointestinal disease
 Pancreatitis
 Cholecystitis
 Penetrating ulcer

Adapted from Deyo RO, Weinstein JN. Low back pain. *N Engl J Med.* 2001;344:363-370.
Percentages indicate the estimated incidence of these conditions in adult patients.

intervention is indicated in patients with persistent radiculopathy or neurologic deficits. Patients who have persistent back pain after 30 days of conservative treatment (NSAIDs) should be evaluated for systemic illness.

LUMBAR SPINAL STENOSIS

Lumbar spinal stenosis is a narrowing of the spinal canal or its lateral recesses. It typically results from hypertrophic degenerative changes in spinal structures (extensive degenerative disc disease and/or osteophyte formation) and occurs most often in elderly patients with chronic back pain and sciatica.

Symptoms include pain, numbness, and weakness in the buttocks that can extend down one or both legs. Symptoms often worsen with standing or walking and improve in the flexed or supine position. The diagnosis of lumbar spinal stenosis is confirmed by magnetic resonance imaging or myelography. Conservative measures may be helpful in some patients, but surgical decompression and fusion are needed for those with progressive functional deterioration.

Rheumatoid Arthritis

Rheumatoid arthritis, the most common chronic inflammatory arthritis, affects approximately 1% of adults. The incidence is two to three times higher in women than in men. The etiology of rheumatoid arthritis is unknown, but it is suspected to be a complex interaction between genetic and environmental factors and the immune system. The disease is characterized by symmetrical polyarthropathy and significant systemic involvement (Table 21-7). Involvement of the proximal interphalangeal and metacarpophalangeal joints of the hands and feet helps distinguish rheumatoid arthritis from osteoarthritis, which typically affects weight-bearing joints and distal interphalangeal joints. The course of the disease is characterized by exacerbations and remissions. Rheumatoid nodules are typically present at pressure points, particularly below the elbows. Rheumatoid factor is an immunoglobulin G antibody that is present in the serum of up to 90% of patients with rheumatoid arthritis but is not present in osteoarthritis. However, the presence of rheumatoid factor is not specific to rheumatoid arthritis. It is also present in patients with viral hepatitis, systemic lupus erythematosus, bacterial endocarditis, sarcoidosis, and Sjögren's syndrome.

SIGNS AND SYMPTOMS

The onset of rheumatoid arthritis in adults may be acute, involving single or multiple joints, or insidious with symptoms such as fatigue, anorexia, and weakness preceding overt arthritis. In some patients, the onset of rheumatoid arthritis coincides with trauma, a surgical procedure, childbirth, or exposure to extremes of temperature.

Morning stiffness is a hallmark of rheumatoid arthritis. Several joints, often the hands, wrists, knees, and feet, are affected in a symmetrical distribution. Fusiform swelling is typical when there is involvement of the proximal interphalangeal joints. These joints are swollen and painful and remain stiff for several hours after the start of daily activity. Synovitis of the temporomandibular joint can produce marked limitation of mandibular motion. When the disease is progressive and unremitting, nearly every joint is affected except for the thoracic and lumbosacral spine.

Cervical spine involvement is frequent and may result in pain and neurologic complications. The most significant abnormality of the cervical spine is atlantoaxial subluxation and consequent separation of the atlantoodontoid articulation. This deformity is best seen on a lateral radiograph of the neck. With the neck flexed, the separation of the anterior margin of the odontoid process from the posterior margin of the

TABLE 21-7 ■ **Comparison of rheumatoid arthritis and ankylosing spondylitis**

Characteristic	Rheumatoid arthritis	Ankylosing spondylitis
Family history	Rare	Common
Gender	Female (30-50 yr)	Male (20-30 yr)
Joint involvement	Symmetrical polyarthropathy	Asymmetrical oligoarthropathy
Sacroiliac involvement	No	Yes
Vertebral involvement	Only cervical	Total (*ascending from lumbosacral region*)
Cardiac changes	Pericardial effusion, aortic regurgitation, cardiac conduction abnormalities, cardiac valve fibrosis, coronary artery arteritis	Cardiomegaly, aortic regurgitation, cardiac conduction abnormalities
Pulmonary changes	Pulmonary fibrosis, pleural effusion	Pulmonary fibrosis
Eyes	Keratoconjunctivitis sicca	Conjunctivitis, uveitis
Rheumatoid factor	Positive	Negative
HLA-B27	Negative	Positive

anterior arch of the atlas can exceed 3 mm. When this separation is severe, the odontoid process can protrude into the foramen magnum and exert pressure on the spinal cord or impair blood flow through the vertebral arteries. Since the odontoid process is often eroded, effects on the spinal cord may be minimized. Subluxation of other cervical vertebrae can also occur. Magnetic resonance imaging has confirmed the frequency of cervical spine involvement in rheumatoid arthritis.

Cricoarytenoid arthritis is common in patients with generalized rheumatoid arthritis. With acute cricoarytenoid arthritis, hoarseness, pain on swallowing, dyspnea, and stridor may accompany tenderness over the larynx. Redness and swelling of the arytenoids can be seen on direct laryngoscopy. With chronic cricoarytenoid arthritis, patients may be asymptomatic or manifest variable degrees of hoarseness, dyspnea, and upper airway obstruction. Cricoarytenoid arthritis may make endotracheal intubation difficult.

Osteoporosis is ubiquitous in patients with rheumatoid arthritis.

Many of the systemic manifestations of rheumatoid arthritis are a result of small and medium-sized artery vasculitis due to deposition of immune complexes. Systemic involvement is usually most obvious in patients with severe arthritis.

In the cardiovascular system, rheumatoid arthritis may manifest as pericarditis, myocarditis, coronary artery arteritis, accelerated coronary atherosclerosis, cardiac valve fibrosis, and formation of rheumatoid nodules in the cardiac conduction system. Aortitis with dilation of the aortic root may result in aortic regurgitation. Pericardial thickening or effusion is present in approximately one third of patients.

Vasculitis in small synovial blood vessels is an early finding in patients with rheumatoid arthritis, but more widespread vascular inflammation may occur, especially in older men. Patients may demonstrate a neuropathy (*mononeuritis multiplex*), skin ulcerations, and purpura. The neuropathy is presumed to be caused by deposition of immune complexes in the vasa nervorum. Manifestations of visceral ischemia, including bowel perforation, myocardial infarction, and cerebral infarction, are possible.

The most common pulmonary manifestation is pleural effusion. Many of these effusions are small and asymptomatic. Rheumatoid nodules can develop in the pulmonary parenchyma and on pleural surfaces and may mimic tuberculosis or cancer on chest radiographs. Progressive pulmonary fibrosis, associated with cough, dyspnea, and diffuse honeycomb changes on chest radiographs, is rare. Costochondral involvement may affect chest wall motion and produce restrictive lung changes with decreased lung volumes and vital capacity. This may result in ventilation/perfusion mismatching and decreased arterial oxygenation.

Neuromuscular involvement can be seen with loss of strength in skeletal muscles adjacent to joints with active synovitis. Peripheral neuropathies resulting from nerve compression, carpal tunnel syndrome, and tarsal tunnel syndrome are common.

The most common hematologic abnormality in patients with rheumatoid arthritis is anemia of chronic disease, the severity of which usually parallels the severity of the rheumatoid arthritis. Felty's syndrome consists of rheumatoid arthritis with splenomegaly and leukopenia. Keratoconjunctivitis sicca (dry eyes) occurs in approximately 10% of patients with rheumatoid arthritis. The cause is lack of tear formation due to impaired lacrimal gland function. A similar pathologic process may involve the salivary glands, resulting in xerostomia (dry mouth). These are both manifestations of Sjögren's syndrome.

Mild abnormalities of liver function are common in patients with rheumatoid arthritis. Renal dysfunction may be secondary to amyloidosis, vasculitis, or drug therapy.

TREATMENT

Treatment of rheumatoid arthritis includes measures to relieve pain, preserve joint function and strength, prevent deformities, and attenuate systemic complications. These objectives may be met by a combination of drugs, physical therapy, occupational therapy, and orthopedic surgery.

Drug therapy is used to provide analgesia, control inflammation, and produce immunosuppression.

NSAIDs are important for symptomatic relief of rheumatoid arthritis but have little role in changing the underlying disease process. They should not be used without the concomitant use of *disease-modifying antirheumatic drugs* (DMARDs). Aspirin remains an important drug for the initial treatment of rheumatoid arthritis, but its use has decreased because of the availability of newer NSAIDs. These drugs decrease swelling in affected joints and relieve stiffness, but associated gastrointestinal irritation and inhibition of platelet cyclooxygenase 1 (COX-1) may necessitate discontinuation of these drugs. Selective COX-2 inhibitors are as effective as COX-1 inhibitors in producing analgesia and reducing inflammation, and they evoke fewer gastrointestinal side effects and do not interfere with platelet function. It appears, however, that some COX-2 inhibitors increase the risk of cardiac ischemic events. Both COX-1 and COX-2 drugs can adversely affect renal blood flow and glomerular filtration rate.

Corticosteroids are potent antiinflammatory drugs that decrease joint swelling, pain, and morning stiffness in patients with rheumatoid arthritis. However, the dosages of systemic corticosteroids necessary to maintain desirable effects are often associated with significant long-term side effects, including osteoporosis, osteonecrosis, increased susceptibility to infection, myopathy, hyperglycemia, and poor wound healing. Intraarticular corticosteroids produce beneficial effects lasting about 3 months, but repeated injections may result in cartilage destruction and osteonecrosis.

Corticosteroids are indicated as bridge therapy, that is, as therapy to decrease inflammation rapidly while DMARDs are starting to work in controlling the disease process. Prednisone dosages greater than 10 mg/day are rarely indicated for joint disease, but higher dosages may be needed to treat other manifestations of rheumatoid arthritis, especially vasculitis.

DMARDs are a group of drugs that have the potential to modify or change the course of rheumatoid arthritis. They can slow or halt the progression of the disease. Included in this group are methotrexate, sulfasalazine, leflunomide, antimalarials, D-penicillamine, azathioprine, and minocycline. These drugs generally take 2 to 6 months to achieve their effects. Patients who show no response to one drug may respond to another.

Methotrexate is the preferred DMARD in the treatment of rheumatoid arthritis. It is given in a once-a-week dosing regimen. Methotrexate is primarily antiinflammatory. Monitoring of hematologic parameters and liver function test results is necessary in individuals being treated with methotrexate because of the risks of bone marrow suppression and cirrhosis. Daily folic acid therapy can decrease methotrexate toxicities.

It appears that cytokines, especially TNF-α and interleukin-1, play a central role in the pathogenesis of rheumatoid arthritis. Interference with the function of TNF either by drug-induced receptor blockade or by monoclonal antibodies is effective in treating rheumatoid arthritis. Drugs such as infliximab and etanercept, TNF inhibitors, are quite effective in treating rheumatoid arthritis and act more rapidly than other DMARDs. Long-term toxicities such as infection (tuberculosis) and demyelinating syndromes are a concern. Anakinra, an interleukin-1 receptor antagonist, is effective against the signs and symptoms of rheumatoid arthritis, but its onset of action is slower and its overall effect is less than that of the TNF-α inhibitors.

Gold, the traditional DMARD, is extremely effective therapy for some patients with rheumatoid arthritis, but it is not commonly used because of its toxicities.

Indications for surgery in patients with rheumatoid arthritis include intractable pain, impairment of joint function, and the need for joint stabilization. Eroded cartilage, ruptured ligaments, and progressive bone destruction can lead to impairment that is amenable only to surgical treatment. Arthroscopic surgery is used to remove cartilaginous fragments and to perform partial synovectomy. When joints are destroyed by the disease process, total replacement of large and small joints can be considered.

MANAGEMENT OF ANESTHESIA

The multiorgan involvement and side effects of drugs used to treat rheumatoid arthritis must be appreciated when planning anesthetic management. Preoperatively, patients should be evaluated for airway involvement by this disease process. Compromise of the airway may occur at the cervical spine, temporomandibular joints, and cricoarytenoid joints. Flexion deformity of the cervical spine may make it difficult if not impossible to straighten the neck. Atlantoaxial subluxation may be present. Radiographic demonstration that the distance from the anterior arch of the atlas to the odontoid process exceeds 3 mm confirms the presence of atlantoaxial subluxation. This abnormality is important, because the displaced odontoid process can compress the cervical spinal cord or medulla or occlude the vertebral arteries. When atlantoaxial subluxation is present, care must be taken to minimize movement of the head and neck during direct laryngoscopy to avoid further displacement of the odontoid process and damage to the spinal cord. It is helpful to evaluate preoperatively whether there is interference with vertebral artery blood flow during flexion, extension, or rotation of the head and cervical spine. This can be accomplished by having the awake patient demonstrate head movement or positioning that can be tolerated without discomfort or other symptoms.

Limitation of temporomandibular joint movement must be recognized before induction of anesthesia. The combination of limited mobility of these joints plus cervical spine stiffness may make visualizing the glottic opening by direct laryngoscopy difficult or impossible. Endotracheal intubation by fiberoptic laryngoscopy or by use of a videolaryngoscope may be indicated if preoperative evaluation suggests that direct visualization of the glottic opening will be difficult. Involvement of the cricoarytenoid joints by arthritic changes is suggested by the preoperative presence of hoarseness or stridor or by the observation of erythema or edema of the vocal cords during direct laryngoscopy. Diminished movement of these joints can result in narrowing of the glottic opening and interference with passage of the tracheal tube or an increased risk of cricoarytenoid joint dislocation.

Preoperative pulmonary function studies plus measurement of arterial blood gases may be indicated if severe rheumatoid lung disease is suspected. Postoperative ventilatory support might be needed in the subset of patients with such disease. The effect of aspirin or NSAIDs on platelet function must be considered. Corticosteroid supplementation may be indicated in patients being treated long term with these drugs. Postextubation laryngeal obstruction may occur in patients with cricoarytenoid arthritis.

Systemic Lupus Erythematosus

Systemic lupus erythematosus (SLE) is a multisystem chronic inflammatory disease characterized by antinuclear antibody production. However, these antinuclear antibodies have not been documented to be directly involved in the pathogenesis of this disease. SLE typically occurs in young women and may affect as many as 1 in 1000 women. Stresses such as infection, pregnancy, or surgery may exacerbate SLE. The onset of SLE can also be drug induced, with procainamide, hydralazine, isoniazid, D-penicillamine, and α-methyldopa being the most frequently associated drugs. Susceptibility to the development of SLE with exposure to hydralazine or procainamide is related to acetylator phenotype. The disease is more likely to develop in those who metabolize these drugs slowly (slow acetylators). The clinical presentation of drug-induced SLE is similar to that of the naturally occurring form of the disease, but the progression is usually slower and the symptoms are usually mild and consist of arthralgias, a maculopapular rash, fever, anemia, and leukopenia. The natural history of SLE is highly variable. The presence of nephritis and hypertension heralds a worse prognosis. Pregnancy in patients with SLE, especially those with nephritis or hypertension, is associated with a substantial risk of disease exacerbation and poor fetal outcome.

DIAGNOSIS

Detection of antinuclear antibodies is a sensitive screening test for SLE. These antibodies occur in more than 95% of SLE patients. The diagnosis is very likely if patients have three of four typical manifestations: antinuclear antibodies, characteristic rash, thrombocytopenia, serositis, and nephritis. However, presentation may not always be so clear, and features such as arthralgias, vague central nervous system symptoms, rash, Raynaud's phenomenon, and/or a weakly positive antinuclear antibody test may make the diagnosis more difficult.

SIGNS AND SYMPTOMS

Clinical manifestations of SLE can be categorized as articular or systemic. Polyarthritis and dermatitis are the most common signs and symptoms. Many of the clinical manifestations of SLE are the result of tissue damage from a vasculopathy mediated by immune complexes. Others, such as thrombocytopenia and antiphospholipid syndrome, are the direct result of antibodies to cell surface molecules or serum components.

Symmetrical arthritis involving the hands, wrists, elbows, knees, and ankles is common and occurs in 90% of patients. This arthritis is characteristically episodic and migratory, with pain that is out of proportion to the apparent degree of synovitis present. Lupus arthritis does not involve the spine. Another form of skeletal involvement is avascular necrosis, which most often involves the head or condyle of the femur.

Systemic manifestations of SLE appear in the central nervous system, heart, lungs, kidneys, liver, neuromuscular system, and skin. Neurologic complications can affect any part of the central nervous system. Cognitive dysfunction occurs in approximately one third of individuals. Psychologic changes ranging from depression and anxiety to psychosomatic complaints to signs of organic psychosis with deterioration of intellectual capacity are seen in more than half of patients. Most serious central nervous system manifestations appear to be the result of vasculitis. Fluid and electrolyte disturbances, fever, hypertension, uremia, infection, and drug-induced effects may contribute to central nervous system dysfunction. Atypical migraine headaches are common and may be accompanied by cortical visual disturbances.

Pericarditis resulting in chest pain, a friction rub, electrocardiographic changes, and pericardial effusion is the most common cardiac manifestation of SLE. Myocarditis may result in abnormalities of cardiac conduction. Congestive heart failure can develop with extensive cardiac involvement. Valvular abnormalities can be identified by echocardiography. These include verrucous endocarditis (Libman-Sacks endocarditis) that can involve the aortic and/or mitral valves.

Pulmonary involvement can manifest as lupus pneumonia characterized by diffuse pulmonary infiltrates, pleural effusion, dry cough, dyspnea, and arterial hypoxemia. Pulmonary function test results in these patients show restrictive lung disease. Recurrent atelectasis can result in shrinking or vanishing lung syndrome. This may be a result of diaphragmatic weakness or elevation caused by phrenic neuropathy. Pulmonary angiitis with lung hemorrhage may complicate severe SLE. Pulmonary hypertension is present in some patients.

The most common renal abnormality is glomerulonephritis with proteinuria, which can result in hypoalbuminemia. Hematuria is a frequent finding. The glomerular filtration rate can decrease dramatically and result in oliguric renal failure.

Liver function test findings are abnormal in approximately 30% of patients. Severe liver disease is most likely due to infection or to undiagnosed autoimmune hepatitis or primary biliary cirrhosis.

Neuromuscular manifestations include myopathy with proximal skeletal muscle weakness and increased serum creatine kinase concentration. Tendinitis is common and can result in tendon rupture.

Hematologic abnormalities may be present. Thromboembolism associated with antiphospholipid antibodies can be an important cause of central nervous system dysfunction. Leukopenia, granulocyte dysfunction, decreased complement levels, and functional asplenia have been implicated in an increased risk of infection. Thrombocytopenia and hemolytic anemia are seen in some patients. The presence of circulating anticoagulants is reflected in a prolonged activated partial thromboplastin time. Patients with circulating anticoagulants often manifest a false-positive test result for syphilis.

Some patients with lupus have cutaneous manifestations. The classic butterfly-shaped malar rash occurs in approximately half of patients. This rash can be transient and is often exacerbated by sunlight. Discoid lesions on the face, scalp, and upper trunk develop in approximately 25% of patients with SLE but may occur in the absence of any other features of SLE. Alopecia is common.

TREATMENT

Treatment is determined by individual disease manifestations. Arthritis and serositis can often be controlled with aspirin or NSAIDs. Antimalarial drugs such as hydroxychloroquine and quinacrine are also effective in treating the dermatologic and arthritic manifestations of SLE. Patients should use sunscreens and avoid intense sun exposure. Thrombocytopenia and hemolytic anemia usually respond to corticosteroid therapy. Danazol, vincristine, cyclophosphamide, or splenectomy can be used if thrombocytopenia does not respond to glucocorticoid administration. In view of the increased susceptibility to infection, the risk/benefit ratio of splenectomy must be carefully considered.

Corticosteroids are the principal treatment for severe manifestations of SLE. Corticosteroids effectively suppress glomerulonephritis and cardiovascular abnormalities. However, corticosteroid therapy can be a major cause of morbidity in patients with SLE. Death during the course of SLE may be due to coronary atherosclerosis. The development and progression of coronary atherosclerosis is accelerated by treatment with corticosteroids. Immunosuppressive treatment with alternative drugs such as methotrexate, cyclophosphamide, azathioprine, or mycophenolate mofetil may be preferable to prolonged treatment with high-dose corticosteroids.

MANAGEMENT OF ANESTHESIA

Management of anesthesia is influenced by the magnitude of organ system dysfunction and the drugs used to treat SLE. Laryngeal involvement, including mucosal ulceration, cricoarytenoid arthritis, and recurrent laryngeal nerve palsy, may be present in as many as one third of patients.

Spondyloarthropathies

Spondyloarthropathies are a group of nonrheumatic arthropathies that include ankylosing spondylitis, reactive arthritis (Reiter's syndrome), juvenile chronic polyarthropathy, psoriatic arthritis, and enteropathic arthritis. These diseases are characterized by involvement of the spine, especially the sacroiliac joints; asymmetrical peripheral arthritis and synovitis; and absence of rheumatoid nodules or detectable circulating rheumatoid factor (see Table 21-7). There is a shared predilection for new bone formation at sites of chronic inflammation, and joint ankylosis often results. There is also a predilection for ocular inflammation. Causes of these seronegative spondyloarthropathies are unknown, but there is a strong association with HLA-B27.

ANKYLOSING SPONDYLITIS

Ankylosing spondylitis is a chronic, usually progressive, inflammatory disease involving the articulations of the spine and adjacent soft tissues. Spinal disease begins in the sacroiliac joints and moves cranially. The degree of spinal disease can range from just sacroiliac involvement to complete ankylosis of the spine. Hip involvement occurs in approximately one third of patients. Back pain characterized by morning stiffness that improves with activity and exercise plus radiographic evidence of sacroiliitis is highly suggestive of this diagnosis. The disease occurs predominantly in men and often begins in young adulthood. The strong familial incidence is supported by the finding that 90% of patients with ankylosing spondylitis are HLA-B27 positive compared with only 6% of the general population. Ankylosing spondylitis is often erroneously diagnosed as back pain caused by lumbar disc degeneration. Examination of the spine may demonstrate skeletal muscle spasm, loss of lordosis, and decreased mobility of the vertebral column.

Systemic involvement can manifest as weight loss, fatigue, and low-grade fever. Conjunctivitis and uveitis occur in approximately 40% of patients. The uveitis is usually unilateral and presents as visual impairment, photophobia, and eye pain. Distinctive pulmonary abnormalities associated with ankylosing spondylitis include apical cavitary lesions and pleural thickening that mimic tuberculosis. Cardiovascular involvement, such as aortic regurgitation or bundle branch block, is observed in 40% of patients. Arthritic involvement of the thoracic spine and costovertebral articulations can result in a decrease in chest wall compliance and, consequently, a decrease in vital capacity.

Treatment

Treatment of ankylosing spondylitis consists of exercises designed to maintain joint mobility and posture plus antiinflammatory drugs. NSAIDs are commonly used. Infliximab and etanercept may cause profound improvement in this disease, but patients often experience relapse when treatment is discontinued. For uveitis, topical corticosteroid eye drops are an integral part of management.

Management of Anesthesia

Management of anesthesia in patients with ankylosing spondylitis is influenced by the magnitude of spinal involvement. The spinal column can be stiff and deformed and prevent appropriate cervical spine motion for endotracheal intubation. Fiberoptic or videolaryngoscope assistance may be needed for endotracheal intubation. Restrictive lung disease from costochondral rigidity and flexion deformity of the thoracic spine must be appreciated. Sudden or excessive increases in systemic vascular resistance are poorly tolerated if significant aortic regurgitation is present. Management of aortic regurgitation includes keeping the heart rate at 90 beats per minute or higher and the systemic vascular resistance lower than normal. Neurologic monitoring is a consideration for patients undergoing corrective spinal surgery. Epidural or spinal anesthesia is an acceptable alternative to general anesthesia for perineal or lower limb surgery, but regional anesthesia may be technically difficult due to limited joint mobility and closed interspinous spaces. Ossification of the ligamentum flavum is uncommon, however. A paramedian approach for spinal or epidural anesthesia may be easier than a midline approach.

REACTIVE ARTHRITIS

Reactive arthritis is an *aseptic* arthritis that occurs after an extraarticular infection, especially infection with *Chlamydia, Salmonella,* and *Shigella* species. When reactive arthritis is accompanied by extraarticular features such as urethritis, uveitis or conjunctivitis, and skin lesions, the term Reiter's syndrome is often used. Predisposing factors include genetic makeup (HLA-B27 positivity). Most of the signs of Reiter's syndrome persist for only a few days, but arthritis progresses to sacroiliitis and spondylitis in approximately 20% of patients. Cricoarytenoid arthritis can also occur. Hyperkeratotic skin lesions cannot be distinguished from those of psoriasis, and the two diseases frequently overlap. Management consists of antibiotic treatment for the initial infection and NSAIDs or sulfasalazine for symptomatic relief of the arthritis.

CHRONIC JUVENILE POLYARTHROPATHY

The pathologic process in chronic juvenile polyarthropathy is similar to that in adult rheumatoid arthritis. Growth abnormalities may occur if arthritis appears before puberty. Hepatic dysfunction may be present, but cardiac involvement is unusual. An acute form of polyarthritis, which presents as fever, rash, lymphadenopathy, and splenomegaly in young children who test negative for rheumatoid factor and HLA-B27, is designated *Still's disease.* Aspirin is commonly used to treat this disorder. Corticosteroids can effectively control the disease, but their use is limited because of concerns about drug-induced growth retardation in these young patients.

ENTEROPATHIC ARTHRITIS

Approximately 10% to 20% of patients with Crohn's disease and 2% to 7% of patients with ulcerative colitis have an inflammatory polyarthritis, most often involving the large joints of the lower extremities. In general, the arthritis activity parallels the activity of the gastrointestinal inflammation, and measures that control the gut disease usually control the joint disease as well. This arthritis is not linked to the presence of HLA-B27.

Inflammatory bowel disease can also be associated with sacroiliitis and spondylitis, which follow a pattern in which the joint inflammation waxes and wanes independently of the gastrointestinal inflammation. HLA-B27 is found in 50% of these patients. This arthritis is usually chronic and may become ankylosing spondylitis. Treatment is as described for ankylosing spondylitis.

Paget's Disease

Paget's disease of bone is characterized by excessive *osteoblastic* and *osteoclastic* activity, which results in abnormally thick but weak bones. The cause is unknown but may involve an excess of parathyroid hormone or a deficiency of calcitonin.

A familial tendency is present, with white men older than 40 years of age affected most often. Bone pain is the most common symptom. Complications of Paget's disease involve bones (fractures and neoplastic degeneration), joints (arthritis), and the nervous system (nerve compression, paraplegia). Hypercalcemia and renal calculi may also occur. The most characteristic radiographic feature of Paget's disease is localized bone enlargement. Lytic and sclerotic bone changes may involve the skull. If the skull is affected, it may be grossly enlarged, and irreversible hearing loss may occur. A radionuclide bone scan is the most reliable test to identify lesions caused by Paget's disease. Serum alkaline phosphatase concentration (reflecting *bone formation*) and urinary hydroxyproline excretion (reflecting *bone resorption*) are usually increased.

Treatment of Paget's disease is designed to alleviate bone pain and to minimize or prevent progression of the disease. Calcitonin is a hormone secreted by the thyroid gland that inhibits osteoclastic activity and decreases bone resorption. Treatment with calcitonin decreases pain and the biochemical and radiographic abnormalities associated with Paget's disease. It may also stabilize the hearing loss caused by Paget's disease. Bisphosphonates can induce marked and prolonged inhibition of bone resorption by decreasing osteoclastic activity. Whereas the effects of calcitonin are short lived, disease activity remains low for many months, sometimes years, after treatment with bisphosphonates is discontinued. Radiographically confirmed repair of osteolytic lesions may occur in response to treatment with bisphosphonates.

Conservative treatment of fractures in patients with Paget's disease is associated with a high risk of delayed union. Patients with Paget's disease who have severe arthritis of the hips or knees often benefit from joint replacement. Rarely, osteotomy must be performed to correct bowing deformities of long bones. Patients with evidence of peripheral nerve compression, radiculopathy, or spinal cord compression require decompressive surgery.

Dwarfism

Dwarfism can occur in two forms: *proportionate* dwarfism, in which the limbs, trunk, and head size are in the same relative proportions as those in a normal adult, and *disproportionate* dwarfism, in which the limbs, trunk, and head size are not in the usual proportions of those in a normal adult.

ACHONDROPLASIA

Achondroplasia is the most common cause of disproportionate dwarfism. It occurs predominantly in females with an incidence of 1.5 per 10,000 births. Transmission is by an autosomal dominant gene, although an estimated 80% of cases represent spontaneous mutations. The basic defect is a decrease in the rate of endochondral ossification that, when coupled with normal periosteal bone formation, produces short tubular bones. The anticipated height of achondroplastic males is 132 cm

(52 inches) and that of females is 122 cm (48 inches). Kyphoscoliosis and genu varum are common. Premature fusion of the bones at the base of the skull can result in a shortened skull base and a stenotic foramen magnum. In addition, there may be functional fusion of the atlantooccipital joint with odontoid hypoplasia, atlantoaxial instability, bulging discs, and severe cervical kyphosis. These changes may result in hydrocephalus or damage to the cervical spinal cord. Central sleep apnea in individuals with achondroplasia may be a result of brainstem compression due to foramen magnum stenosis. Pulmonary hypertension leading to cor pulmonale is the most common cardiovascular disturbance that develops in individuals with dwarfism. Mental and skeletal muscle development are normal, as is life expectancy for those who survive the first year of life.

Management of Anesthesia

Management of anesthesia in patients with achondroplastic dwarfism is influenced by potential airway difficulties, cervical spine instability, and the potential for spinal cord trauma with neck extension (Table 21-8).

Patients with achondroplasia may undergo a number of specific operations, including suboccipital craniectomy for foramen magnum stenosis, laminectomy for spinal column stenosis or nerve root compression, and ventriculoperitoneal shunt placement. A history of obstructive sleep apnea may predispose to development of upper airway obstruction after sedation or induction of anesthesia. Abnormal bone growth can result in several potential anesthetic problems. Facial features, including a large protruding forehead, short maxilla, large mandible, flat nose, and large tongue, may result in difficulty obtaining a good mask fit and in maintaining a patent upper airway. Despite these anatomic characteristics, clinical experience has not confirmed difficulty with upper airway patency or endotracheal intubation in most of these patients.

In achondroplastic patients with cervical kyphosis, tracheal intubation may be difficult because of inability to align the axes of the airway. Hyperextension of the neck during direct laryngoscopy should be avoided because of the likely presence of foramen magnum stenosis. Fiberoptically guided tracheal

TABLE 21-8	Characteristics of achondroplastic dwarfism that may influence management of anesthesia

Difficulty exposing the glottic opening
Foramen magnum stenosis
Odontoid hypoplasia with cervical instability
Kyphoscoliosis
Restrictive lung disease
Obstructive sleep apnea
Central sleep apnea
Pulmonary hypertension
Cor pulmonale
Hydrocephalus

intubation may be considered in selected patients. Weight rather than age is the best guide for selecting the proper size of endotracheal tube.

Excess skin and subcutaneous tissue may make peripheral venous access technically difficult. Patients with achondroplastic dwarfism undergoing suboccipital craniectomy, especially in the sitting position, are at risk of venous air embolism. Insertion of a right atrial catheter is desirable should an air embolism occur, but placing such a catheter may be technically difficult because of the short neck and the difficulty of identifying landmarks, which may be obscured by excess soft tissue. Evoked potential monitoring is useful during surgery that may be associated with brainstem or spinal cord injury. Achondroplastic patients respond normally to anesthetic drugs and neuromuscular blockers. Anesthetic techniques that permit rapid awakening may be desirable for prompt evaluation of neurologic function.

Delivery by cesarean section is necessary in women with achondroplasia because a small, contracted maternal pelvis combined with an infant of near-normal birth weight leads to cephalopelvic disproportion. Regional anesthesia might be considered, but technical difficulties may occur due to kyphoscoliosis and a narrow epidural space and spinal canal. The small epidural space may make it difficult to introduce an epidural catheter. Osteophytes, prolapsed intervertebral discs, or deformed vertebral bodies can also contribute to difficulties with neuraxial blockade. There are no data confirming appropriate doses of local anesthetics for epidural or spinal anesthesia in these patients. Epidural anesthesia may be preferable to spinal anesthesia because it permits titration of the local anesthetic drug to achieve the desired level of sensory blockade.

RUSSELL-SILVER SYNDROME

Russell-Silver syndrome is a form of dwarfism characterized by intrauterine growth retardation with subsequent severe postnatal growth impairment, dysmorphic facial features (including mandibular and facial hypoplasia), limb asymmetry, congenital heart defects, and a constellation of endocrine abnormalities including hypoglycemia, adrenocortical insufficiency, and hypogonadism. Developmental and hormonal abnormalities tend to normalize with age, and individuals with this syndrome can achieve adult heights near 150 cm (approximately 60 inches). Rapid depletion of limited hepatic glycogen stores, especially in small-for-gestational-age neonates, may predispose to hypoglycemia. The risk of hypoglycemia diminishes as the child grows and usually disappears after about 4 years of age.

Management of Anesthesia

Preoperative evaluation should consider the serum glucose concentration, especially in neonates at risk of hypoglycemia. Intravenous infusions containing glucose may be indicated preoperatively. Facial manifestations of this syndrome (similar to those in Goldenhar's and Treacher-Collins syndromes) may make direct laryngoscopy and exposure of the glottic opening difficult. An endotracheal tube smaller than the predicted size may be needed. Obtaining a good mask fit may also be difficult because of facial asymmetry. Administration of some drugs, such as muscle relaxants, based on body weight rather than body surface area may result in relative underdosing. Infants with Russell-Silver syndrome may be especially prone to intraoperative hypothermia because of their large surface-to-volume ratio. Unexplained tachycardia, diaphoresis, or somnolence after emergence from anesthesia may indicate hypoglycemia.

OTHER MUSCULOSKELETAL DISORDERS

Tumoral Calcinosis

Tumoral calcinosis is a rare genetic disorder that presents as metastatic calcifications adjacent to large joints. Joint motion is unaffected, but the masses may enlarge and interfere with skeletal muscle function. Treatment consists of complete excision of the masses. The principal anesthetic consideration is the rare involvement of the hyoid bone, hypothyroid ligament, or cervical intervertebral joints by this disease process, which leads to difficulty exposing the glottic opening during direct laryngoscopy.

Disorders of the Shoulder

Rotator cuff tear is the most common pathologic entity involving the shoulders. The prevalence of partial- or full-thickness rotator cuff tears is 5% to 40% as determined at postmortem examinations of adults older than 40 years of age. The incidence of rotator cuff tears increases with age. As many as half of individuals older than 55 years of age have arthrographically detectable rotator cuff tears. Other pathologic shoulder conditions are less common. Adhesive capsulitis (frozen shoulder) occurs in approximately 2% of the adult population and in 11% of the adult diabetic population. The incidence of calcific tendinitis ranges from 3% to 7%. Shoulder pain ranks just behind back and neck pain as a cause of disability in workers.

Corticosteroid injection into the subacromial space may provide symptomatic relief in patients with impingement syndromes with or without rotator cuff tears, adhesive capsulitis, or supraspinatus tendinitis. Arthroscopic release or manipulation under anesthesia may be used in an attempt to restore shoulder motion. Total shoulder replacement (replacement of humeral and glenoid articular surfaces) reduces shoulder pain in most patients.

MANAGEMENT OF ANESTHESIA

Brachial plexus anesthesia via the interscalene approach with continuous infusion of local anesthetic can provide anesthesia for shoulder surgery and postoperative analgesia. Ipsilateral hemidiaphragmatic paralysis virtually always occurs with an interscalene block because the phrenic nerve lies close to the area into which the local anesthetic is injected for this block.

For this reason, interscalene block may be problematic and is best avoided in patients with severe chronic obstructive pulmonary disease or with neuromuscular diseases associated with weakness of the respiratory muscles. Wound infiltration or lavage with solutions containing a long-acting local anesthetic such as bupivacaine or ropivacaine can also provide postoperative analgesia following major shoulder surgery.

Floppy Infant Syndrome

Floppy infant syndrome is a term used to describe weak, hypotonic skeletal muscles in infants. A diminished cough reflex and difficulty swallowing predispose to aspiration, and recurrent pneumonia is common. Progressive weakness and atrophy of skeletal muscles leads to contractures and kyphoscoliosis.

MANAGEMENT OF ANESTHESIA
Anesthesia may be associated with increased sensitivity to nondepolarizing muscle relaxants and hyperkalemia with cardiac arrest after administration of succinylcholine. These infants are also susceptible to malignant hyperthermia. Ketamine can be useful for anesthesia because it does not cause significant respiratory depression.

Tracheomegaly

Tracheomegaly is characterized by marked dilation of the trachea and bronchi resulting from a congenital defect in elastin and smooth muscle fibers in the tracheobronchial tree or to their destruction after radiotherapy. The diagnosis is confirmed by measuring a tracheal diameter of more than 30 mm on a chest radiograph. Symptoms include a chronic productive cough and frequent pulmonary infection, perhaps related to chronic aspiration. The tracheal and bronchial walls are abnormally flaccid and may collapse during vigorous coughing. Aspiration during general anesthesia is possible, especially if maximal inflation of the endotracheal tube cuff does not produce a seal.

Alcoholic Myopathy

Acute and chronic forms of proximal skeletal muscle weakness occur frequently in alcoholic patients. Differentiation of alcoholic myopathy from alcoholic neuropathy is based on the presence of proximal rather than distal skeletal muscle involvement, an increased serum creatine kinase concentration, myoglobinuria in acute cases, and rapid recovery after cessation of alcohol consumption.

Prader-Willi Syndrome

Prader-Willi syndrome manifests at birth as hypotonia, which may be associated with a weak cough, swallowing difficulties, and upper airway obstruction. Nasogastric feeding may be necessary during infancy. The syndrome progresses during childhood and is characterized by hyperphagia leading to obesity plus endocrine abnormalities including hypogonadism and diabetes mellitus. Pickwickian syndrome may develop in some patients. There is little growth in height and patients remain short. Mental retardation is often severe. There is a deletion in chromosome 15 in this syndrome, and an autosomal recessive mode of inheritance has been proposed.

Micrognathia, a high-arched palate, strabismus, a straight ulnar border, and congenital dislocation of the hip may be present. Dental caries are common and may be related to chronic regurgitation of gastric contents. Seizures are associated with this syndrome, but cardiac dysfunction does not accompany Prader-Willi syndrome.

MANAGEMENT OF ANESTHESIA
The principal anesthetic concerns in these patients center on hypotonia and altered metabolism of carbohydrates and fat. Weak skeletal musculature is associated with a poor cough and an increased incidence of pneumonia. Intraoperative monitoring of blood glucose concentration is necessary and exogenous glucose administration may be needed, because these patients use circulating glucose to manufacture fat rather than to meet basal energy needs. When calculating drug doses, one should consider the decreased skeletal muscle mass and increased fat content in these patients. Muscle relaxant requirements may be decreased in the presence of hypotonia. Succinylcholine has been administered without incident to these patients.

Disturbances in thermoregulation, often characterized by intraoperative hyperthermia and metabolic acidosis, have been observed, but a relationship to malignant hyperthermia has not been established. There is an increased incidence of perioperative aspiration pneumonia.

Prune-Belly Syndrome

Prune-belly syndrome is characterized by congenital agenesis of the lower central abdominal musculature and the presence of urinary tract anomalies, including gross ureteral dilation, hypotonic bladder, prostatic hypoplasia, and bilateral undescended testes. The full syndrome appears only in males, but up to 3% of patients with an incomplete syndrome are female. Recurrent respiratory tract infections are seen and reflect an impaired ability to cough effectively. It is unlikely that muscle relaxants will be necessary during the management of anesthesia in these patients.

Mitochondrial Myopathies

Mitochondrial myopathies are a heterogeneous group of disorders of skeletal muscle energy metabolism. Mitochondria produce the energy required by skeletal muscle cells through the oxidation-reduction reactions of the electron transfer chain and oxidative phosphorylation, thereby generating adenosine triphosphate. Defects in this process result in abnormal fatigability with sustained exercise, skeletal muscle pain, and progressive weakness. The hallmark lesions are large subsarcolemmal accumulations of abnormal mitochondria that appear as red-staining granules (ragged-red fibers) on histologic analysis. Disorders of mitochondrial metabolism may also involve other organ systems with high energy demands, such as the brain, heart, liver, and kidneys.

KEARNS-SAYRE SYNDROME

Kearns-Sayre syndrome is a rare mitochondrial myopathy accompanied by progressive external ophthalmoplegia, retinitis pigmentosa, heart block, hearing loss, short stature, peripheral neuropathy, and impaired ventilatory drive. Dilated cardiomyopathy and congestive heart failure may be present.

Management of Anesthesia

Management of general anesthesia in these patients must consider the risk of drug-induced myocardial depression, development of cardiac conduction defects, and hypoventilation during the early postoperative period.

Multicore Myopathy

Multicore myopathy is a heterogeneous group of diseases characterized by proximal skeletal muscle weakness, a decrease in muscle mass, and musculoskeletal abnormalities such as scoliosis and high-arched palate. Recurrent pulmonary infection is common and may be related to the severity of the associated kyphoscoliosis. Cardiomyopathy may accompany this myopathy. Unlike in other myopathies, serum creatine kinase concentration is usually normal in these individuals. Intelligence is normal, and the myopathy may have a benign course.

MANAGEMENT OF ANESTHESIA

Preoperative assessment of respiratory function is necessary in the presence of kyphoscoliosis and recurrent lung infection. Difficulty swallowing and an inability to clear secretions may reflect pharyngeal and laryngeal muscle involvement. Postoperative aspiration may be associated with impaired upper airway reflexes and the lingering effects of drugs administered during anesthesia. It is important to recognize the potential relationship between multicore myopathy and malignant hyperthermia.

Centronuclear Myopathy

Centronuclear myopathy is a rare congenital myopathy characterized by progressive muscle weakness of extraocular, facial, neck, and limb muscles. The defect is a mutation in a gene important for muscle cell growth and differentiation. There are severe neonatal forms of this disease as well as slowly progressive forms that can begin anytime from birth to adulthood. Development of scoliosis with restrictive lung disease is an important manifestation of disease severity. Serum creatine kinase concentration is usually normal. The association of ptosis and strabismus with this myopathy

increases the likelihood that affected children will undergo surgery.

MANAGEMENT OF ANESTHESIA

Management of anesthesia is influenced by the degree of skeletal muscle weakness, the presence of restrictive lung disease, and gastroesophageal reflux. Muscle relaxants are often avoided and a nontriggering general anesthetic technique used.

Meige's Syndrome

Meige's syndrome is an idiopathic dystonic disorder that manifests as blepharospasm and oromandibular dystonia. It most often affects middle-aged to elderly women. Facial muscle spasms are characterized by symmetrical dystonic contractions of the facial muscles. Dystonia is aggravated by stress and disappears during sleep. The pathophysiology of this disease is unknown but may be related to dopamine hyperactivity or dysfunction of the basal ganglia. Drug therapy (antidopaminergics, anticholinergics, acetylcholine agonists, γ-aminobutyric acid agonists) may have some effect, and facial nerve block has been reported to provide sustained relief.

Spasmodic Dysphonia

Spasmodic dysphonia is a laryngeal disorder characterized by adductor or abductor dystonic spasms of the vocal cords. This syndrome typically manifests as abnormal phonation but on rare occasions is associated with respiratory distress. Stress can exacerbate it, and associated neurologic symptoms (tremors, weakness, dystonia of other skeletal muscle groups) are present in most patients. Botulinum toxin, which blocks neuromuscular transmission, may be effective for treating the spasms of torticollis, blepharospasm, and spasmodic dysphonia.

MANAGEMENT OF ANESTHESIA

Preoperative fiberoptic or direct laryngoscopy may be necessary to define anatomic abnormalities and to estimate airway dimensions. The presence of laryngeal stenosis may necessitate the use of smaller than usual tracheal tubes. The risk of pulmonary aspiration may be increased by vocal cord dysfunction caused by therapeutic interventions such as botulinum toxin injection or recurrent laryngeal nerve interruption. Continued monitoring during the postoperative period is important, because these patients may experience respiratory difficulties.

Juvenile Hyaline Fibromatosis

Juvenile hyaline fibromatosis is a rare syndrome characterized by the presence of numerous dermal and subcutaneous nodules. Patients may have hypertrophic gingivae, osteolytic bone lesions, and stunted growth with normal mental development. Resistance to the effects of succinylcholine has been described in patients with juvenile hyaline fibromatosis.

Chondrodysplasia Calcificans Punctata

Chondrodysplasia calcificans punctata is a rare congenital syndrome caused by dysfunctional peroxisomes. It manifests as erratic cartilage calcification resulting in bone and skin lesions, cataracts, and cardiac malformations. In surviving children, abnormal growth leads to dwarfism, kyphoscoliosis, and subluxation of the hips. There is no available treatment. Orthopedic procedures are often necessary to offset functional limitations of the disease and to stabilize spine and limb malformations. Tracheal cartilage may be involved by the disease process; this results in tracheal stenosis, which may complicate perioperative airway management.

Erythromelalgia

Erythromelalgia literally means "red, painful extremities." Erythema, intense burning pain, and increased temperature of the involved extremities are hallmarks of the disease. The feet, especially the soles, are most often involved, and males are affected twice as often as females. Primary erythromelalgia occurs more frequently than secondary erythromelalgia, which is associated with myeloproliferative disorders such as polycythemia vera. Intravascular platelet aggregation may be prominent. Aspirin is the most effective treatment for secondary erythromelalgia resulting from myeloproliferative diseases. Patients may seek relief by exposing the affected extremity to a cooler environment, such as immersing the extremity in cold water. Neuraxial opioids and local anesthetics may provide some pain relief.

Farber's Lipogranulomatosis

Farber's lipogranulomatosis is an inherited disorder caused by a deficiency of ceramidase that results in accumulation of ceramide in tissues (pleura, pericardium, synovial lining of joints, liver, spleen, lymph nodes). Progressive arthropathy, psychomotor retardation, and nutritional failure are present, and most affected individuals die by 2 years of age as a result of airway and respiratory problems. Acute renal and hepatic failure may reflect accumulation of ceramide in these organs. Difficulty in airway management is a common problem because of granuloma formation in the pharynx or larynx. Tracheal intubation is best avoided in patients with upper airway involvement, because laryngeal edema or bleeding from laryngeal granulomas is possible.

McCune-Albright Syndrome

McCune-Albright syndrome consists of a triad of physical signs: osseous lesions (polyostotic fibrous dysplasia), melanotic cutaneous macules (café au lait spots), and sexual precocity (autonomous ovarian steroid secretion). Conductive and neural deafness occur when osseous lesions involve the temporal bone and impinge on the cochlea. Bony fractures are likely during childhood. Some patients show other endocrine dysfunction, especially hyperthyroidism, acromegaly, and hypophosphatemia.

MANAGEMENT OF ANESTHESIA

An important anesthetic implication of McCune-Albright syndrome is the presence of endocrine abnormalities, especially hyperthyroidism. Perioperative steroid supplementation may be a consideration when adrenal hyperactivity is present, because these patients may exhibit an altered cortisol response to stress. Vascular fragility may make venous access difficult. These patients may have fragile bones, and particular care is needed during intraoperative positioning. Tracheal intubation may be difficult because of airway distortion associated with acromegaly or hypertrophy of soft tissue in the upper airway.

Klippel-Feil Syndrome

Klippel-Feil syndrome is characterized by a short neck resulting from a reduced number of cervical vertebrae or fusion of several vertebrae. Movement of the neck is limited. Associated skeletal abnormalities include spinal stenosis and kyphoscoliosis. Mandibular malformations and micrognathia may be present. There is an increased incidence of cardiac and genitourinary anomalies. Management of anesthesia must consider the risk of neurologic damage during direct laryngoscopy resulting from cervical spine instability. Preoperative lateral neck radiographs help in evaluating the stability of the cervical spine.

Osteogenesis Imperfecta

Osteogenesis imperfecta is a rare, autosomal dominant, inherited disease of connective tissue that affects bones, the sclera, and the inner ear. Bones are extremely brittle because of defective collagen production. The incidence of osteogenesis imperfecta is higher in females. Osteogenesis imperfecta can manifest in two forms: osteogenesis imperfecta congenita and osteogenesis imperfecta tarda. With the congenital form, fractures occur in utero and death often occurs during the perinatal period. The tarda form typically manifests during childhood or early adolescence with blue sclerae fractures after minor trauma, kyphoscoliosis, bowing of the femur and tibia, and gradual onset of otosclerosis and deafness. Impaired platelet function may produce a mild bleeding tendency. Hyperthermia with hyperhidrosis can occur in patients with osteogenesis imperfecta. An increased serum thyroxine concentration associated with an increase in oxygen consumption occurs in at least 50% of patients with this disease.

MANAGEMENT OF ANESTHESIA

Management of anesthesia is influenced by the co-existing orthopedic deformities and the potential for additional fractures during the perioperative period. Patients with osteogenesis imperfecta often have a decreased range of motion of the cervical spine resulting from remodeling of bone. Tracheal intubation must be accomplished with as little manipulation and trauma as possible, because cervical and mandibular fractures may easily occur. Awake fiberoptic intubation or videolaryngoscopy may be prudent if orthopedic deformities suggest that it will be difficult to visualize the glottic opening with direct laryngoscopy. Dentition is often defective, and teeth are vulnerable to damage during direct laryngoscopy. Succinylcholine-induced fasciculations may produce fractures. Kyphoscoliosis and pectus excavatum decrease vital capacity and chest wall compliance and can result in arterial hypoxemia caused by ventilation/perfusion mismatching. Use of automated blood pressure cuffs may be hazardous, since inflation can result in fractures. Regional anesthesia is acceptable in selected patients because it avoids the need for endotracheal intubation, but it may be technically difficult because of kyphoscoliosis. The coagulation status should be evaluated before a regional anesthetic technique is selected, because osteogenesis imperfecta may be associated with a prolonged bleeding time despite a normal platelet count. Desmopressin may be effective in normalizing platelet function. These patients may have mild hyperthermia intraoperatively, but it is not a forerunner of malignant hyperthermia.

Fibrodysplasia Ossificans

Fibrodysplasia ossificans is a rare inherited autosomal dominant disease that usually presents before 6 years of age and is characterized by myositis and proliferation of connective tissue. The term *myositis ossificans* is also applied to this disease, but *fibrodysplasia ossificans* may be a more correct term because this is principally a disease of connective tissue rather than of skeletal muscle. Connective tissue undergoes cartilaginous and osteoid transformation, which eventually leads to displacement of skeletal muscles by ectopic bone. Body parts become rigid. Ectopic bone formation typically affects the muscles of the elbows, hips, and knees, leading to serious limitations of joint movement. Cervical spine involvement is common. There may be varying degrees of cervical fusion, and atlantoaxial subluxation is possible. Temporomandibular joint involvement may also occur. Muscles of the face, larynx, eyes, anterior abdominal wall, diaphragm, and heart usually escape involvement.

During the early stages of the disease, fever may occur at the same time that localized lumps appear in affected skeletal muscles. Alkaline phosphatase activity is increased during active phases of the disease. A restrictive breathing pattern can result from limitation of rib movement, but progression to respiratory failure is rare. Pneumonia, however, is a common complication. Abnormalities on electrocardiogram include ST-segment changes and right bundle branch block. Deafness may occur, but mental retardation is unlikely. There is no effective therapy.

Deformities of the Sternum

Pectus carinatum (outward protuberance of the sternum) and *pectus excavatum* (inward concavity of the sternum) produce cosmetic problems, but functional impairment is unusual. Considerable narrowing of the distance between the posterior sternum and the anterior border of the vertebral bodies can be tolerated with little effect on cardiopulmonary function. Rarely is pectus excavatum associated with increased cardiac filling pressures or dysrhythmias. Obstructive sleep apnea may be more common in young children with pectus excavatum, perhaps because of greater inward movement of the sternum and the pliable costochondral apparatus.

Macroglossia

Macroglossia is an infrequent but potentially lethal postoperative complication that is most often associated with posterior fossa craniotomy performed in the sitting position. Possible causes of macroglossia include arterial compression, venous compression resulting from excessive neck flexion or a head-down position, and mechanical compression of the tongue by the teeth, an oral airway, or an endotracheal tube. Macroglossia may also have a neurogenic origin. When the onset of macroglossia is immediate, it is easily recognized and airway obstruction does not occur because tracheal extubation is delayed. In some patients, however, obstruction to venous outflow from the tongue leads to development of regional ischemia from compression of the lingual arteries. This is followed by a reperfusion injury that does not occur until the outflow obstruction is relieved. As a result, the development of macroglossia may be delayed for 30 minutes or longer. There is then the risk of complete airway obstruction occurring at an unexpected time during the postoperative period.

KEY POINTS

- Epidermolysis bullosa and pemphigus are characterized by bulla formation (blistering) that can involve extensive areas of skin and mucous membranes. Even minor frictional trauma can result in bulla formation. Airway management may be difficult because of bullae in the oropharynx. Airway manipulation, including direct laryngoscopy and endotracheal intubation, can result in acute bulla formation, upper airway obstruction, and bleeding.
- Patients with scleroderma can present several problems in anesthetic management. Decreased mandibular motion and narrowing of the oral aperture caused by taut skin may make endotracheal intubation difficult. Oral or nasal telangiectasias may bleed profusely if traumatized. Intravenous access may be impeded by dermal thickening. Systemic or pulmonary hypertension may be present. Hypotonia of the lower esophageal sphincter puts patients at risk of regurgitation and aspiration.
- Muscular dystrophy is characterized by progressive, symmetrical skeletal muscle weakness and wasting but no evidence of skeletal muscle denervation. Sensation and reflexes are intact. Increased permeability of skeletal muscle membranes precedes clinical evidence of muscular dystrophy. Patients with muscular dystrophy are susceptible to malignant hyperthermia.

■ The term *myotonic dystrophy* designates a group of hereditary degenerative diseases of skeletal muscle characterized by persistent contracture (myotonia) after voluntary contraction of a muscle or electrical stimulation of the muscle. Peripheral nerves and the neuromuscular junction are not affected. This inability of skeletal muscle to relax after voluntary contraction or stimulation results from abnormal calcium metabolism.

■ The clinical course of myasthenia gravis is marked by periods of exacerbation and remission. Muscle strength may be normal in well-rested patients, but weakness occurs promptly with exercise. Ptosis and diplopia resulting from extraocular muscle weakness are the most common initial signs. Weakness of pharyngeal and laryngeal muscles results in dysphagia, dysarthria, and difficulty handling saliva. Patients with myasthenia gravis are at high risk of pulmonary aspiration.

■ The acetylcholine receptor–binding antibodies of myasthenia gravis decrease the number of functional acetylcholine receptors, and this results in an increased *sensitivity* to nondepolarizing muscle relaxants. However, patients with myasthenia gravis demonstrate *resistance* to the effects of succinylcholine.

■ Myasthenic syndrome (Eaton-Lambert syndrome) is a disorder of neuromuscular transmission that resembles myasthenia gravis. Myasthenic syndrome is an acquired autoimmune disease characterized by the presence of immunoglobulin G antibodies to voltage-sensitive calcium channels that causes a deficiency of these channels at the motor nerve terminal. Anticholinesterase drugs effective in the treatment of myasthenia gravis do *not* produce an improvement in patients with myasthenic syndrome.

■ Cervical spine involvement is frequent in patients with rheumatoid arthritis and may result in pain and neurologic complications. The most significant abnormality of the cervical spine is atlantoaxial subluxation and consequent separation of the atlantoodontoid articulation. When this separation is severe, the odontoid process may protrude into the foramen magnum and exert pressure on the spinal cord or impair blood flow through the vertebral arteries.

■ Involvement of the cricoarytenoid joints by rheumatoid arthritis is suggested by the presence of hoarseness or stridor or by the observation of erythema or edema of the vocal cords during direct laryngoscopy. Diminished movement of these joints can result in narrowing of the glottic opening and interference with passage of the endotracheal tube or an increased risk of cricoarytenoid joint dislocation.

■ The spondyloarthropathies are a group of nonrheumatic arthropathies characterized by involvement of the spine, especially the sacroiliac joints; asymmetrical peripheral arthritis; synovitis; and absence of rheumatic nodules or detectable circulating rheumatoid factor. These diseases have a shared predilection for new bone formation at sites of chronic inflammation, and joint ankylosis often results. Ocular inflammation is frequently present.

■ Osteoarthritis is by far the most common joint disease, one of the leading chronic diseases of the elderly and a major cause of disability. Osteoarthritis is a degenerative process that affects articular cartilage. Both the cervical and lumbar spine may be involved. This process is different from rheumatoid arthritis because there is minimal inflammatory reaction in the joints with osteoarthritis. The pathogenesis is likely related to joint trauma from biomechanical stresses, joint injury, or abnormal joint loading resulting from neuropathy, ligamentous injury, or muscle atrophy. Pain is usually present on motion but is relieved by rest.

■ Kyphoscoliosis is a spinal deformity characterized by anterior flexion (kyphosis) and lateral curvature (scoliosis) of the vertebral column. Spinal curvature of more than 40 degrees is considered severe and is likely to be associated with physiologic derangements in cardiac and pulmonary function. Restrictive lung disease and pulmonary hypertension progressing to cor pulmonale are the principal causes of death in patients with kyphoscoliosis. During corrective surgery for scoliosis or kyphosis, spinal cord monitoring now utilizes measurement of evoked potentials (sensory and motor) much more frequently than the wake-up test.

RESOURCES

Almahroos M, Kurban AK. Management of mastocytosis. *Clin Dermatol.* 2003;21:274-277.

Ben-Menachem E. Systemic lupus erythematosus: a review for anesthesiologists. *Anesth Analg.* 2010;111:665-676.

Berman BM, Langevin HM, Witt CM, et al. Acupuncture for chronic low back pain. *N Engl J Med.* 2010;363:454-461.

Dalakas MC, Hohlfeld R. Polymyositis and dermatomyositis. *Lancet.* 2003;362:971-982.

Dillon FX. Anesthesia issues in the perioperative management of myasthenia gravis. *Semin Neurol.* 2004;24:83-94.

Hirsch NP. The neuromuscular junction in health and disease. *Br J Anaesth.* 2007;99:132-138.

Kuczkowski KM. Labor analgesia for the parturient with an uncommon disorder: a common dilemma in the delivery suite. *Obstet Gynecol Surv.* 2003;58:800-803.

Nandi R, Howard R. Anesthesia and epidermolysis bullosa. *Dermatol Clin.* 2010;28:319-324.

O'Neill GN. Acquired disorders of the neuromuscular junction. *Int Anesthesiol Clin.* 2006;44:107-121.

Whyte MP. Paget's disease of bone. *N Engl J Med.* 2006;355:593-600.

Infectious Diseases

ANTONIO HERNANDEZ CONTE ■

Epidemic, pandemic, contagious, evasive, virulent, deadly, resistant, evolutionary—these words illustrate the nature of infectious diseases and the impact they have had since their first appearance as well as the continuing scourge they impose on humankind. On December 4, 1967, Dr. William H. Stewart, the U.S. surgeon general, informed a meeting of state and territorial health officials that infectious diseases were now conquered. He extolled the findings of the Centers for Disease Control and Prevention (CDC) a year earlier. Epidemic diseases such as smallpox and bubonic plague were declared things of the past. Typhoid fever, polio, and diphtheria were ostensibly heading in the same direction. Although syphilis, gonorrhea, and tuberculosis were not quite so readily eradicated, it was felt to be only a matter of time before every plague that had ever struck fear into the hearts of decent Americans would be a distant memory.

With the wisdom of hindsight, the irony of these proclamations is clearly evident. The premature declaration of "mission accomplished" appears naive and even foolhardy. The grim reality is that we have probably experienced only a temporary reprieve from the devastation of plagues and infectious diseases. The twenty-first century has already been marked by a resurgence of infectious diseases, most notably of viral origin. Between 1973 and 2003, more than 36 new infectious diseases were identified.

Despite past declarations of medical victory in eradicating microbial organisms responsible for a wide array of pestilence, the presence of infectious agents as a comorbid condition in patients coming for surgery remains a significant issue for the perioperative physician.

Infectious diseases are different from other co-existing illnesses in several respects. First, patients may have co-existing infectious diseases that impact perioperative care when they come for surgery. These infections may be manifest or occult. Preexisting infectious diseases may be the reason for the surgery or may alter the risks associated with the surgery. Second, every patient undergoing surgery is at risk of acquiring an infectious disease during the perioperative period. Patients undergoing surgery are vulnerable to infection both at the surgical site and where natural defenses are breached, such as the respiratory tract, the urinary tract, the bloodstream, and sites of invasive monitoring. These infectious diseases can be passed on to other patients and to health professionals in the perioperative period, and health care workers themselves may serve as active agents in transmitting infectious diseases to patients.

INFECTION PREVENTION OVERVIEW

Antibiotic Resistance

Before modern times, humans had little understanding of infection and were subject to many devastating pandemics, such as the Black Death of the fourteenth century. Since the discovery of penicillin in 1928, bacteria have undergone thousands of mutations resembling a darwinian "survival of the fittest" evolutionary response to antibiotic exposure, which has perpetuated the need for new antibiotics. Most classes of antibiotics were discovered in the 1940s and 1950s, and these drugs are directed at a few specific aspects of bacterial physiology: biosynthesis of the cell wall, DNA, and proteins. During the past 40 years, only two new chemical classes of antibiotics have been developed. One reason for widespread drug resistance among bacterial pathogens is the limited choice of antibiotics that manipulate only a narrow range of bacterial functions.

Infectious diseases that were presumably eradicated, such as tuberculosis, are demonstrating a resurgence. Some reemerging pathogens, such as multidrug-resistant tuberculosis and extensively drug-resistant tuberculosis, have resistance to previously successful antimicrobial therapies.

Multidrug-resistant organisms cause an increasing number of bacterial infections in hospitals, and bacteria are emerging with resistance to *all* available antibiotics. Much of the attention is presently focused on resistant *gram-positive organisms,* such as methicillin-resistant *Staphylococcus aureus.* New drugs are in development to combat gram-positive organisms. However, there is virtually no development of antibiotics active against resistant *gram-negative pathogens.*

Surgical Site Infections

Surgical site infections (SSIs) have been the focus of much attention during the past 30 years, and the major emphasis has been on completely preventing the occurrence of surgery-related infections and their associated morbidity and mortality. In 2002, the Centers for Medicare and Medicaid Services (CMS), in collaboration with the CDC, implemented the national Surgical Infection Prevention Project (SIPP). The key measures being monitored by this project are: (1) the proportion of patients who receive parenterally administered antibiotics within 1 hour before incision (within 2 hours for vancomycin and fluoroquinolones), (2) the proportion of patients who receive prophylactic antimicrobial therapy consistent with published guidelines, and (3) the proportion of patients whose prophylactic antibiotic is discontinued within 24 hours after surgery.

Despite the implementation of numerous sets of drug and policy guidelines, SSIs continue to occur at a rate of 2% to 5% for extraabdominal surgery and up to 20% for intraabdominal surgery. SSIs are among the most common causes of nosocomial infection, accounting for 14% to 16% of all nosocomial infections in hospitalized patients. SSIs are a major source of morbidity and mortality, rendering patients 60% more likely

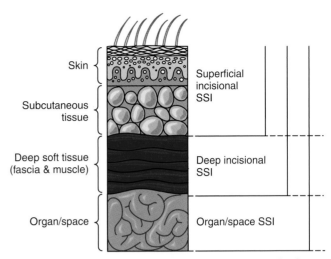

FIGURE 22-1 Cross-section of abdominal wall showing the Centers for Disease Control and Prevention classification of surgical site infection (SSI). *(Adapted from Horan TC, Gaynes RP, Martone WJ, et al. CDC definitions of nosocomial surgical site infections, 1992: a modification of CDC definitions of surgical wound infections.* Infect Control Hosp Epidemiol. *1992;13:606-608.)*

to spend time in the intensive care unit (ICU), five times more likely to require hospital readmission, and twice as likely to die. A recent resurgence in SSIs may be attributable to bacterial resistance, the increased implantation of prosthetic and foreign materials, as well as the poor immune status of many patients undergoing surgery. The universal adoption of simple measures, including frequent hand washing and appropriate administration of prophylactic antibiotics, has been emphasized as a method of decreasing the incidence of SSIs.

SSIs are divided into superficial infections (involving skin and subcutaneous tissues), deep infections (involving fascial and muscle layers), and infections of organs or tissue spaces (any area opened or manipulated during surgery) (Figure 22-1). *S. aureus,* including methicillin-resistant *S. aureus,* is the predominant cause of SSIs. The increased proportion of SSIs caused by resistant pathogens and *Candida* species may reflect the increasing numbers of severely ill and immunocompromised surgical patients and the impact of widespread use of broad-spectrum antimicrobial drugs.

RISK FACTORS FOR SURGICAL SITE INFECTIONS

The risk of developing an SSI is affected by patient-related, microbe-related, and wound-related factors.

Patient-related factors include chronic illness, extremes of age, baseline immunocompetence or inherent or acquired immunocompromise, diabetes mellitus, and corticosteroid therapy. These factors are associated with an increased risk of developing an SSI.

Microbial factors include enzyme production, possession of a polysaccharide capsule, and the ability to bind to fibronectin in blood clots. These are some of the mechanisms by which microorganisms exploit weakened host defenses and initiate infection. *Biofilm* formation is particularly important

TABLE 22-1 ■ Risk factors for surgical site infection

Patient-related factors	Microbial factors	Wound-related factors
Extremes of age	Enzyme production	Devitalized tissue
Poor nutritional status	Polysaccharide capsule	Dead space
American Society of Anesthesiologists physical status score > 2	Ability to bind to fibronectin	Hematoma
Diabetes mellitus	Biofilm and slime formation	Contaminated surgery
Smoking		Presence of foreign material
Obesity		
Co-existing infections		
Colonization		
Immunocompromise		
Longer preoperative hospital stay		

TABLE 22-2 ■ Criteria for diagnosis of a surgical site infection (SSI)

Type of SSI	Time course	Criteria (at least one must be present)
Superficial incisional SSI	Within 30 days of surgery	Superficial pus drainage; Organisms cultured from superficial tissue or fluid; Signs and symptoms (pain, redness, swelling, heat)
Deep incisional SSI	Within 30 days of surgery or within 1 yr if prosthetic implant present	Deep pus drainage; Dehiscence or wound opened by surgeon (for temperature > 38° C, pain, tenderness); Abscess (e.g., radiographically diagnosed)
Organ/space SSI	Within 30 days of surgery or within 1 yr if prosthetic implant present	Pus from a drain in the organ/space; Organisms cultured from aseptically obtained specimen of fluid or tissue in the organ/space; Abscess involving the organ/space

in the development of prosthetic material infections (i.e., prosthetic joint infection). Coagulase-negative staphylococci produce glycocalyx and an associated component called *slime* that physically shield bacteria from phagocytes or inhibit antimicrobial agents from binding with or penetrating into the bacteria.

Devitalized tissue, dead space, and hematomas are wound-related features associated with the development of SSIs. Historically, wounds have been described as *clean, contaminated,* and *dirty* according to the expected number of bacteria entering the surgical site. The presence of a foreign body (i.e., sutures or mesh) reduces the number of organisms required to induce an SSI. Interestingly, the implantation of major devices such as prosthetic joints and cardiac devices is not associated with a higher risk of SSIs. Risk factors for SSI are summarized in Table 22-1.

SIGNS AND SYMPTOMS

SSIs typically present within 30 days of surgery with localized inflammation of the surgical site and evidence of poor wound healing. Systemic features of infection, such as fever and malaise, may occur soon thereafter.

DIAGNOSIS

There may be nonspecific evidence of infection, such as an elevated white blood cell count, poor blood glucose control, and elevated levels of inflammatory markers, such as C-reactive protein. However, surgery is a great confounder, because surgery itself causes inflammation and thus renders surrogate markers of infection less reliable. Purulence at the wound sight is highly suggestive of infection. The gold standard in documenting a wound infection is growth of organisms in an aseptically obtained culture specimen. Approximately one third of organisms cultured are staphylococci (*Staphylococcus aureus* and *Staphylococcus epidermidis*), *Enterococcus* species makes

up more than 10%, and *Enterobacteriaceae* make up the bulk of the remaining culprits. Table 22-2 lists the criteria for diagnosing an SSI.

MANAGEMENT OF ANESTHESIA

Preoperative

Active infections should be treated aggressively before surgery, and when possible, surgery should be postponed until infection has resolved. If a localized area of infection is present at the intended surgical site, surgery should be postponed until the localized infection is treated and/or resolves spontaneously. If a patient has clinical evidence of infection, such as fever, chills, or malaise, efforts should be made to identify the source of the infectious process. Several studies have shown that smoking may increase not only the incidence of respiratory tract infection but also the incidence of wound infections. Preoperative cessation of smoking for 4 to 8 weeks before orthopedic surgery decreases the incidence of wound-related complications. Significant preoperative alcohol consumption may result in generalized immunocompromise. One month of preoperative alcohol abstinence reduces postoperative morbidity in alcohol users.

Diabetes mellitus is an independent risk factor for infection, and optimization of preoperative diabetes treatment may decrease perioperative infection. Malnutrition, whether manifesting as cachexia or obesity, is associated with an increased perioperative infection rate. Appropriate diet and/or weight loss may be beneficial before major surgery.

S. aureus is the organism most commonly implicated in SSIs, and many individuals are carriers of *S. aureus* in the anterior nares. This carrier state has been identified as a risk factor for *S. aureus* wound infections. Topical mupirocin applied to the anterior nares has been successful in eliminating *S. aureus* and decreasing the risk of infection. However, there is concern that this practice may promote development of mupirocin-resistant *S. aureus*. Active surveillance programs to eliminate nasal colonization in hospital surgical personnel have controlled outbreaks of *S. aureus* SSIs.

Hair clipping at the planned surgical site is acceptable, but shaving increases the risks of SSI, probably because microcuts serve as entry portals for microorganisms. Preoperative skin cleansing with chlorhexidine has been shown to reduce the incidence of SSIs.

Intraoperative

Prophylactic Antibiotics. It was recognized many years ago that prophylactic administration of antimicrobial agents prevents postoperative wound infections. This is particularly true when the inoculum of bacteria is high, such as in colon, rectal, or vaginal surgery, or when the procedure involves insertion of an artificial implant, for example, a hip prosthesis or heart valve. The organisms that are implicated in SSIs are usually those that are carried by the patient in the nose or on the skin. Unless the patient has been in the hospital for some time before surgery, these are usually community organisms that have not developed multiple drug resistance. Timing of antibiotic prophylaxis (within 1 hour of surgical incision) is important, since these organisms are introduced into the bloodstream at the time of incision. For most procedures, a single dose of antibiotic is adequate. Prolonged surgery (>4 hours) may necessitate a second dose. Prophylaxis should be discontinued within 24 hours of the procedure. For cardiac surgery, the Joint Commission (formerly the Joint Commission on Accreditation of Healthcare Organizations) has recommended that the duration of prophylaxis be increased to 48 hours. A first-generation cephalosporin such as cefazolin is effective for many types of surgery. In general, the spectrum of bacteria against which cephalosporins are effective, their low incidence of side effects, and the tolerability of these drugs have made them the ideal choice for prophylaxis. For high-risk patients and procedures, the selection of another appropriate antibiotic plays a critical role in decreasing the incidence of SSIs.

When the small bowel is entered, coverage for gram-negative organisms is important, and for procedures involving the large bowel and the female genital tract, the addition of coverage against anaerobic organisms is appropriate. Infections associated with *clean* surgery are caused by staphylococcal species, whereas infections associated with *contaminated* surgery are polymicrobial and involve the flora of the viscus entered. Guidelines for antimicrobial prophylaxis for those considered at risk of infective endocarditis are published by the American Heart Association. Additional considerations are listed in Table 22-3.

Physical and Physiologic Preventive Measures. Several simple physical measures have been studied to determine their effects on the incidence of postoperative infection. Much

TABLE 22-3 ■ Surgical infection prevention guidelines

1. Give prophylactic antibiotics within 1 hr of surgical incision.
2. Stop prophylactic antibiotics at 24 hr (or 48 hr for cardiac surgery).
3. Increase dose of antibiotics for larger patients.
4. Repeat dose when surgery exceeds 4 hr.
5. Administer antibiotic(s) appropriate for local resistance patterns.
6. Follow American Heart Association guidelines for patients at risk of infective endocarditis.
7. Adhere to procedure-specific antibiotic recommendations.

of the work has focused on the oxygen tension at the wound site. Destruction of organisms by oxidation, or oxidative killing, is the most important defense against surgical pathogens and depends on the partial pressure of oxygen in contaminated tissue. In patients with normal peripheral perfusion, the subcutaneous oxygen tension is linearly related to the arterial oxygen tension. An inverse correlation has been demonstrated between subcutaneous tissue oxygen tension and the rate of wound infections Tissue hypoxia appears to increase the vulnerability to infection.

Hypothermia has been shown to increase the incidence of SSI. In a study in which patients were randomly assigned to hypothermia and normothermia groups, SSI was found in 19% of patients in the hypothermia group, but in only 6% of those in the normothermia group. Radiant heating to 38° C increases subcutaneous oxygen tension. This may be one of the mechanisms for the decreased infection risk associated with increased body temperature.

Oxygen. An easy method of improving oxygen tension is to increase the concentration of inspired oxygen. Studies of patients undergoing colorectal resection have demonstrated that perioperative administration of 80% oxygen decreases the incidence of SSI in this patient group. It is unknown whether perioperative administration of 80% oxygen decreases the incidence of SSI in other surgical settings. The universal adoption of this treatment protocol remains controversial, since a prolonged period of high inspired oxygen tension might cause pulmonary damage.

Analgesia. Superior treatment of surgical pain is associated with increased postoperative subcutaneous oxygen partial pressures at wound sites. Adequate analgesia may therefore be associated with a decreased incidence of SSI.

Carbon Dioxide. Hypocapnia occurs frequently during anesthesia and can be deleterious for many reasons, particularly because of the vasoconstriction it causes. Such vasoconstriction could impair perfusion of vital organs. *Hypercapnia* causes vasodilation and increases skin perfusion. Intriguing research has shown that mild intraoperative hypercapnia increases the oxygen tension in subcutaneous tissue and in the colon.

Glucose. The results of studies to date suggest that in the perioperative period, the ideal blood glucose goal should be a narrow physiologic range with minimal variability. A high blood glucose concentration is thought to inhibit leukocyte function and to provide a favorable environment for bacterial growth. Interestingly, the therapy for hyperglycemia may itself have beneficial effects. The administration of glucose, insulin, and potassium stimulates lymphocytes to proliferate and attack pathogens. Glucose, insulin, and potassium may play an important role in restoring immunocompetence to patients with immunocompromise.

Wound-Probing Protocols. Current studies suggest that infection of contaminated wounds can be decreased by following wound-probing protocols. Wound probing is a bedside technique that combines the benefits of primary and secondary wound closure. Use of this technique has been shown to decrease length of stay and SSIs, but the exact mechanism of its effect is not clearly understood.

BLOOD-BORNE INFECTIONS

Bloodstream Infections

Bloodstream infections (BSIs) are among the top three nosocomial infections. Anesthesiologists may play an important role in the prevention and often the treatment of BSIs. Central venous catheters are the major cause of nosocomial bacteremia and fungemia. Catheter-related bloodstream infections are common, costly, and potentially lethal. These infections are monitored by the National Nosocomial Infections Surveillance (NNIS) System of the CDC. A total of 80,000 cases of central venous catheter–associated BSI are estimated to occur annually in the United States, and the attributable mortality risk is estimated to be 12% to 25% for each infection. The NNIS System recommends that the rate of catheter-associated BSIs be expressed as the number of catheter-associated BSIs per 1000 days of central venous catheter exposure.

SIGNS AND SYMPTOMS

Patients typically have nonspecific signs of infection with no obvious source. There is no cloudy urine, purulent sputum, pus drainage, or wound inflammation. There is only an indwelling catheter. Inflammation at the catheter insertion site is suggestive. A sudden change in a patient's condition, such as mental status changes, hemodynamic instability, altered tolerance for nutrition, and generalized malaise, can indicate a BSI.

DIAGNOSIS

Catheter-associated BSIs are defined as bacteremia or fungemia in a patient with an intravascular catheter with at least one blood culture positive for a recognized pathogen not related to another separate infection, clinical manifestations of infection, and no other apparent source for the BSI except the catheter. BSIs are considered to be associated with a central line if the line was in use during the 48-hour period before the

TABLE 22-4   Most common pathogens associated with bloodstream infections (1992-1999)
Pathogen (% of total)
Coagulase-negative staphylococci (37%)
Staphylococcus aureus (13%)
Enterococci (13%)
Gram-negative bacilli (14%)
Escherichia coli (2%)
Enterobacter species (5%)
Pseudomonas aeruginosa (4%)
Klebsiella pneumoniae (3%)
Candida species (8%)

From National Nosocomial Infections Surveillance (NNIS) System report, data summary from January 1990–May 1999, issued June 1999. *Am J Infect Control.* 1999;27(6):520-532.

development of the BSI. If the time interval between the onset of infection and device use is longer than 48 hours, then other sources of infection must be considered. The diagnosis is more compelling if, after catheter removal, the same organisms that grew in the blood culture grow from the catheter tip. Table 22-4 lists pathogens commonly associated with BSI.

TREATMENT

The best "treatment" of central venous catheter–related BSIs is prevention. However, if infection is suspected, the source of the infection should be removed as soon as possible and broad-spectrum antimicrobial therapy should be initiated. Once culture results are available, antibiotic therapy can be targeted to the specific organism. Because of antibiotic resistance patterns, it is difficult to strike a compromise between providing appropriate initial empirical coverage and not exhausting the last-line antimicrobial agents with the first salvo of antibiotic therapy. Treatment of patients with BSIs is similar to treatment of patients with sepsis.

MANAGEMENT OF ANESTHESIA

Preoperative

Many central venous catheters are placed by anesthesiologists who may not be informed about BSIs that develop days later. Preventing BSIs related to central venous catheter use can be minimized by implementing a series of evidence-based steps shown to reduce catheter-related infection. A recent interventional study targeted *five* evidence-based procedures recommended by the CDC and identified as having the greatest effect in reducing the rate of catheter-related BSIs and the fewest barriers to implementation. The five interventions are (1) hand washing with soap and water or an alcohol cleanser before catheter insertion or maintenance, (2) using full-barrier precautions (hat, mask and sterile gown, sterile area covering) during central venous catheter insertion, (3) cleaning the skin with chlorhexidine, (4) avoiding the femoral site and peripheral arms if possible, and (5) conducting routine daily inspection of catheters and removing them as soon as they are deemed unnecessary. In this study, use of these evidence-based interventions resulted in a large and sustained reduction (up to 66%) in rates of catheter-related BSIs that was maintained throughout the 18-month study period. The subclavian and internal jugular venous routes carry less risk of infection than the femoral route, but the decision regarding anatomic location also has to consider the higher risk of pneumothorax with a subclavian catheter. During insertion, catheter contamination rates can be further reduced by rinsing gloved hands in a solution of chlorhexidine in alcohol before handling the catheter. Sterility must be maintained with frequent hand decontamination and cleaning of catheter ports with alcohol before accessing them. The same high standards of sterility should be applied with regional anesthetic catheters. Central venous catheters may be coated or impregnated with antimicrobial or antiseptic agents. These catheters have been associated with a lower incidence of BSIs. Concerns about widespread adoption of drug-impregnated catheters center on increased costs and promotion of antimicrobial resistance. However, use of such catheters may be indicated for the most vulnerable patients, such as those with severe immunocompromise.

Intraoperative

Transfusion of red blood cells and blood components increases the incidence of postoperative infection via two mechanisms: direct transmission of organisms and immunosuppression. Even autologous blood transfusion results in natural killer cell inhibition and is intrinsically immunosuppressive. The mechanisms of immunosuppression may be related to the infusion of donor leukocytes or their byproducts. Blood transfusion–associated immunosuppression may be decreased by leukodepletion.

Transfusion of cellular blood components has been implicated in transmission of viral, bacterial, and protozoal diseases. Over the past 20 years, reductions in the risk of viral infection from blood components have been achieved. Minipool nucleic acid amplification testing detects human immunodeficiency virus, and hepatitis B and C virus during the time before antibodies develop. This sensitive and specific test has decreased the risk of human immunodeficiency virus 1 (HIV-1) and hepatitis C virus transmission to 1 in 2 million blood transfusions.

Because of the success in detecting viral infection, bacterial contamination of blood products has emerged as the greatest residual source of transfusion-transmitted disease. Each year, approximately 9 million units of platelet concentrates are transfused in the United States. An estimated 1 in 1000 to 3000 platelet units is contaminated with bacteria. Platelets, to maintain viability and function, must be stored at room temperature, which creates an excellent growth environment for bacteria. The prevalence of severe episodes of transfusion-associated bacterial sepsis is approximately 1 in 50,000 for platelet units and 1 in 500,000 for red blood cell units. Implementation of bacterial detection methods will improve the safety and extend the shelf life of platelets. The best way to avoid infectious complications related to transfusion is simply to avoid or minimize the use of transfusions.

Postoperative

Several postoperative management strategies can decrease the incidence of catheter-related BSI: (1) removal of central lines and pulmonary artery catheters as soon as possible, and (2) avoidance of unnecessary parenteral nutrition and even administration of dextrose-containing fluid, since these may be associated with an increased risk of BSI. Food and glucose can usually be withheld for a short period or delivered into the gut rather than into a vein.

Sepsis

Sepsis is an umbrella term encompassing those conditions in which there are pathogenic microorganisms in the body. Sepsis may be life threatening because of complications precipitated by an organism, its toxins, and the body's own defensive inflammatory response. (A similar response may occur in the absence of infection, and this is sometimes called *systemic inflammatory response syndrome*.) Sepsis is a spectrum of disorders on a continuum with localized inflammation at one end and a severe generalized inflammatory response with multiorgan failure at the other (Figure 22-2). *Severe sepsis* is defined as acute organ

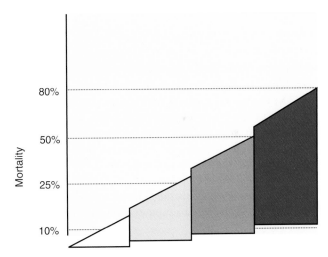

	Infection	Sepsis	Severe sepsis	Septic shock
Definition	Pathogens detected in blood or tissue	Infection plus systemic inflammatory response syndrome (SIRS)	Sepsis plus organ dysfunction: Lactic acidosis Oliguria Confusion Hepatic dysfunction	Severe sepsis plus hypotension (systolic BP < 90 mm Hg despite adequate fluid resuscitation)
Estimated mortality	0%-10%	10%-25%	25%-50%	50%-80%

FIGURE 22-2 Continuum of sepsis with definitions and approximate mortality rates. *BP,* Blood pressure. (*Adapted from Bone RC. Toward an epidemiology and natural history of systemic inflammatory response syndrome.* JAMA. 1992;268:3452-3455.)

dysfunction secondary to infection, and *septic shock* is severe sepsis with hypotension not reversed by fluid resuscitation.

Surgery and anesthesia should ideally be postponed until sepsis is at least partially treated. However, sometimes the underlying cause of sepsis requires urgent surgical intervention. Such surgery may be termed *source control* surgery. Examples of septic sources are abscesses, infective endocarditis, bowel perforation or infarction, infected prosthetic device (e.g., intravenous catheter, intrauterine device, or pacemaker), endometritis, and necrotizing fasciitis.

Bacterial components such as endotoxin, through their action on neutrophils and macrophages, can induce a wide range of proinflammatory factors and counterregulatory host responses that turn off production of proinflammatory cytokines. As a result of sepsis, the proinflammatory reaction (systemic inflammatory response syndrome) can become exaggerated by associated activation of the complement system and coagulation cascade, widespread arterial vasodilation, and altered capillary permeability. This may result in multiorgan dysfunction and death.

SIGNS AND SYMPTOMS

Signs and symptoms of sepsis are often nonspecific, and presentation varies according to the initial source of infection. The systemic inflammatory response syndrome is an important component of sepsis (Table 22-5).

Sepsis may result in multiple organ system failure. Features of infection, including fever, altered mental status, encephalopathy, and hyperglycemia, may be present. *Septic shock* refers to hemodynamic instability that may accompany sepsis along with perfusion abnormalities that may include but are not limited to lactic acidosis, oliguria, or a change in mental status. Classically, hypotension, bounding pulses, and a wide pulse pressure are present. These are characteristic signs of high-output cardiac failure and distributive shock, both of which may occur with sepsis. Patients who are receiving inotropic agents or vasopressor support may not be hypotensive.

DIAGNOSIS

A diagnosis of sepsis is surmised from history, signs, and symptoms. Confirmation is based on the isolation of a specific causative pathogen. It is important to identify the culprit microbe to ensure that antimicrobial therapy is appropriate and targeted. Specimens for culture should be sent from all sources where organism growth is suspected. Blood, urine, and sputum specimens are a minimum. Tissue sampling from specific sources such as heart valves, bone marrow, and cerebrospinal fluid can also be important.

TREATMENT

The initial treatment of sepsis is provision of broad antimicrobial coverage coupled with supportive care of failing organs. The speed and appropriateness of therapy administered in the initial hours of sepsis can dramatically influence outcome. The replication of virulent bacteria can be so rapid that every minute may be crucial. As soon as specific microbiologic information is available, therapy should be tailored to the specific organism and its sensitivities. Choice of an antibiotic must also take into account the ability of the drug to penetrate various tissues, including bone, cerebrospinal fluid, lung tissue, and abscess cavities.

In addition to targeted antimicrobial therapy, supportive treatment relating to organ system dysfunction is essential. Early goal-directed optimization that targets oxygen delivery and cardiac output might improve outcome in sepsis.

PROGNOSIS

Prognosis in sepsis depends on the virulence of the infecting pathogen(s), the stage at which appropriate treatment is initiated, the inflammatory response of the patient, the immune status of the patient, and the extent of organ system dysfunction. It is impossible to predict the outcome for any individual patient.

MANAGEMENT OF ANESTHESIA

Preoperative

The most important considerations for a patient with sepsis requiring surgery are whether the surgery may be postponed pending treatment of sepsis and whether the patient's condition may be improved before surgery. A treatment algorithm for septic patients (Figure 22-3) suggests goal-directed optimization of the condition of patients with sepsis. Resuscitation should be targeted to achieve mean arterial pressure greater than 65 mm Hg, central venous pressure of 8 to 12 mm Hg, adequate urine output, a "normal" pH without a metabolic (lactic) acidosis, and a mixed venous oxygen saturation above 70%.

Intraoperative

Intraoperative management of patients with sepsis is challenging. Patients with sepsis may have limited physiologic reserve, which renders them vulnerable to hypotension and hypoxemia with induction of anesthesia. Invasive monitoring, such as intraarterial blood pressure and central venous pressure monitoring, is usually indicated. Establishment of sufficient intravenous access to allow for volume resuscitation as well as transfusion of blood and blood components is essential. Antimicrobial prophylaxis appropriate for surgery is indicated. Ideally, this would be combined with the treatment regimen for the pathogen thought to be responsible for the sepsis. Prophylactic antibiotics should ideally be administered within 30 minutes of skin incision.

TABLE 22-5	**Systemic inflammatory response syndrome**

Diagnosis of systemic inflammatory response syndrome requires fulfillment of two or more of the following criteria in a variety of clinical scenarios, not necessarily involving infection:

White blood cell count > 12,000/mm^3 or < 4000/mm^3 or more than 10% band forms

Heart rate > 90 beats/min

Temperature > 38° C or < 36° C

Respiratory rate > 20 breaths/min or $Paco_2$ < 32 mm Hg

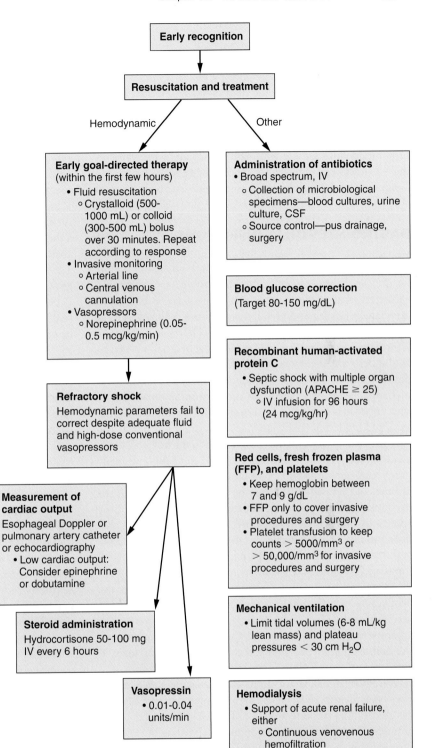

FIGURE 22-3 Management of sepsis. *APACHE,* Acute Physiology and Chronic Health Evaluation II (score); *CSF,* cerebrospinal fluid; *DVT,* deep vein thrombosis; *IV,* intravenous(ly).

Postoperative

Patients with sepsis invariably merit ICU admission after surgery. In the ICU, the priorities are to support failing organ systems, to target antimicrobial therapy, and to try to minimize the likelihood of new infection, such as fungal infection, infection with *Clostridium difficile,* or the emergence of a resistant organism. Another important postoperative priority is to continue antimicrobial therapy only for as long as it is indicated. Broad guidelines for the treatment of patients with sepsis in the ICU have been published in the Surviving Sepsis Campaign Guidelines for Management of Severe Sepsis and Septic Shock.

GASTROINTESTINAL INFECTIONS

Clostridium difficile Infection

C. difficile is an anaerobic, gram-positive, spore-forming bacterium that is the major identifiable cause of antibiotic-associated diarrhea and pseudomembranous colitis. It is clear today that most antibiotics can alter bowel flora facilitating the growth of *C. difficile.* With the frequent use of broad-spectrum antibiotics, the incidence of *C. difficile* diarrhea has risen dramatically.

C. difficile infection is also the most common cause of diarrhea in health care settings, resulting in increased hospital stays and higher morbidity and mortality among patients. The prevalence of asymptomatic colonization in the hospital, especially in older people, is more than 20%. *C. difficile* is extremely hardy, can survive in the environment for prolonged periods of time, and is resistant to common disinfectants, which leads to transmission from contaminated surfaces and airborne spores. In approximately one third of those colonized, *C. difficile* produces toxins that cause diarrhea. The two principal toxins are toxin A and toxin B. Toxin B is approximately 1000 times more cytotoxic than toxin A. Toxin A activates macrophages and mast cells. Activation of these cells causes the production of inflammatory mediators, which leads to fluid secretion and increased mucosal permeability. Toxin A is also an enterotoxin in that it loosens the tight junctions between the epithelial cells that line the colon, which helps toxin B enter into epithelial cells.

A number of risk factors for *C. difficile*–associated diarrhea have been identified: advanced age, severe underlying disease, gastrointestinal surgery, presence of a nasogastric tube, use of antiulcer medications, admission to an ICU, long duration of hospital stay, long duration of antibiotic administration (risk doubles after 3 days), use of multiple antibiotics, immunosuppressive therapy or general immunocompromise, recent surgery, and sharing of a hospital room with a *C. difficile*–infected patient.

SIGNS AND SYMPTOMS

The most frequent symptoms of *C. difficile* infection are diarrhea and abdominal pain. Patients may be febrile with abdominal tenderness and distention. With perforation, patients may have an acute abdomen.

DIAGNOSIS

The gold standard for diagnosis of *C. difficile* infection is detection of *C. difficile* via enzyme-linked immunoassay for *C. difficile* toxins A and B in stool.

TREATMENT

Therapy for patients with *C. difficile*–associated diarrhea consists of fluid and electrolyte replacement, withdrawal of current antibiotic therapy if possible, and institution of targeted antibiotic treatment to eradicate *C. difficile.* Antibiotic treatment should be given orally, if possible. The first-line regimen is oral metronidazole 400 mg three times daily. An alternative is oral vancomycin 125 mg four times daily. Vancomycin has a theoretical advantage over metronidazole, since it is not well absorbed and may therefore reach the site of infection better. The major downside to vancomycin is that it may promote the growth of vancomycin-resistant enterococci.

Additional therapies may include probiotics such as *Saccharomyces boulardii* and *Lactobacillus rhamnosus.* These may be useful in restoring normal bowel flora.

PROGNOSIS

C. difficile infection accounts for considerable increases in length of hospital stays and more than $1.1 billion in health care costs each year in the United States. The condition is a common cause of significant morbidity and even death in elderly, debilitated, and immunocompromised patients.

MANAGEMENT OF ANESTHESIA

Preoperative

It is generally the sickest patients with *C. difficile* colitis, including those whose infection does not improve with conventional therapy, who come for surgery such as subtotal colectomy and ileostomy. If the patient is in hemodynamically unstable condition, major surgery should be deferred and an ileostomy, cecostomy, or colostomy performed as a temporizing intervention. Surgery is associated with high mortality. Resuscitation and preoperative treatment of metabolic derangements may be beneficial. Patients with *C. difficile* infection should be scheduled for surgery at the end of the surgical day so that the operating room can undergo additional cleaning to minimize the risk of transmission to subsequent patients.

Intraoperative

Patients with fulminant *C. difficile* colitis are very ill, and hemodynamic instability is likely during anesthesia. Invasive monitoring, including an intraarterial catheter and central venous catheter, may guide fluid administration and the use of inotropes and vasopressors. Dehydration, acid base abnormalities, and electrolyte imbalances occur because of diarrhea. Opiates decrease intestinal motility, which may exacerbate toxin-mediated disease.

Postoperative

One of the most important considerations is to prevent the spread of *C. difficile.* The spores are hardy and are not destroyed by alcohol. Strict contact and isolation precautions are essential, routine use of disposable gloves and gowns is important, and vigorous hand washing with soap and water may remove spores. Stethoscopes and neckties are potential repositories for spores.

CUTANEOUS INFECTIONS

Necrotizing Soft Tissue Infection

Necrotizing soft tissue infection is a nonspecific term that may encompass such diagnoses as gas gangrene, Fournier's gangrene, severe cellulitis, and "flesh-eating" infections. One of the most important aspects of these infections is that the severity may be underappreciated at the time of presentation. The responsible organisms are highly virulent, the clinical course is fulminant, and mortality is high (up to 75%). Fournier's gangrene was eponymously named for the French physician Jean Alfred Fournier, who described scrotal gangrene in five young men. He noted a sudden onset, rapid progression to gangrene, and absence of a definite cause. Necrotizing soft tissue infections are surgical emergencies and represent a subclass of severe sepsis.

SIGNS AND SYMPTOMS

At presentation patients may have general features of infection, including malaise, fever, sweating, and altered mental status. Pain is invariable and may be out of proportion to the physical signs. Specific features may include scrotal swelling and erythema, vaginal discharge, tissue inflammation, pus, or subcutaneous air (crepitus). The cutaneous signs are often surprisingly mild and do not reflect the extent of tissue necrosis, because necrotizing skin infections begin in *deep* tissue planes. Hypotension is an ominous sign and may presage progression to septic shock. The resolution of pain may also be ominous, since this may occur with the progression to gangrene.

DIAGNOSIS

History is important in suggesting a diagnosis. Older patients and patients with a history of alcohol use, malnutrition, obesity, trauma, cancer, burns, vascular disease, and diabetes are more susceptible, as are patients taking immunosuppressant therapy or those infected with HIV. There may be a high white blood cell count, thrombocytopenia, coagulopathy, electrolyte abnormalities, acidosis, hyperglycemia, elevated levels of markers of inflammation such as C-reactive protein, and radiographic evidence of extensive necrotic inflammation/necrosis with subcutaneous air. Ultrasonography, computed tomography, or magnetic resonance imaging may be used to delineate the extent of tissue necrosis. Blood, urine, and tissue samples should be sent to the laboratory for culture. Organisms most frequently grown from necrotic tissue include *Streptococcus pyogenes, S. aureus, S. epidermidis, Bacteroides* species, *Clostridium perfringens,* and gram-negative organisms, especially *Escherichia coli.* Polymicrobial infection is common.

TREATMENT

The definitive treatment is extensive débridement of necrotic tissue coupled with antimicrobial therapy, which typically includes coverage of gram-positive, gram-negative, and anaerobic organisms. Empirical broad-spectrum antibiotic coverage is provided initially, and treatment can subsequently be targeted to the specific organism(s) based on culture results.

PROGNOSIS

Necrotizing soft tissue infection is associated with a high mortality. If patients survive the initial insult, they may remain vulnerable to secondary infection. They may also require repeated anesthesia for débridements, skin grafts, and reconstructive surgery.

MANAGEMENT OF ANESTHESIA

Preoperative

The anesthesiologist should treat patients with necrotizing soft tissue infection as having severe sepsis and should resuscitate preoperatively with goal-directed therapy, including administration of intravenous fluids and optimization of global oxygen delivery, with success reflected by resolution of lactic acidosis or an increase in mixed venous oxygen saturation. However, surgical débridement should not be postponed, because delay is associated with increased mortality.

Intraoperative

Concern has been raised about the use of etomidate for induction of anesthesia in patients with septic shock, since they may already have adrenal insufficiency, which theoretically may be worsened by even a single dose of etomidate. Major fluid shifts, blood loss, and release of cytokines occur intraoperatively. Good intravenous access is essential, and invasive intraarterial and central venous monitoring may provide valuable information. Blood should be cross-matched and readily available. Patients are at risk of developing both hypovolemic and septic shock.

Postoperative

Like patients with sepsis, patients with necrotizing soft tissue infection are at risk of developing multiple organ failure. Postoperative admission to an ICU is prudent. Antibiotic therapy and fluid resuscitation should be continued in the postoperative period.

Tetanus

Tetanus is caused by the gram-negative bacillus *Clostridium tetani* and occurs when a wound or entry site becomes contaminated with bacterial spores. Production of the neurotoxin *tetanospasmin* is responsible for the clinical manifestations of tetanus. With the exception of botulinum toxin, tetanospasmin is the most powerful microbe-produced poison known. Tetanospasmin, when absorbed into wounds, spreads centrally along motor nerves to the spinal cord or enters the systemic circulation to reach the central nervous system. The toxin migrates into synapses, where it binds to presynaptic nerve terminals and inhibits or stops the release of certain inhibitory neurotransmitters such as glycine and γ-aminobutyric acid. Because the motor nerve has no inhibitory signals from other nerves, the chemical signal to the motor nerve of the muscle intensifies, which causes the muscle to tighten up in a continuous contraction or spasm.

Tetanospasmin affects the nervous system in several areas: in the spinal cord, tetanospasmin suppresses inhibitory internuncial neurons, which results in generalized skeletal muscle contractions (spasms), and in the brain, there is fixation of toxin by gangliosides. The fourth cerebral ventricle is believed to have selective permeability for tetanospasmin, which results in early manifestations of trismus and neck rigidity. Sympathetic nervous system hyperactivity may manifest as the disease progresses.

SIGNS AND SYMPTOMS

Trismus is the presenting symptom of tetanus in most patients. The greater strength of the masseter muscles, compared with the opposing digastric and mylohyoid muscles, results in lockjaw, and these patients may initially seek dental attention. Rigidity of the facial muscles results in the characteristic appearance described as *risus sardonicus.* Spasm of laryngeal muscles can occur at any time. Intractable pharyngeal spasms following tracheal extubation have been described in patients with unrecognized tetanus. Dysphagia may be due to spasm of the pharyngeal muscles. Spasm of the intercostal muscles and the diaphragm interferes with adequate ventilation. The rigidity of abdominal and lumbar muscles accounts for the opisthotonic posture. Skeletal muscle spasms are tonic and clonic in nature and are excruciatingly painful. The increased skeletal muscle work is associated with dramatic increases in oxygen consumption, and peripheral vasoconstriction can contribute to hyperthermia.

External stimulation, including sudden exposure to bright light, unexpected noise, or tracheal suction, can precipitate generalized skeletal muscle spasms, leading to inadequate ventilation and death. Hypotension has been attributed to myocarditis. Isolated and unexplained tachycardia may be an early manifestation of hyperactivity of the sympathetic nervous system, but more often this hyperactivity manifests as systemic hypertension. Sympathetic nervous system responses to external stimuli are exaggerated, as demonstrated by tachydysrhythmias and labile blood pressure. In addition, excessive sympathetic nervous system activity is associated with intense peripheral vasoconstriction and diaphoresis.

TREATMENT

Treatment of patients with tetanus is directed toward controlling the skeletal muscle spasms, preventing sympathetic hyperactivity, supporting ventilation, neutralizing circulating toxin, and surgically débriding the affected area to eliminate the source of the toxin. Diazepam (40 to 100 mg/day IV) is useful for controlling skeletal muscle spasms. Occasionally, administration of nondepolarizing muscle relaxants and mechanical ventilation are necessary. Indeed, early protection of the upper airway is important, since laryngospasm may accompany generalized skeletal muscle spasms. Overactivity of the sympathetic nervous system can be managed with intravenous administration of β-blockers such as propranolol and esmolol. The circulating exotoxin may be neutralized by intrathecal or intramuscular administration of human antitetanus immunoglobulin. This neutralization does not alter the symptoms already present but does prevent additional exotoxin from reaching the central nervous system. Penicillin and metronidazole can destroy the toxin-producing vegetative forms of *C. tetani.*

MANAGEMENT OF ANESTHESIA

General anesthesia including tracheal intubation is a useful approach for surgical débridement. Surgical débridement is delayed until several hours after the patient has received antitoxin, because tetanospasmin is mobilized into the systemic circulation during surgical resection. Invasive monitoring is indicated and should include continuous recording of systemic blood pressure and measurement of central venous pressure. Volatile anesthetics are useful for maintenance of anesthesia if excessive sympathetic nervous system activity is present. Drugs such as lidocaine, esmolol, metoprolol, magnesium, nicardipine, and nitroprusside should be readily available to treat excessive sympathetic nervous system activity during the perioperative period.

RESPIRATORY INFECTIONS

Pneumonia

COMMUNITY-ACQUIRED PNEUMONIA

Combined with influenza, community-acquired pneumonia is one of the 10 leading causes of death in the United States. *Streptococcus pneumoniae* is by far the most frequent cause of bacterial pneumonia in adults. *S. pneumoniae* causes *typical* pneumonia. Influenza virus, *Mycoplasma pneumoniae,* chlamydia, legionella, adenovirus, and other microorganisms may cause *atypical* pneumonia. The pneumonia is considered atypical because these organisms are not commonly pneumonia-producing bacteria, do not respond to common antibiotics, and can cause uncommon symptoms.

ASPIRATION PNEUMONIA

Patients with depressed consciousness may experience aspiration, which, in the presence of underlying diseases that impair host defense mechanisms, may manifest as aspiration pneumonia. Alcohol- and drug-induced alterations of consciousness, head trauma, seizures, other neurologic disorders, and administration of sedatives are most often responsible for the development of aspiration pneumonia. Patients with abnormalities of deglutition or esophageal motility resulting from placement of nasogastric tubes, esophageal cancer, bowel obstruction, or repeated vomiting are also prone to aspiration. Poor oral hygiene and periodontal disease predispose to development of pneumonia after aspiration because of the presence of increased bacterial flora. Induction and recovery from anesthesia may place patients at increased risk of aspiration.

Clinical manifestations of pulmonary aspiration depend on the nature and volume of aspirated material. Aspiration of large volumes of acidic gastric fluid produces fulminant pneumonia and arterial hypoxemia. Aspiration of particulate material may result in airway obstruction, and smaller particles may produce atelectasis. Infiltrates are most common in dependent areas of the lungs. Penicillin-sensitive anaerobes are the most likely cause of aspiration pneumonia. Hospitalization or antibiotic therapy alters the usual oropharyngeal flora, so aspiration pneumonia in hospitalized patients often involves pathogens that are uncommon in community-acquired pneumonia.

POSTOPERATIVE PNEUMONIA

Postoperative pneumonia occurs in approximately 20% of patients undergoing major thoracic, esophageal, or upper abdominal surgery but is rare after other procedures in previously fit patients. Chronic lung disease increases the incidence of postoperative pneumonia threefold. Other risk factors include obesity, age older than 70 years, and operations lasting longer than 2 hours.

LUNG ABSCESS

Lung abscess may develop after bacterial pneumonia. Alcohol abuse and poor dental hygiene are important risk factors. Septic pulmonary embolization, which is most common in intravenous drug abusers, may also result in the formation of a lung abscess. The finding of an air-fluid level on the chest radiograph signifies rupture of the abscess into the bronchial tree. Foul-smelling sputum is characteristic. Antibiotics are the mainstay of treatment of a lung abscess. Surgery is indicated only when complications such as empyema occur. Thoracentesis is necessary to establish the diagnosis of empyema, and treatment requires chest tube drainage and antibiotics. Surgical drainage is necessary to treat chronic empyema.

DIAGNOSIS

An initial chill followed by abrupt onset of fever, chest pain, dyspnea, fatigue, rigors, cough, and copious sputum production often characterize bacterial pneumonia Nonproductive cough is a feature of atypical pneumonia. A detailed history may suggest possible causative organisms. Hotels and whirlpools are associated with outbreaks of Legionnaires disease. Fungal pneumonia may occur with cave exploration and diving. *Chlamydia psittaci* pneumonia may follow contact with birds, and Q fever may follow contact with sheep. Alcoholism increases the risk of aspiration. Patients who are immunocompromised, such as those with acquired immunodeficiency syndrome (AIDS), are at risk of fungal pneumonia, such as *Pneumocystis* pneumonia.

Chest radiography may be extremely helpful in diagnosing pneumonia. Diffuse infiltrates are suggestive of an atypical pneumonia, whereas a lobar opacification is suggestive of a typical pneumonia. Atypical pneumonia occurs more frequently in young adults. Radiography is useful for detecting pleural effusions and multilobar involvement. Leukocytosis is typical, and arterial hypoxemia may occur in severe cases of bacterial pneumonia. Arterial hypoxemia reflects intrapulmonary shunting of blood resulting from perfusion of alveoli filled with inflammatory exudates.

Microscopic examination of sputum plus cultures and sensitivity testing may be helpful in suggesting the cause of the pneumonia and in guiding antibiotic treatment. Unfortunately, sputum specimens are frequently inadequate, and organisms do not always grow from sputum. Interpretation of sputum culture results may be challenging. If there is suspicion of tuberculosis, sputum specimens should be sent for testing for acid-fast bacilli. Antigen detection in urine is a good test for *Legionella,* whereas blood antibody titers are helpful in diagnosing *Mycoplasma* pneumonia. Sputum polymerase chain reaction testing is useful for diagnosing *Chlamydia* infection. Blood cultures usually yield negative results, but are important to rule out bacteremia. HIV infection is an important risk factor for pneumonia and should be ruled out when pneumonia is suspected.

TREATMENT

For severe pneumonia, empirical therapy is typically a combination of antibiotic agents. However, local patterns of antibiotic resistance should always be considered before initiating therapy.

Therapy is advised for 10 days for pneumonia caused by *S. pneumoniae* and for 14 days for that caused by *M. pneumoniae* or *Chlamydia pneumoniae.* When symptoms resolve, therapy can be switched from intravenous to oral. The inappropriate prescription of antibiotics for nonbacterial respiratory tract infections is common and promotes antibiotic resistance. It has recently been demonstrated that even brief administration of a macrolide antibiotic such as azithromycin to healthy subjects promotes resistance of oral streptococcal flora that lasts for months. Resistance of *S. pneumoniae* is becoming a problem.

PROGNOSIS

The Pneumonia Severity Index (Table 22-6) is a useful tool for aiding clinical judgment, guiding appropriate management, and suggesting prognosis. Old age and co-existing organ dysfunction have a negative impact. Physical examination findings associated with worse outcome are the following:

T temperature $\leq 35°$ C or $\geq 40°$ C
R respiratory rate ≥ 30 breaths/min
A altered mental status
S systolic blood pressure < 90 mm Hg
H heart rate ≥ 125 beats/min

Laboratory findings and other test results that are indicative of a poorer prognosis are the following:

H hypoxia ($Po_2 < 60$ mm Hg or saturation $< 90\%$ on room air)
E effusion
A anemia (hematocrit $< 30\%$)
R renal: blood urea nitrogen > 64 mg/dL
G glucose > 250 mg/dL
A acidosis (pH < 7.35)
S sodium < 130 mmol/L

TABLE 22-6 ■ Elements of the Pneumonia Severity Index

Age in years
Gender
Nursing home resident
Neoplastic disease history
Liver disease
Congestive heart failure
Cerebrovascular disease
Renal disease
Altered mental status
Respiratory rate > 29 breaths/min
Systolic blood pressure < 90 mm Hg
Temperature < 35° C or > 39.9° C
Pulse > 124 beats/min
pH < 7.35
Blood urea nitrogen > 29 mg/dL
Sodium < 130 mmol/L
Glucose > 249 mg/dL
Hematocrit < 30%
Pao_2 < 60 mm Hg
Pleural effusion on radiograph

TABLE 22-7 ■ Calculation of the Clinical Pulmonary Infection Score

Parameter	Options	Score
Temperature (° C)	≥36.5 and ≤38.4	0
	≥38.5 and ≤38.9	1
	≥39 or ≤36	2
Blood leukocytes (per mm³)	≥4000 and ≤11,000	0
	<4000 or >11000	1
	+ Band forms ≥50%	Add 1
Tracheal secretions	No tracheal secretions	0
	Nonpurulent tracheal secretions	1
	Purulent tracheal secretions	2
Oxygenation: Pao_2/Fio_2 (mm Hg)	>240 or ARDS	0
	≤240 and no ARDS	2
Pulmonary radiograph	No infiltrate	0
	Diffuse (or patchy) infiltrate	1
	Localized infiltrate	2
Progression of pulmonary infiltrate	No radiographic progression	0
	Radiographic progression (after cardiac failure and ARDS excluded)	2
Culture of tracheal aspirate	Pathogenic bacteria present rarely or in light quantity	0
	Pathogenic bacteria present in moderate or heavy quantity	1
	Same pathogenic bacteria seen with Gram's stain	Add 1

Data from Luyt CE, Chastre J, Fagon JY. Value of the clinical pulmonary infection score for the identification and management of ventilator-associated pneumonia. *Intensive Care Med*. 2004;30:844-852.
ARDS, Acute respiratory distress syndrome; *Pao₂/Fio₂*, ratio of arterial oxygen pressure to fraction of inspired oxygen.

MANAGEMENT OF ANESTHESIA

Anesthesia and surgery should ideally be deferred if acute pneumonia is present. Patients with acute pneumonia are often dehydrated and may have renal insufficiency. Fluid management can be challenging, since overhydration may worsen gas exchange and morbidity. If general anesthesia is used, a protective ventilation strategy is appropriate with tidal volumes of 6 to 8 mL/kg ideal body mass and mean airway pressures of less than 30 cm H_2O. The anesthesiologist can perform pulmonary hygiene including actively removing secretions during the period of intubation, even via bronchoscopy if needed. Endotracheal intubation offers the opportunity to obtain distal sputum specimens for Gram's staining and culture.

Ventilator-Associated Pneumonia

Ventilator-associated pneumonia (VAP) is the most common nosocomial infection in the ICU and makes up one third of all nosocomial infections. VAP is defined as pneumonia developing more than 48 hours after the patient has been intubated and mechanical ventilation initiated. Between 10% and 20% of patients who have endotracheal tubes and undergo mechanical ventilation for longer than 48 hours acquire VAP, with mortality rates ranging from 5% to 50%. Several simple interventions may decrease the occurrence of VAP, including ensuring meticulous hand hygiene, providing oral care, limiting patient sedation, positioning patients semi-upright, performing repeated aspiration of subglottic secretions, limiting

intubation time if feasible, and considering the appropriateness of noninvasive ventilatory support.

DIAGNOSIS

VAP is difficult to differentiate from other common causes of respiratory failure, such as acute respiratory distress syndrome and pulmonary edema. VAP is usually suspected when a patient develops a new or progressive infiltrate on chest radiograph, leukocytosis, and purulent tracheobronchial secretions. An endotracheal tube or a tracheostomy tube provides a foreign surface that rapidly becomes colonized with upper airway flora. However, the mere presence of potentially pathogenic organisms in tracheal secretions is not diagnostic of VAP. A standardized diagnostic algorithm for VAP employing clinical and microbiologic data is used in the NNIS System and in the clinical pulmonary infection score to promote diagnostic consistency among clinicians and investigators. A Clinical Pulmonary Infection Score greater than 6 is consistent with a diagnosis of VAP (Table 22-7). In approximately half of patients suspected on clinical grounds of having VAP, the diagnosis remains in doubt and cultures of specimens from the distal airway do not grow organisms. The accurate diagnosis of VAP can be elusive.

TREATMENT AND PROGNOSIS

The treatment of VAP includes supportive care for respiratory failure plus antibiotics against the organism most likely to be implicated. The most common pathogens are *Pseudomonas aeruginosa* and *S. aureus*. Prognosis is improved if treatment is initiated early. Therefore, despite the high rate of false-positive diagnoses, broad-spectrum antibiotic therapy should be initiated to cover resistant organisms such as methicillin-resistant *S. aureus* and *P. aeruginosa*. Treatment should be narrowed to target specific organisms once results of culture and sensitivity testing are available and should be stopped at 48 hours if culture results are negative. Figure 22-4 presents an algorithm to guide treatment.

MANAGEMENT OF ANESTHESIA

Patients with VAP frequently require anesthesia for tracheostomy. Major surgery should be deferred until the pneumonia has resolved and respiratory function has improved. Tracheostomy is not an emergency procedure, and it may be ill advised to proceed when the patient has minimal pulmonary reserve. One of the major goals for the anesthesiologist in this situation is to ensure that patients with VAP do not experience a setback following anesthesia and tracheostomy. Because patients with respiratory failure may be PEEP dependent, a PEEP valve should be used to decrease the likelihood of "de-recruitment" of alveoli during transport to the operating room. In the operating room, protective mechanical ventilation should be used. Ideally, the same ventilator settings, mode of ventilation, and PEEP that were used in the ICU should be continued.

Severe Acute Respiratory Syndrome and Influenza

Influenza pandemics have been described throughout history and typically occur several times each century. The influenza pandemic of 1918 was one of the major plagues to have affected humankind. It is estimated that this "Spanish flu" infected as many as 500 million people worldwide and led to the death of as many as 50 to 100 million people around the world in just 25 weeks. The Spanish flu was caused by an H1N1 strain of influenza virus, which continues to cause human influenza pandemics. The 1957 and 1968 pandemics did not approach the catastrophic level of the 1918 pandemic.

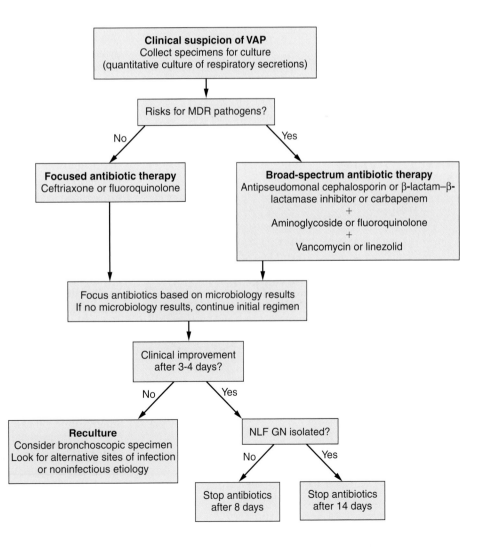

FIGURE 22-4 Management of ventilator-associated pneumonia (VAP). *GN*, Gram-negative (organism); *NLF*, non–lactose fermenting; *MDR*, multidrug-resistant. (*Adapted from Porzecanski I, Bowton DL. Diagnosis and treatment of ventilator-associated pneumonia.* Chest. *2006;130:597-604.*)

H1N1 influenza (so named based on the specific types of the capsular peptides hemagglutinin and neuraminidase that are found on the virus) continues to impact society to this day, and CDC estimates for the 2009 pandemic of influenza A (H1N1) in the United States from April 2009 to January 2010 was 57 million cases, 257,000 hospitalizations, and 11,700 deaths. In seasonal influenza, the greatest mortality is among the very young and the very old. In contrast, the 1918 and 2009 epidemics affected children and younger adults.

Influenza A virus and the virus causing severe acute respiratory syndrome (SARS) are examples of respiratory viruses that may be associated with rampant courses, high virulence, and high mortality. From 2002 to 2003, SARS occurred without any warning and was a grim reminder of our vulnerability to new infectious diseases (Figure 22-5). SARS affected populations in Asia, the Pacific Rim, and Canada. The causative agent for SARS is thought to be an RNA coronavirus that is passed along through direct contact and droplet spread. This virus is viable ex vivo for 24 to 48 hours. Twenty percent of the victims of the 2003 SARS coronavirus outbreak were health care workers. There were over 8000 documented cases of SARS coronavirus infection and approximately 700 deaths in 29 countries.

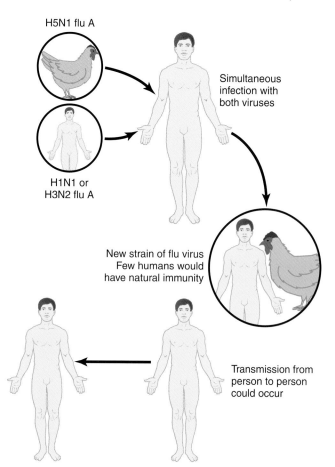

FIGURE 22-5 How a pathogenic and contagious new strain of influenza could theoretically emerge.

A new strain of avian influenza or "bird flu," the H5N1 strain, which is a subtype of influenza A, is now threatening humankind. Influenza is an RNA orthomyxovirus that, like other RNA viruses, mutates at an alarming rate. The World Health Organization (WHO) has reported that 478 human cases of avian influenza occurred between 2003 and 2010 with 286 deaths. Many cases were in young children. Currently, H5N1 influenza A is passed from bird to human. This virus has not developed a high affinity for human respiratory tract receptors. Therefore, human-to-human transmission is not sustained, and cases have occurred only in small clusters.

SIGNS AND SYMPTOMS

Symptoms include nonspecific complaints of viral infection such as cough, sore throat, headache, diarrhea, arthralgias, and muscle pain. In more severe cases, patients may show respiratory distress, confusion, and hemoptysis. Signs may include fever, tachycardia, sweating, conjunctivitis, rash, tachypnea, use of accessory respiratory muscles, cyanosis, and pulmonary features of pneumonia, pleural effusion, or pneumothorax. A chest radiograph may show patchy infiltrates, areas of opacification, pneumothoraces, and/or evidence of pleural effusion. Both H5N1 influenza A virus and SARS coronavirus infection may cause acute lung injury and acute respiratory distress syndrome. These viruses exhibit a propensity to bind to receptors in the lower respiratory tract. Therefore, they may create primary hemorrhagic bronchitis and pneumonia with diffuse alveolar damage and destruction. Complications include multiple organ failure and severe sepsis.

DIAGNOSIS

In the context of an outbreak, history, symptoms, and presentation are usually sufficient to suggest the diagnosis. A definitive diagnosis is made by detection of the virus in sputum. The problem with serologic testing is that it may take 2 to 3 weeks for seroconversion (development of antibodies) after infection. Reverse-transcriptase polymerase chain reaction test kits are available and are useful for diagnosing both SARS coronavirus infection and H5N1 influenza A.

TREATMENT

Vaccine development is a key component in the prevention of widespread viral infection and in the reduction of morbidity and mortality associated with viral infection. Thus far, there is no vaccine for the SARS coronavirus or for the H5N1 influenza A virus. For H5N1 influenza, neuraminidase inhibitors have been developed, including zanamivir and oseltamivir. These drugs may decrease the severity of infection, but insufficient quantities of these drugs may be available in the event of a major outbreak. Other pharmacologic treatments for influenza include amantadine and rimantadine. Antiviral drugs are of modest benefit and help only if administered within the first 48 hours of symptoms. There is no proven drug therapy that attenuates the course of SARS.

The mainstay of treatment for influenza and SARS is supportive care.

PROGNOSIS

Prognosis depends on the virulence of the infecting virus as well as the susceptibility of the infected person. Influenza and SARS may trigger a marked inflammatory response and a cytokine storm. A clinical picture indistinguishable from severe bacterial sepsis may result. Superinfection with bacteria has been described and considerably worsens the outcome.

MANAGEMENT OF ANESTHESIA

Preoperative

The anesthesiologist should assess the patient with an appreciation of the potential lethality of the infection. Both patient and family should be counseled about the high risks associated with SARS coronavirus infection. Since primary transmission is via direct and indirect respiratory droplet spread, these viruses are highly contagious. Strict patient isolation should be enforced, and precautions to protect health care workers must be taken. Contact precautions are also necessary because the viruses can be spread via fomites such as clothing, contaminated surfaces, and exposed skin.

Ideally, infected patients should be cared for in rooms with negative pressure to decrease aerosolized spread and contagion. Barrier precautions include the use of full-body disposable oversuits, double gloves, goggles, and powered air-purifying respirators with high-efficiency particulate air filters. If these are not available, N95 masks (which block 95% of particles) should be used rather than regular surgical masks.

Intraoperative

Aerosolized particles may be generated during all invasive airway procedures, ventilation with noninvasive and positive pressure ventilator support modes, suctioning, sputum induction, high-flow oxygen delivery, aerosolized or nebulized medication delivery, and interventions that stimulate coughing. If mechanical ventilation is required, protective ventilation as for acute respiratory distress syndrome is indicated. Tidal volumes should be limited to 6 to 8 mL/kg lean body mass, and mean airway pressure should be less than 30 cm H_2O. Sudden cardiorespiratory compromise could indicate an expanding pneumothorax. Draining of pleural effusions may improve ventilation and gas exchange.

Postoperative

Precautions to prevent spread of infection should be ongoing. The same treatment principles as for acute respiratory distress syndrome and sepsis should apply.

Tuberculosis

Mycobacterium tuberculosis is the obligate aerobe responsible for tuberculosis (TB). This organism survives and thrives in tissues with high oxygen concentrations, which is consistent with the increased presentation of TB in the apices of the lungs.

In the past, many cases of TB in the United States were due to reactivation of infection, especially in elderly individuals. However, from 1985 to 1992, the United States was confronted with an unprecedented resurgence in TB. This resurgence was accompanied by a rise in multidrug-resistant (MDR) TB, defined as TB caused by *M. tuberculosis* strains resistant to the most effective first-line drugs, that is, isoniazid and rifampin. In addition, virtually untreatable strains of the TB organism are emerging worldwide. Extensively drug-resistant (XDR) strains of *M. tuberculosis* are resistant to second-line therapeutic agents, including fluoroquinolones and at least one of three injectable second-line drugs used to treat TB (amikacin, kanamycin, or capreomycin). Mortality rates for patients with XDR TB are similar to those for TB patients in the preantibiotic era. Unfortunately, drug-resistant TB is a human-created problem resulting from poor adherence of infected patients to the medical regimen or improper treatment regimen design. Worldwide, approximately 2 billion persons are infected with *M. tuberculosis*. In 2008, WHO estimated that 440,000 new cases of MDR TB occurred worldwide with 150,000 deaths.

At present, most cases of TB in the United States occur in minority racial and ethnic groups, foreign-born individuals from areas where TB is endemic (Asia and Africa), intravenous drug abusers, and patients who are HIV seropositive or have AIDS. Any patient with TB should be tested for HIV, since there is a high association between the two infections. However, even in patients who are HIV negative, MDR TB has a 26% mortality rate. The epidemiologic rise in the incidence of TB coincided with the initial AIDS epidemic in the early 1980s.

Almost all *M. tuberculosis* infections result from inhalation of aerosolized droplets. It has been estimated that up to 600,000 droplet nuclei are expelled with each cough and that the expelled organisms remain viable for several days. Although a single infectious unit is capable of causing infection in susceptible individuals, prolonged exposure in closed environments is optimal for transmission of infection. It is estimated that 90% of patients infected with *M. tuberculosis* never become symptomatic and are identified only by conversion of the tuberculin skin test or by results on an interferon release assay. Often patients who acquire the infection early in life do not become symptomatic until much later. Patients who are HIV seropositive or immunocompromised with AIDS are at much higher risk of becoming symptomatic, especially after initiation of highly active antiretroviral therapy.

DIAGNOSIS

The diagnosis of TB is based on the presence of clinical symptoms, the epidemiologic likelihood of infection, and the results of diagnostic tests. Symptoms of pulmonary TB often include persistent nonproductive cough, anorexia, weight loss, chest pain, hemoptysis, and night sweats. The most common test for TB is the tuberculin skin test (Mantoux's test). The skin reaction is read in 48 to 72 hours, and a positive reaction is generally defined as induration of more than 10 mm. For patients with severe immunocompromise, including but not limited to AIDS, a reaction of 5 mm or more is considered positive. Because the skin test is nonspecific, the utility of the skin test is limited. The tuberculin skin test result may be positive if the individual has received a bacille Calmette-Guérin (BCG) vaccine or if the individual has been exposed to TB, or to other mycobacteria, even if no viable mycobacteria are present at the time of the skin test. The CDC and WHO have now accepted two interferon release assays as equivalent to, and possibly even better than, the tuberculin skin test in sensitivity and specificity. These are the QuantiFERON TB Gold In-Tube test and the T-SPOT.*TB* test. Both are blood tests that measure release of interferon-γ from sensitized lymphocytes that are incubated with two peptides from the TB bacillus. Results of these tests are not affected by prior BCG immunization, nor do the tests cross-react with common environmental mycobacteria or *Mycobacterium avium-intracellulare.*

Chest radiographs are important for the diagnosis of TB. Apical or subapical infiltrates are highly suggestive of TB. Bilateral upper lobe infiltration with cavitation is also common. Patients with AIDS may demonstrate a less classic picture on chest radiography, which may be further confounded by the presence of *Pneumocystis* pneumonia. Tuberculous vertebral osteomyelitis (Pott's disease) is a common manifestation of extrapulmonary TB.

Sputum smears and cultures are used to diagnose TB. Smears are examined for the presence of acid-fast bacilli. This test is based on the ability of mycobacteria to take up and retain neutral red stains after an acid wash. It is estimated that 50% to 80% of individuals with active TB have positive sputum smear results. Although the absence of acid-fast bacilli does not rule out TB, a sputum culture positive for *M. tuberculosis* provides a definitive diagnosis.

Health care workers are at increased risk of occupational acquisition of TB, and TB is twice as prevalent in physicians as in the general population. Nosocomial outbreaks of TB have occurred especially among patients with AIDS. Anesthesiologists are at increased risk of nosocomial TB by virtue of events surrounding the induction and maintenance of anesthesia that may induce coughing (tracheal intubation, tracheal suctioning, mechanical ventilation). Bronchoscopy is a particularly high-risk procedure for anesthesiologists and has been associated with conversion of the tuberculin skin test. As a first step in preventing occupational acquisition of TB, anesthesia personnel should participate in annual tuberculin screening so that those who develop a positive skin test result may be offered chemotherapy. The decision to initiate TB chemotherapy is not trivial, since treatment carries serious toxicity. A baseline chest radiograph is indicated when a positive tuberculin skin test result first occurs.

TREATMENT

Antituberculous chemotherapy has decreased mortality from TB by more than 90%. With adequate treatment, more than 90% of patients who have susceptible strains of *M. tuberculosis* have bacteriologically negative sputum smears within 3 months.

Some argue that, for the protection of the community, people who have positive results on a skin test should receive chemotherapy with isoniazid. However, isoniazid is a potentially toxic drug. The toxicity of isoniazid manifests in the peripheral nervous system, liver, and possibly the kidneys. Neurotoxicity may be prevented by daily administration of pyridoxine. Hepatotoxicity is most likely to be related to metabolism of isoniazid by hepatic acetylation. Depending on genetically determined traits, patients may be characterized as slow or rapid acetylators. Hepatitis appears to be more common in rapid acetylators, consistent with their greater production of hydrazine, a potentially hepatotoxic metabolite of isoniazid. Persistent elevations of serum transaminase concentrations mandate that isoniazid be discontinued, but mild, transient increases do not.

Other first-line drugs used to treat TB include rifampicin, pyrazinamide, streptomycin, and ethambutol. Adverse effects of rifampicin include thrombocytopenia, leukopenia, anemia, and renal failure. Hepatitis associated with increases in serum transaminase concentrations occurs in approximately 10% of patients being treated with rifampicin. To be curative, treatment for pulmonary TB should continue for 6 months. Extrapulmonary TB usually requires a longer course of antituberculous therapy.

MANAGEMENT OF ANESTHESIA

The preoperative assessment of patients considered to be at risk of having TB includes taking a detailed history, with questions concerning the presence of a persistent cough and tuberculin test status. Patients with HIV or AIDS should undergo a thorough review of systems to elicit a possible history of TB.

Elective surgical procedures should be postponed until patients are no longer considered infectious. Patients are considered noninfectious if they have received antituberculous chemotherapy, are improving clinically, and have had three consecutive negative findings on sputum smears. If surgery cannot be delayed, it is important to limit the number of involved personnel, and high-risk procedures (bronchoscopy, tracheal intubation, and suctioning) should be performed in a negative-pressure environment whenever possible. Patients should be transported to the operating room wearing a tight-fitting N95 face mask to prevent casual exposure of others to airborne bacilli. Staff should also wear N95 masks.

A high-efficiency particulate air filter should be placed in the anesthesia delivery circuit between the Y connector and the mask, laryngeal mask airway, or tracheal tube. Bacterial filters should be placed on the exhalation limb of the anesthesia delivery circuit to decrease the discharge of tubercle bacilli into the ambient air. Anesthesia equipment should be sterilized with standard methods using a disinfectant that destroys tubercle bacilli. Use of a dedicated anesthesia machine and ventilator is recommended. Postoperative care should, if possible, take place in a negative-pressure isolation room.

INFECTIOUS DISEASES IN SOLID ORGAN TRANSPLANT RECIPIENTS

Each year, over 16,000 patients in the United States receive solid organ transplants, and this number is expected to continue rising. Patients who have received solid organ transplants (liver, kidney, heart, or lung) present unique perioperative challenges to the anesthesiologist. Because of advances in surgical technique, immunosuppressive therapy, and medical management, this patient population has a 1-year survival rate of 80% to 90%, so these patients are coming for additional surgical procedures not necessarily related to their organ transplant.

To prevent allograft rejection, solid organ transplant recipients commonly receive a combination of immunosuppressive agents. The mechanisms of action of immunosuppressants include blunting of general antibody responses, depression of cell-mediated immunity, downmodulation of lymphocyte and macrophage function, inhibition of cell proliferation, blocking of T-cell activation, and depletion of T-cells. Regardless of the effect, immunosuppression is variable and depends on dosage, duration of therapy, and time since transplantation. Immunosuppression is most intense in the first few months immediately after transplantation and becomes progressively less intense as immunosuppressive therapy is gradually withdrawn over time.

Immunosuppression in transplant recipients can also be affected by metabolic abnormalities, damage to mucocutaneous barriers, foreign bodies that interrupt these barriers (such as surgical incisions, chest tubes, biliary drains, endotracheal tubes, urinary catheters), and the possible presence of immunomodulating viruses such as cytomegalovirus and HIV. Therefore, the resultant state of immunosuppression in the posttransplantation patient is a dynamic condition that impacts the development of infectious diseases and/or cancer.

Infectious Disease Occurrence

The best approach to infection control in the solid organ transplant recipient is prevention. If prevention is not possible, immediate diagnosis and treatment is essential. The challenges in managing infectious diseases in organ transplant recipients are many and include the following: (1) the spectrum of infective organisms is diverse and unusual, (2) the inflammatory response is blunted because of immunosuppressive therapy so that clinical and radiologic findings may be limited, and (3) antimicrobial coverage is complex and typically empirically based. There are three major time periods during which specific infectious disease processes occur in the posttransplantation patient: the first month, the second through sixth months, and beyond the sixth month after transplantation. In addition, these periods may be influenced by surgical factors, the net level of immunosuppression present, and environmental exposures. Defining the time period after transplantation will assist the clinician in determining likely infectious processes.

During the first month after transplantation, active infections can be harbored within the allograft and are typically bacterial or fungal. In addition, anatomic defects related to surgery must be addressed if they foster infection, such as devitalized tissue and undrained fluid collections that are at high risk for microbial seeding. The only common viral infection during the first month after transplantation is reactivated herpes simplex virus infection in individuals positive for this virus before transplantation.

The period from the second through the sixth month after transplantation may be marked by unusual infections. These may be either community-acquired or opportunistic infections. Opportunistic pathogens possess very little virulence in healthy hosts, but can cause serious infections in patients with immunocompromise or immune defects. Trimethoprim-sulfamethoxazole is commonly given as prophylaxis for *Pneumocytis* pneumonia during the first 6 months after transplantation in all solid organ graft recipients and for longer periods in heart and lung transplant recipients.

In addition, high-dose immunosuppression may lead to reactivation disease syndromes caused by organisms present in the recipient before transplantation. TB has become especially common and occurs in 1% of the posttransplant population.

From 6 months after transplantation onward, most transplant recipients do fairly well from an infectious disease standpoint and usually only sustain infections paralleling those seen in the community at large. However, another group of patients may have chronic or progressive viral infections with hepatitis B virus, hepatitis C virus, cytomegalovirus, or Epstein-Barr virus. The most commonly occurring viral infection is varicella-zoster virus infection manifesting as herpes zoster.

Patients with chronic or recurrent rejection are generally taking high dosages of immunosuppressants and are predisposed to acquiring the opportunistic infections typically seen in posttransplantation patients during the second to sixth months. In addition, posttransplantation patients with HIV and/or AIDS must be more closely followed for evidence of infections, both common and opportunistic. HIV highly active antiretroviral therapeutic regimens must be maintained and can complicate immunosuppressive drug dosing.

Management of Anesthesia

PREOPERATIVE

Patients who have received solid organ transplants comprise a wide clinical spectrum, and it is difficult to make any generalizations about this patient population. Overall, the preoperative assessment should focus on determining the degree of immunosuppression and allograft function, examining for the presence of any infection, and evaluating any co-existing medical diseases. Laboratory evaluation should include a complete blood count, full metabolic panel, liver function tests, viral panels with viral loads as indicated, chest radiograph, and electrocardiogram. If patients are currently receiving immunosuppressants, blood levels of immunosuppressive agents should also be obtained when possible. Findings elicited on history taking, review of systems, and physical examination may serve as indicators for additional laboratory testing or further specialist evaluations. Evidence of active rejection is a contraindication to elective surgery. However, one may be faced with managing anesthesia in a posttransplantation patient with active rejection who requires explantation of the transplanted organ. This is considered an urgent or emergent procedure.

All additional medications and antimicrobial agents taken by the patient should be ascertained and maintained during the perioperative period. If the posttransplantation patient manifests any active infection, surgery should be delayed or cancelled until additional consultation is obtained.

INTRAOPERATIVE

All anesthetic techniques—general anesthesia, regional anesthesia, and sedation—have been used successfully in posttransplantation patients. Selection of anesthetic technique should be based on the type of surgery to be performed, the patient's associated comorbid conditions, the presence of contraindications for specific anesthetic techniques, and the potential for interactions between immunosuppressant drugs and anesthetic drugs.

Use of regional anesthesia in immunosuppressed patients remains controversial, since studies have demonstrated that infections may occur secondary to neuraxial blockade. However, few studies have evaluated the frequency of epidural abscesses or meningitis in the immunocompromised population. Information on the incidence of infection during peripheral nerve blockade and pain procedures in immunocompromised posttransplantation patients is scant. With regard to general anesthesia, nasal intubation should be avoided, because it may introduce nasal bacterial flora into the systemic circulation. Overall, general anesthesia is considered to create more generalized immunosuppressant effects than regional anesthesia, although levels of specific and nonspecific biologic markers indicating immune suppression are not consistently depressed. Cyclosporine may delay the metabolism of neuromuscular blockers, specifically pancuronium and vecuronium. Invasive monitoring may be warranted, but strict use of aseptic technique is critical in this patient population.

POSTOPERATIVE

Because of the high potential for further immunosuppression secondary to anesthesia and surgery, the posttransplantation patient must be observed for any clinical deterioration in graft function or a potential infectious disease process. All antibiotics regimens must be strictly followed and monitored closely. Because of the blunted inflammatory response in immunosuppressed patients, signs and symptoms of active infection are often difficult to detect.

HUMAN IMMUNODEFICIENCY VIRUS INFECTION AND ACQUIRED IMMUNODEFICIENCY SYNDROME

The disease syndrome now known as *AIDS* was first described in 1981 and was initially termed *gay-related immune disorder* because it was identified in a group of homosexual men in Los Angeles, California. The etiologic mechanism was unknown at that time. However, severe immune dysfunction was present and was clinically manifested by the occurrence of unusual malignancies and opportunistic infections in previously healthy individuals. The disease was later reclassified as *acquired immunodeficiency syndrome* (AIDS). In 1984, the cause of AIDS was elucidated and was found to be a retrovirus, which was named *human immunodeficiency virus (HIV) type 1* and *type 2*.

Thirty years later, HIV infection and the associated AIDS pandemic continue to pose a major threat to global health. It is estimated that more than 50 million people worldwide (or approximately 0.6% of the world's population) are infected with HIV, and AIDS is thought to have caused more than 26 million deaths worldwide. There are approximately 1.2 million people in the United States living with HIV infection and/or AIDS. HIV infection continues to spread. The most rapid increases are being observed in southern and central Africa and in Southeast Asia. Throughout the world, the predominant mode of HIV transmission is by heterosexual sex, with women representing a large proportion of the new infections. In the United States, the primary means of transmission is via sex in men who have sex with men. However, the mechanism for disease transmission is variable and may also include spread via heterosexual sex, intravenous drug use, vertical transmission from pregnant mother to child, and blood transfusion. Although HIV antiretroviral therapy has decreased the rate of disease progression, there is no cure available and almost 600,000 people have died of AIDS in the United States since the epidemic began. Research continues into development of a vaccine to prevent the acquisition of HIV infection.

Recent treatment modalities known as *highly active antiretroviral therapy* (HAART) have been effective in halting HIV replication and thereby delaying the transition from HIV infection to AIDS or delaying the progression of AIDS itself. An increasing number of patients coming for surgery are HIV seropositive or have AIDS. Therefore, anesthesiologists should be familiar with this infectious disease and syndrome and its impact on anesthetic management. An understanding of the pathogenesis of HIV, the multiple organ system involvement of HIV and AIDS, the possible drug interactions occurring with HIV therapy, side effects related to HAART, and associated opportunistic infections will serve to better guide preoperative assessment and anesthetic planning.

Signs and Symptoms

Acute seroconversion illness occurs approximately 2 to 3 weeks after inoculation with the HIV virus. The acute viral phase is typically marked by a flulike illness associated with fever, fatigue, headache, night sweats, pharyngitis, myalgias, and arthralgias. Therefore, signs and symptoms during the period after the initial infection may mimic those of any common flulike illness. Within 1 to 2 weeks after inoculation with HIV, the virus initiates rapid replication. After several months, there is a gradual decrease in the viremia. As the immune system responds, viral replication decelerates, and a balance develops between host immune defenses and viral replication. The resulting viral level can be described as a steady-state rate of viral production equal to the rate of viral destruction and suppression. Generalized lymphadenopathy is a hallmark of HIV infection and may persist until HAART is initiated. An HIV-positive individual is *not* considered to have AIDS unless one of the AIDS-defining diagnoses is present.

As noted earlier, HIV belongs to the family of retroviruses. It is characteristically cytopathic (cell damaging) with a long latency period and a chronic course of infection. When the first cases of AIDS appeared, its pathogenesis was frustratingly elusive because the disease does not appear immediately after infection with HIV. It has been shown that the steady-state viral level is a reliable predictor of the rate of progression from simple HIV positivity to the development of AIDS. In general, higher basal viral levels correspond to more rapid disease progression. Weight loss and failure to thrive are among the first manifestations patients display as HIV infection progresses from the chronic latent phase to the development of AIDS.

Diagnosis

With the advent of HAART, the prognosis of those infected with HIV has been dramatically improved. Therefore, it is important that the stigma attached to HIV infection be removed so that high-risk individuals feel comfortable undergoing testing. The standard test to diagnose HIV infection is an enzyme-linked immunosorbent assay (ELISA), the results of which become positive when antibodies to HIV are present. This is typically 4 to 8 weeks after infection. This test is not a measure of viral load but simply indicates the presence of antibodies to HIV. During the initial period of infection, there is significant viremia and patients are highly infectious, but antibodies may *not* be present. Therefore, a false-negative test result may occur. If a positive diagnosis is made, infection is confirmed with a Western blot test or by direct measurement of HIV viral load in the blood. HIV viral load is measured via polymerase chain reaction RNA analysis. If a patient is tested within a very short period after the initial infection, the ELISA test result may be negative or inconclusive. Nucleic acid testing of HIV RNA is the most specific and sensitive test for HIV.

Since HIV is lymphotropic and has a particular affinity for CD4+ cells, measurement of these cells is useful in assessing the degree of HIV progression. CD4+ cell levels are measured as cells per cubic millimeter. Ninety-eight percent of helper T lymphocytes (CD4+ T cells) are located in lymph nodes, which are the major site of viral replication and T-cell destruction. During the acute infectious period, CD4+ cell counts decline dramatically then rise again. Over the course of 8 to 12 years, there is a gradual involution of lymph nodes with a concomitant slow decrease in CD4+ T cell counts that is accompanied by an increase in viral load as the inexorable onset of AIDS occurs (Figure 22-6).

After the diagnosis of HIV infection is confirmed, a patient will undergo further testing to determine viral genotype and phenotype. In addition, HIV sensitivity and resistance to existing HAART agents as well as coreceptor usage will be determined. These new testing modalities have been extremely effective in minimizing resistance when HAART is initiated, because selection of HAART agents is tailored to each individual patient. For the purposes of disease surveillance and disease severity estimation and management, patients who are HIV positive are classified as having AIDS *only* when at least *one* of the AIDS-defining diagnoses is present (Table 22-8).

Human Immunodeficiency Virus Infection Clinical Continuum

Patients who are HIV positive are typically asymptomatic and will not demonstrate any external evidence of clinical immunosuppression. However, HIV infection is a disease

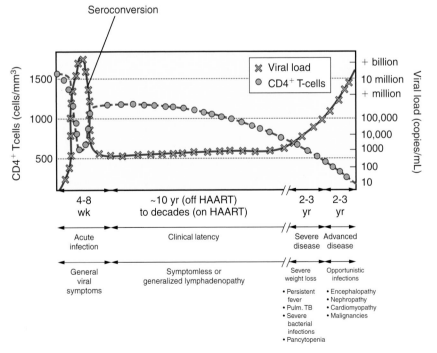
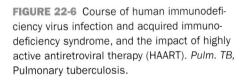

FIGURE 22-6 Course of human immunodeficiency virus infection and acquired immunodeficiency syndrome, and the impact of highly active antiretroviral therapy (HAART). *Pulm. TB,* Pulmonary tuberculosis.

that encompasses a continuum of clinical signs from acute infection to clinical latency, then to clinical progression, and eventually to development of AIDS with associated opportunistic infections and ultimately death. However, the clinical continuum from HIV infection to AIDS can be interrupted, delayed, or distorted by the institution of HAART. Opportunistic infections are caused by pathogens with no intrinsic virulence and require a compromised immune system or defect to proliferate. Because subclinical and clinical multiple organ system involvement is a hallmark of HIV infection, the anesthesiologist should be adept at eliciting a history and reviewing systems to detect any of the myriad co-existing diseases that could be present, as well as performing a thorough physical examination to detect pertinent pathologic conditions.

CARDIAC MANIFESTATIONS

Cardiac involvement in the course of HIV infection is common, but often subclinical. Up to 50% of HIV-positive patients have abnormal echocardiographic findings at some point during their disease. HIV is an extremely trophic virus with a high affinity for the myocardium, and evidence has demonstrated

---

TABLE 22-8   AIDS-defining diagnoses in HIV-seropositive patients

Bacterial infection, multiple or recurrent

Burkitt's lymphoma

Candidiasis of the bronchi, trachea, lungs, or esophagus

CD4+ T-lymphocyte cell count <200 cells/mm³

Cervical cancer, invasive

Coccidiomycosis, disseminated or extrapulmonary

Cryptococcosis, extrapulmonary

Cryptosporidiosis, chronic intestinal (>1 mo)

Cytomegalovirus retinitis or cytomegalovirus infection (with loss of vision)

Herpes simplex with chronic ulcers (>1 mo), bronchitis, pneumonitis, or esophagitis

HIV-related encephalopathy

Histoplasmosis, disseminated or extrapulmonary

Isosporiasis, chronic (>1 mo)

Kaposi's sarcoma

Immunoblastic lymphoma

Lymphoma of the brain, primary

Mycobacterium avium-intracellulare complex or *Mycobacterium kansasii* infection, disseminated or extrapulmonary

Mycobacterium tuberculosis infection, any site

Mycobacterium infection, any other species, pulmonary or extrapulmonary

Pneumocystis jiroveci (*Pneumocystis carinii*) pneumonia (PCP)

Pneumonia, recurrent

Progressive multifocal leukoencephalopathy (PML)

Recurrent *Salmonella* septicemia

Toxoplasmosis of the brain

Wasting syndrome due to HIV

AIDS, Acquired immunodeficiency syndrome; *HIV,* human immunodeficiency virus.

---

the presence of HIV in myocardial cells. Left ventricular dilatation and cardiac dysfunction may result. In addition, pulmonary hypertension is present in about 1% of patients with HIV infection or AIDS. Cardiac disease may be exacerbated by HAART, especially when protease inhibitors are utilized. Protease inhibitors may cause premature atherosclerosis and diastolic dysfunction leading to heart failure. Myocardial infarction has been reported even in young patients with HIV infection. Approximately 25% of patients with HIV infection have pericardial effusions. Myocarditis, which is more common in advanced disease, may be caused by toxoplasmosis, disseminated cryptococcosis, coxsackievirus B infection, cytomegalovirus infection, lymphoma, aspergillosis, and HIV infection itself. In addition, HIV is trophic for vascular structures and has been implicated in the development of multifocal abdominal aortic aneurysms in adults and children, as well as aortic arch, aneurysms, and aortic dissection in adults.

CENTRAL AND PERIPHERAL NERVOUS SYSTEM MANIFESTATIONS

Neurologic disease, ranging from AIDS dementia to infectious and neoplastic involvement, may be common, especially as AIDS progresses. HIV enters the central nervous system early in the course of infection, and the central nervous system is considered a reservoir for HIV. Three diagnoses comprise the majority of predominantly focal cerebral diseases complicating AIDS: cerebral toxoplasmosis, primary central nervous system lymphoma, and progressive multifocal leukoencephalopathy. *Cryptococcus neoformans,* HIV, and the TB bacillus can cause meningitis. Aggressive generalized cerebrovascular disease may occur as a complication of HAART. Increased intracranial pressure may develop with active HIV infection resulting from the presence of intracranial masses or opportunistic infections. Peripheral neuropathy is the most frequent neurologic complication in HIV-positive patients. Approximately 35% of patients with AIDS show clinical evidence of polyneuropathy or myopathy, Autonomic nervous dysfunction may also appear with or without the presence of central nervous system involvement.

PULMONARY MANIFESTATIONS

The pulmonary manifestations in HIV-positive patients are typically caused by opportunistic infections. Complications include respiratory failure, pneumothorax, and chronic pulmonary disease. Cavitary lung disease can be due to pyogenic bacterial lung abscess, pulmonary TB, fungal infections, and *Nocardia* infection. Kaposi's sarcoma and lymphoma can also affect the lungs. Adenopathy can lead to tracheobronchial obstruction or compression of the great vessels. Endobronchial Kaposi's sarcoma may cause massive hemoptysis. HIV directly affects the lungs and may cause a destructive pulmonary syndrome similar to emphysema.

Pneumocytis jiroveci pneumonia (PCP), formerly called *Pneumocytis carinii* pneumonia, does not usually occur until the CD4+ count falls below 200 cells/mm³ and fortunately has become less common with the use of HAART. With PCP, an

AIDS-defining illness, the chest radiograph can be normal but typically shows bilateral ground-glass opacities. Pneumothoraces may be evident or there may be several pneumatoceles. High-resolution computed tomographic scans reveal a ground-glass appearance, even when chest radiograph findings are normal. Pulmonary function tests show reduced lung volumes with decreased compliance and diminished diffusing capacity. Measurements of oxygen saturation during exercise may be more helpful than lung function tests. If PCP is suspected, fiberoptic bronchoscopy and bronchoalveolar lavage should be performed. The advantage of an early diagnosis compensates for the high frequency of negative examination findings.

Disseminated TB is a potential cause of severe respiratory failure, and respiratory secretions should be examined routinely for acid-fast bacilli in HIV/AIDS patients with pulmonary infiltrates. Bacterial pneumonia may also be the cause of severe acute respiratory failure. Bacteria may be detected in sputum or bronchial washings.

ENDOCRINE MANIFESTATIONS

Adrenal insufficiency should be considered since this may occur with advanced HIV infection. Random measurement of cortisol levels and tests of adrenal stimulation may reveal absolute or relative adrenal insufficiency, and this is the most serious endocrine complication in HIV-positive patients. In HIV-positive patients taking protease inhibitor therapy, glucose intolerance, disorders of lipid metabolism, and fat redistribution are common.

HEMATOLOGIC MANIFESTATIONS

The hematopoietic system is widely affected by HIV infection, and the most common early finding of HIV infection is anemia. Lymphocytosis, with an increase mainly in CD8+ T lymphocytes, may appear within 2 weeks of initial HIV infection. Bone marrow involvement can occur secondary to HIV infection itself and/or to opportunistic infection. This can produce leukopenia, lymphopenia, and thrombocytopenia. In addition, bone marrow suppression may develop after initiation of zidovudine therapy. Thrombocytopenia typically worsens as CD4+ counts diminish to less than 250 cells/mm^3. HIV-positive patients may be prone to either hypercoagulable states or coagulation abnormalities.

RENAL MANIFESTATIONS

HIV-positive patients may develop renal diseases secondary to HIV infection, viral hepatitis, associated drug use, or HAART. Protease inhibitor therapy has been specifically implicated in both toxic acute tubular necrosis and nephrolithiasis. In addition, nephrotic syndrome may occur as a result of HIV-associated nephropathy. HIV-associated nephropathy is especially common in African American men and commonly leads to end-stage renal disease.

Treatment

HAART targets the various steps in the HIV replication cycle (Figure 22-7). Six major classes of antiretroviral drugs are

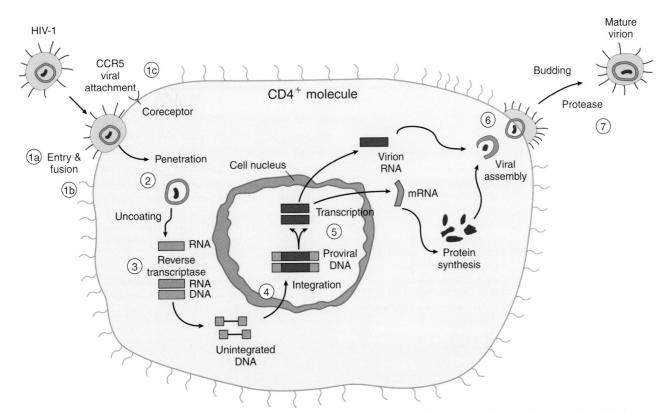

FIGURE 22-7 Life cycle of human immunodeficiency virus (HIV) and targets of action of antiretroviral therapy (indicated by circled numbers). *1a,* Fusion inhibitors; *1b,* entry inhibitors; *1c,* chemokine receptor 5 (CCR5) antagonists/blockers; *2,* no antivirals available for "uncoating"; *3,* nucleoside and non-nucleoside reverse transcriptase inhibitors; *4,* integrase strand transfer inhibitors; *5,* no antivirals available for RNA transcription; *6,* maturation inhibitors; *7,* protease inhibitors; *mRNA,* messenger RNA.

currently in use, and two groups of agents are undergoing clinical investigations.

There is continued interest in developing treatment regimens that have a higher safety profile, lower rate of side effects or complications, and easier dosing regimens. Antiretroviral drugs used to treat HIV infection are *always* employed in combinations of at least three agents. Patients who have developed resistance to commonly used HAART regimens or have advanced AIDS may require four agents and possibly additional booster medications designed to increase drug bioavailability.

The decision to initiate HAART is based on multiple factors, and once begun, treatment entails a lifelong commitment. Nonadherence to the medical regimen for any reason is one of the main causes of the development of viral resistance and treatment failure. Initiation of HAART is not necessarily a benign process, and implementation of HAART may result in a myriad of drug-related complications. Some patients who are in the early phase of HIV infection may decide, in conjunction with their physicians, *not* to immediately implement therapy and choose simply to be monitored.

Patients begin HAART immediately when there is evidence that CD4$^+$ cell counts are diminishing rapidly, counts have already fallen below 200 cells/mm^3, or a patient with newly diagnosed HIV infection already meets AIDS-defining criteria. New recommendations advocate that HAART be instituted when CD4$^+$ cell counts approach 500 cells/mm^3 or soon after the initial HIV diagnosis when the patient can realistically begin HAART. Early institution of HAART is linked to greater long-term survival and lower morbidity.

As noted earlier, a typical antiretroviral regimen consists of at least three drugs, and drug selection is based on viral sensitivity, resistance patterns, coreceptor subtypes, and virulence subtypes. In some circumstances, combinations of four or more drugs are used, such as when drug resistance patterns are evident when the patient is undergoing a rapid clinical decline. The aim of therapy in treatment-naive patients is to achieve an undetectable viral load by 24 weeks of therapy and to improve and extend the length and quality of life. Numerous side effects and drug interactions complicate such regimens and decrease adherence. Patients may develop a myriad of adverse drug reactions, and some are potentially fatal (Table 22-9).

Patients who begin HAART may also develop a reaction known as *immune reconstitution inflammatory syndrome* (IRIS). IRIS occurs as a result of restoration of basic immune competence with HAART and the gradual improvement and strengthening of the immune system. IRIS leads to a paradoxical deterioration of general clinical symptoms in the context of improving CD4$^+$ counts and a reduced viral load. IRIS is marked by the appearance and/or exacerbation of previously silent clinical diseases such as hepatitis A, B, and C; PCP; TB; and any other dormant opportunistic infection.

Concurrent use of zidovudine and corticosteroids may result in severe myopathy and respiratory muscle dysfunction. In addition, reports have documented several cases of respiratory failure related to HAART initiation. Of particular

TABLE 22-9 ■ Highly active antiretroviral therapy (HAART) drug interactions

Class	Common drug-HAART interactions	Anesthetic-specific drug-HAART interactions
Nucleoside reverse transcriptase inhibitors (NRTIs)	Interactions with: *Anticonvulsant:* phenytoin *Antifungals:* ketoconazole, dapsone Alcohol *H$_2$ blocker:* cimetidine	HAART potentially changes drug clearance and effects of: *Opiate:* methadone
Nonnucleoside reverse transcriptase inhibitors (NNRTIs)	Interactions with: *Anticoagulant:* warfarin *Anticonvulsants:* carbamazepine, phenytoin, phenobarbital *Anti-TB drug:* rifampin, *Herbal:* St. John's wort	HAART prolongs half-life and/or effects of: *Sedatives:* diazepam, midazolam, triazolam *Opiates:* fentanyl, meperidine, methadone
Protease inhibitors (PIs)	Interactions with: *Anticoagulant:* warfarin *Anticonvulsants:* carbamazepine, phenytoin, phenobarbital *Antidepressant:* sertraline *Calcium channel blockers* *Anti-TB drug:* rifampin, *Herbal:* St. John's wort *Immunosuppressant:* cyclosporine	HAART prolongs half-life and/or effects of: *Antiarrhythmics:* amiodarone, digoxin, quinidine *Sedatives:* diazepam, midazolam, triazolam *Opiates:* fentanyl, meperidine, methadone *Local anesthetic:* lidocaine
Integrase strand transfer inhibitors (INSTIs)	Interactions with: *Proton pump inhibitor:* omeprazole *Anti-TB drug:* rifampin	None
Entry inhibitors	Interactions with: *Anticonvulsant:* carbamazepine *Anti-TB drug:* rifampin *Oral contraceptives* *Proton pump inhibitor:* omeprazole *Herbal:* St. John's wort	HAART potentially changes drug clearance and effects of: *Sedative:* midazolam

TB, Tuberculosis.

importance to anesthesiologists is that patients receiving HAART are subject to long-term metabolic complications, including lipid abnormalities and glucose intolerance, which may result in the development of diabetes, coronary artery disease, and cerebrovascular disease. HAART has also been implicated in fat redistribution to the neck, back of the neck, and abdomen. This phenomenon may make airway management more difficult or increase intraabdominal pressure.

Protease inhibitors, particularly ritonavir and saquinavir, act as inhibitors of cytochrome P-450. In contrast, drugs such as nevirapine are inducers of hepatic microsomal enzymes. These variable effects on liver enzyme mechanics further complicate the dosing of HAART drugs and other drugs that undergo hepatic metabolism, including anesthetic and analgesic drugs. Therefore, caution must be used when administering pharmacologic agents that may be metabolized via these pathways, because drug duration and anticipated effect may be highly variable.

Prognosis

Before 1995, the prospects for treatment of HIV infection were dismal, and a diagnosis of HIV infection was inevitably followed by death. Today, the situation has changed dramatically as a result of several independent factors: (1) an improved understanding of the pathogenesis of HIV infection; (2) the availability of surrogate markers of immune function and plasma viral burden, specifically CD4+ cell counts and HIV viral load quantification, to determine if HAART is effective; (3) the use of CD4+ cell counts and viral load determinations by researchers to determine minimal effective concentrations of HAART and thereby improve its risk/benefit profile; (4) the development of viral genotypic-phenotypic profiling, coreceptor subtyping, and sensitivity and resistance pattern analysis, which has enabled optimal selection of specific HAART regimens; (5) the continued development of new and more powerful drugs; (6) the completion of several large clinical end-point trials that have conclusively demonstrated that antiretroviral combinations significantly delay the progression of HIV disease and improve long-term survival.

Management of Anesthesia

PREOPERATIVE

Patients with HIV infection and/or AIDS are usually managed by an internist, primary care provider, or infectious disease specialist. Although a medical evaluation by one of these physicians immediately before surgery is not mandatory, it may be helpful to obtain a consultation if the patient is unable to delineate pertinent medical history and management specifically related to HIV infection and/or AIDS. Additional information from primary care and infectious disease specialists may be especially pertinent in patients in advanced stages of AIDS.

Not all patients with HIV/AIDS are receiving HAART, and it is important to understand what current treatment strategies are being utilized for each specific patient. Some patients may

be waiting for further deterioration in clinical and immune status before initiating HAART, whereas a subset of patients may be on physician-approved "drug holidays," and other patients may simply be unable to tolerate the adverse effects of HAART. Regardless of whether a patient is receiving HAART and has an undetectable viral load, patients with HIV/AIDS should always be considered a potential source of disease transmission. In patients who are not receiving HAART, initiating HAART to minimize viral load to improve overall clinical condition in the period immediately before surgery is not indicated, Studies have indicated that HAART has no protective effect in reducing perioperative risk, and the initiation of HAART within 6 months of surgery actually increases overall morbidity and mortality in patients with HIV infection. In addition, the occurrence of IRIS after HAART is begun may paradoxically worsen the patient's overall condition and further delay surgery.

Since HIV infection, AIDS, and HAART can potentially impact multiple organ systems, it is advisable to order a complete blood count, basic metabolic panel including renal function studies, liver function tests, and coagulation studies. A chest radiograph and electrocardiogram are also useful preoperatively regardless of age or lack of related disease. If a patient with HIV infection or AIDS has any signs or symptoms of possible cardiac dysfunction, echocardiography or stress testing may also be indicated with additional consultation by a cardiologist as indicated.

There is little specific information concerning the overall risk of anesthesia and surgery in the HIV-positive patient. The American Society of Anesthesiologists (ASA) physical status assessment and the inherent surgical risk probably provide a measure of global risk assessment. An ASA status of 2 is typically assigned to HIV-positive patients *without* any clinical evidence of immunocompromise or acute deterioration; these patients *may* or *may not* be receiving HAART. Patients with AIDS may be classified as having an ASA status of either 3 or 4 depending on the severity of co-existing disease processes related or unrelated to HIV infection. In addition, patients with advanced AIDS may be receiving HAART but for all practical purposes may be minimally responsive to it; CD4+ cell counts may be low and viral load may range from undetectable to low, moderate, or high. This information, when combined with the stage of the HIV infection, the degree of clinical immunosuppression, and the presence and severity of opportunistic infections or neoplasms, may offer the best predictor of global perioperative risk in the HIV-positive patient.

The specific utility of obtaining a CD4+ cell count and viral load determination before surgery has not been demonstrated. Various studies have shown that there is no significant difference in perioperative outcomes in HIV-positive or AIDS patients whose CD4+ cell counts are higher than 50 cells/mm^3 compared with outcomes in patient populations without HIV/AIDS matched for the same surgery, comorbid conditions, and ASA status. Viral load level is also not a predictor of perioperative outcome unless viral load exceeds 30,000 copies/mL. HAART does not offer any real protective effects or decrease the overall morbidity and mortality associated with surgery and anesthesia. However, patients with HIV infection and AIDS do demonstrate a higher overall mortality 1 year after surgery than similar cohorts without HIV/AIDS. This has been attributed to HIV infection and/or AIDS itself and not to the surgical procedure performed or the anesthetic used.

In general, if a patient is HIV positive and has never met AIDS-defining criteria, one can presume the patient's CD4+ cell count is higher than 200 cells/mm³. However, patients with AIDS-defining diagnoses or a history of AIDS (with or without HAART) may have widely varying CD4+ cell counts. Not all HIV-positive patients receiving HAART have undetectable viral loads, so viral load quantification does not assist the anesthesiologist in any meaningful manner during the perioperative period. In addition, even if viral load is undetectable, universal precautions must continue to be employed since this does not imply that HIV cannot be transmitted. HIV persistence is a known phenomenon, and HIV remains dormant in lymph nodes and central nervous system reservoirs.

Since patients with HIV infection or AIDS can manifest a wide array of co-existing diseases, every patient should undergo a thorough history taking, review of systems, and physical examination particularly focused on subclinical or clinical manifestations of cardiac, pulmonary, neurologic, renal, and hepatic disorders related to HIV or AIDS. With regard to selection of anesthetic method, any anesthetic technique is acceptable unless there is a specific contraindication to regional anesthesia. Consideration should be given to addressing potential HAART-drug interactions when using pharmacologic agents in the perioperative period.

Overall, HIV infection and AIDS do not increase the risk of postsurgical complications, including death, up to 30 days postoperatively. Thus, surgical intervention should not be limited because of HIV status and concern for subsequent complications. However, during anesthesia, tachycardia is more frequently seen in HIV-positive patients, and postoperatively high fever, anemia, and tachycardia are more frequent.

INTRAOPERATIVE

Selection of a particular anesthetic technique should take into account both HIV/AIDS-related comorbidities and any other clinical issues. Overall, no specific anesthetic technique has been shown to be superior or inferior in patients with HIV infection or AIDS. Specifically in patients with AIDS, focal neurologic lesions may increase intracerebral pressure, which precludes neuraxial anesthesia. Spinal cord involvement, peripheral neuropathy, and myopathy may occur with cytomegalovirus or HIV infection itself. Therefore, succinylcholine could conceivably be hazardous in this setting. HIV infection is associated with autonomic neuropathy, and this can manifest perioperatively as hemodynamic instability during anesthesia or in the ICU. Invasive hemodynamic monitoring may be helpful in patients with severe autonomic dysfunction. Steroid supplementation may decrease hemodynamic instability and should be considered in cases of unexplained, persistent hypotension.

Several studies indicate that general anesthesia and opiates may have a negative effect on immune function. Although this immunosuppressive effect is probably of little clinical importance in healthy individuals, the implications for the HIV-infected patient are unknown. Immunosuppression resulting from general anesthetics occurs within 15 minutes of induction and may persist for as long as 3 to 11 days. The psychological stress of undergoing anesthesia and surgery may also lead to some degree of generalized immunosuppression. However, no studies have been undertaken to determine specific effects in HIV-positive patients. Aside from CD4+ cell count and viral load, there are no specific markers of immune status in this patient population.

HIV infection and AIDS are increasing in women of childbearing age, and there has been much study of this patient population. Although research has demonstrated the effectiveness of zidovudine in parturient women, monotherapy has limited long-term benefit, because HIV resistance develops rapidly. Therefore, in pregnancy, combination therapy is preferable, and acceptable multidrug regimens are available. Data suggests that cesarean section decreases the incidence of vertical transmission of HIV from mother to child. A combination of antiretroviral therapy and elective cesarean section reduces the rate of vertical transmission to 2%. However, cesarean section is a major surgical intervention that has well-reported complications. Many practitioners in the past did not recommend elective cesarean section for HIV-infected women who were adherent to antiretroviral treatment regimens and had undetectable HIV viral loads. However, studies demonstrate that cesarean section can proceed safely. Unfortunately, HIV-positive women with low CD4+ lymphocyte counts whose infants would likely benefit most from caesarean delivery are also the women who are most likely to experience perioperative complications.

HIV-positive parturient women who are given regional anesthesia have not had neurologic or infectious complications related to the anesthetic or obstetric course. In the immediately postpartum period, immune function status has remained essentially unchanged, as has the severity of the pre-existing HIV disease. There have been concerns that epidural and lumbar puncture in HIV-positive patients might allow entry of the virus into the central nervous system. However, the natural history of HIV infection includes central nervous system involvement early in the clinical course. The central nervous system is known to be a reservoir of HIV. The safety of epidural blood patches for treatment of post–dural puncture headache has been reported in HIV-positive patients. Fear of disseminating HIV from the bloodstream into the central nervous system is not warranted.

POSTOPERATIVE

A limited number of retrospective studies have evaluated the long-term consequences of undergoing anesthesia and surgery in HIV-positive and AIDS patients, but many of the studies conducted in the pre-HAART era yielded conflicting results. Newer studies are now examining surgical and anesthetic-related morbidity and mortality in HIV-positive patients who had been receiving HAART. Therefore, it is important to understand the impact that HAART has had on overall well-being in the HIV-positive population.

It appears that patients with HIV infection and AIDS do not experience any statistically significant increases in perioperative complications compared with similar cohorts who are not HIV positive. No statistically significant differences have been noted with regard to wound healing, SSI rates, wound dehiscence, number of complications, length of hospital stay, number of follow-up visits to the surgeon, or need for further operative procedures to treat surgical complications. However, 1-year mortality is higher overall in patients who are HIV positive and/or have AIDS. This is hypothesized to be due to HIV infection itself. Patients with CD4+ cell counts of less than 50 cells/mm³ and patients with viral loads of more than 30,000 copies/mL fare the worst in terms of postoperative mortality. Patients with HIV infection may have a higher incidence of postoperative pneumonia than non-HIV+ patients. Proper diagnosis and treatment typically leads to resolution of the pulmonary infection without sequelae.

Acute Physiology and Chronic Health Evaluation II (APACHE II) scoring significantly underestimates mortality risk in HIV-positive patients admitted to the ICU with a total lymphocyte count of less than 200 cells/mm³. This is particularly true of patients admitted with pneumonia or sepsis. There is a diverse range of indications for critical care in patients with HIV infection. Historically, respiratory failure caused by PCP was the most common reason for ICU admission and accounted for a third of ICU admissions in HIV-positive patients. The need for mechanical ventilation for PCP and other pulmonary disorders is associated with a mortality rate of more than 50%. In contrast, admission to the ICU and mechanical ventilation for nonpulmonary disorders is associated with a mortality rate of less than 25%. In patients with septic shock, however, HIV infection is an independent predictor of poor outcome. In the era of HAART, fewer patients with HIV infection are admitted to the ICU with AIDS-defining illnesses. Many patients are now admitted to the ICU with unrelated critical illnesses and are found coincidentally to be infected with HIV.

Initiation of HAART has improved overall outcomes regardless of the clinical stage of HIV infection. However, HAART does not offer any protective effect during surgery and anesthesia. As noted earlier, patients who begin HAART within 6 months of surgery experience a higher incidence of perioperative complications, perhaps because of IRIS.

KEY POINTS

- The twenty-first century is likely to be marked by a proliferation of infectious viral illnesses.
- There is a paucity of new antibiotics under development to combat resistant gram-negative organisms.
- Multidisciplinary protocols focusing on preoperative, intraoperative, and postoperative prevention of SSI do decrease the likelihood of patients' developing such infections.

- Frequent hand decontamination with alcohol may be the single most effective intervention in decreasing nosocomial infection.
- Administration of antibiotics at the right time, in the right dosage, and for an appropriate duration of time effectively treats infection and retards the development of antibiotic drug resistance.
- There is a growing epidemic of virulent C. difficile–associated diarrhea among hospitalized patients, which may be associated with the widespread use of broad-spectrum antibiotics.
- To minimize widespread resistance of organisms to all antimicrobial agents, therapy *must* be narrowed as soon as organisms are identified and susceptibility testing is completed.
- Specimens for culture should be obtained from all likely sources if sepsis is suspected.
- With necrotizing soft tissue infections, the superficial cutaneous signs typically do not reflect the extent of tissue necrosis.
- Between 10% and 20% of patients requiring endotracheal intubation and mechanical ventilation for longer than 48 hours develop VAP, which is associated with significant mortality.
- Respiratory viruses may have high virulence, a fulminant infectious course, and high lethality.
- Allogeneic red blood cell transfusion creates generalized immunosuppression and can reactivate latent viruses.
- The development of XDR TB, caused by *M. tuberculosis* strains that not only are resistant to antibiotic therapy but also are more virulent and frequently lethal, has become a large public health concern.
- Posttransplantation patients are especially susceptible to infectious diseases, and strict adherence to immunosuppressant regimens, antimicrobial prophylaxis, and surgical infection prophylaxis is critical in preventing new infections.
- HIV infection is a modern pandemic and has acute, latent, and end-stage phases. HAART has transformed HIV into a manageable chronic disease; however, significant HAART-induced and/or HIV-related morbidity continues to exist.
- Health care workers must recognize that they are potential agents of infection transmission.

RESOURCES

Bartlett JG. Narrative review: the new epidemic of *Clostridium difficile*–associated enteric disease. *Ann Intern Med*. 2006;145:758-764.

Bartzler DW, Hunt DR. The Surgical Infection Prevention and Surgical Care Improvement projects: national initiatives to improve outcomes for patients having surgery. *Clin Infect Dis*. 2006;43:322-330.

Dellinger EP. Prophylactic antibiotics: administration and timing before operation are more important than administration after operation. *Clin Infect Dis*. 2007;44:928-930.

Dellinger RP, Levy MM, Carlet JM, et al. Surviving Sepsis Campaign: international guidelines for management of sever sepsis and shock. *Intensive Care Med*. 2008;34:17-60.

Diagnosis of HIV infection and AIDS in the United States and dependent areas, 2009. Centers for Disease Control and Prevention. *MMWR Morb Mortal Wkly Rep*. 2009;57(30):1073-1076.

Horberg MA, Hurley LB, Klein DB, et al. Surgical outcomes in human immunodeficiency virus–infected patients in the era of highly active antiretroviral therapy. *Arch Surg.* 2006;141:1238-1245.

Hughes SC. HIV and anesthesia. *Anesthesiol Clin North Am.* 2004;22:379-404.

Lutfiyya MN, Henley E, Chang LF, et al. Diagnosis and treatment of community-acquired pneumonia. *Am Fam Physician.* 2006;73:442-450.

Luyt CE, Chastre J, Fagon JY. Value of the clinical pulmonary infection score for the identification and management of ventilator-associated pneumonia. *Intensive Care Med.* 2004;30:844-852.

Mauermann WJ, Nemergut EC. The anesthesiologist's role in the prevention of surgical site infections. *Anesthesiology.* 2006;105:413-421.

Plan to combat extensively drug-resistant tuberculosis: recommendations of the Federal Tuberculosis Task Force. *MMWR Recomm Report.* 2009;58(RR-3):1-43.

Pronovost P, Needham D, Berenholtz S, et al. An intervention to decrease catheter-related bloodstream infections in the ICU. *N Engl J Med.* 2006;355:2725-2732.

Sander RD, Hussel T, Maze M. Sedation and immunomodulation. *Crit Care Clin.* 2009;25:551-570.

Webster RG, Govorkova EA. H5N1 influenza—continuing evolution and spread. *N Engl J Med.* 2006;355:2174-2177.

Cancer

NATALIE F. HOLT ■

Cancer is the second leading cause of death in the United States, superseded only by heart disease. The lifetime risk of developing cancer is estimated to be one in two for men and one in three for women. The lifetime risk of dying from cancer is one in four for men and one in five for women. About 90% of patients with cancer require surgery for reasons both related and unrelated to the cancer diagnosis. Furthermore, approximately 65% of patients diagnosed with cancer survive for at least 5 years, which means that a growing number of patients will come to surgery after successful cancer treatment.

The anesthetic implications of cancer stem not only from the cancer itself, but also from the therapies employed for its treatment. In addition, since the median age at diagnosis is 65 years, patients with cancer often have comorbid conditions that affect their perioperative course.

MECHANISM

Cancer results from an accumulation of genetic mutations that causes dysregulation of cellular proliferation. Genes are involved in carcinogenesis by virtue of inherited traits that predispose to cancer (e.g., altered metabolism of potentially carcinogenic compounds), mutation of a normal gene into an oncogene that promotes the conversion of normal cells into cancer cells, or inactivation of a tumor suppressor gene, which triggers malignant transformation. A critical gene related to cancer in humans is the tumor suppressor *p53*. This gene is not only essential for cell viability, but critical for monitoring damage to DNA. Inactivation of *p53* is an early step in the development of many types of cancer. Stimulation of oncogene formation by carcinogens (tobacco, alcohol, sunlight) is estimated to be responsible for 80% of cancers in the United States. Tobacco accounts for more cases of cancer than all other known carcinogens combined.

The fundamental event that causes cells to become malignant is an alteration in their DNA structure. These mutations occur in cells of target tissues, and these cells then become ancestors of the entire future tumor cell population. Evolution to more undifferentiated cells reflects high mutation rates and contributes to the development of tumors that are resistant to therapy.

Cancer cells must evade the host's immune surveillance system, which is designed to seek out and destroy tumor cells. Most mutant cancer cells stimulate the host's immune system to form antibodies. This protective role of the immune system is apparent in those with acquired immunodeficiency syndrome and recipients of organ transplants who are maintained on long-term immunosuppressive drugs. These groups have a higher incidence of cancer.

DIAGNOSIS

Most cancers produce solid tumors. Cancer often becomes clinically evident when tumor bulk compromises vital organ function. The initial diagnosis is frequently made by aspiration cytology or biopsy. Monoclonal antibodies that recognize antigens for specific cancers may aid in the diagnosis of cancer. A commonly used staging system for solid tumors is the TNM system based on tumor size (T), lymph node involvement (N), and distant metastases (M). This system groups cancers into stages ranging from I (best prognosis) to IV (poorest prognosis). Tumor invasiveness is related to the release of various tumor mediators that modify the surrounding microenvironment in such a way as to permit cancer cells to spread along the lines of least resistance. Lymphatics lack a basement membrane, so local spread of cancer is influenced by the anatomy of the regional lymphatics. For example, regional lymph node involvement occurs late in squamous cell cancer of the vocal cords because these structures have few lymphatics, whereas regional lymph node involvement is an early manifestation of supraglottic cancer because this region is rich in lymphatics. Imaging techniques including computed tomography (CT) and magnetic resonance imaging (MRI) are used for further delineation of tumor presence and spread.

TREATMENT

Most cancers are treated by a multimodal approach involving surgery, radiation therapy, and/or chemotherapies that vary by tumor type and stage. The development of more effective cancer treatments has dramatically improved survival. However, use of these more powerful therapies is associated with toxicities and adverse effects that have the potential to affect nearly every organ system. Some of these effects are transient; others produce permanent sequelae. All of them have important potential consequences in the perioperative care of cancer patients.

Traditional Chemotherapy

Traditional chemotherapy involves the use of cytotoxic agents that target rapidly dividing cells and interfere with replication. They are divided into classes based on mechanism of action: alkylating agents, antimetabolites, antibiotics, microtubule assembly inhibitors, hormonal agents, and various miscellaneous or mixed-mechanism drugs. *Alkylating agents* form reactive molecules that cause DNA cross-linking problems such as abnormal base pairing and strand breaks that interfere primarily with DNA but also with RNA and protein synthesis and replication. *Antimetabolites* are structural analogues of folic acid, purines, or pyrimidines that block enzymes necessary for nucleic acid and protein synthesis. *Antitumor antibiotics* form complexes with DNA or RNA that inhibit their subsequent synthesis. *Microtubule assembly inhibitors* include the vinca alkaloids and taxanes, both of which act on the mitotic process by interfering with microtubule assembly or disassembly. The growth of certain tumor types, notably breast and prostate, is responsive to *hormonal agents*. Hormones are not cytotoxic, so they often stimulate tumor regression but do not cause cell death. Several other drugs have been shown to have anticancer properties. The epipodophyllotoxins act by inhibiting the topoisomerase II enzyme, which causes DNA strand breaks that lead to apoptotic cell death. The topoisomerase I inhibitors work by a similar mechanism but on a different enzyme.

Targeted Chemotherapy

Targeted chemotherapy utilizes a new set of chemotherapeutic agents directed against specific processes involved in tumor cell proliferation and migration. The first targeted therapy was that developed for estrogen receptors present in certain types of breast cancers. Binding of estrogen to estrogen receptors is an important step in the growth of these tumor cells, and estrogen receptor blockade turned out to be an effective way to reduce tumor spread.

Other targeted therapies have been developed against a number of cell processes, including secretion of growth factors that facilitate gene expression, angiogenesis (creation of new blood vessels), cell migration, and tumor growth. Growth factors such as endothelial growth factor (EGF), vascular endothelial growth factor (VEGF), and matrix metalloproteinases are involved in growth and differentiation of normal cells, but they are usually overexpressed or mutated on cancer cells. Binding of growth factors to receptors on the cell membrane induces a cascade of signal transduction events that often involve activation of the enzyme tyrosine kinase. Absence of these signals may lead to apoptosis. Drugs have now been developed that block these growth factors, their receptors, or their associated tyrosine kinases. Included among the targeted therapies are monoclonal antibodies that act on extracellular receptors such as EGF and VEGF, as well as small molecules that penetrate cell membranes and block intracellular signaling pathways. Cancer cells have the ability to mutate and develop resistance to targeted therapies, so targeted therapies are often used in conjunction with other drugs.

Radiation Therapy

Radiation induces cell death by causing damage to DNA. The sensitivity of a cell to radiation injury is influenced by its phase in the cell cycle and its ability to repair DNA damage. For the treatment of cancer, radiation timing and delivery are adjusted to maximize therapeutic benefit and minimize damage to surrounding tissue. Radiation can be administered through external beam technology or through radioactive pellets implanted into a target organ (e.g., radioactive "seeds" for treatment of prostate cancer). Technologic advances such as three-dimensional imaging and conformal radiotherapy that allow radiation energy to be matched to tumor shape have helped minimize damage to surrounding tissue.

Adverse Effects of Cancer Treatment

Bone marrow suppression, cardiovascular and pulmonary toxicity, and central and peripheral nervous system damage are among the most serious adverse effects of cancer treatment. However, dysfunction of nearly every organ system has been described. The following sections present a system-specific review of toxicities related to cancer treatment. Tables 23-1 and 23-2 summarize the adverse effects of selected chemotherapies and radiation treatment.

CARDIOVASCULAR SYSTEM

Anthracyclines like doxorubicin (Adriamycin) and idarubicin are the chemotherapeutic drugs most often associated with cardiotoxicity. These drugs are commonly used to treat

TABLE 23-1 ▪ Toxicities of commonly used chemotherapeutic agents

Agent	Adverse effects	Agent	Adverse effects
Doxorubicin	Cardiac toxicity, myelosuppression	Fluorouracil	Acute cerebellar ataxia, cardiac toxicity, gastritis, myelosuppression
Arsenic	Leukocytosis, pleural effusion, QT interval prolongation	Ifosfamide	Cardiac toxicity, hemorrhagic cystitis, renal insufficiency, SIADH
Asparaginase	Coagulopathy, hemorrhagic pancreatitis, hepatic dysfunction, thromboembolism	Methotrexate	Encephalopathy, hepatic dysfunction, mucositis, platelet dysfunction, pulmonary toxicity, renal failure, myelosuppression
Bevacizumab	Bleeding, congestive heart failure, gastrointestinal perforation, hypertension, impaired wound healing, pulmonary hemorrhage, thromboembolism	Mitomycin	Myelosuppression, pulmonary toxicity
		Mitoxantrone	Cardiac toxicity, myelosuppression
Bleomycin	Pulmonary hypertension, pulmonary toxicity	Paclitaxel	Ataxia, autonomic dysfunction, myelosuppression, peripheral neuropathy, arthralgias, bradycardia
Busulfan	Cardiac toxicity, myelosuppression, pulmonary toxicity	Sorafenib	Cardiac ischemia, hypertension, impaired wound healing, thromboembolism
Carmustine	Myelosuppression, pulmonary toxicity		
Chlorambucil	Myelosuppression, pulmonary toxicity, SIADH	Sunitinib	Adrenal insufficiency, cardiac ischemia, hypertension, thromboembolism
Cisplatin	Dysrhythmias, magnesium wasting, mucositis, ototoxicity, peripheral neuropathy, SIADH, renal tubular necrosis, thromboembolism	Tamoxifen	Thromboembolism
		Thalidomide	Bradycardia, neurotoxicity, thromboembolism
Cyclophosphamide	Encephalopathy/delirium, hemorrhagic cystitis, myelosuppression, pericarditis, pericardial effusion, SIADH, pulmonary fibrosis	Tretinoin	Myelosuppression, retinoic acid syndrome
		Vinblastine	Cardiac toxicity, hypertension, myelosuppression, pulmonary toxicity, SIADH
Erlotinib	Deep vein thrombosis, pulmonary toxicity		
Etoposide	Cardiac toxicity, myelosuppression, pulmonary toxicity	Vincristine	Autonomic dysfunction, cardiac toxicity, peripheral neuropathy, SIADH, pulmonary toxicity

SIADH, Syndrome of inappropriate secretion of antidiuretic hormone.

cancers such as leukemias and lymphomas. Anthracyclines impair myocyte function via the formation of free radicals, which interfere with mitochondrial activation and cause lipid peroxidation. Cardiotoxicity may be acute or chronic. Acute toxicity begins early in treatment with the development of dysrhythmias, QT prolongation, and cardiomyopathy and then reverses with discontinuation of therapy. Chronic toxicity (left ventricular dysfunction and cardiomyopathy) can occur in an early-onset form that usually appears within 1 year of treatment and a late-onset form that can emerge several years or decades after completion of therapy. Risks factors for cardiotoxicity include a large cumulative dose of drug (for doxorubicin, >300 mg/m^2), a history of high-dose bolus administration, and a history of concomitant radiation therapy or use of other cardiotoxic drugs. The cardiotoxicity of doxorubicin may be decreased by the use of free radical scavengers such as dexrazoxane or liposomal preparations.

Mitoxantrone, which is structurally similar to the anthracyclines, has also been associated with cardiomyopathy, as have other drugs including cyclophosphamide, clofarabine, and certain of the tyrosine kinase inhibitors. Baseline echocardiography is recommended for all patients before anthracycline treatment. Periodic echocardiography is advised in patients receiving high-dose therapy and those with underlying cardiac impairment or significant risk factors for heart disease.

Pericarditis, angina, coronary artery vasospasm, ischemia-related electrocardiographic changes, and conduction defects are other cardiac complications related to cancer chemotherapy. Fluorouracil and capecitabine cause the highest incidence of chemotherapy-related ischemia. Estimates vary widely from 1% to 68% for fluorouracil and from 3% to 9% for capecitabine. Paclitaxel and thalidomide can cause severe bradycardia requiring pacemaker implantation. Arsenic, lapatinib, and nilotinib frequently cause QT prolongation.

Hypertension has emerged as a relatively common adverse effect of treatment with newer targeted chemotherapeutic drugs such as bevacizumab, trastuzumab, sorafenib, and sunitinib, and occurs in as many as 35% to 45% of patients. The pathophysiology of the cardiac damage associated with these drugs is probably directly related to inhibition of EGF and VEGF. Although important to tumor cell proliferation, these growth factors also play a role in normal myocyte growth, repair, and adaptation to pressure loads.

Patients who receive radiation to the mediastinum are at risk for developing myocardial fibrosis, pericarditis, valvular fibrosis, conduction abnormalities, and accelerated development of coronary artery disease. Incidence is related to cumulative radiation exposure as well as concomitant administration of cardiotoxic chemotherapeutic agents.

RESPIRATORY SYSTEM

Pulmonary toxicity is a well-recognized complication of bleomycin therapy. Other agents associated with pulmonary damage include busulfan, cyclophosphamide, methotrexate, lomustine, carmustine, mitomycin, and the vinca alkaloids. The mechanism of injury differs for each drug. In the case of bleomycin, free radical formation seems to be a factor. EGF receptor blockade is the postulated mechanism reported with erlotinib and gefitinib, both of which are EGF receptor blockers. Type II pneumocytes possess EGF receptors that play a role in alveolar repair.

Pneumonitis or bronchiolitis obliterans with organizing pneumonia occurs in 3% to 20% of patients treated with bleomycin, depending on dose. Pulmonary fibrosis can develop decades after treatment. Risk factors include preexisting lung disease, smoking, and radiation exposure. Baseline and serial pulmonary function testing and chest radiography are often performed. Of note, evidence suggests that intraoperative exposure to high concentrations of oxygen may exacerbate preexisting bleomycin-induced lung injury and contribute to postoperative ventilatory failure. Perioperative corticosteroid administration may be of benefit in treating bleomycin-induced pneumonitis.

Interstitial pneumonitis and pulmonary fibrosis are complications of radiation to the thorax or total body irradiation. Symptoms typically begin within the first 2 to 3 months of treatment and generally regress within 12 months of treatment completion. However, subclinical abnormalities revealed by pulmonary function testing reportedly occur in up to 50% of patients exposed to radiation for treatment of childhood cancers. *Radiation recall pneumonitis* is a recognized clinical syndrome in which patients with prior radiation exposure manifest symptomatic pneumonitis after exposure to a second pulmonary toxin.

TABLE 23-2	Common adverse effects of radiation therapy	
System	Acute	Chronic
Skin	Erythema, rash, hair loss	Fibrosis, sclerosis, telangiectasias
Gastrointestinal	Malnutrition, mucositis, nausea, vomiting	Adhesions, fistulas, strictures
Cardiac		Conduction defects, pericardial effusion, pericardial fibrosis, pericarditis
Respiratory		Airway fibrosis, pulmonary fibrosis, pneumonitis, tracheal stenosis
Renal	Glomerulonephritis	Glomerulosclerosis
Hepatic	Sinusoidal obstruction syndrome	
Endocrine		Hypothyroidism, panhypopituitarism
Hematologic	Bone marrow suppression	Coagulation necrosis

RENAL SYSTEM

Many of the chemotherapeutic agents can be nephrotoxic; among the most commonly cited are cisplatin, high-dose methotrexate, and ifosfamide. Renal insufficiency and hypomagnesemia are the typical presenting signs of cisplatin-related nephrotoxicity. Ifosfamide usually causes proximal tubule dysfunction marked by proteinuria and glucosuria. Leucovorin, a folic acid precursor, can be helpful in treating methotrexate-related renal failure. Renal insufficiency usually resolves with cessation of treatment and supportive therapy. Prehydration and avoidance of other nephrotoxins limit the risk of renal toxicity.

Cyclophosphamide is often associated with the syndrome of inappropriate secretion of antidiuretic hormone (SIADH) via a direct effect on renal tubules, but this condition is usually benign. The most serious adverse effect of cyclophosphamide is hemorrhagic cystitis, which can cause hematuria severe enough to produce obstructive uropathy.

Induction chemotherapy or high-dose radiation therapy can induce tumor cell lysis that causes the release of large amounts of uric acid, phosphate, and potassium. Hyperuricemia can cause uric acid crystals to precipitate in renal tubules, which leads to acute renal failure. Calcium phosphate deposition may exacerbate the condition. Radiation exposure can cause glomerulonephritis or glomerulosclerosis with permanent injury marked by chronic renal insufficiency and systemic hypertension.

HEPATIC SYSTEM

Antimetabolites such as methotrexate, as well as asparaginase, arabinoside, plicamycin, and streptozocin, have been associated with acute liver dysfunction. However, chronic liver disease is uncommon. Radiation-induced liver injury is also typically dose dependent and reversible.

The most severe form of liver dysfunction in cancer patients is *sinusoidal obstruction syndrome*. This usually occurs in patients receiving total body irradiation in preparation for hematopoietic stem cell transplantation; however, several chemotherapeutic agents have also been associated with this syndrome, including busulfan, cyclophosphamide, vincristine, and dactinomycin. Mortality ranges from 19% to 50%.

AIRWAY AND ORAL CAVITY

Mucositis is a painful inflammation and ulceration of the mucous membranes of the digestive tract. Oral lesions begin as mucosal whitening followed by the development of erythema and tissue friability. Oral mucositis is a relatively common adverse effect of high-dose chemotherapy and radiation to the head and neck. Mucositis can also occur in the context of hematopoietic stem cell transplantation. Chemotherapeutic drugs associated with mucositis include the anthracyclines, taxanes, and platinum-based compounds, as well as antimetabolites such as methotrexate and fluorouracil. Mucositis associated with chemotherapy often begins during the first week of treatment and typically resolves after treatment is terminated. Mucositis associated with radiation therapy usually has a more delayed onset. Patients with mucositis are at risk of infection from spread of oral bacteria. Narcotics are frequently required to achieve adequate analgesia. In its most severe form, pseudomembrane formation, edema, and bleeding may cause airway compromise or risk of aspiration.

Radiation to the head and neck can result in permanent tissue fibrosis that may limit mouth opening and neck and tongue mobility. Airway fibrosis and tracheal stenosis may result in difficulty in ventilation and intubation that is not recognized on physical examination.

GASTROINTESTINAL SYSTEM

Almost all chemotherapy and radiation therapy produce gastrointestinal adverse effects. Nausea, vomiting, diarrhea, and enteritis are common. Diarrhea is frequent with fluorouracil, melphalan, anthracyclines, and the topoisomerase inhibitors. In the short term, these symptoms can produce dehydration, electrolyte abnormalities, and malnutrition, but these effects are usually transient. Radiation, however, may produce permanent sequelae such as adhesions and stenotic lesions anywhere along the gastrointestinal tract. Hemorrhagic pancreatitis is a unique complication associated with asparaginase.

ENDOCRINE SYSTEM

Hyperglycemia is a common adverse effect of glucocorticoid therapy, as is suppression of the hypothalamic-pituitary-adrenal axis, which may become evident during stress or surgery. Adrenal suppression is reversible, but it may take up to a year for adrenal function to return to normal. SIADH can be seen with cyclophosphamide, ifosfamide, cisplatin, and melphalan, although symptomatic hyponatremia is uncommon.

Total body irradiation in the context of hematopoietic stem cell transplantation and radiation therapy for head and neck cancers can cause panhypopituitarism and/or hypothyroidism, which typically becomes symptomatic during the first few *years* following treatment. Patients with a history of radiation exposure to the neck are also at increased risk of thyroid cancer.

HEMATOLOGIC SYSTEM

Myelosuppression is the most frequent adverse effect associated with chemotherapy. In most cases, this effect is transient, and blood cell counts return to normal within a week following therapy.

Bleeding is relatively common in patients on chemotherapy and may be the result of thrombocytopenia and/or platelet dysfunction. Depletion of vitamin K–dependent coagulation factors contributes to this problem. Bleeding has also been associated with the angiogenesis inhibitor bevacizumab as well as several of the tyrosine kinase inhibitors, particularly when used in conjunction with other drugs. For this reason, it has been recommended that bevacizumab therapy be withheld before major surgery.

Tumors release procoagulants such as tissue factor that create a hypercoagulable state. Some chemotherapeutic drugs can exacerbate this condition. Thalidomide and the related drug lenalidomide pose an especially high risk of venous thromboembolism, particularly when used in combination with glucocorticoids and doxorubicin. Other drugs associated with an increased risk of thromboembolism include cisplatin and tamoxifen.

Radiation-induced coagulation disorders occur as a delayed effect and involve coagulation necrosis of vascular endothelium. Postradiation bleeding in the rectum, vagina, bladder, lung, and brain have been reported.

NERVOUS SYSTEM

Chemotherapy can cause a number of neurotoxic adverse effects, including peripheral neuropathy and encephalopathy. Virtually all patients treated with vincristine develop paresthesias in their hands and feet. Autonomic neuropathy may accompany the paresthesias. These changes are usually reversible. Cisplatin causes dose-dependent large fiber neuropathy by damaging dorsal root ganglia. Loss of proprioception may be sufficiently severe to interfere with ambulation. Consideration of regional anesthesia in patients being treated with cisplatin must take into account the fact that subclinical neurotoxicity is present in a large percentage of these patients and cisplatin neurotoxicity may extend several months beyond discontinuation of treatment. Paclitaxel causes dose-dependent ataxia that may be accompanied by paresthesias in the hands and feet and proximal skeletal muscle weakness. Corticosteroids (prednisone or its equivalent at 60 to 100 mg/day) may cause a myopathy characterized by weakness of the neck flexors and proximal weakness of the extremities. The first sign of corticosteroid-induced neuromuscular toxicity is difficulty rising from the sitting position. Respiratory muscles may also be affected. Corticosteroid-induced myopathy usually resolves when the drug is discontinued.

Cancer chemotherapeutic drugs can cause encephalopathy, delirium, and/or cerebellar ataxia. Examples include high-dose cyclophosphamide and methotrexate. Prolonged administration of methotrexate, especially in conjunction with radiation therapy, can lead to progressive irreversible dementia.

Tumor Lysis Syndrome

Tumor lysis syndrome is caused by sudden destruction of tumor cells by chemotherapy or radiation, leading to the release of large amounts of uric acid, potassium, and phosphate. This syndrome occurs most often after induction treatment for hematologic neoplasms, such as acute lymphoblastic leukemia. Acute renal failure can develop because of uric acid crystal formation and/or calcium phosphate deposition in the kidney. Hyperkalemia and cardiac dysrhythmias are more likely in the presence of renal dysfunction. Hyperphosphatemia can lead to secondary hypocalcemia, which increases the risk of cardiac dysrhythmias from hypokalemia and can cause neuromuscular symptoms such as tetany.

CANCER IMMUNOLOGY

Diagnosis

The use of monoclonal antibodies to detect proteins encoded by oncogenes or other types of tumor-associated antigens (TAs) is a common method for identifying cancer. TAs (α-fetoprotein, prostate-specific antigen, carcinoembryonic antigen) are present on cancer cells and normal cells, but concentrations are higher on tumor cells. Monoclonal antibodies to various TAs can be labeled with radioisotopes and injected to monitor the spread of cancer. Because TAs are present on normal tissues, measurement of these antigens may be less useful for the diagnosis of cancer than for monitoring disease in patients with known malignancies.

Immunomodulators

Tumor cells are antigenically different from normal cells, and evidence now confirms that the body is able to mount an immune response against TAs in a process similar to that which causes allograft rejection. However, because TAs also exist on normal cells, they are only weakly antigenic. Adjuvants are compounds that potentiate the immune response. Examples include bacille Calmette-Guérin (BCG) and naturally occurring interferons such as interleukin-2 (IL-2), interferon-α (INF-α), and granulocyte-macrophage colony-stimulating factor (GM-CSF). These agents are used to augment the host's intrinsic anticancer capabilities.

Cancer Vaccines

Appreciation of the role of TAs in eliciting an immune response is now driving the development of cancer vaccines. Two types of cancer vaccines exist: preventive and therapeutic. The preventive vaccines target infectious agents know to contribute to cancer development. Two preventive vaccines are currently marketed, one against human papillomavirus (HPV) types 6, 11, 16, 18 and another against hepatitis B virus (HBV). HPV types 16 and 18 are responsible for approximately 70% of cervical cancers and are also a causal factor in some cancers of the vagina, vulva, anus, penis, and oropharynx. Chronic HBV infection is a major risk factor for the development of hepatocellular carcinoma. HBV vaccination is now recommended in childhood as part of a strategy to reduce not only the risk of HBV infection but also the incidence of hepatocellular cancer.

The premise behind therapeutic cancer vaccines is that injection of tumor antigen can be used to stimulate an immune system response against tumor cells. In 2010, the U.S. Food and Drug Administration approved the first therapeutic cancer vaccine, sipuleucel-T (Provenge) for the treatment of some cases of metastatic prostate cancer. Sipuleucel-T is an autologous vaccine produced by isolating antigen-presenting cells from the patient's own immune system, then culturing them with a protein consisting of prostatic acid phosphatase linked to GM-CSF. Treatment elicits an immune response that has shown efficacy in reducing tumor progression. Vaccines are in development for a number of other cancers. Some of these are made from weakened or killed cancer cells that contain TAs, others from immune cells that have been modified to express TAs. Still others are being made synthetically. A novel type of cancer vaccine uses "naked" DNA or RNA that codes for TAs. Injection of the vaccine either directly or via a virus carrier induces massive TA production, which in turn promotes a robust immune response that is intended to halt tumor progression.

PARANEOPLASTIC SYNDROMES

Paraneoplastic syndromes are pathophysiologic disturbances that affect an estimated 8% of patients with cancer. Sometimes, symptoms of a paraneoplastic syndrome manifest before the cancer diagnosis and may actually result in cancer detection. Certain of these conditions (superior vena cava obstruction, increased intracranial pressure) may manifest as life-threatening medical emergencies.

Fever and Cachexia

Fever may occur with any type of cancer but is particularly likely with metastases to the liver. Increased body temperature may accompany rapidly proliferating tumors such as leukemias and lymphomas. Fever may reflect tumor necrosis, inflammation, the release of toxic products by cancer cells, or the production of endogenous pyrogens.

Cancer cachexia is a frequent occurrence in cancer patients. In addition to the psychologic effects of cancer on appetite, cancer cells compete with normal tissues for nutrients and may eventually cause nutritive death of normal cells. Tumor factors such as proteolysis-inducing factor and host response factors such as tumor necrosis factor-α, IFN-γ, and IL-6 also contribute to muscle atrophy and lipolysis. Hyperalimentation is indicated for nutritional support when malnutrition is severe, especially if surgery is planned.

Neurologic Abnormalities

Paraneoplastic neurologic syndromes are the result of antibody-mediated damage to the nervous system. Antibodies produced by the host in response to TAs cross-react with elements of the nervous system, which leads to neurologic dysfunction. The vast majority of paraneoplastic neurologic syndromes (80%) manifest *before* the diagnosis of cancer. They can affect both the central and peripheral nervous systems. They are relatively rare—occurring in about 1% of cancer patients—but are seen disproportionately in those with small cell lung cancer, lymphoma, and myeloma. Examples are limbic encephalitis, paraneoplastic cerebellar degeneration, Lambert-Eaton myasthenia syndrome, and myasthenia gravis. Lambert-Eaton syndrome is caused by antibodies to voltage-gated calcium channel receptors and is commonly associated with small cell lung cancer. Myasthenia gravis is caused by antibodies to the acetylcholine receptor and is often present in

TABLE 23-3 ■ **Ectopic hormone production**

Hormone	Associated cancer	Manifestations
Adrenocorticotropic hormone	Carcinoid, lung (small cell), thymoma, thyroid (medullary)	Cushing's syndrome
Antidiuretic hormone	Duodenal, lung (small cell), lymphoma, pancreatic, prostate	Water intoxication
Erythropoietin	Hemangioblastoma, hepatic, renal cell, uterine myofibroma	Polycythemia
Human chorionic gonadotropin	Adrenal, breast, lung (large cell), ovarian, testicular	Gynecomastia, galactorrhea, precocious puberty
Insulin-like substances	Retroperitoneal tumors	Hypoglycemia
Parathyroid hormone	Lung (small cell, squamous cell), ovary, pancreas, renal	Hyperparathyroidism, hypercalcemia, hypertension, renal dysfunction, left ventricular dysfunction
Thyrotropin	Choriocarcinoma, testicular (embryonal)	Hyperthyroidism, thrombocytopenia
Thyrocalcitonin	Thyroid (medullary)	Hypocalcemia, hypotension, muscle weakness

patients with thymoma. Potentiation of neuromuscular blocking agents may be observed in these myasthenic disorders.

These paraneoplastic neurologic syndromes often present a diagnostic challenge because symptoms are nonspecific and the underlying cancer diagnosis is usually unknown. Antibodies to tumor-associated material (called *onconeural antibodies*) are present in the serum of some but not all patients. Immunosuppression is the mainstay of treatment of these syndromes. Corticosteroids and immunoglobulin therapies are frequently employed. Plasmapheresis may also be required to reduce the antibody burden. Once the condition is diagnosed, screening for an underlying malignancy is indicated.

Endocrine Abnormalities

Paraneoplastic endocrine syndromes arise from hormone or peptide production within tumor cells (Table 23-3). Most occur after the diagnosis of cancer has been established. Treatment of the underlying tumor is the preferred management.

SYNDROME OF INAPPROPRIATE SECRETION OF ANTIDIURETIC HORMONE

SIADH affects approximately 1% to 2% of cancer patients, with most cases related to small cell lung cancer. Headache and nausea are early symptoms that may progress to confusion, ataxia, lethargy, and seizures. Symptoms depend on the degree of hyponatremia and the rapidity with which it develops. SIADH resolves with treatment of the underlying tumor. Vasopressin receptor antagonists and demeclocycline are the pharmacologic therapies available if symptoms are severe.

HYPERCALCEMIA

Cancer is the most common cause of hypercalcemia in hospitalized patients and is considered a poor prognostic indicator. There are several different mechanisms for the hypercalcemia seen in cancer patients. The most common is secretion of a parathyroid hormone–related protein by tumor cells that binds to parathyroid hormone receptors in the bone and kidney. This type occurs commonly with squamous cell cancers of the kidneys, lungs, pancreas, and ovaries. Hypercalcemia can also be caused by local osteolytic activity associated with bone metastases, especially from breast cancer, multiple myeloma, and some lymphomas. Occasionally, tumors secrete vitamin D.

The rapid onset of hypercalcemia that occurs in patients with cancer may present as lethargy or coma. Polyuria accompanies hypercalcemia and may lead to dehydration. Treatment includes hydration with normal saline. Intravenous bisphosphonates or calcitonin may also be indicated.

CUSHING'S SYNDROME

Cushing's syndrome is most commonly associated with neuroendocrine tumors of the lung such as small cell lung cancer and carcinoid. It is caused by tumor secretion of either adrenocorticotropic hormone (ACTH) or corticotropin-releasing factor (CRF). Clinical symptoms include hypertension, weight gain, central obesity, and edema. The diagnosis can be confirmed by measuring serum concentrations of ACTH or CRF and by performing a dexamethasone suppression test, which involves administration of dexamethasone followed by measurement of urinary cortisol levels. Normally administration of dexamethasone causes a marked reduction in urinary cortisol concentration. In patients with paraneoplastic Cushing's syndrome, however, there is no reduction in urinary cortisol level after dexamethasone administration. Treatment includes agents that block steroid production such as ketoconazole and mitotane. Antihypertensives and diuretics may also be needed for symptom management.

HYPOGLYCEMIA

Intermittent hypoglycemic episodes can occur with insulin-producing islet cell tumors in the pancreas or with non–islet cell tumors outside of the pancreas that secrete insulin-like growth factor 2 (IGF-2). Patients with islet cell tumors demonstrate a *high* serum insulin level. In contrast, those with non–islet cell tumors that secrete insulin-like substances demonstrate a *low* serum insulin level and an elevated level of IGF-2.

Renal Abnormalities

Paraneoplastic glomerulopathies occur in a variety of different forms, including membranous glomerulonephritis, nephrotic syndrome, and amyloidosis. Many involve renal deposition of immunoglobulins or immune complexes containing tumor antigens with host antibodies. Amyloidosis is marked by deposition of a unique protein called *amyloid* and is most often associated with renal cell carcinoma. Glomerulopathies are relatively common in lymphoma and leukemia.

Dermatologic and Rheumatologic Abnormalities

Paraneoplastic dermatologic and rheumatologic conditions can occur without overt evidence of malignancy, but their appearance should initiate screening for an underlying cancer. Acanthosis nigricans is a thickening and hyperpigmentation of the skin. It usually occurs in the axilla or neck and is most commonly related to insulin resistance or other non–cancer-related conditions. When found on the palms, it is almost always associated with cancer, most often an adenocarcinoma. Dermatomyositis is an inflammatory condition that causes proximal muscle weakness as well as characteristic skin changes, including a rash on the eyelids and hands. It can be seen with ovarian, breast, lung, prostate, and colorectal cancers. Hypertrophic osteoarthropathy—commonly known as *clubbing*—involves subperiosteal bone deposition that causes a characteristic remodeling of the phalangeal shafts. It is classically associated with intrathoracic tumors or metastases to the lungs.

Hematologic Abnormalities

Paraneoplastic hematologic syndromes are rarely symptomatic but are usually present with advanced cancer. Paraneoplastic eosinophilia is related to production of specific interleukins that promote eosinophilic differentiation and is most often seen in leukemia and lymphoma. Eosinophilia can sometimes cause wheezing or occasionally end-organ damage resulting from eosinophilic infiltration. Granulocytosis usually occurs with solid tumors, particularly large cell lung cancer. Pure red cell aplasia is commonly associated with thymoma, but also occurs with leukemia and lymphoma. Underlying malignancy is the diagnosis in about a third of patients with thrombocytosis (platelet count >400,000/mm^3). It appears to be caused by tumor-released cytokines such as IL-6.

LOCAL EFFECTS OF CANCER AND METASTASES

Superior Vena Cava Syndrome/Superior Mediastinal Syndrome

Obstruction of the superior vena cava is caused by spread of cancer into the mediastinum or directly into the caval wall and is most often associated with lung cancer. Veins above the level of the heart, particularly the jugular veins and veins in the arms, become engorged. Edema of the face and upper extremities is usually prominent. Increased intracranial pressure manifests as nausea, seizures, and decreased levels of consciousness and is most likely due to the increase in cerebral venous pressure. Compression of the great vessels may cause syncope.

Superior mediastinal syndrome is the combination of superior vena cava syndrome and tracheal compression. Hoarseness, dyspnea, and airway obstruction may be present because of tracheal compression. Treatment consists of prompt radiation therapy or chemotherapy for symptomatic relief. Bronchoscopy and/or mediastinoscopy to obtain a tissue diagnosis can be very hazardous, especially in the presence of co-existing airway obstruction and increased pressure in the mediastinal veins.

Spinal Cord Compression

Spinal cord compression results from the presence of metastatic lesions in the epidural space, most often breast, lung, or prostate cancer or lymphoma. Symptoms include pain, skeletal muscle weakness, sensory loss, and autonomic dysfunction. CT and MRI can visualize the limits of compression. Radiation therapy is a useful treatment when neurologic deficits are only partial or in development. Corticosteroids are often administered to minimize the inflammation and edema that can result from radiation directed at tumors in the epidural space. Once total paralysis has developed, the results of surgical laminectomy or radiation treatment to decompress the spinal cord are poor.

Increased Intracranial Pressure

Metastatic brain tumors, most often from lung and breast cancer, present initially as mental deterioration, focal neurologic deficits, or seizures. Treatment of an acute increase in intracranial pressure caused by a metastatic lesion includes corticosteroids, diuretics, and mannitol. Radiation therapy is the usual palliative treatment, but surgery can be considered for patients with only a single metastatic lesion. Intrathecal administration of chemotherapeutic drugs is usually necessary when the tumor involves the meninges.

CANCER PAIN

Cancer patients may experience acute pain associated with pathologic fractures, tumor invasion, surgery, radiation treatment, and chemotherapy. Pain is frequently related to metastatic spread of the cancer, especially to bone. Nerve compression or infiltration may also cause pain. Patients with cancer who experience frequent and significant pain often exhibit signs of depression and anxiety.

Pathophysiology

Cancer pain resulting from organic causes may be subdivided into nociceptive and neuropathic pain. Nociceptive pain includes somatic and visceral pain and refers to pain caused by the peripheral stimulation of nociceptors in somatic or visceral structures. Somatic pain is related to tumor involvement of somatic structures such as bones or skeletal muscles and is often described as aching, stabbing, or throbbing. Visceral pain is related to lesions in a hollow or solid viscus and is described as diffuse, gnawing, or crampy if a hollow viscus is involved and as aching or sharp if a solid viscus is involved. Nociceptive pain is typically responsive to both nonopioid and opioid medication. Neuropathic pain involves peripheral or central afferent neural pathways and is commonly described as burning or lancinating pain. Patients experiencing neuropathic pain often respond poorly to opioids.

Trauma associated with surgery for removal of cancerous tissue may also be a cause of chronic pain. Scars and injury of soft tissue and of sensory afferents that innervate the surgical area may contribute to the development of chronic pain.

Drug Therapy

Drug therapy is the cornerstone of cancer pain management because of its efficacy, rapid onset of action, and relatively low cost. Mild to moderate cancer pain is initially treated with nonsteroidal antiinflammatory drugs (NSAIDs) and acetaminophen. NSAIDs are especially effective for managing bone pain, which is the most common type of cancer pain. The next step in management of cancer pain is the addition of codeine or one of its analogues. When cancer pain is severe, more potent opioids are employed. Morphine is commonly selected and can be administered orally. When the oral route of administration is inadequate, alternative routes (intravenous, subcutaneous, epidural, intrathecal, transmucosal, transdermal) are considered. Fentanyl is available in transdermal and transmucosal delivery systems. Tolerance to opioids does occur and may necessitate dosage adjustment. Fear of addiction is a major reason why opioids are underutilized, but addiction is rare when these drugs are correctly managed.

Tricyclic antidepressant drugs are indicated for patients with depressive symptoms. These drugs may also exhibit analgesic properties by potentiating the effects of opioids. Anticonvulsants are useful for the management of chronic neuropathic pain. Corticosteroids can decrease pain perception, have a sparing effect on opioid requirements, improve mood, increase appetite, and lead to weight gain. Multimodal analgesia with local anesthetics and adjunctive agents such as gabapentin and ketamine may be effective in preventing both acute and chronic pain and reducing analgesic use after surgery.

Neuraxial Analgesia

Neuraxial analgesia is an effective way to control pain in cancer patients undergoing surgery and may play a role in providing preemptive analgesia. Neuraxial analgesia with local anesthetics provides immediate pain relief in patients whose pain cannot be alleviated with oral or intravenous analgesics and is frequently employed for the treatment of cancer pain.

Neuraxial analgesia is not used in patients with local infection, bacteremia, and systemic infection because of the increased risk of epidural abscess. However, in the setting of intractable cancer pain, there may be a role for epidural analgesia despite the risk of meningeal infection. Morphine may be administered intrathecally or epidurally for management of acute and chronic cancer pain. Spinal opioids may be delivered for weeks to months via a long-term, subcutaneously tunneled, exteriorized catheter or an implanted drug delivery system. The implantable systems can be intrathecal or epidural and typically feature a drug reservoir and the capability for external programming. Patients are typically considered for neuraxial opioid administration when systemic opioid administration has failed because of the occurrence of intolerable adverse effects or inadequate analgesia. Neuraxial administration of opioids is usually successful, but some patients may require the addition of a dilute concentration of local anesthetic to the infusate to achieve adequate pain control.

Neurolytic Procedures

Neurolytic procedures intended to destroy sensory components of nerves cannot be used without also destroying motor and autonomic nervous system fibers. Important considerations in determining the suitability of a destructive nerve block are the location and quality of the pain, the effectiveness of less destructive treatment modalities, the inherent risks associated with the block, the availability of experienced anesthesiologists to perform the procedures, and the patient's anticipated life expectancy. In general, constant pain is more amenable to destructive nerve block than is intermittent pain. Neurolytic celiac plexus block with alcohol or phenol has been used to treat pain originating from abdominal viscera, especially in the context of pancreatic cancer. The block is associated with significant adverse effects, but analgesia usually lasts 6 months or longer.

Neuroablative or neurostimulatory procedures for managing cancer pain are reserved for patients whose pain is unresponsive to other less invasive procedures. Cordotomy involves interruption of the spinothalamic tract in the spinal cord and is considered for treatment of unilateral pain involving the lower extremity, thorax, or upper extremity. Dorsal rhizotomy involves interruption of sensory nerve roots and is used when pain is localized to specific dermatomal levels. Dorsal column stimulators or deep brain stimulators may be used in select patients.

MANAGEMENT OF ANESTHESIA

Preoperative evaluation of patients with cancer includes consideration of the pathophysiologic effects of the disease and recognition of the potential adverse effects of cancer treatments (Table 23-4). In addition, the patient's underlying medical comorbidities must not be overlooked. Correction of nutrient deficiencies, electrolyte abnormalities, anemia, and coagulopathies may be needed preoperatively. In most cases,

laboratory evaluation should include complete blood count, coagulation profile, serum electrolyte concentrations, and transaminase levels. Chest radiography, echocardiography, pulmonary function evaluation, and other specialized testing should be used if clinical suspicion warrants. There are no specific rules regarding the preoperative management of chemotherapeutic drugs. However, most of them have the potential to impair wound healing, especially the growth factor and angiogenesis inhibitors. It has been suggested that surgery be delayed for 4 to 8 weeks after treatment with bevacizumab because of an increased risk of bleeding and postoperative wound complications.

Potential pulmonary or cardiac toxicity is a consideration in patients being treated with chemotherapeutic drugs known to be associated with these complications. The myocardial-depressant effects of anesthesia can unmask cardiac dysfunction related to cardiotoxic chemotherapeutic drugs such as doxorubicin. Therefore, when major surgery is planned, preoperative echocardiography may be indicated. Since several chemotherapeutic agents can cause electrocardiographic abnormalities such as QT prolongation, a baseline electrocardiogram should be reviewed.

A preoperative history of drug-induced pulmonary fibrosis (dyspnea, nonproductive cough) or congestive heart failure will influence the subsequent management of anesthesia. In patients treated with bleomycin, it may be helpful to perform arterial blood gas monitoring in addition to oximetry and to carefully titrate intravascular fluid replacement, since these patients are at risk of developing interstitial pulmonary edema, presumably because of impaired lymphatic drainage in the lung. Bleomycin-associated pulmonary injury may be exacerbated by high oxygen concentrations; therefore, it is prudent to adjust the delivered oxygen concentration to the minimum that provides adequate oxygen saturation. Nitrous oxide may augment the toxicity of methotrexate, so it is best avoided.

The presence of hepatic or renal dysfunction should influence the choice and dose of anesthetic drugs and muscle relaxants. Although it is not consistently observed, the possibility of a prolonged response to succinylcholine is a consideration in patients being treated with alkylating chemotherapeutic drugs like cyclophosphamide. The presence of paraneoplastic syndromes such as myasthenia gravis and Eaton-Lambert syndrome may also affect the patient's response to muscle relaxants.

Attention to aseptic technique is important, because immunosuppression occurs with most chemotherapeutic agents and is exacerbated by malnutrition. Immunosuppression produced by anesthesia, surgical stress, or blood transfusion during the perioperative period could have deleterious effects on the patient's subsequent response to his or her cancer. Adrenal suppression may be present in patients who are being treated with steroids. Those who have been receiving more than 20 mg of prednisone (or its equivalent) per day for longer than 3 weeks are considered most at risk. Recovery of the hypothalamic-pituitary-adrenal axis may take up to a year. A typical steroid replacement regimen is hydrocortisone 100 mg IV

TABLE 23-4 ■ **Preanesthetic evaluation of the cancer patient**

System	Risk factors	Investigations	Anesthetic considerations
Cardiovascular	Doxorubicin exposure Radiation to the mediastinum Anterior mediastinal mass	Chest radiograph Chest CT scan Echocardiogram	Left ventricular dysfunction Dysrhythmias Engorgement of great vessels
Pulmonary	Bleomycin, busulfan, chlorambucil exposure Radiation to the thorax	Arterial blood gas analysis Chest radiograph Chest CT scan Flow-volume loops Pulmonary function tests	Obstructive/restrictive disease Avoid high concentrations of oxygen with history of bleomycin exposure
Renal and hepatic	Induction chemotherapy or radiation therapy Tumor lysis syndrome	Renal and liver function tests Coagulation profile Uric acid level	Acute renal failure with tumor lysis syndrome Adjust dosage based on end-organ damage
Hematologic	Metastatic disease Exposure to most chemotherapeutic drugs and radiation	Complete blood count Coagulation profile	Infection risk Bleeding risk Thromboembolism prophylaxis
Neurologic	Cisplatin, vincristine, fluorouracil exposure Metastatic disease Paraneoplastic syndromes (myasthenia gravis, Eaton-Lambert syndrome)	Physical examination and documentation of preexisting sensorimotor defects	Elevated intracranial pressure, papilledema, spinal cord compression due to metastases Phrenic nerve palsy in presence of metastases or superior vena cava syndrome Exercise caution with peripheral nerve blocks, neuraxial anesthesia
Gastrointestinal	Exposure to all chemotherapeutic drugs and radiation Advanced cancer	Physical examination Serum electrolyte and prealbumin levels	Hypovolemia Electrolyte abnormalities Metabolic acidosis/alkalosis Mucositis/oral ulcerations that may predispose to bleeding with airway instrumentation Increased aspiration risk in presence of nausea/vomiting Increased infection risk, poor wound healing
Endocrine	Steroid exposure Paraneoplastic syndromes—SIADH, hypercalcemia	Preoperative medication history Serum electrolyte levels	Risk of electrolyte abnormalities (hyponatremia, hypercalcemia, hypocalcemia) Consider stress-dose steroids with adrenal insufficiency
Airway	Radiation to head/neck Anterior mediastinal mass	Physical examination Chest radiograph Chest CT scan Flow-volume loops	Difficult airway precautions Tracheal compression Airway collapse with cessation of spontaneous ventilation

Adapted from Latham GJ, Greenberg RS. Anesthetic considerations for the pediatric oncology patient—part 3: pain, cognitive dysfunction, and preoperative evaluation. *Paediatr Anaesthes*. 2010;20(6):486, Fig 2.
CT, Computed tomography; *SIADH,* syndrome of inappropriate antidiuretic hormone secretion.

administered at induction of anesthesia followed by 100 mg IV every 8 hours for the first 24 hours after surgery.

Intubation in the presence of oral mucositis may cause bleeding. Patients with cancers of the head, neck, and anterior mediastinum may exhibit airway compromise. Patients with a history of radiation exposure may have airway deformities that are difficult to recognize on physical examination.

Recent evidence suggests that anesthetics and analgesics have immunomodulatory properties (see Chapter 24). Intravenous opioids tend to blunt natural killer cell activity, producing an immunosuppressive effect that supports the proliferation of tumor cells. The use of neuraxial anesthesia may preserve the host's intrinsic anticancer defenses better than general anesthesia. However, coagulopathies may prevent the use of these techniques in some cancer patients. Peripheral nerve blocks may be utilized, but baseline peripheral neuropathies related to chemotherapeutic drugs such as vincristine and cisplatin should be well documented.

Postoperative care must include adequate attention to pain management. Many cancer patients have been treated for pain related to their underlying diagnosis. Therefore, narcotic dosing must be adjusted to account for possible drug tolerance. Prophylaxis against infection and thromboembolism must also be considered.

COMMON CANCERS ENCOUNTERED IN CLINICAL PRACTICE

The most common cancers in adults encountered by anesthesiologists in the surgical setting are lung cancer, breast cancer, colon cancer, and prostate cancer. Lung cancer is the second most common malignancy in men, surpassed only by prostate cancer; in women the incidence of lung cancer is increasing and it is now exceeded only by breast cancer.

Lung Cancer

Lung cancer is the leading cause of cancer death among men and women. It is largely a preventable disease, since about 90% of lung cancer deaths are related to cigarette smoking. Five-year survival varies significantly based on stage at diagnosis: 50% of patients with only local disease may survive 5 years, but only 2% of those with distant metastases evident at the time of diagnosis will be alive 5 years later.

ETIOLOGY

The strong association between cigarette smoking and lung cancer is well established. Smoking marijuana produces a greater carbon monoxide and tar burden than smoking a similar quantity of tobacco, and thus its use may pose an additional risk factor for lung cancer in cigarette smokers. The mutagens and carcinogens present in cigarette smoke may cause chromosomal damage and over time may cause malignancy. Other carcinogens that cause lung cancer are ionizing radiation (byproduct of coal and iron mining), asbestos (increases the incidence of lung cancer in nonsmokers and acts as a synergistic cocarcinogen with tobacco smoke), and naturally occurring radon gas. Adjuvant radiation therapy for breast cancer following mastectomy is also associated with an increased risk of lung cancer.

There is a familial risk of lung cancer that is related to genetic and ecogenetic factors and to exposure to passive smoking. Inhalation of second-hand smoke increases the risk of lung cancer and contributes to the development of childhood respiratory infections and asthma. Cigarette smokers who develop emphysema are at increased risk of developing lung cancer. Acquired immunodeficiency syndrome may be associated with an increased incidence of lung cancer. Following cessation of cigarette smoking, the risk and incidence of lung cancer decreases to that of nonsmokers after approximately 10 to 15 years.

SIGNS AND SYMPTOMS

Patients with lung cancer have features related to the extent of the disease, including local and regional manifestations, signs and symptoms of metastatic disease, and various paraneoplastic syndromes related indirectly to the cancer. Cough, hemoptysis, wheezing, stridor, dyspnea, or pneumonitis from airway obstruction may be presenting clinical signs. Mediastinal metastases may cause hoarseness (recurrent laryngeal nerve compression), superior vena cava syndrome, cardiac dysrhythmias, or congestive heart failure from pericardial effusion and tamponade. Pleural effusion results in increasing dyspnea and often chest pain. Generalized weakness, fatigue, anorexia, and weight loss are common.

HISTOLOGIC SUBTYPES

Clinical manifestations of lung cancer vary with the histologic subtype. Non–small cell lung cancer, which includes squamous cell carcinoma, adenocarcinoma, and large cell carcinoma, accounts for about 85% of all new cases of lung cancer.

Squamous cell cancers arise in major bronchi or their primary divisions (central origin) and are usually detected by cytologic analysis of sputum. These tumors tend to grow slowly and may reach a large size before they are finally detected. Hemoptysis, bronchial obstruction with associated atelectasis, dyspnea, and fever from pneumonia are common presenting signs. Cavitation may be evident on chest radiography.

Adenocarcinomas most often originate in the lung periphery. These tumors commonly present as subpleural nodules and have a tendency to invade the pleura and induce pleural effusions that contain malignant cells. Lung adenocarcinomas may be difficult to differentiate morphologically from malignant mesothelioma or adenocarcinoma that has metastasized from other sites such as breast, gastrointestinal tract, or pancreas.

Large cell carcinomas are usually peripheral in origin and present as large, bulky tumors. Like adenocarcinomas, these tumors metastasize early and preferentially to the central nervous system.

Small cell carcinomas are usually of central bronchial origin and have a high frequency of early lymphatic invasion, especially to lymph nodes in the mediastinum, and metastases to liver, bone, central nervous system, adrenal glands, and pancreas. Prominent mediastinal lymphadenopathy may lead to the erroneous diagnosis of malignant lymphoma. Superior vena cava syndrome may result from mediastinal compression. Small cell tumors have a marked propensity to produce polypeptides and ectopic hormones, which results in metabolic abnormalities. The tumors are not usually detected in these patients until the disease process is widespread.

DIAGNOSIS

Cytologic analysis of sputum is often sufficient for the diagnosis of lung cancer, especially when the cancer arises in proximal endobronchial locations where shedding of cells is likely to occur. Peripheral lesions as small as 3 mm can be detected by high-resolution CT. Lung cancer screening has been recommended for patients who are at highest risk, such as cigarette smokers with chronic obstructive lung disease.

Flexible fiberoptic bronchoscopy, in combination with biopsy, brushings, or washings, is a standard procedure for initial evaluation of lung cancer. Peripheral lung lesions can be diagnosed by percutaneous fine-needle aspiration guided by fluoroscopy, ultrasonography, or CT. Video-assisted thoracoscopic surgery is useful for diagnosing peripheral lung lesions and pleura-based tumors. CT is sensitive for detecting pulmonary metastases. Brain MRI and head CT are useful for detecting metastases even in patients without neurologic abnormalities. Mediastinoscopy and video-assisted thoracoscopy provide the opportunity to biopsy lymph nodes and stage the tumor.

TREATMENT

Treatments for lung cancer include surgery, radiation therapy, and chemotherapy. The preferred treatment depends on cell type, stage, and the patient's underlying health.

Pulmonary function testing is used to evaluate the patient's candidacy for lung resection. Forced expiratory volume in 1 second (FEV_1) and diffusing capacity for carbon monoxide (D_{LCO}) are considered among the most useful predictors of postoperative complications. If FEV_1 is more than 2 L and D_{LCO} is more than 80%, patients are at low risk of postoperative respiratory complications. When patients are not clearly in a low-risk category, predicted postoperative pulmonary function can be evaluated. Predicted postoperative pulmonary function takes into consideration preoperative lung function, the amount of lung tissue that will be resected, and the relative contribution of that tissue to overall lung function. Ideally, its calculation is based on preoperative pulmonary function test results as well as some quantitative measure of differential lung function, such as ventilation-perfusion scanning. Predicted postoperative FEV_1 can also be estimated using a formula that takes into account the number of lung segments expected to be removed: predicted postoperative FEV_1 = preoperative $FEV_1 \times$ (number of segments remaining postoperatively/total number of lung segments). In general, if predicted postoperative FEV_1 is less than 0.8 L, patients are considered poor candidates for pneumonectomy. Cardiopulmonary exercise testing with measurement of maximum oxygen consumption is another test that can be used to evaluate patients at high risk.

Surgery has little effect on survival when the disease has spread to mediastinal lymph nodes or when metastases are present. Even among those considered to have surgically curable disease, recurrent metastatic disease develops in half of patients within 5 years. For these reasons, many patients with non–small cell lung cancers are candidates for chemotherapy alone or in combination with surgery or radiation therapy. Video-assisted thoracoscopy is the preferred surgical approach, especially for wedge resection and lobectomy. Standard thoracotomy is needed for more complex procedures or pneumonectomy. In most patients, radiation therapy is effective in palliating symptoms from tumor invasion.

Radiation therapy is the preferred treatment for small cell carcinoma because it is particularly radiosensitive and the cancer is not detected in most patients until disease is extensive. Chemotherapy is used as an adjunct.

MANAGEMENT OF ANESTHESIA

Management of anesthesia in patients with lung cancer includes preoperative consideration of tumor-induced effects such as malnutrition, pneumonia, pain, and ectopic hormone production leading to imbalances like hyponatremia

or hypercalcemia. When resection of lung tissue is planned, it is important to evaluate underlying pulmonary and cardiac function.

Hemorrhage and pneumothorax are the most frequently encountered complications of mediastinoscopy. The mediastinoscope can also exert pressure on the right innominate artery, causing loss of the radial pulse and an erroneous diagnosis of cardiac arrest. Likewise, unrecognized compression of the right innominate artery, of which the right carotid artery is a branch, may manifest as a postoperative neurologic deficit. Bradycardia during mediastinoscopy may be due to stretching of the vagus nerve or tracheal compression by the mediastinoscope. Lung resection requires the ability to perform differential lung ventilation, such as with a double-lumen tube or bronchial blocker.

Colorectal Cancer

Colon cancer is second only to lung cancer as a cause of cancer deaths in the United States. Almost all colorectal cancers are adenocarcinomas, and the disease generally occurs in adults older than 50 years.

ETIOLOGY

Most colorectal cancers arise from premalignant adenomatous polyps. Although adenomatous polyps are common (present in >30% of patients aged >50 years), fewer than 1% become malignant. Large polyps, especially those larger than 1.5 cm in diameter, are more likely to contain invasive cancer. It is thought that adenomatous polyps require 5 to 10 years of growth before they develop into a cancer. The evolution of normal colonic mucosa to a benign adenomatous polyp that contains cancer and then to life-threatening invasive cancer is associated with a series of genetic events that involve the mutational activation of a proto-oncogene and the loss of several genes that normally suppress tumorigenesis.

Most colorectal cancers appear to be related to diet. There is a direct correlation between colorectal cancer incidence and the amount of calories, animal fat, and meat protein consumed. Family history of colorectal cancer, inflammatory bowel disease, and cigarette smoking for longer than 35 years are also risk factors.

DIAGNOSIS

The rationale for colorectal cancer screening is that early detection and removal of localized superficial tumors and precancerous lesions in asymptomatic individuals increases the cure rate. Screening programs (digital rectal examination, examination of the stool for occult blood, colonoscopy) appear to be particularly useful for persons who have first-degree relatives with a history of the disease, especially if these relatives developed colorectal cancer before 55 years of age.

SIGNS AND SYMPTOMS

The presenting signs and symptoms of colorectal cancer reflect the anatomic location of the cancer. Because stool is relatively liquid as it passes into the right colon through the ileocecal valve, tumors in the cecum and ascending colon can become large and markedly narrow the bowel lumen without causing obstructive symptoms. Ascending colon cancers frequently ulcerate, which leads to chronic blood loss in the stool. These patients experience symptoms related to anemia, including fatigue and, in some patients, angina pectoris.

Stool becomes more concentrated as it passes into the transverse colon. Transverse colon cancers cause abdominal cramping, occasional bowel obstruction, and even perforation. Abdominal radiographs reveal characteristic abnormalities in the colonic gas pattern, reflecting narrowing of the lumen ("napkin ring lesion"). Colon cancers developing in the rectosigmoid portion of the large intestine result in tenesmus and thinner stools. Anemia is unusual despite the passage of bright red blood from the rectum (often attributable to hemorrhoids).

Colorectal cancers initially spread to regional lymph nodes and then through the portal venous circulation to the liver, which represents the most common visceral site of metastases. Colorectal cancers rarely spread to lung, bone, or brain in the absence of liver metastases. A preoperative increase in the serum concentration of carcinoembryonic antigen suggests that the tumor will recur following surgical resection. Carcinoembryonic antigen is a glycoprotein that is also increased in the presence of other cancers (stomach, pancreas, breast, lung) and certain nonmalignant conditions (alcoholic liver disease, inflammatory bowel disease, cigarette smoking, pancreatitis).

TREATMENT

The prognosis for patients with adenocarcinoma of the colorectum depends on the depth of tumor penetration into the bowel wall and the presence or absence of regional lymph node involvement and distant metastases (liver, lung, bone). Radical surgical resection, which includes the blood vessels and lymph nodes draining the involved bowel, offers the best potential for cure. Surgical management of cancers that arise in the distal rectum may necessitate a permanent colostomy (abdominoperineal resection). Because most recurrences occur within 3 to 4 years, the cure rate for colorectal cancer is often estimated by 5-year survival rates.

Radiation therapy is considered for patients with rectal tumors, since the risk of recurrence following surgery is significant. Postoperative radiation therapy causes transient diarrhea and cystitis, but permanent damage to the small intestine and bladder is uncommon.

MANAGEMENT OF ANESTHESIA

Management of anesthesia for surgical resection of colorectal cancers may be influenced by anemia and the effects of metastatic lesions in liver, lung, bone, or brain. Chronic large bowel obstruction probably does not increase the risk of aspiration during induction of anesthesia, although abdominal distention could interfere with adequate ventilation and oxygenation. Blood transfusion during surgical resection of colorectal cancers has been alleged to be associated with a decrease in the length of patient survival. This could reflect immunosuppression produced by transfused blood. For this reason, careful review of the risks and benefits of blood transfusions in these patients is prudent.

Prostate Cancer

The reported number of cases of prostate cancer has increased dramatically in recent years, which presumably reflects the widespread use of prostate-specific antigen (PSA) testing. The incidence of prostate cancer is highest in African Americans and lowest in Asians. The presence of the hereditary prostate cancer gene mutation (*HPC1*) greatly increases the risk of developing prostate cancer. The possibility that vasectomy may be associated with an increased risk of prostate cancer has not been substantiated. Prostate cancer is almost always an adenocarcinoma.

DIAGNOSIS

The use of PSA-based screening has changed the way prostate cancer is diagnosed. An increased serum PSA concentration may indicate the presence of prostate cancer in asymptomatic men and prompt a digital rectal examination. Detection of a discrete nodule or diffuse induration on digital rectal examination raises suspicion of prostate cancer, especially in the presence of impotence or symptoms of urinary obstruction (frequency, nocturia, hesitancy, urgency). However, the rectal examination can evaluate only the posterior and lateral aspects of the prostate. If the rectal examination indicates the possible presence of cancer, transrectal ultrasonography and biopsy are needed regardless of the PSA concentration. There is a much greater likelihood of detecting cancer if the PSA level is higher than 10 ng/mL, regardless of the findings on rectal examination. Infrequently, patients have symptoms of metastatic disease, such as bone pain and weight loss, at presentation.

TREATMENT

Focal, well-differentiated prostate cancers are usually cured by transurethral resection. However, recurrent disease may develop in up to 16% of these patients within 8 years. For this reason, more aggressive treatment such as radical prostatectomy or radiation therapy may be indicated in subsets of these patients, especially those younger than 65 years of age. If lymph nodes are involved, radical prostatectomy or definitive radiation therapy may be recommended. Radical prostatectomy can be performed via a retropubic or perineal approach. Use of the retropubic approach permits the surgeon to take lymph node samples for frozen section before beginning the prostatectomy. Radiation therapy can be delivered either by an external beam or by implantation of radioactive seeds. The decision to select surgery or radiation therapy is based on the adverse effects of each treatment and the patient's overall health. Impotence and urinary incontinence are risks of radical prostatectomy. Preservation of the neurovascular bundles on each side of the prostate may decrease the risk of impotence following surgery. Radiation therapy produces impotence less often, but debilitating cystitis or proctitis may develop.

Hormone therapy is indicated for management of metastatic prostate cancer, because these tumors are under the trophic influence of androgens. Androgen deprivation therapy dramatically reduces testosterone levels and causes tumor regression. Androgen deprivation can be accomplished by surgical castration, administration of exogenous estrogens such as diethylstilbestrol, use of analogues of gonadotropin-releasing hormone (GNRH) that inhibit the release of pituitary gonadotropins, use of antiandrogens such as flutamide that block the action of androgens at target tissues, and use of combination therapy, such as an antiandrogen in combination with a GNRH agonist or bilateral orchiectomy.

When advanced prostate cancers become resistant to hormone therapy, incapacitating bone pain often develops. Systemic chemotherapy with mitoxantrone plus corticosteroids or estramustine plus a taxane may be effective in palliating pain. In the terminal phases of the disease, administration of high doses of prednisone for short periods may produce subjective improvement.

Breast Cancer

Women in the United States have a 12% lifetime risk of developing breast cancer. The risk of death from breast cancer is approximately 3%. Most women in whom breast cancer is diagnosed do not die of the disease.

RISK FACTORS

The principal risk factors for development of breast cancer are increasing age (75% of cases occur in patients >50 years of age) and family history (a first-degree relative diagnosed with breast cancer before age 50 increases the risk threefold to fourfold). Reproductive risk factors that increase the risk of breast cancer include early menarche, late menopause, late first pregnancy, and nulliparity, all of which are presumed to prolong exposure of the breasts to estrogen. Two breast cancer susceptibility genes (*BRCA1* and *BRCA2*) are mutations that are inherited as autosomal dominant traits.

SCREENING

Recommended screening strategies for breast cancer include the triad of breast self-examination, clinical breast examination by a professional, and screening mammography. Clinical breast examination by a professional and regular mammography appear to decrease mortality from breast cancer by approximately one third in women older than age 50. Annual screening mammography is generally recommended for all women beginning between the ages of 40 and 50 years. A small percentage of breast cancers are not detected by mammography, so alternative screening methods such as ultrasonography and/or MRI may be of value in selected patients.

PROGNOSIS

Axillary lymph node invasion and tumor size are the two most important determinants of outcome in patients with early breast cancer. Other established prognostic factors include the estrogen and progesterone receptor content of the primary tumor and its histologic grade. The absence of estrogen and progesterone receptor expression is associated with a worse prognosis. Most tumors that express receptors are responsive to endocrine therapy.

TREATMENT

Although radical mastectomy (removal of the involved breast, axillary contents, and underlying chest wall musculature) was the principal treatment for invasive breast cancer in the past, it is seldom used in current practice. Breast conservation therapy, including lumpectomy with radiation therapy, simple mastectomy, and modified radical mastectomy provide similar survival rates. Because the likelihood of distant micrometastases is highly correlated with the number of lymph nodes invaded by tumor, axillary lymph node dissection provides prognostic information. Sentinel lymph node mapping involves injection of a radioactive tracer or isosulfan blue dye into the area around the primary breast tumor. The injected substance tracks rapidly to the dominant axillary lymph node (sentinel node). If the sentinel node is tumor free, the remaining lymph nodes are also likely to be tumor free, and further axillary surgery can be avoided. The morbidity associated with breast cancer surgery is now largely related to adverse effects of lymph node dissection such as lymphedema and restricted arm motion. Obesity, weight gain, and infection in the arm are additional risk factors for development of lymphedema. To minimize the risk of lymphedema, it is reasonable to protect the ipsilateral arm from venipuncture, compression, infection, and exposure to heat.

Radiation treatment is an important component of breast conservation therapy, since lumpectomy alone is associated with a high incidence of recurrence. Radiation therapy after a mastectomy is reserved for women with extensive local disease, such as skin and chest wall invasion and extensive lymph node involvement.

Systemic Treatment

Many women with early-stage breast cancer already have distant micrometastases at the time of diagnosis. Systemic therapy is intended to prevent or delay recurrence of the disease. Tamoxifen and other chemotherapeutic agents as well as ovarian ablation are the most commonly used modes of systemic therapy.

Tamoxifen. Tamoxifen is a mixed estrogen agonist-antagonist often referred to as a *selective estrogen receptor modulator*. It acts as an estrogen antagonist on tumor cells but has agonist properties on some other targets. Five years of tamoxifen therapy in patients with estrogen receptor–positive tumors is associated with a significant reduction in the risk of recurrence. Benefits of tamoxifen therapy are similar for patients with node-positive and node-negative disease. However, tamoxifen does not alter outcome in patients with minimal or no estrogen receptor expression on their tumors.

Tamoxifen can cause body temperature disturbances (hot flashes), vaginal discharge, and an increased risk of developing endometrial cancer. Megestrol (progestin) may be administered to decrease the severity of the hot flashes associated with tamoxifen treatment. Tamoxifen lowers serum cholesterol and low-density lipoprotein concentrations, but the importance of these effects in reducing the risk of ischemic heart disease is unclear. Tamoxifen preserves bone density in postmenopausal women by its proestrogenic effects and may decrease the incidence of osteoporosis-related fractures of the hip, spine, and radius. There is an increased risk of thromboembolic events, including deep vein thrombosis, pulmonary embolism, and stroke, with tamoxifen therapy.

Chemotherapy. Combination chemotherapy decreases the rate of recurrence and mortality from breast cancer in patients with both node-positive and node-negative disease. The maximum benefit seems to be in women younger than 50 years of age with node-positive disease. A commonly used combination chemotherapy regimen includes cyclophosphamide, methotrexate, and fluorouracil. The chemotherapy dose is an important determinant of cell kill. Conventional adjuvant chemotherapy usually begins within a few months of surgery. Chemotherapy or radiation therapy may be administered before surgery to selected patients in an attempt to decrease tumor size and improve breast conservation. In women at high risk who have multiple positive lymph nodes, high-dose chemotherapy with alkylating drugs combined with autologous bone marrow transplantation may be considered.

Chemotherapy for breast cancer has adverse effects such as nausea and vomiting, hair loss, and bone marrow suppression that typically resolve following treatment. The most serious late sequelae of chemotherapy are leukemia and doxorubicin-induced cardiac impairment. Patients with symptoms of cardiac disease or congestive heart failure should be evaluated with electrocardiography and echocardiography. Myelodysplastic syndromes or acute myeloid leukemia can occur after chemotherapy, but the incidence is low (0.2% to 1.0%). High-dose radiation therapy may be associated with brachial plexopathy or nerve damage, pneumonitis, and/or pulmonary fibrosis.

Supportive Treatment

Palliation of symptoms and prevention of complications are primary goals when treating advanced breast cancer. The most common site of breast cancer metastasis is bone. Regular administration of bisphosphonates in addition to hormone therapy or chemotherapy can decrease bone pain and lower the incidence of bone complications by inhibiting osteoclastic activity. Adequate pain control is usually achieved with sustained-release oral and/or transdermal opioid preparations.

MANAGEMENT OF ANESTHESIA

Preoperative evaluation includes a review of potential adverse effects related to chemotherapy. Placement of intravenous catheters in the arm at risk of lymphedema is avoided because of the potential to exacerbate lymphedema and the susceptibility to infection. It is also necessary to protect that arm from compression (as from a blood pressure cuff) and heat

exposure. The presence of bone pain and pathologic fractures is noted when considering regional anesthesia and when positioning the patient during surgery. Selection of anesthetic drugs, techniques, and special monitoring is influenced more by the planned surgical procedure than by the presence of breast cancer. Of note, if isosulfan blue dye is injected during the surgical procedure, it is likely that pulse oximetry will demonstrate a transient spurious decrease in the measured oxygen saturation, usually a 3% decrease.

LESS COMMON CANCERS ENCOUNTERED IN CLINICAL PRACTICE

Less commonly encountered cancers include cardiac tumors, head and neck cancers, and cancers involving the endocrine glands, liver, gallbladder, genitourinary tract, and reproductive organs. Lymphomas and leukemias are examples of cancers that involve the lymph glands and blood-forming elements.

Cardiac Tumors

Cardiac tumors may be primary or secondary, benign or malignant. Metastatic cardiac involvement—usually from adjacent lung cancer—occurs 20 to 40 times more often than primary malignant cardiac tumors. Cardiac myxomas account for 40% to 50% of benign cardiac tumors in adults. About three quarters of cardiac myxomas occur in the left atrium, and the remaining 25% occur in the right atrium. Myxomas often demonstrate considerable movement within the cardiac chamber during the cardiac cycle.

Signs and symptoms of cardiac myxomas reflect interference with filling and emptying of the involved cardiac chamber. Left atrial myxoma may mimic mitral valve disease with development of pulmonary edema. Right atrial myxoma often mimics tricuspid disease and can be associated with impaired venous return and evidence of right-sided heart failure. Emboli occur in about a third of patients with cardiac myxomas. These emboli are composed of myxomatous material or thrombi that have formed on the tumor. Because most myxomas are located in the left atrium, systemic embolism is particularly frequent and often involves the retinal and cerebral arteries. Cardiac myxomas may occur as part of a syndrome that includes cutaneous myxomas, myxoid fibroadenomas of the breast, pituitary adenomas, and adrenocortical hyperplasia with Cushing's syndrome. Echocardiography can determine the location, size, shape, attachment, and mobility of cardiac myxomas.

Surgical resection of cardiac myxomas is usually curative. After the diagnosis has been established, prompt surgery is indicated because of the possibility of embolic complications and sudden death. In most cases, cardiac myxomas can be removed easily because they are pedunculated. Intraoperative fragmentation of the tumor must be avoided. All chambers of the heart are examined to rule out the existence of multifocal disease. Mechanical damage to a heart valve or adhesion of the tumor to valve leaflets may necessitate valvuloplasty or valve replacement.

Anesthetic considerations in patients with cardiac myxomas include the possibility of low cardiac output and arterial hypoxemia resulting from obstruction at the mitral or tricuspid valve. Symptoms of obstruction may be exacerbated by changes in body position. The presence of a right atrial myxoma prohibits placement of right atrial or pulmonary artery catheters. Supraventricular dysrhythmias may follow surgical removal of atrial myxomas. In some patients, permanent cardiac pacing may be required because of atrioventricular conduction abnormalities.

Head and Neck Cancers

Head and neck cancers account for approximately 5% of all cancers in the United States, with a predominance in men older than 50 years of age. Most patients have a history of excessive alcohol use and cigarette smoking. The most common sites of metastases are lung, liver, and bone. Hypercalcemia may be associated with bony metastases, and altered liver function test results presumably reflect alcohol-induced disease. Preoperative nutritional therapy may be indicated before surgical resection. The goal of chemotherapy, if selected, is to decrease the bulk of the primary tumor or known metastases and thereby enhance the efficacy of subsequent surgery or radiation treatment. A secondary goal is eradication of occult micrometastases.

Anesthetic considerations in patients with head and neck cancers include the possibility of distorted airway anatomy that may not be appreciated on external airway examination. Available diagnostic images and the report of nasal fiberoptic examination should be reviewed preoperatively. Preparation must be made for the possibility of difficult ventilation and/or intubation.

Thyroid Cancer

Papillary and follicular thyroid carcinomas are among the most curable of all cancers. Thyroid cancers are more frequent in women. External radiation to the neck during childhood increases the risk of papillary thyroid cancer, as does a family history of the disease. Medullary thyroid cancers may be associated with pheochromocytomas in an autosomal dominant disorder known as *multiple endocrine neoplasia type II*. This type of thyroid cancer typically produces large amounts of thyrocalcitonin, which provides a sensitive measure of the presence of the disease as well as its successful cure.

Subtotal and total thyroidectomy result in lower recurrence rates than more limited partial thyroidectomy. Even with total thyroidectomy, some thyroid tissue remains, as detected by postoperative scanning with radioactive iodine. Risks of total thyroidectomy include recurrent laryngeal nerve injury (2%) and permanent hypoparathyroidism (2%). Patients with papillary thyroid cancers require dissection of paratracheal and tracheoesophageal lymph nodes. The growth of papillary and follicular tumor cells is controlled by thyrotropin, and inhibition of thyrotropin secretion with thyroxine improves

long-term survival. External beam radiation can be used for palliative treatment of obstructive and bony metastases.

Esophageal Cancer

Esophageal cancer has two histologic subtypes: squamous cell and adenocarcinoma. Excessive alcohol consumption and long-term cigarette smoking are independent risk factors for the development of squamous cell carcinoma of the esophagus. The risk of adenocarcinoma is highest in people with Barrett's esophagus, a complication of gastroesophageal reflux disease. Dysphagia and weight loss are the initial symptoms of esophageal cancer in most patients. The dysphagia may be associated with malnutrition. Difficulty swallowing may result in regurgitation and increase the risk of aspiration. The disease has usually metastasized by the time clinical symptoms are present. The lack of a serosal layer around the esophagus and the presence of an extensive lymphatic system are responsible for the rapid spread of tumor to adjacent lymph nodes. However, in patients with Barrett's esophagus who undergo routine endoscopic surveillance, the disease can be diagnosed at a very early stage.

Even with aggressive treatment, the 5-year survival rate for patients with squamous cell carcinoma is only 15% to 20%. Esophagectomy is often performed for carcinoma of the esophagus and is associated with significant morbidity and mortality. Chemotherapy and radiation therapy may be instituted before surgical resection is attempted. Adenocarcinomas are radioinsensitive, but chemotherapy and surgery may improve survival. Palliation may include surgical placement of a feeding tube, bougienage, or endoscopic stent placement.

The likelihood of underlying alcohol-induced liver disease, chronic obstructive pulmonary disease from cigarette smoking, and cross-tolerance of anesthetic drugs in patients who abuse alcohol are considerations during anesthetic management of patients with esophageal cancer. Extensive weight loss often parallels a decrease in intravascular fluid volume and manifests as hypotension during induction and maintenance of anesthesia.

Gastric Cancer

The incidence of gastric cancer has decreased dramatically since 1930, when it was the leading cause of cancer-related death among men in the United States. Achlorhydria (loss of gastric acidity), pernicious anemia, chronic gastritis, and *Helicobacter* infection contribute to the development of gastric cancer. The presenting features of gastric cancer (indigestion, epigastric distress, anorexia) are indistinguishable from those of benign peptic ulcer disease. Approximately 90% of gastric cancers are adenocarcinomas, and approximately half of them occur in the distal portion of the stomach. Gastric cancer is usually far advanced when signs and symptoms such as weight loss, palpable epigastric mass, jaundice, and ascites appear.

Complete surgical eradication of gastric tumors with resection of adjacent lymph nodes is the only treatment that may be curative. Resection of the primary lesion also offers the best palliation. Gastric cancer is relatively resistant to radiation therapy, but it is one of the few gastrointestinal tumors that may have some response to chemotherapy.

Liver Cancer

Liver cancer occurs most often in men with liver disease caused by hepatitis B or hepatitis C virus, alcohol consumption, or hemochromatosis. Initial manifestations are typically abdominal pain, palpable abdominal mass, and constitutional symptoms such as anorexia and weight loss. There may be compression of the inferior vena cava and/or portal vein, lower extremity edema, ascites, and jaundice. Laboratory findings reflect the abnormalities associated with underlying chronic liver disease. Liver function test results are likely to be abnormal. CT and MRI can determine the anatomic location of the tumor, although angiography may be more useful for distinguishing hepatocellular cancer (hypervascular) from hepatic metastases (hypovascular) and for determining whether a tumor is resectable. Radical surgical resection or liver transplantation offers the only hope for survival, but most patients with liver cancer are not surgical candidates because of extensive cirrhosis, impaired liver function, and the presence of extrahepatic disease. Chemotherapy and radiation therapy are of limited value.

Pancreatic Cancer

Pancreatic cancer, despite its low incidence, is the fourth most common cause of cancer-related death in men and women in the United States. There is no evidence linking this cancer to caffeine ingestion, cholelithiasis, or diabetes mellitus, but cigarette smoking, obesity, and chronic pancreatitis show a positive correlation. Approximately 95% of pancreatic cancers are ductal adenocarcinomas, with most occurring in the head of the pancreas. Abdominal pain, anorexia, and weight loss are the usual initial symptoms. Pain suggests retroperitoneal invasion and infiltration of splanchnic nerves. Jaundice reflects biliary obstruction in patients with tumor in the head of the pancreas. Diabetes mellitus is rare in patients who develop pancreatic cancer.

Pancreatic cancer may appear as a localized mass or as diffuse enlargement of the gland. Biopsy is needed to confirm the diagnosis. Complete surgical resection is the only effective treatment. Patients most likely to have resectable lesions are those with tumors in the head of the pancreas that cause painless jaundice. Extrapancreatic spread eliminates the possibility of surgical cure. The two most commonly employed surgical resection techniques are total pancreatectomy and pancreaticoduodenectomy (Whipple's procedure). Total pancreatectomy is technically easier but has the disadvantage of producing diabetes mellitus and malabsorption. Even when surgical resection can be performed, only about 10% of patients survive for 5 years. The median survival for patients with unresectable tumors is 5 months. Palliative procedures

include radiation therapy, chemotherapy, and surgical diversion of the biliary system to relieve obstruction. Celiac plexus block with alcohol or phenol is the most effective intervention for treating the pain associated with pancreatic cancer. A complication of celiac plexus block is hypotension resulting from sympathetic denervation in these often hypovolemic patients. CT guidance of a celiac plexus block may be used to confirm proper needle placement before any neurolytic solution is injected into the celiac plexus.

Renal Cell Cancer

Renal cell cancer most often manifests as hematuria, mild anemia, and flank pain. Risk factors include a family history of renal cancer and cigarette smoking. Renal ultrasonography can help identify renal cysts, and CT and MRI are useful for determining the presence and extent of disease. Laboratory testing may reveal eosinophilia and renal function abnormalities. Paraneoplastic syndromes, especially hypercalcemia caused by ectopic parathyroid hormone secretion and erythrocytosis resulting from ectopic erythropoietin production, are not uncommon. The only curative treatment for renal cell carcinoma confined to the kidneys is radical nephrectomy with regional lymphadenectomy. Radical nephrectomy is not helpful in patients with distant metastases, but chemotherapy may have some benefit.

Bladder Cancer

Bladder cancer occurs more often in men and is associated with cigarette smoking and long-term exposure to chemicals used in the dye (aniline), leather, and rubber industries. The most common presenting feature is hematuria.

Treatment of noninvasive bladder cancer includes endoscopic resection and intravesical chemotherapy, often with BCG. Carcinoma in situ of the bladder often behaves aggressively and may require cystectomy to help prevent muscle invasion and metastatic spread. In men, radical cystectomy includes removal of the bladder, prostate, and proximal urethra. In women, a hysterectomy, oophorectomy, and partial vaginectomy are required. Urinary diversion is either by ureteroileostomy (ileal conduit) or creation of an artificial bladder (neobladder) from segments of small bowel. Traditional treatments for metastatic disease include radiation therapy and chemotherapy.

Testicular Cancer

Although testicular cancer is rare, it is the most common cancer in young men and represents a tumor that can be cured even when distant metastases are present. Orchiopexy before 2 years of age is recommended for cryptorchidism to decrease the risk of testicular cancer. Testicular cancer usually presents as a painless testicular mass. When the diagnosis is suspected, an inguinal orchiectomy is performed and the diagnosis is histologically confirmed. A transscrotal biopsy is not performed because disruption of the scrotum may predispose to local recurrence and/or metastatic spread to inguinal lymphatics. Germ cell cancers, which account for 95% of testicular cancers, can be subdivided into seminomas and nonseminomas. Seminomas metastasize through regional lymphatics to the retroperitoneum and mediastinum, and nonseminomas spread hematogenously to viscera, especially the lungs.

Patients with seminomas that do not extend beyond the retroperitoneal lymph nodes are treated with radiation. Chemotherapy is recommended when seminomas are large, present with several anatomic levels of nodal involvement, or have spread above the diaphragm. Nonseminomas are not radiation sensitive and are treated with retroperitoneal lymph node dissection and combination chemotherapy.

Cervical and Uterine Cancer

Cancer of the uterine cervix is the most common gynecologic cancer in females aged 15 to 34 years. Infection with HPV types 16 and 18 are responsible for approximately 70% of cervical cancers. Vaccination against these viruses is expected to reduce the incidence of cervical cancers in future generations. Carcinoma in situ detected by Papanicolaou's test is treated with cone biopsy, whereas more extensive local disease or disease that has metastasized is treated with some combination of surgery, radiation therapy, and chemotherapy.

Cancer involving the uterine endometrium occurs most frequently in women 50 to 70 years of age and may be associated with estrogen replacement therapy at menopause, more than 5 years of tamoxifen treatment for breast cancer, obesity, hypertension, and diabetes mellitus. Endometrial cancer is often diagnosed at an early stage because more than 90% of patients have postmenopausal or irregular bleeding. The initial evaluation of these patients often includes fractional dilation and curettage. In the absence of metastatic disease, a total abdominal hysterectomy and bilateral salpingo-oophorectomy with or without radiation to the pelvic and periaortic lymph nodes is usually the treatment of choice. Hormone therapy with progesterone may be useful for metastatic disease. Metastatic endometrial cancer responds poorly to traditional chemotherapy.

Ovarian Cancer

Ovarian cancer is the most deadly of the gynecologic malignancies. Ovarian cancer is most likely to develop in women who experience early menopause or who have a family history of ovarian cancer. Early ovarian cancer is usually asymptomatic, so advanced disease is often present by the time the cancer is discovered. Widespread intraabdominal metastases to lymph nodes, omentum, and peritoneum are frequently present. Surgery is the treatment of choice for both early-stage and advanced ovarian cancer. Aggressive tumor debulking, even if all cancer cannot be removed, improves the length and quality of survival. Intraperitoneal chemotherapy is indicated postoperatively in most women and is usually well tolerated.

Skin Cancer

Skin cancer is a very common cancer in the United States. Skin cancers are either melanomas or nonmelanomas. Nonmelanonas include basal cell carcinomas and squamous cell carcinomas. Basal cell carcinoma is the most common type of skin cancer. Most of these cancers grow superficially and rarely metastasize, so local treatment (excision, topical chemotherapy, cryotherapy) is usually curative.

Melanoma accounts for only about 5% of all skin cancers, but 75% of skin cancer deaths. The incidence of cutaneous melanoma is increasing. Sunlight (ultraviolet light) is an important environmental factor in the pathogenesis of melanoma. The initial treatment of a suspected lesion is wide and deep excisional biopsy, often with sentinel node mapping. Melanoma can metastasize to virtually any organ. Treatment of metastatic melanoma focuses on palliation and can include resection of a solitary metastasis, simple or combination chemotherapy, and/or immunotherapy.

Bone Cancer

Bone cancers include multiple myeloma, osteosarcoma, Ewing's sarcoma, and chondrosarcoma.

MULTIPLE MYELOMA

Multiple myeloma (plasma cell myeloma) is a malignant neoplasm characterized by poorly controlled growth of a single clone of plasma cells that produce a monoclonal immunoglobulin. Multiple myeloma accounts for approximately 10% of hematologic cancers and 1% of all cancers in the United States. The disease is more common in elderly patients (median age at time of diagnosis is 65 years), and it occurs twice as often in African Americans as in Caucasians. The cause of multiple myeloma is unknown. Its extent, complications, sensitivity to drugs, and clinical course vary greatly.

The most frequent manifestations of multiple myeloma are bone pain (often from vertebral collapse), anemia, thrombocytopenia, neutropenia, hypercalcemia, renal failure, and recurrent bacterial infection reflecting bone marrow invasion by tumor cells. Extramedullary plasmacytomas can produce compression of the spinal cord. This occurs in approximately 10% of patients. Other extramedullary sites of tumor invasion include the liver, spleen, ribs, and skull. Inactivation of plasma procoagulants by myeloma proteins may interfere with coagulation. These proteins coat the platelets and interfere with platelet function. The presence of hypercalcemia from excessive bone destruction should be suspected in patients with myeloma who develop nausea, fatigue, confusion, or polyuria. Renal insufficiency occurs in approximately 25% of patients with multiple myeloma resulting from either deposition of an abnormal protein (Bence Jones protein) in renal tubules or the development of acute renal failure. Amyloidosis or immunoglobulin deposition can cause nephrotic syndrome or contribute to renal failure. The combination of hypogammaglobulinemia, granulocytopenia, and depressed cell-mediated immunity increases the risk of infection. Development of fever in patients with multiple myeloma is an indication for antibiotic therapy. In an estimated 20% of patients, multiple myeloma is diagnosed by chance in the absence of symptoms when screening laboratory studies reveal increased serum protein concentrations.

Treatment of overt symptomatic multiple myeloma most often includes autologous stem cell transplantation and chemotherapy. Palliative radiation therapy is limited to patients who have disabling pain and a well-defined focal process that has not responded to chemotherapy. The median duration of remission is approximately 2 years and the median survival time approximately 3 years, but these vary depending on the cytogenetic characteristics of the myeloma cells. Signs of spinal cord compression resulting from an extramedullary plasmacytoma require early confirmation and prompt radiation therapy. Urgent decompressive laminectomy to avoid permanent paralysis may be needed if radiation treatment is not effective. Chemotherapy reverses mild renal failure in many patients with multiple myeloma, but temporary hemodialysis may be necessary until chemotherapy becomes effective. Erythropoietin therapy may be indicated to treat anemia. Hypercalcemia requires prompt treatment with volume expansion and saline diuresis. Bed rest is avoided, because inactivity leads to further mobilization of calcium from bone and increased risk of deep vein thrombosis.

The presence of compression fractures requires caution when positioning patients during anesthesia and surgery. Fluid therapy depends on the degree of renal insufficiency and/or hypercalcemia. Pathologic fractures of the ribs may impair ventilation and predispose to the development of pneumonia.

OSTEOSARCOMA

Osteosarcoma occurs most often in adolescents and typically involves the distal femur and proximal tibia. A genetic predisposition is suggested by the association of this tumor with retinoblastoma. MRI is used to assess the extent of the primary lesion and the existence of metastatic disease, especially in the lungs. Serum alkaline phosphatase concentrations are likely to be increased, and the levels correlate with prognosis. Treatment consists of combination chemotherapy followed by surgical excision or amputation. Successful chemotherapy may permit limb salvage procedures in selected patients. Pulmonary resection may be indicated in patients with solitary metastatic lesions. Nonmetastatic disease is associated with an 85% to 90% survival rate.

EWING'S SARCOMA

Ewing's sarcoma usually occurs in children and young adults and most often involves the pelvis, femur, or tibia. Ewing's sarcoma is highly malignant, and metastatic disease is often present at the time of diagnosis. Treatment consists of surgery, local radiation therapy, and combination chemotherapy.

CHONDROSARCOMA

Chondrosarcoma usually involves the pelvis, ribs, or upper end of the femur or humerus in young or middle-aged adults.

This tumor often grows slowly and can be treated by radical surgical excision of larger lesions and irradiation of smaller lesions.

LYMPHOMAS AND LEUKEMIAS

Hodgkin's Lymphoma

Hodgkin's disease is a lymphoma that seems to have infective (Epstein-Barr virus), genetic, and environmental associations. Another factor that appears to predispose to the development of lymphoma is impaired immunity as seen in patients after organ transplantation or in patients infected with the human immunodeficiency virus. The most useful diagnostic test in patients with suspected lymphoma is lymph node biopsy.

Hodgkin's lymphoma is a lymph node–based malignancy, and presentation consists of lymphadenopathy in predictable locations, including the neck and anterior mediastinum. Characteristic systemic symptoms also occur, including pruritus, night sweats, and unexplained weight loss. Moderately severe anemia is often present. Peripheral neuropathy and spinal cord compression may occur as a direct result of tumor growth. Bone marrow and central nervous system involvement is unusual in Hodgkin's lymphoma but not in other lymphomas.

Staging of the disease is accomplished by CT and positron emission tomographic scanning of the chest, abdomen, and pelvis; biopsy of available nodes; and bone marrow biopsy. Precise definition of the extent of nodal and extranodal disease is necessary to select the proper treatment strategy. Radiation therapy is curative for localized early-stage Hodgkin's lymphoma. Bulkier or more advanced Hodgkin's disease is treated by combination chemotherapy. Cure can be achieved, with 20-year survival rates approaching 90%.

Non-Hodgkin's Lymphoma

Non-Hodgkin's lymphomas are divided into subtypes based on cell type and immunophenotypic and genetic features. They can be of B-cell, T-cell, or natural killer cell origin. Treatment and prognosis vary widely depending on subtype. Chemotherapy is the first-line treatment for most non-Hodgkin's lymphomas. Hematopoietic stem cell transplantation can be used in refractory cases.

Leukemia

Leukemia is the uncontrolled production of leukocytes owing to cancerous mutation of lymphogenous or myelogenous cells. Lymphocytic leukemias begin in lymph nodes and myeloid leukemias begin as cancerous production of myelogenous cells in bone marrow with spread to extramedullary organs. The principal difference between normal hematopoietic stem cells and leukemia cells is the ability of the latter to continue to divide. The result is an expanding mass of cells that infiltrates the bone marrow, and renders patients functionally aplastic.

Anemia may be profound. Eventually, bone marrow failure leads to fatal infection or hemorrhage caused by thrombocytopenia. Leukemia cells may also infiltrate the liver, spleen, lymph nodes, and meninges, producing signs of dysfunction at these sites. Extensive use of nutrients by rapidly proliferating cancerous cells depletes amino acid stores, which leads to patient fatigue and metabolic starvation of normal tissues.

ACUTE LYMPHOBLASTIC LEUKEMIA

Acute lymphoblastic leukemia—also known as *acute lymphocytic leukemia*—is the most common leukemia in children but also occurs in adults. Central nervous system dysfunction is common. Affected patients are highly susceptible to life-threatening opportunistic infections, including infections caused by *Pneumocystis jiroveci* (formerly *Pneumocystis carinii*) and cytomegalovirus. Chemotherapy can cure as many as 80% of children and 40% of adults.

CHRONIC LYMPHOCYTIC LEUKEMIA

Chronic lymphocytic leukemia usually occurs in adults older than 55 years and is more common in men than in women. This form of leukemia rarely occurs in children. The diagnosis of chronic lymphocytic leukemia is confirmed by the presence of lymphocytosis and lymphocytic infiltrates in bone marrow. Signs and symptoms are highly variable, with the extent of bone marrow infiltration often determining the clinical course. Autoimmune hemolytic anemia and hypersplenism that results in pancytopenia may be prominent. Lymph node enlargement may obstruct the ureters. Corticosteroids may be useful in treating the hemolytic anemia, but splenectomy may occasionally be necessary. Single or combination chemotherapy is the usual treatment, with radiation therapy reserved for treatment of localized nodal masses or an enlarged spleen. Five-year survival is approximately 75%.

ACUTE MYELOID LEUKEMIA

Acute myeloid leukemia (AML) is characterized by an increase in the number of myeloid cells in bone marrow and arrest of their maturation, which frequently results in hematopoietic insufficiency (granulocytopenia, thrombocytopenia, anemia). Clinical signs and symptoms of AML are diverse and nonspecific, but they are usually attributable to leukemic infiltration of the bone marrow. Approximately one third of patients with AML have significant or life-threatening infection when initially seen. Other patients present with complaints of fatigue, bleeding gums or nosebleeds, pallor, and/or headache. Dyspnea on exertion is common due to severe anemia. Leukemic infiltration of various organs (hepatomegaly, splenomegaly, lymphadenopathy), bones, gingiva, and the central nervous system can produce a variety of signs. Hyperleukocytosis (>100,000 cells/mm^3) can result in signs of leukostasis with ocular and cerebrovascular dysfunction or bleeding. Metabolic abnormalities may include hyperuricemia and hypocalcemia.

Chemotherapy is administered to induce remission. Five-year survival varies from 15% to 70% depending on tumor cell cytogenics and age at diagnosis. Bone marrow transplantation may be a consideration in patients who do not have an initial remission or who experience relapse after chemotherapy.

Retinoic acid syndrome is a unique, potentially lethal complication of induction therapy in patients with acute promyelocytic leukemia. It is often but not exclusively associated with treatment with all-*trans* retinoic acid (tretinoin). Respiratory distress, pulmonary infiltrates, fever, and hypotension are common presenting symptoms. The etiology is unclear, but it may be related to release of cytokines from myeloid cells, which causes capillary leak syndrome. High-dose corticosteroid administration is the most commonly employed treatment for retinoic acid syndrome.

CHRONIC MYELOGENOUS LEUKEMIA

Chronic myelogenous leukemia (also known as *chronic myeloid leukemia*) manifests as myeloid leukocytosis with splenomegaly. In most cases, there is a prolonged dormant phase in which patients are asymptomatic. The disease then progresses through an accelerated phase followed by blast crisis. This latter condition resembles acute leukemia and signals a poor prognosis. High leukocyte counts may predispose to vascular occlusion. Hyperuricemia is common and is treated with allopurinol. Cytoreduction therapy with hydroxyurea, chemotherapy, leukapheresis, and splenectomy may be necessary. Chronic myelogenous leukemia is treated with chemotherapeutic agents such as imatinib, which are targeted to the BCR-ABL tyrosine kinase inhibitor. This drug is successful in the vast majority of patients. Hematopoietic stem cell transplantation or other combined chemotherapies are alternatives if primary treatment is unsuccessful.

HEMATOPOIETIC STEM CELL TRANSPLANTATION

Hematopoietic stem cell transplantation offers an opportunity for cure for several otherwise fatal diseases. Hematopoietic stem cells can be obtained from peripheral blood or from bone marrow. Autologous bone marrow transplantation entails collection of the patient's own bone marrow for subsequent reinfusion, whereas allogeneic transplantation uses bone marrow or peripheral blood elements from an immunocompatible donor. Regardless of the type of bone marrow transplantation, recipients must undergo a preprocedural regimen designed to achieve functional bone marrow ablation. This is produced by a combination of total body irradiation and chemotherapy.

Bone marrow is usually harvested by repeated aspirations from the posterior iliac crest. For allogeneic bone marrow transplantation with major AB incompatibility between donor and recipient, it is necessary to remove mature erythrocytes from the graft to avoid a hemolytic transfusion reaction. Removal of T cells from the allograft can decrease the risk of graft-versus-host disease. Processing of the harvested bone marrow may take 2 to 12 hours. The condensed volume of bone marrow (approximately 200 mL) is then infused into the recipient through a central venous catheter. From the systemic circulation, the bone marrow cells pass into the recipient's bone marrow, which provides the microenvironment necessary for maturation and differentiation of the cells. The time necessary for bone marrow engraftment is usually 10 to 28 days, during which time protective isolation of the patient is required.

Anesthesia for Bone Marrow Transplantation

General or regional anesthesia is used during aspiration of bone marrow from the iliac crests. Use of nitrous oxide might be avoided in the donor because of potential bone marrow depression associated with this drug. However, there is no evidence that nitrous oxide administered during bone marrow harvesting adversely affects marrow engraftment and subsequent function. Substantial fluid losses may accompany this procedure. Blood replacement may be necessary, either by autologous blood transfusion or by reinfusion of separated erythrocytes obtained during the harvest. Perioperative complications are rare, although discomfort at bone puncture sites is predictable.

Complications of Bone Marrow Transplantation

In addition to prolonged myelosuppression, bone marrow transplantation is associated with several specific complications.

GRAFT-VERSUS-HOST DISEASE

Graft-versus-host disease (GVHD) is a life-threatening complication of bone marrow transplantation manifesting as organ system dysfunction that most often involves the skin, liver, and gastrointestinal tract (Table 23-5). Severe rash, jaundice, and diarrhea are usually seen. This response occurs when immunologically competent T lymphocytes from the donor graft target proteins on the recipient's cells. These proteins are usually human leukocyte antigens (HLAs), which are encoded by the major histocompatibility complex. Even when the patient and host are matched for HLAs, minor histocompatibility antigens can provoke GVHD.

GVHD can be divided into two somewhat distinct clinical entities: acute disease, which usually occurs during the first 30 to 60 days after bone marrow transplantation, and chronic disease, which develops at least 100 days after transplantation. The incidence of acute GVHD is directly associated with the degree of incompatibility between HLA proteins. It ranges from 35% to 45% in fully matched sibling donors to 60% to 80% in patients with a single HLA mismatch. Patients undergoing allogeneic bone marrow transplantation receive prophylaxis to prevent acute GVHD. These treatments are mainly directed at minimizing the host's immune response. Examples of agents used are tacrolimus and cyclosporine, which inhibit calcineurin, an enzyme that is important for T-cell activation. When it occurs, acute GVHD is usually treated with high-dose steroids. Extracorporeal photopheresis is an emerging treatment for acute GVHD that involves removal of a patient's white blood cells and their exposure to ultraviolet light, followed by reinfusion into the patient. This process induces cellular apoptosis, which in turn prompts an acute antiinflammatory response that appears to reduce the risk of graft rejection.

TABLE 23-5	Manifestations of acute graft-versus-host disease
Desquamation, erythroderma, maculopapular rash	
Interstitial pneumonitis	
Gastritis, diarrhea, abdominal cramping	
Mucosal ulceration and mucositis	
Hepatitis with coagulopathy	
Glomerulonephritis, nephrotic syndrome	
Immunodeficiency and pancytopenia	

Chronic GVHD shares features typical of autoimmune diseases. Symptoms include sclerosis of the skin, xerostomia, fasciitis, myositis, transaminitis, pericarditis, nephritis, and restrictive lung disease. The pathophysiology of chronic GVHD is poorly understood, so treatments are limited. Prophylaxis against acute GVHD appears to reduce the risk of chronic GVHD. Extracorporeal photopheresis has shown benefit in some studies. Steroids remain the mainstay of treatment.

GRAFT REJECTION

Graft rejection occurs when immunologically competent cells of host origin destroy the cells of donor origin. This is rarely seen with transplants from well-matched related donors but can occur with transplants from other donors.

PULMONARY COMPLICATIONS

Pulmonary complications following hematopoietic stem cell transplantation include infection, adult respiratory distress syndrome, chemotherapy-induced lung damage, and interstitial pneumonitis. When interstitial pneumonitis occurs 60 days or longer after bone marrow transplantation, it is most likely due to cytomegalovirus or fungal infection.

SINUSOIDAL OBSTRUCTION SYNDROME

Sinusoidal obstruction syndrome—formerly called *venoocclusive disease of the liver*—may occur following allogeneic and autologous hematopoietic stem cell transplantation and appears to be related to high-dose radiation exposure. Primary symptoms include jaundice, tender hepatomegaly, ascites, and weight gain. The syndrome can manifest within days or as late as a year after hematopoietic stem cell transplantation. Progressive hepatic and multiorgan failure can develop, and the mortality rate approaches 50%.

KEY POINTS

- Stimulation of oncogene formation by carcinogens (tobacco, alcohol, sunlight) is estimated to be responsible for 80% of cancers in the United States. Tobacco accounts for more cases of cancer than all other known carcinogens combined. The fundamental event that causes cells to become malignant is an alteration in the structure of their DNA. The responsible mutations occur in cells of target tissues, with these cells then becoming the ancestors of the entire future tumor cell population.

- A commonly used staging system for solid tumors is the TNM system based on tumor size (T), lymph node involvement (N), and distant metastasis (M). This system further groups cancers into stages ranging from I (best prognosis) to IV (poorest prognosis).

- Drugs administered for cancer chemotherapy may produce significant adverse effects, including cardiomyopathy, pulmonary fibrosis, and peripheral neuropathy. These adverse effects may have important implications for the management of anesthesia during surgical procedures for cancer treatment as well as during operations unrelated to the cancer.

- Many patients with cancer exhibit paraneoplastic syndromes, some of which are related to ectopic hormone production and others of which are caused by the host's immune response to the tumor cells. Examples include SIADH, Cushing's syndrome, and Eaton-Lambert syndrome.

- Mass effects of tumors or metastases can cause life-threatening oncologic crises. Superior vena cava syndrome results from spread of cancer into the mediastinum or caval wall that causes engorgement of the jugular and upper extremity veins and diminished venous return to the heart. Increased intracranial pressure as a result of increased cerebral venous pressure can lead to nausea, seizures, and/or diminished consciousness. Superior mediastinal syndrome exists when tracheal compression accompanies superior vena cava syndrome. Other examples of mass-effect conditions are spinal cord compression and increased intracranial pressure resulting from metastases to the central nervous system.

- Cancer is the most common cause of hypercalcemia in hospitalized patients. It reflects local osteolytic activity from bone metastases (especially in breast cancer) or ectopic parathyroid hormonal activity associated with tumors that arise from the kidneys, lungs, pancreas, or ovaries. The rapid onset of hypercalcemia that occurs in patients with cancer may manifest as lethargy or coma. Polyuria and dehydration may accompany hypercalcemia.

- Induction chemotherapy or high-dose radiation therapy can destroy large numbers of tumor cells and result in tumor lysis syndrome, a major feature of which is acute hyperuricemic nephropathy resulting from precipitation of uric acid crystals and calcium phosphate in the renal tubules.

- Hematopoietic stem cell transplantation is a potentially lifesaving treatment for many types of cancer, but it has serious potential complications. GVHD occurs when immunologically competent T lymphocytes from a donor graft target proteins on the recipient's cells and incite a profound immune response. GVHD manifests as organ system dysfunction, most often involving the skin, liver, and gastrointestinal tract. Sinusoidal obstruction syndrome is marked by sudden onset of jaundice, tender hepatomegaly, ascites, and weight gain. The syndrome can manifest within days or as late as a year after hematopoietic stem cell transplantation. Progressive hepatic and multiorgan failure can develop, and mortality is high.

- Cancer patients may experience acute pain associated with surgery, chemotherapy, radiation therapy, pathologic fractures, and tumor invasion. A frequent source of pain is metastatic spread of the cancer, especially to bone. Nerve compression or infiltration may be a cause of pain. Patients with cancer who experience frequent and significant pain often exhibit signs of depression and anxiety.

- Drug therapy is the cornerstone of cancer pain management because of its efficacy, rapid onset of action, and relatively low cost. Mild to moderate cancer pain is initially treated with acetaminophen and/or NSAIDs. NSAIDs are particularly effective for managing bone pain. The next step in management is the addition of codeine or one of its analogues. When cancer pain is severe, more potent opioids are employed.

- Spinal opioids may be delivered for weeks to months via a long-term, subcutaneously tunneled, exteriorized catheter or an implanted drug delivery system. Implantable systems can be intrathecal or epidural. Patients are typically considered for neuraxial opioid administration when systemic opioid administration has failed as a result of intolerable adverse effects or inadequate analgesia. Neuraxial administration of opioids is usually successful, but some patients require the addition of a dilute concentration of local anesthetic to the neuraxial infusion to achieve adequate pain control.

- Important aspects of determining the suitability of a destructive nerve block are the location and quality of the pain, the effectiveness of less destructive treatment modalities, life expectancy, the inherent risks associated with the block, and the availability of experienced anesthesiologists to perform the procedure. In general, constant pain is more amenable to destructive nerve block than intermittent pain.

RESOURCES

Arain MR, Buggy DJ. Anaesthesia for cancer patients. *Curr Opin Anaesthesiol.* 2007;20:247-253.

Chang VT, Janjan N, Jain S, et al. Update in cancer pain syndromes. *J Palliat Med.* 2006;9:1414-1434.

Ferrara JLM, Levine JE, Reddy P, et al. Graft-versus-host disease. *Lancet.* 2009;373:1550-1561.

Latham GJ, Greenberg RS. Anesthetic considerations for the pediatric oncology patient—part 2: systems-based approach to anesthesia. *Paediatr Anaesthes.* 2010;20:396-420.

Libert N, Tourtier J-P, Védrine L, et al. Inhibitors of angiogenesis: new hopes for oncologists, new challenges for anesthesiologists. *Anesthesiology.* 2010;113:704-712.

Pelosof LC, Gerber DE. Paraneoplastic syndromes: an approach to diagnosis and treatment. *Mayo Clin Proc.* 2010;85:838-854.

Sahai SK, Zalpour A, Rozner MA. Preoperative evaluation of the oncology patient. *Med Clin North Am.* 2010;94:403-419.

Vahid B, Marik PE. Pulmonary complications of novel antineoplastic agents for solid tumors. *Chest.* 2008;133:528-538.

Yeh ET, Bickford CL. Cardiovascular complications of cancer therapy: incidence, pathogenesis, diagnosis, and management. *J Am Coll Cardiol.* 2009;53:2231-2247.

CHAPTER 24

Diseases Related to Immune System Dysfunction

NATALIE F. HOLT ∎

The human immune system is traditionally viewed as consisting of two pathways: *innate immunity* and *adaptive immunity* (also known as *acquired immunity*). Each is comprised of a series of unique components, all of which function to protect the host against invading microorganisms. The innate immune response is rapid and nonspecific, that is, it recognizes targets that are common to many pathogens and requires no prior exposure to a target antigen. Its noncellular elements include physical barriers (epithelial and mucous membrane surfaces), complement factors, acute phase proteins, and proteins of the contact activation pathway. Cellular elements include neutrophils, macrophages, monocytes, and a subset of lymphocytes called *natural killer (NK) cells* (Figure 24-1). The adaptive immune response is an evolutionarily more mature system present only in vertebrates. Adaptive immunity has a more delayed onset of activation, but is capable of developing memory and more specific antigenic responses. It consists of a humoral component mediated by B lymphocytes that produce antibodies and a cellular component composed of T lymphocytes. T cells are divided into two main subsets—cytotoxic (T_C) cells and helper-modulatory (T_H) cells—and are distinguished by their different combinations of surface antigens. T_C cells express a predominance of CD8 antigen, whereas T_H cells express a predominance of CD4 antigen. Precursor helper T lymphocytes differentiate into four distinct cell lines: T_H1, T_H2, T_H17, and regulatory T (T_{reg}) cells. T_H1 cells produce interferon and promote cell-mediated immune responses. T_H2 cells produce specific interleukins (ILs), including IL-4 and IL-10, which favor a humoral immune response and suppress cell-mediated immunity. T_H17 cells are proinflammatory and appear to play a role in chronic inflammatory conditions, including some cell-mediated autoimmune diseases. In contrast, T_{reg} cells promote tolerance and minimize autoimmune and allergic or inflammatory responses. As a general rule, cytotoxic and helper T-cell responses are most important in mounting an effective response to trauma, infection, and tumorigenesis. IL-4, IL-10, and T_H2 cells tend to promote the humoral immune system and help to protect against immune-mediated tissue injury; however, they may also activate immunoglobulin E (IgE) and contribute to hypersensitivity reactions (Table 24-1).

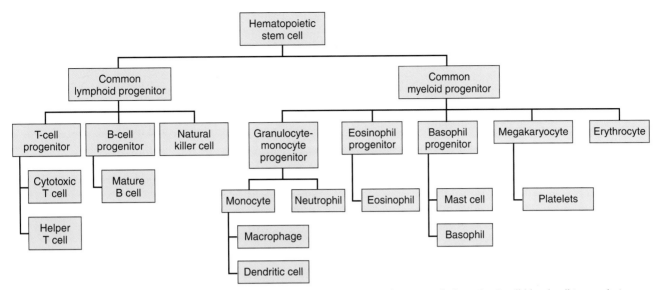

FIGURE 24-1 Hematopoietic stem cell differentiation. A pluripotent hematopoietic stem cell gives rise to all blood cell types via two main lineages: lymphoid and myeloid. A common myeloid progenitor differentiates into the granule-containing cells of the immune system (monocytes, macrophages, neutrophils, eosinophils, basophils), as well as megakaryocytes and erythrocytes. A common lymphoid progenitor differentiates into the non–granule-containing cells of the immune system (T cells, B cells, and natural killer cells).

Immune dysfunction can be divided into three categories: (1) an inadequate immune response; (2) an excessive immune response; and (3) a misdirection of the immune response.

INADEQUATE INNATE IMMUNITY

Neutropenia

Neutropenia is defined as a neutrophil granulocyte count of less than 1500/mm³. Normal neutrophil counts vary somewhat by age and ethnicity. For example, newborns tend to have higher granulocyte counts in the first few days of life, and African Americans tend to have lower average granulocyte counts in general compared with whites. It is not until the granulocyte count decreases to less than 500/mm³ that a patient is at significantly increased risk of pyogenic infections. Common infecting organisms include *Staphylococcus aureus, Pseudomonas aeruginosa, Escherichia coli,* and *Klebsiella* species, which frequently produce infections of the skin, mouth, pharynx, and lung. Broad-spectrum parenteral antibiotics are indicated in the management of these patients.

NEUTROPENIA IN PEDIATRIC PATIENTS

Several neutropenic syndromes can be observed in newborns and children. Neonatal sepsis is the most common cause of severe neutropenia within the first few days of life. A transient neutropenia may be seen in children born to mothers with autoimmune diseases and may also occur as a result of maternal hypertension or drug ingestion. Persistent neutropenia can occur as a result of defects in neutrophil production, maturation, or survival.

The autosomal dominant disorder *cyclic neutropenia* is a particularly well-studied cause of childhood neutropenia. It is characterized by recurrent episodes of neutropenia that are

TABLE 24-1   T-lymphocyte differentiation

Subset	Main functions	Cytokines
HELPER T CELLS		
T_H1	Macrophage activation	INF-γ
	Cellular cytotoxicity	IL-2
	Protection against intracellular microorganisms	IL-10
		TNF-β
T_H2	IgE production	IL-4
	Eosinophil proliferation	IL-5
	Protection against parasitic infection	IL-6
		IL-9
		IL-10
		IL-13
T_H17	Protection against extracellular bacteria and fungi	IL-17
		IL-21
		IL-22
	Aberrant regulation leads to chronic inflammation, allergy, autoimmune diseases	
T_{reg}	Maintenance of tolerance	IL-19
	Downregulation of immune response	TGF-β
		IL-35
CYTOTOXIC T CELLS	Induction of apoptosis in infected or tumor cells	INF-γ
		TNF-β
	Inhibition of microbial replication	

Ig, Immunoglobulin; *IL,* interleukin; *INF,* interferon; *TNF,* tumor necrosis factor; *TGF,* transforming growth factor; T_{reg}, regulatory T cell.

not always associated with infection but that occur in regular cycles every 3 to 4 weeks. Each episode is characterized by 1 week of reduced granulocyte production, followed by a period of reactive mastocytosis and then spontaneous recovery of normal granulocyte production. The granulocytopenia can be severe enough to result in recurrent, severe bacterial infection that requires antibiotic therapy. As the child grows up, chronic, persistent granulocytopenia may result. The postulated mechanism of this disorder is a defect in a feedback mechanism that normally stimulates precursor cells to respond to growth factors such as granulocyte colony-stimulating factor (G-CSF).

Kostmann's syndrome is an autosomal recessive disorder of neutrophil maturation. Patients with Kostmann's syndrome appear to have a normal population of early progenitor cells that somehow become suppressed, which inhibits normal maturation. If the disorder is left untreated, mortality in the first year of life approaches 70%. Treatment with G-CSF is effective in 90% of patients; in patients who show no response to G-CSF, bone marrow transplantation may be considered.

NEUTROPENIA IN ADULTS

Acquired defects in the production of neutrophils in adults are very common. Typical causes include cancer chemotherapy and treatment of human immunodeficiency virus (HIV) infection with zidovudine. Neutropenia usually reflects the impact of a drug on proliferation of stem cells and early myelocytic progenitors. In most cases, the marrow recovers once the drug is withdrawn. Many drugs have been associated with neutropenia. Among the most prominent of these are injectable gold salts, chloramphenicol, antithyroid medications (carbimazole and propylthiouracil), analgesics (indomethacin, acetaminophen, and phenacetin), tricyclic antidepressants, and phenothiazines. However, virtually any drug can, on occasion, produce severe life-threatening neutropenia. Therefore, when neutropenia occurs in the course of medical treatment, the possibility that it is drug induced must be considered.

Autoimmune-related neutropenia can be observed as an isolated disorder or in the context of another known autoimmune condition. Antineutrophil antibodies are sometimes present. The two most common associations are with systemic lupus erythematosus (in which the neutropenia can occur alone or be accompanied by thrombocytopenia) and rheumatoid arthritis. Conditions associated with splenomegaly often lead to granulocytopenia resulting from white cell sequestration. *Felty's syndrome* is the triad of rheumatoid arthritis, splenomegaly, and neutropenia. Other causes of splenomegaly and neutropenia include lymphoma, myeloproliferative disease, and severe liver disease with portal hypertension. In these latter situations, it is often difficult to decide whether the granulocytopenia is caused simply by splenic sequestration or whether it also has an autoimmune component. In some patients, splenectomy has been reported to significantly improve neutrophil production.

Acute, life-threatening granulocytopenia can occur as a result of certain infections. A decreasing white cell count in a patient with sepsis is a bad prognostic sign. It reflects a rate of granulocyte use that exceeds the marrow's ability to produce

new cells. Alcoholic patients are especially susceptible to infection-induced granulocytopenia. Both folic acid deficiency and direct toxic effects of ethanol on marrow precursor cells compromise the host's ability to produce new neutrophils in response to infection. HIV infection is a common cause of T-cell dysfunction. In these patients, loss of the T_H subset and overexpression of the T_{reg} subset is associated with abnormalities of neutrophil production and function.

Chronic benign neutropenia is a condition characterized by markedly reduced neutrophil counts, often as low as 200 to 500/mm^3. Although the clinical course is variable, most patients have a benign course.

Abnormalities of Phagocytosis

Chronic granulomatous disease is a genetic disorder in which granulocytes lack the ability to generate reactive oxygen species. The granulocytes can migrate to a site of infection and ingest organisms but are unable to kill them. *S. aureus* and certain gram-negative bacteria such as *Serratia marcescens* and *Burkholderia cepacia* that are normally killed by phagocytosis and lysosomal digestion are responsible for most infections in patients with this disorder. The condition is usually diagnosed during childhood or early adult life when patients have recurrent microabscesses and chronic granulomatous inflammation. Persistent inflammation and granuloma formation can lead to multiorgan dysfunction, including intestinal obstruction, glomerulonephritis, and chorioretinitis. Aggressive treatment of infectious complications, prophylaxis with antibiotics and antifungal agents, and use of recombinant interferon-γ has significantly improved survival in patients with this disease.

The primary substrate for the enzymatic generation of reactive oxygen species is the reduced form of nicotinamide adenine dinucleotide phosphate (NADPH). Patients with *neutrophil glucose-6-phosphate dehydrogenase (G6PD) deficiency* are unable to generate large amounts of NADPH, which limits their ability to produce the oxidase needed to kill ingested microorganisms. Like patients with chronic granulomatous disease, neutrophil G6PD-deficient patients are at lifelong risk of infection with catalase-positive microorganisms.

Leukocyte adhesion deficiency is a relatively rare deficiency of a subunit of the integrin family of leukocyte adhesion molecules. This subunit is critical for cellular adhesion and chemotaxis. Although clinical severity varies, patients with leukocyte adhesion deficiency experience a higher risk of recurrent bacterial infections. Persistent granulocytosis is often present; however, the absence of pus is the most characteristic feature of this disease.

Chédiak-Higashi syndrome is a rare multisystem disease characterized by partial oculocutaneous albinism, frequent bacterial infections, a mild bleeding diathesis, progressive neuropathy, and cranial nerve defects. The neutrophils of these patients contain characteristic giant granules. Patients exhibit multiple defects of immune function, including impairment in neutrophil chemotaxis, phagocytosis, NK cell activity, and T-cell cytotoxicity. Many white blood cells are destroyed before leaving the bone marrow. In most patients, an accelerated lymphoproliferative syndrome leads to death. However, bone marrow transplantation can reverse immunologic dysfunction in some patients.

Specific granule deficiency syndrome is another rare congenital disorder characterized by neutrophils that exhibit impaired chemotaxis and bactericidal activity. Patients are prone to recurrent bacterial and fungal infections with abscess formation. Skin and pulmonary infections appear to predominate, and most of these respond well to aggressive antibiotic therapy. Affected patients frequently survive into their adult years.

Management of Patients with Neutropenia or Abnormalities of Phagocytosis

Patients with neutropenia or a qualitative disorder of granulocyte function often benefit significantly from treatment with G-CSF. Recombinant G-CSF therapy reduces the duration of absolute neutropenia in patients receiving ablative chemotherapy and autologous bone marrow transplantation. It also shortens the length of antibiotic therapy and reduces the risk of life-threatening bacteremia and fungal infections. G-CSF therapy has been approved for the reversal of the neutropenia associated with HIV infection and the prevention of worsening neutropenia in patients receiving HIV therapy. Neutropenic patients undergoing elective surgery may benefit from a course of G-CSF preoperatively to reduce the risk of perioperative infection.

Deficiencies in Components of the Complement System

Complement refers to a family of serum proteins that are critical to the host response to infection. Complement activation may occur by pathogen-dependent (classical or lectin) or pathogen-independent (alternative) pathways (Figure 24-2). Complement proteins assist in clearing microorganisms by coating infectious agents with proteins that facilitate phagocytosis. Complement proteins also promote the inflammatory response. Certain complement components are unique to a particular pathway, but all pathways lead to the formation of C3 and the membrane-attack complex. Deficiencies in virtually all of the soluble complement components have been described. Defects in early components of the classical pathway of complement activation (C1q, C1r, C2, and C4) predispose to autoimmune inflammatory disorders resembling systemic lupus erythematosus. Deficiencies in the common pathway component C3 are usually fatal in utero. Deficiencies in the terminal complement components C5 through C8 are associated with recurrent infection and rheumatic diseases. Patients with deficiencies in C9 and components of the alternative pathway (factor D and properdin) are predisposed to neisserial infection. Factor H deficiency is associated with familial relapsing hemolytic uremic syndrome. The liver is the primary organ of complement protein synthesis. Therefore, patients with advanced liver disease are often at increased risk of infection, especially pneumonia and sepsis caused by *Streptococcus pneumoniae*, *S. aureus*, and *E. coli*. Prompt recognition and treatment of infection and careful maintenance of routine immunizations are the hallmarks of treating these patients.

Tight regulation of complement activation prevents misdirected activation of the inflammatory and immune response. The main inhibitor compound is C1 esterase inhibitor. Deficiency of C1 esterase inhibitor is responsible for hereditary angioedema, an autosomal dominant condition marked by episodes of subcutaneous and submucosal edema caused primarily by excessive concentrations of bradykinin, which increases vascular permeability.

Hyposplenism

Splenectomy is the most common cause of splenic dysfunction, although various clinical conditions may lead to impaired splenic functioning. Perhaps the most common of these is sickle cell anemia, which causes autoinfarction of the spleen as a result of vasoocclusive disease. *S. pneumoniae* is the most common cause of bacterial sepsis in postsplenectomy patients. Splenic dysfunction also increases the risk of infection with *Neisseria meningitidis*, *E. coli*, *Haemophilus influenzae*, and malaria. As recommended for patients with complement deficiencies, management of hyposplenic patients relies heavily on prevention, mainly through immunization against *S. pneumoniae*, *H. influenzae* type b, and *N. meningitidis* in particular. Penicillin prophylaxis was once widely recommended after splenectomy in children younger than age 5. However, this practice is falling out of favor because of concern over the spread of penicillin-resistant species and the effectiveness of immunization in most patients.

EXCESSIVE INNATE IMMUNITY

Neutrophilia

The earliest response to an infection is the migration of granulocytes out of the circulation and into the site of bacterial invasion. The rapidity and magnitude of the increase in the number of circulating granulocytes in response to infection is remarkable. Within hours of the onset of a severe infection, the granulocyte count increases twofold to fourfold. This increase represents a change in the marginated and circulating pools of granulocytes as well as the delivery of new granulocytes from the bone marrow. *Neutrophilia* is defined as an absolute neutrophil count higher than 7000/mm^3. Major causes of neutrophilia are listed in Table 24-2.

An increase in the granulocyte count does not produce specific symptoms or signs unless the count exceeds 100,000/mm^3. Such marked leukocytosis can produce leukostasis resulting in infarction of the spleen and a reduction in the oxygen-diffusing capacity of the lungs. Granulocytes can also accumulate in the skin to produce nontender, purplish nodules called *chloromas*. Unlike immature blasts, mature granulocytes do not invade brain tissue, so neurologic complications do not result from reactive granulocytosis.

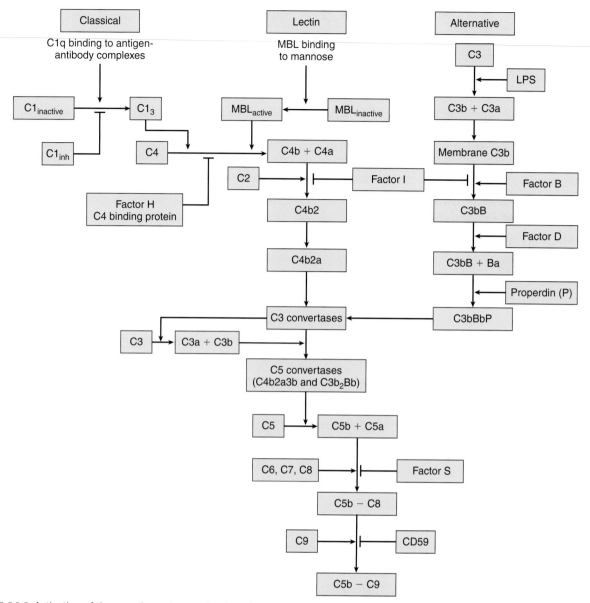

FIGURE 24-2 Activation of the complement cascade. Complement activation can occur via classical and lectin pathways or by alternative pathways. In the classical pathway, binding of an antigen-antibody complex to C1q is the triggering event. In the lectin pathway, mannose residues on bacteria bind to mannose binding lectin (MBL), setting off complement activation. The alternative pathway can be activated by microbes or tumor cells. All pathways lead to the formation of C3, which is important in immune complex modification, opsonization, and lymphocyte activation. The terminal common pathway that flows from all three activation pathways leads to production of the membrane-attack complex C5b-9, which lyses cells. *C1$_{inh}$*, C1 inhibitor; *LPS*, lipopolysaccharide.

The clinical features associated with moderate granulocytosis vary depending on the primary disease underlying the condition. Deep-seated infections and peritonitis are associated with granulocyte counts of 10,000 to 30,000/mm^3 or more. Reactive monocytosis is seen in patients with tuberculosis, subacute bacterial endocarditis, or severe granulocytopenia. Parasitic infestations are typically associated with an elevated eosinophil count, whereas basophilia is seen in patients with chronic myelogenous leukemia. As a general rule, sustained granulocyte counts of 50,000/mm^3 or higher indicate a noninfectious, malignant disease process such as a myeloproliferative disorder. The appearance of very immature myelocytic cells in the circulation and accompanying changes in other cell lines (increased or decreased platelets or red blood cells) are also signs of hematologic malignancy.

Granulocytosis is an expected side effect of glucocorticoid therapy, because glucocorticoids interfere with the egress of granulocytes from the circulation into tissues. Patients receiving prednisone 60 to 100 mg/day often have white blood cell counts of 15,000 to 20,000/mm^3. Other causes of granulocytosis include physiologic stress, exposure to certain drugs, and cigarette smoking.

TABLE 24-2 ■ Clinical conditions associated with neutrophilia

Condition	Mechanism
Infection/inflammation	Increased neutrophil production and bone marrow release
Stress	Increased neutrophil production
Metabolic disorders such as preeclampsia and diabetic ketoacidosis	Increased neutrophil production
Steroid treatment	Demargination of neutrophils
Myeloproliferative disorders	Increased marrow neutrophil release and demargination of neutrophils
Splenectomy	Decrease in splenic trapping of neutrophils

Monocytosis

Monocytosis occurs in conjunction with inflammatory disorders such as systemic lupus erythematosus, rheumatoid arthritis, and sarcoidosis and in the context of certain infections, including tuberculosis, syphilis, and subacute bacterial endocarditis. Monocytosis can also be seen in patients with primary neutropenic disorders or hematologic malignancies. Although monocytes are important components of the immune system, the association between the circulating monocyte count and the propensity for infection is not as clear as in the case of neutrophils.

Asthma

Asthma is characterized by an exaggerated bronchoconstrictor response to certain stimuli (see Chapter 9). Triggers for bronchospasm unrelated to the immune system produce *intrinsic* asthma. Placement of an endotracheal tube may trigger this type of asthma; other common triggers are cold, exercise, stress, and inhaled irritants. Mediators of intrinsic asthma are components of the innate immune system. By contrast, triggers that activate the immune system and release IgE produce *extrinsic* asthma and are part of adaptive immunity. Inhaled allergens such as pollen and pet dander are common causes of extrinsic asthma. Symptoms of extrinsic or allergic asthma are highly variable and can include cough, dyspnea, and wheezing. Treatment consists of administration of β-agonists, anticholinergics, corticosteroids, and leukotriene inhibitors.

MISDIRECTED INNATE IMMUNITY

Angioedema

Angioedema may be hereditary or acquired and is characterized by episodic subcutaneous and submucosal edema formation, often involving the face, extremities, and gastrointestinal tract. Two types of angioedema can be distinguished. One is caused by release of mast cell mediators and is associated with urticaria, bronchospasm, flushing, and even hypotension. The other results from bradykinin release and does not cause allergic symptoms. The most common hereditary form of angioedema results from an autosomal dominant deficiency or dysfunction of *C1 esterase inhibitor*. This serine protease inhibitor (serpin) regulates complement, contact activation, and fibrinolytic pathways. The absence of C1 esterase inhibitor also leads to release of vasoactive mediators that increase vascular permeability and produce edema via bradykinin. Patients deficient in this regulatory enzyme experience repeated bouts of facial and/or laryngeal edema lasting 24 to 72 hours. These episodes usually begin in the second decade of life and may be triggered by menses, trauma, infection, stress, or estrogen-containing oral contraceptives. Dental surgery can be an important trigger of laryngeal attacks. Abdominal attacks usually present with excruciating pain, nausea, vomiting, and/or diarrhea.

C1 esterase inhibitor deficiency can be acquired by patients with lymphoproliferative disorders. These patients have antibodies to C1 inhibitor, and this gives rise to a syndrome that closely mimics hereditary angioedema. Angiotensin-converting enzyme (ACE) inhibitors used for the treatment of hypertension and heart failure can also precipitate angioedema in about 0.5% of patients. This drug-induced angioedema is thought to result from increased availability of bradykinin made possible by the ACE inhibitor–mediated blockade of bradykinin catabolism. Interestingly, angioedema provoked by ACE inhibitors may develop unexpectedly after prolonged drug use.

Androgens such as danazol and stanozolol have been the mainstay of prophylactic therapy, both long term and preoperatively, in patients with angioedema. Antifibrinolytic therapy (e.g., ε-aminocaproic acid, tranexamic acid, or aprotinin) has also been used. Anabolic steroids (androgens) are believed to increase hepatic synthesis of C1 esterase inhibitor, whereas antifibrinolytics are thought to act by inhibiting plasmin activation. The preferred treatment for an acute episode of angioedema is C1 inhibitor concentrate (25 units/kg) or fresh frozen plasma (2 to 4 units) to replace the deficient enzyme. It is important to note that androgens, catecholamines, antihistamines, and antifibrinolytics are *not* useful in the treatment of acute episodes of angioedema. Should upper airway obstruction develop during acute attacks, tracheal intubation until the edema subsides may be lifesaving. When laryngoscopy is undertaken, it is important to have personnel and equipment available to perform tracheostomy if needed, but tracheostomy itself may be extremely difficult or impossible in the face of massive airway edema.

MANAGEMENT OF ANESTHESIA

Patients experiencing recurrent angioedema, whether hereditary or acquired, require prophylaxis before a stimulating procedure such as dental surgery or any surgery requiring endotracheal intubation. It is prudent to ensure the ready availability of C1 inhibitor concentrates for intravenous infusion should an acute attack occur. Incidental trauma to the oropharynx, such as that produced by suctioning, should be minimized. Regional anesthetic techniques and intramuscular injections are well tolerated by these patients.

INADEQUATE ADAPTIVE IMMUNITY

Defects of Antibody Production

X-linked agammaglobulinemia is an inherited defect in the maturation of B cells. Mature B cells are missing or reduced in the circulation and lymphoid tissues have no plasma cells; therefore, functional antibody is not produced. Affected boys have recurrent pyogenic infections during the latter half of their first year of life as maternal antibodies wane. Treatment with intravenous immunoglobulin every 3 to 4 months to maintain plasma IgG levels near 500 mg/dL allows the majority of these children to survive into adulthood.

Selective IgA deficiency occurs in 1 in every 600 to 800 adults. In this condition, plasma IgA concentrations are less than 5 mg/dL, but the concentrations of other immunoglobulins are normal. Recurrent sinus and pulmonary infections are common, although many patients remain asymptomatic. About 40% of affected patients produce IgA antibodies. This subset of patients may experience life-threatening anaphylaxis when transfused with blood products containing IgA. Therefore, these patients should receive blood or blood components obtained from IgA-deficient donors.

Waldenström's macroglobulinemia is due to proliferation of a malignant plasma cell clone that secretes IgM, which results in marked increases in plasma viscosity. The bone marrow is infiltrated with malignant lymphocytes, as are the liver, spleen, and lungs. Anemia and an increased incidence of spontaneous hemorrhage are common findings in these patients. In contrast to multiple myeloma, Waldenström's macroglobulinemia rarely involves the skeletal system. As a result, renal dysfunction resulting from hypercalcemia is uncommon. Treatment consists of plasmapheresis to remove the abnormal proteins and reduce plasma viscosity. Chemotherapy may be instituted to decrease proliferation of the cells responsible for the production of abnormal immunoglobulins.

Cold autoimmune diseases are characterized by the presence of abnormal circulating proteins (usually IgM or IgA antibodies) that agglutinate in response to a decrease in body temperature. These disorders include *cryoglobulinemia* and *cold hemagglutinin disease*. Hyperviscosity of the plasma is prominent, and microvascular thrombosis may cause acute end-organ damage during a period of hypothermia. Symptoms normally do not occur until body temperature falls below 33° C. Management of anesthesia in these patients includes strict maintenance of normothermia. Patients scheduled for surgery requiring cardiopulmonary bypass present significant challenges. Use of systemic hypothermia may be contraindicated, and cold cardioplegia solutions may precipitate intracoronary hemagglutination with consequent thrombosis, ischemia, or infarction. Alternatives to cold cardioplegia include fibrillatory arrest for brief time periods. Plasmapheresis may also be helpful in reducing plasma concentrations of these immunoglobulins.

Amyloidosis encompasses several disorders characterized by the accumulation of insoluble fibrillar proteins (amyloid) in various tissues, including the heart, vascular smooth muscle, kidneys, adrenal glands, gastrointestinal tract, peripheral nerves, and skin. Primary amyloidosis is a plasma cell disorder marked by the accumulation of immunoglobulin light chains. Secondary amyloidosis is observed in association with several other conditions, including multiple myeloma, rheumatoid arthritis, and a prolonged antigenic challenge, such as may be produced by chronic infection.

Macroglossia is a classic feature of patients with amyloidosis, occurring in about 20% of patients. The enlarged, stiff tongue may impair swallowing and speaking. Involvement of the salivary glands and adjacent tissue may cause upper airway obstruction that mimics angioedema. Cardiac involvement is fairly common and may cause intraventricular conduction delays, including heart block. Sudden death is not uncommon. Cardiac dysfunction classically involves right-sided heart failure, with relative sparing of left-sided heart function until late in the disease. Accumulation of amyloid in the kidneys may produce nephrotic syndrome. Deposition in joint spaces may lead to limited range of motion as well as peripheral nerve entrapments such as carpal tunnel syndrome. Amyloidosis of the gastrointestinal tract may lead to malabsorption, ileus, and impaired gastric emptying. Hepatomegaly is common, although hepatic dysfunction is rare. The diagnosis is based on clinical suspicion confirmed by tissue biopsy. The frequent presence of amyloid deposits in the rectum makes rectal biopsy a common initial diagnostic procedure.

Treatment of amyloidosis is generally directed toward symptomatic improvement rather than cure. Airway management may be challenging due to an enlarged tongue. Perioperative management of these patients requires careful preoperative evaluation for signs of end-organ dysfunction such as renal insufficiency and heart failure or conduction defects. Gastric motility drugs may be useful in some patients. Of note, amyloid deposits have the potential to trap factor X or evoke fibrinolysis, which predisposes these patients to hemorrhagic complications.

Defects of T Lymphocytes

DiGeorge syndrome (thymic hypoplasia) is the result of a gene deletion. Features include absent or diminished thymus development, hypoplasia of the thyroid and parathyroid glands, cardiac malformations, and facial dysmorphisms. The degree of immunocompromise correlates with the amount of thymic tissue present. Complete absence of the thymus produces a severe combined immunodeficiency syndrome–like phenotype, and bacterial, fungal, and parasitic infections can all be problems. Complete DiGeorge syndrome is treated by thymus transplantation or infusion of mature T cells. Partial DiGeorge syndrome requires no therapy.

Combined Immune System Defects

Severe combined immunodeficiency syndromes are caused by a number of genetic mutations that affect T, B, or NK cell functions. The most common form of severe combined immunodeficiency syndrome is the *X-linked form,* which has a prevalence of approximately 1 in 50,000 live births and accounts for approximately half of severe combined immunodeficiency syndrome cases in the United States. The disease is caused by a mutation in a gene that encodes for a protein subunit shared by several of the interleukin receptors. Absence of these receptors results in defective interleukin signaling, which in turn blocks normal differentiation of NK, B, and T cells. The only treatment that substantially prolongs life expectancy is bone marrow or stem cell transplantation from an HLA-compatible donor.

Adenosine deaminase deficiency is another form of severe combined immunodeficiency syndrome, accounting for approximately 15% of cases. The adenosine deaminase enzyme is most abundant in lymphocytes, and deficiency allows toxic levels of purine intermediates to accumulate, which leads to T-cell death. There is profound lymphopenia together with skeletal abnormalities of the ribs and hips. Bone marrow or stem cell transplantation or enzyme replacement with bovine adenosine deaminase enzyme is of benefit in increasing life expectancy.

Ataxia-telangiectasia is a syndrome consisting of cerebellar ataxia, oculocutaneous telangiectasias, chronic sinopulmonary disease, and immunodeficiency. The genetic basis of this disorder is a gene mutation in the surveillance system that monitors DNA for double-strand breaks. In this syndrome, DNA damage that occurs during cell division is missed, and defective cells are released into the circulation. One consequence of this defect is the production of dysfunctional lymphocytes. These patients also have a significant predisposition to malignancy, especially leukemia and lymphoma. Patients with ataxia-telangiectasia are so susceptible to radiation-induced injury that bone marrow transplantation is not possible. Supportive therapy includes intravenous administration of immunoglobulin.

EXCESSIVE ADAPTIVE IMMUNITY

Allergic Reactions

Immune-mediated allergic reactions are classified according to their mechanism. *Type I* allergic reactions are IgE mediated and involve mast cells and basophils. The majority of cases of anaphylaxis are IgE-mediated events. *Type II* reactions mediate cytotoxicity via IgG, IgM, and complement. Type II reactions usually manifest as hemolytic anemia, thrombocytopenia, or neutropenia, since these are the cell types that are most often affected. Clinical presentation and severity vary widely, and presentation may be delayed for several days. *Type III* reactions produce tissue damage via immune complex formation and deposition, and often lead to glomerulonephritis, urticaria, vasculitis, and arthralgias. *Type IV* reactions are marked by T lymphocyte–mediated delayed hypersensitivity. Cutaneous symptoms are the most common physical manifestation of drug allergy. Clinical severity ranges from simple contact dermatitis to Stevens-Johnson syndrome and toxic epidermal necrolysis, two types of severe exfoliative dermatitis that can be life threatening. Drug-induced hypersensitivity syndrome (DIHS), also called *drug rash with eosinophilia and systemic symptoms* (DRESS), is another severe form of type IV delayed drug hypersensitivity marked by eosinophilia, rash, fever, and multiple organ system failure. Patients with certain viral infections such as Epstein-Barr virus or cytomegalovirus infection experience an increased incidence of some type IV drug reactions.

Not all drug allergies are mediated by the immune system. Nonimmune anaphylaxis (formerly called *anaphylactoid* reactions) occurs when mediator is released from mast cells and basophils as a result of direct interaction with the offending drug rather than immune system activation.

Anaphylaxis

Anaphylaxis is a life-threatening condition marked by cardiovascular collapse, interstitial edema, and bronchospasm. Anaphylaxis may occur by immune-mediated or non–immune-mediated mechanisms. The most common type of immune-mediated anaphylaxis results when previous exposure to antigens in drugs or foods evokes production of antigen-specific IgE antibodies. Subsequent exposure to the same or a chemically similar antigen results in antigen-antibody interactions that initiate marked degranulation of mast cells and basophils. Approximately 60% of anaphylactic reactions are mediated by IgE antibodies. Less commonly, IgG or IgM antibody reactions are to blame. Non–immune-mediated anaphylaxis results from direct release of histamine and other mediators from mast cells and basophils. Initial manifestations of anaphylaxis usually occur within 5 to 10 minutes of exposure to the antigen. Vasoactive mediators released by degranulation of mast cells and basophils are responsible for the clinical indicators of anaphylaxis (Table 24-3). Urticaria and pruritus are common. Primary vascular collapse occurs in approximately 25% of cases of fatal anaphylaxis. Laryngeal edema, bronchospasm, and arterial hypoxemia may accompany anaphylaxis. Extravasation of up to 50% of the intravascular fluid volume into the extracellular space reflects the extent of microvascular permeability that can accompany anaphylaxis. Indeed, hypovolemia is a likely cause of hypotension in these patients, although leukotriene-mediated negative inotropism may also be a factor.

The estimated incidence of all immune- and non–immune-mediated episodes of anaphylaxis during anesthesia is between 1 in 5000 and 1 in 20,000 anesthetic cases. The wide variability reflects the difficulty in determining the denominator (total

TABLE 24-3 ■ Vasoactive mediators released during anaphylaxis

Mediator	Physiologic effect
Histamine	Increased capillary permeability Peripheral vasodilation Bronchoconstriction Urticaria
Leukotrienes	Increased capillary permeability Bronchoconstriction Negative inotropy Coronary artery vasoconstriction
Prostaglandins	Bronchoconstriction
Eosinophil chemotactic factor	Attraction of eosinophils
Neutrophil chemotactic factor	Attraction of neutrophils
Platelet-activating factor	Platelet aggregation Release of vasoactive amines

number of anesthetic cases) as well as inconsistencies in event reporting. Estimated mortality from perioperative anaphylaxis ranges from 3% to 6%. Risk factors include asthma, longer duration of anesthesia, female sex (especially for neuromuscular blocking drugs and hypnotic induction drugs), multiple past surgeries or procedures (especially for incidents involving latex and ethylene dioxide), and the presence of other allergic conditions or systemic mastocytosis.

DIAGNOSIS

The diagnosis of anaphylaxis can be suggested by the often dramatic nature of the clinical manifestations in close temporal relationship to exposure to a particular antigen. Cardiovascular, respiratory, and cutaneous manifestations are most common. Typical signs include tachycardia, bronchospasm, and laryngeal edema. Recognition of an allergic reaction that occurs during anesthesia may be compromised by inability of the patient to communicate early symptoms such as pruritus. Covering of the patient by surgical drapes may obscure recognition of cutaneous signs. Consequently, cardiovascular collapse may be the first detectable signal of the event.

Immunologic and biochemical evidence of anaphylaxis is provided by an increased plasma tryptase concentration within 1 to 2 hours of the suspected event. Tryptase, a neutral protease stored in mast cells, is liberated into the systemic circulation during immune-mediated but not non–immune-mediated reactions. Its presence verifies that mast cell activation and mediator release have occurred, and thus it serves to distinguish immunologic from chemical reactions. Plasma histamine concentration returns to baseline within 30 to 60 minutes of an anaphylactic reaction, so plasma histamine concentration must be measured immediately after treatment of anaphylaxis to capture the change in plasma histamine concentration.

In cases of IgE-mediated anaphylaxis, identification of the offending agent can be established by a positive response to a skin prick or intradermal test (wheal and flare response), which confirms the presence of specific IgE antibodies. Skin testing should not be performed within 6 weeks of an anaphylactic reaction because mast cell and basophil mediator depletion may lead to a false-negative result. Because of the risk of inducing a systemic reaction, testing must be done with a dilute, preservative-free solution of suspected antigen and performed only by trained personnel with appropriate resuscitation equipment available. In vitro immunoassays for allergen-specific IgE are commercially available for some drugs. This type of testing is most commonly used in the evaluation of potential reactions to neuromuscular blockers, latex, penicillin, and other β-lactam antibiotics. Skin testing remains the more sensitive and preferred method of testing in the majority of cases.

TREATMENT

The immediate goals of treatment of anaphylaxis are reversal of hypotension and hypoxemia, replacement of intravascular volume, and inhibition of further cellular degranulation and release of vasoactive mediators (Table 24-4). Several liters of crystalloid and/or colloid solution must be infused to restore intravascular fluid volume and blood pressure. Epinephrine is indicated in doses of 10 to 100 mcg IV. Early intervention with epinephrine is critical for reversing the life-threatening events characteristic of anaphylaxis. Epinephrine, by increasing intracellular concentrations of cyclic adenosine monophosphate, restores membrane permeability and decreases the release of vasoactive mediators. The β-agonist effects of epinephrine relax bronchial smooth muscle and reverse bronchospasm. The dose of epinephrine can be doubled and repeated every 1 to 2 minutes until a satisfactory blood pressure response has been obtained. If anaphylaxis is not life threatening, subcutaneous rather than intravenous epinephrine may be used in a dose of 0.3 to 0.5 mg. In cases where cardiovascular collapse is unresponsive to epinephrine, the use of alternative vasopressors such as vasopressin, glucagon, or norepinephrine should be considered.

Antihistamines such as diphenhydramine compete with membrane receptor sites normally occupied by histamine and may decrease some manifestations of anaphylaxis, including pruritus and bronchospasm. However, administration of an antihistamine is not effective in treating anaphylaxis once vasoactive mediators have been released. $β_2$-Agonists such as albuterol delivered by metered-dose inhaler or nebulizer are useful for the treatment of bronchospasm associated with anaphylaxis.

Corticosteroids are often administered intravenously to patients experiencing life-threatening anaphylaxis. These drugs have no known effect on degranulation of mast cells or antigen-antibody interactions, and the favorable impact observed with corticosteroid therapy may reflect enhancement of the β-agonist effects of other drugs or inhibition of the release of arachidonic acid responsible for the production of leukotrienes and prostaglandins. Corticosteroids may

TABLE 24-4 ■ Management of anaphylactic reactions during anesthesia

PRIMARY TREATMENT

General measures

Inform the surgeon
Request immediate assistance
Stop administration of all drugs, colloids, blood products
Maintain airway with 100% oxygen
Elevate the legs, if practical

Epinephrine administration

Titrate dose according to symptom severity and clinical response
Adults: 10 mcg to 1 mg by bolus, repeat every 1-2 min as needed
IV infusion starting at 0.05-1 mcg/kg/min
Children: 1-10 mcg/kg by bolus, repeat every 1-2 min as needed

Fluid therapy

Crystalloid: normal saline 10-25 mL/kg over 20 min, more as needed
Colloid: 10 mL/kg over 20 min, more as needed

Anaphylaxis resistant to epinephrine

Glucagon: 1-5 mg bolus followed by 1-2.5 mg/hr IV infusion
Norepinephrine: 0.05-0.1 mcg/kg/min IV infusion
Vasopressin: 2-10 unit IV bolus followed by 0.01-0.1 unit/min IV infusion

SECONDARY TREATMENT

Bronchodilator

β_2-Agonist for symptomatic treatment of bronchospasm

Antihistamines

Histamine 1 antagonist: diphenhydramine 0.5-1 mg/kg IV
Histamine 2 antagonist: ranitidine 50 mg IV

Corticosteroids

Adults: hydrocortisone 250 mg IV or methylprednisolone 80 mg IV
Children: hydrocortisone 50-100 mg IV or methylprednisolone 2 mg/kg IV

AFTERCARE

Patient may experience relapse; admit for observation
Obtain blood samples for diagnostic testing
Arrange allergy testing at 6-8 wk postoperatively

Adapted from Mertes PM, Tajima K, Regnier-Kimmoun MA, et al. Perioperative anaphylaxis. *Med Clin North Am.* 2010;94:780.

be uniquely helpful in patients experiencing life-threatening allergic reactions resulting from activation of the complement system.

Drug Allergy

EPIDEMIOLOGY

Drug sensitivity has been implicated in 3.4% to 4.3% of anesthesia-related deaths. The incidence of allergic and anaphylactic drug reactions during anesthesia may be increasing, probably because of the frequent administration of several drugs to a patient and cross-sensitivity among drugs. It is not possible to reliably predict which patients are likely to experience anaphylaxis after administration of drugs that are usually innocuous. However, patients with a history of allergy (extrinsic asthma, allergy to tropical fruits or drugs) have an increased incidence of anaphylaxis, possibly related to a genetic predisposition to form increased amounts of IgE antibodies. Patients allergic to penicillin have a threefold to fourfold greater risk of experiencing an allergic reaction to *any* drug. A history of allergy to specific drugs elicited during the preoperative evaluation is helpful, but previous uneventful exposure to a drug does not eliminate the possibility of anaphylaxis on subsequent exposure. In addition, anaphylaxis can occur on first exposure to a drug because of cross-reactivity with other environmental agents.

Allergic drug reactions must be distinguished from drug intolerance, idiosyncratic reactions, and drug toxicity. The occurrence of undesirable pharmacologic effects at a low dose of drug reflects intolerance, whereas idiosyncratic reactions are undesirable responses to a drug independent of the dose administered. Evidence of histamine release along veins into which drugs are injected indicates localized and nonimmunologic release of histamine insufficient to evoke systemic symptoms. Patients manifesting such a localized response should not be categorized as allergic to a drug.

ALLERGIC DRUG REACTIONS DURING THE PERIOPERATIVE PERIOD

Allergic drug reactions have been reported to almost any drug that may be administered during anesthesia. Most drug-induced allergic reactions manifest within 5 to 10 minutes of exposure. An important exception is the allergic response to latex, which is typically delayed for as long as 30 minutes. When signs appear during maintenance of anesthesia, attention should be directed to the possibility of allergy to latex, volume expanders, or dyes (Table 24-5).

Muscle Relaxants

Muscle relaxants are responsible for approximately 60% of drug-induced allergic reactions during the perioperative period. Cross-sensitivity among muscle relaxants emphasizes the structural similarities of these drugs. Approximately half of patients who experience an allergic reaction to one muscle relaxant are also allergic to other muscle relaxants. IgE antibodies develop to quaternary or tertiary ammonium ions. Many over-the-counter drugs and cosmetics contain these ammonium ions and are capable of sensitizing an individual. Consequently, anaphylaxis may develop on the first exposure to a muscle relaxant in a patient sensitized by one of these products. Neostigmine and morphine contain ammonium ions that are also capable of cross-reacting with antibodies to muscle relaxants. Antibodies that develop against muscle relaxants remain present for decades. Therefore, a patient with a history of anaphylaxis to any muscle relaxant should be skin tested preoperatively for all drugs that are likely to be used in future anesthetic management, and ideally an alternative

TABLE 24-5 ◻ Perioperative allergic drug reactions

Drug	Estimated incidence (%)	Mechanism(s)	Comments
Muscle relaxants	50%-60%	Mostly IgE Nonspecific histamine release	Frequent cross-sensitization between drugs, mainly due to quaternary and tertiary ammonium ions
Latex	15%	IgE	Commonly occurs as a delayed clinical reaction
Antibiotics: β-lactam drugs, quinolones, sulfonamides, vancomycin	10%-15%	IgE, IgG Nonspecific histamine release	<1% cross-reactivity between penicillins and cephalosporins
Hypnotics: barbiturates, propofol	<3%	IgE	
Synthetic colloids: dextran, hydroxyethyl starch	<3%	IgE, IgG	
Opioids: morphine, codeine, fentanyl	<3%	IgE, Nonspecific histamine release	
Radiocontrast media	<2%	IgE, IgG Nonspecific histamine release	
Protamine, aprotinin	<2%	IgE, IgG	
Blood and blood products	<2%	IgA	
Local anesthetics (esters more than amides)	<2%	IgG	

Ig, Immunoglobulin.

agent to which the patient has been skin tested and found to be nonallergic should be utilized. Avoidance is preferred if an alternative means of providing anesthesia is available. Desensitization is theoretically possible but is not practical given that it would require prolonged exposure to a paralytic agent.

Nonimmune reactions to muscle relaxants include direct mast cell degranulation that causes release of histamine and other mediators. Benzyl isoquinolinium compounds such as D-tubocurarine, metocurine, atracurium, and mivacurium are more likely to cause direct mast cell degranulation than aminosteroid compounds like pancuronium, vecuronium, and rocuronium. Skin testing is not useful in the investigation of non–immune-mediated allergic reactions. Reactions that are not IgE mediated may be reduced in frequency or intensity by pretreatment with antihistamines and glucocorticoids.

Induction Drugs

Approximately 5% of perioperative anaphylactic events are caused by hypnotic induction agents, more commonly by barbiturates than by nonbarbiturates. Most reported cases of barbiturate allergy have occurred in patients with a history of previous uneventful exposure to a barbiturate. Cross-reactivity among barbiturates is possible, but there is no evidence of cross-reactivity between barbiturate and nonbarbiturate agents. Propofol has been implicated in allergic reactions both on first and repeated exposure. It has been advised that propofol be used with caution in patients with a history of egg or soy allergy because of the presence of lecithins in the propofol emulsion that may elicit allergic responses. Allergic reactions to midazolam, etomidate, and ketamine are extremely rare.

Local Anesthetics

True allergy to local anesthetics is rare, despite the common labeling of patients as allergic to drugs in this class. It is estimated that only about 1% of purported allergic reactions to local anesthetics are in fact truly allergic; the remainder represent adverse but known responses to inadvertent intravascular injection (hypotension and seizure) or systemic absorption of epinephrine added to local anesthetic (hypertension and tachycardia). Careful history and review of past medical records are most useful in discerning the true mechanism responsible for the event. Urticaria, laryngeal edema, and bronchoconstriction suggest a true allergic response.

Ester-type local anesthetics more commonly cause allergic reactions than amide-type anesthetics. Ester-type local anesthetics are metabolized to compounds related to para-aminobenzoic acid, which is a highly antigenic compound. Preservatives used in local anesthetic solutions such as methylparaben, propylparaben, and metabisulfite also produce allergic reactions. As a result, anaphylaxis may actually be due to stimulation of antibody production to the preservative rather than to the local anesthetic itself.

It is not uncommon to be presented with the question of the safety of administering a local anesthetic to a patient with a purported history of allergy to this class of drugs. It is generally agreed that cross-sensitivity does not exist between ester-type and amide-type compounds. It is also advisable to use only preservative-free local anesthetic solutions, since preservatives may evoke allergic reactions. It is reasonable to recommend intradermal testing with preservative-free local anesthetic in the occasional patient with a convincing history of allergy in whom failure to document a safe local anesthetic drug would prevent the use of local or regional anesthesia when clinically indicated.

Opioids

Anaphylaxis after administration of opioids is very rare, which perhaps reflects the similarity of these drugs to naturally occurring endorphins. Certain opioids, including morphine, codeine, and meperidine, may directly evoke the release of histamine from mast cells and basophils, which mimics an allergic response. These reactions are usually limited to cutaneous manifestations such as pruritus and urticaria, consistent with the fact that opioid receptors have been found on dermal mast cells but not on mast cells from any other organs. Fentanyl is unique among narcotics in that it lacks the ability to stimulate mast cell degranulation; this makes it a good option for patients with cutaneous reactions to other narcotics.

Aspirin and Other Nonsteroidal Antiinflammatory Drugs

Pseudoallergic reactions after administration of aspirin and other nonsteroidal antiinflammatory drugs (NSAIDs) are well documented. Patients with a history of asthma, hyperplastic sinusitis, and nasal polyps are at increased risk of experiencing these reactions. Common symptoms include rhinorrhea and bronchospasm; airway compromise and severe angioedema may also occur. For the most part, these reactions are attributable to inhibition of the cyclooxygenase-1 (COX-1) enzyme that promotes the synthesis of leukotrienes and the subsequent release of mediators from basophils and mast cells. This is substantiated by the fact the reactions are far less severe when selective COX-2 inhibitors are employed.

Volatile Anesthetics

Clinical features of halothane-induced hepatitis suggest a drug-induced allergic reaction. These include eosinophilia, fever, rash, and previous exposure to halothane. The plasma of patients with a clinical diagnosis of halothane hepatitis may contain antibodies that react with halothane-induced liver antigens (neoantigens). These neoantigens are formed by the covalent interaction of reactive oxidative trifluoroacetyl halide metabolites with hepatic microsomal proteins. Acetylation of liver proteins changes these metabolites so that they are no longer recognized as "self" but rather are regarded as "nonself." As a result antibodies are formed against these now foreign proteins. It is postulated that subsequent antigen-antibody interactions are responsible for the liver injury associated with halothane hepatitis. Similar oxidative halide metabolites are produced after exposure to enflurane, isoflurane, and desflurane, which indicates the possibility of cross-sensitivity to volatile anesthetics in susceptible patients. Based on the degree of metabolism of these volatile anesthetics, it is predictable that the likelihood of anesthetic-induced allergic hepatitis would be greatest for halothane, intermediate for enflurane, minimal for isoflurane, and remote for desflurane. Unlike the other volatile agents, sevoflurane does not produce these oxidative halide metabolites.

Radiocontrast Media

Contrast media injected intravenously for radiographic studies evoke allergic reactions in approximately 3% of patients. The risk of an allergic reaction is increased in patients with a history of asthma or allergies to other drugs or foods. However, the pathogenesis of allergy to contrast material is unrelated to that of "seafood" allergy, which is attributed to high concentrations of iodine. Most reactions to contrast material appear to be non–immune mediated. Therefore, in patients with a history of contrast agent allergy, pretreatment with corticosteroids and histamine antagonists is usually effective. A common regimen is oral prednisone 50 mg administered at 13, 7, and 1 hour before exposure and diphenhydramine 50 mg administered 1 hour before contrast agent administration. Allergic reactions are most common with the use of ionic contrast agents; use of nonionic agents substantially reduces the incidence of allergic reactions.

Although rare, severe progressive nephrogenic fibrosis has been reported in patients exposed to gadolinium-based contrast agents. An immunologic reaction to gadolinium chelates appears to be involved; delayed gadolinium excretion resulting from preexisting renal failure is an important predisposing factor.

Latex

Latex is a saplike substance produced by the commercial rubber tree, *Hevea brasiliensis*. Several different *Hevea* proteins may cause an IgE-mediated antibody response that can lead to cardiovascular collapse during anesthesia and surgery. A feature that distinguishes latex-induced allergic reactions from other drug-induced allergic reactions is its delayed onset, typically longer than 30 minutes after exposure to the latex. This may reflect the time needed for the responsible antigen to be eluted from rubber gloves and absorbed across mucous membranes into the systemic circulation in amounts sufficient to cause an allergic reaction. Contact with latex at mucosal surfaces is the most significant route of latex exposure. However, inhalation of latex antigens is an alternative route. Cornstarch powder in gloves is not immunogenic but can act as an airborne vehicle for latex antigens.

Sensitized patients develop IgE antibodies directed specifically against latex antigens. Skin testing can confirm latex hypersensitivity, but anaphylaxis has occurred during skin testing, so this test must be performed with great caution. A radioallergosorbent test and an enzyme-linked immunosorbent assay are available for in vitro detection of latex-specific IgE antibodies. These tests are virtually equal in sensitivity and specificity and avoid the risk of anaphylaxis associated with skin testing.

Questions about itching, conjunctivitis, rhinitis, rash, or wheezing after inflating balloons or wearing latex gloves or after undergoing dental or gynecologic examinations performed using latex gloves may be helpful in identifying sensitized patients. Operating room personnel and patients with spina bifida have an increased incidence of latex allergy that is thought to reflect frequent exposure to latex devices such as bladder catheters and protective outerwear. The incidence of latex sensitivity in anesthesiologists may exceed 15%. Latex sensitivity most often manifests as contact dermatitis or bronchospasm resulting from inhalation of latex allergens. Prevalence of latex allergy peaked in the 1990s and has declined since then. Factors responsible for the increase during that period probably include the widespread adoption of universal precautions in the 1990s so that latex gloves were worn much more often than before. In addition, the tapping of younger rubber trees and the use of stimulant chemicals to increase latex production probably increased the amount of allergenic protein in the raw material and ultimately in the finished goods of production, which also contributed to the increase in allergic responses. The reduction in the frequency of latex allergy over the past several years is probably a result of the transition to the use of latex-free products and avoidance of powdered latex gloves.

Patients at high risk of latex sensitivity (those with spina bifida, multiple previous operations, or history of fruit allergy, as well as health care workers) should be questioned for symptoms related to exposure to natural rubber during their daily routines or previous surgical procedures. Intraoperative management of these patients includes strict maintenance of a latex-free environment, including the use of nonlatex gloves (styrene, neoprene) by all personnel in contact with the patient. In addition, medications should not be drawn up through latex caps or injected through latex ports on intravenous delivery tubing.

Protamine

Protamine is capable of causing direct histamine release from mast cells and activating the complement pathway to produce thromboxane, which causes bronchoconstriction, pulmonary artery hypertension, and systemic hypotension. This is a predictable response and is directly related to the rate of injection. It is not an allergic reaction.

Immune-mediated anaphylactic reactions to protamine are rare. The presence of serum antiprotamine IgE and IgG antibodies can be demonstrated in these patients. Protamine allergy is more likely to occur in patients who are allergic to seafood, which reflects the fact that protamine is derived from salmon sperm. After vasectomy, men may be at increased risk of allergic reactions to protamine because they develop circulating antibodies to spermatozoa. Diabetic patients treated with protamine-containing insulin preparations such as neutral protamine Hagedorn (NPH) are also at increased risk. Patients known to be allergic to protamine present a therapeutic challenge when neutralization of heparin is required, because no effective alternative to protamine is commonly available. In the rare instances when patients with protamine allergy require anticoagulation, the use of a direct thrombin inhibitor such as bivalirudin instead of heparin can be considered. Heparinase, a heparin-neutralizing enzyme from the gram-negative bacterium *Flavobacterium heparinum*, has also been used as a substitute for protamine.

Antibiotics

Antibiotics are the second most common cause of anaphylaxis in the perioperative period, accounting for approximately 10% to 15% of all episodes. Penicillin allergy is most common, and in the general population, penicillin accounts for most fatal anaphylactic drug reactions. Approximately 10% of patients report a penicillin allergy; however, it has been estimated that up to 90% of these patients are in fact able to tolerate penicillin. This is due in part to an initial misattribution of clinical signs to a penicillin reaction rather than to the underlying medical illness being treated with penicillin. In addition, IgE antibodies to penicillin wane over time; therefore many patients diagnosed as penicillin allergic in childhood are able to tolerate penicillin as adults. Elective skin testing should be considered for any patient with a convincing history of IgE-mediated penicillin allergy to avoid inappropriate avoidance of β-lactam antibiotics and unnecessary use of more expensive and broader-spectrum antibiotics. The negative predictive value of penicillin skin testing is high; that is, a negative skin test result for penicillin does reliably indicate that the patient is not allergic to penicillin. Patients with a positive skin test result are candidates for drug desensitization. This is accomplished by administration of escalating challenge doses of an allergen or drug to an allergic patient so that the patient eventually becomes desensitized to the allergen or drug.

The structural similarity between penicillin and the cephalosporins (both contain β-lactam rings) suggests the possibility of cross-sensitivity. However, the incidence of life-threatening allergic reactions following administration of cephalosporins is low (0.05%). Historically, the incidence of allergic reaction to cephalosporins in patients with a history of penicillin allergy was reported to be in the range of 7%. More recent research suggests a much lower rate of cross-reactivity (0.2%). Cross-reactivity is seen most often in patients reporting an allergy to amoxicillin who are given first-generation cephalosporins or cefamandole. Cross-reactivity is seen less often if later-generation cephalosporins are administered.

Allergy to sulfonamide antibiotics is the second most commonly reported antibiotic allergy. These reactions manifest most often as delayed cutaneous rashes, and sulfonamides are the most common cause of Stevens-Johnson Syndrome. In HIV-positive patients, the incidence of skin rash to sulfonamides is approximately ten times higher than that in HIV-negative patients. Because trimethoprim-sulfamethoxazole is the drug of choice for the treatment and prophylaxis of *Pneumocystis jiroveci* (formerly called *Pneumocystis carinii*) pneumonia in HIV-positive patients, drug desensitization is advised.

Most purported cases of vancomycin allergy are non–IgE-mediated reactions involving direct histamine release from mast cells and basophils, and are directly related to the rate of drug infusion. In most cases, these patients are able to tolerate repeat administration utilizing slower infusion rates and antihistamine premedication. However, in rare cases IgE-mediated allergy has been reported on repeat exposure to this drug.

Blood, Blood Products, and Synthetic Volume Expanders

Minor urticarial allergic reactions to properly cross-matched blood products may occur in 1% to 3% of patients. The cause is unknown, but may involve soluble antigens in the donor unit to which the recipient has been previously sensitized.

Anaphylactic reactions are rare, occurring in approximately 1 in 20,000 to 50,000 transfusions. These may result from antibodies against IgA, HLA, or complement proteins.

The leading cause of transfusion-related morbidity and mortality is transfusion-related acute lung injury (TRALI). Diagnostic criteria for TRALI include hypoxia and bilateral pulmonary edema that occur within 6 hours of transfusion and in the absence of intravascular fluid overload or heart failure. The pathogenesis of TRALI appears to be activation of neutrophils on the pulmonary vascular endothelium as a result of donor leukocyte antibodies, particularly anti-HLA and anti-neutrophil antibodies. These antibodies are contained in the plasma component of transfused blood products. Therefore, TRALI is most commonly seen after transfusion of plasma-rich components such as fresh frozen plasma and platelets. The reported incidence of TRALI varies significantly since diagnostic criteria have only recently been agreed upon. Treatment is supportive, and most patients recover spontaneously within a few days. Neither steroid therapy nor diuresis is beneficial.

Hemolytic transfusion reactions occur in 1 in 10,000 to 50,000 blood component transfusions. These reactions appear to be mediated by immunoglobulins, particularly IgM and IgG.

The estimated incidence of allergic reactions to plasma volume expanders is between 0.03% and 0.22%. All synthetic colloids have been implicated, but reactions are more common with dextrans and gelatins than with albumin and hydroxyethyl starch. Both immune- and non–immune-mediated mechanisms have been implicated, with manifestations ranging from rash and modest hypotension to bronchospasm and shock.

Other Agents

Several other drugs have been implicated in cases of perioperative drug allergy. These include the serine protease inhibitor aprotinin, formerly used in cardiac surgery to reduce blood loss, as well as antiseptic solutions such as chlorhexidine, vital dyes, heparin, and insulin. This underscores the importance of including drug allergy as part of the differential diagnosis of any case of cardiovascular collapse that occurs during the perioperative period.

Eosinophilia

Clinically significant eosinophilia is defined as a sustained absolute eosinophil count of more than 1000 to 1500/mm^3. Moderate eosinophilia is commonly seen in a wide spectrum of disorders, including parasitic infestations, systemic allergic disorders, collagen vascular diseases, various forms of dermatitis, drug reactions, and tumors. Hodgkin's disease and both B- and T-cell non-Hodgkin's lymphomas can present with eosinophilia. Even when there is no obvious sign of an underlying lymphoma, up to 25% of patients with apparent idiopathic eosinophilia have an expanded clone of aberrant T cells that produce high levels of IL-5.

Hypereosinophilia is associated with tissue damage secondary to release of basic protein by the eosinophil.

Irreversible endomyocardial fibrosis producing a restrictive cardiomyopathy is common in patients who maintain eosinophil counts higher than 5000/mm^3. In patients with eosinophilic leukemia or idiopathic hypereosinophilic (Löffler's) syndrome, eosinophil counts can reach 20,000 to 100,000/mm^3. Widespread organ dysfunction and rapidly progressive heart disease are associated with these conditions. These patients need aggressive treatment with both corticosteroids and hydroxyurea. Leukapheresis can be used to acutely lower eosinophil counts.

MISDIRECTED ADAPTIVE IMMUNITY

Autoimmune Disorders

The challenge of adaptive immunity is the need for immune cells to be capable of responding efficiently to a wide variety of foreign antigens yet still be able to recognize and tolerate "self" antigens. There is growing evidence that major immunologic stimuli, such as certain infections, can activate self-reactive lymphocytes. In general, these primed self-reactive lymphocytes tend to undergo apoptotic elimination once the immunologic challenge has been controlled. Indeed, transient autoimmunity appears to be a relatively common byproduct of major immune system activation. The specific defects that cause autoimmunity to persist and develop into a chronic, self-destructive immune disorder are not well understood. Genetic predisposition may play a role. Table 24-6 lists some diseases with a known autoimmune basis.

The anesthetic implications of autoimmune disorders can be divided into three categories. The first includes the anesthetic considerations involving certain vulnerable organs specific to the particular immune disorder. Examples include cervical instability with rheumatoid arthritis, renal injury with systemic lupus erythematosus, and liver failure with chronic autoimmune hepatitis. The second category is related to the consequences of therapy used to treat the autoimmune disorder. The potential for addisonian crisis in patients treated long term with corticosteroids is well recognized. Newer therapies for autoimmune disorders inhibit specific facets of the immune response, which places patients who take these medications at increased risk of perioperative infection. The third category, especially in patients with long-standing autoimmune disorders, concerns the risk of accelerated atherosclerosis and associated cardiovascular complications such as heart disease and stroke. Some studies suggest that the risk of cardiovascular morbidity and mortality is increased by as much as 50-fold in the presence of an autoimmune disease. Some of this added risk may be due to the agents used to treat the autoimmune disease itself. For example, long-term steroid therapy is associated with hypertension and diabetes mellitus, both of which are powerful risk factors for cardiovascular disease. Therefore, patients with long-standing autoimmune conditions warrant thorough cardiovascular evaluation and consideration of the increased risk of perioperative cardiovascular complications.

TABLE 24-6 ▪ Examples of autoimmune diseases

RHEUMATIC
Rheumatoid arthritis
Scleroderma
Sjögren's syndrome
Systemic lupus erythematosus

GASTROINTESTINAL
Chronic active hepatitis
Crohn's disease
Primary biliary cirrhosis
Ulcerative colitis

ENDOCRINE
Graves' disease
Hashimoto's thyroiditis
Type 1 diabetes mellitus

NEUROLOGIC
Multiple sclerosis
Myasthenia gravis

HEMATOLOGIC
Autoimmune hemolytic anemia
Idiopathic thrombocytopenic purpura
Pernicious anemia

RENAL
Goodpasture's syndrome

MULTIPLE ORGAN SYSTEM
Ankylosing spondylitis
Polymyositis
Psoriasis
Sarcoidosis
Vasculitis

ANESTHESIA AND IMMUNOCOMPETENCE

Many perioperative factors affect immunocompetence and therefore may alter the incidence of perioperative infection or the body's response to cancer.

Transfusion-Related Immunomodulation

In recent years, it has come to be appreciated that transfusion of allogeneic blood products has a measurable impact on immune function. Such transfusion-related immunomodulatory (TRIM) effects include increased susceptibility to infection and promotion of tumor growth. Conversely, a TRIM effect is likely to explain improved renal allograft survival in transplant patients. Specific TRIM effects include decreased NK cell and phagocytic function, impaired antigen presentation, and suppression of lymphocyte production. The mechanism underlying TRIM effects remains unclear but may involve donor leukocytes present in transfused blood products and soluble HLA class I peptides. Partial HLA compatibility between donor leukocytes and the recipient induces a state of microchimerism that prompts the release of IL-4, IL-10, and other inflammatory mediators that impair cell-mediated immunity and cytotoxicity. An extreme manifestation of microchimerism is the development of transfusion-associated graft-versus-host disease, a rare but often fatal condition in which immunocompetent donor (graft) cells attack the recipient's cells, which leads to pancytopenia and liver failure. Application of leukoreduction techniques to stored blood appear to mitigate some but not all TRIM effects. The presence in stored blood of other soluble mediators such as histamine and other proinflammatory cytokines that are not removed by leukoreduction may account for the incomplete effect of leukoreduction.

The Neuroendocrine Stress Response

By far the most important influence on immune function in the perioperative period is the neuroendocrine stress response initiated by activation of the autonomic nervous system and the hypothalamic-pituitary axis. Surgical stress induces release of catecholamines, corticotropin, and cortisol. Monocytes, macrophages, and T cells possess β_2-adrenergic and glucocorticoid receptors. Activation of these receptors results in net inhibition of T_H1 cytokine production and promotion of T_H2 antiinflammatory cytokine release. Monocyte and macrophage activation lead to the release of cytokines such as IL-1, IL-6, and tumor necrosis factor-α, which further stimulate the hypothalamic-pituitary axis. The benefit of this immunosuppression is to minimize the inflammatory response caused by surgical trauma. The downside of this immunosuppression is an increased vulnerability to infection and tumor proliferation.

Numerous other perioperative factors weaken the immune system. Acute pain suppresses NK cell activity, probably as a result of activation of the hypothalamic-pituitary axis and autonomic nervous system. Hypothermia exacerbates the neuroendocrine stress response and induces thermoregulatory vasoconstriction. Tissue hypoxia impairs oxidative killing by neutrophils and prolongs wound healing. Hypothermia has also been shown to suppress NK cell activity and lymphocyte function. Elevated plasma cortisol and catecholamine concentrations during surgery result in hyperglycemia, which can provide a medium for bacterial growth. Hyperglycemia itself also has deleterious effects on the immune system. Hyperglycemia induces changes in the vascular endothelium that impede lymphocyte migration. It also reduces immune cell proliferation by interfering with critical enzymatic functions, and it impairs neutrophil phagocytosis.

Effects of Anesthetics on the Immune Response

It is well established that immunocompetence is essential for a host to resist cancer. For example, recipients of solid organ transplants who have a history of cancer experience a higher rate of cancer recurrence following the initiation of immunosuppressive therapy. Surgical excision remains the treatment of choice for most locally contained solid organ cancers, but there is concern that exposure to surgery and anesthesia may actually promote tumor progression.

Several mechanisms are likely at play. Surgical disruption of the tumor may release tumor cells into the circulation, which provides the seeds for micrometastases. The presence of a primary tumor may itself inhibit angiogenesis; therefore, tumor removal may paradoxically favor the survival of minimal residual disease. Release of growth factors and suppression of antiangiogenic factors may also contribute. In addition, tissue injury depresses cell-mediated immunity, including the function of cytotoxic T cells and NK cells. Allogeneic red blood cell transfusion in the perioperative period may also play a role in increasing the risk of tumor recurrence. Laboratory investigation of TRIM has demonstrated a reduction in T_H and NK cell counts and decreased levels of the $T_H 1$ cytokines IL-2 and interferon.

Considerable in vitro and in vivo evidence from animal studies suggest that anesthetics and analgesics also have an impact on the immune response (Table 24-7). The magnitude of this effect is probably considerably less than that of the surgical stress itself, but an additive effect may be important. Ketamine, thiopental, and all of the volatile anesthetics appear to reduce NK cell activity and/or number. Volatile anesthetics also impair neutrophil function by inhibiting the respiratory oxidative burst mechanism and reducing lymphocyte proliferation. Nitrous oxide impairs DNA and nucleotide synthesis and has been observed to depress hematopoietic and mononuclear cell synthesis and depress neutrophil chemotaxis. The impact of propofol on immune function is less clear, but propofol bears a chemical resemblance to the antioxidant α-tocopherol and may possess antiinflammatory and antioxidative properties that tend to inhibit neutrophil, monocyte, and macrophage activity. Recently interest has focused on propofol conjugates in the treatment of breast cancer since they have been shown to inhibit cellular adhesion and promote apoptosis of breast cancer cells.

The immunosuppressive effects of opiates have been known for decades. Opioid receptors in the hypothalamic-pituitary axis promote the release of corticotropin and cortisol. Sympathetic nervous system activation and catecholamine release further suppress NK cell, lymphocyte, neutrophil, and macrophage functions. Immune cells also possess a specific subset of μ receptors, the activation of which leads to increased intracellular calcium gradients and activation of nitric oxide synthase. Elevated nitric oxide concentrations appear to mediate many of the antiinflammatory effects of naturally occurring opioids. Morphine also impairs antibody formation and the synthesis of proinflammatory cytokines. As expected, many of the immunomodulatory effects of opioids can be blocked by administration of the μ-receptor antagonist naloxone. There is some evidence to suggest that synthetic opioids such as fentanyl and remifentanil have less of an impact on immune function, possibly related to their differential activation of specific opioid receptors.

Nonopioid analgesics seem to have less effect on immune function than opiates. In fact, there is some evidence to

TABLE 24-7	Effects of anesthetic drugs on immune system function
Drug	**Effect on immune system**
Thiopental	Reduces NK cell activity and number in animal models
Propofol	Reduces NK cell number in animal models
Volatile agents	Inhibit stimulation of NK cell cytotoxicity in animal models
	Reduce NK cell number in humans
Nitrous oxide	Associated with acceleration in development of lung and liver metastases in animal models
	Inhibits hematopoietic cell formation
Local anesthetic drugs	Inhibit tumor cell proliferation
Morphine	Inhibits cellular and NK cell immunity in animal models
Fentanyl	Inhibits NK cell activity in humans
Tramadol	Stimulates NK cell activity in animal and human models
Cyclooxygenase-2 inhibitors	Display antiangiogenic and antitumor effects in animal models

Data from Snyder GL, Greenberg S. Effect of anaesthetic technique and other perioperative factors on cancer recurrence. *Br J Anaesth.* 2010;105:109.
NK, Natural killer.

suggest that tramadol, which has noradrenergic and serotoninergic activity in addition to μ-receptor affinity, may promote NK cell activity. NSAIDs that inhibit the COX enzyme have been shown in an animal model to possess antitumor and antiangiogenic properties. COX-2 inhibitors such as etodolac and celecoxib may attenuate the deleterious effects of opioid-induced tumor growth.

Some retrospective studies have shown that the use of regional anesthesia instead of intravenous morphine for postoperative pain control is associated with measurable reductions in cancer recurrence. Several mechanisms may account for this observation. Regional anesthesia attenuates the neuroendocrine surgical stress response by blocking afferent transmission to the hypothalamic-pituitary axis. In addition, patients who receive regional anesthesia or regional analgesia have reduced requirements for drugs with known immunosuppressive effects, such as general anesthetics and opioids. Local anesthetic agents may also possess intrinsic antitumor properties. Both lidocaine and ropivacaine have been shown to exert antiproliferative effects on tumor cells. Not all research has supported a benefit of regional anesthesia over general anesthesia in terms of cancer prognosis. The impact may differ depending on tumor type. Therefore, despite these promising findings, more research is needed before definitive conclusions can be drawn about the optimal anesthetic choice in cancer patients.

KEY POINTS

- The immune system is divided into *innate* and *adaptive* or *acquired* pathways.
- The innate immune pathway mounts the initial response to any infection, recognizes targets that are common to many pathogens, and has no specific memory. Its cellular components are neutrophils, macrophages, monocytes, and NK cells, and its main noncellular elements are the complement proteins.
- The adaptive immune pathway has a more delayed onset of action and may take days to activate when challenged by an unfamiliar antigen. However, adaptive immunity is capable of developing memory and is more rapidly induced by antigen when memory is present. Adaptive immunity consists of a humoral component mediated by B lymphocytes that produce antibodies and a cellular component dominated by T lymphocytes.
- Angioedema may be hereditary or acquired and is characterized by episodic edema resulting from increased vascular permeability. The condition commonly involves swelling of the face and mucous membranes and may lead to airway compromise. The most common hereditary form results from an autosomal dominant deficiency of C1 esterase inhibitor, which results in a build-up of the vasoactive compound bradykinin. Treatment of acute episodes involves administration of C1 inhibitor concentrate or fresh frozen plasma to replace the deficient enzyme. Androgens, catecholamines, antihistamines, and antifibrinolytics are *not* useful in the treatment of acute episodes of angioedema.
- Anaphylaxis is a life-threatening condition caused by massive release of vasoactive mediators via degranulation of mast cells and basophils through either immune- or non–immune-mediated mechanisms. Treatment requires reversal of hypotension through replacement of intravascular fluid volume and inhibition of further release of vasoactive mediators. Early intervention with epinephrine is critical. Epinephrine increases intracellular cyclic adenosine monophosphate and thereby reduces vasoactive mediator release. It also relaxes bronchial smooth muscle and relieves bronchospasm.
- Muscle relaxants are responsible for more than 60% of drug-induced allergic reactions in the perioperative period, and cross-sensitization among different muscle relaxants is common. Reaction may occur on first exposure (presumably caused by sensitization from other environmental agents) or after previous uneventful exposure.
- Almost all allergic reactions occur within 5 to 10 minute of exposure to an antigen. An important exception to this rule is the allergic response to latex, which typically occurs at least 30 minutes after exposure. Preoperative referral for skin testing is appropriate for patients with a strong clinical history of previous latex allergic reaction. Latex sensitivity is an occupational hazard for health care workers. Other groups with a higher than average risk of latex allergy are patients with a history of spina bifida, multiple prior surgeries, or fruit allergy.
- Autoimmune disorders result in immune-mediated end-organ dysfunction because of inappropriate activation of antibody against self-antigens. Each disorder is accompanied by a distinct set of multisystem features. Patients with autoimmune disorders also have an increased risk of cardiovascular disease. Therefore, careful preoperative evaluation is imperative to prevent excess perioperative morbidity and mortality. Many of these patients are treated with exogenous glucocorticoids and may require "stress-dose" steroids prior to major surgery to prevent addisonian crisis.
- Many factors related to surgery and anesthesia impair immune function, which may precipitate infection and cancer progression in susceptible patients. The principal factor appears to be the neuroendocrine response to surgical stress, which includes release of catecholamines and glucocorticoids that impair both innate and adaptive immune responses. Anesthetic agents, including volatile anesthetics and opioids, also impair immune function. Regional and neuraxial anesthesia with local anesthetics may help preserve immune system function.

RESOURCES

Bonilla FA, Oettgen HC. Adaptive immunity. *J Allergy Clin Immunol.* 2010;125:S33-S40.

Chaplin DD. Overview of the immune response. *J Allergy Clin Immunol.* 2010;125:S3-S23.

Frank MM. Complement disorders and hereditary angioedema. *J Allergy Clin Immunol.* 2010;125:S262-S271.

Lekstrom-Himes JA, Gallin JI. Immunodeficiency diseases caused by defects in phagocytes. *N Engl J Med.* 2000;343:1703-1714.

Mertes PM, Tajima K, Regnier-Kimmoun MA, et al. Perioperative anaphylaxis. *Med Clin North Am.* 2010;94:761-789.

Snyder GL, Greenberg S. Effect of anaesthetic technique and other perioperative factors on cancer recurrence. *Br J Anaesth.* 2010;105:106-115.

Walport MJ. Complement. *N Engl J Med.* 2001;344:1058-1066:1140-1151.

Zuraw BL. Hereditary angioedema. *N Engl J Med.* 2010;359:1027-1036.

Psychiatric Disease, Substance Abuse, and Drug Overdose

ROBERTA L. HINES ■
KATHERINE E. MARSCHALL ■

The prevalence of mental disorders and substance use disorders in the United States is about 30%, so these conditions will often be present in patients undergoing anesthesia and surgery. Effects of and potential drug interactions with psychotropic medications are important perioperative considerations. In addition, substance abuse and suicide represent significant occupational hazards for anesthesiologists.

MOOD DISORDERS

Mood disorders are characterized by disturbances in the regulation of mood, behavior, and affect. They are typically divided into three classes: (1) depressive disorders, (2) bipolar disorders, and (3) depression associated with medical illness or substance abuse.

Depression

Depression is a common psychiatric disorder, affecting 2% to 4% of the population. It is distinguished from normal sadness and grief by the severity and duration of the mood disturbances. There is a familial pattern to major depression, and females are affected more often than males. Approximately 15% of patients with *major* depression commit suicide. Pathophysiologic causes of major depression are unknown, although abnormalities of amine neurotransmitter pathways are the most likely etiologic factors.

DIAGNOSIS

The diagnosis of major depression is based on the persistent presence of at least five of the symptoms noted in Table 25-1 for a period of at least 2 weeks. There is a profound loss of pleasure in previously enjoyable activities (anhedonia). Organic causes of irritability or mood changes and the normal reaction to a major loss such as the death of a loved one or loss of a job must be excluded. Depressive symptoms often are present

TABLE 25-1 Characteristics of severe depression

Depressed mood
Markedly diminished interest or pleasure in almost all
  activities
Fluctuations in body weight and appetite
Insomnia or hypersomnia
Restlessness
Fatigue
Feelings of worthlessness or guilt
Decreased ability to concentrate
Suicidal ideation

TABLE 25-2 Commonly used antidepressant medications

Drug class	Generic name	Trade name
SSRIs	Fluoxetine	Prozac
	Paroxetine	Paxil
	Sertraline	Zoloft
	Fluvoxamine	Luvox
	Citalopram	Celexa
Tricyclics	Amitriptyline	Elavil
	Imipramine	Tofranil
	Protriptyline	Vivactil
	Doxepin	Sinequan
MAOIs	Phenelzine	Nardil
	Tranylcypromine	Parnate
Atypical	Bupropion	Wellbutrin
	Trazodone	Desyrel
	Nefazodone	Serzone
	Venlafaxine	Effexor

MAOIs, Monoamine oxidase inhibitors; *SSRIs,* selective serotonin reuptake inhibitors.

in patients with cardiac disease, cancer, neurologic diseases, diabetes mellitus, hypothyroidism, and human immunodeficiency virus (HIV) infection. Even if it is not directly related to the medical illness, the depression can be a side effect of medication used to treat the medical illness.

All patients with depression should be evaluated for the potential to commit suicide. Suicide is the eighth leading cause of death among Americans. About 5% of depressed patients will commit suicide. Interestingly, physicians have moderately higher (men) to much higher (women) suicide rates than the general population. Most individuals who commit suicide have been under the care of a physician (not necessarily a psychiatrist) within the month before their death, which emphasizes the need for physicians in all specialties to recognize patients at risk. Hopelessness is the most important aspect of depression associated with suicide.

TREATMENT

Depression can be treated with antidepressant medications, psychotherapy, and/or electroconvulsive therapy (ECT). An estimated 70% to 80% of patients respond to pharmacologic therapy, and at least 50% who do not respond to antidepressants do respond favorably to ECT. ECT is usually reserved for patients with depression resistant to antidepressant drugs or those with medical contraindications to treatment with these drugs. Patients with depression plus psychotic symptoms (delusions, hallucinations, catatonia) require both antidepressant and antipsychotic drugs.

Approximately 50 years ago, neurochemical hypotheses regarding depression postulated that decreased availability of norepinephrine and serotonin at specific synapses in the brain is associated with depression and, conversely, that an increased concentration of these neurotransmitters is associated with mania. Subsequent studies have generally supported the hypotheses that norepinephrine and serotonin metabolism are important in mood states, although the exact mechanisms remain to be elucidated. Almost all drugs with antidepressant properties affect the availability of catecholamine and/or serotonin in the central nervous system (Table 25-2).

The selective serotonin reuptake inhibitors (SSRIs) block reuptake of serotonin at presynaptic membranes but have relatively little effect on adrenergic, cholinergic, histaminergic, or other neurochemical systems. As a result, they are associated with few side effects.

Tricyclic antidepressants are thought to affect depression by inhibiting synaptic reuptake of norepinephrine and serotonin. However, they also affect other neurochemical systems, including histaminergic and cholinergic systems. Consequently, they have a large range of adverse effects, including postural hypotension, cardiac dysrhythmias, and urinary retention.

Monoamine oxidase inhibitors (MAOIs) are inhibitors of both the A and B forms of brain monamine oxidase and change the concentration of neurotransmitters by preventing breakdown of catecholamines and serotonin. They are not considered first-line drugs in treatment of depression because of their adverse effect profile, which includes the risk of hypertensive crises from consumption of tyramine-containing foods and the risk of serotonin syndrome if they are used concomitantly with SSRIs.

Venlafaxine is a methylamine antidepressant that selectively inhibits reuptake of norepinephrine and serotonin without affecting other neurochemical systems. Other atypical antidepressants have more diverse effects, including inhibition of reuptake of serotonin and dopamine, antagonism of specific serotonin receptors, dopamine receptor blockade, presynaptic α_2-blockade resulting in increases in norepinephrine and serotonin release, and histamine receptor blockade.

There has been a resurgence in the use of amphetamine and its congeners in treating depression. Typically these drugs are used in small dosages in combination with SSRIs. The effects on mood can be remarkable. However, because of their status as class II controlled substances, it is unlikely that they will be widely used.

Selective Serotonin Reuptake Inhibitors
Serotonin is produced by hydroxylation and decarboxylation of L-tryptophan in presynaptic neurons, then stored in

vesicles that are released and bound to postsynaptic receptors when needed for neurotransmission. A reuptake mechanism allows for return of serotonin to the presynaptic vesicles. Metabolism is by monoamine oxidase type A. Serotonin-specific reuptake inhibitors, as their name implies, inhibit the reuptake of serotonin from the neuronal synapse without having significant effects on reuptake of norepinephrine and dopamine.

SSRIs comprise the most widely prescribed class of antidepressants and are the drugs of choice to treat mild to moderate depression. These drugs are also effective for treating panic disorders, posttraumatic stress disorder, bulimia, dysthymia, obsessive-compulsive disorder, and irritable bowel syndrome. Common side effects of SSRIs are insomnia, agitation, headache, nausea, diarrhea, dry mouth, and sexual dysfunction. Appetite suppression is associated with fluoxetine therapy. Abrupt cessation of SSRI use, especially use of paroxetine and fluvoxamine, which have short half-lives and no active metabolites, can result in a discontinuation syndrome that can mimic serious illness and can be distressing and uncomfortable. Discontinuation symptoms typically begin 1 to 3 days after abrupt cessation of SSRI use and may include dizziness, irritability, mood swings, headache, nausea and vomiting, dystonia, tremor, lethargy, myalgias, and fatigue. Symptoms are relieved within 24 hours of restarting SSRI therapy.

Among SSRIs, fluoxetine is a potent inhibitor of certain hepatic cytochrome P-450 enzymes. As a result, this drug may increase plasma concentrations of drugs that depend on hepatic metabolism for clearance. For example, the addition of fluoxetine to treatment with tricyclic antidepressant drugs may result in twofold to fivefold increases in the plasma concentrations of tricyclic drugs. Some cardiac antidysrhythmic drugs and some β-adrenergic antagonists are also metabolized by this enzyme system, and fluoxetine inhibition of enzyme activity may result in potentiation of their effects.

Serotonin Syndrome. Serotonin syndrome is a potentially life-threatening adverse drug reaction that may occur with therapeutic drug use, overdose, or interaction between serotoninergic drugs. A large number of drugs have been associated with serotonin syndrome. These include SSRIs, atypical and cyclic antidepressants, MAOIs, opiates, cough medicine, antibiotics, weight reduction drugs, antiemetic drugs, antimigraine drugs, drugs of abuse (especially "ecstasy" [3,4-methylenedioxymethamphetamine]), and herbal products (Table 25-3).

Typical symptoms of serotonin syndrome include agitation, delirium, autonomic hyperactivity, hyperreflexia, clonus, and hyperthermia (Figure 25-1). Additional syndromes to consider in the differential diagnosis of serotonin syndrome are listed in Table 25-4. Treatment includes supportive measures and control of autonomic instability, excess muscle activity, and hyperthermia. Cyproheptadine, a 5-hydroxytryptamine (serotonin) type 2A (5-HT$_{2A}$) antagonist, can be used to bind serotonin receptors. It is available only for oral use.

TABLE 25-3 ■ Drug and drug interactions associated with serotonin syndrome

DRUGS ASSOCIATED WITH SEROTONIN SYNDROME

SSRIs
Atypical and cyclic antidepressants
Monoamine oxidase inhibitors
Anticonvulsant drugs: valproate
Analgesics: meperidine, fentanyl, tramadol, pentazocine
Antiemetic drugs: ondansetron, granisetron, metoclopramide
Antimigraine drugs: sumatriptan
Bariatric medications: sibutramine
Antibiotics: linezolid, ritonavir
Over-the-counter cough medicine: dextromethorphan
Drugs of abuse: ecstasy, lysergic acid diethylamide (LSD), 5-methoxy-diisopropyltryptamine ("foxy methoxy"), Syrian rue
Dietary supplements: St. John's wort, ginseng
Other: lithium

DRUG INTERACTIONS ASSOCIATED WITH SEVERE SEROTONIN SYNDROME

Phenelzine and meperidine
Tranylcypromine and imipramine
Phenelzine and SSRIs
Paroxetine and buspirone
Linezolid and citalopram
Moclobemide and SSRIs
Tramadol, venlafaxine, and mirtazapine

Modified from Boyer EW, Shannon M. The serotonin syndrome. *N Engl J Med*. 2005;352:1112-1120. Copyright 2005 Massachusetts Medical Society. All rights reserved.
SSRIs, Selective serotonin reuptake inhibitors.

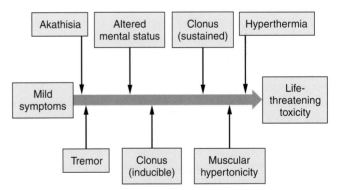

FIGURE 25-1 Spectrum of clinical findings in serotonin syndrome. Manifestations range from mild to life threatening. The vertical arrows suggest the approximate point at which clinical findings initially appear in the spectrum of the disease. *(Adapted from Boyer EW, Shannon M. The serotonin syndrome.* N Engl J Med. *2005;352:1112-1120. Copyright 2005 Massachusetts Medical Society. All rights reserved.)*

Tricyclic Antidepressants

Before the availability of SSRIs, tricyclic antidepressants were the most commonly prescribed drugs for treatment of depression. Now they are used in selected patients with depression and as adjuvant therapy for patients with chronic pain syndromes. Advantages include low cost and, for nortriptyline, imipramine, and desipramine, the existence of

TABLE 25-4   Drug-induced hyperthermic syndromes

Syndrome	Time to onset	Causative drugs	Outstanding features	Treatment
Malignant hyperthermia	Within minutes	Succinylcholine, inhalation anesthetics	Muscle rigidity, severe hypercarbia	Dantrolene, supportive care
Neuroleptic malignant syndrome	24-72 hr	Dopamine antagonist antipsychotic drugs	Muscle rigidity, stupor or coma, bradykinesia	Bromocriptine or dantrolene, supportive care
Serotonin syndrome	Up to 12 hr	Serotoninergic drugs including SSRIs, MAOIs, and atypical antidepressants	Clonus, hyperreflexia, agitation; possible muscle rigidity	Cyproheptadine, supportive care
Sympathomimetic syndrome	Up to 30 min	Cocaine, amphetamines	Agitation, hallucinations, myocardial ischemia, dysrhythmias, no rigidity	Vasodilators, α- and β-blockers, supportive care
Anticholinergic poisoning	Up to 12 hr	Atropine, belladonna	Toxidrome of hot, red, dry skin; dilated pupils; delirium; no rigidity	Physostigmine, supportive care
Cyclic antidepressant overdose	Up to 6 hr	Cyclic antidepressants	Hypotension, stupor or coma, wide-complex dysrhythmias, no rigidity	Serum alkalinization, magnesium

MAOIs, Monoamine oxidase inhibitors; *SSRIs,* selective serotonin reuptake inhibitors.

well-defined correlations between dosage, plasma concentration, and therapeutic responses. Adverse effects influence drug choice, because all these drugs are equally effective if administered in equivalent dosages. In addition to causing sedative and anticholinergic effects, tricyclic antidepressants can cause cardiovascular abnormalities, including orthostatic hypotension and cardiac dysrhythmias.

Management of Anesthesia. Patients being treated with tricyclic antidepressants may have altered responses to drugs administered during the perioperative period. Increased availability of neurotransmitters in the central nervous system can result in increased anesthetic requirements. Likewise, increased availability of norepinephrine at postsynaptic receptors in the sympathetic nervous system can be responsible for exaggerated blood pressure responses following administration of indirect-acting vasopressors, such as ephedrine. The potential for significant hypertension is greatest during acute treatment with tricyclic antidepressants (first 14 to 21 days); long-term treatment is associated with downregulation of receptors.

Long-term treatment with tricyclic antidepressants may alter the response to pancuronium. Tachydysrhythmias have been observed following administration of pancuronium to patients who were also receiving imipramine. Presumably, there is an interaction between tricyclic antidepressants and the anticholinergic- and sympathetic-stimulating effects of pancuronium. Ketamine, meperidine, and epinephrine-containing local anesthetic solutions might produce adverse responses similar to those seen with pancuronium and are best avoided.

Monoamine Oxidase Inhibitors

Patients whose depression does not respond to other antidepressant drugs may benefit from treatment with MAOIs.

TABLE 25-5   Adverse effects of monoamine oxidase inhibitors

Sedation
Blurred vision
Orthostatic hypotension
Tyramine-induced hypertensive crisis
Excessive effects of sympathomimetic drugs
Potential for serotonin syndrome

MAOIs inhibit norepinephrine and serotonin breakdown, so there is more norepinephrine and serotonin available for release. The principal clinical problem associated with use of these drugs is the occurrence of significant systemic hypertension if patients ingest foods containing tyramine (cheeses, wines) or receive sympathomimetic drugs. Both tyramine and sympathomimetic drugs are potent stimuli for norepinephrine release. Orthostatic hypotension is the most common adverse effect observed in patients being treated with MAOIs (Table 25-5). The mechanism for this hypotension is unknown, but it may involve accumulation of false neurotransmitters such as octopamine, which are less potent than norepinephrine. This mechanism may also explain the antihypertensive effects observed with long-term use of MAOIs.

As noted earlier, adverse interactions between MAOIs and other serotoninergic drugs have been observed. In the anesthetic environment, the interaction with the opioid meperidine has been the most notable.

Management of Anesthesia. Anesthesia can be safely conducted in patients being treated with MAOIs despite earlier recommendations that these drugs be discontinued 14 days before elective operations to permit time for regeneration of new enzyme. Proceeding with anesthesia and surgery in patients being treated with MAOIs influences the selection and doses of drugs to be administered. Benzodiazepines are acceptable for pharmacologic treatment of preoperative anxiety. Induction of anesthesia can be safely accomplished with most intravenous induction agents, but it should be kept in mind that central nervous system effects and depression of ventilation may be exaggerated. Ketamine, a sympathetic stimulant, should be avoided. Serum cholinesterase activity may decrease in patients treated with phenelzine, so the dose of succinylcholine may need to be reduced. Nitrous oxide combined with a volatile anesthetic is acceptable for maintenance of anesthesia. Anesthetic requirements may be increased because of increased concentrations of norepinephrine in the central nervous system. Fentanyl has been administered intraoperatively to patients being treated with MAOIs without apparent adverse effects. The choice of nondepolarizing muscle relaxants is not influenced by treatment with MAOIs, with the possible exception of pancuronium. Spinal or epidural anesthesia is acceptable, although the potential of these anesthetic techniques to produce hypotension and the consequent need for vasopressors may argue in favor of general anesthesia. The addition of epinephrine to local anesthetic solutions should probably be avoided.

During anesthesia and surgery, it is important to avoid stimulating the sympathetic nervous system as, for example, by light anesthesia, topical application of cocaine spray, or injection of indirect-acting vasopressors to decrease the incidence of systemic hypertension. If hypotension occurs and vasopressors are needed, use of direct-acting drugs such as phenylephrine is recommended. The dose should probably be decreased to minimize the likelihood of an exaggerated hypertensive response.

Postoperative Care. Provision of analgesia during the postoperative period is influenced by the potential adverse interactions between opioids, especially meperidine and MAOIs, which can result in severe serotonin syndrome (see Table 25-3). If opioids are needed for postoperative pain management, morphine is a preferred drug. Alternatives to opioid analgesics such as nonopioid analgesics, nonsteroidal antiinflammatory drugs, and peripheral nerve blocks should be considered. Neuraxial opioids provide effective analgesia, but experience is too limited to permit recommendations regarding use of this approach in patients being treated with MAOIs.

Electroconvulsive Therapy

Despite many decades of use of ECT, the exact mechanism for its therapeutic effect remains unknown. Alterations in neurophysiologic, neuroendocrinologic, and neurochemical systems are thought to be involved but have not been clearly elucidated. What is evident is that electrically induced seizures of at least 25 seconds' duration are necessary for a therapeutic effect. ECT is indicated for treatment of severe depression in patients who show no response to drug therapy, cannot tolerate the adverse effects of psychotropic drug therapy, or are suicidal. The electrical current may be administered to both

TABLE 25-6	Adverse effects of electroconvulsive therapy

Parasympathetic nervous system stimulation
   Bradycardia
   Hypotension
Sympathetic nervous system stimulation
   Tachycardia
   Hypertension
Dysrhythmias
Increased cerebral blood flow
Increased intracranial pressure
Increased intraocular pressure
Increased intragastric pressure

hemispheres or only to the nondominant hemisphere, which may reduce memory impairment. The electrical stimulus produces a grand mal seizure consisting of a brief tonic phase followed by a more prolonged clonic phase. The electroencephalogram shows changes similar to those present during spontaneous grand mal seizures. Typically, patients undergo 6 to 12 induction treatments during hospitalization and then may continue weekly, biweekly, or monthly maintenance therapy. More than two thirds of patients receiving ECT show significant improvement in their depressive symptoms.

In addition to the seizure and its neuropsychiatric effects, ECT produces significant cardiovascular and central nervous system effects (Table 25-6). The typical cardiovascular response to the ECT stimulus consists of 10 to 15 seconds of parasympathetic stimulation producing bradycardia with a reduction in blood pressure, followed by sympathetic nervous system activation resulting in tachycardia and hypertension lasting several minutes. These changes may be undesirable in patients with ischemic heart disease. Indeed, the most common causes of death associated with ECT are myocardial infarction and cardiac dysrhythmias, although overall mortality rates are low, approximately 1 in 5000 treatments. Transient myocardial ischemia, however, is not an uncommon event. Other cardiovascular changes in response to ECT are decreased venous return caused by the increased intrathoracic pressure that accompanies the seizure and/or positive pressure ventilation and ventricular premature beats that presumably reflect excess sympathetic nervous system activity. Patients with acute coronary syndromes, decompensated congestive heart failure, significant dysrhythmias, and severe valvular heart disease require cardiologic consultation before initiation of ECT.

Cerebrovascular responses to ECT include marked increases in cerebral blood flow (up to sevenfold) and blood flow velocity (more than double) compared with pretreatment values. Cerebral oxygen consumption increases as well. The rapid increase in systemic blood pressure may transiently overwhelm cerebral autoregulation and result in a dramatic increase in intracranial pressure. Thus, the use of ECT is prohibited in patients with known space-occupying lesions or head injury. The cerebral hemodynamic changes are also associated with increased wall stress on cerebral aneurysms, and intracranial aneurysm disease is another contraindication to ECT.

Increased intraocular pressure is an inevitable side effect of electrically induced seizures. Increased intragastric pressure also occurs during seizure activity. Transient apnea, postictal confusion or agitation, nausea and vomiting, and headache may follow the seizure. The most common long-term effect of ECT is memory impairment.

Management of Anesthesia. Anesthesia for ECT must be brief, provide the ability to monitor and limit the physiologic effects of the seizure, and minimize any interference with seizure activity or duration. Patients must fast before the procedure. Administration of glycopyrrolate intravenously 1 to 2 minutes before induction of anesthesia and delivery of the electrical current may be useful in decreasing excessive salivation and bradycardia. The magnitude of treatment-induced hypertension can be ameliorated by the use of nitroglycerin intravenously, sublingually, or transcutaneously. Likewise, esmolol 1 mg/kg IV administered just before induction of anesthesia can attenuate the tachycardia and hypertension associated with ECT, and it does so better than labetalol. Many other drugs, including calcium channel blockers, ganglionic blockers, α_2-agonists and antagonists, and direct-acting vasodilators, have been used to treat the sympathetic overactivity during ECT, but they do not appear to offer any specific advantages over esmolol or nitroglycerin therapy.

Methohexital (0.5 to 1.0 mg/kg IV) is the traditional drug used for induction of anesthesia for ECT. It has a rapid onset, short duration of action, and minimal anticonvulsant effects, and recovery is rapid. Thiopental offers no advantage over methohexital and may be associated with longer recovery times.

Because of shortages of barbiturates in the United States, other induction drugs are now commonly used for ECT. Propofol is an alternative to methohexital and is associated with a lower blood pressure and heart rate response to ECT. Recovery time is similar after administration of methohexital and propofol, but the anticonvulsant effect of propofol can be manifested as shortened seizure duration. Ketamine and etomidate improve the quality and duration of the electrically induced seizure, but ketamine is associated with a prolonged reorientation time after the procedure, and etomidate is associated with more hypertension after the seizure and the possibility of spontaneous seizures before the electrical stimulus is delivered.

Intravenous injection of succinylcholine promptly after induction is intended to attenuate the potentially dangerous skeletal muscle contractions and bone fractures that can result from seizure activity. Doses of 0.3 to 0.5 mg/kg IV are sufficient to attenuate skeletal muscle contractions and still permit visual confirmation of seizure activity. The most reliable method to confirm electrically induced seizure activity is the electroencephalogram. Alternatively, tonic and clonic movements in an extremity that has been isolated from the circulation by applying a tourniquet before administration of succinylcholine are evidence that a seizure has occurred. Succinylcholine-induced myalgias are remarkably uncommon, occurring in approximately 2% of patients undergoing ECT. There is no evidence that succinylcholine-induced release of potassium is increased by ECT. Ventilatory support and oxygen supplementation are continued as necessary until there is complete recovery to pretreatment cardiopulmonary status. Because repeated administration of anesthetics is necessary, it is possible to establish the doses of the anesthetic induction drug and succinylcholine that produce the most predictable and desirable effects in each patient.

Occasionally, ECT is necessary in a patient with a permanent cardiac pacemaker or cardioverter-defibrillator. Fortunately, most of these devices are shielded and are not adversely affected by the electrical currents necessary to produce seizures, but it is prudent to have an external magnet available to ensure that the pacemaker can be converted to asynchronous modes should malfunction occur in response to the externally delivered electrical current or myopotentials from the succinylcholine or the seizure. Monitoring the electrocardiogram (ECG) and the plethysmographic waveform of the pulse oximeter, and palpation of peripheral arterial pulses document the uninterrupted function of cardiac pacemakers. Implantable cardioverters-defibrillators should be turned off before ECT and reactivated when the treatment is finished.

Safe and successful use of ECT has been described in patients following cardiac transplantation. In such patients, the lack of vagal innervation to the heart eliminates the risk of bradydysrhythmias. However, the sympathetic responses still occur.

Bipolar Disorder

Bipolar disorder, previously called *manic-depressive disorder,* is characterized by marked mood swings from depressive episodes to manic or hypomanic episodes with normal behavior often seen in between these episodes. Between 8% and 10% of patients with bipolar disorder commit suicide. The manic phase of bipolar disorder is manifested clinically by sustained periods of expansive euphoric mood in which the patient expresses grandiose ideas and plans. The mood disturbance is sufficiently severe to cause impairment in occupational functioning and in social activities and relationships, so there is risk of harm to self and others. Irritability and hyperactivity are also present, and in severe cases psychotic delusions and hallucinations may appear that are indistinguishable from those of schizophrenia (Table 25-7).

TABLE 25-7 ■ Manifestations of mania
Expansive, euphoric mood
Inflated self-esteem
Decreased need for sleep
Flight of ideas
Greater talkativeness than usual
Distractibility
Psychomotor agitation

The genetic pattern in bipolar disorder suggests autosomal dominance with variable penetrance. Presumably, there are abnormalities in neuroendocrine pathways that result in aberrant regulation of one or more amine neurotransmitter systems. Thus, the pathophysiology of bipolar disorder, to the extent that it is known, is similar to that of major depressive illness. The evaluation of mania must exclude the effects of substance abuse drugs, medications, and concomitant medical conditions.

TREATMENT

Mania necessitates prompt treatment, usually in a hospital setting to protect patients from potential harmful actions. Lithium remains a mainstay of treatment, but antiepileptic drugs such as carbamazepine and valproate are often used. Olanzapine is another treatment option. When manic symptoms are severe, lithium may be administered in combination with an antipsychotic drug until the acute symptoms abate.

Lithium

Lithium is an alkali metal, a monovalent cation, and is minimally protein bound. It does not undergo biotransformation and is excreted renally. Lithium is efficiently absorbed after oral administration. Its therapeutic serum concentration for acute mania and for prophylaxis is approximately 0.8 to 1.2 mEq/L. Because of its narrow therapeutic window, serum lithium concentration must be monitored to prevent toxicity. The therapeutic effects of lithium are most likely related to actions on second messenger systems based on phosphatidylinositol turnover. Lithium also affects transmembrane ion pumps and has inhibitory effects on adenylate cyclase.

Common adverse effects of lithium therapy include cognitive dysfunction, weight gain, and tremor. Lithium inhibits release of thyroid hormone and results in hypothyroidism in approximately 5% of patients. Long-term administration of lithium may also result in polyuria due to a form of vasopressin-resistant diabetes insipidus. Cardiac problems may include sinus bradycardia, sinus node dysfunction, atrioventricular block, T-wave changes, and ventricular irritability. Leukocytosis in the range of 10,000 to 14,000 cells/mm^3 is common.

Toxicity occurs when the serum lithium concentration exceeds 2 mEq/L, with signs of skeletal muscle weakness, ataxia, sedation, and widening of the QRS complex. Atrioventricular heart block, hypotension, and seizures may accompany severe lithium toxicity. Hemodialysis may be necessary in this medical emergency.

Lithium is excreted entirely by the kidneys. Reabsorption of lithium occurs in the proximal tubule in exchange for sodium. Diuretic use can affect the serum lithium concentration. Thiazide diuretics trigger an increase in lithium reabsorption in the proximal tubule, whereas loop diuretics do not promote lithium reabsorption. Administration of sodium-containing solutions or osmotic diuretics enhances renal excretion of lithium and results in lower lithium levels. Concomitant administration of nonsteroidal antiinflammatory drugs and/or angiotensin-converting enzyme inhibitors increases the risk of lithium toxicity.

Management of Anesthesia. Evidence of lithium toxicity is important to consider during the preoperative evaluation. The most recent serum lithium concentration should be reviewed, and inclusion of lithium level in measurements of the patient's serum electrolyte concentrations during the perioperative period is very useful. To prevent significant renal reabsorption of lithium, it is reasonable to administer sodium-containing intravenous solutions during the perioperative period. Stimulation of urine output with thiazide diuretics must be avoided. The ECG should be monitored for evidence of lithium-induced conduction defects or dysrhythmias. The association of sedation with lithium therapy suggests that anesthetic requirements may be decreased in these patients. Monitoring the effects of neuromuscular blockade is indicated, because the duration of action of both depolarizing and nondepolarizing muscle relaxants may be prolonged in the presence of lithium.

SCHIZOPHRENIA

Schizophrenia (Greek for "split mind") is the major psychotic mental disorder. It is characterized by abnormal reality testing or thought processes. The essential features of the illness include two broad categories of symptoms. Positive symptoms are those that reflect distortion or exaggeration of normal behavior and include delusions and hallucinations. Negative symptoms represent a loss or diminution in normal function and include flattened affect, apathy, social or occupational dysfunction including withdrawal, and changes in appearance and hygiene. Subtypes of schizophrenia include the paranoid type, the disorganized type, the catatonic type, and the undifferentiated type. In some patients, the disorder is persistent, whereas in others, there are exacerbations and remissions.

Treatment

The dopamine hypothesis concerning the etiology of schizophrenia suggests that the disorder is a result of neurotransmitter dysfunction, specifically dysfunction of the neurotransmitter dopamine. This hypothesis is based on the discovery that agents that diminish dopaminergic activity also reduce the acute signs and symptoms of psychosis, especially agitation, anxiety, and hallucinations. Drugs that affect dopaminergic function by blocking dopamine receptors, especially D_2 and D_4 receptors, have demonstrated the ability to improve a variety of psychotic symptoms, especially positive symptoms. Conventional antipsychotic drugs have broad-spectrum dopamine receptor–blocking properties, affecting all dopamine receptor subtypes. As a result, these drugs have significant motor adverse effects. These troubling adverse effects include tardive dyskinesia (choreoathetoid movements), akathisia (restlessness), acute dystonia (contraction of skeletal muscles of the neck, mouth, and tongue), and parkinsonism. Some of these effects diminish over time, but some persist even after drug discontinuation. Concurrent administration of anticholinergic medication may lessen some of these motor

TABLE 25-8   Commonly used antipsychotic medications

Class	Generic name	Trade name	EPSEs	Special side effects
TRADITIONAL DRUGS				
Phenothiazines	Chlorpromazine	Thorazine	Common	
	Perphenazine	Trilafon		
	Fluphenazine	Prolixin		
	Trifluoperazine	Stelazine		
	Thioridazine	Mellaril		
Butyrophenones	Haloperidol	Haldol	Common	Retinal pigmentation
Thioxanthenes	Thiothixene	Navane	Common	
ATYPICAL DRUGS				
	Risperidone	Risperdal	Uncommon	
	Clozapine	Clozaril	Rare	Agranulocytosis
	Quetiapine	Seroquel	Uncommon	Cataracts
	Olanzapine	Zyprexa	Uncommon	Neutropenia
	Ziprasidone	Geodon	Uncommon	Prolonged QT interval

EPSEs, Extrapyramidal side effects.

abnormalities. Acute dystonia resolves with administration of diphenhydramine 25 to 50 mg IV.

Newer antipsychotic drugs, also called *atypical* antipsychotic drugs, have variable effects on dopamine receptor subtypes and serotonin receptors, especially the $5\text{-}HT_{2A}$ receptor. These newer drugs appear to be quite effective in relieving the negative symptoms of schizophrenia and have fewer extrapyramidal adverse effects than the traditional drugs (Table 25-8).

MANAGEMENT OF ANESTHESIA

For the anesthesiologist, important effects of antipsychotic medications include β-adrenergic blockade causing postural hypotension, prolongation of the QT interval potentially producing torsade de pointes, seizures, elevations in hepatic enzyme levels, abnormal temperature regulation, and sedation. Drug-induced sedation may decrease anesthetic requirements.

Neuroleptic Malignant Syndrome

Neuroleptic malignant syndrome is a rare, potentially fatal complication of antipsychotic drug therapy that is presumed to reflect dopamine depletion in the central nervous system. This syndrome can occur anytime during the course of antipsychotic treatment but often is manifest during the first few weeks of therapy or following an increase in drug dosage. Clinical manifestations usually develop over 24 to 72 hours and include hyperpyrexia, severe skeletal muscle rigidity, rhabdomyolysis, autonomic hyperactivity (tachycardia, hypertension, cardiac dysrhythmias), altered consciousness, and acidosis. Skeletal muscle spasm may be so severe that mechanical ventilation becomes necessary. Renal failure may occur as a result of myoglobinuria and dehydration.

Treatment of neuroleptic malignant syndrome requires immediate cessation of antipsychotic drug therapy and supportive therapy (ventilation, hydration, cooling). Bromocriptine (5 mg PO every 6 hours) or dantrolene (up to 6 mg/kg daily as a continuous infusion) may decrease skeletal muscle rigidity. Mortality rates approach 20% in untreated patients, with death resulting from cardiac dysrhythmias, congestive heart failure, hypoventilation, or renal failure. Patients who have this syndrome are likely to experience a recurrence when treatment with antipsychotic drugs is resumed, so a switch is usually made to a less potent antidopaminergic drug or to an atypical antipsychotic drug.

Because there are similarities between neuroleptic malignant syndrome and malignant hyperthermia, the possibility that patients with a history of neuroleptic malignant syndrome are vulnerable to developing malignant hyperthermia is an important issue to consider (see Table 25-4). At the present time, there is no evidence of a pathophysiologic link between the two syndromes, and there is no familial pattern or evidence of inheritance in neuroleptic malignant syndrome. However, until any association between neuroleptic malignant syndrome and malignant hyperthermia is clearly disproved, careful metabolic monitoring during general anesthesia is recommended. Note that succinylcholine has been used without problems for ECT in patients with a history of neuroleptic malignant syndrome.

ANXIETY DISORDERS

Anxiety disorders are the most prevalent form of psychiatric illness in the general community. Anxiety is defined as a subjective sense of unease, dread, or foreboding. It can be a primary psychiatric illness, a reaction to or a result of a medical illness, or a medication side effect. Anxiety is associated with distressing symptoms such as nervousness, insomnia, hypochondriasis, and somatic complaints. It is useful clinically to consider anxiety disorders as occurring in two different patterns: (1) generalized anxiety disorder, and (2) episodic, often situation-dependent, anxiety. The γ-aminobutyric acid (GABA) neurotransmitter system has been implicated in the pathogenesis of anxiety disorders.

Anxiety resulting from identifiable stresses is usually self-limited and rarely requires pharmacologic treatment. Performance anxiety (stage fright) is a type of situational anxiety that is often treated with β-blockers, which do not produce sedation or allay anxiety but do eliminate the motor and autonomic manifestations of anxiety. The presence of unrealistic or excessive worry and apprehension may be cause for drug therapy. Buspirone, a partial 5-HT_{2A} receptor antagonist, is a nonbenzodiazepine anxiolytic drug that is not sedating and does not produce tolerance or drug dependence. However, its slower onset of action (several weeks until full effect is reached) and the need for thrice-daily dosing have limited its use. Short-term and often dramatic relief is afforded by almost any benzodiazepine, which is not surprising since these drugs bind to GABA receptors. Other drugs with GABAergic properties such as gabapentin, pregabalin, and divalproex may also be effective in treating anxiety disorders. Supplemental cognitive-behavioral therapy, relaxation techniques, hypnosis, and psychotherapy are also very useful in treating anxiety disorders.

Panic disorders are qualitatively different from generalized anxiety. The patient typically experiences recurrent and *unprovoked* episodes of intense fear and apprehension associated with physical symptoms and signs such as dyspnea, tachycardia, diaphoresis, paresthesias, nausea, chest pain, and fear of impending doom or dying. Such episodes can be confused with or indeed caused by certain medical conditions such as angina pectoris, epilepsy, pheochromocytoma, thyrotoxicosis, hypoglycemia, or cardiac dysrhythmias. Several classes of medications are effective in reducing panic attacks, including SSRIs, benzodiazepines, cyclic antidepressants, and MAOIs. These drugs have approximately comparable efficacy. Psychotherapy and education increase the effectiveness of drug treatment.

EATING DISORDERS

Eating disorders are traditionally classified as anorexia nervosa, bulimia nervosa, and binge-eating disorder (Table 25-9). Bulimia nervosa and binge-eating disorder are more common than anorexia nervosa. All of these disorders are characterized by serious disturbances in eating (fasting or binging) and excessive concerns about body weight. Eating disorders typically occur in adolescent girls or young women, although 5% to 15% of cases of anorexia nervosa and bulimia and 40% of binge-eating disorders occur in boys and young men.

Anorexia Nervosa

Anorexia nervosa is a relatively rare disorder, with an incidence of 5 to 10 cases per 100,000 and a mortality rate of 5% to 10%. Approximately one half of deaths result from medical

TABLE 25-9 ■ Diagnostic criteria for eating disorders
ANOREXIA NERVOSA
Body mass index < 17.5 kg/m²
Fear of weight gain
Inaccurate perception of body shape and weight
Amenorrhea
BULIMIA NERVOSA
Recurrent binge eating (twice weekly for 3 mo)
Recurrent purging, excessive exercise, or fasting
Excessive concern about body weight or shape
BINGE-EATING DISORDER
Recurrent binge eating (2 days/wk for 6 mo)
Eating rapidly
Eating until uncomfortably full
Eating when not hungry
Eating alone
Guilt feelings after a binge
No purging or excessive exercise

Adapted from Becker AE, Grinspoon SK, Klibanski A, et al. Eating disorders. *N Engl J Med*. 1999;340:1092-1098.

complications associated with malnutrition and the remainder are due to suicide. The disease is characterized by a dramatic decrease in food intake and excessive physical activity in the obsessive pursuit of thinness. Bulimic symptoms may be part of the syndrome. Weight loss often exceeds 25% of normal body weight, but patients perceive that they are still obese despite this dramatic weight loss.

SIGNS AND SYMPTOMS

Marked, unexplained weight loss in adolescent girls is suggestive of anorexia nervosa. Among the more serious medical complications seen in these patients are those that affect the cardiovascular system. Such changes include a decrease in cardiac muscle mass and depressed myocardial contractility. Cardiomyopathy secondary to starvation or to abuse of ipecac (used to induce vomiting) may be present. Sudden death has been attributed to ventricular dysrhythmias presumably reflecting the effects of starvation or associated hypokalemia. ECG findings may include low QRS amplitude, nonspecific ST-T wave changes, sinus bradycardia, U waves, and a prolonged QT interval (another possible association with sudden death). Hyponatremia, hypochloremia, and hypokalemia can be present along with metabolic alkalosis from vomiting and laxative and diuretic abuse.

Amenorrhea is often seen in patients with anorexia. Physical examination reveals emaciation, dry skin that may be covered with fine body hair, and cold, cyanotic extremities. Decreased body temperature, orthostatic hypotension, bradycardia, and cardiac dysrhythmias may reflect alterations in autonomic nervous system activity. Bone density is decreased as a result of poor nutrition and low estrogen concentrations, and long bones or vertebrae may fracture as a result of osteoporosis. Gastric emptying may be slowed, which leads to complaints of gastric distress after eating. In addition, starvation may impair cognitive function. Occasionally patients develop a fatty liver and altered results on liver function tests. Renal complications may reflect long-term dehydration resulting in damage to the renal tubules. Parturient women are at increased risk of delivering low-birth-weight infants. Anorexic patients are often anemic, neutropenic, and thrombocytopenic.

TREATMENT

Treatment of patients with anorexia nervosa is complicated by the patient's denial of the condition. Psychopharmacologic treatment with tricyclic antidepressants, lithium, and antipsychotic drugs has not been predictably successful. SSRIs that are effective in treating obsessive-compulsive disorder, particularly fluoxetine, may have some value in treating patients with anorexia nervosa.

MANAGEMENT OF ANESTHESIA

There is a paucity of information relating to the management of anesthesia in patients with this eating disorder. Preoperative evaluation is based on the known pathophysiologic effects of starvation. The ECG is useful for detecting evidence of cardiac dysfunction. Electrolyte abnormalities, hypovolemia, and delayed gastric emptying are important preanesthetic considerations. The risk of perioperative cardiac dysrhythmias is present. Reversal of neuromuscular blockade and respiratory alkalosis could contribute to the risk of development of dysrhythmias. Experience is too limited to permit recommendations regarding specific anesthetic drugs, muscle relaxants, and anesthetic techniques.

Bulimia Nervosa

Bulimia nervosa is characterized by episodes of binge eating (a sense of loss of control over eating), purging, and dietary restriction. Binges are most often triggered by a negative emotional experience. Purging usually consists of self-induced vomiting that may be facilitated by laxatives and/or diuretics. In most patients, this disorder is chronic, with relapses and remissions. Depression, anxiety disorders, and substance abuse commonly accompany bulimia nervosa.

SIGNS AND SYMPTOMS

Findings on physical examination that suggest the presence of bulimia nervosa are dry skin, evidence of dehydration, and bilateral painless hypertrophy of the salivary glands. Resting bradycardia is often present. The most common laboratory finding is an increased serum amylase concentration, presumably of salivary gland origin. Metabolic alkalosis secondary to purging is frequently seen. Dental complications are common, especially enamel loss from repeated vomiting and exposure of the lingual surface of the teeth to gastric acid.

TREATMENT

The most effective treatment of bulimia nervosa is cognitive-behavioral therapy. Pharmacotherapy with tricyclic antidepressants and SSRIs may be helpful. Potassium supplementation may be necessary in the presence of hypokalemia caused by recurrent self-induced vomiting.

Binge-Eating Disorder

Binge-eating disorder resembles bulimia nervosa, but in contrast to patients with bulimia, those with binge-eating disorder do not purge and the periods of dietary restriction are shorter. The diagnosis of binge-eating disorder should be suspected in morbidly obese patients, particularly obese patients with continued weight gain or marked weight cycling. The disease is chronic and accompanied by weight gain. Like anorexia nervosa and bulimia nervosa, this disorder is frequently accompanied by depression, anxiety disorders, and personality disorders. The principal medical effects of binge-eating disorder are severe clinical obesity and its associated complications: hypertension, diabetes mellitus, hypercholesterolemia, and degenerative joint disease. Antidepressant medications may be useful for treating those with binge-eating disorders.

SUBSTANCE ABUSE

Substance abuse may be defined as self-administration of drugs that deviates from accepted medical or social use, which, if sustained, can lead to physical and psychologic dependence. The incidence of substance abuse and drug-related deaths is high among physicians, especially during the first 5 years after medical school graduation. Dependence is diagnosed when patients manifest at least three of nine characteristic symptoms and the symptoms have persisted for at least 1 month or have occurred repeatedly (Table 25-10). Physical dependence develops when the presence of a drug in the body is *necessary* for normal physiologic function and prevention of withdrawal symptoms. Typically, the withdrawal syndrome consists of a rebound in the physiologic systems modified by the drug. Tolerance is a state in which tissues become accustomed to

TABLE 25-10 Characteristic symptoms of psychoactive drug dependence
Use of drug in higher dosages or for longer periods than intended
Unsuccessful attempts to reduce use of the drug
Increased time spent obtaining the drug
Frequent intoxication or withdrawal symptoms
Restricted social or work activities because of drug use
Continued drug use despite social or physical problems related to drug use
Evidence of tolerance to the effects of the drug
Characteristic withdrawal symptoms
Drug use to avoid withdrawal symptoms

the presence of a drug so that increased dosages of that drug become necessary to produce effects similar to those experienced initially with smaller dosages. Substance abusers can manifest cross-tolerance to drugs, which makes it difficult to predict analgesic or anesthetic requirements. Most often, *long-term* substance abuse results in increased analgesic and anesthetic requirements, whereas additive or even synergistic effects may occur in the presence of *acute* substance abuse. It is important to recognize the signs of drug withdrawal during the perioperative period. Certainly, a detoxification program should not be attempted during the perioperative period.

Diagnosis

Substance abuse is often first suspected or recognized during the medical management of other conditions, such as hepatitis, acquired immunodeficiency syndrome, and pregnancy. Patients almost always have a concomitant personality disorder and may display antisocial traits. Sociopathic characteristics (school dropout, criminal record, abuse of multiple drugs) seem to predispose to, rather than result from, drug addiction. Approximately 50% of patients admitted to hospitals with factitious disorders are drug abusers, as are some patients with chronic pain. Psychiatric consultation is recommended in all cases of substance abuse.

Drug overdose is the leading cause of unconsciousness in patients brought to emergency departments. Often more than one class of drug as well as some alcohol has been ingested. Conditions other than drug overdose may result in unconsciousness, which emphasizes the importance of laboratory testing (electrolyte levels, blood glucose concentration, arterial blood gas analysis, renal and liver function tests) to confirm the diagnosis. The depth of central nervous system depression can be estimated based on the response to painful stimulation, activity of the gag reflex, presence or absence of hypotension, respiratory rate, and size and responsiveness of the pupils.

Treatment

Regardless of the drug(s) ingested, the manifestations are similar. Assessment and treatment proceed simultaneously. The first step is to secure the airway and support ventilation and circulation. Absence of a gag reflex is confirmatory evidence that protective laryngeal reflexes are dangerously depressed. In this situation, a cuffed endotracheal tube should be placed to protect the lungs from aspiration. Body temperature is monitored, since hypothermia frequently accompanies unconsciousness as a result of drug overdose. Decisions to attempt removal of ingested substances (gastric lavage, forced diuresis, hemodialysis) depend on the drug ingested, the time since ingestion, and the degree of central nervous system depression. Gastric lavage may be beneficial if less than 4 hours have elapsed since ingestion. Gastric lavage or pharmacologic stimulation of emesis is not recommended when the ingested substances are hydrocarbons or corrosive materials or when protective laryngeal reflexes are not intact. After gastric lavage

or emesis, activated charcoal can be administered to adsorb any drug remaining in the gastrointestinal tract. Hemodialysis may be considered when potentially fatal doses of drugs have been ingested, when there is progressive deterioration of cardiovascular function, or when normal routes of metabolism and excretion are impaired. Treatment with hemodialysis is of little value when the ingested drugs are highly protein bound or are avidly stored in tissues because of high lipid solubility.

Alcohol

Alcoholism is defined as a primary chronic disease whose development and manifestations are influenced by genetic, psychosocial, and environmental factors. Alcoholism affects at least 10 million Americans and is responsible for 200,000 deaths annually. Up to one third of adult patients have medical problems related to alcohol (Table 25-11). The diagnosis of alcoholism requires a high index of suspicion combined with

TABLE 25-11   Medical problems related to alcoholism
CENTRAL NERVOUS SYSTEM EFFECTS
Psychiatric disorders (depression, antisocial behavior)
Nutritional disorders (Wernicke-Korsakoff syndrome)
Withdrawal syndrome
Cerebellar degeneration
Cerebral atrophy
CARDIOVASCULAR EFFECTS
Cardiomyopathy
Cardiac dysrhythmias
Hypertension
GASTROINTESTINAL AND HEPATOBILIARY EFFECTS
Esophagitis
Gastritis
Pancreatitis
Hepatic cirrhosis
Portal hypertension
SKIN AND MUSCULOSKELETAL EFFECTS
Spider angiomata
Myopathy
Osteoporosis
ENDOCRINE AND METABOLIC EFFECTS
Decreased serum testosterone concentrations (impotence)
Decreased gluconeogenesis (hypoglycemia)
Ketoacidosis
Hypoalbuminemia
Hypomagnesemia
HEMATOLOGIC EFFECTS
Thrombocytopenia
Leukopenia
Anemia

nonspecific but suggestive symptoms such as gastritis, tremor, history of falling, or unexplained episodes of amnesia. The possibility of alcoholism is often overlooked in the elderly.

Male gender and family history of alcohol abuse are the two major risk factors for alcoholism. Adoption studies indicate that male children of alcoholic parents are more likely to become alcoholic, even when raised by nonalcoholic adoptive parents. Other forms of psychiatric disease such as depression and sociopathy are *not* increased in the children of alcoholic parents.

Although alcohol appears to produce widespread nonspecific effects on cell membranes, there is evidence that many of its neurologic effects are mediated by actions at receptors for the inhibitory neurotransmitter GABA. When GABA binds to receptors, it causes chloride channels in the receptors to open, which hyperpolarizes the neurons and makes the occurrence of depolarization less likely. Alcohol appears to increase GABA-mediated chloride ion conductance. A shared site of action for alcohol, benzodiazepines, and barbiturates would be consistent with the ability of these different classes of drugs to produce cross-tolerance and cross-dependence.

TREATMENT

Treatment of alcoholism mandates total abstinence from alcohol. Disulfiram may be administered as an adjunctive drug along with psychiatric counseling. The unpleasantness of the symptoms that accompany alcohol ingestion in the presence of disulfiram (flushing, vertigo, diaphoresis, nausea, vomiting) is intended to serve as a deterrent to the urge to drink. These symptoms reflect the accumulation of acetaldehyde from oxidation of alcohol, which cannot be further oxidized because of disulfiram-induced inhibition of aldehyde dehydrogenase activity. Adherence to long-term disulfiram therapy is often poor, and this drug has not been documented to have advantages over placebo for achieving total alcohol abstinence. Medical contraindications to disulfiram use include pregnancy, cardiac dysfunction, hepatic dysfunction, renal dysfunction, and peripheral neuropathy. Emergency treatment of an alcohol-disulfiram interaction includes intravenous infusion of crystalloids and, occasionally, transient maintenance of systemic blood pressure with vasopressors.

OVERDOSE

The intoxicating effects of alcohol parallel its blood concentration. In patients who are not alcoholics, blood alcohol levels of 25 mg/dL are associated with impaired cognition and coordination. At blood alcohol concentrations higher than 100 mg/dL, signs of vestibular and cerebellar dysfunction (nystagmus, dysarthria, ataxia) are likely. Autonomic nervous system dysfunction may result in hypotension, hypothermia, stupor, and coma. Intoxication with alcohol is often defined as a blood alcohol concentration of more than 80 to 100 mg/dL, and levels above 500 mg/dL are usually fatal as a result of respiratory depression. Long-term tolerance from prolonged excessive alcohol ingestion may cause alcoholic patients to remain sober despite potentially fatal blood alcohol concentrations. The critical aspect of treating life-threatening alcohol overdose is maintenance of ventilation. Hypoglycemia may be profound if excessive alcohol consumption is associated with food deprivation. It must be appreciated that other central nervous system–depressant drugs are often ingested simultaneously with alcohol.

WITHDRAWAL SYNDROME

Physiologic dependence on alcohol produces a withdrawal syndrome when the drug is discontinued or when there is decreased intake.

The earliest and most common *alcohol withdrawal syndrome* is characterized by generalized tremors that may be accompanied by perceptual disturbances (nightmares, hallucinations), autonomic nervous system hyperactivity (tachycardia, hypertension, cardiac dysrhythmias), nausea, vomiting, insomnia, and mild confusional states with agitation. These symptoms usually begin within 6 to 8 hours after a substantial decrease in blood alcohol concentration and are typically most pronounced at 24 to 36 hours. These withdrawal symptoms can be suppressed by the resumption of alcohol ingestion or by administration of benzodiazepines, β-blockers, or α_2-agonists. In clinical situations, diazepam is usually administered to produce sedation. A β-blocker is added if tachycardia is present. The ability of sympatholytic drugs to attenuate these symptoms suggests a role for autonomic nervous system hyperactivity in the etiology of alcohol withdrawal syndrome.

Approximately 5% of patients experiencing alcohol withdrawal syndrome exhibit *delirium tremens*, a life-threatening medical emergency. Delirium tremens occurs 2 to 4 days after the cessation of alcohol ingestion and manifests as hallucinations, combativeness, hyperthermia, tachycardia, hypertension or hypotension, and grand mal seizures. Treatment of delirium tremens must be aggressive, with administration of diazepam (5 to 10 mg IV every 5 minutes) or another benzodiazepine until the patient becomes sedated but remains awake. Administration of β-blockers such as propranolol and esmolol is useful to suppress manifestations of sympathetic hyperactivity. The goal of β-blocker therapy is to decrease the heart rate to less than 100 beats per minute. Protection of the airway with a cuffed endotracheal tube is necessary in some patients. Correction of fluid, electrolyte (magnesium, potassium), and metabolic (thiamine) derangements is also important. Lidocaine is usually effective if dysrhythmias occur despite correction of electrolyte abnormalities. Physical restraints may be necessary to decrease the risk of self-injury or injury to others. Even with aggressive treatment, mortality from delirium tremens is approximately 10%, principally resulting from hypotension, dysrhythmias, or seizures.

Wernicke-Korsakoff syndrome reflects a loss of neurons in the cerebellum (*Wernicke's encephalopathy*) and a loss of memory (*Korsakoff's psychosis*) resulting from the lack of thiamine (vitamin B_1), which is required for the intermediary metabolism of carbohydrates. This syndrome is not an alcohol withdrawal syndrome, but its occurrence establishes that a patient is, or has been, physically dependent on alcohol.

In addition to ataxia and memory loss, many patients exhibit global confusional states, drowsiness, nystagmus, and orthostatic hypotension. An associated peripheral polyneuropathy is almost always present.

Treatment of Wernicke-Korsakoff syndrome consists of intravenous administration of thiamine, with normal dietary intake when possible. Because carbohydrate loads may precipitate this syndrome in thiamine-depleted patients, it may be useful to administer thiamine before initiation of glucose infusions in malnourished or alcoholic patients.

Alcohol crosses the placenta and may result in decreased infant birth weight. High blood alcohol concentrations (>150 mg/dL) may lead to *fetal alcohol syndrome,* characterized by craniofacial dysmorphology, growth retardation, and mental retardation. The incidence of cardiac malformations, including patent ductus arteriosus and septal defects, is increased in the children of alcoholic mothers.

MANAGEMENT OF ANESTHESIA

Management of anesthesia in patients being treated with disulfiram should consider the potential presence of disulfiram-induced sedation and hepatotoxicity. Decreased drug requirements could reflect additive effects from co-existing sedation or the ability of disulfiram to inhibit metabolism of drugs other than alcohol. For example, disulfiram may potentiate the effects of benzodiazepines. Acute, unexplained hypotension during general anesthesia could reflect inadequate stores of norepinephrine as a result of disulfiram-induced inhibition of dopamine β-hydroxylase. This hypotension might respond to ephedrine, but direct-acting sympathomimetics such as phenylephrine produce a more predictable response in the presence of norepinephrine depletion. Use of regional anesthesia may be influenced by the presence of disulfiram-induced or alcohol-induced polyneuropathy. Alcohol-containing solutions, such as those used for skin cleansing, should probably be avoided in disulfiram-treated patients.

Cocaine

Cocaine use for nonmedical purposes is a public health problem with important economic and social consequences. Myths associated with cocaine abuse are that the drug is sexually stimulating, nonaddictive, and physiologically benign. In fact, cocaine is *highly* addictive. Casual use is not possible once addiction occurs, and life-threatening adverse effects accompany cocaine use. Cocaine produces sympathetic stimulation by blocking the presynaptic uptake of norepinephrine and dopamine, and thereby increases the postsynaptic concentrations of these neurotransmitters. Because of this effect, dopamine is present in high concentrations in synapses, which produces the characteristic "cocaine high."

Acute cocaine administration has been known to cause coronary vasospasm, myocardial ischemia, myocardial infarction, and ventricular dysrhythmias, including ventricular fibrillation. Associated systemic hypertension and tachycardia further increase myocardial oxygen requirements at a time when coronary oxygen delivery is decreased by the effects of cocaine on coronary blood flow. Cocaine use can cause myocardial ischemia and hypotension that lasts as long as 6 weeks after discontinuation of cocaine use. The excessive sensitivity of the coronary vasculature to catecholamines after long-term exposure to cocaine may be due in part to cocaine-induced depletion of dopamine stores. Lung damage and pulmonary edema have been observed in patients who smoke cocaine. Cocaine-abusing parturient women are at higher risk of spontaneous abortion, abruptio placentae, and fetal malformations. Cocaine causes a dose-dependent decrease in uterine blood flow. It may also produce hyperpyrexia, which can contribute to seizures. There is a temporal relationship between the recreational use of cocaine and cerebrovascular accidents. Long-term cocaine abuse is associated with nasal septal atrophy, agitated behavior, paranoid thinking, and heightened reflexes. Symptoms associated with cocaine withdrawal include fatigue, depression, and increased appetite. Death due to cocaine use has occurred with all routes of administration (intranasal, oral, intravenous, inhalational) and is usually due to apnea, seizures, or cardiac dysrhythmias. Persons with decreased plasma cholinesterase activity (elderly individuals, parturient women, those with severe liver disease) may be at risk of sudden death when using cocaine, because this enzyme is essential for metabolizing the drug.

Cocaine overdose evokes overwhelming sympathetic stimulation of the cardiovascular system. Uncontrolled hypertension may result in pulmonary and cerebral edema, and the effects of increased circulating catecholamines may include coronary artery vasoconstriction, coronary artery vasospasm, and platelet aggregation, all of which can lead to myocardial infarction.

TREATMENT

Treatment of cocaine overdose includes administration of nitroglycerin to manage myocardial ischemia. Although esmolol has been recommended for treating the tachycardia caused by cocaine overdose, there is evidence that β-blockade can accentuate cocaine-induced coronary artery vasospasm. α-Adrenergic blockade is quite effective in the treatment of coronary vasoconstriction caused by cocaine. Administration of intravenous benzodiazepines such as diazepam is effective in controlling seizures associated with cocaine toxicity. Active cooling may be necessary if hyperthermia is significant.

MANAGEMENT OF ANESTHESIA

Management of anesthesia in patients acutely intoxicated with cocaine must consider the vulnerability of these patients to myocardial ischemia and dysrhythmias. Any event or drug likely to increase already enhanced sympathetic activity must be avoided. It seems prudent to have nitroglycerin readily available to treat signs of myocardial ischemia associated with tachycardia or hypertension. Increased anesthetic requirements may be present in *acutely* intoxicated patients, which presumably reflects increased concentrations of catecholamines in the central nervous system. Thrombocytopenia associated with cocaine abuse may influence the selection of regional anesthesia. Unexpected agitation during the postoperative period may reflect the effects of cocaine ingestion.

In the absence of acute intoxication, long-term abuse of cocaine has not been shown to be associated with adverse anesthetic interactions, although the possibility of cardiac dysrhythmias remains a constant concern. The rapid metabolism of cocaine probably decreases the likelihood that an acutely intoxicated patient will come to the operating room.

Administration of topical cocaine for medically indicated purposes followed by administration of a volatile anesthetic that sensitizes the myocardium may exaggerate the cardiac-stimulating effects of cocaine. Cocaine use for medically indicated purposes should be avoided in patients with hypertension or coronary artery disease and in patients receiving drugs that potentiate the effects of catecholamines, such as MAOIs.

Opioids

Contrary to common speculation, opioid dependence rarely develops from the use of these drugs to treat acute postoperative pain. It is possible to become addicted to opioids in less than 14 days, however, if the drug is administered daily in ever-increasing dosages. Opioids are abused orally, subcutaneously, or intravenously for their euphoric and analgesic effects. Numerous medical problems are encountered in patients addicted to opioids, especially those who take the drugs intravenously (Table 25-12). Evidence of these medical problems in patients addicted to opioids should be sought during the preoperative evaluation. Tolerance may develop to some of the effects of opioids (analgesia, sedation, emesis, euphoria, hypoventilation) but not to others (miosis, constipation). Fortunately, as tolerance increases, so does the lethal dose of the opioid. In general, there is a high degree of cross-tolerance among drugs with morphinelike actions, although tolerance wanes rapidly when opioids are withdrawn.

OVERDOSE

The most obvious manifestation of overdose of an opioid (usually heroin) is a slow breathing rate with an increased tidal volume. Pupils are typically miotic, although mydriasis

TABLE 25-12   Medical problems associated with chronic opioid abuse

Hepatitis
Cellulitis
Superficial skin abscesses
Septic thrombophlebitis
Endocarditis
Systemic septic emboli
Acquired immunodeficiency syndrome
Aspiration pneumonitis
Malnutrition
Tetanus
Transverse myelitis

may occur if hypoventilation results in severe hypoxemia. Central nervous system manifestations range from dysphoria to unconsciousness. Seizures are unlikely. Pulmonary edema occurs in a large proportion of patients with heroin overdose. The cause of this pulmonary edema is poorly understood, but hypoxemia, hypotension, neurogenic mechanisms, drug-related pulmonary endothelial damage, or the effects of other materials (contaminants) injected with the heroin may be responsible. Gastric atony is a predictable accompaniment of acute opioid overdose. Fatal opioid overdose is most often an outcome of fluctuations in the purity of street products or the combination of opioids with other central nervous system depressants. Naloxone is the specific opioid antagonist administered to maintain an acceptable respiratory rate.

WITHDRAWAL SYNDROME

Although withdrawal from opioids is rarely life threatening, it is unpleasant and may complicate management during the perioperative period. In this regard, it is useful to consider the time to onset, peak intensity, and duration of withdrawal symptoms after abrupt withdrawal of opioids. Opioid withdrawal symptoms develop within seconds after intravenous administration of naloxone. Conversely, it is usually possible to abort the withdrawal syndrome by reinstituting administration of the abused opioid or by substituting methadone (2.5 mg equivalent to 10 mg of morphine). Clonidine may also attenuate opioid withdrawal symptoms, presumably by replacing opioid-mediated inhibition with α_2-agonist–mediated inhibition of the sympathetic nervous system in the brain.

Opioid withdrawal symptoms include manifestations of excess sympathetic activity, such as diaphoresis, mydriasis, hypertension, and tachycardia. Craving for the drug and anxiety are followed by yawning, lacrimation, rhinorrhea, piloerection (origin of the term *cold turkey*), tremors, skeletal muscle and bone discomfort, and anorexia. Insomnia, abdominal cramps, diarrhea, and hyperthermia may also develop. Skeletal muscle spasms and jerking of the legs (origin of the term *kicking the habit*) follow, and cardiovascular collapse is possible. Seizures are rare, and their occurrence should raise suspicion of other causes of seizures, such as unrecognized barbiturate withdrawal or underlying epilepsy.

Rapid opioid detoxification using high doses of an opioid antagonist (nalmefene) administered during general anesthesia followed by naltrexone maintenance has been proposed as a cost-effective alternative to conventional detoxification approaches. There is evidence that opioid withdrawal, primarily involving the locus caeruleus, peaks and then recovers to near baseline within 4 to 6 hours after administration of high doses of opioid antagonists. Subsequent administration of naloxone to patients who have undergone rapid detoxification under general anesthesia should produce no evidence of opioid withdrawal, which confirms that rapid opioid detoxification has been achieved. Unlike in conventional detoxification accomplished by the gradual tapering of opioid doses, the unpleasant aspects of opioid withdrawal are compressed into a few hours, during which time the patient is anesthetized. This is thought to contribute to an increased success rate.

Profound increases in serum catecholamine concentrations during anesthesia-assisted opioid detoxification have been described, manifesting as changes in systolic blood pressure and tachycardia. Previous administration of clonidine may blunt these changes. During anesthesia, manifestations of sympathetic nervous system hyperactivity may be treated with pharmacologic interventions such as administration of β-blockers. Deep general anesthesia with skeletal muscle paralysis and controlled ventilation is recommended. Although general anesthesia seems to be safely tolerated during rapid opioid detoxification, there is some concern regarding the occurrence of cardiac dysrhythmias (prolonged QT interval) and postoperative mortality. Naltrexone is often administered in the postanesthesia care unit along with adjunctive medications such as midazolam, ketorolac, and clonidine. The occurrence of mild to moderate withdrawal symptoms for 3 to 4 days after rapid opioid detoxification is expected.

Buprenorphine is a semisynthetic alkaloid derived from brain tissue. It is a long-acting, lipid-soluble, mixed μ agonist-antagonist opioid. Continued interest in buprenorphine has been attributed to its unique pharmacologic effects. It is a partial μ opioid agonist having moderate intrinsic activity, with high affinity to and slow dissociation from μ opioid receptors. Buprenorphine has a very low abuse potential and has become a widely used therapeutic agent in patients with opioid dependence.

Pharmacotherapy for opioid dependence has included μ opiate agonists, such as methadone and levomethadyl, and partial agonists. Levomethadyl is a congener of methadone that is biotransformed to active metabolites with long durations of action. The advantage of levomethadyl over methadone is the option for every other day dosing. Buprenorphine has pharmacodynamic effects very similar to those of typical opioid agonists such as morphine and heroin. Buprenorphine is an effective intervention for use in the maintenance treatment of heroin dependence. However, if used as the sole drug, it appears to offer no advantages over methadone. Buprenorphine-carbamazepine, however, may be more effective than methadone-carbamazepine in detoxification strategies for patients addicted to opioids who also abuse other drugs. The U.S. Food and Drug Administration (FDA) has approved the marketing of buprenorphine in sublingual tablets or liquids containing buprenorphine alone (Subutex) or in combination with naloxone (Suboxone) for treatment of opioid dependence. The naloxone is added to the compound to prevent patients from dissolving the pills and then injecting them intravenously. If they do this, they will experience withdrawal symptoms. Buprenorphine may also have a ceiling effect that is useful in controlling opioid dependence. The FDA reclassified buprenorphine from a Schedule V drug to a Schedule III drug. This imposed the regulatory controls and criminal sanctions of a Schedule III narcotic on those persons who handle buprenorphine or buprenorphine-containing products. Schedule III substances by definition have less abuse potential than substances in Schedules I and II, including morphine or fentanyl. Methadone is a schedule II drug. Because of the pharmacology of buprenorphine, transfer from methadone to buprenorphine may precipitate withdrawal symptoms.

The unique pharmacologic properties of buprenorphine, with its high patient acceptance, favorable safety profile, and ease of administration, should facilitate its use in the treatment of opioid dependence. Opiate detoxification with buprenorphine occurs with a minimum of discomfort. Detoxification occurs without the fatigue, sweats, unpleasant tactile sensations, aches, seizures, and confused thought processes common during traditional detoxification procedures. Buprenorphine 8 to 12 mg is roughly equivalent to 35 to 60 mg of oral methadone. Buprenorphine can be used to treat pregnant addicted patients. However, it is secreted in breast milk and should not be used by nursing mothers.

Recent comparisons of rapid opioid detoxification with naltrexone under general anesthesia and buprenorphine-assisted detoxification indicate that there are more potentially life-threatening complications with rapid detoxification under general anesthesia.

MANAGEMENT OF ANESTHESIA

In patients addicted to opioids, the opioids or methadone should be maintained during the perioperative period. Preoperative medication may also include an opioid. Opioid agonist-antagonist drugs are not recommended for perioperative use because they can precipitate acute withdrawal reactions. There is no advantage to trying to maintain anesthesia with opioids, since dosages greatly in excess of normal are likely to be required. Furthermore, *long-term* opioid use leads to cross-tolerance to other central nervous system depressants. This may manifest as a decreased analgesic effect from inhaled anesthetics or nitrous oxide. Conversely, *acute* opioid administration *decreases* anesthetic requirements. Maintenance of anesthesia is most often accomplished with a volatile anesthetic. There is a tendency for perioperative hypotension to occur, which may reflect inadequate intravascular fluid volume secondary to chronic infection, fever, malnutrition, or adrenocortical insufficiency. Chronic liver disease may be present.

Management of anesthesia in patients rehabilitated from opioid addiction and in patients receiving agonist-antagonist therapy often includes a volatile anesthetic. Regional anesthesia may have a role in some patients, but it is important to remember the tendency for hypotension to occur, the increased incidence of positive results on serologic testing for HIV, the occasional presence of peripheral neuritis, and the rare occurrence of transverse myelitis.

Patients addicted to opioids often seem to experience exaggerated degrees of postoperative pain. For reasons that are not clear, satisfactory postoperative analgesia may often be achieved when average doses of meperidine are administered in addition to the usual daily maintenance dose of methadone or other opioid. Methadone and buprenorphine have minimal analgesic activity with respect to management of postoperative pain, so they are typically administered in addition to other opioids for postoperative analgesia. Alternative methods of postoperative pain relief include continuous regional anesthesia with local anesthetics, neuraxial opioid analgesia, and transcutaneous electrical nerve stimulation.

Barbiturates

Long-term barbiturate abuse is not associated with major pathophysiologic changes. These drugs are most commonly abused orally to produce euphoria, to counter insomnia, and to antagonize the stimulant effects of other drugs. There is tolerance to most of the actions of these drugs as well as cross-tolerance to other central nervous system depressants. Although the barbiturate doses required to produce sedative or euphoric effects increase rapidly, lethal doses do not increase at the same rate or to the same magnitude. Thus, the margin of error for individuals who abuse barbiturates, in contrast to that for those who abuse opioids or alcohol, *decreases* as barbiturate doses are increased to achieve the desired effect.

OVERDOSE

Central nervous system depression is the principal manifestation of barbiturate overdose. Barbiturate blood levels correspond to the degree of central nervous system depression (slurred speech, ataxia, irritability), with excessively high blood levels resulting in loss of pharyngeal and deep tendon reflexes and the onset of coma. No specific pharmacologic antagonist exists to reverse barbiturate-induced central nervous system depression, and the use of nonspecific stimulants is not encouraged. Depression of ventilation may be profound. Maintenance of a patent airway, protection from aspiration, and support of ventilation using a cuffed endotracheal tube may be necessary. Barbiturate overdose may be associated with hypotension because of central vasomotor depression, direct myocardial depression, and increased venous capacitance. This hypotension usually responds to fluid infusion, although occasionally vasopressors or inotropic drugs are required. Hypothermia is frequent. Acute renal failure resulting from hypotension and rhabdomyolysis may occur. Forced diuresis and alkalinization of the urine promote elimination of phenobarbital but are of lesser value for many of the other barbiturates. Induced emesis or gastric lavage followed by administration of activated charcoal may be helpful in awake patients who ingested barbiturates less than 6 hours previously.

WITHDRAWAL SYNDROME

In contrast to opioid withdrawal, the abrupt cessation of excessive barbiturate ingestion is associated with potentially life-threatening responses. The time of onset, peak intensity, and duration of symptoms of withdrawal from barbiturates are delayed compared with those for opioids (Table 25-13). Barbiturate withdrawal manifests initially as anxiety, skeletal muscle tremors, hyperreflexia, diaphoresis, tachycardia, and orthostatic hypotension. Cardiovascular collapse and hyperthermia may occur. The most serious problem associated with

TABLE 25-13	Time course of barbiturate withdrawal syndrome		
Drug	**Onset (hr)**	**Peak intensity (days)**	**Duration (days)**
Pentobarbital	12-24	2-3	7-10
Secobarbital	12-24	2-3	7-10
Phenobarbital	48-72	6-10	10+

barbiturate withdrawal is the occurrence of grand mal seizures. Seizures are likely to be caused by an abrupt decrease in the circulating concentration of the barbiturate. Many of the manifestations of barbiturate withdrawal, particularly seizures, are difficult to abort once they develop. Pentobarbital may be administered to treat barbiturate withdrawal. Typically, the initial oral dose is 200 to 400 mg, with subsequent doses titrated to effect. Phenobarbital and diazepam may also be useful for suppressing evidence of barbiturate withdrawal.

MANAGEMENT OF ANESTHESIA

Although there are few data concerning management of anesthesia in patients who habitually abuse barbiturates, it is predictable that cross-tolerance to the depressant effects of anesthetic drugs occurs. Anecdotal reports describe the need for increased barbiturate doses for induction of anesthesia in long-term barbiturate abusers. Although acute administration of barbiturates has been shown to decrease anesthetic requirements, there are no reports of increased anesthetic requirements in long-term barbiturate abusers. Long-term barbiturate abuse leads to induction of hepatic microsomal enzymes, which introduces the potential for drug interactions with concomitantly administered medications (warfarin, digitalis, phenytoin, volatile anesthetics). Venous access is a likely problem in patients who abuse intravenous barbiturates, since the alkalinity of the self-injected solutions is likely to sclerose veins.

Benzodiazepines

Benzodiazepine addiction requires ingestion of *large* dosages of drug. As with barbiturates, tolerance and physical dependence occur with long-term benzodiazepine abuse. Benzodiazepines do not significantly induce microsomal enzymes. Symptoms of withdrawal generally occur later than with barbiturates and are less severe because of the prolonged elimination half-lives of most benzodiazepines and the fact that many of these drugs are metabolized to pharmacologically active metabolites that also have prolonged elimination half-lives. Anesthetic considerations in patients who habitually abuse benzodiazepines are similar to those described for patients who abuse barbiturates.

Acute benzodiazepine overdose is *much less likely* to produce ventilatory depression than barbiturate overdose. It must be recognized, however, that the combination of benzodiazepines and other central nervous system depressants, such as alcohol, has proved to be life threatening. Supportive treatment usually suffices for treatment of a benzodiazepine overdose. Flumazenil, a specific benzodiazepine antagonist, is useful for managing severe or life-threatening overdose. Seizure activity suppressed by benzodiazepines could be unmasked by administration of flumazenil.

Amphetamines

Amphetamines stimulate the release of catecholamines, which results in increased alertness, appetite suppression, and decreased need for sleep. Approved medical uses of amphetamines are treatment of narcolepsy, attention-deficit disorders, significant depression, and hyperactivity associated with minimal brain dysfunction in children. Tolerance to the appetite-suppressant effects of amphetamines develops within a few weeks, which makes these drugs poor substitutes for proper dieting techniques. Physiologic dependence on amphetamines is profound, and dosages may be increased to several hundred times the therapeutic dosage. Long-term abuse of amphetamines results in depletion of body stores of catecholamines. Such depletion may manifest as somnolence and anxiety or a psychotic state. Other physiologic abnormalities reported with long-term amphetamine abuse include hypertension, cardiac dysrhythmias, and malnutrition. Amphetamines are most often abused orally but, in the case of methamphetamine, abuse is via the intravenous route.

OVERDOSE

Amphetamine overdose causes anxiety, a psychotic state, and progressive central nervous system irritability manifesting as hyperactivity, hyperreflexia, and occasionally seizures. Other physiologic effects include hypertension and tachycardia, dysrhythmias, decreased gastrointestinal motility, mydriasis, diaphoresis, and hyperthermia. Metabolic imbalances such as dehydration, lactic acidosis, and ketosis may occur.

Treatment of oral amphetamine overdose includes induced emesis or gastric lavage followed by administration of activated charcoal and a cathartic. Phenothiazines may antagonize many of the acute central nervous system effects of amphetamines. Similarly, diazepam may be useful for controlling amphetamine-induced seizures. Acidification of the urine promotes elimination of amphetamines.

WITHDRAWAL SYNDROME

Abrupt cessation of amphetamine use is accompanied by extreme lethargy, depression that may be suicidal, an increased appetite, and weight gain. Benzodiazepines are useful in the management of withdrawal if sedation is needed, and β-blockers may be administered to control sympathetic nervous system hyperactivity. Postamphetamine depression may last for months and may require treatment with antidepressant drugs.

MANAGEMENT OF ANESTHESIA

Pharmacologic doses of amphetamines that have been administered long term for medically indicated uses (narcolepsy, attention-deficit disorder) need not be discontinued before elective surgery. Patients who require emergency surgery and who are acutely intoxicated from ingestion of amphetamines may exhibit hypertension, tachycardia, hyperthermia, and increased requirements for volatile anesthetics. Intraoperative intracranial hypertension and cardiac arrest have been attributed to amphetamine abuse. In animals, *acute* intravenous administration of dextroamphetamine produces dose-related increases in body temperature and anesthetic requirements. For these reasons, it is prudent to monitor body temperature during the perioperative period. *Long-term* amphetamine abuse may be associated with markedly decreased anesthetic requirements, presumably as a result of catecholamine depletion in the central nervous system. Refractory hypotension can reflect depletion of catecholamine stores. Direct-acting vasopressors, including phenylephrine and epinephrine, should be available to treat hypotension, because the response to indirect-acting vasopressors such as ephedrine may be attenuated by the amphetamine-induced catecholamine depletion. Intraoperative monitoring of blood pressure using an intra-arterial catheter should be considered. Postoperatively, there is the potential for orthostatic hypotension once the patient begins to ambulate.

Hallucinogens

Hallucinogens, as represented by lysergic acid diethylamide (LSD) and phencyclidine, are usually ingested orally. Although there is a high degree of psychologic dependence, there is no evidence of physical dependence or withdrawal symptoms when LSD is abruptly discontinued. Long-term use of hallucinogens is unlikely. The effects of these drugs develop within 1 to 2 hours and last 8 to 12 hours. They consist of visual, auditory, and tactile hallucinations and distortions of the surroundings and body image. The ability of the brain to suppress relatively unimportant stimuli is impaired by LSD. Evidence of sympathetic nervous system stimulation includes mydriasis, increased body temperature, hypertension, and tachycardia. Tolerance to the behavioral effects of LSD occurs rapidly, whereas tolerance to the cardiovascular effects is less pronounced.

OVERDOSE

Overdose of LSD has not been associated with death, although patients may experience unrecognized injuries, which reflects the intrinsic analgesic effects of the drug. On rare occasions, LSD produces seizures and apnea. It can lead to an acute panic reaction characterized by hyperactivity, mood lability, and, in extreme cases, overt psychosis. Patients should be placed in a calm, quiet environment with minimal external stimuli. No specific antidote exists, although benzodiazepines may be useful for controlling agitation and anxiety reactions. Supportive care in the form of airway management, mechanical ventilation, treatment of seizures, and control of the manifestations of sympathetic nervous system hyperactivity may be needed. Forced diuresis and acidification of the urine promotes elimination of phencyclidine but also introduces the risk of fluid overload and electrolyte abnormalities, especially hypokalemia.

MANAGEMENT OF ANESTHESIA

Anesthesia and surgery have been reported to precipitate panic responses in these patients. If such an event occurs, midazolam or diazepam is likely to be a useful treatment. Exaggerated responses to sympathomimetic drugs are likely. The analgesia and ventilatory-depressant effects of opioids are prolonged by LSD.

Marijuana

Marijuana is usually abused via smoking, which leads to higher bioavailability of the primary psychoactive component, tetrahydrocannabinol (THC), than with oral ingestion. Inhalation of marijuana smoke produces euphoria, with signs of increased sympathetic nervous system activity and decreased parasympathetic nervous system activity. The most consistent cardiac change is an increased resting heart rate. Orthostatic hypotension may occur. Long-term marijuana abuse leads to increased tar deposits in the lungs, impaired pulmonary defense mechanisms, and decreased pulmonary function. An increased incidence of sinusitis and bronchitis is likely. In predisposed persons, marijuana may evoke seizures. Conjunctival reddening is evidence of vasodilation. Drowsiness is a common side effect. Tolerance to most of the psychoactive effects of THC has been observed. Although physical dependence on marijuana is not believed to occur, abrupt cessation after long-term use is characterized by mild withdrawal symptoms, such as irritability, insomnia, diaphoresis, nausea, vomiting, and diarrhea. The one medical use for marijuana is as an antiemetic in patients receiving cancer chemotherapy.

The pharmacologic effects of inhaled THC occur within minutes but rarely persist longer than 2 to 3 hours, which decreases the likelihood that acutely intoxicated patients will be seen in the operating room. Management of anesthesia includes consideration of the known effects of THC on the heart, lungs, and central nervous system. Animal studies have demonstrated drug-induced drowsiness and decreased dose requirements for volatile anesthetics following *intravenous* administration of THC. Barbiturate and ketamine sleep times are prolonged in THC-treated animals, and opioid-induced respiratory depression may be potentiated.

Substance Abuse as an Occupational Hazard in Anesthesiology

Anesthesiologists represent 3.6% of all physicians in the United States. However, they are overrepresented in addiction treatment programs, enrolling at a rate approximately three times higher than that of any other physician group. In addition, anesthesiologists are at highest risk of relapse after drug addiction treatment. At the present time, 12% to 15% of all physicians in treatment are anesthesiologists. The encouraging news is that a survey covering 1994 and 1995 revealed that the apparent incidence of substance abuse among anesthesiology residents was 0.4% with a faculty incidence of 0.1%. Both rates represented a decline in incidence since 1986.

WHY ANESTHESIOLOGISTS?

Numerous factors have been proposed to explain the high incidence of substance abuse among anesthesiologists. These include the following:

- Easy access to potent drugs, particularly opioids
- High addictive potential of accessible drugs, particularly fentanyl and sufentanil
- Relative simplicity of diversion of these agents, since only small doses will initially provide the effect desired by the abusing physician
- Curiosity about patients' experiences with these substances
- Control-oriented personality

DEMOGRAPHIC CHARACTERISTICS OF ANESTHESIOLOGISTS WHO ABUSE DRUGS

The curriculum on drug abuse and addiction compiled by the American Society of Anesthesiologists Committee on Occupational Health is a highly recommended in-depth source of information on this important topic. This curriculum notes the following demographic characteristics of anesthesiologists who are addicted to drugs:

- Fifty percent are younger than 35 years of age, but this may reflect the age distribution within the specialty.
- Residents are overrepresented. It may be that, because of increased awareness of the high risk of substance abuse among anesthesiologists, training programs are looking more carefully for signs of addiction in this group. Interestingly, a higher proportion of anesthesiology residents who are addicted are members of the Alpha Omega Alpha Honor Society.
- Sixty-seven percent to 88% are male, and 75% to 96% are white.
- Seventy-six percent to 90% use opiates as the drug of choice.
- Thirty-three percent to 50% are polydrug users.
- Thirty-three percent have a family history of addictive disease, most frequently alcoholism.
- Sixty-five percent of anesthesiologists with a documented history of addiction are associated with academic departments.

MOST FREQUENTLY ABUSED DRUGS

Traditionally, opioids are the drugs selected for abuse by anesthesiologists. Fentanyl and sufentanil are the most commonly abused drugs, followed by meperidine and morphine. This choice is particularly evident among anesthesiologists younger than 35 years of age. Alcohol is the abused substance in older anesthesiologists, probably because the time to produce impairment is significantly longer than that observed with opiate addiction. The data also suggest that opiates are the substance of choice for abuse early in an anesthesiologist's career, whereas alcohol abuse is more frequently detected in anesthesia practitioners who have been out of residency for longer than 5 years.

Other agents that have been abused include cocaine, benzodiazepines (midazolam), and, more recently, propofol. Over the past 5 years, there has been a major switch to "needleless" delivery of commonly abused drugs. This approach provides a cleaner alternative to the more traditional intravenous or intramuscular routes. Every possible route of administration has been tried, including unusual intravenous sites (hidden veins in the feet, groin, thigh, and penis), oral-nasal administration (benzodiazepines), and sublingual and rectal routes. Volatile anesthetics are now entering the abuse arena as well. Sevoflurane has been reported as the drug of choice among inhalational agents. Regardless of the drug initially abused, after 6 months there is an increasing incidence of polydrug abuse.

METHODS OF OBTAINING DRUGS FOR ABUSE

Anesthesiologists have developed numerous and often creative methods for obtaining drugs for abuse. The most frequently employed methods are falsely recording drug administration, improperly filling out the anesthesia record, and keeping rather than wasting leftover drugs. In addition, recent reports have highlighted a new practice involving secretly accessing multidose vials and then refilling and resealing them with other substances. It is important to be wary of the faculty member or resident who is too anxious to give breaks to others or who volunteers to take late cases. One of the most frequently reported retrospective markers of addictive behavior was the desire to work overtime, particularly during periods when supervision might be reduced, such as evenings and weekends.

SIGNS AND SYMPTOMS OF ADDICTIVE BEHAVIOR

Regardless of which drugs are abused, any unusual and persistent changes in behavior should be cause for alarm. Classically, these behaviors include wide mood swings, such as periods of depression, anger, and irritability alternating with periods of euphoria. Key points to remember about addictive behavior include the following:

- Denial is universal.
- Symptoms at work are the last to appear (symptoms appear first in the community and then at home).
- The pathognomonic sign is self-administration of drugs.
- Addiction is often detected when an individual is found comatose.
- Individuals whose addiction remains untreated are often found dead!

The following is a list of the most frequently overlooked symptoms of addictive behavior:

- Desire to work alone
- Refusal of lunch relief or breaks
- Frequent offers to relieve others

- Volunteering for extra cases or call
- Patient pain needs in the postanesthetic care unit that are disproportionately high given the narcotics recorded as administered
- Weight loss
- Frequent bathroom breaks

ASSOCIATED RISKS OF PHYSICIAN DRUG ADDICTION

Although traditionally the risks related to substance abuse were assigned to the individual physician-abuser, it is clear that there are also significant risks to patients and potential risks to the hospital staff and administration when a physician becomes impaired or addicted.

Physician

The principal risks to the anesthesia provider with addictive disease are an increased risk of suicide by drug overdose and drug-related death. Unfortunately, the relapse rate for anesthesiologists is the highest among all physicians with a history of narcotic addiction. The risk of relapse is greatest in the first 5 years and decreases as time in recovery increases. The positive news is that 89% of anesthesiologists who complete treatment and commit to aftercare remain abstinent for longer than 2 years. However, death is the primary presenting sign of relapse in opiate-addicted anesthesiologists!

Patient

Patients can be affected by addictive behavior. The data show that impaired physicians (those who are actively abusing drugs) are at increased risk of malpractice suits. Data from both California and Oklahoma revealed a dramatic decrease in both the number and dollar value of claims filed after treatment for substance abuse.

Hospital or Institution

Most states have laws requiring that hospital and medical staff report any suspected addictive behavior. Failure to report may have significant consequences depending on individual state statutes.

PROCESS FOR DEALING WITH SUSPECTED SUBSTANCE ABUSE

The process for dealing with suspected substance abuse by an anesthesiologist will be significantly affected by the presence or absence of a physician assistance committee. If an institution does not have such a committee, one should be formed and policies developed so that the support required by an impaired physician is in place when it is needed. The membership of this committee should include an anesthesiologist. In addition, this group should have a consulting agreement with local addiction specialists with experience in treating and referring physicians. Ideally, this treatment group would include a physician-counselor with experience and expertise in treating anesthesiologists. Finally, this committee should have a help line telephone number and a point of contact with at least one preselected addiction treatment program.

Admission to an alcohol or drug addiction treatment program is not considered a reportable event by state or national agencies. It can be dealt with as a medical leave of absence. However, intervention must be initiated as soon as there is firm evidence that substances of abuse are being diverted for personal use. This evidence needs to be clear and convincing to the physician assistance committee.

The primary goal of intervention is to get the addicted individual into a multidisciplinary medical evaluation process conducted by a team of experts at an experienced residential treatment program. *One-on-one intervention must be avoided.* The expertise of the hospital physician assistance committee and county or state medical society can be called upon to help with the intervention. After an individual has been confronted and is awaiting final disposition of his or her case, it is important not to leave the individual alone, because newly identified addicted physicians are at increased risk of suicide following the initial confrontation.

TREATMENT

The specifics of substance abuse treatment for physicians are beyond the scope of this chapter. However, it is important that a member of the faculty, group, or impairment committee keep in contact with the addicted physician and his or her treatment team. There is no cure for addiction and recovery is a lifelong process. The most effective treatment programs are multidisciplinary and are able to provide long-term follow-up for the impaired physician.

DRUG OVERDOSE

Tricyclic Antidepressant Overdose

Deliberate overdose of antidepressant medication is a common cause of death due to drug ingestion. The tricyclic antidepressant drugs account for most of this mortality. Potentially lethal doses of these drugs may be only 5 to 10 times the daily therapeutic doses. Overdose principally affects the central nervous system, parasympathetic nervous system, and cardiovascular system. Inhibition of neuronal uptake of norepinephrine and/or serotonin, anticholinergic effects, peripheral α-adrenergic blockade, and membrane-depressant effects account for the toxicity. Evidence of intense anticholinergic effects include delirium, fever, tachycardia, mydriasis, flushed dry skin, ileus, and urinary retention (see Table 25-4). Cardiovascular toxicity consists of sinus tachycardia with prolongation of the PR interval, QRS complex, and QT interval; ventricular dysrhythmias (especially polymorphic ventricular tachycardia); and myocardial depression and may be lethal. Seizures are not uncommon. The likelihood of seizures and cardiac dysrhythmias is very low when the maximal limb lead QRS duration is less than 100 milliseconds. Plasma concentrations of cyclic antidepressants are not usually measured because of the reliability of the limb lead QRS duration in predicting the risk of neurologic and cardiac complications.

The obtundation-coma-seizure phase of cyclic antidepressant overdose lasts 24 hours or longer. Even after this phase passes, the risk of life-threatening cardiac dysrhythmias may persist for several days, which necessitates prolonged ECG monitoring.

Initial treatment of tricyclic antidepressant overdose in the presence of preserved upper airway reflexes includes gastric lavage and administration of activated charcoal. Emesis should not be induced, because progression from being alert with mild symptoms to being obtunded with life-threatening changes (seizures, hypoventilation, hypotension, coma) may be very rapid, and pulmonary aspiration may result. Depressed ventilation or coma may require tracheal intubation and mechanical ventilation. Serum alkalinization is the principal treatment and results in an increase in protein-bound drug, less free drug, and thereby less toxicity. Intravenous administration of sodium bicarbonate or hyperventilation to a pH between 7.45 and 7.55 should be performed to a clinical end point such as narrowing of the QRS complex or cessation of dysrhythmias. If polymorphic ventricular tachycardia (torsade de pointes) is present, magnesium should be administered. Patients who remain hypotensive after volume expansion and alkalinization may benefit from vasopressor or inotropic support. Diazepam is useful for seizure control. Hemodialysis and hemoperfusion are ineffective in removing cyclic antidepressants because of the high lipid solubility and high degree of protein binding of these drugs.

Salicylic Acid Overdose

Once aspirin is ingested, it is converted to its active metabolite, salicylic acid. At toxic levels, salicylates are metabolic poisons that affect many organs by uncoupling oxidative phosphorylation and interfering with the Krebs cycle. This uncoupling of oxidative phosphorylation leads to accumulation of lactic acid and ketoacids.

Manifestations of salicylic acid overdose include tinnitus, nausea and vomiting, fever, seizures, obtundation, hypoglycemia, low cerebrospinal fluid glucose concentrations, coagulopathy, hepatic dysfunction, and direct stimulation of the respiratory center. The respiratory alkalosis resulting from this respiratory center stimulation assists in renal elimination of the drug by increasing the water-soluble ionized fraction of salicylic acid. Metabolic acidosis, on the other hand, favors the lipid-soluble nonionized fraction of the drug, which enhances the passage of drug into tissues and brain where toxic effects are produced. Noncardiogenic pulmonary edema often occurs during the first 24 hours after aspirin overdose.

Initial treatment of acute salicylic acid overdose includes administration of activated charcoal. Serum salicylate concentration should be measured initially and reassessed at a later time for evidence of continued absorption of drug, such as might be seen with enteric-coated or sustained-release formulations of aspirin. Empirical administration of dextrose will help prevent low cerebrospinal fluid glucose concentrations. Administration of sodium bicarbonate to increase arterial blood pH to 7.45 to 7.55 alkalinizes the urine, which dramatically increases renal clearance of salicylate. In addition, alkalemia promotes the movement of salicylate away from the brain and other tissues into the blood. Potential complications of this therapy include fluid overload and hypokalemia. Endotracheal intubation and mechanical ventilation, if undertaken, must be done very cautiously, because an abrupt decrease in salicylate-induced hyperventilation and hyperpnea may lead to life-threatening acidosis. Hemodialysis is indicated for potentially lethal concentrations of salicylic acid (>100 mg/dL) and for refractory acidosis, coma, seizures, volume overload, or renal failure.

Acetaminophen Overdose

Acetaminophen overdose is the most common medicinal overdose reported to poison control centers in the United States. Patients typically have nausea and/or vomiting and abdominal pain at presentation. Acetaminophen toxicity is due to centrilobular hepatic necrosis caused by N-acetyl-p-benzoquinoneimine (NAPQI), which reacts with and destroys hepatocytes. Normally, this metabolite constitutes only 5% of acetaminophen metabolic products and is inactivated by conjugation with endogenous glutathione. In overdose, the supply of glutathione becomes depleted and NAPQI is not detoxified.

Treatment of acetaminophen overdose begins with determination of the time of drug ingestion and with administration of activated charcoal to impede drug absorption. At 4 hours after drug ingestion, plasma acetaminophen concentration is measured and plotted on the Rumack-Matthew nomogram, which stratifies patients into those who are not at risk of hepatotoxicity, those who are possibly at risk, and those who are probably at risk (Figure 25-2). All patients who are possibly or probably at risk of hepatotoxicity and anyone for whom the time of ingestion is not known are treated with N-acetylcysteine, which repletes glutathione, combines directly with N-acetyl-p-benzoquinoneimine, and enhances sulfate conjugation of acetaminophen. Administration of N-acetylcysteine is virtually 100% effective in preventing hepatotoxicity when administered within 8 hours of drug ingestion.

POISONING

Methyl Alcohol Ingestion

Methyl alcohol (methanol) is found in paint remover, gasoline antifreeze, windshield washing fluid, and camper fuel. Methanol is a weak toxin, but it has very toxic metabolites. It is metabolized by alcohol dehydrogenase to formaldehyde and formic acid, which results in an anion gap metabolic acidosis. It is formic acid that is primarily responsible for the metabolic acidosis and visual disturbances that are associated with methanol toxicity. The target organs for its toxic effects are the retina, the optic nerve, and the central nervous system. Blurred vision, optic disk hyperemia, and blindness are hallmarks of

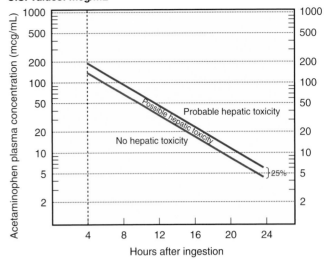

U.S. values: mcg/mL

FIGURE 25-2 Rumack-Matthew nomogram for acetaminophen toxicity. The plasma concentration of acetaminophen is measured and plotted on the nomogram according to the time the blood sample was drawn relative to the time of ingestion of the overdose. The position on the nomogram indicates whether hepatotoxicity is probable, possible, or unlikely. Concentrations are expressed as mcg/mL. *(Adapted from Rumack BH, Matthew H. Acetaminophen poisoning and toxicity. Pediatrics. 1975;55[6]:871-876.)*

methanol intoxication. Severe abdominal pain that mimics a surgical emergency may also occur.

Treatment of methyl alcohol poisoning includes providing supportive care and ensuring a secure airway. Activated charcoal *does not* adsorb alcohols. Intravenous administration of ethyl alcohol, which is preferentially metabolized by the enzyme alcohol dehydrogenase, will decrease the metabolism of methanol. Alternatively, the activity of alcohol dehydrogenase may be competitively inhibited by administration of fomepizole. Folic acid and/or folinic acid will provide cofactors to assist in formic acid elimination. Hemodialysis may be indicated for refractory acidosis or visual impairment.

Ethylene Glycol Ingestion

Ingestion of as little as 4 fl oz of ethylene glycol may be fatal. Ethylene glycol (found in antifreeze, de-icers, and industrial solvents) is metabolized by alcohol dehydrogenase to glycolic acid, which leads to metabolic acidosis. Glycolic acid is then metabolized to oxalate. Accumulation and precipitation of calcium oxalate crystals in the renal tubules can produce acute tubular necrosis. Myocardial dysfunction, pulmonary edema, cerebral edema, and hypocalcemia resulting from oxalate chelation of calcium are additional features of ethylene glycol poisoning. Treatment of ethylene glycol ingestion is similar to that described for methyl alcohol ingestion. Formation of toxic metabolites can be inhibited by administration of ethyl alcohol or fomepizole. Thiamine, pyridoxine, and sufficient calcium to reverse the hypocalcemia are also given. Urgent hemodialysis may be necessary.

Organophosphate Overdose

Organophosphate pesticides, carbamate pesticides, and organophosphorus compounds (nerve agents developed for chemical warfare and used in terrorist attacks) all inhibit acetylcholinesterase, which results in cholinergic overstimulation. These chemicals are absorbed by inhalation, by ingestion, and through the skin. There are several important differences between the nerve agents and the insecticides. The insecticides are oily, less volatile liquids with a longer time to onset of toxicity but longer-lasting effects. Nerve agents are typically watery and volatile, acting rapidly and severely but for a shorter period of time. Carbamate insecticides have a more limited penetration of the central nervous system, bind acetylcholinesterase reversibly, and result in a shorter, milder course of toxicity than organophosphates. All can be aerosolized and vaporized. The manifestations of pesticide and nerve agent poisoning are influenced by the route of absorption, with the most severe effects occurring after inhalation (Table 25-14). Muscarinic signs and symptoms of organophosphate exposure include profuse exocrine secretions (tearing, rhinorrhea, bronchorrhea, salivation), gastrointestinal signs, and ophthalmic signs such as miosis. Exposure to larger doses results in stimulation of nicotinic receptors, which produces skeletal muscle weakness, fasciculations, and paralysis. Cardiovascular findings may include tachycardia or bradycardia, hypertension or hypotension. Central nervous system effects include cognitive impairment, convulsions, and coma. Acute respiratory failure is the primary cause of death and is mediated by bronchorrhea, bronchospasm, respiratory muscle and diaphragmatic weakness or paralysis, and inhibition of the medullary respiratory center.

Treatment of organophosphate overdose involves administration of three types of drugs: an anticholinergic drug to counteract the acute cholinergic crisis, an oxime drug to reactivate inhibited acetylcholinesterase, and an anticonvulsant drug to prevent or treat seizures (Table 25-15). Atropine in 2-mg doses repeated every 5 to 10 minutes as needed is the main antidote for this poisoning. The clinical end point of atropine therapy is ease of breathing without significant airway secretions. Pralidoxime is an oxime that complexes with the organophosphate, which results in its removal from the acetylcholinesterase enzyme and splitting of the organophosphate into rapidly metabolizable fragments. The removal of the organophosphate from acetylcholinesterase reactivates the enzyme, and its normal functions can be resumed. Benzodiazepines are the only effective anticonvulsants for the treatment of patients with organophosphate exposure. All patients with severe intoxication by these compounds should be given diazepam or midazolam. Respiratory muscle weakness may require mechanical ventilation.

Carbon Monoxide Poisoning

Carbon monoxide (CO) poisoning is a common cause of morbidity and the leading cause of poisoning mortality in

TABLE 25-14   Signs of organophosphate poisoning

MUSCARINIC EFFECTS

Copious secretions
    Salivation
    Tearing
    Diaphoresis
    Bronchorrhea
    Rhinorrhea
Bronchospasm
Miosis
Hyperperistalsis
Bradycardia

NICOTINIC EFFECTS

Skeletal muscle fasciculations
Skeletal muscle weakness
Skeletal muscle paralysis

CENTRAL NERVOUS SYSTEM EFFECTS

Seizures
Coma
Central apnea

TABLE 25-15   Goals of treatment of organophosphate poisoning

Reverse the acute cholinergic crisis created by the poison
    Atropine 2 mg IV every 5-10 min as needed until ventilation improves
Reactivate the functioning of acetylcholinesterase
    Pralidoxime 600 mg IV
Prevent or treat seizures
    Diazepam or midazolam as needed
Provide supportive care

IV, Intravenously.

the United States. Exposure may be accidental (inhalation of fire-related smoke, motor vehicle exhaust, fumes from a poorly functioning heating system, tobacco smoke) or intentional.

PATHOPHYSIOLOGY

CO is a colorless, odorless, nonirritating gas that is easily absorbed through the lungs. The amount of CO absorbed depends on minute ventilation, duration of exposure, and ambient CO and oxygen concentrations. CO toxicity appears to result from a combination of tissue hypoxia and direct CO-mediated cellular damage. CO competes with oxygen for binding to hemoglobin. The affinity of hemoglobin for CO is more than 200 times greater than its affinity for oxygen. The consequence of this competitive binding is a shift of the oxyhemoglobin dissociation curve to the left, which results in impaired release of oxygen to tissues (Figure 25-3). However, the binding of CO to hemoglobin does not account for all of the pathophysiologic consequences of CO poisoning. CO also disrupts oxidative metabolism, increases nitric oxide concentrations, causes brain lipid peroxidation, generates oxygen free radicals, and produces other metabolic changes that may result in neurologic and cardiac toxicity. CO binds more tightly to fetal hemoglobin than to adult hemoglobin, so that infants are particularly vulnerable to its effects. Children, because of their higher metabolic rate and oxygen consumption, are also very susceptible to CO toxicity. CO exposure has uniquely deleterious effects in pregnant women because CO readily crosses the placenta, and fetal carboxyhemoglobin concentration may exceed maternal carboxyhemoglobin concentration and fetal elimination of CO is slower than that of the mother.

SIGNS AND SYMPTOMS

The initial signs and symptoms of CO exposure are nonspecific. Headache, nausea, vomiting, weakness, difficulty concentrating, and confusion are common. The highly oxygen-dependent organs—the brain and the heart—show the major signs of injury. Tachycardia and tachypnea reflect cellular hypoxia. Angina pectoris, cardiac dysrhythmias, and pulmonary edema may result from the increased cardiac output necessitated by the hypoxia. Syncope and seizures may result from cerebral hypoxia and cerebral vasodilation, Of note, the degree of systemic hypotension in CO poisoning is correlated with the severity of central nervous system structural damage. The classic finding of cherry-red lips is not commonly seen.

The effects of CO poisoning are not confined to the period immediately after exposure. Persistent or delayed neurologic effects may be seen. *Delayed neuropsychiatric syndrome*, which may include cognitive dysfunction, memory loss, seizures, personality changes, parkinsonism, dementia, mutism, blindness, and psychosis, may occur following apparent recovery from the acute phase of CO intoxication. No clinical findings or laboratory test results reliably predict which patients are at risk of delayed neuropsychiatric syndrome, but patients who are comatose at presentation, older patients, and those with prolonged exposure seem to be at greater risk.

DIAGNOSIS

Serum carboxyhemoglobin concentrations should be obtained for patients suspected of CO exposure. Arterial blood sampling is not necessary since arterial and venous carboxyhemoglobin levels correlate well. Measurement requires a CO-oximeter, which, by spectrophotometry, can detect and quantify all normal and abnormal hemoglobins. Routine blood gas analysis does not recognize the presence of abnormal hemoglobins, and pulse oximetry cannot distinguish carboxyhemoglobin from oxyhemoglobin. Oxygen saturation values measured by pulse oximetry may therefore be quite misleading.

TREATMENT

Treatment consists of removal of the individual from the source of the CO production, immediate administration of

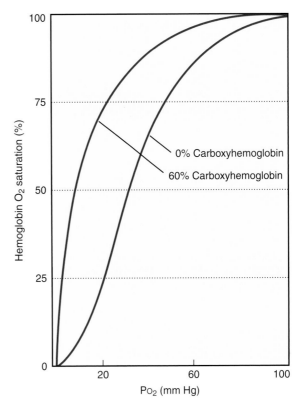

FIGURE 25-3 Carboxyhemoglobin shifts the oxyhemoglobin dissociation curve to the left and changes it to a more hyperbolic shape. This results in decreased oxygen-carrying capacity and impaired release of oxygen at the tissue level. *(Adapted from Ernst A, Zibrak JD. Carbon monoxide poisoning. N Engl J Med. 1998;339:1603-1608. Copyright 1998 Massachusetts Medical Society. All rights reserved.)*

supplemental oxygen, and aggressive supportive care: airway management, blood pressure support, and cardiovascular stabilization. Oxygen therapy shortens the elimination half-time of CO by competing at the binding sites on hemoglobin and improves tissue oxygenation. Oxygen administration is continued until the carboxyhemoglobin concentrations have returned to normal. The half-life of carboxyhemoglobin is 4 to 6 hours when patients are breathing room air, 40 to 80 minutes when they are breathing 100% oxygen, and approximately 15 to 30 minutes when they are breathing hyperbaric oxygen. Hyperbaric oxygen therapy consists of delivery of 100% oxygen within a pressurized chamber, which results in huge increases in the amount of oxygen dissolved in blood. Hyperbaric oxygen therapy accelerates the elimination of CO and may decrease the frequency of the neurologic sequelae that can result from severe CO exposure. Hyperbaric oxygen therapy is controversial, is not universally available, and has some risks. However, it may be indicated in selected patients: those who are comatose or have neurologic abnormalities at presentation, those who have carboxyhemoglobin concentrations in excess of 40%, and those who are pregnant and have carboxyhemoglobin concentrations above 15%.

KEY POINTS

- Serotonin syndrome is a potentially life-threatening adverse drug reaction that results from overstimulation of central serotonin receptors. It can be caused by an excess of precursors, increased release, reduced reuptake, or reduced metabolism of serotonin. Many drugs are serotoninergic (i.e., involved in these serotonin processes), including SSRIs, atypical and cyclic antidepressants, MAOIs, lithium, drugs of abuse, and narcotic analgesics.

- In addition to the seizure and its neuropsychiatric effects, ECT produces significant cardiovascular effects. The typical cardiovascular response to the electrically induced seizure consists of 10 to 15 seconds of parasympathetic stimulation producing bradycardia and a reduction in blood pressure. This is followed by sympathetic nervous system activation resulting in tachycardia and hypertension lasting several minutes.

- Substance abuse may be defined as self-administration of drugs that deviates from accepted medical or social use, which, if sustained, can lead to physical and psychologic dependence. Physical dependence has developed when the presence of a drug in the body is necessary for normal physiologic function and prevention of withdrawal symptoms. Tolerance is the state in which tissues become accustomed to the presence of a drug so that increased dosages of that drug become necessary to produce effects similar to those observed initially with smaller dosages.

- Although alcohol appears to produce widespread nonspecific effects on cell membranes, there is evidence that many of its neurologic effects are mediated by actions at receptors for the inhibitory neurotransmitter GABA. Alcohol appears to increase GABA-mediated chloride ion conductance. A shared site of action for alcohol, benzodiazepines, and barbiturates would be consistent with the ability of these different classes of drugs to produce cross-tolerance and cross-dependence.

- Acute cocaine administration is known to cause coronary vasospasm, myocardial ischemia, myocardial infarction, and ventricular cardiac dysrhythmias, including ventricular fibrillation. Associated systemic hypertension and tachycardia further increase myocardial oxygen requirements at a time when oxygen delivery to the heart is decreased by the effects of cocaine on coronary blood flow. Cocaine use can cause myocardial ischemia and hypotension for as long as 6 weeks after discontinuance of the drug.

- Anesthesiologists comprise 3.6% of all physicians in the United States but they are overrepresented in addiction treatment programs, enrolling at a rate approximately three times higher than that of any other physician group. In addition, anesthesiologists are at highest risk of relapse of all physician specialists.

- Fentanyl and sufentanil are the drugs most commonly abused by anesthesiologists. This drug choice is particularly evident among anesthesiologists younger than 35 years of age. Alcohol abuse is seen primarily among older anesthesiologists, because the time to produce impairment is significantly longer than that observed with opiate addiction. It appears that opiates are the substances of choice for abuse early in an anesthesiologist's career.

- The primary goal of intervention is to get the addicted physician into a multidisciplinary medical evaluation process conducted by a team of experts at an experienced residential treatment program. One-on-one intervention must be avoided. After an individual has been confronted and is awaiting final disposition of his or her case, it is important not to leave the individual alone, because newly identified addicted physicians are at increased risk of suicide following the initial confrontation.

- Acetaminophen overdose is the most common medicinal overdose reported to poison control centers in the United States. Patients typically have nausea and/or vomiting and abdominal pain. Acetaminophen hepatic toxicity is caused by a metabolite of acetaminophen that reacts with and destroys hepatocytes. Normally, this metabolite constitutes only 5% of acetaminophen metabolic products and is inactivated by conjugation with endogenous glutathione. In overdose, the supply of glutathione becomes depleted and the destructive metabolite is not detoxified.

- Nerve agents are organophosphate poisons that have been used in warfare and in terrorist attacks. They inactivate acetylcholinesterase and create an acute, severe cholinergic crisis. Emergency management of this poisoning consists of administration of repeated large doses of atropine.

- Routine blood gas analysis does not recognize the presence of abnormal hemoglobins, and pulse oximetry cannot distinguish carboxyhemoglobin from oxyhemoglobin. Therefore, in the presence of CO poisoning, these methods provide erroneous readings.

- The effects of CO are not confined to the period immediately following exposure. Delayed neuropsychiatric syndrome, which may include cognitive dysfunction, memory loss, seizures, personality changes, parkinsonism, dementia, mutism, blindness, and psychosis, may occur after apparent recovery from the acute phase of CO intoxication. Patients who are comatose at presentation, older patients, and those with prolonged exposure seem to be at greater risk.

RESOURCES

Alapat PM, Zimmerman JL. Toxicology in the critical care unit. *Chest.* 2008;133:1006-1013.

American Association of Poison Control Centers. http://www.aapcc.org. Accessed January 12, 2012. National Poison Control Center Hotline: 800-222-1222.

American Society of AnesthesiologistsCommittee on Occupational Health. Model curriculum on drug abuse and addiction for residents in anesthesiology. http://www.asahq.org. Accessed January 18, 2012.

Breen CL, Harris SJ, Lintzeris N, et al. Cessation of methadone maintenance treatment using buprenorphine: transfer from methadone to buprenorphine and subsequent buprenorphine reductions. *Drug Alcohol Depend.* 2003;71(1):49-55.

Deiner S, Frost EA. Electroconvulsive therapy and anesthesia. *Int Anesthesiol Clin.* 2009;47:81-92.

Gold MS, Byars JA, Frost-Pineda K. Occupational exposure and addiction in physicians: case studies and theoretical implications. *Psychiatr Clin North Am.* 2004;27:745-753.

Kales SH, Christiani DC. Acute chemical emergencies. *N Engl J Med.* 2004;350:800-808.

May JA, White HC, Leonard-White A, et al. The patient recovering from alcohol and drug addiction: special issues for the anesthesiologist. *Anesth Analg.* 2001;92:1608-1610.

Rumack BH, Matthew H. Acetaminophen poisoning and toxicity. *Pediatrics.* 1975;55:871-876.

Sadock BJ, Sadock VA. *Kaplan and Sadock's Pocket Handbook of Clinical Psychiatry.* 5th ed. Philadelphia, PA: Lippincott Williams & Wilkins; 2010.

Smith FA, Wittmann CW, Stern TA. Medical complications of psychiatric treatment. *Crit Care Clin.* 2008;24:635-656.

Weaver LK. Carbon monoxide poisoning. *N Engl J Med.* 2009;360:1217-1225.

CHAPTER 26

Pregnancy-Associated Diseases

DENIS SNEGOVSKIKH ■
FERNE R. BRAVEMAN ■

Pregnancy as well as labor and delivery are accompanied by physiologic changes in multiple organ systems that may influence maternal responses to anesthesia and the choice of anesthetic techniques. These normal physiologic changes of pregnancy may negatively interact with preexisting maternal conditions. Medical diseases unique to parturient women may influence management of anesthesia, especially during labor and delivery.

PHYSIOLOGIC CHANGES ASSOCIATED WITH PREGNANCY

Cardiovascular System

Most changes in the cardiovascular system are caused by the hormonal changes of pregnancy. Increased activity of progesterone results in increased production of nitric oxide and prostacyclin, which together with a decreased response to norepinephrine and angiotensin result in vasodilation. Increased concentrations of relaxin lead to renal artery dilation and, through reduction in aortic stiffness, aortodilation (an approximately 0.5-cm increase in the diameter of the aorta is seen at term). The decrease in systemic vascular resistance during the initial weeks after conception causes a compensatory elevation of cardiac output (initially resulting from an increase in heart rate) and an increase in renin activity. The increased renin activity results in retention of sodium and, by osmotic gradient, water. About 1000 mEq of sodium will be retained by term, which results in the retention of an extra 7 to 10 L of water. Plasma volume begins to rise in the fourth week of pregnancy, is increased by 10% to 15% at 6 to 12 weeks, and reaches a maximum (30% to 50% increase) at 28 to 34 weeks. The increase in plasma volume, combined with a 20% to 30% increase in total red blood cell mass, results in significantly elevated total blood volume, which reaches 100 mL/kg at term. Cardiac output rises in parallel with plasma volume, increasing by 15% at 8 weeks' gestation and reaching a maximum increase of 50% by 28 to 32 weeks. Plasma volume and cardiac output remain stable from approximately 32 weeks until labor begins. In labor, cardiac output rises as a result of sympathetic stimulation (pain and stress) and "autotransfusion," the displacement of blood from the contracting uterus into the circulation. Compared with prelabor output, cardiac output is increased by 20% during the first stage and 50% during the second stage of labor. Just after delivery of the placenta (the end of the third stage of labor), cardiac output is elevated 80% above prelabor levels. Cardiac output falls to the prelabor level in 24 to 48 hours and returns to the prepregnancy level in the next 12 to 24 weeks. Twin pregnancy results in a 20% greater increase in cardiac output than with single gestation.

Such an increase in cardiac workload results in ventricular hypertrophy. According to one echocardiographic study, the left ventricle increases in size by 6% and the right ventricle increases by 15% to 20% by term. Increases in the size and dilation of the cardiac chamber result in a mild degree of insufficiency of all the valves except the aortic valve; it is not normal to see aortic insufficiency at any stage of pregnancy. Enlargement of the heart and cephalic displacement of the diaphragm cause a horizontal shift in and rotation of the heart, which results in changes in the cardiac axis on the electrocardiogram. It is not abnormal to see a deep S wave in lead I and a large Q wave with negative T waves in leads III and IVF. The decline in systemic vascular resistance in early pregnancy reaches a nadir of 35% decrease at 20 weeks. Systemic vascular resistance slowly rises later, but remains 20% lower at term than the prepregnancy level. Central venous pressure, pulmonary artery pressure, and pulmonary capillary wedge pressure remain stable throughout the pregnancy.

A mechanical change in the cardiovascular system during pregnancy is inferior vena cava compression. By term, femoral vein pressure is elevated 2.5-fold in the supine position. Compression of the aorta by the gravid uterus results in aortocaval compression or supine hypotension syndrome. At term, about 15% of pregnant patients in the supine position develop a short period of tachycardia, followed by bradycardia and profound hypotension that is resistant to treatment with pressors. To prevent and treat this syndrome, left displacement of the uterus is recommended.

Respiratory System

Changes in the respiratory system are also caused by the hormonal changes of pregnancy. Increased activity of relaxin results in a relaxation of the ligaments of the rib cage, which allows displacement of the ribs into a more horizontal position. This leads to upward displacement of the diaphragm very early in pregnancy, before the gravid uterus shifts the abdominal contents. Elevation of the diaphragm and the more horizontal position of the ribs modify the shape of the chest into a barrel-like form; this decreases the vertical dimension of the chest by about 4 cm, but increases the diameter of the chest by more than 5 cm, which significantly increases the volume of the lungs available for gas exchange during normal spontaneous respiration. Tidal volume increases up to 40% by term. Increased activity of progesterone, a potent respiratory stimulant, leads to an increase in tidal volume and more rapid respiratory rate, so that minute ventilation is increased by 50% at term. Chronic hyperventilation results in respiratory alkalosis with a pH of 7.44, $Paco_2$ of 28 to 32 mm Hg, and HCO_3 concentration of 20 mmol/L. Secondary to a diminished

physiologic shunt during pregnancy Pao_2 rises slightly to 104 to 108 mm Hg. These changes increase the gradient between mother and fetus and improve maternal-fetal gas exchange.

The decrease in the vertical size of the chest secondary to elevation of the diaphragm leads to a 25% decrease in the expiratory reserve volume and a 15% decrease in the residual volume, which results in a 20% decrease in functional residual capacity. A 20% increase in oxygen consumption caused by an elevated basal metabolic rate, combined with the decrease in functional residual capacity, produces more rapid desaturation during periods of apnea. In a fully preoxygenated healthy nonpregnant patient desaturation from 100% to lower than 90% occurs in approximately 9 minutes; in a healthy patient at term, desaturation occurs in only 3 to 4 minutes; and in a morbidly obese pregnant patient, desaturation occurs in 98 seconds.

Edema and hyperemia of the oropharyngeal mucosa, glandular hyperactivity, and capillary engorgement secondary to elevated activity of estrogen, progesterone, and relaxin result in nasal stiffness, epistaxis, and upper airway narrowing. The rates of difficult and failed intubation in pregnant women are increased—3.3% and 0.4%, respectively—which are more than eight times higher than in nonpregnant patients. When providing general anesthesia, the anesthesiologist is thus faced with a potentially difficult airway in a patient who will undergo desaturation more rapidly than a nonpregnant patient. This is one of the factors contributing to a 17-times higher mortality rate among parturient women who undergo general anesthesia than among those who undergo regional anesthesia. Prophylactic placement of an epidural catheter in patients assessed to have a difficult airway may help to avoid airway manipulation and minimize maternal morbidity and mortality. Even when this approach was used, however, the rate of failed intubation was 1 in 98 obstetric general anesthesia cases over a 5-year period at Brigham and Women's Hospital.

Hematologic System

Normal pregnancy is associated with substantial changes in hemostasis resulting in a relatively hypercoagulable state. The activity of the majority of coagulation factors (I, VII, VIII, IX, X, XII) is increased, whereas the activity of physiologic anticoagulants is decreased. The latter includes a significant reduction in protein S activity and acquired activated protein C resistance. Deep vein thrombosis occurs in 1 per 1000 deliveries, which is 5.5 to 6 times higher than the rate in the general female population of childbearing age. Procoagulant changes during normal pregnancy are counterbalanced by a significant activation of the fibrinolytic system and deactivation of natural antifibrinolytics via a decrease in the activity of factors XI and XIII. A relative deficiency of factors XI and XIII causes decreased polymerization of fibrin monomers into fibrin and diminishes the cross-links of α_2-antiplasmin to fibrin, which makes fibrin much less resistant to degradation. The relatively low levels of factors XI and XIII decrease the activation of thrombin-activatable fibrinolysis inhibitor, which results in a decrease in antifibrinolytic potential. Increased activity of the coagulation system and fibrinolytic system, and decreased activity of the anticoagulation and antifibrinolytic systems predispose pregnant patients to the development of consumption coagulopathy (increased fibrin generation following its degradation). Levels of D-dimers and fibrin degradation products increase during normal pregnancy with rapid depletion of fibrinogen and factor XIII.

Gastrointestinal System

Lower esophageal sphincter tone is decreased in pregnancy as a result of two factors: the displacement of the stomach upward and muscle relaxation caused by the effects of progestins. Heartburn is a frequent occurrence among pregnant women. Gastric emptying is not altered in pregnancy, although it is slowed during labor.

Bile secretion is increased during pregnancy. Stasis resulting from the effect of progesterone together with changes in the composition of bile acids results in increased gallstone formation. Cholecystectomy is the second most frequent surgery during pregnancy with a reported incidence as high as 1 in 1600 pregnancies.

Endocrine System

Pregnancy is characterized by insulin resistance, caused by increased activity of hormones such as progesterone, estrogen, cortisol (2.5-fold increase at term), and placental lactogen. This insulin resistance resolves rapidly after delivery. Fasting glucose levels are lower in pregnant than in nonpregnant patients because of high glucose utilization by the fetus.

Estrogen increases the level of thyroxin-binding globulin, which results in an elevation of total triiodothyronine (T_3) and thyroxine (T_4) levels, but levels of free T_3 and T_4 remain stable.

Other Changes

Increased levels of progesterone and endorphins elevate the pain threshold. Studies using bispectral index monitoring do not support the previous belief that pregnant patients show increased sensitivity to the effect of inhalational anesthetics.

Cerebrospinal fluid volume is decreased during pregnancy, but intracranial pressure remains stable.

Renal blood flow is increased in pregnancy. Glomerular filtration rate increases by 50% at 12 weeks of gestation, which results in a decrease in blood urea nitrogen and creatinine concentrations. Usual blood urea nitrogen and creatinine values at term are abnormal and indicate renal dysfunction (Table 26-1).

ANESTHETIC CONSIDERATIONS

Nonobstetric Surgery

Between 1% and 2% of all pregnant women in the United States will undergo surgery unrelated to their pregnancy (>80,000 procedures requiring anesthesia per year). The most frequent nonobstetric procedures are excision of ovarian cysts, appendectomy, breast biopsy, and surgery required because of trauma. Until recently, the use of laparoscopic surgery in pregnancy was controversial because of concerns that the required pneumoperitoneum would decrease maternal lung compliance, leading to hypercarbia and fetal acidosis. Analysis of data from case registries has provided reassurance that laparoscopic procedures can be safely carried out during pregnancy. Treatment of an incompetent cervix (cervical cerclage) typically occurs early in pregnancy. Cardiac surgery in pregnancy is associated with a maternal mortality of 3% to 15% and a fetal mortality of 20% to 35%. Pulsatile flow during bypass is preferred, and fetal survival is better if maternal temperature remains above 29.3° C. Fetal surgery, first performed in 1981, is now being carried out in many hospitals. Ex utero intrapartum treatment (EXIT) procedures are performed at cesarean delivery. Fetal manipulations and minor surgeries on the fetus are being conducted earlier in pregnancy and require uterine relaxation and, at times, fetal immobility.

TABLE 26-1 ■ **Physiologic changes accompanying pregnancy**

Parameter	Average change from nonpregnancy value (%)
Intravascular fluid volume	+35
Plasma volume	+45
Erythrocyte volume	+20
Cardiac output	+40
Stroke volume	+30
Heart rate	+15
Peripheral circulation	
Systolic blood pressure	No change
Systemic vascular resistance	−15
Diastolic blood pressure	−15
Central venous pressure	No change
Femoral venous pressure	+15
Minute ventilation	+50
Tidal volume	+40
Breathing rate	+10
Pao_2	+10 mm Hg
$Paco_2$	−10 mm Hg
Arterial pH	No change
Total lung capacity	No change
Vital capacity	No change
Functional residual capacity	−20
Expiratory reserve volume	−20
Residual volume	−20
Airway resistance	−35
Oxygen consumption	+20
Renal blood flow and glomerular filtration rate	−50
Serum cholinesterase activity	−25

The objective of anesthetic management in patients undergoing nonobstetric operative procedures is maternal safety, safe care of the fetus, and prevention of premature labor related to the surgical procedure or to drugs administered during or as part of the anesthesia care. To achieve these goals, the effects of the patient's altered physiology must be recognized and incorporated into the anesthetic plan. Induction of and emergence from anesthesia are more rapid than in the nonpregnant state because of increased minute ventilation and decreased functional residual capacity. Supine hypotensive syndrome can occur as early as the second trimester.

It is important to remember that the effects of pregnancy-related physiologic changes are not limited to general anesthesia. Local anesthetics have an increased effect during pregnancy; thus, the amount of local anesthetic administered for regional anesthesia should be reduced by 25% to 30% during any stage of pregnancy. Local anesthetic toxicity, especially cardiovascular toxicity, is also seen at lower plasma concentrations of these drugs.

Teratogenicity may occur at any stage of gestation. However, most of the critical organogenesis occurs in the first trimester. Although many commonly used anesthetics are teratogenic at high dosages in animals, few, if any, studies support teratogenic effects of anesthetic or sedative medications at the dosages used for anesthesia care in humans. There is some evidence of a link between maternal high-dose diazepam injection in the first trimester and cleft palate. Medicinal dosages of benzodiazepines are safe when used to treat perioperative anxiety. In fact, teratogenicity has been shown only with high-dose diazepam and not with other benzodiazepines.

Nitrous oxide has been suggested to be teratogenic in animals when administered for prolonged periods (1 to 2 days). Of concern regarding its use in humans is its effect on DNA synthesis. Although teratogenesis has been seen in animals only under extreme conditions that are not likely to be reproduced in clinical care, some believe that nitrous oxide use is contraindicated in the first two trimesters of pregnancy. Recent studies suggest that volatile anesthetics stimulate neuronal apoptosis in rats, but it is not obvious whether these data can be extrapolated to humans. Widespread neuronal apoptosis is associated with memory and learning deficits in laboratory animals, but again this has not been examined in humans.

Intrauterine fetal asphyxia can be avoided by maintaining maternal PaO_2 and $PaCO_2$, and uterine blood flow. $PaCO_2$ can affect uterine blood flow, because maternal alkalosis may cause direct vasoconstriction. Alkalosis shifts the oxyhemoglobin dissociation curve, which results in the release of less oxygen to the fetus at the placenta. Maternal hypotension leads to a reduction in uterine blood flow and thus fetal hypoxia. Uterine hypertension, as occurs with increased uterine irritability, also decreases uterine blood flow.

Anesthesia and surgery may result in preterm labor during the intraoperative and postoperative periods. Abdominal and pelvic procedures are associated with the greatest incidence of preterm labor.

Generally, elective surgery should be delayed until the patient is no longer pregnant and has returned to her nonpregnant physiologic state (approximately 2 to 6 weeks post partum). Procedures that can be scheduled with some flexibility but that cannot be delayed until after delivery are best performed in the middle trimester. This lessens the risk of teratogenicity (greater with first-trimester medication administration) and preterm labor (greater risk in the third trimester) (Figure 26-1).

There are no data to support the preference of any anesthetic technique over another when emergency surgery is required, provided oxygenation and blood pressure are maintained and hyperventilation is avoided. Nevertheless, regional

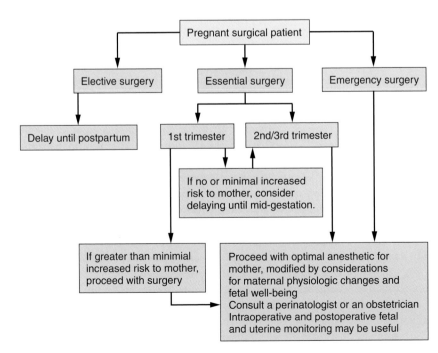

FIGURE 26-1 Recommendations for management of pregnant women undergoing surgery. (Adapted from Rosen MA. Management of anesthesia for the pregnant surgical patient. Anesthesiology. 1999;91:1159-1163. © 1999, Lippincott Williams & Wilkins.)

anesthesia should be considered because it minimizes fetal exposure to medications. If general anesthesia is needed, then, as emphasized previously, normal oxygenation and blood pressure must be maintained and hyperventilation avoided. Left uterine displacement should be used during the second and third trimesters and aspiration prophylaxis implemented in all pregnant patients. For monitoring, at a minimum preoperative and postoperative fetal heart rate and uterine activity must be assessed. The statement of the American College of Obstetricians and Gynecologists Committee on Obstetric Practice titled "Nonobstetric Surgery During Pregnancy" recommends that an obstetric consult be obtained before surgery and that use of fetal monitoring be individualized.

Obstetric Anesthesia Care

REGIONAL ANALGESIC TECHNIQUES

The use of regional techniques in parturient patients requires an understanding of the neural pathways responsible for the transmission of pain during labor and delivery. The pain of labor arises primarily from receptors in uterine and perineal structures. Afferent pain impulses from the cervix and uterus travel in nerves that accompany sympathetic nervous system fibers and enter the spinal cord at T10 to L1. Pain pathways from the perineum travel to S2 to S4 via the pudendal nerves. Pain during the first stage of labor (onset of regular contractions) results from dilation of the cervix, contraction of the uterus, and traction on the round ligament. The pain is visceral and is referred to dermatomes supplied by spinal cord segments T10 to L1. During the second stage of labor (complete dilation of the cervix to delivery of the fetus), pain is somatic and is produced by distention of the perineum and stretching of fascia, skin, and subcutaneous tissues.

LUMBAR EPIDURAL ANALGESIA

When an epidural catheter is placed for the provision of analgesia during labor and delivery or anesthesia for cesarean delivery, it is important to confirm that the catheter is not in an intravascular or subarachnoid position. For this purpose, it is common to administer a test dose of a solution containing the local anesthetic and epinephrine (15 mcg). An epinephrine-induced increase in the maternal heart rate alerts the anesthesiologist to the possibility of an intravascular catheter placement. A rapid onset of analgesia suggests subarachnoid placement. Hypotension may require administration of small doses of ephedrine (5 to 10 mg IV) or phenylephrine (20 to 100 mcg IV). Use of neuraxial analgesia, specifically combined spinal-epidural analgesia, in early labor does not increase the incidence of cesarean delivery and may shorten labor compared with systemic analgesia. See Table 26-2 for analgesic choices.

COMBINED SPINAL-EPIDURAL ANALGESIA

Combined spinal-epidural analgesia has been advocated as an alternative to epidural analgesia during labor. Advantages

TABLE 26-2   Epidural labor analgesia

Bolus (10 mL)	Infusion	
	Local anesthetic	Opioid
Bupivacaine 0.125% with hydromorphone 10 mcg/mL	Bupivacaine 0.0625%-0.125%	Hydromorphone 3 mcg/mL
Bupivacaine 0.125% with fentanyl 5 mcg/mL	Bupivacaine 0.0625%-0.125%	Fentanyl 2 mcg/mL
Bupivacaine 0.125% with sufentanil 1 mcg/mL	Bupivacaine 0.0625%-0.125%	Sufentanil 2 mcg/mL
(Ropivacaine 0.075% may be used with opioid as above)	(Ropivacaine 0.075%-0.125% may be used)	(Any of the above)

cited for the combined technique include more rapid onset of analgesia, increased reliability, effectiveness when instituted in a rapidly progressing labor, and minimal motor block. Subarachnoid administration of low doses of opioids such as fentanyl (12.5 to 25 mcg) or sufentanil (5 to 10 mcg) results in rapid (5 minutes), nearly complete pain relief during the first stage of labor. Low doses of local anesthetics such as 2.5 mg of bupivacaine may also be added to the opioid solution. Disadvantages of the combined technique include the risk of fetal bradycardia, which is usually benign and very short lasting. Increased risk of postdural puncture headache has not been cited as a concern in the literature. This technique should be considered especially when neuraxial analgesia is requested in very early labor or in a rapidly progressing multiparous labor.

ANESTHESIA FOR CESAREAN DELIVERY

A large and growing minority (>30%) of parturient women deliver by cesarean section. If epidural analgesia is used for labor, this technique can then be converted to provide surgical anesthesia by changing the quantity and concentration of drug administered. Most elective cesarean deliveries and many urgent cesarean deliveries are performed under spinal anesthesia. Hyperbaric bupivacaine solutions provide reliable anesthesia, often with the addition of morphine or meperidine for postoperative analgesia. General anesthesia is reserved for the most emergent cases and for cases in which the condition of the mother contraindicates regional anesthesia. For unscheduled cesarean deliveries, the consensus of the American College of Obstetricians and Gynecologists and the American Society of Anesthesiologists is that hospitals *should have the capability* to begin a cesarean delivery within 30 minutes of the decision to operate. However, not all indications for cesarean delivery require a 30-minute response time. Ironically, a time interval of longer than 18 minutes, not 30 minutes, from the onset of *severe* fetal heart rate decelerations to delivery is associated with poor neonatal outcome. The anesthesiologist must consider the indication for unscheduled cesarean delivery (e.g., arrest of labor, nonreassuring fetal heart rate, maternal illness) as well as the maternal risks and benefits when choosing the anesthetic. Maternal safety and well-being are paramount in selecting an anesthetic for nonscheduled cesarean delivery.

Ideally, all patients should be assessed by the anesthesiology team on admission for labor and delivery. At a minimum, the anesthesiology staff should be informed in advance and the patient evaluated when a complicated delivery is anticipated, when patient characteristics indicate increased anesthetic risk (Table 26-3), and at the first indication of a nonreassuring fetal heart rate pattern. Obviously, preanesthetic assessment must include evaluation for co-existing diseases as well as a thorough airway examination. Pulmonary aspiration and failed intubation account for three fourths of all maternal deaths related to anesthesia care. The incidence of aspiration of gastric contents is 1 in 661 patients undergoing cesarean delivery under general anesthesia compared with 1 in 2131 in the general surgical population. Between 15% and 20% of patients who experience aspiration pneumonitis require mechanical ventilation or prolonged hospitalization. To decrease the risk of significant aspiration pneumonitis, the patient should receive appropriate premedication with histamine 2 (H_2) blockers, a nonparticulate antacid, and/or metoclopramide, famotidine, or both. General anesthesia should be avoided whenever possible; cricoid pressure and an endotracheal tube should be used if general anesthesia is required. During labor, oral intake should be restricted to clear fluids, because one cannot predict which patients in labor will progress to cesarean delivery. The incidence of failed intubation in the obstetric population is 1 in 250, which is 10 times that in the general surgical population. Urgent cesarean delivery for a nonreassuring fetal heart rate pattern does not necessarily preclude the use of regional anesthesia. Rapid induction of spinal anesthesia is appropriate in many situations in which there is fetal compromise. Parturient patients at high risk of airway complications should undergo early induction of labor analgesia in hopes of precluding the need for general anesthesia should emergent cesarean delivery become necessary, because labor analgesia can rapidly be converted to surgical anesthesia for cesarean section.

HYPERTENSIVE DISORDERS OF PREGNANCY

Hypertensive disorders of pregnancy encompass a range of disorders that include chronic hypertension, chronic hypertension with superimposed preeclampsia, gestational hypertension, preeclampsia, and eclampsia. These disorders complicate 8% to 12% of all pregnancies. Hypertensive disorders are second only to thromboembolic disorders as the leading cause of maternal mortality in developed countries. Hypertensive disorders result in 70 maternal deaths a year in the United States and 50,000 maternal deaths a year worldwide. The only curative treatment for hypertensive disorders that develop during pregnancy is delivery. Deteriorating maternal

TABLE 26-3 ■ Factors associated with increased anesthesia risk
Obesity
Facial and neck edema
Extremely short stature
Difficulty opening mouth
Arthritis of neck, short neck, small mandible
Abnormalities of face, mouth, or teeth
Large thyroid
Pulmonary disease
Cardiac disease

condition mandates urgent delivery of the fetus regardless of gestational age. The risk of developing essential hypertension later in life is thought to be increased in women who experience gestational hypertension.

Gestational Hypertension

Gestational hypertension or pregnancy-induced hypertension is defined as an elevation of blood pressure above 139/89 mm Hg in a previously healthy woman after the first 19 weeks of pregnancy if the elevated blood pressures were recorded at least twice with the readings taken a minimum of 6 hours apart and no proteinuria is present. Gestational hypertension may develop into preeclampsia if proteinuria develops or may be redefined as chronic hypertension if hypertension persists longer than 12 weeks after delivery.

Pregnancy-induced hypertension may be classified as severe when blood pressure remains elevated above 159/109 mm Hg for longer than 6 hours.

Preeclampsia

Preeclampsia is a complex multisystem disorder of unknown etiology that is characterized by combined development of new-onset hypertension (see earlier) and new-onset proteinuria (>300 mg/24 hours) after the first 20 weeks of pregnancy. Edema is no longer a diagnostic criterion for preeclampsia; preeclampsia is a clinical diagnosis. Tables 26-4 and 26-5 list the diagnostic criteria and clinical manifestations of preeclampsia.

Risk factors for preeclampsia include obesity, nulliparity, and advanced maternal age (Table 26-6). Of interest, smoking during pregnancy is protective against preeclampsia.

PATHOPHYSIOLOGY

Preeclampsia is specific to human pregnancy. It is a disease of the placenta and occurs in molar pregnancies (pregnancy without the presence of fetal tissue). The hallmark of preeclampsia is an abnormal placentation-implantation. Normally, cytotrophoblasts invade the uterine wall, reaching decidual arteries and interacting with the endothelium. As a result of that interaction cytotrophoblasts acquire an endothelial phenotype and decidual arteries become low-resistance vessels. In preeclampsia, shallow endovascular invasion

TABLE 26-4   Criteria for the diagnosis of preeclampsia

Blood pressure > 139/89 mm Hg after 20 wk of gestation in a woman with previously normal blood pressure

Proteinuria of ≥0.3 g protein in a 24-hr urine specimen

TABLE 26-5   Manifestations and complications of preeclampsia

Systemic hypertension
Congestive heart failure
Decreased colloid osmotic pressure
Pulmonary edema
Arterial hypoxemia
Laryngeal edema
Cerebral edema (headaches, visual disturbances, changes in levels of consciousness)
Grand mal seizures
Cerebral hemorrhage
Hypovolemia
HELLP syndrome (*h*emolysis, *e*levated *l*iver enzymes, *l*ow *p*latelets)
Disseminated intravascular coagulation
Proteinuria
Oliguria
Acute tubular necrosis
Epigastric pain
Decreased uterine blood flow
Intrauterine growth retardation
Premature labor and delivery
Abruptio placentae

TABLE 26-6   Risk factors for the development of preeclampsia

Factor	Relative risk
Nulliparity	3
African American race	1.5
Age < 15 yr or > 35 yr	3
Multiple gestation	4
Family history of preeclampsia	5
Chronic hypertension	10
Chronic renal disease	20
Diabetes mellitus	2
Collagen vascular disease	2-3
Angiotensinogen T235 allele	
Homozygosity	20
Heterozygosity	4

preclude this cytotrophoblast-endothelium interaction. Spiral arteries remain constricted, high-resistance blood vessels that fail to provide adequate oxygen and nutrients for the growing placenta and fetus. The abnormal placenta releases vasoactive substances, which cause severe endothelial dysfunction of the maternal vasculature. This injured or hyperactivated endothelium further compromises placental blood flow. The plasma concentrations of vasoconstrictive substances, markers of oxidative stress, and inflammatory cytokines are increased, and the concentrations of vasodilators such as nitric oxide and prostacyclin are decreased. Severe proangiogenic and antiangiogenic imbalance has been described in patients with preeclampsia. It is unclear whether this imbalance is a cause or a consequence of abnormal implantation. Antiangiogenic proteins cause endothelial damage, especially in blood vessels with fenestrated endothelium as is found in kidney, liver, and brain.

The sensitivity of vascular receptors to angiotensin II is significantly decreased during normal pregnancy. In preeclampsia, the sensitivity increases, which contributes to vasoconstriction and placental insufficiency.

Hypoalbuminemia secondary to proteinuria and, sometimes, impairment of synthetic liver function results in low oncotic pressure. Endothelial injury and low oncotic pressure lead to third spacing of fluid and intravascular volume depletion.

TREATMENT

The definitive treatment for preeclampsia is delivery. At term, a patient diagnosed with preeclampsia should be delivered. If the preeclampsia is mild and the patient remote from term, conservative management with bed rest and monitoring until 37 weeks of gestation or until the status of the mother or fetus deteriorates is recommended.

In women with severe preeclampsia (Table 26-7) the fetus should be delivered immediately regardless of gestational age. Expectant management of patients with severe preeclampsia is possible in the following circumstances:

- The pregnancy is early preterm (24 to 28 weeks' duration).
- The diagnosis is based only on a high level of proteinuria.
- The diagnosis is based on intrauterine growth retardation before 32 weeks of gestation and results of fetal testing are good.
- The diagnosis is based only on a blood pressure of higher than 159/109 mm Hg, before 32 weeks of gestation.

The mode of delivery depends on fetal gestational age, the findings on cervical examination, assessment of fetal well-being, and the fetal presenting part. Only 14% to 20% of women with severe preeclampsia are delivered vaginally.

Magnesium sulfate is administered for seizure prophylaxis. It is the anticonvulsant of choice because it is 50% more effective in the prevention of new and recurrent seizures than diazepam or phenytoin. The precise mechanism of action is not known. Possible explanations for its anticonvulsant effect include competitive blockade of N-methyl-d-aspartate receptors, prevention of calcium ion entry into ischemic cells, protection of endothelial cells from free radical injury, and selective dilation of the cerebral blood vessels. Other beneficial effects include a decrease in systemic vascular resistance and an increase in cardiac index.

TABLE 26-7 ◼ **Diagnostic features of severe preeclampsia**

Blood pressure > 159/109 mm Hg on two occasions at least 6 hr apart
Proteinuria of ≥5 g protein in 24-hr urine specimen or dipstick reading of ≥3+ on two samples taken at least 4 hr apart
Oliguria (<500 mL in 24 hr)
Pulmonary edema or cyanosis
Abnormal liver function
Right upper quadrant or epigastric pain
Cerebral disturbances
Thrombocytopenia

There is no need to treat hypertension in women with mild preeclampsia. Indications for antihypertensive treatment during pregnancy are chronic hypertension, severe hypertension during labor and delivery, and expectant management of severe preeclampsia. There are only two benefits from such a treatment: prevention of abruptio placentae and prevention of cerebrovascular accident (which accounts for 15% to 20% of maternal deaths). The goal of therapy is to maintain blood pressure below 160/110 mm Hg.

Hydralazine, labetalol, and nifedipine are all effective antihypertensives in these patients. Refractory hypertension may necessitate continuous infusion of an antihypertensive. Nitroglycerin, sodium nitroprusside, and fenoldopam all are useful as short-term therapy (Table 26-8).

Invasive hemodynamic monitoring may be useful, especially during cesarean delivery. Catheterization of the internal jugular vein during the peripartum period is associated with a higher overall risk of complications, especially infectious complications, in parturient patients compared with nonpregnant medical or surgical patients (25% vs. 15% to 20%, respectively). The internal jugular vein overlies the carotid artery to a greater extent in pregnant than in nonpregnant patients, so the standard landmark approach is associated with a higher risk of carotid puncture (19% in pregnant patients vs. 10% in nonpregnant patients with the landmark approach and 6% vs. 3%, respectively, with the palpatory technique).

MANAGEMENT OF ANESTHESIA

Fluid management in the patient with preeclampsia is complicated by the conflict between the need to give fluids to an intravascularly depleted patient (the degree of depletion may be reflected by a rising hematocrit) and the obligation to avoid administration of fluids to a patient with "leaky" vasculature. As mentioned earlier, endothelial damage and low oncotic pressure make preeclamptic patients prone to third spacing of fluids and thus may lead to pulmonary edema. Invasive hemodynamic monitoring may help to guide fluid therapy in patients with preeclampsia. It should be remembered, however, that catheterization of the internal jugular vein during the peripartum period carries a higher risk of complications than in nonpregnant medical or surgical patients.

TABLE 26-8 ◼ **Treatment of systemic hypertension associated with preeclampsia**

Maintain diastolic blood pressure < 110 mm Hg
  Hydralazine 5-10 mg IV every 20-30 min
  Hydralazine 5 mg IV followed by 5-20 mg/hr IV as a continuous infusion
  Labetalol 50 mg IV or 100 mg PO
  Labetalol 20-160 mg/hr IV as a continuous infusion
  Nitroglycerin 10 mcg/min IV, titrated to response
  Nitroprusside 0.25 mcg/kg/min IV, titrated to response
  Fenoldopam 0.1 mcg/kg/min IV, increase by 0.05-0.2 mcg/kg/min until desired response reached; average dose is 0.25-0.5 mcg/kg/min
Seizure prophylaxis
  Magnesium 4-6 g IV followed by 1-2 g/hr IV as a continuous infusion (goal is to maintain serum concentrations of 2.0-3.5 mEq/L)
  Toxicity
    4.0-6.5 mEq/L is associated with nausea, vomiting, diplopia, somnolence, loss of patellar reflex
    6.5-7.5 mEq/L is associated with skeletal muscle paralysis, apnea
    ≥10 mEq/L is associated with cardiac arrest

IV, Intravenous; *PO,* by mouth.

Labor Analgesia

In addition to providing the common benefits of epidural labor analgesia, use of neuraxial techniques in preeclamptic patients can facilitate blood pressure control during labor. Epidural analgesia will also increase intervillous blood flow in preeclampsia, which will improve uteroplacental performance and, as a result, fetal well-being.

Because these patients are at high risk of requiring cesarean delivery, early placement of an epidural catheter can be considered to facilitate the use of epidural anesthesia for cesarean delivery and thus avoid the risks of general anesthesia.

Spinal Anesthesia. Spinal anesthesia is an anesthetic choice for patients with preeclampsia, unless it is contraindicated because of hypocoagulation. Neuraxial blockade causes sympathectomy and may lead to hypotension in healthy patients. In preeclamptic patients hypertension and vasoconstriction are the result of hyperactivity of the angiotensin II receptors. Spinal anesthesia does not influence the angiotensin system and thus may result in a lesser degree of hypotension in preeclamptic patients than in healthy parturient patients.

General Anesthesia. Not only are patients with preeclampsia subject to the common risks of general anesthesia during pregnancy, but these patients also have a higher risk of difficult intubation resulting from severe upper airway edema and a higher risk of aspiration because of the increased likelihood of difficulty in airway management. They also have an exaggerated response to sympathomimetics and methylergonovine. They have a greater sensitivity to the action of nondepolarizing muscle relaxants secondary to magnesium therapy. Finally, these patients have a higher risk of uterine atony and peripartum hemorrhage resulting from the smooth muscle–relaxant effects of magnesium therapy.

HELLP Syndrome

SIGNS AND SYMPTOMS

Hemolysis, elevated liver transaminase levels, and low platelet counts are the characteristic features of HELLP syndrome, a severe form of preeclampsia. Some 26% of patients with preeclampsia demonstrate one sign, 12% have two signs, and 10% show all three signs of the syndrome. Approximately 30% of cases present post partum. The most frequent clinical symptoms are right upper quadrant pain (80% of patients) and edema (50% to 60% of patients). Hemolysis is diagnosed by abnormalities on peripheral blood smear (presence of schistocytes), elevated bilirubin concentration (>1.2 mg/dL), decreased haptoglobin level (<25 mg/dL), and elevated lactate dehydrogenase level (>600 units/L). Plasma concentrations of transaminases are more than twice the normal levels. The platelet count is often lower than 100,000/mm^3. Maternal and perinatal morbidity and mortality is increased. Formation of a subcapsular hematoma of the liver may complicate HELLP syndrome, and hepatic rupture with a very high incidence of mortality can occur.

TREATMENT

The definitive treatment of HELLP syndrome is the delivery of the fetus. The American College of Obstetricians and Gynecologists recommends that women with HELLP syndrome be delivered regardless of fetal gestational age. Patients must receive seizure prophylaxis with magnesium sulfate and correction of coagulopathy. Dexamethasone increases platelets count to a greater degree than does betamethasone.

MANAGEMENT OF ANESTHESIA

Coagulopathy, risk of disseminated intravascular coagulation (DIC), and risk of severe intraabdominal bleeding resulting from the rupture of a subcapsular hematoma of the liver are specific concerns in patients with HELLP. These are in addition to the general problems of anesthetic management in parturient patients with severe preeclampsia.

Eclampsia

SIGNS AND SYMPTOMS

Eclampsia is seizures or coma in the setting of preeclampsia in the absence of any other pathologic brain condition. It is by definition considered severe preeclampsia and has an incidence of 1 in 2000 pregnancies. The majority of patients are diagnosed with preeclampsia before development of seizures; however, eclampsia is the first manifestation of preeclampsia in 20% to 38% of cases. The magnitude of hypertension does not correlate with the risk of eclampsia. Of patients with preeclampsia who develop seizures, approximately half report prodromal symptoms such as headache or visual changes.

Between 38% and 50% of eclamptic seizures occur before term. Sixteen percent of seizures occur longer than 48 hours after delivery. Seventy-five percent of seizures occurring at term take place during labor or within 48 hours of delivery.

Typical eclamptic seizures last less than 10 minutes and are neither recurrent nor associated with focal neurologic signs. Mortality related to eclampsia is about 2%.

About one third of eclamptic patients develop respiratory failure (with 23% of cases requiring mechanical ventilation), kidney failure, coagulopathy, cerebrovascular accident, or cardiac arrest. Fetal perinatal mortality is approximately 7% and is primarily related to issues associated with prematurity.

MANAGEMENT OF ANESTHESIA

Eclampsia is not an indication for cesarean delivery.

Management of the patient with eclampsia is directed at prevention of aspiration, maintenance of airway patency, control of seizures and prevention of their recurrence, control of hypertension, and evaluation for delivery. Eclamptic seizures are self-limiting.

Magnesium sulfate is the anticonvulsant of choice because it is more effective and has a better safety profile than benzodiazepines, phenytoin, or lytic cocktails. The standard intravenous regimen is a loading of magnesium sulfate of 2 g every 15 minutes to a maximum of 6 g. If the patient develops seizures while receiving a magnesium infusion for seizure prophylaxis, administration of a 1- to 2-g bolus recommended, after which plasma magnesium level should be measured.

If the patient and fetus are in stable condition following an eclamptic seizure, the management of the patient will proceed as it would for a patient with preeclampsia, and immediate delivery is not indicated unless that had been the plan before the seizure.

OBSTETRIC CONDITIONS AND COMPLICATIONS

Conditions that complicate delivery include hemorrhagic complications, amniotic fluid embolism, uterine rupture, trial of labor after cesarean delivery, vaginal birth after cesarean delivery, abnormal presentations, and multiple births.

Obstetric Hemorrhage

Obstetric hemorrhage remains a serious complication, contributing to maternal and prenatal morbidity and mortality. Although bleeding can occur at any time during pregnancy, third-trimester hemorrhage is the most threatening to maternal and fetal well-being (Table 26-9). Obstetric hemorrhage is one of the leading causes of all pregnancy-related deaths and accounts for a significant portion of perinatal morbidity and mortality. Placenta previa and abruptio placentae are the major causes of bleeding during the third trimester. Uterine rupture can be responsible for uncontrolled hemorrhage that manifests during active labor. Postpartum hemorrhage occurs after 3% to 5% of all vaginal deliveries. Uterine atony and placenta accreta are two leading cause of peripartum hemorrhage. Placenta accreta is the most common indication for cesarean hysterectomy. Retained products of conception and cervical or vaginal lacerations may also lead to postpartum hemorrhage.

Because of the increased blood volume and relative good health of the average pregnant patient, parturient women tolerate mild to moderate hemorrhage with few clinical signs or symptoms. This can lead to an underestimation of blood loss.

PLACENTA PREVIA

Signs and Symptoms

The cardinal symptom of placenta previa is painless vaginal bleeding. The first episode usually stops spontaneously. Bleeding typically manifests at approximately week 32 of gestation, when the lower uterine segment begins to form. When this diagnosis is suspected, the position of the placenta needs to be confirmed via ultrasonography or radioisotope scan.

Diagnosis

Placenta previa occurs in up to 1% of full-term pregnancies. The cause of placenta previa is not known, although there may be an association with advanced maternal age and with high parity. The greatest risk factor is previous cesarean section. Placenta previa is classified as *complete* when the entire cervical os is covered by placental tissue, *partial* when the internal cervical os is covered by placental tissue when closed but not when fully dilated, and *marginal* when placental tissue encroaches on or extends to the margin of the internal cervical os. Approximately 50% of parturient women with placenta previa have marginal implantations. The availability of more sophisticated obstetric ultrasonography has eliminated the need for a double setup cervical examination to diagnose placenta previa. Magnetic resonance imaging and color flow mapping during an ultrasonographic examination may identify, or at least raise suspicion for, placenta accreta.

Treatment

Once the diagnosis is made, the obstetrician will determine timing and mode of delivery. Expectant management will be chosen if the bleeding stops and the fetus is immature. When fetal lung maturity is achieved, or at 37 weeks, delivery should proceed. Obviously, delivery will occur at any time that the mother exhibits cardiovascular instability. Except for patients with a marginal previa who might elect vaginal delivery, patients will be delivered by cesarean section.

Prognosis

Maternal mortality is rare. Infant perinatal mortality is 12 per 1000 births. The risk that cesarean hysterectomy will be required increases with the number of previous cesarean deliveries.

Management of Anesthesia

Anesthetic management depends on the obstetric plan and the condition of the parturient patient.

Preoperative. Mild to moderate blood loss is well tolerated by the patient and thus may be underestimated by the anesthesiologist. Adequate volume resuscitation is thus paramount to the patient's care. Typing and cross-matching should be performed for all patients to ensure continuous availability of packed red blood cells (PRBCs) and component products.

Intraoperative. Parturient patients with complete or partial placenta previa will be delivered by cesarean section. Anesthetic management will depend on maternal and fetal status and the urgency of the surgery. If the patient has not had recent bleeding and is scheduled for an elective procedure, regional anesthesia is preferred, as it is for all patients undergoing cesarean delivery. Large-bore intravenous access should be established, because the patient is at greater risk of intraoperative bleeding. Cross-matched blood should be immediately

TABLE 26-9 Differential diagnosis of third-trimester bleeding

Parameter	Placenta previa	Abruptio placentae	Uterine rupture
Signs and symptoms	Painless vaginal bleeding	Abdominal pain Bleeding partially or wholly concealed Uterine irritability Shock Coagulopathy Acute renal failure Fetal distress	Abdominal pain Vaginal pain Recession of presenting part Disappearance of fetal heart tones, fetal bradycardia Hemodynamic instability
Predisposing conditions	Advanced age Multiple parity	High parity Advanced age Cigarette smoking Cocaine abuse Trauma Uterine anomalies Compression of the inferior vena cava Chronic systemic hypertension	Previous uterine incision Rapid spontaneous delivery Excessive uterine stimulation Cephalopelvic disproportion Multiple parity Polyhydramnios

available, and if the patient is in unstable condition, component products should also be available.

If hemorrhage necessitates emergency delivery, general anesthesia is the anesthetic technique of choice. Ketamine and etomidate are the preferred induction agents in the hypovolemic patient. Drug selection for maintenance of anesthesia will be determined by the hemodynamic status of the mother.

PLACENTA ACCRETA

Placenta accreta refers to a placenta that is abnormally adherent to the myometrium. Placenta accreta is an adherent placenta that has not invaded the myometrium. In placenta increta, the placenta has invaded the myometrium. Placenta percreta is invasion through the serosa. Massive hemorrhage may occur when removal of the placenta is attempted after delivery.

Signs and Symptoms

Retained placenta and postpartum hemorrhage occur in patients with placenta accreta.

Diagnosis

The majority of patients with placenta accreta have no symptoms; therefore, recognizing known risk factors is essential to early diagnosis. Risk factors include placenta previa and/or previous cesarean delivery, with the risk increasing with placenta previa in patients with multiple cesarean deliveries. Placenta implantation anteriorly in patients with previous cesarean deliveries also increases the risk. Additional risk factors include a short interval from cesarean delivery to conception, advanced maternal age, and female gender of the fetus. Magnetic resonance imaging and ultrasonography with Doppler flow mapping have identified placenta accreta antenatally. However, because the predictive value of these tests is poor, this diagnosis is often made at the time of surgery.

Treatment

The management of placenta accreta requires close coordination among the anesthesiologist, obstetrician, interventional radiologist, gynecologic oncologist, blood bank, and specialized surgical teams. Thorough planning decreases blood loss, requirements for blood products, and perioperative morbidity and mortality. Elective cesarean delivery at 34 weeks to avoid emergent delivery is recommended.

Cesarean hysterectomy used to be the traditional expectation. Now, with advances in endovascular procedures, uterine-sparing management can be offered to selected patients. In this approach, the placenta is left in place after delivery of the fetus without further surgical intervention, and inflation of angio-balloons or repeated selective uterine artery embolization is performed. Resorption of the poorly perfused placenta may be augmented by concurrent treatment with methotrexate.

Selective uterine artery embolization for the treatment of postpartum hemorrhage was initially described in 1979. Interventions include prophylactic selective catheterization of the internal iliac arteries with either temporary balloon occlusion or embolotherapy, selective embolization of collateral pelvic vessels in the setting of surgical ligation of the internal iliac arteries and/or delivery-related injuries to the genital tract, and transarterial embolization for the management of abnormal placentation. Prophylactic pelvic artery catheterization and embolization in women with placenta accreta can decrease perioperative blood loss and potentially allow hysterectomy to be avoided. Embolization of the uterine arteries as an alternative to hysterectomy has the advantage of being a minimally invasive treatment that preserves the uterus.

In the absence of data from large randomized controlled trials, controversy still exists about the safety and efficacy of endovascular interventions.

Prognosis

Maternal prognosis is good if the patient does not experience significant hemorrhage. As noted earlier, there has been some success with uterine preservation in selected cases; however, the majority of women still undergo cesarean hysterectomy. If an attempt is made to extract the placenta manually, profound hemorrhage may occur.

Management of Anesthesia

Preoperative. Significant hemorrhage should be anticipated, and thus at least two large-bore intravenous catheters should be placed. Insertion of an arterial catheter should be considered. PRBCs and component products should be immediately available. As soon as it is known that a patient with suspected placenta accreta will be undergoing surgical delivery, the anesthesiologist should communicate directly with the blood bank, request blood products, and provide information about the possibility of massive transfusion. The amount and type of requested products depends on the predicted severity of bleeding (i.e., accreta vs. percreta), baseline patient condition (i.e., presence of severe anemia or thrombocytopenia), and expected limitations in supply (e.g., rare blood group or difficult match because of the presence of antibodies). In routine placenta accreta cases it is recommended that 4 units of matched RBCs and 4 units of fresh frozen plasma (FFP) be available in the operating room before the beginning of surgery. In complicated cases availability of 10 units of matched RBCs, 10 units of FFP, and 10 units of platelets is recommended.

In emergency cases, when the diagnosis of placenta accreta is made intraoperatively, the anesthesiologist should initiate the massive transfusion protocol. At Yale–New Haven Hospital, this protocol is as follows: the blood bank immediately releases 6 units of O-negative RBCs and 4 units of AB FFP. Within 20 minutes, the blood bank releases an additional 10 units of O-negative RBCs, 10 units of AB FFP, 10 units of platelets, and 10 units of cryoprecipitate, and provides recombinant factor VIIa if requested. If further therapy is needed, the listed components are again be provided. It is strongly recommended that a massive transfusion protocol be established at any institution that provides obstetric care.

Intraoperative. Intraoperative management of a patient at risk of hemorrhage and/or cesarean hysterectomy is controversial. Many believe that all patients should undergo general anesthesia (as discussed for patients with a placenta previa). Others argue that, if needed, a cesarean hysterectomy can be performed under epidural anesthesia. There is general agreement that if a patient is deemed potentially to have a difficult airway, it is prudent to use general anesthesia.

Management of blood loss is the major issue in patients with placenta accreta. The blood flow through each uterine artery increases from 100 mL/min to 350 mL/min during pregnancy. Arteries at the site of the placenta accreta are large in diameter. In the event that an attempt is made to remove the placenta, these arteries are torn, which leads to uncontrolled hemorrhage.

Hemorrhagic shock occurs in over half of patients who undergo emergency postpartum hysterectomy, and coagulopathy or DIC occurs in approximately one quarter of these patients.

Autologous RBC salvage can decrease the transfusion of allogenic blood. Use of the intraoperative cell salvage machine ("cell saver") began in the 1970s in nonobstetric cases. Unfortunately, no prospective trials have confirmed the safety of its use in obstetric practice. Concerns include the risk of amniotic fluid embolism and maternal alloimmunization. Theoretically, the washing process and leukocyte-reducing filter should eliminate this risk of contamination. Several studies showed that the level of contamination of the maternal circulatory system by amniotic fluid is similar during caesarean delivery with and without the use of the cell saver. These studies, however, did not involve transfusion of salvaged blood back into the parturient patient. In the absence of solid evidence caution is recommended if cell salvage is used during cesarean delivery, and the risk of severe hypotension must be kept in mind.

DAMAGE CONTROL RESUSCITATION. In 2005 the U.S. Army Institute of Surgical Research offered a new strategy for the transfusion of severely injured military patients: the decreased use of crystalloids and colloids and the matching of PRBC transfusion in a 1:1:1 ratio with FFP and platelets. Results of this new strategy, called *damage control resuscitation,* appear remarkable. With an increase in the FFP/PRBC ratio from 1:8 to 1:1.4, mortality dropped from 65% to 19%. The number needed to treat to save one life was only two patients.

Extrapolation of data from military and civilian trauma centers to massively bleeding parturient women should be viewed with caution. The pathophysiologic mechanisms of dilutional and consumption coagulopathy, and the harmful effects of metabolic acidosis and hypothermia are present in both populations. However, some physiologic mechanisms are different or even opposite, such as early activation of the thrombomodulin–protein C anticoagulation system in trauma patients in contrast with protein C resistance in parturient patients.

To avoid development of dilutional coagulopathy and further exacerbation of the discrepancy in activity of the coagulation factors, transfusion of colloids and crystalloids should be minimized during massive resuscitation of bleeding parturient patients. Also important to consider is that colloids may impair platelet function, inhibit fibrin polymerization, and increase the fibrinolytic tendency.

RATIO OF FRESH FROZEN PLASMA TO RED BLOOD CELLS. A higher ratio of FFP and platelets to RBCs is believed to significantly decrease the risk of coagulation abnormalities during massive peripartum resuscitation. This opinion is based on the literature discussed earlier on damage control resuscitation and the fact that a mixture of 1 unit of PRBCs, 1 unit of FFP, and 1 unit of platelets has a hematocrit of 29%, a platelet count of 85,000/mm^3, and coagulation factor activity of 62%.

CRYOPRECIPITATE AND ANTIFIBRINOLYTICS. A recent review of clinical data in postpartum hemorrhage suggested that a higher than previously recommended level of fibrinogen is necessary for adequate hemostasis (2 to 3 g/L vs. 1 g/L). Factor XIII activity should be kept above 50% to 60% to reduce bleeding after major surgery. As much as 30 mL/kg of FFP is required to increase fibrinogen level by 1 g/L, so even when transfusing at a high FFP/RBC ratio, early administration of cryoprecipitate is recommended. Cryoprecipitate is rich in fibrinogen, as well as in factors XIII and VIII. Only 3 mL/kg of cryoprecipitate is enough to raise the fibrinogen level by 1 g/L.

FACTOR VII. A dose of 80 to 95 mcg/kg of factor VII may stop or reduced hemorrhage without an increase in the incidence of thromboembolic events. Failure of this therapy to correct coagulopathy may be due to hypothermia, acidosis, or low fibrinogen level.

Monitoring. PTT, PT, platelet count, and fibrinogen level should be measured at baseline and every hour after the initiation of massive transfusion to guide therapy. PT is more sensitive than PTT for indicating a nonhemostatic level of at least one clotting factor. Unfortunately, none of these tests assesses platelet function, factor XIII level, clot stability, or level of fibrinolysis, all of which show abnormalities in obstetric patients. Use of point-of care devices such as a thromboelastograph or thromboelastometer may improve assessment of hemostasis and provide goal-directed hemostatic therapy.

Plasma electrolyte levels should also be measured at baseline and every hour after the initiation of massive transfusion, with specific assessment for hyperkalemia, hypomagnesemia, hypocalcemia, and hyperchloremia.

ABRUPTIO PLACENTAE

Signs and Symptoms

Signs and symptoms of abruptio placentae depend on the site and extent of the placental separation, but abdominal pain is always present. When the separation involves only the placental margins, the escaping blood can appear as vaginal bleeding. On the other hand, large volumes of extravasated blood can remain concealed within the uterus. Severe blood loss from abruptio placentae presents as maternal hypotension, uterine irritability and hypertonus, and fetal distress or demise. Clotting abnormalities can occur. The classic hemorrhagic picture includes thrombocytopenia, depletion of fibrinogen, and prolonged plasma thromboplastin times. DIC can occur and may be accompanied by acute renal failure resulting from fibrin deposition in renal arterioles. Fetal distress reflects the loss of functional placenta and decreased uteroplacental perfusion because of maternal hypotension.

Diagnosis

Abruptio placentae is defined as premature separation of a normally implanted placenta after 20 weeks of gestation. The precise causes are unknown, but the incidence is increased with high parity, uterine anomalies, compression of the inferior vena cava, gestational hypertension, and cocaine abuse. Abruptio placentae accounts for approximately one third of third-trimester hemorrhages and occurs in 0.5% to 1% of all pregnancies. Diagnosis is made before delivery using ultrasonography and at delivery by examination of the placenta.

Treatment

Definitive treatment of abruptio placentae is delivery of the fetus and placenta. Delivery may be vaginal if the abruption is not jeopardizing maternal or fetal well-being. Otherwise, delivery is by cesarean section.

Prognosis

Maternal complications associated with abruptio placentae include DIC, acute renal failure, and uterine atony, which may lead to postpartum hemorrhage. DIC occurs in approximately 10% of patients with abruptio placentae.

Neonatal complications are significant. Perinatal mortality is 25-fold higher if a term pregnancy is complicated by abruption. Fetal distress is also common due to the disruption of placental blood flow.

Management of Anesthesia

If maternal hypotension is absent, clotting study results are acceptable, and there is no evidence of fetal distress due to uteroplacental insufficiency; epidural analgesia is useful to provide analgesia for labor and vaginal delivery. When the magnitude of placental separation and resulting hemorrhage are severe, emergency cesarean delivery is necessary; most often, general anesthesia is used, because regional anesthesia may be unwise in a patient with hemodynamic instability. Anesthetic management is similar to that in patients with placenta previa. Blood and blood products should be readily available because of the risk of bleeding and DIC.

It is not uncommon for blood to dissect between layers of the myometrium after premature separation of the placenta. As a result, the uterus is unable to contract adequately after delivery, and postpartum hemorrhage occurs. Uncontrolled hemorrhage may require an emergency hysterectomy. Bleeding may be exaggerated by coagulopathy, in which case infusion of FFP and platelets may be indicated to replace deficient clotting factors. Clotting parameters usually revert to normal within a few hours after delivery of the fetus.

POSTPARTUM HEMORRHAGE

Uterine Atony

Uterine atony after vaginal delivery is a common cause of postpartum bleeding and a potential cause of maternal mortality. Complete atony of the uterus may result in a 2000-mL blood loss in 5 minutes. Conditions associated with uterine atony include multiple parity, multiple births, polyhydramnios, a large fetus, and a retained placenta. Uterine atony may occur immediately after delivery or may manifest itself several hours later. Treatment is with intravenous oxytocin, which results in contraction of the uterus. Methylergonovine, administered intravenously or intramuscularly, or intramuscular or intrauterine carboprost tromethamine (or misoprostol) may also be used to control hemorrhage. In rare instances, it may be necessary to perform an emergency hysterectomy.

Retained Placenta

Retained placenta occurs in approximately 1% of all vaginal deliveries and usually necessitates a manual exploration of the uterus. If epidural analgesia has been used for vaginal delivery, manual removal of the retained placenta may be attempted under epidural anesthesia. Spinal anesthesia (saddle block) or low-dose intravenous ketamine may provide adequate analgesia if an epidural catheter is not in place. In rare cases, a general anesthetic may be needed. Low doses of intravenous nitroglycerin (40-mcg boluses, as needed) are used to relax the uterus for placental removal when indicated.

Uterine Rupture

Uterine rupture occurs in up to 0.1% of full-term pregnancies and may be associated with separation of previous uterine surgical scars, rapid spontaneous delivery, excessive oxytocin stimulation, or multiple parity with cephalopelvic disproportion or unrecognized transverse presentation. Uterine rupture and dehiscence represent a spectrum ranging from incomplete rupture or gradual dehiscence of surgical scars to explosive rupture with intraperitoneal extrusion of uterine contents.

SIGNS AND SYMPTOMS

Uterine rupture may present with severe abdominal pain, often referred to the shoulder because of subdiaphragmatic irritation by intraabdominal blood, as well as maternal hypotension and disappearance of fetal heart tones.

DIAGNOSIS

An ultrasonographic examination is useful in making the diagnosis of uterine rupture. Visual examination of the uterus at cesarean delivery will detect rupture or dehiscence. Manual examination with vaginal delivery will also detect dehiscence.

TREATMENT

Uterine rupture with maternal and/or fetal distress mandates immediate laparotomy, delivery, and surgical repair or hysterectomy.

PROGNOSIS

Maternal mortality is rare. Fetal mortality is approximately 35%.

MANAGEMENT OF ANESTHESIA

Anesthetic management is similar to that for patients with placenta previa who are in unstable condition.

Trial of Labor after Cesarean Delivery

Women with a history of one or two low transverse cesarean deliveries may attempt a vaginal birth (trial of labor after cesarean delivery, or TOLAC), with the goal of achieving vaginal birth after cesarean delivery (VBAC). TOLAC decreases the rate of cesarean deliveries, reduces maternal morbidity and mortality (from 13 per 100,000 to 4 per 100,000 live births), and diminishes risk of complications in future pregnancies. Seventy-four percent of appropriately chosen candidates for TOLAC will successfully accomplish vaginal delivery. Unfortunately, many medical and nonmedical factors may increase the risk of failure of TOLAC and lead to increased maternal and perinatal morbidity.

Factors associated with a lower rate of successful VBAC include African American or Hispanic ethnicity, advanced maternal age, single motherhood, fewer than 12 years of maternal education, delivery at low-volume hospitals, and maternal comorbid conditions, including hypertension, diabetes, asthma, seizure disorders, renal disease, heart disease, and obesity. Also, induction of labor, fetal gestational age of more than 40 weeks, fetal weight of more than 4000 g, and poor cervical dilation may be predictive of failure.

The most feared obstetric emergency related to TOLAC is uterine rupture. (See earlier section.) Factors that may increase the risk of uterine rupture among parturient women with a history of previous cesarean delivery include a classical uterine scar; induction of labor, especially after 40 weeks; two or more cesarean deliveries; maternal obesity; fetal weight of more than 4000 g; and delivery at a low-volume facility. In a retrospective analysis of 1787 cases of TOLAC, Bujold found only two risk factors for uterine rupture: interdelivery interval of less than 18 month (which increased the risk threefold) and use of a single-layer closure during prior cesarean section. Careful selection of candidates for TOLAC with consideration of all risk factors is necessary.

The American College of Obstetricians and Gynecologists practice bulletin for VBAC recommends that the potential complications of VBAC be thoroughly discussed with the patient and that they be documented before the patient is offered the option for VBAC. Both the American College of Obstetricians and Gynecologists and the American Society of Anesthesiologists recommend that personnel including the obstetrician, anesthetist, and operating staff be immediately available at all times to perform an emergency cesarean delivery when VBAC is being attempted. Despite the concern for uterine rupture in this patient population, the risk of uterine rupture in patients undergoing VBAC following one cesarean delivery is approximately 2%. Women who undergo VBAC rather than elective repeat cesarean delivery have reduced morbidity associated with their delivery. However, there may be a higher incidence of perinatal death in patients undergoing VBAC.

MANAGEMENT OF ANESTHESIA

Neuraxial labor analgesia provides all the same benefits for parturient women attempting TOLAC as for women without a history of cesarean delivery.

The suggestion that neuraxial analgesia will mask the signs and symptoms of uterine rupture is unfounded. The pain of uterine rupture is constant (does not resolve between contractions), is much more intense, and has a different quality than the pain of contractions. Worsening of the fetal heart rate tracing will alert obstetric and anesthesiology teams to abnormality as well. The opioid-based epidural solutions used for labor provide only analgesia and cannot mask the pain of uterine rupture because these solutions do not provide anesthesia.

Amniotic Fluid Embolism

Amniotic fluid embolism is a rare catastrophic and life-threatening complication of pregnancy that occurs when there is a disruption in the barrier between the amniotic fluid and the maternal circulation. The three most common sites for entry of amniotic fluid into the maternal circulation are the endocervical veins, the placenta, and a uterine trauma site. Multiparous parturient women experiencing tumultuous labors are at increased risk of amniotic fluid embolism.

SIGNS AND SYMPTOMS

The onset of the signs and symptoms of amniotic fluid embolism is dramatic and abrupt, classically manifesting as dyspnea, arterial hypoxemia, cyanosis, seizures, loss of consciousness, and hypotension that is disproportionate to the blood loss. Fetal distress is present at the same time. More than 80% of these parturient women experience cardiopulmonary arrest. Coagulopathy resembling DIC with associated bleeding is common and may be the only presenting symptom.

PATHOPHYSIOLOGY

The principal defect created by amniotic fluid embolism is a mechanical blockage of part of the pulmonary circulation accompanied by vasoconstriction of the remaining vessels resulting from release of undefined chemicals such as prostaglandins, leukotrienes, serotonin, and histamine. As a result, pulmonary artery pressures increase, arterial hypoxemia develops owing to ventilation/perfusion mismatching, and hypotension occurs, reflecting decreased cardiac output and congestive heart failure caused by right ventricular outflow obstruction and acute cor pulmonale.

DIAGNOSIS

The diagnosis of amniotic fluid embolism is based largely on clinical signs and symptoms. These include increased pulmonary artery pressures and decreased cardiac output as determined by measurements from invasive monitors. Ultimately, the presence of amniotic fluid material is confirmed in the parturient patient's blood aspirated from a central venous or pulmonary artery catheter. Findings of fetal squamous cells, fat, and mucin in samples of the patient's blood are indicative of amniotic fluid embolism.

Conditions that can mimic amniotic fluid embolism include inhalation of gastric contents, pulmonary embolism, venous air embolism, and local anesthetic toxicity. Pulmonary aspiration is more likely when bronchoconstriction accompanies the clinical signs and symptoms. Indeed, bronchospasm is rare in parturient women who experience amniotic fluid embolism. Pulmonary embolism is usually accompanied by chest pain. High sensory levels produced by spinal or epidural anesthesia may be confused with amniotic fluid embolism.

TREATMENT

Treatment of amniotic fluid embolism includes tracheal intubation and mechanical ventilation of the lungs with 100% oxygen, inotropic support as guided by central venous or pulmonary artery catheter monitoring, and correction of coagulopathy. The use of positive end-expiratory pressure is often helpful for improving oxygenation. Dopamine, dobutamine, and norepinephrine have been recommended as inotropes to treat acute left ventricular dysfunction and associated hypotension. Fluid therapy is guided by central venous pressure monitoring, but it must be kept in mind that these patients are vulnerable to developing pulmonary edema. Treatment of DIC may include administration of FFP, cryoprecipitate, and platelets. Even with immediate and aggressive treatment, mortality resulting from amniotic fluid embolism remains higher than 80%.

Abnormal Presentations and Multiple Births

The presentation of the fetus is determined by the presenting part and the anatomic portion of the fetus felt through the cervix by manual examination. The description of the fetal position is based on the relationship of the fetal occiput, chin, or sacrum to the left or right side of the parturient patient. Approximately 90% of deliveries are cephalic presentations in either the occiput transverse or occiput anterior position. All other presentations and positions are considered abnormal.

BREECH PRESENTATION
Diagnosis
Breech, rather than cephalic, presentations characterize approximately 3.5% of all pregnancies. The cause of breech presentation is unknown, but factors that seem to predispose to this presentation include prematurity, placenta previa, multiple gestations, and uterine anomalies. Fetal abnormalities, including hydrocephalus and polyhydramnios, are also associated with breech presentations.

Treatment
Fetuses in breech presentations are delivered by elective cesarean section. Vaginal breech delivery is rare and necessitates

the immediate availability of anesthetic care, because serious complications can occur.

Prognosis
Breech vaginal deliveries result in increased maternal morbidity. Compared with cephalic presentations, there is a greater likelihood of cervical lacerations, perineal injury, retained placenta, and shock resulting from hemorrhage. Morbidity and mortality of the neonate are also increased. These infants are more likely to experience arterial hypoxemia and acidosis during delivery because of umbilical cord compression. Prolapse of the umbilical cord occurs with increased frequency in breech presentations and is presumed to reflect failure of the presenting part to fill the lower uterine segment.

Management of Anesthesia
In parturient patients undergoing elective cesarean delivery for breech presentation spinal anesthesia is generally used, as is routine for elective cesarean delivery.

Vaginal delivery may be complicated by umbilical cord prolapse or fetal head entrapment, which necessitates emergency anesthesia for cesarean or instrumented vaginal delivery. Dense perineal anesthesia is needed for vaginal instrumentation and must be administered rapidly, either by using 3% 2-chloroprocaine if an epidural catheter is in place, or by inducing general anesthesia.

MULTIPLE GESTATIONS
The increasing use of assisted reproductive technologies has resulted in a markedly greater frequency of multiple gestations. Twin pregnancies comprise approximately 3% of all pregnancies. Triplet and higher-order gestations increased by 500% from 1980 to 2001 and continue to increase in conjunction with the increase in the availability and use of assisted reproductive technologies.

Treatment
In all triplet and higher-order gestations, delivery is by cesarean section. For twin gestations, the presentation of the twins is considered when determining the mode of delivery. If both are in vertex position, vaginal delivery is appropriate. If twin A is in breech position, cesarean delivery is recommended. The route of delivery for vertex-nonvertex twins is controversial, but often cesarean delivery is recommended.

Prognosis
Maternal morbidity and mortality are increased with multiple gestations because many obstetric complications are more common in this setting. Fetal perinatal mortality and morbidity are also increased, with preterm delivery the most common cause.

Management of Anesthesia
Preoperative. The physiologic changes associated with pregnancy may be exaggerated with multiple gestations. The larger size of the uterus causes a greater decrease in functional

residual capacity. Maternal blood volume is 500 mL greater with twins, and cardiac output is greater. Supine hypotension syndrome is also more significant because of the larger uterus.

Intraoperative. Epidural analgesia is preferred for labor analgesia because it will facilitate instrumented vaginal delivery or allow rapid induction of surgical anesthesia, if needed. Particular attention must be paid to left uterine displacement. The risk of intrapartum and postpartum hemorrhage is increased; thus, large-bore intravenous access should be established and current blood typing and screening results should be available. The anesthesiologist must be prepared for vaginal (forceps) or abdominal operative delivery of twin B if that twin has a nonvertex presentation.

For planned cesarean delivery, maternal and fetal status will dictate anesthetic choice. Severe aortocaval compression despite left uterine displacement may lead to profound hypotension, which should be treated aggressively.

CO-EXISTING MEDICAL CONDITIONS

Co-existing medical diseases may accompany pregnancy and thus assume importance out of proportion to the implications of the disease in the absence of pregnancy.

Heart Disease

Because of the cardiovascular changes of pregnancy, women with congenital heart disease have increased risk of peripartum cardiac complications ("cardiac events"). According to the Cardiac Disease in Pregnancy (CARPREG) study, which reviewed data for 562 patients with heart disease who had 599 pregnancies and were treated in 13 Canadian hospitals, such cardiac events include pulmonary edema (documented by findings on chest radiograph or the auscultation of crackles over more than one third of the posterior lung fields), sustained symptomatic tachyarrhythmia or bradyarrhythmia requiring treatment, stroke, cardiac arrest, and death.

The likelihood of occurrence of a cardiac event can be estimated using a scale based on the presence of certain risk factors. These risk factors are a history of a previous cardiac event, a baseline New York Heart Association (NYHA) class II rating, or cyanosis; left heart obstruction (mitral valve area of 2 cm², aortic valve area of <1.5 cm², or peak left ventricular outflow tract gradient of >30 mm Hg by echocardiography); and reduced systemic ventricular systolic function (ejection fraction of <40%). One point is assigned for each risk factor. The risk of an event is estimated to be 5% with no points, 27% with 1 point, and 75% with 2 or more points.

Pulmonary hypertension is a significant risk factor for poor maternal and neonatal outcome. Patients with pulmonary hypertension are usually advised against pregnancy. Pulmonary insufficiency has been shown to increase the risk of peripartum complications.

The ZAHARA study identified similar risk factors: a history of arrhythmia, use of cardiac medication before pregnancy,

NYHA class higher than II, aortic stenosis, moderate or severe mitral and/or tricuspid regurgitation, presence of a mechanical valve, and cyanotic heart disease. A new risk score calculation for cardiac complications was offered. Among all the cardiac events observed during pregnancy, the most frequent were arrhythmia and congestive heart failure. Of note, patients who died during the peripartum period were excluded from the ZAHARA study (Table 26-10).

CARDIOMYOPATHY OF PREGNANCY

Diagnosis

Left ventricular failure late in the course of pregnancy or during the first 6 weeks post partum has been termed the *cardiomyopathy of pregnancy.* The precise etiology remains unknown. Suggested causes include myocarditis or an autoimmune response. Patients have signs and symptoms of left ventricular failure, frequently after delivery or in the postpartum period.

Treatment

Medical treatment of peripartum cardiomyopathy is similar to the treatment of other dilated cardiomyopathies. This includes preload optimization, afterload reduction, and

TABLE 26-10 ■ Multivariable model for the composite end points of cardiac and neonatal complications corrected for maternal age and parity

	Odds ratio	P value
CARDIAC COMPLICATIONS		
History of arrhythmia	4.3	.0011
Cardiac medication use before pregnancy	4.2	<.0001
NYHA functional class	2.2	.0298
Left-sided heart obstruction (peak gradient > 50 mm Hg, aortic valve area < 1.0 cm²)	12.9	<.0001
Moderate to severe AI	2.0	.0427
Moderate to severe PI	2.3	.0287
Mechanical prosthetic valve	74.7	.0014
Cyanotic heart disease (corrected or not)	3.0	<.0001
NEONATAL COMPLICATIONS		
Twin or multiple gestation	5.4	.0014
Smoking during pregnancy	1.7	.0070
Cyanotic heart disease (corrected or not)	2.0	.0003
Mechanical prosthetic valve	13.9	.0331
Cardiac medication use before pregnancy	2.2	.0009

Adapted from ZAHARA investigators. Predictors of pregnancy complications in women with congenital heart disease. *Eur Heart J.* 2010;31(17):2124-2132. Epub Jun 28, 2010.
AI, Aortic insufficiency; *NYHA,* New York Heart Association; *PI,* pulmonary insufficiency.

improvement of myocardial contractility. In addition, these patients may require anticoagulant therapy because of the increased risk of thromboembolism. It is important to remember that angiotensin-converting enzyme inhibitors, which are routinely used for afterload reduction in nonpregnant patients, are contraindicated during pregnancy. However, nitroglycerin or nitroprusside can be used for afterload reduction in pregnant patients.

Collaboration among the obstetrician, cardiologist, and anesthesiologist is essential to optimize care of these patients. Induction of labor is usually recommended if the patient's cardiac status can be stabilized with medical therapy. However, if acute cardiac decompensation occurs, cesarean delivery may be required because of the inability of the mother to tolerate the stresses of labor.

Prognosis

In approximately one half of these parturient patients, heart failure is transient, resolving within 6 months of delivery. In the remaining patients, idiopathic congestive cardiomyopathy persists, and the mortality rate is as high as 25% to 50%.

Management of Anesthesia

Parturient patients with peripartum cardiomyopathy will likely require invasive monitoring, including intraarterial catheterization and pulmonary artery catheterization to assess the patient's hemodynamic status and guide intrapartum management. Acute cardiac decompensation during labor may require the administration of intravenous nitroglycerin or nitroprusside for preload and afterload reduction and dopamine or dobutamine for inotropic support. Early initiation of epidural labor analgesia is essential to minimize the cardiac stress associated with the pain of labor. The invasive monitoring will guide fluid management, the titration of vasoactive drugs, and the induction of epidural analgesia.

If cesarean delivery is required, epidural or spinal anesthesia may be used, with fluid management guided by the use of the invasive monitors. If spinal anesthesia is selected, a continuous technique should be implemented, because use of a single-shot technique, which produces rapid hemodynamic changes, will not be well tolerated. If general anesthesia is required, the high-dose opioid remifentanil is often preferred. Neonatal depression from the opioid is expected, and thus personnel must be available to perform neonatal resuscitation.

Diabetes Mellitus

Diabetes mellitus is one of the most common co-existing medical conditions in pregnancy, occurring in approximately 2% of parturient women. The incidence is increasing because of the epidemic of obesity and the greater number of women becoming pregnant at an advanced maternal age. Ninety percent of diabetic pregnant patients have gestational diabetes, whereas the other 10% have preexisting diabetes. Pregnancy is a state of progressive insulin resistance, as discussed earlier in the chapter. Women who cannot produce enough insulin

to compensate for this resistance develop gestational diabetes. Patients who had diabetes before pregnancy have increased insulin requirements during pregnancy. Patients with type 1 diabetes are at greater risk of diabetic ketoacidosis, because pregnancy is associated with enhanced lipolysis and ketogenesis and diminished ability to buffer overproduced acids. The decreased buffering ability is secondary to the lower HCO_3 concentration that results from compensation for chronic respiratory alkalosis. Diabetic ketoacidosis occurs at lower glucose levels in pregnancy, as low as 130 to 150 mg/dL, because of utilization of glucose by the fetus and placenta. Administration of β-adrenergic drugs and glucosteroids may precipitate diabetic ketoacidosis.

DIAGNOSIS

The possibility of gestational diabetes arises if the results of a routine 1-hour glucose tolerance test are abnormal, and a 3-hour glucose tolerance test is then required. If the results of this test are also abnormal, the diagnosis of gestational diabetes is made. For evaluation of risk, patients with prepregnancy diabetes are classified by the type and duration of the diabetes and the presence of comorbid conditions (Table 26-11).

TREATMENT

Glycemic control is the major focus of the care of pregnant women with diabetes. A blood glucose level of 60 to 120 mg/dL is desirable, which requires frequent changes in insulin dosage during pregnancy. Management of diabetic ketoacidosis is similar to that in nonpregnant patients. In patients with gestational diabetes, dietary control is used initially. If glycemic control cannot be achieved through diet, insulin therapy is initiated.

During the third trimester, antenatal fetal surveillance is conducted using twice-weekly nonstress tests, beginning at 28 weeks. If the nonstress test shows fetal nonreactivity, a biophysical profile is compiled to determine timing and route of delivery. At 38 to 40 weeks, elective induction is commonly

TABLE 26-11	White's classification of diabetes mellitus during pregnancy
Class	**Definition**
A_1	Diet-controlled gestational diabetes
A_2	Gestational diabetes requiring insulin
B	Preexisting diabetes, without complications (duration < 10 yr or onset at age > 20 yr)
C	Preexisting diabetes without complications (duration 10-19 yr or onset at age < 10-19 yr)
D	Preexisting diabetes (duration > 20 yr or onset at age < 10 yr)
F	Preexisting diabetes with nephropathy
R	Preexisting diabetes with retinopathy
T	Preexisting diabetes with prior renal transplantation
H	Preexisting diabetes with heart disease

chosen to avoid risks to the neonate associated with maternal diabetes.

PROGNOSIS

Patients with gestational diabetes are at increased risk of type 2 diabetes later in life. In addition, the incidence of preeclampsia is increased, as is the incidence of polyhydramnios.

Fetal effects of diabetes include a greater risk of anomalies in fetuses of women with preexisting diabetes mellitus. Intrauterine fetal death, including late-trimester stillbirth, occurs more frequently in diabetic mothers, probably secondary to poor uteroplacental blood flow. Macrosomia leads to a higher incidence of cesarean delivery, shoulder dystocia, and birth trauma. Neonates are at risk for hypoglycemia and may be at greater risk of respiratory distress.

MANAGEMENT OF ANESTHESIA

Preoperative

Patients with pregestational diabetes should be assessed for diabetes-related complications. Appropriate evaluation for gastroparesis, autonomic dysfunction, and cardiac, vascular, and renal involvement should be made.

Intraoperative

Epidural labor analgesia decreases pain, which results in decreased maternal plasma catecholamine levels and thus improved uteroplacental blood flow. Patients with autonomic dysfunction are especially prone to hypotension with epidural analgesia, and hypervigilance and rapid treatment are indicated.

Diabetic parturient patients are at increased risk of requiring emergent cesarean delivery; therefore epidural analgesia may be preferred to spinal-epidural analgesia, because the catheter should be known to be functioning to minimize the need for general anesthesia in the event that cesarean section is required.

The choice of anesthetic for cesarean delivery, as in other parturient patients, depends on the status of the mother and fetus. As for all diabetic patients undergoing surgery, blood glucose level should be checked intraoperatively.

Myasthenia Gravis

Myasthenia gravis is a disorder characterized by skeletal muscle fatigability and weakness caused by autoantibody destruction or blockade of postsynaptic nicotinic acetylcholine receptors. Muscle weakness may involve only the eye muscles, predominantly the limb and axial muscles, or bulbar and respiratory muscles.

The course of myasthenia gravis during gestation is highly variable and unpredictable. Exacerbations are most likely to occur during the first trimester or within the first 10 days post partum. Anticholinesterase drugs should be continued during pregnancy and labor. Theoretically, these drugs increase uterine contractility but without increasing the incidence of spontaneous abortion or premature labor.

Skeletal muscles are greatly involved in the second stage of labor. Myasthenia gravis causes weakness and fatigue of the skeletal muscles, resulting in impairment of the second stage of labor and sometimes in respiratory distress. Outlet forceps may be used to shorten the second stage of labor and thereby minimize skeletal muscle fatigue.

An effectively working epidural catheter for labor anesthesia provides excellent pain control and alleviates the stress of labor, which diminishes fatigue and prevents exacerbation of myasthenia gravis. Instrumented vaginal delivery is easier to perform in the presence of good neuraxial analgesia. Presence of a properly placed and functioning epidural catheter should allow general anesthesia to be avoided in case of an unplanned cesarean delivery. Early initiation of epidural analgesia is preferable.

Important considerations regarding the use of general anesthesia in patients with myasthenia gravis are the following: First, nondepolarizing muscle relaxants are likely to have a prolonged effect. Second, the reversal of nondepolarizing muscle relaxants may cause cholinergic crisis. Finally, larger doses of succinylcholine may be necessary to achieve relaxation unless adequate muscle relaxation can be achieved with an inhalation agent only.

Neonatal myasthenia gravis occurs transiently in 20% to 30% of infants born to mothers with this disorder. Manifestations usually occur within 24 hours of birth and are characterized by generalized skeletal muscle weakness and expressionless facies. When breathing efforts are inadequate, tracheal intubation and mechanical ventilation of the infant's lungs should be initiated. Anticholinesterase therapy in neonates is usually necessary for approximately 21 days after birth.

Maternal Obesity

Obesity in the United States has become a national epidemic and is a major contributor to maternal morbidity. Nearly half of U.S. women of childbearing age are overweight or obese. The pathophysiologic features associated with obesity result in a greater incidence of pregnancy-related complications for both mother and infant than for nonobese patients and has lifelong health implications for offspring.

PROGNOSIS

The presence of obesity during pregnancy has significant consequences for both mother and fetus. Hypertensive disorders including chronic hypertension and preeclampsia are increased in these patients. Obese patients are more likely to develop gestational diabetes and are at increased risk of thromboembolic disease. Obese patients are more likely to have an abnormal labor, and failed induction is more likely to occur. These patients are also at greater risk of postpartum hemorrhage, regardless of the route of delivery The overall cesarean delivery rate and emergency cesarean delivery rate are increased in obese patients. Factors that lead to these increased rates include preeclampsia and diabetes as well as an increased incidence of fetal macrosomia. Soft tissue dystocia may also be a contributing factor. Duration of surgery can be expected to be prolonged in these patients.

Obesity has been found to increase the risk of maternal death, related to the increased incidence of preeclampsia, diabetes, pulmonary embolism, and infection. Anesthesia-related maternal mortality is also increased in the obese parturient, with airway difficulties being a major cause.

Perinatal outcome is adversely affected by obesity. The increased incidence of fetal macrosomia leads to a greater risk of birth trauma and shoulder dystocia. Meconium aspiration occurs more frequently in infants of obese women, and these infants are at greater risk of neural tube defects and other congenital abnormalities. In addition, fetal exposure to hyperglycemia in utero may result in an increased risk of developing diabetes, hypertension, and premature coronary artery disease.

OBSTETRIC MANAGEMENT

Obesity presents specific technical problems in management of labor and delivery in that external fetal and contraction monitoring is difficult, which necessitates internal monitoring of these parameters. As noted earlier, obesity is associated with a higher incidence of cesarean delivery, and the obesity itself creates greater technical problems related to the surgery. Thus, the duration of surgery in these patients is longer than in nonobese patients.

MANAGEMENT OF ANESTHESIA

Preanesthetic Evaluation

The high incidence of medical disease associated with obesity as well as the difficulties encountered because of the patient's body habitus present a significant challenge in the management of obese parturient patients. Preanesthetic evaluation and preparation should include a thorough airway examination and assessment of the patient's pulmonary and cardiac status. Arterial blood gas analysis to assess for carbon dioxide retention, electrocardiography, and echocardiography may be indicated. An appropriately sized blood pressure cuff designed to fit the patient's arm must be available for management.

Labor Analgesia

Epidural analgesia is a reasonable choice for labor analgesia. It provides excellent pain relief, reduces oxygen consumption, and may attenuate the cardiac responses to labor and delivery. Because obese women have a higher likelihood of requiring cesarean delivery and the risk of general anesthesia is substantial in this patient population, early epidural analgesia offers another advantage—the ability to extend the block for surgical anesthesia.

The technical challenge of performing epidural analgesia in the obese parturient patient cannot be underestimated. Long needles may be required to reach the epidural space and should be readily available in the labor and delivery unit. Placement of the patient in the sitting, rather than the lateral, position should facilitate successful identification of the epidural space. Because the failure rate for epidural analgesia is increased in obese patients, these patients must be monitored frequently

and the epidural catheter replaced promptly if inadequate analgesia occurs.

Continuous spinal analgesia is an option for labor analgesia and may provide advantages over epidural analgesia in morbidly obese patients. Correct placement of the catheter is confirmed by aspiration of cerebrospinal fluid, and thus initial failure rates will be lower than with epidural analgesia. A dislodged catheter will also be more readily identified than with epidural analgesia. Continuous spinal anesthesia is associated with a small but significant risk of postural puncture headache, which may require treatment in the postpartum period.

Cesarean Delivery

The incidence of cesarean delivery is higher in obese women than in nonobese women. Longer duration of surgery and increased blood loss must be anticipated by the anesthesiologist because of the patient's obesity and because the obstetrician frequently requires cephalad retraction of the patient's panniculus. The anesthesiologist must be vigilant for signs and symptoms of maternal respiratory compromise caused by increased chest wall compliance related to this retraction. These patients are at high risk of aspiration and thus should receive aspiration prophylaxis with sodium citrate and metoclopramide in combination with an H_2-receptor antagonist. Finally, the anesthesiologist must realize that technical difficulties are more likely to occur in obese parturient patients regardless of the type of anesthetic chosen. Regional anesthesia is preferred whenever possible in obese patients. This is primarily because of the even higher risks associated with general anesthesia and the greater likelihood of airway difficulty in obese parturient patients. One significant factor in the use of regional anesthesia is that the exaggerated spread of local anesthetic which occurs in obese patients may result in a high spinal anesthesia when a single-shot spinal anesthetic is used. For this reason, a continuous technique, spinal or epidural, may be considered in morbidly obese patients. The continuous technique also has the advantage of maintaining anesthesia for what may be an extended period of surgery.

If general anesthesia is unavoidable, emergency airway equipment must be immediately available. If difficult intubation is anticipated, awake fiberoptic intubation should be elected.

Advanced Maternal Age

In 2002, approximately 14% of all births in the United States were to women 35 years or older. In Canada in 2002, 30% of all births were to women 30 to 34 years of age, and 14% were to women 35 to 39 years of age. In 2008, births to women older than 40 years made up 3% of births in the United States, triple the rate of two decades earlier. Patients and health care professionals believe that advanced maternal age results in poor outcomes. The rationale for this view is the higher incidence of chronic medical conditions in older patients. Indeed, advanced maternal age is independently associated with maternal morbidities, including gestational diabetes, preeclampsia, abruptio placentae, and cesarean delivery. In addition, older parturient women are more likely to weigh more than 70 kg and have preexisting hypertension or diabetes. Thus, these medical problems will complicate the pregnancy and its management.

PROGNOSIS

The prognosis in patients of advanced maternal age is related to the presence of comorbid conditions, not to the patient's age. Healthy women of advanced maternal age would be expected to have uneventful pregnancies and deliveries. However, almost half of patients of advanced maternal age have preexisting medical conditions or develop pregnancy-related illness. Their pregnancy outcomes are related to these illnesses.

Perinatal complications are significant in patients of advanced maternal age. Multiple gestations are more common in older pregnant women, as are miscarriage, preterm delivery, and fetal complications such as congenital anomalies, low birth weight, and intrauterine and neonatal death.

OBSTETRIC MANAGEMENT

The focus of obstetric management is on the patient's comorbid conditions. Prenatal care should concentrate on early diagnosis of pregnancy-related illnesses to allow early and aggressive management of these problems.

Cesarean delivery is performed more frequently in women of advanced maternal age. In some, the need for cesarean delivery is related to confounding problems. However, advanced maternal age is also independently associated with an increased likelihood of cesarean delivery, and rates of patient-requested cesarean delivery are much higher in women older than 34 years of age than in women 25 years of age or younger.

MANAGEMENT OF ANESTHESIA

As with obstetric management, anesthetic care of the parturient patient of advanced maternal age is related to the patient's comorbid conditions, the most frequent of which have been discussed in other sections of this chapter.

Substance Abuse

DIAGNOSIS

Diagnosis of substance abuse is often by history. Many commonly abused substances are mind altering or affect the cardiovascular system when the patient is in an acutely toxic state. Diagnosis of substance abuse in a patient who is not under the influence of a substance at admission may be made when that patient, or her infant, develops withdrawal symptoms or the newborn is diagnosed with a syndrome related to in utero exposure.

Substances abused in pregnancy parallel those abused in society at large: alcohol, tobacco, opioids, and cocaine are frequently abused.

ALCOHOL ABUSE

Signs and Symptoms

Approximately 4% of pregnant women are heavy alcohol users. Maternal signs and symptoms may include abnormal results on liver function tests, but often the diagnosis is not made until delivery, when fetal alcohol syndrome is diagnosed in the neonate. Fetal alcohol syndrome occurs in approximately one third of infants born to mothers who drink more than 3 oz of alcohol per day during pregnancy. However, studies have reported neurobehavioral deficit, intrauterine growth retardation, and other congenital abnormalities in infants of moderate alcohol consumers. Current recommendations reflect the view that there is no safe level of alcohol consumption during pregnancy.

Management of Anesthesia

Management of anesthesia in pregnant patients who abuse alcohol entails the same considerations as anesthetic care of nonpregnant alcohol abusers (see Chapter 25).

TOBACCO ABUSE

Signs and Symptoms

Cigarettes are the most commonly abused drug during pregnancy. Because pregnant smokers are relatively young, often there are minimal signs and symptoms associated with tobacco abuse in this population. A strong association is found between cigarette smoking and low infant birth rate, abruptio placentae, and impaired respiratory function in newborns. In those who smoke more than 20 cigarettes per day, the incidence of premature delivery doubles. Sudden infant death syndrome occurs much more frequently in infants of mothers who smoke. Smoking has a protective effect against the development of preeclampsia.

Management of Anesthesia

As with alcohol abuse, the anesthetic considerations for care of tobacco-abusing parturient patients are similar to those for care of nonpregnant patients who smoke.

OPIOID ABUSE

There are numerous medical complications of injected drug use. These include infectious complications such as human immunodeficiency virus infection and hepatitis. Patients may develop local abscesses or, more significantly, may have endocarditis or thrombophlebitis. A pregnant patient admitted while receiving long-term opioid therapy should be maintained on that therapy during her pregnancy and into the postpartum period. It is not recommended that these patients undergo detoxification during the pregnancy. In fact, withdrawal from opioids during the third trimester can result in perinatal asphyxia or death of the neonate. Withdrawal of the neonate from opioids can present as respiratory distress, seizures, hyperthermia, and sudden infant death syndrome. Neonates should be observed and treated for withdrawal symptoms as necessary.

Management of Anesthesia

Considerations for the anesthetic care of opioid-dependent parturient women are similar to those for nonpregnant opioid-dependent patients.

COCAINE ABUSE

Signs and Symptoms

Cocaine abuse among parturient women affects multiple organs, including the cardiovascular, respiratory, neurologic, and hematologic systems. Cocaine is associated with maternal cardiovascular complications such as systemic hypertension, myocardial ischemia and infarction, cardiac dysrhythmias, and sudden death. Sudden increases in systemic blood pressure may be the primary cause of cerebral hemorrhage. Alternatively, cerebrovascular spasm can produce local ischemia and infarction. Subarachnoid hemorrhage, intracerebral bleeding, aneurysmal rupture, and seizures have been associated with cocaine use during pregnancy. Thrombocytopenia may occur following cocaine use and result in prolonged bleeding times. The maternal use of cocaine may lead to metabolic and endocrine changes in both the fetus and the mother, which presumably reflects cocaine-induced release of catecholamines. Pulmonary complications (asthma, chronic cough, dyspnea, pulmonary edema) occur most often in parturient women who smoke free-base cocaine.

An increased incidence of significant obstetric complications is seen in parturient women who abuse cocaine during pregnancy (Table 26-12). The incidence of spontaneous abortion, stillbirth, and preterm labor is increased. High spontaneous abortion rates may be related to cocaine-induced vasoconstriction, enhanced uterine contractions, and abrupt changes in systemic blood pressure.

Diagnosis

Identification of parturient women abusing cocaine is difficult, because urine checks detect metabolites of cocaine for only 14 to 60 hours after use. One of the single most important predictors of cocaine abuse is the absence of prenatal care.

Prognosis

Cocaine use during the third trimester may result in immediate uterine contractions, increased fetal activity, abruptio placentae, and preterm labor. Uteroplacental insufficiency results in fetal intrauterine growth retardation, microcephaly, prematurity, and decreased birth weight. Use of cocaine during organogenesis is associated with fetal anomalies. Maternal systemic hypertension and vasoconstriction may be the cause of the increased incidence of abruptio placentae in cocaine-abusing parturient women. Cocaine effects on the fetus may manifest as an increased incidence of meconium staining and low Apgar score at birth.

Management of Anesthesia

Preoperative. Evaluation of parturient patients suspected of cocaine abuse includes electrocardiography and possibly echocardiography to check for the presence of valvular heart disease. In parturient patients who have severe cocaine-induced cardiovascular toxicity, hemodynamic stabilization must be established before induction of anesthesia.

Intraoperative. Cocaine-induced thrombocytopenia must be excluded if regional anesthesia is planned. Epidural

TABLE 26-12	Obstetric complications associated with cocaine abuse during pregnancy

Spontaneous abortion
Preterm labor
Premature rupture of membranes
Abruptio placentae
Precipitous delivery
Stillbirth
Maternal hypertension
Meconium aspiration
Low Apgar scores at birth

anesthesia is instituted gradually, with attention to hydration and left uterine displacement to prevent hypotension. Hypotension caused by rapid-sequence induction of general anesthesia or institution of regional anesthesia usually responds to ephedrine, although long-term cocaine abuse can deplete catecholamines and theoretically blunt responses to indirect-acting vasopressors. Thus, phenylephrine may be the better choice for treatment of hypotension in these patients. Ester-based local anesthetics, which undergo metabolism by plasma cholinesterase, may compete with cocaine, so that metabolism may be decreased for both drugs. Body temperature increases and sympathomimetic effects associated with cocaine may mimic malignant hyperthermia.

FETAL ASSESSMENT AND NEONATAL PROBLEMS

Electronic Fetal Monitoring

Electronic fetal monitoring permits evaluation of fetal welfare by following changes in fetal heart rate, as recorded using an external (Doppler) monitor or fetal scalp electrode. The basic principle of electronic fetal monitoring is to correlate changes in fetal heart rate with fetal well-being and uterine contractions. In 2009 the American College of Obstetricians and Gynecologists published a revised practice bulletin updating the nomenclature for intrapartum fetal monitoring. A three-tier interpretation system was established that combines the assessment of baseline rate, beat-to-beat variability, accelerations, and periodic decelerations.

BASELINE HEART RATE

Normal fetal heart rate is 110 to 160 beats per minute.
Bradycardia is less than 110 beats per minute for longer than 10 minutes.
Tachycardia is more than 160 beats per minute for longer than 10 minutes.

BEAT-TO-BEAT VARIABILITY

The fetal heart rate varies by 5 to 20 beats per minute in a manner that is irregular in amplitude and frequency. This normal heart rate variability is thought to reflect the integrity of neural pathways from the fetal cerebral cortex through the medulla, vagus nerve, and cardiac conduction system. Fetal well-being is confirmed when beat-to-beat variability is present. Conversely, fetal distress resulting from arterial hypoxemia, acidosis, or central nervous system damage is associated with minimal to absent beat-to-beat variability.

Drugs administered to parturient patients may blunt or eliminate fetal heart rate variability, even in the absence of fetal distress. Drugs most frequently associated with loss of beat-to-beat variability are benzodiazepines, opioids, barbiturates, anticholinergics, and local anesthetics, as used for continuous lumbar epidural analgesia. These drug-induced effects do not appear to be deleterious but may cause difficulty in interpreting the results of fetal heart rate monitoring. In addition, lack of heart rate variability may be present normally in the premature fetus and during fetal sleep cycles.

Terms used to describe fetal heart rate variability are defined as follows:

Absent: variability undetectable
Minimal: 5 beats per minute or less
Moderate: 6 to 25 beats per minute
Marked: more than 25 beats per minute

ACCELERATIONS

An acceleration is a visually apparent abrupt increase in the fetal heart rate. A prolonged acceleration lasts longer than 2 minutes but less than 10 minutes. If an acceleration lasts 10 minutes or longer, it is a change in baseline.

DECELERATIONS

Early Decelerations

Early decelerations are characterized by a slowing of the fetal heart rate that begins with the onset of uterine contractions. Slowing is maximum at the peak of the contraction, with a return to near baseline at its termination. Decreases in heart rate are usually not more than 20 beats per minute or below an absolute rate of 100 beats per minute. This deceleration pattern is thought to be caused by vagal stimulation secondary to compression of the fetal head. Early decelerations are not prevented by increasing fetal oxygenation but are blunted by the administration of atropine. Traditionally, this fetal heart rate pattern is not associated with fetal distress.

Late Decelerations

Late decelerations are characterized by a slowing of the fetal heart rate that begins 10 to 30 seconds after the onset of uterine contractions. Maximum slowing occurs after the peak intensity of the contraction. A mild late deceleration is defined as a decrease in heart rate of less than 20 beats per minute; profound slowing is present when the decrease is more than 40 beats per minute. Late decelerations may be associated with fetal distress and most likely reflect myocardial hypoxia secondary to uteroplacental insufficiency. Primary factors contributing to the appearance of late decelerations include maternal hypotension, uterine hyperactivity, and chronic uteroplacental insufficiency, such as may be seen with maternal diabetes mellitus or hypertension. When this pattern persists, there is a predictable correlation with the development of fetal acidosis. Late decelerations can be corrected by improving fetal oxygenation. When beat-to-beat variability persists despite late decelerations, the fetus is still likely to be born vigorous.

Variable Decelerations

Variable decelerations are the most common pattern of fetal heart changes observed during the intrapartum period. As the term indicates, these decelerations are variable in magnitude, duration, and time of onset relative to uterine contractions. For example, this pattern may begin before, with, or after the onset of uterine contractions. Characteristically, deceleration patterns are abrupt in onset and cessation. The fetal heart rate almost invariably decreases to less than 100 beats per minute. Variable decelerations are thought to be caused by umbilical cord compression. Atropine diminishes the severity of variable decelerations, but administration of oxygen to the mother is without effect. If deceleration patterns are not severe and repetitive, there are usually only minimal alterations in the fetal acid-base status. Severe variable deceleration patterns that persist for 15 to 30 minutes are associated with fetal acidosis.

Prolonged Decelerations

A prolonged deceleration is a decrease in the fetal heart rate from baseline of more than 15 beats per minute that lasts longer than 2 minutes and less than 10 minutes. If the deceleration lasts longer than 10 minutes, it represents a baseline change.

SINUSOIDAL PATTERN

Sinusoidal heart rate variability is a visually smooth, undulating sine wave–like pattern with a cyclical frequency of 3 to 5 minutes persisting for 20 minutes or longer.

THREE-TIERED CLASSIFICATION OF FETAL HEART RATE TRACINGS

Table 26-13 presents a three-tiered system for categorizing the tracings obtained in fetal heart rate monitoring based on baseline rate, degree of variability, and pattern of decelerations and/or accelerations.

Category 1 tracings are normal. These tracings are strongly predictive of normal acid-base status. No specific action is required.

Category 2 tracings are indeterminate. Although they are not predictive of abnormal acid-base status, there is not enough evidence to classify them as normal or abnormal. Ancillary testing or intrauterine resuscitation may be indicated.

Category 3 tracings are abnormal and are associated with abnormal fetal acid-base status. Evaluation of the fetus and measures to resolve the abnormal pattern are required. If the tracing does not improve with intervention, delivery should be expedited.

TABLE 26-13 ▪ Three-tiered system for interpretation of electronic fetal heart rate (FHR) monitoring

Category	Characteristics
Category I *(Must include all characteristics listed)*	**Rate:** 110-160 beats/min **Variability:** moderate **Late or variable decelerations:** absent **Early decelerations:** present or absent **Accelerations:** present or absent

Category II
 (All FHR tracings not classified as category I or III; must include all characteristics listed)
	Baseline rate
	   Bradycardia not accompanied by
	     absence of variability
	   Tachycardia
	 Baseline FHR variability
	   Minimal variability
	   Absence of variability not
	     accompanied by recurrent
	     decelerations
	   Marked baseline variability
	 Accelerations
	   Absence of induced accelerations
	     after fetal stimulation
	 Periodic or episodic decelerations
	   Recurrent variable decelerations
	     accompanied by minimal or
	     moderate baseline variability
	   Prolonged deceleration of ≥2 min
	     but <10 min
	   Recurrent late decelerations with
	     moderate baseline variability
	   Variable decelerations with other
	     characteristics, such as slow
	     return to baseline, overshoots,
	     or "shoulders"

Category III
 (Includes either of the characteristics listed)
	***Absence* of baseline FHR variability *and* any of the following:**
	   Recurrent late decelerations
	   Recurrent variable decelerations
	   Bradycardia
	 Sinusoidal pattern

TABLE 26-14 ▪ Determination of the Apgar score for evaluating neonates

Parameter	POINTS		
	0	**1**	**2**
Heart rate (beats/min)	Absent	<100	>100
Respiratory effort	Absent	Slow Irregular	Crying
Reflex irritability	No response	Grimace	Crying
Muscle tone	Limp	Flexion of extremities	Active
Color	Pale Cyanotic	Body pink Extremities cyanotic	Pink

Points assigned for each parameter are summed to obtain the Apgar score.

oxygen saturations range between 30% and 70%. Saturations less than 30% are suggestive of fetal acidemia.

ULTRASONOGRAPHY

Ultrasonographic examination of the fetus when the mother is in labor may be useful to determine the fetal presenting part. Also, if fetal heart tones are undetectable using Doppler scanning, ultrasonography may confirm intrauterine fetal health or demise. Ultrasonography may also be used to determine the quantity of amniotic fluid present in the uterus and to diagnose abruptio placentae and placenta previa.

Evaluation of the Neonate

Assessment of the infant immediately after birth is important so that neonates in distress who require active resuscitation can be identified promptly. As a guide to identifying and treating neonates with depressed function, the Apgar score has not been surpassed.

The Apgar score assigns a numerical value to five signs measured or observed in neonates 1 minute and 5 minutes after delivery (Table 26-14). Of the five factors, heart rate and quality of respiratory effort are the most important; color is the least informative in identifying neonates in distress. A heart rate of less than 100 beats per minute generally signifies arterial hypoxemia. Disappearance of cyanosis is often rapid when ventilation and circulation are normal. Nevertheless, many healthy neonates still have cyanosis at 1 minute owing to peripheral vasoconstriction in response to cold ambient temperatures in the delivery room. Acidosis and pulmonary vasoconstriction are the most likely causes of persistent cyanosis.

Apgar scores correlate well with acid-base measurements performed immediately after birth. When scores are higher than 7, neonates have either normal blood gas concentrations or mild respiratory acidosis. Infants with scores of 4 to 6 have moderately depressed function; those with scores of 3 or below have combined metabolic and respiratory acidosis. Infants with mild to moderately depressed function (Apgar scores of

FETAL SCALP SAMPLING

Fetal scalp sampling may be indicated to evaluate a fetus with an abnormal fetal heart rate pattern. Based on the results, suspected fetal hypoxia may be confirmed, which establishes a need for urgent delivery. Good neonatal outcomes are associated with a pH 7.20 or greater, whereas a pH of 7.20 or lower suggests fetal compromise necessitating immediate delivery.

FETAL PULSE OXIMETRY

Fetal pulse oximetry is a newer technique evaluating intrapartum fetal oxygenation. It is currently employed as an adjunct to electronic fetal heart rate monitoring and may be used when the heart rate monitoring produces a nonreassuring tracing. The fetal pulse oximeter provides continuous fetal arterial oxygen saturation readings when placed through the cervix to lie alongside the fetal cheek or temple. Normal fetal

3 to 7) frequently improve in response to oxygen administration by face mask, with or without positive pressure ventilation of the lungs. Tracheal intubation and perhaps external cardiac massage are indicated when Apgar scores are less than 3. Apgar scores are not sufficiently sensitive to detect drug-related changes reliably or to provide data necessary to evaluate the subtle effects of obstetric anesthetic techniques on neonates.

PERIOD IMMEDIATELY AFTER BIRTH

Major changes in the neonatal cardiovascular system and respiratory system occur immediately following delivery. For example, with clamping of the umbilical cord at birth, systemic vascular resistance increases, left atrial pressure increases, and flow through the foramen ovale ceases. Expansion of the lungs decreases pulmonary vascular resistance, and the entire right ventricular output is diverted to the lungs. In normal newborns, the increase in Pao_2 to more than 60 mm Hg causes vasoconstriction and functional closure of the ductus arteriosus. When adequate oxygenation and ventilation are not established after delivery, a fetal circulation pattern persists that is characterized by increased pulmonary vascular resistance and decreased pulmonary blood flow. Furthermore, the ductus arteriosus and foramen ovale remain open, which results in large right-to-left intracardiac shunts with associated arterial hypoxemia and acidosis.

A high index of suspicion must be maintained for serious abnormalities that can be present at birth or manifest shortly after delivery. These include meconium aspiration, choanal stenosis and atresia, diaphragmatic hernia, hypovolemia, hypoglycemia, tracheoesophageal fistula, and laryngeal anomalies.

Hypovolemia

Newborns with mean arterial pressures of less than 50 mm Hg at birth are likely to be hypovolemic. Poor capillary refill, tachycardia, and tachypnea will be present. Hypovolemia frequently follows intrauterine fetal distress during which larger than normal portions of fetal blood are shunted to the placenta and remain there after delivery and clamping of the umbilical cord. Umbilical cord compression is also frequently associated with hypovolemia.

Hypoglycemia

Hypoglycemia can manifest as hypotension, tremors, and seizures. Infants with intrauterine growth retardation and those born to diabetic mothers or after severe intrauterine fetal distress are vulnerable to hypoglycemia.

Meconium Aspiration

Meconium is the breakdown product of swallowed amniotic fluid, gastrointestinal cells, and secretions. It is seldom present before 34 weeks of gestation. After approximately 34 weeks, intrauterine arterial hypoxemia can result in increased gut motility and defecation. Gasping associated with arterial hypoxemia causes the fetus to inhale amniotic fluid and debris into the lungs. If delivery is delayed, meconium

is broken down and excreted from the lungs. If birth occurs within 24 hours of aspiration, the meconium is still present in the major airways and is distributed to the lung periphery with the onset of spontaneous breathing. Obstruction of small airways causes ventilation/perfusion mismatching. The breathing rate may be more than 100 breaths per minutes and lung compliance decreases to levels seen in infants with respiratory distress syndrome. In severe cases, pulmonary hypertension and right-to-left shunting through the patent foramen ovale and ductus arteriosus (persistent fetal circulation) lead to severe arterial hypoxemia. Pneumothorax is also a common problem in the presence of meconium aspiration.

In the past, treatment of meconium aspiration consisted of placing a tracheal tube immediately after delivery and attempting to suction meconium from the newborn's airways. Currently, a more conservative approach is recommended, because routine tracheal intubation of all infants with meconium staining (approximately 10% of all newborns) may cause unnecessary airway complications. Routine oropharyngeal suctioning is recommended at the time of delivery, but tracheal intubation and suctioning is performed selectively, depending on the infant's condition (those with Apgar scores of >7 are managed conservatively). Infants who have low Apgar scores or who have clinical signs of meconium obstruction require active resuscitation, including tracheal intubation and attempted removal of meconium via suctioning.

Choanal Stenosis and Atresia

Nasal obstruction should be suspected in neonates who have good breathing efforts but in whom air entry is absent. Cyanosis develops if these infants are forced to breathe with their mouths closed. Unilateral or bilateral choanal stenosis is diagnosed based on the inability to pass a small catheter through each naris. Such failure may reflect congenital (anatomic) obstruction or, more commonly, functional atresia resulting from obstruction by blood, mucus, or meconium. The congenital form of choanal atresia must be treated surgically during the neonatal period. Use of an oral airway may be necessary until surgical correction can be accomplished. Functional choanal atresia is treated by nasal suctioning. Opioids often cause congestion of the nasal mucosa and obstruction. Such congestion can be treated with phenylephrine nose drops.

Diaphragmatic Hernia

Severe respiratory distress at birth, in association with cyanosis and a scaphoid abdomen, suggests a diaphragmatic hernia. Chest radiographs demonstrate abdominal contents in the thorax. Initial treatment in the delivery room includes tracheal intubation and ventilation of the lungs with oxygen. A pneumothorax on the side opposite the hernia is likely if attempts are made to expand the ipsilateral lung.

Tracheoesophageal Fistula

A tracheoesophageal fistula should be suspected when polyhydramnios is present (see Chapter 27). An initial diagnosis in the delivery room is suggested when a catheter inserted into the esophagus cannot be passed into the stomach. Copious amounts of oropharyngeal secretions are usually present. Chest radiographs taken with the catheter in place confirm the diagnosis.

Laryngeal Anomalies

Stridor is present at birth as a manifestation of laryngeal anomalies and subglottic stenosis. Insertion of a tube into the trachea beyond the obstruction alleviates the symptoms. Vascular rings are anomalies of the aorta that may compress the trachea, producing both inspiratory and expiratory obstruction. It may be difficult to advance a tracheal tube beyond the obstruction produced by vascular rings.

KEY POINTS

- Physiologic changes of pregnancy affect all organ systems. They influence maternal compensation for comorbid conditions and maternal responses to anesthesia.
- There is less fetal drug exposure with regional anesthesia. Any well-managed anesthetic is safe.
- Blood pressure, oxygenation, and normocarbia should be maintained during delivery.
- Delivery is the definitive treatment for pregnancy-induced hypertension. Delivery should be delayed only if the risk of neonatal immaturity outweighs maternal risk.
- Co-existing medical diseases may result in maternal decompensation related to the physiologic changes of pregnancy.
- Fetal assessment permits evaluation of fetal well-being and guides neonatal management.

RESOURCES

American College of Obstetricians and Gynecologists. ACOG practice bulletin No. 106: intrapartum fetal heart rate monitoring: nomenclature, interpretation, and general management principles. *Obstet Gynecol.* 2009;114:192-202.

American College of Obstetricians and Gynecologists. ACOG practice bulletin No. 115: vaginal birth after previous cesarean delivery. *Obstet Gynecol.* 2010;116(2 pt 1):450-463.

American College of Obstetricians and Gynecologists. Committee on Practice Bulletins—Obstetrics. ACOG practice bulletin No. 33: diagnosis and management of preeclampsia and eclampsia. *Obstet Gynecol.* 2002;99(1):159-167.

Bolliger D, Gorlinger K, Tanaka KA. Pathophysiology and treatment of coagulopathy in massive hemorrhage and hemodilution. *Anesthesiology.* 2010;113(5):1205-1219.

Centre for Maternal and Child Enquiries (CMACE). *Maternal obesity in the UK: findings from a national project.* London, England: CMACE; 2010.

Cheek TG, Baird E. Anesthesia for nonobstetric surgery: maternal and fetal considerations. *Clin Obstet Gynecol.* 2009;52:535-545.

Hull D, Resnik R. Placenta accreta and postpartum hemorrhage. *Clin Obstet Gynecol.* 2010;53(1):228-236.

NIH. Consensus Development conference statement: vaginal birth after cesarean: new insights. *Obstet Gynecol.* 2010;115(6):1279-1290.

Ouyang DW, Khairy P, Fernandes SM, et al. Obstetric outcomes in pregnant women with congenital heart disease. *Int J Cardiol.* 2010;144(2):195-199:Epub May 2, 2009.

Pereira L. Surgery in the obese pregnant patient. *Clin Obstet Gynecol.* 2009;52:546-556.

Sihler KC, Napolitano LM. Complications of massive transfusion. *Chest.* 2010;137(1):209-220.

ZAHARA investigators. Predictors of pregnancy complications in women with congenital heart disease. *Eur Heart J.* 2010;31(17):2124-2132:Epub June 28, 2010.

Pediatric Diseases

MICHELLE W. DIU ■
THOMAS J. MANCUSO ■

UNIQUE CONSIDERATIONS IN PEDIATRIC PATIENTS

Much of the focus in pediatrics is on growth and development. Not only are children different from adults, they are also very different from one another. Newborn medicine and adolescent medicine are two different subspecialties within pediatrics, each requiring an extensive medical fellowship, yet the anesthesiologist is called upon to care for patients from a preterm newborn who could weigh less than 1 kg to a vigorous adolescent athlete tipping the scales at 100 kg. Although it is quite obvious that special considerations apply in caring for preterm newborns, there are also many unique aspects of adolescents that should be borne in mind when caring for them despite their physical and physiologic similarities to adults.

Psychology

Although the physical and physiologic differences between children and adults are paramount and are reviewed in detail, the perianesthetic experience of pediatric patients and their parents is undoubtedly influenced by how the anesthesiologist manages the psychologic assessment and preparation of the child and family. All patients experience anxiety before undergoing anesthesia and surgery. Quite frequently, children undergo anesthesia so that a diagnostic and not a surgical procedure can be performed. In these cases, nearly all of the preprocedure anxiety is focused on the anesthesia. An appreciation of circumstances that contribute to preanesthetic anxiety is an important first step in designing an approach that minimizes apprehension and potential psychologic trauma. Factors associated with a greater likelihood and degree of perianesthetic anxiety in children include the following:

- Age of 1 to 5 years
- Unsatisfactory prior medical experiences
- Shy temperament
- Anxious parents
- A noisy and busy preoperative environment

Children and adolescents all have some degree of anxiety, but specific fears will differ depending on age group and the related developmental stage (Table 27-1). Toddlers and young children fear separation from their caretakers. Separation anxiety typically begins at 8 to 10 months of age. Preschool-aged children still fear separation, but they have enough understanding of medical procedures also to fear pain and discomfort, particularly needles. They also fear a loss of control. Allowing them to choose a hospital gown color or a favorite mask scent may help them regain a small sense of control of an unfamiliar environment. Younger children have a concrete thought process, and they cannot put it into perspective that any discomfort is temporary and that their lives will soon return to normal. In addition to the aforementioned concerns, adolescents also fear death but are often afraid to ask questions about the risk of mortality. An explicit delineation of the expected perioperative course, from induction to emergence

TABLE 27-1 ■ Age-related perianesthetic anxiety	
Age group	**Psychologic assessment**
Neonate (0-30 days of life)	Parental anxiety may be extreme
Infant (1-12 mo)	Separation anxiety begins at 8-10 mo
Toddler (1-3 yr)	Loss of control
Children (4-12 yr)	Preschool age: concrete thoughts School age: desire to meet adult's expectations
Teenager/adolescent (13-19 yr)	Fears death, hides emotions

and recovery in the postanesthesia care unit (PACU), is often helpful to allay their fears.

Preanesthetic programs including play and simulation of the anesthetic induction, videos, or separate preanesthetic visits scheduled ahead of time all can help to alleviate anxiety. The timing of these visits should take into account the child's age and developmental stage. Patient-centered approaches involve a preanesthetic interview with the child and parents, the use of anxiolytic premedication, and the choice of induction of anesthesia with a parent present. Although many parents report increased satisfaction with such a process, data are conflicting regarding the effect on the child's own anxiety. Discussion must be held and preparations made for cases in which parents become overly emotional during the induction or the induction does not proceed as smoothly as planned.

Finally, allowing parental visits in the PACU can often contribute to a positive perioperative experience for both the child and family. As with parental presence during the induction of anesthesia, parental presence in the PACU should be permitted only after careful consideration of the viewpoints of all involved caregivers. Educating the parents regarding potential emergence delirium and probable postoperative-postanesthetic problems is also important.

Anatomy and Physiology

BODY SIZE AND THERMOREGULATION

Pediatric patients can weigh from less than 1 kg to more than 100 kg. Physical aspects of the care of larger adolescents are similar to those encountered in the care of adult patients. The younger, smaller patients present different challenges. Neonates and infants are vulnerable to becoming hypothermic during the perioperative period. Body heat is lost more rapidly in this age group than in older children or adults because of the high ratio of body surface area to body weight and volume, the thin layer of insulating subcutaneous fat, and the decreased ability to produce heat. Shivering plays little or no role in heat production in neonates, whose primary mechanism of heat generation is nonshivering thermogenesis mediated by brown fat. Brown fat is a specialized type of adipose tissue located in the posterior neck and interscapular and vertebral areas, as well as surrounding the kidneys and adrenal glands. Metabolism of brown fat is stimulated by norepinephrine and results in triglyceride hydrolysis and thermogenesis.

For all patients, children as well as adults, general anesthesia is associated with some degree of heat loss as a result of exposure to the cold environment and the anesthetic effects of central thermoregulatory inhibition and reduction of metabolic rate. It is very difficult to reestablish normothermia once hypothermia develops in newborns and infants. Because of this, prevention of hypothermia is essential. Hypothermia may be protective in selected circumstances, but normothermia should be maintained in general. Complications that have been associated with intraoperative hypothermia include surgical wound infection, negative nitrogen balance, delayed wound healing, delayed postoperative anesthetic recovery, impaired coagulation, and prolonged hospitalization.

To minimize oxygen consumption, newborns should be in a neutral thermal environment (one in which heat is neither gained nor lost). The temperature required for a newborn to have the lowest oxygen consumption is quite warm and is rarely achieved in the operating room. For example, the neutral thermal environment for an unclothed 3-kg newborn is 32° to 33° C. Steps aimed at decreasing loss of body heat include transporting neonates in heated isolettes; increasing the ambient temperature of operating rooms; using a heating mattress, radiant warmer, or convective forced-air warming device; and humidifying and warming inspired gases.

CENTRAL NERVOUS SYSTEM

A newborn's brain comprises approximately 10% of the total body weight. In comparison, an adult's brain constitutes only 2% of total body weight. Myelinization and synaptic connections are not complete until the child reaches the third or fourth birthday. From birth to 2 years of age, a child's brain undergoes the most rapid phase of growth, achieving 75% of its adult size. The location of the spinal cord within the vertebrae changes with growth. At birth, the spinal cord reaches the level of the third lumbar vertebra but migrates to the normal adult level at L1 and L2 by the third year of life.

AIRWAY

The airway of a term newborn differs in several ways from that of an adult. The larynx has a higher position in the neck. Newborns have a proportionately larger head and tongue, a short and mobile epiglottis, and vocal cords whose anterior commissure is slanted inferiorly. Airway obstruction occurs more readily in the newborn and infant because of the larger tongue size relative to the oral cavity. The cricoid cartilage (as opposed to the vocal cords in adults) is the narrowest portion of the larynx in pediatric patients. As in adults, angulation of the right main bronchus favors right endobronchial intubation if the tracheal tube is inserted beyond the carina. The importance of the smaller absolute dimensions of the upper and lower airways in newborns and infants cannot be overemphasized. In the equations describing turbulent (upper

TABLE 27-2 ■ Mean pulmonary function values

Parameter	Neonates (3 kg)	Adults (70 kg)
Oxygen consumption (mL/kg/min)	6.5	3.5
Alveolar ventilation (mL/kg/min)	130	60
Carbon dioxide production (mL/kg/min)	6	3
Tidal volume (mL/kg)	6	6
Breathing frequency (breaths/min)	35	15
Vital capacity (mL/kg)	35	70
Functional residual capacity (mL/kg)	30	35
Tracheal length (cm)	5.5	12
Pao_2 (room air, mm Hg)	65-85	85-95
$Paco_2$ (room air, mm Hg)	30-36	36-44
pH	7.34-7.40	7.36-7.44

airway) and laminar (lower airway) flow, airflow is directly proportional to the airway radius raised to the fifth and fourth power, respectively. As the newborn grows into infancy and young childhood, the relative size of the head and tongue decreases, and the location of the larynx in the neck shifts to the lower position seen in adults.

RESPIRATORY SYSTEM

The functional aspects of the respiratory system, such as respiratory rate, tidal volume, and minute ventilation, reflect a crucial physiologic difference between children and adults. Oxygen consumption ($\dot{V}o_2$) is much greater on a per-kilogram basis in children than in adults (Table 27-2). This is due to the difference in the ratio of surface area to volume. The higher $\dot{V}o_2$ explains the speed with which infants and children exhibit hypoxemia (by pulse oximetry) with interruption in oxygen supply. In addition, the high compliance of both lung parenchyma and chest wall in newborns and infants predisposes to alveolar collapse with resultant $\dot{V}/\overline{V}$ mismatching and hypoxemia. Recall also that the $\dot{V}o_2$ noted in Table 27-2 is *resting* consumption. $\dot{V}o_2$ increases 15% for every 1° C rise in body temperature and also increases dramatically with anxiety and/or struggling as may occur during a difficult inhalation induction.

CARDIOVASCULAR SYSTEM

Significant adaptations occur at birth with respect to the cardiovascular system. The lungs take over the role of gas exchange from the placenta. Pulmonary vascular resistance gradually decreases over the first several months of life but remains reactive and can increase dramatically under conditions of acidosis, hypoxemia, and hypercarbia. The foramen ovale and ductus arteriosus can reopen under these circumstances, and the circulation can revert to fetal patterns with significantly decreased pulmonary blood flow and profound hypoxemia. Anatomic closure of the foramen ovale occurs between 3 months and 1 year of age, although 20% to 30% of adults have probe-patent foramen ovale. Functional closure of the ductus arteriosus normally occurs 10 to 15 hours after birth, with anatomic closure taking place in 4 to 6 weeks. Constriction of the ductus arteriosus occurs in response to the increased arterial oxygenation that develops after birth. Nevertheless, the ductus arteriosus may reopen during periods of arterial hypoxemia.

Heart rate is the main determinant of cardiac output and systemic blood pressure in neonates and young infants. Contractility of the myocardium is lower in neonates than in older children and adults because of a relative decrease in contractile elements. Stroke volume is also relatively fixed due to a paucity of elastic elements. The Frank-Starling mechanism is not operational under most circumstances. Because of this, increase in cardiac output in the newborn is dependent on increases in heart rate for the most part. At very high heart rates, however, cardiac output will decrease because of reduced diastolic filling times. An approximation of stroke volume for the newborn and children is 1 mL/kg.

FLUIDS AND RENAL SYSTEM

Total body water content and extracellular fluid (ECF) volume are increased proportionately in neonates. The ECF volume is equivalent to approximately 40% of body weight in neonates compared with approximately 20% in adults. By 18 to 24 months of age, the proportion of ECF volume relative to body weight is similar to that in adults. In addition to fluid replacement (usually with Ringer's lactate or normal saline), newborns and young infants may also require glucose supplementation. The maintenance glucose requirement for newborns is 6 to 8 mg/kg/min. Term newborns are capable of maintaining normoglycemia for up to 10 hours with no exogenous glucose administration. However, since the signs and symptoms of hypoglycemia such as jitteriness, lethargy, and poor tone are masked by general anesthesia, most practitioners supply some of the required glucose to infants while they are anesthetized. Five percent dextrose in normal saline at maintenance (Table 27-3) will supply approximately 50% of the requirement. In surgical procedures of any significant length, glucose measurements should be used to guide the rate of administration.

Perioperative fluid administration for pediatric patients can be divided into several components:

- Replacement of fluid deficits from fasting
- Maintenance fluid requirement
- Replacement of blood loss
- Replacement of evaporative losses

Fluid maintenance and replacement of deficits are based on the Holliday and Segar formula for caloric expenditure of children of different sizes. Caloric expenditure based on weight and water requirement is approximately 1 mL per kcal expended per day. This is the basis for the 4:2:1 rule used by anesthesiologists (see Table 27-3).

TABLE 27-3 ■ Holliday-Segar formula for caloric expenditure

Weight	Caloric expenditure	Water requirement	Fluid maintenance*
0-10 kg	100 kcal/kg/day	100 mL/kg/day	4 mL/kg/hr (for first 10 kg)
11-20 kg	50 kcal/kg/day	50 mL/kg/day	2 mL/kg/hr (for second 10 kg)
>20 kg	20 kcal/kg/day	20 mL/kg/day	1 mL/kg/hr (for each additional kg above 20 kg)

*Fluid maintenance rates are additive. For example, a 25-kg child requires 4 mL/kg/hr for the first 10 kg (40 mL/hr) plus 2 mL/kg/hr for the second 10 kg (20 mL/hr) plus 1 mL/kg/hr for each additional kg above 20 kg (5 mL/hr), for a total of 65 mL/hr (40 + 20 + 5) for the hourly fluid maintenance rate.

TABLE 27-4 ■ Intraoperative fluid therapy for pediatric patients

Procedure	NORMAL SALINE OR LACTATED RINGER'S SOLUTION (mL/kg/hr)		
	Maintenance	Replacement	Total
Minor surgery (e.g., herniorrhaphy)	4	2	6
Moderate surgery (e.g., pyloromyotomy)	4	4	8
Extensive surgery (e.g., bowel resection)	4	6	10

Blood loss is generally replaced 3:1 for each milliliter of blood loss with isotonic crystalloid, and replenishment for evaporative loss is guided by estimations based on type of procedure and associated area of surgical exposure (Table 27-4).

The glomerular filtration rate is greatly decreased in term newborns but increases nearly fourfold by 3 to 5 weeks. Preterm newborns may show delayed increases in glomerular filtration rate. Newborns are obligate sodium losers and cannot concentrate urine as effectively as adults. Therefore, adequate exogenous sodium and water must be provided during the perioperative period. Conversely, newborns excrete volume loads more slowly than adults and are therefore more susceptible to fluid overload. Decreased renal function can also delay excretion of drugs dependent on renal clearance for elimination.

HEPATIC SYSTEM

At term, the liver actually has significant glycogen stores that can be converted to glucose for use by the neonate. The newborn's glycogen stores, on a per-kilogram basis, are at least equal to the stores in most adults. Details regarding administration

TABLE 27-5 ■ Hematologic values in infancy and childhood

Age	Hemoglobin (g/dL)	Hematocrit (%)	Leukocytes (1000/mm³)
Cord blood	14-20	45-65	9-30
Newborn	13-20	42-66	5-20
3 mo	10-14	31-41	6-18
6 mo to 12 yr	11-15	33-42	6-15
Young adult male	14-18	42-52	5-10
Young adult female	12-16	37-47	5-10

TABLE 27-6 ■ Estimated blood volumes for neonates, infants, and children

Age group	Estimated blood volume (mL/kg)
Premature neonates	90-100
Term neonates	80-90
Infants	75-80
Children >1 yr	70-75

TABLE 27-7 ■ Estimation of maximal allowable blood loss*

A 3-kg term neonate is scheduled for intraabdominal surgery. The preoperative hematocrit (Hct) is 50%. What is the maximum allowable blood loss (MABL) to maintain the hematocrit at 40%?

$$MABL = EBV \times [(Hct_{high} - Hct_{low}) / Hct_{average}]$$

$$EBV = 3 \text{ kg} \times 85 \text{ mL} / \text{kg} = 255 \text{ mL}$$
$$Hct_{high} - Hct_{low} = 50\% - 40\% = 10\%$$
$$Hct_{average} = (50\% + 40\%) / 2 = 45\%$$

$$MABL = 255 \text{ mL} \times [(50\% - 40\%) / 45\%] = 56.1 \text{ mL}$$

EBV, Estimated blood volume.

*These calculations are only guidelines and do not consider the potential impact of intravenous infusion of crystalloid or colloid solutions on the hematocrit.

of intravenous glucose have already been discussed in the previous section on fluids and renal physiology. Hepatic capacity for biotransformation and metabolism of drugs, however, is diminished until several months of postnatal life. Even though vitamin K–dependent and other coagulation factors are at approximately 50% of adult levels, significant bleeding is uncommon in newborns who have adequate vitamin K levels.

HEMATOLOGIC SYSTEM

The hematologic system undergoes significant changes after birth. In fetal life, fetal hemoglobin (Hb) has a lower P_{50} (partial pressure of oxygen at which Hb is 50% saturated), which is adaptive and allows the fetus to extract oxygen from maternal Hb. In the first 2 months of life, as fetal Hb is replaced by adult Hb, the P_{50} increases from 19 mm Hg to 22 mm Hg and then eventually to the typical adult level of 26 mm Hg. Not only does the Hb type change (fetal to adult), but the Hb concentration changes as well. Physiologic anemia occurs between 2 and 3 months of age. This decrease in Hb concentration is a result of several physiologic changes. Because of rapid postnatal growth, shortened neonatal red blood cell (RBC) survival (70 to 90 days compared with the adult RBC life span of 120 days), and transient cessation of erythropoiesis (decreased erythropoietin release upon exposure to higher arterial oxygen content), there is a progressive decrease in RBC mass and Hb level. The nadir is typically seen between the eighth and tenth weeks of life. In view of the decreased cardiovascular reserve of neonates and the leftward shift of the oxyhemoglobin dissociation curve, it may be useful to maintain the neonate's hematocrit closer to 40% than 30%, as is often accepted for older children. Typical blood cell values are delineated in Table 27-5.

Whether or not routine preoperative Hb determination is needed is controversial. Routine preoperative Hb measurement in children younger than 1 year of age results in the detection of only a small number of patients with Hb concentrations of less than 10 g/dL, which rarely influences management of anesthesia or delays planned surgery. However, preoperative Hb measurement may be prudent in young infants coming for surgery at a time coincident with the typical period of physiologic anemia. Based on the estimated blood volume (Table 27-6), calculation of the maximal allowable blood loss is useful to guide intraoperative blood replacement (Table 27-7).

Pharmacology

Pharmacologic responses to drugs may differ in pediatric patients and adults. These manifest as differences in anesthetic requirements, responses to muscle relaxants, and pharmacokinetics.

ANESTHETIC REQUIREMENTS

Full-term neonates require *lower* concentrations of volatile anesthetics than do infants 1 to 6 months of age. Furthermore, minimal alveolar concentration (MAC) in preterm neonates decreases with decreasing gestational age. Lowered anesthetic requirements in neonates may be related to immaturity of the central nervous system (CNS) and to increased circulating concentrations of progesterone and β-endorphins. MAC steadily increases until 2 to 3 months of age, but after 3 months, the MAC steadily declines with age, although there are slight increases at puberty.

Sevoflurane is unique among the currently used volatile anesthetics. The MAC of sevoflurane in neonates and infants younger than 6 months (3.2%) and in infants older than 6 months and children up to 12 years (2.5%) remains constant. The reason that the MAC of sevoflurane does not decline with advancing age in childhood, as is seen with the other volatile anesthetics, is unclear.

Morphologic and functional maturation of the neuromuscular junctions are not complete until approximately 2 months of age, but the implications of this initial immaturity on the pharmacodynamics of muscle relaxants are not clear. Because of immature muscle composition, the infant's diaphragm is paralyzed at the same time as the peripheral muscles (as opposed to later, as in adults). This has led to the suggestion that infants may be more sensitive to the effects of nondepolarizing muscle relaxants, but the relatively large volume of distribution requires induction doses that are similar on a per-kilogram basis to those for adults. Duration of action may be prolonged because of immature hepatic and renal drug handling and excretion. Antagonism of neuromuscular blockade is generally unaffected in infants, and requirements for anticholinergics may be decreased because of longer clearance times than in adults.

Neonates and infants require more succinylcholine on a per-kilogram basis than do older children to produce similar degrees of neuromuscular blockade because of the increased ECF volume and larger volume distribution characteristic of this age group. Most practitioners limit the use of succinylcholine to cases requiring rapid-sequence induction and to the treatment of laryngospasm because of the risks of severe bradycardia and potential malignant hyperthermia and other associated adverse effects (rhabdomyolysis, hyperkalemia) in children (especially those younger than age 5) with undiagnosed myopathies and dystrophinopathies.

PHARMACOKINETICS

Pharmacokinetics differs in neonates and infants compared with adults. For example, uptake of inhaled anesthetics is more rapid in infants than in older children or adults because of the infant's high alveolar ventilation relative to functional residual capacity. More rapid uptake may unmask negative inotropic effects of volatile anesthetics, resulting in an increased incidence of hypotension in neonates and infants upon inhalation induction of anesthesia.

An immature blood–brain barrier and decreased ability to metabolize drugs could increase the sensitivity of neonates to the effects of hypnotics. As a result, neonates might require lower doses of intravenous agents for induction of anesthesia. On the other hand, older children and adolescents generally require a higher dose of intravenous induction agents than adults (up to 3 mg/kg of propofol in children and teenagers compared with 1.5 to 2 mg/kg in adults).

Decreased hepatic and renal clearance of drugs, which is characteristic of neonates, can produce prolonged drug effects. Clearance rates increase to adult levels by 5 to 6 months of age and during early childhood may even exceed adult rates. Protein binding of many drugs is decreased in infants, which can result in high circulating concentrations of unbound and pharmacologically active drugs.

Pediatric Cardiac Arrest during Anesthesia

The majority of children tolerate general anesthesia without incident. However, cardiac arrests do occur during anesthesia in children, although data are incomplete regarding the precise incidence. Many of these cardiac arrests are not due to poor or inadequate anesthetic care but rather result from either the critical health condition of the patient or complications of the surgical procedure. Data on the incidence of anesthesia-related cardiac arrest are not available for neonates as a separate group. The incidence of anesthesia-related cardiac arrest reported in *infants* is 15 in 10,000 anesthetics, with a range of 9.2 to 19 in 10,000. Overall, *children* experience anesthesia-related cardiac arrest at a rate of 3.3 in 10,000 anesthetics with a range of 0 to 4.3 in 10,000. The incidence of anesthesia-related cardiac arrest reported for *all pediatric age groups* is 1.8 in 10,000.

CAUSES OF CARDIAC ARREST

The causes of cardiac arrest in children gathered from the Pediatric Perioperative Cardiac Arrest Registry are summarized in Table 27-8. One hundred and fifty cases of anesthesia-related cardiac arrest from 1994 to 1997 were analyzed. More than 50% of arrests occurred among infants. Medications accounted for 37% of all arrests. The most common medication-related cause was cardiovascular depression resulting from volatile anesthetic agents. During this reporting period, it is likely that halothane was the offending agent in many of these cases. In present times, anesthetic overdose has decreased as halothane has been replaced by sevoflurane, and related cardiovascular sequelae (arrhythmias, hypotension, cardiac arrest) have also decreased accordingly. Other medication-related causes included syringe swaps and succinylcholine-induced hyperkalemia. In a follow-up period from 1998 to 2003, the registry analyzed data for more than 300 cases of perioperative cardiac arrest. More than half (163) were related to anesthetic causes.

Accidental intravenous injection of local anesthetic and/or local anesthetic toxicity resulting from overdose remain persistent problems. The promise of a significantly increased margin of safety with ropivacaine and L-bupivacaine has not been borne out. Until a local anesthetic with a much lower cardiovascular toxicity profile becomes available, only meticulous care and constant vigilance in the administration of bupivacaine will lessen the incidence of its cardiotoxicity.

MANAGEMENT

Management of cardiac arrest in the perioperative period depends, of course, on the cause. Initial management of a cardiac arrest that occurs in the perianesthetic period is guided by the same principles used in the management of any pediatric cardiac arrest. Certification in pediatric advanced life

TABLE 27-8	Pediatric Perioperative Cardiac Arrest Registry reported causes for anesthesia-related cardiac arrest	
Primary cause	1994-1997 (n = 150)	1998-2003 (n = 163)
Cardiovascular	32%	36%
Medication	37%	20%
Respiratory	20%	27%
Equipment	7%	4%

support (PALS) is recommended for anesthesiologists who regularly care for infants and children. The reader is referred to the latest PALS algorithm as published by the American Heart Association (http://www.heart.org/HEARTORG/). An underlying respiratory cause of cardiac arrest should always be sought.

THE PRETERM NEWBORN

The Committee on Fetus and Newborn of the American Academy of Pediatrics has recently revised the classification of preterm newborns using gestational age instead of birth weight. This change was made because of advances in technology that allow very exact determination of gestational age. Preterm morbidity also correlates better with gestational age than with birth weight. A preterm newborn is classically defined as one born before 37 weeks of gestation. Table 27-9 illustrates the traditional classification of preterm newborns by weight and the related approximate gestational age. Currently, the term *extremely low gestational age newborn* is used to refer to a newborn delivered at 23 to 27 weeks of gestation regardless of birth weight. As a group, extremely low gestational age newborns have immaturity of all organ systems and represent the most vulnerable of all pediatric patients with the highest morbidity and mortality. Terms related to the age of preterm neonates and infants are defined in Table 27-10.

Although newborns are categorized by gestational age, weight is still considered. Newborns are classified as small, appropriate, or large for gestational age, based on normal values established for weight at various gestational stages. In general, newborns who are small for gestational age have experienced some sort of placental insufficiency. Other causes for a newborn to be small for gestational age are congenital infection, maternal chronic disease, and maternal nicotine abuse. These newborns are also called *growth restricted*. Affected infants may have lower liver glycogen stores, which predisposes them to hypoglycemia, and less subcutaneous fat, which predisposes them to hypothermia. They may also have polycythemia, which predisposes them to problems of hyperviscosity such as necrotizing enterocolitis and CNS injury. Paradoxically, these infants, having been stressed in utero, may have advanced lung maturity compared with appropriate for gestational age newborns of the same gestational age. Large for gestational age newborns are at risk of hypoglycemia, because they have often been born to diabetic mothers and have been exposed to higher levels of the growth-promoting hormone insulin in utero.

Respiratory Distress Syndrome

Lack of the appropriate type of surface-active material or surfactant leads to the development of neonatal respiratory distress syndrome (RDS). The incidence is inversely proportional to the gestational age and birth weight. Mature levels of pulmonary surfactant are present in most cases by 35 weeks of gestation. Five percent of newborns with the diagnosis of RDS are born at term, however.

PATHOGENESIS

Surfactant, produced by type II pneumocytes, helps maintain alveolar stability by reducing alveolar surface tension. Without surfactant, some alveoli collapse and others become overdistended. Functional residual capacity and residual volume are decreased, and $\dot{V}/\dot{Q}$ mismatching develops with resultant arterial hypoxemia and metabolic acidosis.

SIGNS AND SYMPTOMS

RDS usually becomes apparent within minutes of birth. Respiratory distress is evidenced by tachypnea, prominent grunting, intercostal and subcostal retractions, and nasal flaring. Grunting is the newborn's effort to keep open collapsing alveoli. Cyanosis and dyspnea progressively worsen. Before surfactant preparations became available, treatment included administering higher inspired fractions of oxygen and providing distending airway pressure. If RDS is untreated, apnea and irregular respirations, signs of impending respiratory failure, develop. Without adequate treatment, hypotension, hypothermia, a mixed respiratory-metabolic acidosis, edema, ileus, and oliguria may ensue. The clinical course, chest radiograph, and blood gas analysis help to establish the clinical diagnosis of RDS. The typical radiographic appearance of the lungs is a fine reticular granularity of the parenchyma and air bronchograms. Blood gas findings are characterized by progressive hypoxemia, hypercarbia, and variable metabolic acidosis.

TABLE 27-9 Classification of preterm newborns

Weight-based category*	Birth weight (g)	Estimated gestational age (wk)
Low birth weight	<1500-2499	31-35
Very low birth weight	1000 to <1499	26-30
Extremely low birth weight	<1000	<26

*Very-low-birth-weight and extremely-low-birth-weight newborns are considered "micropreemies."

TABLE 27-10 Age terminology for preterm newborns and infants

Term	Definition
Gestational age (GA)	First day of last menstrual period to birth in weeks
Chronologic age (CA)	Time since birth in weeks or months
Postmenstrual age	GA + CA in weeks or months
Corrected postconceptual age	CA − (40 − GA) in weeks or months

TREATMENT

Surfactant is now administered to preterm newborns, either immediately in the delivery room or later as a rescue treatment. Various types of naturally derived and synthetic preparations are used. Surfactant increases lung compliance and stabilizes the alveoli at end exhalation. Surfactant administration decreases the need for high concentrations of inspired oxygen, ventilatory support, and high ventilatory pressures. Unfortunately, it has not decreased the incidence of subsequent chronic lung disease or bronchopulmonary dysplasia. In addition to administration of surfactant, newborns with RDS are being treated with nasal continuous positive airway pressure (CPAP) in the delivery room in an effort to minimize the loss of lung volume and obviate the need for both surfactant and endotracheal intubation and mechanical ventilation. If CPAP therapy fails, the newborn is intubated and surfactant administered. In centers that successfully employ this technique, surfactant use is decreased, but the long-term effect, if any, on the incidence of chronic lung disease is yet unknown.

MANAGEMENT OF ANESTHESIA

During anesthesia, the arterial oxygen saturation should be maintained near its preoperative levels. Placement of an arterial catheter (ideally in a preductal artery) is useful to monitor oxygenation, avoid hyperoxia (because these are preterm neonates predisposed to developing retinal damage), and prevent respiratory and metabolic acidosis during the intraoperative and postoperative periods. Some patients may arrive with an in-situ umbilical artery catheter, which generally suffices for monitoring purposes for brief procedures. Pneumothorax from barotrauma is an ever-present danger and should be considered if there is sudden cardiorespiratory decompensation. Maintaining the patient's hematocrit near 40% helps to optimize systemic oxygen delivery. Excessive hydration should be avoided; therefore, smaller total volumes of colloids such as 5% albumin (in 10 to 20 mL/kg increments) should be used over crystalloids in case of hypovolemia. Postoperative mechanical ventilation is needed in most cases, but when extubation is possible, the patient must be monitored closely for postoperative respiratory distress and apnea.

Bronchopulmonary Dysplasia

Bronchopulmonary dysplasia (BPD) is a form of chronic lung disease of infancy. As already mentioned, the incidence of chronic lung disease in children who were born preterm has not decreased despite the widespread use of surfactant in the treatment of neonatal RDS.

PATHOGENESIS

The pathogenesis of BPD is complex and remains poorly understood. Nonetheless, the cause is likely multifactorial involving insults sustained in both prenatal and postnatal life with resultant arrest of normal lung (alveolar) development.

The clinical entity of BPD is different in newborns treated with surfactant, however. The lung damage, as opposed to

TABLE 27-11 Factors that contribute to the pathogenesis of bronchopulmonary dysplasia

FACTORS ASSOCIATED WITH PREMATURITY

Positive pressure ventilation
High inspired oxygen concentration
Inflammation (alone or associated with infection)
Pulmonary edema (resulting from patent ductus arteriosus or excess fluid administration)
Pulmonary air leak
Poor nutrition
Airway hyperreactivity
Adrenal insufficiency

OTHER FACTORS

Meconium aspiration pneumonia
Neonatal pneumonia
Congestive heart failure

being variable as was the case in the presurfactant era, is more uniform throughout. Airway injury and hyperreactivity with smooth muscle hyperplasia, alternating areas of overinflation, fibrosis, and atelectasis, seen in the presurfactant era, are not present in patients with the so-called new BPD. Although they may not exhibit the same degree of respiratory distress as infants with classic BPD, these patients still do have decreased compliance, impaired gas exchange, and increased oxygen consumption caused by increased work of breathing.

Preterm infants likely to develop BPD are born during the canalicular phase of lung development at 24 to 26 weeks. Despite the different clinical and radiographic picture of new BPD, this condition is thought to have causes similar to those of the classic form, including the use of mechanical ventilation and supplemental oxygen that initiates a cascade of cellular damage and inflammation. Other factors that may play a role in the development of BPD are listed in Table 27-11.

SIGNS AND SYMPTOMS

BPD is a clinical diagnosis defined as oxygen dependence at 36 weeks' postconceptual age or oxygen requirement (to maintain $Pao_2 > 50$ mm Hg) beyond 28 days of life in infants with birth weights of less than 1500 g. The radiographic appearance of the lungs gradually changes from a picture of almost complete opacification with air bronchograms and interstitial emphysema to one of small, round, radiolucent areas alternating with areas of irregular density resembling a sponge. Pulmonary dysfunction in patients with BPD is most marked during the first year of life. Infants with mild BPD may eventually become asymptomatic, but airway hyperreactivity may persist.

TREATMENT

Maintenance of adequate oxygenation (with $Pao_2 > 55$ mm Hg and oxygen saturation by pulse oximetry > 94%) is necessary to prevent or treat cor pulmonale and to promote growth of lung tissue and remodeling of the pulmonary vascular bed. Reactive airway bronchoconstriction is treated with bronchodilating agents. Diuretic administration is often needed for treatment of interstitial fluid retention and pulmonary edema to improve gas exchange.

MANAGEMENT OF ANESTHESIA

Preoperative assessment of the child with BPD should focus on any recent respiratory decompensation and need for intervention. Ongoing drug therapy (bronchodilators, diuretics) as well as baseline oxygen saturation measurements provide valuable clues to the severity of BPD and the child's clinical stability. The choice of drugs for anesthesia is not as important as management of the airway. In children with a history of mechanical ventilation, an endotracheal tube one to one half size smaller than that predicted for age should be used because subglottic stenosis may be present. Tracheomalacia and bronchomalacia may also present as sequelae of previous prolonged intubation. Airway hyperreactivity is likely; thus, a deep plane of anesthesia must be established before airway instrumentation. Indeed, children who have or have had BPD can be assumed to have reactive airway disease and should be treated similarly to those with asthma. Often, increased peak inspiratory pressures are required, which reflects decreased pulmonary compliance. Adequate oxygen should be delivered to maintain a PaO_2 of 50 to 70 mm Hg. Patients with metabolic alkalosis from furosemide therapy may exhibit a compensatory retention of carbon dioxide. Fluid should be administered judiciously to avoid pulmonary edema.

Laryngomalacia and Bronchomalacia

Laryngomalacia is a congenital or acquired condition of excessive flaccidity of the laryngeal structures, especially the epiglottis and arytenoids. It can be caused by the lack of neural control of laryngeal muscles or result from pressure on the laryngeal cartilage, which leads to inadequate laryngeal rigidity and thus structural collapse during inspiration and exhalation. Laryngomalacia accounts for more than 70% of persistent stridor in neonates and young infants. A congenital cause is found in 85% of cases of stridor in children who come to medical attention before the third birthday. After laryngomalacia, which accounts for the majority of cases, congenital vocal cord paralysis is the most common cause and is seen in approximately 10% of infants with congenital stridor.

Bronchomalacia is seen in infants who have had a prolonged stay in the neonatal intensive care unit (NCU). Risk factors include long periods of mechanical ventilation, poor nutrition, intercurrent infections, and other impediments to normal growth and development. The cartilage of the major airways is weakened, and when affected infants bear down, these airways can become partially or completely compressed. Infants with bronchomalacia generally also have a component of BPD. These two conditions together lead to significant respiratory difficulties. When the infant breathes more forcefully, the higher negative inspiratory forces cause further collapse of the airways affected with bronchomalacia, which leads

to worsening respiratory distress. Any mild viral respiratory infection may worsen the situation to the point that hospitalization will be needed. With time and good nutrition, both bronchomalacia and laryngomalacia usually resolve.

Retinopathy of Prematurity

Retinopathy of prematurity (ROP), formerly known as *retrolental fibroplasia,* is a vasoproliferative retinopathy of multifactorial etiology that occurs almost exclusively in preterm infants in whom retinal vasculogenesis is incomplete. It is the second leading cause of childhood blindness in the United States. The risk of retinopathy is inversely related to birth weight and gestational age. ROP occurs in up to 70% of newborns who weigh less than 1000 g at birth, but fortunately in many of these cases the condition regresses spontaneously. The first few weeks of life seem to be the period of greatest vulnerability to the development of ROP.

PATHOGENESIS

The most cited cause of ROP is exposure to elevated tension of oxygen with resultant injury to the developing retinal capillaries. The development of ROP is roughly divided into two phases. In phase 1, oxygen toxicity to the immature retina causes an arrest of normal vascularization. In phase 2, the increased metabolic demand of the growing retina is met with relative hypoxia caused by the paucity of blood vessels. Because of this, the retina undergoes reactive abnormal neovascularization that extends into the vitreous humor. Retinal and vitreal fibrous tissue formation also ensues. Retinal vasculogenesis normally begins at the sixteenth week of gestation and is complete by 44 weeks, after which time the risk of ROP is negligible.

SIGNS AND SYMPTOMS

ROP is classified into five stages of disease severity. In stage 1, the mildest form, there is simply a more clear demarcation between vascular and avascular portions of the retina. In the most severe form, stage 5, there is total detachment of the retina.

The risk factors associated with ROP are not fully known. Hyperoxia is a major risk factor. However, oxygen alone is not sufficient to produce ROP, because cases have been reported to occur even in the absence of oxygen therapy. Concentration, duration, timing, and fluctuation of oxygen delivery may all play a role in the development of ROP. The one risk factor that outweighs all others is prematurity. Other identified risk factors for ROP are sepsis, congenital infections, congenital heart disease, mechanical ventilation, RDS, blood transfusions, intra ventricular hemorrhage, hypoxia, hypercapnia and hypocapnia, asphyxia, and vitamin E deficiency. Approximately 80% to 90% of mild cases of ROP undergo spontaneous regression with little or no residual visual disability. However, infants who develop ROP are at higher risk of experiencing ophthalmologic problems later in life, including retinal tears, retinal detachment, myopia, strabismus, amblyopia, and glaucoma.

TREATMENT

Primary treatments for ROP include transscleral cryotherapy and laser photocoagulation. The goal is to destroy the peripheral avascular areas of the retina, which slows or even reverses the abnormal vasculogenesis and thus reduces the risk of retinal detachment. However, in those with severe ROP, laser treatment reduces the risks of retinal detachment and blindness by only approximately 25%. Central vision is preserved at the expense of some peripheral vision. Surgical options aimed at relieving cicatrix-induced traction on the retina allow the retina to relax and reattach and may be considered in cases that do not respond to laser therapy or cryotherapy. A scleral buckle procedure may be performed on infants if a shallow retinal detachment develops as a result of traction from fibrovascular scar tissue.

MANAGEMENT OF ANESTHESIA

Since oxygen toxicity is recognized as a major risk factor for the development of ROP, the anesthesiologist is often faced with the challenge of limiting supplemental oxygen while maximizing oxygen delivery in this group of vulnerable patients. The benefit of low oxygen saturation for ROP is often at odds with the potential ill effects of hypoxemia on other immature organ systems such as the CNS. Currently, there are no established guidelines for specific intraoperative oxygen saturation goals for preterm infants undergoing surgery. There is also no published evidence to indicate that high oxygen saturation increases ROP risk *after 32 weeks' postconceptual age.* However, use of supplemental oxygen likely has different implications depending on the infant's postconceptual age because it correlates with different phases of ROP as described previously. In phase 1, high oxygen saturation is likely to promote cessation of normal vasculogenesis and thus will increase the risk of and worsen ROP. In the second phase, however, in which abnormal neovascularization is driven by hypoxia, a higher oxygen saturation may be preferred. Several multicenter studies (Benefits of Oxygen Saturation Targeting [BOOST], Supplemental Therapeutic Oxygen for Prethreshold Retinopathy of Prematurity [STOP-ROP]) showed that higher oxygen saturation (between 96% and 99%) did not worsen preexisting ROP and was associated with a nonsignificant reduction in disease severity. It must be recognized that these studies included mostly infants who were well into the second phase of ROP, in which higher oxygen saturation may be potentially protective.

Because the optimal intraoperative oxygen saturation for these patients is yet to be determined, it remains prudent to limit oxygen supplementation to preterm infants without a diagnosis of ROP, especially to those of less than 32 weeks' postconceptual age. This must be balanced with the need to maintain hemodynamic stability and neurologic function, and thus oxygen should not be withheld in these circumstances. Although it is desirable to avoid hyperoxia, arterial hypoxemia can be life threatening and more deleterious. Infants undergoing peripheral retinal ablation have an increased incidence of apnea and bradycardia, both during the procedure and in the following 1 to 3 days.

Apnea of Prematurity

Just as RDS is a result of immaturity of the pulmonary system, apnea of prematurity (AOP) is a result of immaturity of the respiratory control centers in the newborn brainstem. The severity of AOP is inversely proportional to the gestational age of the newborn at birth.

SIGNS AND SYMPTOMS

Affected newborns exhibit both primary (or central) apnea, in which there is simply lack of effort to breathe in the absence of any obstruction, and obstructive apnea. In obstructive apnea of the preterm newborn, there is immaturity of both the mechanisms that maintain airway patency and the mechanisms that detect physiologic sequelae of obstruction (hypercarbia, hypoxemia) to bring about arousal and correct the obstruction. Mixed episodes of central and obstructive apnea are also seen. The carbon dioxide response of infants with AOP has been measured and is decreased compared with that of infants without AOP. AOP is diagnosed on clinical grounds and the criteria are somewhat variable. The diagnosis is made if an infant exhibits apnea of longer than 15 to 20 seconds, apnea associated with a heart rate of less than 80 to 100 beats per minute, or apnea associated with significant decreases in oxygen saturation.

TREATMENT

Treatment of AOP is begun once other causes of apnea such as infection or CNS disorder have been eliminated. Some cases of AOP are associated with lowered hematocrit levels and resolve after transfusion with packed red cells. Other nonpharmacologic treatments include nasal CPAP therapy and, in very severe cases, mechanical ventilation. Methylxanthines are the mainstay of drug therapy for AOP. These central stimulants actually increase the sensitivity of the respiratory centers to carbon dioxide. Various forms of methylxanthines are used, including aminophylline, caffeine, and caffeine citrate.

Postanesthetic Apnea

Postanesthetic apnea has many similarities with AOP. Preterm newborns who are at risk for AOP based on their corrected postconceptual age are also at increased risk for developing postanesthetic apnea. Postanesthetic apnea is seen mostly in infants born preterm (where preterm birth is defined as birth at <37 weeks of gestation). The incidence is inversely related to postconceptual age. One of the most significant risk factors is a hematocrit of less than 30%. Infants who were small for gestational age but were born at term do not have an increased risk of postanesthetic apnea. In general, it is prudent to keep infants whose postconceptual age is less than 52 to 60 weeks for overnight observation because of the risk of this complication. Use of regional anesthesia, without the addition of any systemic sedatives and opioids, appears to decrease the incidence of postanesthetic apnea in infants at risk, but the data are insufficient to recommend against overnight admission and apnea monitoring.

Hypoglycemia

Hypoglycemia is the most common metabolic problem occurring in newborn infants. Inadequate glycogen stores and deficient gluconeogenesis are important risk factors. The incidence of symptomatic hypoglycemia is highest in those born small for gestational age. Infants may be at risk of hypoglycemia as a result of maternal factors or intrinsic neonatal problems such as those related to prematurity and endocrine or metabolic dysfunctions (Table 27-12).

SIGNS AND SYMPTOMS

The absolute serum glucose concentration or duration of hypoglycemia that causes CNS injury in neonates in not known with certainty. Serum glucose levels are rarely less than 35 to 40 mg/dL in the first 24 hours of life or less than 45 mg/dL thereafter. CNS or systemic signs of hypoglycemia such as jitteriness, seizures, apnea, lethargy, or mottling and pallor will usually be observed when serum glucose concentrations decrease to less than 30 to 40 mg/dL in term infants during the first 72 hours and to less than 40 mg/dL thereafter. It may be prudent to keep serum glucose concentrations above 40 mg/dL in all newborns.

Many neonates whose serum glucose levels are at or just below the lower limits of the normal range are asymptomatic. The clinical manifestations of mild hypoglycemia are subtle and nonspecific, and a high index of suspicion must be maintained in neonates at high risk. Hypoglycemia that persists beyond the first week of life is uncommon and is most often due to congenital hyperinsulinism, endocrine deficiency, or other disorders of carbohydrate, amino acid, and fatty acid metabolism.

The prognosis for a normal outcome is good in asymptomatic neonates with transient hypoglycemia. The prognosis for subsequent normal intellectual development is more guarded in symptomatic infants, particularly low-birth-weight infants, those with persistent hyperinsulinemic hypoglycemia, and infants of diabetic mothers.

TREATMENT

Infants with symptoms other than seizures should receive an intravenous bolus of 2 mL/kg (200 mg/kg) of 10% dextrose. If the infant is experiencing convulsions, an intravenous bolus of 4 mL/kg of 10% dextrose is indicated. Following bolus administration, a 10% dextrose infusion should be given at 8 mg/kg/min and titrated to maintain the serum glucose level above 40 to 50 mg/dL.

MANAGEMENT OF ANESTHESIA

In neonates who are less than 48 hours old, premature, or small for gestational age, and in those born to diabetic mothers, the risk of intraoperative hypoglycemia is significant. As in adults, signs and symptoms of hypoglycemia may be

TABLE 27-12 Causes of neonatal hypoglycemia
MATERNAL FACTORS
Intrapartum administration of glucose
Drug treatment
β-Adrenergic antagonists (terbutaline, propranolol)
Oral hypoglycemic agents
Salicylates
Maternal diabetes/gestational diabetes
NEONATAL FACTORS
Depleted glycogen stores
Asphyxia
Perinatal stress
Increased glucose utilization (metabolic demands)
Sepsis
Polycythemia
Hypothermia
Respiratory distress syndrome
Congenital heart disease
Limited glycogen stores
Intrauterine growth retardation
Prematurity
Hyperinsulinism/endocrine disorders
Diabetic mother
Erythroblastosis fetalis, fetal hydrops
Insulinoma
Beckwith-Wiedeman syndrome
Panhypopituitarism
Decreased glycogenolysis/gluconeogenesis/utilization of alternative fuels
Inborn errors of metabolism
Adrenal insufficiency

masked by anesthetic drugs. For this reason, preemptive glucose monitoring is essential in at-risk neonates. Maintenance fluid requirements may be met with a glucose-containing solution of 5% dextrose in 0.2 normal saline 4 mL/kg/hr or 10% dextrose in water 2 to 3 mL/kg/hr to prevent intraoperative hypoglycemia. Hyperglycemia (plasma glucose level ≥ 150 mg/dL) may occur in stressed neonates receiving infusions of glucose-containing solutions intraoperatively or those already receiving parenteral nutrition. Thus, fluid deficits, blood, and third-space losses should be replaced using dextrose-free solutions. Serum glucose concentrations in excess of 125 mg/dL can result in osmotic diuresis from glucosuria with subsequent dehydration as well as further release of insulin leading to rebound hypoglycemia. In addition, a hyperosmolar state in neonates, especially premature very-low-birth-weight neonates, increases the risk of intraventricular hemorrhage.

Hypocalcemia

Neonates at particular risk of hypocalcemia are those born prematurely or with low birth weight, particularly infants with intrauterine growth retardation, infants of mothers with insulin-dependent diabetes, and infants with birth asphyxia associated with prolonged, difficult deliveries. Late neonatal hypocalcemia occurring 5 to 10 days after birth is usually due to ingestion of cow's milk, which contains high levels of phosphorus. It is not seen in breast-fed infants, because human breast milk has a lower phosphate content.

Hypocalcemia occurs in newborns for a variety of reasons, and in many cases, ionized calcium is decreased even as total calcium remains within normal limits. Risk factors for neonatal hypocalcemia include maternal factors and factors intrinsic to the newborn. Examples of maternal factors are use of medications such as anticonvulsants or calcium antacids, and vitamin D deficiency. Factors intrinsic to the newborn include parathyroid hormone abnormalities, malabsorption, hypomagnesemia, inadequate intake, and inadequate calcium replenishment after transfusion of citrated blood products. Other notable causes of hypocalcemia in the newborn include maternal hypercalcemia and DiGeorge's syndrome.

SIGNS AND SYMPTOMS

The clinical manifestations of hypocalcemia include irritability, jitteriness, seizures, and lethargy. The classic signs of hypocalcemic tetany are seen only rarely. Under anesthesia, hypocalcemia manifests as hypotension and depressed cardiac performance. Newborns have little stored calcium within the sarcolemma. Extracellular calcium is a much more important determinant of myocardial contractility than it is in older children and adults. Treatment with intravenous calcium should be considered for newborns who have hypotension without an obvious cause.

The laboratory definition of hypocalcemia varies depending on the specific range of normal values at each institution. Regardless, it is important to evaluate both total and ionized calcium levels.

TREATMENT

Management of hypocalcemia involves correction of hypocalcemia as well as hypomagnesemia and any other metabolic or acid-base abnormalities. An intravenous infusion of calcium is the most effective means to correct symptomatic hypocalcemia in the neonatal ICU and the operating room. The dose used to correct hypocalcemia should be based on the amount of elemental calcium administered. The starting dose is 10 to 20 mg/kg of elemental calcium. Calcium gluconate 10% provides 9 mg/mL of elemental calcium and calcium chloride provides 27.2 mg/mL of elemental calcium. These doses have been shown to increase ionized calcium levels, blood pressure, and cardiac contractility.

Cases of bradycardia and even asystole have been seen with rapid intravenous administration of calcium. Intravenous calcium should be given over 5 to 10 minutes with electrocardiographic monitoring. Extravasation of calcium from a faulty peripheral intravenous catheter can have severe consequences such as tissue sloughing and necrosis. If calcium is given via an umbilical venous line, the tip should be confirmed to be in the inferior vena cava and not too near the right atrium; administration of calcium too close to the heart can result in arrhythmias. Calcium in intravenous preparations will precipitate with solutions containing bicarbonate or phosphorus.

MANAGEMENT OF ANESTHESIA

Intraoperative metabolic derangements such as alkalosis from hyperventilation and sodium bicarbonate administration can lead to hypocalcemia by causing albumin binding of calcium that decreases ionized calcium concentration. Hypocalcemia can also occur during infusions of albumin and citrated blood products resulting from calcium chelation. Hypotensive effects of citrate-induced hypocalcemia can be minimized by administering calcium gluconate (1 to 2 mg IV) for each milliliter of blood transfused.

SURGICAL DISEASES OF THE NEWBORN

Congenital Diaphragmatic Hernia

Congenital diaphragmatic hernia (CDH) is a defect in the diaphragm that is associated with a variable amount of intraabdominal organ extrusion into the thoracic cavity. It has an incidence between 1 in 2500 and 1 in 3000 live births. CDH may be an isolated lesion, or it may be associated with other anomalies or syndromes such as Beckwith-Wiedemann syndrome, CHARGE association (*c*oloboma, *h*eart defects, *a*tresia of the choanae, *r*etardation, *g*enital anomalies, and *e*ar anomalies), and various chromosomal abnormalities such as trisomy 21 or 18.

PATHOGENESIS

CDH is an early gestational event with incomplete closure of the diaphragm. This defect is usually associated with bilateral pulmonary hypoplasia resulting from in utero compression of the developing lungs by the herniated viscera, pulmonary hypertension, and increased airway reactivity. In addition to the effects of lung compression, there may be an underlying primary abnormality in airway branching that results in pulmonary hypoplasia. The most common and largest diaphragmatic defect occurs through the left posterolateral pleuroperitoneal canal (foramen of Bochdalek) and accounts for 75% of all cases. The remainder of defects occur at the right posterolateral foramen of Bochdalek, at the anterior foramen of Morgagni, and in paraesophageal locations.

SIGNS AND SYMPTOMS

Prenatal diagnosis of CDH has increased from approximately 10% of cases in 1985 to nearly 60% in present day. The most common findings include displacement of the heart and fluid-filled gastrointestinal segments into the thorax. Both stomach and small bowel are often present. Ultrasonographic findings that suggest a poorer prognosis include a dilated intrathoracic stomach or the presence of the left lobe of the liver in the chest. However, prenatal ultrasonography can generate a high number of false negatives. Postnatal lung volume is of some prognostic significance and can be estimated from the prenatal ultrasonographic findings. At birth, a newborn with CDH will exhibit cyanosis, dyspnea, and apparent dextrocardia. Physical findings will include decreased breath sounds, distant or right-displaced heart sounds, and bowel sounds in the chest. Because of a reduction in the intraabdominal visceral content, the newborn will have a scaphoid abdomen. A chest radiograph typically shows a bowel gas pattern (and perhaps part of the liver) in the chest and a mediastinal shift.

These infants can have profound hypoxemia, which reflects right-to-left shunting through the ductus arteriosus; the cause is persistent fetal circulation resulting from lung parenchymal and vascular hypoplasia with resultant high pulmonary vascular resistance. A vicious cycle is set in place in which the already elevated pulmonary vascular resistance is further exacerbated by the severe arterial hypoxemia, hypercarbia, and acidosis. The ductus arteriosus remains patent and fetal circulation patterns persist.

TREATMENT

Care of a newborn with a severe CDH starts immediately in the delivery room. If spontaneous respiratory efforts are inadequate, endotracheal intubation with institution of gentle ventilatory support and decompression of the stomach are undertaken. These interventions may prevent further distention of the gastrointestinal tract and further pulmonary compression by the displaced abdominal contents. In contrast to earlier approaches, which considered CHD a surgical emergency, current management is aimed at medically stabilizing the cardiorespiratory status of the newborn as well as possible (correcting hypoxia and acidosis, and achieving cardiovascular stability) before surgical repair.

The specific timing of surgery is not as important as stabilization of the neonate's condition. Specific goals of preoperative medical management include achievement of a preductal oxygen saturation of at least 90% and correction of metabolic acidosis. Crystalloid fluid and blood products are administered to maintain intravascular volume and RBC mass. Adequate sedation is achieved in an effort to minimize increases in pulmonary vascular resistance. Dopamine and milrinone may be needed to maintain hemodynamic stability. When mechanical ventilation is used in the preoperative period, the settings should be as low as possible to allow for moderate permissive hypercarbia to minimize ventilator-induced lung injury. Surgery should be delayed for as long as 5 to 15 days until pulmonary vascular resistance has decreased and ventilation can be maintained with low peak inspiratory pressures and fraction of inspired oxygen (FIO_2). If pulmonary hypertension persists or recurs, then trials of inhaled nitric oxide and high-frequency oscillatory ventilation (HFOV) are initiated. Extracorporeal membrane oxygenation (ECMO) is also considered. These maneuvers have been variably effective in reversing pulmonary hypertension. Although inhaled nitric oxide has been used with good success in infants with pulmonary hypertension associated with meconium aspiration or congenital heart disease, its efficacy in newborns with elevated pulmonary vascular resistance in the setting of CDH has not been conclusively demonstrated.

For newborns with CDH who exhibit clinical deterioration, ECMO and HFOV have been used in different centers; survival rates with these two rescue modalities are nearly identical (53% and 55%, respectively). At some centers, ECMO is used as a rescue therapy for infants who have persistent preductal hypoxemia in spite of inotropic and ventilatory support (including HFOV and inhaled nitric oxide). Significant risks are associated with ECMO, including bleeding at surgical or chest tube insertion sites, intracranial hemorrhage, sepsis, and complications of the extracorporeal circuit, including clotting and embolism. HFOV also can lead to significant morbidity. In view of the improved survival with gentle ventilation, sedation, and pharmacologic cardiovascular support, extraordinary maneuvers such as HFOV and ECMO have assumed a less central role in the management of infants with CDH.

MANAGEMENT OF ANESTHESIA

If mechanical ventilation has not already been initiated, anesthetic care of neonates with CDH begins with either an awake or a rapid-sequence tracheal intubation following preoxygenation. Induction medications appropriate for rapid-sequence intubation in critically ill newborns include propofol or an opioid and succinylcholine. The dose of the induction agent is based on the newborn's cardiovascular condition. Atropine may be added depending on the infant's clinical status. In addition to routine monitoring devices, two pulse oximeters (in preductal and postductal locations) are useful to monitor the degree of shunting. Placement of a preductal arterial cannula (right radial artery) is recommended for monitoring systemic blood pressure, acid-base status, and other blood parameters. Venous access should be avoided in the lower extremities, because venous return may be impaired as a result of compression of the inferior vena cava following reduction of the hernia.

Anesthesia can be induced and maintained with an opioid, a nondepolarizing muscle relaxant, and, if tolerated, low concentrations of inhaled anesthetics. Nitrous oxide should be avoided, because its diffusion into loops of intestine present in the chest may result in distention with subsequent compression of functional lung tissue. If arterial oxygenation is satisfactory, the delivered concentration of oxygen can be diluted by adding air to the gas mixture.

Repair of CDH via minimally invasive techniques is becoming more common, but open repair is still the preferred method. Infants with CDH, almost by definition, have pulmonary dysfunction, and this pathophysiologic condition limits the ability of the newborn to tolerate thoracoscopy and one-lung ventilation. The primary advantage of thoracoscopic repair is the much smaller surgical wounds and the associated reduction in postoperative pain. However, thoracoscopic procedures tend to be lengthier and are very challenging for the anesthesiologist, since compromise of cardiorespiratory functions may be even more significant than with open repairs. For example, carbon dioxide insufflation can cause overwhelming hypercarbia with significant respiratory acidosis requiring intermittent deflation to allow for ventilation. In the open surgical technique, reduction of the diaphragmatic hernia is usually accomplished through a left subcostal abdominal incision, although the repair can be performed through a thoracotomy incision as well. Use of the abdominal approach facilitates the correction of intestinal malrotation. Depending on the size of the defect, prosthetic material may be used to close the diaphragm. During intraoperative mechanical ventilation of the lungs, airway pressures should be monitored and maintained at less than 25 to 30 cm H_2O to minimize the risk of barotrauma and pneumothorax. A sudden decrease in lung compliance or deterioration of oxygenation or blood pressure suggests a pneumothorax. Hypothermia must be avoided. Complications associated with hypothermia include increased pulmonary vascular resistance with resultant right-to-left shunting and increased oxygen consumption; this may result in inadequate oxygen delivery and acidosis, which further increases pulmonary vasoconstriction and worsens arterial hypoxemia.

After the abdominal contents are returned to the abdomen, an attempt to inflate the hypoplastic lung is not recommended, because the lung is unlikely to expand and excessive positive airway pressures may damage the contralateral lung. In addition to a hypoplastic lung, these neonates are likely to have an underdeveloped abdominal cavity; thus, a tight surgical abdominal closure causes increased intraabdominal pressure, with cephalad displacement of the diaphragm, decreased functional residual capacity, and compression of the inferior vena cava. To prevent excessively tight abdominal surgical closures in infants with large defects, it is often necessary to create a ventral hernia (which can be surgically repaired later) and close the skin or to place a silastic pouch. A pulse oximeter applied to a lower extremity may forewarn of abdominal compartment syndrome and circulatory compromise.

In some institutions, surgery for CDH may be performed in the neonatal ICU to avoid the stresses of transport and sudden changes in ventilation parameters. If surgery is performed in the neonatal ICU without a conventional anesthesia machine and/or while the patient is undergoing unconventional modes of ventilation or ECMO, a high-dose intravenous opioid and muscle relaxant technique is chosen. If the newborn is undergoing ECMO, it is crucial to communicate the anesthetic plan to both the ECMO perfusionist and the neonatologist who will care for the patient postoperatively.

POSTOPERATIVE MANAGEMENT

Postoperative management of neonates with CDH presents significant challenges. The long-term outcome for these newborns is ultimately determined by the degree of pulmonary hypoplasia. Unfortunately, there is no effective treatment for pulmonary hypoplasia other than provision of adequate nutrition and oxygen supplementation to allow for remodeling of the pulmonary vasculature and growth of more lung tissue.

Ventilatory support is minimized to the extent possible. Neonatal pressure-support ventilation with low pressures and the lowest safe F_{IO_2} are employed. Sedation and analgesia are provided to allow the infant to tolerate intubation and ventilation. Some centers use epidural analgesia to minimize splinting and any respiratory depression from systemic opioids.

In the long term, infants with CDH face a number of challenges. Gastroesophageal reflux occurs in many infants with CDH and is more common in those with larger defects and those with a synthetic patch repair. Developmental delay, behavioral problems, and hearing deficits, among other neurologic problems, are common in survivors of CDH. In addition, these children often develop chest wall deformities and scoliosis. Recurrence of hernia can occur and is most often seen in those with large defects with a patch in place. Because survivors of CDH have undergone major invasive care in the neonatal ICU and multiple surgical interventions, structured long-term multidisciplinary follow-up care is essential.

Esophageal Atresia and Tracheoesophageal Fistula

Esophageal atresia (EA) is the most frequent congenital anomaly of the esophagus, with an approximate incidence of 1 in 4000 neonates (Figure 27-1). More than 90% of affected individuals have an associated tracheoesophageal fistula (TEF). The most common form of EA/TEF (type C), representing 90% of all cases of this anomaly, manifests as a blind upper esophageal pouch and a distal esophagus that forms a fistula with the trachea. In this variant of EA/TEF, the fistula is connected to the trachea on the posterior aspect near the carina.

In various series, 25% or more of infants with EA have other congenital anomalies, most often the VATER association (vertebral defects, imperforate anus, tracheoesophageal fistula, and renal dysplasia) or VACTERL association (similar to VATER but also including cardiac and limb anomalies). In addition, TEF and EA are known to be common in some chromosomal abnormalities such as trisomy 13, 18, and 21. Approximately 20% of neonates with EA have major co-existing cardiovascular anomalies (atrial septal defect, ventricular septal defect, tetralogy of Fallot, coarctation of the aorta), and 30% to 40% are born prematurely. Survival of neonates with EA and no associated defects approaches 100%. The mortality of infants with EA/TEF varies depending on the birth weight and the presence of a cardiac anomaly. Newborns born weighing more than 1500 g with EA/TEF but without a cardiac anomaly have a survival rate of more than 95%, whereas those with a birth weight of less than 1500 g and a major cardiac anomaly have only a 50% survival rate.

SIGNS AND SYMPTOMS

EA should be suspected if maternal polyhydramnios is present. However, EA is usually diagnosed soon after birth when an oral catheter cannot be passed into the stomach or when the neonate exhibits cyanosis, coughing, and choking during oral feedings. Plain radiographs of the chest and abdomen will reveal coiling of a nasogastric tube in the esophageal pouch and possibly an air-filled stomach in the presence of a co-existing TEF. In contrast, pure EA may present as an airless,

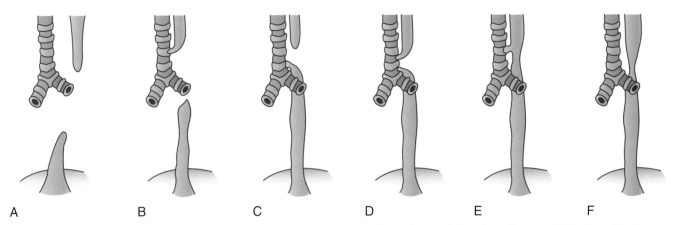

A B C D E F

FIGURE 27-1 Gross classification of congenital anomalies of the trachea and esophagus. **A,** Esophageal atresia (EA) without fistula. **B,** EA with proximal fistula. **C,** EA with distal fistula. **D,** EA with proximal and distal fistulas. **E,** Tracheoesophageal fistula with no EA. **F,** Esophageal stenosis. *(With permission from Holzman RS, Mancuso TJ, Polaner DM. A Practical Approach to Pediatric Anesthesia. 1st ed. Philadelphia, PA: Lippincott Williams & Wilkins; 2008:387, Fig 18.5.)*

scaphoid abdomen. An isolated TEF without EA may elude diagnosis until later in life when the patient may experience recurrent pneumonia and refractory bronchospasm.

TREATMENT

Initial therapeutic measures include maintaining a patent airway and preventing aspiration of secretions. The infant is kept under orders to receive nothing by mouth (NPO), given intravenous fluids, and placed in a head-up position to minimize regurgitation of gastric secretions through the fistula. Continuous suctioning of the proximal esophageal segment prevents aspiration of pharyngeal secretions. Endotracheal intubation is avoided, if possible, because of the potential to worsen distention of the stomach, which can lead to gastric rupture. Gastric distention can be of sufficient magnitude to impair ventilation and venous return, and result in cardiopulmonary arrest. Should life-threatening gastric distention occur, one-lung ventilation may be necessary until the stomach can be decompressed.

Primary repair without initial gastrostomy is routine. Repair of a TEF is urgent. However, neonates with EA, particularly those who are premature, may exhibit significant associated anomalies or have severe lung disease, and in these neonates, a thorough evaluation for associated anomalies, particularly congenital heart disease, should be undertaken. If the newborn's condition is considered too unstable to allow a complete primary repair, a staged surgical approach with an initial gastrostomy created under local anesthesia may be selected. Definitive repair of the TEF can then be delayed until the neonate's condition has improved.

MANAGEMENT OF ANESTHESIA

Awake intubation with spontaneous ventilation allows optimal positioning of the endotracheal tube while minimizing the risk of ventilatory impairment associated with gastric distention resulting from positive pressure ventilation and passage of gases through the fistula. However, awake intubation may be difficult and traumatic in a vigorous infant. If inhalation induction is chosen, the trachea can be intubated without the use of muscle relaxants and the neonate allowed to breath spontaneously. If induction by the intravenous route is chosen, care must be exercised during ventilation to minimize peak inspiratory pressure and potential gastric distention, especially in the absence of a gastrostomy. Proper placement of the tracheal tube is critical; it should be above the carina but below the TEF. It is important that the tracheal tube be above the carina, because the right lung is compressed during thoracotomy. Accidental intubation of the right main bronchus results in precipitous severe hypoxemia, especially during surgical retraction of the lung. The endotracheal tube can be gently advanced into the right main bronchus and then withdrawn until bilateral breath sounds are heard. Alternatively, once induction is completed, the surgeon can perform rigid bronchoscopy to clearly demonstrate the anatomy. Once the fistula is identified, often near the carina, a Fogarty catheter can be passed outside the lumen of the bronchoscope and through the fistula into the stomach. The balloon of the Fogarty catheter is then inflated and pulled back to the stomach wall and fixed in that location to isolate the lungs before positive pressure ventilation is begun.

Selection of anesthetic technique during surgical correction of EA/TEF depends on the physiologic status of the neonate. Low-dose volatile anesthetics in conjunction with air, oxygen, and an opiate are usually well tolerated if the neonate is adequately hydrated. A nondepolarizing muscle relaxant can be administered after the airway is secured and ventilation is deemed satisfactory. In addition to routine monitoring, placement of a catheter in a peripheral artery permits continuous monitoring of systemic blood pressure and measurement of arterial blood gas concentrations. Since pulse oximetry and end-tidal carbon dioxide monitors are standard, precordial stethoscopes are used less often. In these cases, however, a precordial stethoscope placed in the left axillary area can be very helpful in detecting inadvertent right main bronchus migration of the endotracheal tube. Ligation of the TEF and primary esophageal anastomosis is usually performed via a right thoracotomy. During surgery, lung retraction may impair ventilation and surgical manipulation of the trachea may cause airway obstruction. Close communication between the surgeon and anesthesiologist is mandatory. Intermittent release of lung and trachea retraction may be necessary to improve oxygenation and ventilation. Accumulation of secretions and blood may also cause airway obstruction. Frequent tracheal suctioning may be required.

Intraoperative insensible and third-space fluid losses should be replaced with crystalloid at a rate of 6 to 8 mL/kg/hr. Blood loss may be replaced with 5% albumin and packed red cells to maintain a hematocrit of higher than 35%. Hypothermia should be avoided with use of a warming mattress, forced-air warming devices, and warming of all fluids and gases.

Extubation of term infants at the end of surgery is preferable, but is usually not feasible. A full-term infant who has undergone an uneventful simple ligation of a TEF is the best candidate for immediate extubation. Tracheomalacia, resulting from in utero compression by the dilated esophageal pouch, may cause partial upper airway obstruction. Aspiration of gastric secretions may lead to chemical pneumonitis or pneumonia. These and other factors, such as the length of the procedure and possible damage to the airway from rigid bronchoscopy, may influence the decision the continue postoperative mechanical ventilation. Infusions of opioids and/or regional analgesia techniques have been used for pain management.

Omphalocele and Gastroschisis

Omphalocele and gastroschisis are congenital defects of the anterior abdominal wall that permit external herniation of abdominal viscera. They are the most common abdominal wall defects. These conditions have important differences, however (Table 27-13). Approximately 95% of cases can be detected by ultrasonography in the early weeks of gestation. In utero diagnosis allows planned delivery at a medical center with resources for obstetric, surgical, anesthetic, and neonatal care in high-risk cases.

SIGNS AND SYMPTOMS
Omphalocele
Omphalocele manifests as external herniation of abdominal viscera through the base of the umbilical cord. By definition, the defect is larger than 4 cm. A defect smaller than 4 cm is termed an *umbilical hernia*. The abdominal contents are contained within a sac formed by the peritoneal membrane internally and the amniotic membrane externally, without overlying skin. The incidence of herniation of intestines into the cord is approximately 1 in 5000 live births, whereas herniation of liver and intestines occurs in 1 in 10,000 live births. Approximately three quarters of cases are associated with other congenital defects, including cardiac anomalies, trisomy 21, and Beckwith-Wiedemann syndrome (omphalocele, organomegaly, macrosomia, macroglossia, and hypoglycemia). Approximately 33% of neonates with omphaloceles are preterm. Cardiac defects and prematurity are the major causes of mortality (approximately 30%).

TABLE 27-13   Comparison of omphalocele and gastroschisis

Characteristic	Omphalocele	Gastroschisis
Incidence	1 in 3000-10,000	1 in 30,000
Gender distribution	Male > female	Male = female
Preterm birth	30%	60%
Location	Within umbilical cord	Periumbilical cord (right)
Associated anomalies	5%-70% (cardiovascular 20%)	Rare

Gastroschisis
Gastroschisis manifests as external herniation of abdominal viscera through a small (usually less than 5 cm) defect in the anterior abdominal wall. In most cases, the defect occurs laterally, just to the right of the normally inserted umbilical cord. Unlike in omphalocele, a hernia sac does not cover the herniated abdominal viscera. The bowel is exposed to the intrauterine environment without a protective covering, which causes its loops to become matted, thickened, and often covered with an inflammatory coating or peel. In most cases, only intestines are herniated. Gastroschisis is rarely associated with other congenital anomalies. The incidence of preterm birth, however, is higher than in neonates with omphalocele.

Decompressing the stomach with an orogastric or nasogastric tube decreases the risk of regurgitation, aspiration pneumonia, and further bowel distention. Broad-spectrum antibiotics are started along with intravenous fluid therapy with isotonic solution at a rate sufficient to replace the large fluid deficits and ongoing losses (150 to 300 mL/kg/day). These neonates experience considerable protein loss and third-space fluid translocation. To maintain normal oncotic pressure, protein-containing solutions (5% albumin) should constitute approximately 25% of the replacement fluids. Without such vigorous fluid resuscitation, severe hypovolemia and metabolic acidosis may ensue. A urinary catheter should be placed to monitor achievement of the goal of 1 to 2 mL/kg/hr of urine output.

TREATMENT
Gastroschisis requires urgent repair. The sooner the bowel is reduced, the more likely primary closure can be achieved and the less severe the degree of bowel wall edema and accumulation of fibrinous coating. Placing the infant's lower body and exposed intestine into a plastic drawstring bowel bag immediately after delivery reduces evaporative fluid loss and heat loss from the large surface area of exposed bowel. Although omphalocele also requires urgent corrective surgery, the frequency of associated cardiac anomalies warrants preoperative cardiologic evaluation. Primary closure is not always possible. Staged closure is very successful and avoids potential complications of increased abdominal pressure following reduction of herniated viscera. Primary closure may cause respiratory compromise, decreased venous return, and circulatory

dysfunction if the abdomen is too tense. A profound decrease in cardiac output and organ perfusion can result in acidosis, anuria, and bowel necrosis. Lower extremity congestion and cyanosis may also be seen if venous return from the lower body is impaired. If primary closure is deemed not feasible, the viscera should be covered with a prosthetic silo and then slowly reduced over a period of several days to 1 week.

MANAGEMENT OF ANESTHESIA

Important aspects of the anesthetic management for omphalocele and gastroschisis closure include preservation of body temperature and continuation of fluid replacement. After decompression of the stomach and preoxygenation, the airway is best secured by rapid-sequence induction. Opioids or an intravenous hypnotic should be dosed based on the clinical condition of the newborn. The endotracheal tube should allow for ventilation with peak inspiratory pressures of more than 20 cm H_2O. Primary closure may require the ability to provide ventilation with high peak inspiratory pressures into the postoperative period. Repair of a large defect will require maximal relaxation during the procedure and during the initial postoperative period. Anesthesia is maintained with volatile anesthetics and/or opioids (fentanyl or sufentanil) titrated to avoid hypotension. Nitrous oxide is avoided because of its potential to diffuse into the intestinal tract and interfere with the reduction of eviscerated bowel back into the abdomen.

It must be remembered that these neonates have an underdeveloped abdominal cavity; tight surgical abdominal closure can result in compression of the inferior vena cava and decreased diaphragmatic excursion, resulting in impaired abdominal organ perfusion and decreased lung compliance. Monitoring of airway pressures is helpful for detecting changes in pulmonary compliance during abdominal closure. If inspiratory pressures are greater than 25 to 30 cm H_2O or intravesical or intragastric pressures are greater than 20 cm H_2O, primary closure is not recommended. Although measurement of various pressures can be helpful in determining whether or not to close the abdomen, clinical assessment of the neonate's condition is equally important. Any changes in ventilatory parameters and oxygen requirement must be communicated to the surgeon throughout the procedure and will impact the decision to perform primary closure of the abdomen. High ventilatory pressures and excessive FIO_2 are indications for postponing immediate abdominal closure.

Evidence of unacceptable intraabdominal pressure requires removal of fascial sutures and closure of only the skin or addition of a prosthesis, such as a silo chimney or silastic silo. The silo consists of a silastic or Teflon mesh that is sutured to the fascia of the defect. The synthetic material used to cover the lesion and the specific technique for placing the organs into the abdomen vary from center to center. After the silo is in place, the extraabdominal organs are gradually returned to the peritoneal cavity over the ensuing days. This gradual reduction can be done in the neonatal ICU and requires no anesthesia. When the abdominal contents have been largely returned, the infant is brought back to the operating room for complete closure.

Postoperative ICU care is recommended with continuation of direct monitoring of arterial blood gas concentrations to guide fluid replacement and management of mechanical ventilation. Fluid requirements will be less than those in the period before repair or silo placement but still will likely exceed maintenance requirements.

Hirschsprung's Disease

Hirschsprung's disease, or congenital aganglionic megacolon, is the most common cause of lower intestinal obstruction in full-term neonates. The incidence is approximately 1 in 5000 live births, with a pronounced male predominance.

SIGNS AND SYMPTOMS

Hirschsprung's disease may be evident at birth, and the diagnosis is made during the neonatal period in up to 80% of patients. Affected newborns show delayed passage of meconium, irritability, failure to thrive, and abdominal distention. The presentation of Hirschsprung's disease in older children includes constipation, fecal soiling, and diarrhea. Suction rectal biopsy findings confirm the diagnosis. The pathologic features in Hirschsprung's disease include absence of ganglion cells and the presence of hypertrophied nerve bundles that stain positively for acetylcholinesterase.

TREATMENT

The surgical approaches are varied and have undergone many modifications over time; they include the Swenson, Soave, Boley, and Duhamel operations. A primary pull-through procedure in which the diseased portion is removed and the normally innervated bowel segments are reanastomosed is the preferred surgical treatment for affected infants. However, a decompressive colostomy is indicated in infants who have severe enterocolitis or who have a markedly dilated proximal colon that might make a primary pull-through procedure unfeasible. Laparoscopically assisted repairs are becoming more popular and have produced successful outcomes in selected patients.

Affected newborns have partial or complete intestinal obstruction and require early decompression. The infants are kept on NPO status and given intravenous fluid replacement. If the infant has enterocolitis and/or systemic infection, antibiotics and even inotropic support may be needed. The outcomes for patients with surgically treated Hirschsprung's disease are reasonably good. Most patients attain fecal continence. However, in patients with retained aganglionic bowel or acquired aganglionosis, sequelae such as severe strictures, dysfunctional bowel, or intestinal neuronal dysplasia may occur, requiring reoperation.

MANAGEMENT OF ANESTHESIA

In elective procedures, either the inhalational or intravenous route may be used to induce general anesthesia. In urgent cases, such as in the situation of concomitant enterocolitis, full-stomach precautions should be taken. Anesthesia can be maintained with a mixture of air, oxygen, volatile agent, and muscle relaxant. Extra care should be taken in positioning, since these operations can be quite lengthy. A lithotomy position is required for anorectal pull-through procedures that involve both abdominal and perineal incisions. Intravenous catheters should be placed in the upper extremities, because the lower extremities may be included in the surgical field. Intraoperative blood loss is usually low, but third-space fluid losses can be significant. Patients may require an initial intravenous bolus of 10 to 20 mL/kg of crystalloid to offset the volume deficit resulting from bowel preparation and fasting.

Epidural anesthesia provides excellent intraoperative as well as postoperative analgesia in patients undergoing open abdominal procedures. Extubation at the end of surgery is routine. If regional techniques are not used, intravenous opioids are the mainstay of postoperative analgesia. Postoperative fluid requirements may be greater than maintenance requirements in the first 24 hours.

Anorectal Anomalies

The incidence of anorectal malformations is approximately 1 in 5000 live births. Anorectal anomalies include a spectrum of defects, most of which involve a fistula between the lower intestinal tract and the genitourinary structures. Additional genitourinary abnormalities are seen in many of these patients. Imperforate anus without fistula occurs in a small number of patients, especially in association with Down's syndrome and most commonly with the VACTERL association. Spinal and vertebral anomalies also occur in up to 50% of patients with anorectal malformations. Tethered cord is seen in approximately 25% of these patients. Cardiovascular anomalies such as atrial septal defect, patent ductus arteriosus, tetralogy of Fallot, and ventral septal defect are present in approximately one third of patients with imperforate anus.

SIGNS AND SYMPTOMS

Anorectal malformations are apparent upon examination of the perineum. The neonate may fail to pass meconium in the first 24 to 48 hours of life. Male infants with imperforate anus usually require emergent surgery (diverting colostomy) to relieve the obstruction, whereas in females, the presence of a rectovaginal (rectovestibular) fistula will allow passage of stool. Rectovesicular fistula is frequently seen in males and requires antibiotic prophylaxis to prevent urinary tract infection even after decompressive surgery until definitive repair is performed.

Affected newborns have partial or complete intestinal obstruction and require decompression. The infants are kept on NPO status and given intravenous fluids and nutritional supplements (peripheral nutrition and lipids). If the infant has a fistula as well, there may also be obstructive uropathy and associated systemic infection.

TREATMENT

Preliminary treatment for high lesions is a diverting colostomy followed at a later date by a posterior sagittal surgical repair that involves placing the rectum within the pelvic muscles with division and closure of rectourinary or rectovestibular fistulas. Low lesions such as perineal fistulas, on the other hand, may be repaired during the neonatal period without an initial diverting colostomy. The majority of patients with perineal fistula and rectal atresia can attain full urinary and fecal continence after definitive repairs. More severe sacral malformations are associated with a lower rate of full bowel and bladder control.

MANAGEMENT OF ANESTHESIA

Anesthetic management of patients undergoing decompressive colostomy or primary repair should be conducted as for any infant with bowel obstruction. Rapid-sequence induction is often employed, particularly if abdominal distention is significant. Definitive anorectal reconstruction is usually performed 1 to 12 months later. All defects can be repaired through a posterior sagittal approach, although some patients may also require an abdominal incision to mobilize a high rectum or vagina. Extra care should be taken in positioning and padding for these lengthy procedures. Neuromuscular blocking agents should be avoided, because electrical muscle stimulation is used throughout the procedure to identify muscle structures and to define the anterior and posterior limits of the new anus. Blood loss and third-space fluid losses are usually moderate. Intravenous catheters should be placed in upper extremities, because surgical positioning of the legs may impede venous flow or limit access to the intravenous catheter insertion sites.

Patients can usually be extubated at the end of the surgery. Analgesia can be provided with opioids, but these should be given to newborns and young infants in a monitored setting.

Pyloric Stenosis

Pyloric stenosis is one of the most common gastrointestinal abnormalities appearing in the first 6 months of life. This disorder has a polygenic mode of inheritance and occurs four times more commonly in males, more often in first-born infants, and more frequently in white infants. The incidence is approximately 1 in 300 live births. It is usually an isolated finding, and fewer than 10% of affected infants have other anomalies.

SIGNS AND SYMPTOMS

The lesion is a thickening of the circular muscles of the pylorus, with a gradually increasing obstruction of the gastric outlet. Pyloric stenosis presents as relentless postprandial, nonbilious projectile vomiting beginning at 2 to 5 weeks of age. Symptoms may develop as early as the first week and as late as the fifth month of life. Jaundice may occur in some infants. With continued vomiting of gastric contents, which contain sodium, potassium, chloride, and hydrogen, the infant classically develops a hypochloremic, hypokalemic metabolic alkalosis. With persistent vomiting, volume contraction ensues, and the kidneys respond by defending extracellular volume in preference to serum pH by conserving sodium and excreting hydrogen ions. The initially alkaline urine thus becomes acidic, and this paradoxic aciduria worsens the existing metabolic alkalosis. The severity of dehydration can be assessed by physical examination of skin turgor, mucous membranes, and anterior fontanelle, and measurement of resting vital signs. The more severe the fluid and electrolyte loss, the lower the serum chloride concentration. The diagnosis can be confirmed by palpation of an olivelike mass just below the xiphoid process, although this may be difficult to do in a struggling infant. Abdominal ultrasonography is both sensitive and specific in detecting a hypertrophied pylorus.

TREATMENT

The initial therapeutic approach is aimed at repletion of intravascular volume and correction of electrolyte and acid-base abnormalities. Severely dehydrated infants should receive an initial intravenous bolus (20 mL/kg) of isotonic normal saline to reexpand the intravascular volume. Further resuscitation is given as 5% dextrose in 0.45% NaCl at 1.5 times the maintenance rate. Potassium chloride 10 to 40 mEq/L can be added to the fluids if necessary when adequate urine output is demonstrated. Fluid resuscitation should be guided by measurement of serum electrolyte concentrations, which is essential for estimating the degree of dehydration, alkalosis, and metabolic derangements in these patients. Although this condition is considered a medical urgency and the corrective surgery elective once rehydration is complete and electrolyte levels are normalized, pyloromyotomy is done at all hours to minimize the duration of hospitalization.

MANAGEMENT OF ANESTHESIA

All patients with pyloric stenosis should be regarded as having full stomachs. Pulmonary aspiration of gastric fluid is a definite risk in infants with gastric outlet obstruction. Fortunately, barium swallow studies are rarely, if ever, done to confirm the diagnosis, and there is no added risk of contrast aspiration in most cases. The stomach should be emptied as completely as possible with a large-bore orogastric catheter before induction of anesthesia. Often, several passes of the suction catheter are needed to accomplish this. The airway can be secured by awake intubation or by use of a rapid-sequence technique after administration of a hypnotic and succinylcholine. Atropine may be given before induction or kept immediately available in case of bradycardia. Maintenance of anesthesia with volatile agents or low-dose inhaled anesthetics along with an infusion of remifentanil is acceptable. Muscle relaxation may be needed for surgical exposure. After tracheal intubation, an orogastric tube is reinserted and left in place during surgery so that air can be insufflated into the stomach to test for mucosal perforation after the hypertrophied muscle is split. An acetaminophen suppository can be administered after intubation. Alternatively, intravenous acetaminophen may be given if available. Longer-acting opioids are generally not needed.

The traditional open Ramstedt pyloromyotomy is a relatively simple procedure in the hands of skilled pediatric surgeons and completely resolves the problem. The operative mortality is less than 0.5%. Laparoscopic pyloromyotomy has become the dominant approach in most centers. This technique may require longer operative times but produces smaller surgical scars, and the patient may have an even more rapid recovery and resumption of full enteral nutrition. Infiltration of the incision sites with local anesthetics generally provides sufficient postoperative analgesia.

The patient can be extubated once the usual criteria are met at the conclusion of the procedure. However, postoperative respiratory depression often occurs in infants with pyloric stenosis. The cause may be related to cerebrospinal fluid (CSF) alkalosis that persists beyond correction of the serum pH. Infants anesthetized using a remifentanil infusion may have a decreased incidence of postoperative apnea. Occasionally, hypoglycemia may occur 2 to 3 hours after surgical correction of pyloric stenosis. This is most likely due to inadequate liver glycogen stores and cessation of intravenous dextrose infusions. Postoperatively, infants should remain in a monitored environment for several hours. Depending on the preference of the surgeon and the specifics of the procedure, infants usually can begin oral feedings 8 hours after the surgical repair. Hospital discharge often occurs within 24 hours of the end of the procedure.

Necrotizing Enterocolitis

Necrotizing enterocolitis (NEC) is characterized by varying degrees of mucosal or transmural necrosis of the intestine, most frequently involving the terminal ileum and proximal colon. It is the most common neonatal surgical emergency, resulting in substantial perinatal morbidity and mortality. The overall incidence is 1 to 3 in 100 live births, with 90% of cases seen in preterm newborns. The incidence and case fatality rates are inversely related to gestational age and birth weight. Neonates at greatest risk are those who are born at less than 32 weeks' gestation and who weigh less than 1500 g. NEC with bowel perforation carries a mortality rate of 30% to 50%.

SIGNS AND SYMPTOMS

Early signs and symptoms are often nonspecific and include recurrent apnea, lethargy, temperature instability, and glucose level instability. If therapy is not undertaken (and often even after prompt treatment), cardiovascular instability follows. More specific clinical manifestations of NEC are abdominal distention, high gastric residuals after feeding, evidence of malabsorption, and bloody or mucoid diarrhea. Metabolic acidosis is very common secondary to generalized peritonitis and hypovolemia. Neutropenia and thrombocytopenia are usually present and appear to be associated with gram-negative sepsis and platelet binding by endotoxin. The diagnosis of NEC is made clinically in correlation with abdominal plain radiographic findings. Pneumatosis intestinalis (air in the intestinal wall), air within the portal system, or free air within the peritoneal cavity are diagnostic of NEC in newborns. Pneumoperitoneum indicates intestinal perforation. However, perforation is frequently present without evidence of free air in the peritoneal cavity.

TREATMENT

Medical treatment, consisting of cessation of feeding, gastric decompression, and administration of intravenous fluids and antibiotics, can be successful in the management of neonates with NEC. However, there is pressure to resume enteral feeding in these ill preterm newborns, since recovery from the complications of preterm birth requires adequate nutrition. If abdominal distention is significant enough to impair ventilation, endotracheal intubation and mechanical ventilation are indicated. Hypotension is treated with crystalloid and blood products. Ionotropic agents such as dopamine may be required to improve cardiac output and bowel perfusion. Umbilical artery catheters should be removed, if present, to avoid compromising mesenteric blood flow. Placement of percutaneous abdominal drains in the neonatal ICU (without sedation or general anesthesia) is occasionally done. Surgery is reserved for neonates for whom medical management fails, as evidenced by bowel perforation, sepsis (peritonitis), and progressive metabolic acidosis indicating bowel necrosis. As many as 50% of infants with NEC require surgical intervention. The infants who do come to the operating room exhibit significant cardiovascular instability. NEC carries a high mortality, especially when medical management fails, in which case mortality approaches 25%. Some infants may require repeat bowel resections, which predisposes them to short-gut syndrome as well as complications from long-term parenteral nutrition, such as catheter-related infection and sepsis, and total parenteral nutrition cholestasis.

MANAGEMENT OF ANESTHESIA

Intraoperative care of the critically ill newborn is often more a resuscitation effort than management of general anesthesia. Newborns with NEC are usually hypovolemic and require aggressive fluid resuscitation with crystalloid and colloid solutions before induction of anesthesia. Blood and platelet transfusions are often necessary. Adequate monitoring of fluid resuscitation is critical. A peripheral artery catheter provides the ability to measure systemic blood pressure continuously and to monitor arterial blood gas concentrations, hematocrit, and electrolyte levels. It is very important to have adequate vascular access. If postoperative intravenous nutrition is planned, placement of a central venous line before the start of the surgery will provide excellent access for the procedure (although the small catheter diameter and long catheter length preclude rapid fluid or blood administration). It must be appreciated that rapid administration of fluid to preterm neonates may cause intracranial hemorrhage or reopening of the ductus arteriosus.

These infants are usually undergoing mechanical ventilation before surgery. If the infant is not already intubated, induction should proceed with full-stomach precautions and awareness of the infant's depleted intravascular volume and possible impaired contractility. Preoxygenation and, typically,

premedication with atropine should be accomplished before induction and laryngoscopy. An endotracheal tube should be chosen to allow ventilation with peak inflating pressures of more than 20 cm H_2O, because high intraabdominal pressures and decreased pulmonary compliance are likely to be encountered. The ventilator from the neonatal ICU usually allows for more effective ventilation in these tiny patients than most conventional ventilators used in operating rooms. Consideration should be given to bringing the neonatal ICU team (neonatologist, neonatal nurse, respiratory therapist) to help with transportation as well as intraoperative management. Maintenance of anesthesia is generally limited to the use of short-acting intravenous opioids (fentanyl) as tolerated, muscle relaxation, and replenishment of intravascular volume as needed. Inotropes such as dopamine may be required to maintain adequate cardiac output and bowel perfusion. Massive third-space losses necessitate aggressive volume resuscitation. All fluids and the operating room should be appropriately warmed to prevent hypothermia. Postoperative mechanical ventilation is usually required because of abdominal distention and co-existing RDS.

Even if there is minimal cardiovascular instability and fluid administration is not excessive, it is safer to transport the infant with a secure, protected airway until the patient's condition is determined to be stable in the neonatal ICU. Given the risk of bacteremia, neuraxial analgesia is not recommended for these patients. Postoperative pain is usually managed with intravenous opioids, often as continuous infusions in the neonatal ICU.

Biliary Atresia

Biliary atresia is characterized by obliteration or discontinuity of the extrahepatic bile duct system with resultant obstruction to bile flow. It has an overall incidence of 1 in 16,000 live births in Europe and North America but a much higher incidence in east Asian countries (e.g., 1 in 5000 in Taiwan). Associated anomalies such as intestinal malrotation, situs inversus, and polysplenia are seen in 10% to 15% of patients with biliary atresia.

SIGNS AND SYMPTOMS

Biliary atresia typically presents in the early weeks after birth with persistent jaundice accompanied by dark urine and acholic stool. Hepatomegaly and splenomegaly can both be seen, but the latter is usually a late sign. Any term infant who has jaundice for longer than 14 days should be evaluated for underlying hepatobiliary disease. Of note, conjugated hyperbilirubinemia is seen in most biliary diseases, whereas unconjugated hyperbilirubinemia is found in physiologic and breast-milk jaundice. However, a mixed picture of unconjugated and conjugated hyperbilirubinemia can occur in biliary atresia when the obstruction is so severe that bile spills into the systemic circulation before undergoing conjugation. There is relentless bile flow obstruction, and if the condition is left untreated, liver cirrhosis ensues and death occurs by 2 years of age. Initial diagnostic evaluation includes laboratory testing (bilirubin level, transaminase level, liver synthetic function tests, γ-glutamyltransferase level) and ultrasonography. Endoscopic retrograde cholangiopancreatography and even magnetic resonance cholangiopancreatography are occasionally performed, but these are limited in terms of both equipment size and availability at treatment centers. Diagnosis is confirmed by liver biopsy findings.

Early recognition and diagnosis are essential, because the success rate of surgical treatment depends largely on early restoration of bile flow.

TREATMENT

Kasai's operation (portoenterostomy) and liver transplantation are the cornerstones of treatment for biliary atresia. Portoenterostomy involves excision of the porta hepatis to expose microscopic ductular continuity that allows for bile flow, and results are best if it is performed by 8 weeks of age. A jejunal Roux loop is anastomosed to the exposed patent ductules to restore normal bile drainage into the intestinal tract. Although Kasai's portoenterostomy can achieve complete resolution of jaundice and restoration of hepatic metabolic and synthetic functions, progressive inflammation of the hepatobiliary tree may persist, leading to recurrence of bile flow obstruction. Because of this, a significant number of patients redevelop signs and symptoms of liver disease after an initial period of clinical improvement. Cholangitis is another common complication after Kasai's portoenterostomy.

Liver transplantation is a curative treatment for biliary atresia and remains as the last resort for patients in whom Kasai's procedure has failed. Indeed, biliary atresia is the most common indication for liver transplantation in children younger than 2 years of age.

MANAGEMENT OF ANESTHESIA

Preoperative evaluation and correction of coagulopathy is important. Vitamin K may be given 1 to 2 days before the scheduled procedure. A coagulation profile should be obtained, and a complete blood count and electrolyte panel should be performed and any abnormalities corrected accordingly. Most patients will arrive with a functioning intravenous catheter, and an intravenous induction technique is used, with the appropriate dose of a hypnotic agent and nondepolarizing muscle relaxant given to facilitate tracheal intubation. If ascites is present, rapid-sequence induction is indicated. Adequate venous access is important, and if it cannot be obtained, a central venous catheter should be placed. Insertion of a peripheral arterial catheter is recommended for both hemodynamic monitoring and frequent blood sampling to guide anesthetic and fluid management. Anesthesia can be maintained with low doses of inhaled agents along with opioids and muscle relaxants. Nitrous oxide should be avoided. Temperature maintenance is important and can be a challenge in these lengthy procedures with a large area of exposure. A moderate amount of blood loss is to be expected, but there is usually significant evaporative fluid loss. Of note, bleeding can be excessive with

liver transplantation. The reader is referred to Chapter 13 for a detailed discussion of the management of anesthesia for liver transplantation. Severe, sudden hypotension may occur if the inferior vena cava is compressed during surgical manipulation. The importance of keen observation and close communication between the surgeon and anesthesiologist cannot be overemphasized.

The infant should receive postoperative care in the ICU. Management of the patient will vary depending on the details of the procedure. If blood and evaporative losses were small and the infant demonstrates a stable hemodynamic profile, consideration can be given to early extubation. In many cases, postoperative mechanical ventilation is appropriate. Better pain control can also be achieved with more liberal doses of intravenous opioids in infants undergoing mechanical ventilation. Placement of an epidural catheter at the conclusion of the procedure can be considered only when there has been no coagulopathy.

Congenital Lobar Emphysema and Congenital Cystic Adenomatoid Malformation

CONGENITAL LOBAR EMPHYSEMA

Congenital lobar emphysema is the postnatal overdistention of an otherwise normal lobe of the lung that compresses adjacent normal lung units and leads to atelectasis. If this process continues, mediastinal shift with impairment of venous return can occur. Congenital lobar emphysema is a rare cause of respiratory distress in newborns. The affected bronchus allows passage of air on inspiration but limits expulsion of air on exhalation, which leads to air trapping and lobar overexpansion.

Pathologic causes of congenital lobar emphysema include collapse of bronchi resulting from hypoplasia of supporting cartilage, bronchial stenosis, mucous plugs, obstructing cysts, and vascular compression of bronchi. The most frequent site of involvement is the left upper lobe (40% to 50% of cases), followed by the right middle lobe (30% to 40%), and then the right upper lobe (20%). Acquired lobar emphysema may result from barotrauma associated with the treatment of bronchopulmonary dysplasia. Right lower lobe involvement is common in these cases as a result of endotracheal tube positioning. There is an increased incidence of congenital heart disease, particularly ventral septal defect and patent ductus arteriosus, in patients with congenital lobar emphysema. Twenty-five percent of cases of congenital lobar emphysema are diagnosed at birth and 50% of cases are diagnosed by 1 month of age.

The clinical presentation may range from mild tachypnea and wheezing to severe dyspnea and cyanosis. The chest radiograph typically shows faint bronchovascular markings and herniation of the affected lobe across the midline. With pneumothorax or congenital cysts, these marking are absent. Treatment consists of resection of the diseased lobe in infants who are symptomatic or who show disease progression. Long-term outcomes are generally excellent.

CONGENITAL CYSTIC ADENOMATOID MALFORMATION

The clinical presentation of congenital cystic adenomatoid malformation depends on the size of the lesion. Congenital cystic adenomatoid malformations are abnormal congenital cystic pockets that communicate with the tracheobronchial tree and may become overdistended because of air trapping. Up to 80% of affected infants exhibit respiratory distress in the newborn period as a result of compression of adjacent normal lung tissue. In this sense, the pathophysiology is similar to that seen with congenital lobar emphysema as described earlier.

Congenital cystic adenomatoid malformations are structurally similar to bronchioles but do not have alveoli, bronchial glands, or cartilage. The clinical manifestations includes tachypnea, grunting, use of accessory muscles of respiration, and cyanosis. In infants who have multiple cystic adenomatoid malformations, the radiographic appearance may be similar to that in patients with a congenital diaphragmatic hernia. Infants with small lesions may not come to medical attention until early childhood when a chest radiograph is done to evaluate pneumonia. Treatment is surgical resection of the affected lobe, and prognosis depends on the amount and health of the remaining lung tissues, which may be hypoplastic because of compression in utero.

MANAGEMENT OF ANESTHESIA

In the preoperative period, supplemental oxygen is administered and positive pressure should be studiously avoided. Infants in respiratory distress are kept on NPO status to minimize the risk of choking and aspiration.

The recommended induction technique for infants with either congenital lobar emphysema or congenital cystic adenomatoid malformations is inhalation, and induction represents the most critical phase of the perioperative period. In a struggling and distressed infant who may also be crying, the amount of trapped gas can increase. In addition, any positive pressure ventilation of the lungs before the chest is opened may cause abrupt, exaggerated expansion of emphysematous lobes or cystic spaces (gas enters but cannot leave because of a ball-valve effect), with sudden mediastinal shift and cardiac arrest. Because of this, the optimal technique is a smooth inhalation induction with sevoflurane and oxygen without, if possible, any positive pressure ventilation. However, the infant often develops apnea under deep levels of anesthesia, which necessitates the use of some positive pressure. Tracheal intubation without muscle relaxants and maintenance of spontaneous breathing with minimal positive airway pressures is recommended. Use of nitrous oxide is contraindicated because it can lead to rapid and untoward expansion of the emphysematous and cystic areas. The surgeon should be present at induction in the event that sudden cardiopulmonary decompensation necessitates urgent thoracotomy. If the induction goes well, without excessive expansion of the emphysematous lobe or adenomatoid malformation, general anesthesia may be supplemented with local anesthesia until the chest is opened and the pathologic lobe or cyst is delivered through the incision. A peripheral arterial catheter should be placed to monitor hemodynamic changes during surgical lung retraction and to allow for repeat blood gas sampling.

Meticulous attention must be paid to avoidance of nerve and other compression injuries during positioning (usually lateral decubitus with the infant's ipsilateral arm placed directly over the head). If a thoracoscopic approach is planned, one-lung ventilation is needed. In these small patients, lung isolation can be accomplished either with endobronchial intubation or with placement of a bronchial blocker (the smallest bronchial blocker, size 2F, can be placed through endotracheal tubes with an inner diameter as small as 3.5 to 4 mm but may also be placed outside of the endotracheal tube). Once the abnormal lung is resected, these infants may be paralyzed and mechanical ventilation begun. Infants who show sudden deterioration may require emergent needle aspiration or thoracotomy for decompression of the affected lung tissues.

Since the remaining lung tissue in patients with congenital lobar emphysema is normal, many of these infants demonstrate dramatic improvement once the emphysematous lobe is resected. Results are more variable in infants with congenital cystic adenomatoid malformations, since the remaining lung tissue may or may not be hypoplastic. Generally, the patient can be safely extubated at the end of the procedure. Postoperative atelectasis is common, however. Observation in a closely monitored setting is indicated in the immediately postoperative period. Analgesia can be provided with either neuraxial techniques or intermittent administration of intravenous opioids, but only practitioners with expert skills in the placement of infant thoracic epidural catheters should undertake this procedure.

CENTRAL NERVOUS SYSTEM DISORDERS

Cerebral Palsy

Cerebral palsy is a generic term used to describe a group of nonprogressive disorders characterized by kinetic and postural abnormalities. Although causes may differ, they all represent a common phenotype of motor dysfunction resulting from abnormalities that occurred in the *developing* brain. Therefore, clinical pictures similar or identical to cerebral palsy that are due to brain injuries that occurred from age 3 years through adulthood are not considered as cerebral palsy. Since cerebral palsy is a *nonprogressive* disorder of the CNS, it is also termed *static encephalopathy*, the clinical expression of which may vary over the course of the child's lifetime. Additional disturbances of sensation, perception, cognition, behavior, and electrical activity (seizures) are common.

SIGNS AND SYMPTOMS

Cerebral palsy can be generally categorized based on the resting tone, extremities involved, and presence of kinetic abnormalities. For example, *spastic quadriplegia* denotes baseline spasticity with impaired motor function of all four extremities and *spastic diplegia* denotes a spastic resting tone with motor dysfunction of either the two upper or the two lower extremities. Spastic monoplegia, triplegia, and hemiplegia also exist. If dyskinesia (abnormal movement) is the defining feature, then the term *dyskinetic cerebral palsy* is used. The specific movement abnormalities may be athetoid (slow, writhing movements), choreoathetoid (jerky, rhythmic movements alternating with athetosis), or dystonic. Less commonly, cerebellar dysfunction predominates and is categorized as ataxic cerebral palsy.

Spastic cerebral palsy types are the most common. Affected individuals manifest initial hypotonia (usually from age 6 months to 1 year) that later changes into spasticity. True hypotonic cerebral palsy is rare. A history of gross motor delays is almost universal and is commonly associated with delays in reaching other milestones (fine motor skills, language, social interaction). Intelligence can range from normal to severely impaired.

Truncal tone is often affected, which results in spinal curvature deformities such as scoliosis. Patients may experience recurrent aspiration pneumonia as a result of poor pharyngeal muscle tone and a high incidence of gastroesophageal reflux. Spasticity can lead to severe contractures that require medical therapy (baclofen, dantrolene, botulinum toxin A injection) and surgical interventions. Selective dorsal rhizotomy is occasionally performed to decrease the reflexive motor activation that occurs in response to the loss of descending inhibitory input.

Seizure disorder is common, and some children may be given antiepileptic medications even in the absence of seizures for off-label treatment of conditions such as spasticity and behavioral issues.

Diagnosis is mostly based on clinical findings in conjunction with a thorough investigation of the patient's prenatal, perinatal, and postnatal history as well as the intrapartum maternal history. Diagnostic imaging, including cranial ultrasonography (for neonates), computed tomography (CT), and magnetic resonance imaging (MRI), is helpful in identifying associated structural abnormalities.

MANAGEMENT OF ANESTHESIA

Patients with cerebral palsy can come for a variety of surgical procedures that may be simple or complex. Examples are ventriculoperitoneal shunt placement for hydrocephalus, dental restoration for poor dental hygiene, Nissen's fundoplication for severe reflux, posterior spinal fusion for scoliosis, and Achilles tenotomy for contractures. There is no single best anesthetic plan, because each patient will have a different combination of respiratory, gastrointestinal, and neurobehavorial problems.

Almost any anesthetic technique can be used; volatile agents need not be avoided, because cerebral palsy is not associated with malignant hyperthermia. Succinylcholine is not contraindicated but should be used with discretion. In general, children with cerebral palsy require a lower MAC of volatile anesthetics and have a longer emergence time than their healthy counterparts. This may be due in part to the intrinsic brain abnormality, but another contributor is often the sedative effects of many medications used to treat the various complications of cerebral palsy.

Low pharyngeal tone and a high incidence of gastroesophageal reflux disease call for a low threshold of endotracheal intubation to protect against aspiration, even for brief procedures. Administration and dosing of muscle relaxants should be done with caution, because these patients generally have prolonged recovery from neuromuscular blockade. Positioning is often difficult because of severe contractures; avoidance of compression injury to bony and soft tissues requires vigilance from all members of the perioperative team. For patients with seizure disorders, drug-drug interactions (e.g., cytochrome P-450 induction by antiepileptics) and the epileptogenic effects of some anesthetic agents (etomidate, ketamine) must be recognized. Extubation must occur only when the patient has fully recovered from neuromuscular blockade with as little residual anesthesia as possible. This is especially true for those with developmental disabilities, because these children are more likely to develop sedation-related hypoventilation.

Postoperative pain management must be meticulously planned and coordinated, since impaired communication is common and the child may not be able to voice complaints. Diazepam is an important adjunct in managing pain related to muscle spasm. Supplemental regional and epidural continuous analgesia are ideal, since they provide superior pain control and can help limit the use of medications with respiratory-depressant effects.

Hydrocephalus

Hydrocephalus is a disorder of CSF accumulation that results in ventricular dilation resulting from increased intracranial pressure (ICP). This is a different entity from ventricular dilatation resulting from parenchymal loss (periventricular white matter atrophy) with passive filling by CSF. Accumulation of CSF in hydrocephalus is due to an imbalance between CSF production and absorption. Hydrocephalus has many causes and can be congenital or acquired.

PATHOGENESIS

Hydrocephalus results from overproduction, impaired circulation, or underabsorption of CSF (Table 27-14). CSF is produced by the choroid plexus, a collection of highly vascularized and epithelium-lined villous folds located in the lateral, third, and fourth ventricles. CSF flows from the lateral ventricles into the midline third ventricle via the interventricular foramen of Monro. From there, CSF drains through the aqueduct of Sylvius into the midline fourth ventricle, which is connected to the posterior fossa cisterns by a pair of laterally located foramina of Luschka and a midline foramen of Magendie. Cisterns are focally enlarged intracranial subarachnoid spaces that channel CSF from the ventricular system and the spinal subarachnoid space up to the hemispheric convexity, where CSF is absorbed into the systemic circulation by the subarachnoid villi. Any disturbance in the normal production,

TABLE 27-14 ■ Causes of hydrocephalus
EXCESSIVE PRODUCTION OF CSF
Chorioid plexus papilloma
OBSTRUCTION OF CSF PATHWAYS
Obstruction within the ventricular system
Lateral ventricular (atrium, body, foramen of Monro)
Third ventricular
Aqueductal (congenital stenosis, mass lesions)
Fourth ventricular (Dandy-Walker malformation)
Obstruction within the subarachnoid space
Basal cisterns (Chiari I malformation, infection)
Convexity
DECREASED ABSORPTION OF CSF
Arachnoid villi pathologic process (inflammation)
Dural venous sinus obstructions (thrombus, tumor, infection)
Extracranial venous sinus obstruction (achondroplasia)

CSF, Cerebrospinal fluid.

flow, and absorption in the aforementioned pathway will lead to accumulation of CSF and increased ICP with resultant ventriculomegaly. Although hydrocephalus is characterized by ventricular dilation, a significant rise in ICP usually occurs before demonstrable change in ventricular size.

Hydrocephalus is rarely caused by CSF production but can be seen in choroid plexus disorders such as choroid plexus papillomas. The most common cause of congenital hydrocephalus is impaired circulation or obstruction of flow caused by structural abnormalities such as stenosis of the aqueduct of Sylvius, tumors, malformations (Chiari's malformation, Dandy-Walker malformation), and trauma-related defects. The most common genetic cause of congenital hydrocephalus is X-linked hydrocephalus due to aqueductal stenosis, which is associated with other CNS structural abnormalities as well as characteristic adducted thumbs. Hydrocephalus caused by decreased CSF absorption is infrequent and is seen mostly after CNS infections that cause inflammation of the subarachnoid villi. Intrauterine TORCHES infections (*to*xoplasmosis, *r*ubella, *c*ytomegalovirus infection, *h*erpes simplex, *s*yphilis) are classic examples.

SIGNS AND SYMPTOMS

Hydrocephalus can be acute, subacute, or chronic. The rate at which CSF accumulates and the compliance of the CNS determine the clinical presentation. In general, symptoms are nonspecific and are independent of the underlying cause. If hydrocephalus occurs before the closure of cranial sutures (approximately 18 to 24 months of age), the rise in ICP is generally mitigated by expansion of the intracranial space. Once cranial sutures have closed, the noncompliance of the system can lead to a rapid rise in ICP.

In newborns and infants, hydrocephalus most often manifests as an enlarged head resulting from separation of the cranial bone plates. The anterior fontanelle can be full or bulging, and the scalp veins may be prominent because of increased venous pressure. The infant may also display so-called sunsetting eyes, an impaired ability to gaze upward caused by compression of the midbrain. Other signs and symptoms of CNS parenchymal compression include third and sixth nerve palsy, papilledema, bradycardia, systemic hypertension, disturbances in respiratory pattern, endocrine abnormalities, and impaired fluid and electrolyte balance. Headaches along with nausea and vomiting result from stretching of the meninges and intracranial vessels. Infants may be irritable and then become progressively lethargic with increasing ICP. Stretching of the motor cortex can also occur if hydrocephalus is severe, resulting in spasticity. A continued rise in ICP that exhausts ventricular expansion capacity can cause disruption of the ventricular ependymal lining, which leads to parenchymal edema and necrosis with resultant white matter atrophy (periventricular leukomalacia).

Any newborn or infant with an enlarged head should undergo evaluation for hydrocephalus. Serial head circumference measurement is an easy and effective means of monitoring the progression of hydrocephalus. Most infants can be treated conservatively if head circumference increases at a slow and steady rate unless clinical symptoms are present. Rapid increase in size usually requires surgical intervention even if the child is relatively asymptomatic. Diagnosis is confirmed with neuroimaging (head ultrasonography for newborns, CT and MRI for infants and older children).

TREATMENT

Medical therapy mainly consists of diuretic treatment (furosemide and acetazolamide decrease CSF production), although this remains controversial in children. Serial lumbar punctures have also been tried, but are only a temporizing measure and do not significantly reduce the need for subsequent shunt surgery. Hydrocephalus associated with intracranial and intraventricular hemorrhage has been treated with fibrinolysis at some centers, but the benefits have not been shown to outweigh the potential risks.

The majority of children require surgical treatment in the form of either shunt placement or shuntless endoscopic third ventriculostomy (ETV). The former consists of inserting a catheter into the lateral ventricle that is connected to a one-way valved shunt system that drains into the right atrium (ventriculoatrial shunt) or the peritoneal space (ventriculoperitoneal shunt). Shunt malfunction can be due to infection or mechanical failure and occurs most frequently in the first year after placement (approximately 40% failure rate). In ETV, an endoscope is placed via a burr hole first into the lateral ventricle and then into the third ventricle, where a blunt perforation is made through its floor. This allows shuntless CSF drainage from the ventricular system into the cisterns beneath the third ventricle. Choroid plexectomy is sometimes performed at the same time to decrease overall CSF production. ETV is most successful in children older than 1 year of age. Finally, any structural cause of hydrocephalus such as tumor or Chiari's malformation must also be addressed.

MANAGEMENT OF ANESTHESIA

The most important anesthetic considerations in the child with hydrocephalus relate to the presence and severity of increased ICP. Positional change (head down, head flexion), behavioral change (crying), and physiologic change (hypercarbia) all can affect ICP. For this reason, the child should be kept in a head-up position with as few agitating maneuvers as possible. A delicate balance must be maintained between promoting calmness by pharmacologic means and minimizing the risk of hypoventilation. A careful preoperative assessment, consisting of history taking, review of current clinical symptoms, and physical examination, usually provides the most useful information about the severity of ICP and its impact on the child's neurologic status. Specifically, it is important to note the mental status (lethargy, drowsiness) as well as any focal neurologic deficits the child may have.

Inhalation induction may be acceptable in a child without clinical and/or radiographic evidence of severe intracranial hypertension. Volatile agents are potent cerebral vasodilators and increase ICP by increasing cerebral blood flow. This effect can be attenuated by preinduction hyperventilation, but this is not an easily accomplished or feasible task in most children. Children with significantly increased ICP are usually lethargic, which permits easier awake intravenous catheter placement. With the exception of ketamine, virtually all intravenous anesthetic agents lower ICP by decreasing cerebral blood volume and generally preserve cerebral perfusion pressure better than volatile agents. Ketamine is contraindicated because it can precipitate a sudden increase in ICP and rapid neurologic decompensation. The neurophysiologic effects of dexmedetomidine, an α_2-agonist, is not as well understood. Studies show that it generally decreases cerebral blood volume and cerebral blood flow and has minimal effect on the cerebral metabolic rate.

Succinylcholine may be used if necessary. It can increase cerebral blood flow and ICP, but the effects are transient and can be attenuated by premedication with a "defasciculating" dose of a nondepolarizing muscle relaxant.

Normocapnia should be maintained for patients with normal ICP, whereas mild hypocapnia is helpful to prevent further increases in ICP; severe hypocapnia can precipitate cerebral ischemia.

Invasive blood pressure monitoring is not needed in most cases of shunt surgery or ETV, but may be useful to help guide anesthetic management to optimize cerebral perfusion pressure, particularly if an ICP monitor is in place (cerebral perfusion pressure = mean arterial pressure − ICP).

Finally, positional changes can have serious consequences. Extreme positioning of the head (flexion, lateral rotation) can cause further displacement of a structural abnormality (Chiari's malformation) and impair venous drainage, which leads to increased ICP.

Cerebrovascular Anomalies

Cerebrovascular anomalies are uncommon in the pediatric population. However, they are an important cause of pediatric stroke and intracranial hemorrhage, each with significant morbidity and mortality. Stroke, commonly regarded as a problem limited to the adult population, is among the top 10 causes of death in children. Vascular abnormalities such as arteriovenous malformations, cavernous malformations, and aneurysms are the most important causes of hemorrhagic stroke, which accounts for nearly half of all stroke cases in children. Cerebrovascular arteriopathy, such as moyamoya disease, has recently become recognized as a major cause of ischemic stroke in children.

MANAGEMENT OF ANESTHESIA

Minimizing the risk of intracranial bleeding and preventing cerebral ischemia are the most important goals in the perioperative management of children with cerebrovascular anomalies. For children with moyamoya disease, a thorough preoperative assessment, particularly of the neurologic status, is extremely important; any deficits should be noted. It is also important to obtain a baseline trend of blood pressures during both awake and asleep states to determine the lowest pressure that the child may tolerate. The child should not be subjected to prolonged periods of fasting, because dehydration may precipitate cerebral ischemia. Thus, preoperative hydration is prudent to minimize hypotension upon induction of anesthesia. Preoperative anxiolysis is recommended; hyperventilation with anxiety or with crying must be avoided, because hypocarbia will lead to cerebral vasoconstriction, which further compromises cerebral perfusion. If an intravenous catheter is not in place, a slow inhalation induction is acceptable as long as the agent is titrated to minimize change in systemic blood pressure. An arterial line should be placed as soon as possible to establish uninterrupted blood pressure monitoring. Throughout the intraoperative course, blood pressure must be maintained within the child's baseline range. Ventilation parameters should be set to maintain normocarbia. Hypocarbia is detrimental because it will induce cerebral vasoconstriction; hypercarbia should also be avoided because vasodilation of the normal vasculature may create a steal from the affected vessels. Intraoperative electroencephalography is sometimes performed to detect potential ischemia related to surgical manipulation. Any changes in anesthetic level or drug administration should be communicated to the surgical team to avoid misinterpretation of potential anesthetic-related signal changes as ischemia. The child is still at risk for cerebral ischemia even after the completion of the surgery, because several months are required for new collateral formation to become fully established after indirect bypass procedures. Direct bypass procedures may reestablish flow immediately, but there is an attendant risk of reperfusion injury that may lead to cerebral edema. For this reason, a smooth emergence with adequate analgesia is important to avoid extreme hemodynamic changes.

The same principles apply to children with arteriovenous malformations who come for surgery; they are also at risk of ischemia. In addition, it is important to avoid hypertension perioperatively to minimize risk of bleeding or rupture, because the vessels of the malformation have weakened walls and may even have aneurysmal dilatations. Sudden hemorrhage can occur during the dissection and resection of arteriovenous malformations; thus, large-bore intravenous access must be established and reserved blood products arranged. If criteria are met, the child should be extubated as soon as possible to allow for neurologic examination.

Spina Bifida

Spina bifida is the most common form of neural tube defect (Figure 27-2), characterized by a cleft in the spinal column. The defect results from abnormal fusion of one or more vertebral posterior arches. This cleft can be covered by normal-appearing skin, which results in a hidden defect (*spina bifida occulta*) without involvement of the underlying neural structures. Meninges can herniate through the spinal cleft, creating a CSF-filled sac (*meningocele*) with or without skin covering. More often, both the spinal cord and meninges herniate through the spinal cleft (*myelomeningocele*) forming a defect that lacks a skin, and sometimes dural, covering. Overall, spina bifida represents the second most common type of congenital defect.

PATHOGENESIS

Normally, the neuroectoderm invaginates and closes to form the primary neural tube from which the future brain, spinal cord, spinal column, and overlying skin derive. Failure of neural tube closure, an event that normally is completed by 28 days' gestation, results in abnormal formation or fusion of any of the aforementioned elements. The precise causes of neural tube defects are not known. Over the years, multiple teratogens and vitamin deficiencies have been implicated. The clearest causal relationship that has been established is between folic acid deficiency and myelomeningocele. However, the exact mechanism by which folic acid may be protective against myelomeningocele formation is unclear. Valproic acid and carbamazepine have also been strongly associated with neural tube defects. A likely explanation for the effect of valproic acid is that it is a known folate antagonist.

SIGNS AND SYMPTOMS

The clinical presentation varies widely and depends on the elements involved and the severity of the defect. Spina bifida occulta, as its name implies, is sometimes discovered only incidentally, because normal skin hides the defect and the mild spinal cleft does not usually cause neurologic deficits. In most cases, however, the overlying skin displays an abnormal

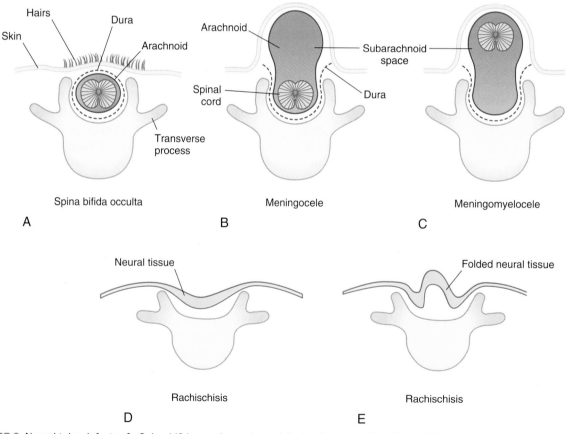

FIGURE 27-2 Neural tube defects. **A,** Spina bifida occulta—a bony defect only, covered by skin or skin with hair. **B,** Meningocele—protrusion of a fluid-filled sac only (no neural tissue present). **C,** Meningomyelocele—protrusion of a fluid-filled sac plus neural tissue. **D** and **E,** Rachischisis—defects characterized by an open neural tube. *(With permission from Holzman RS, Mancuso TJ, Polaner DM. A Practical Approach to Pediatric Anesthesia. 1st ed. Philadelphia, PA: Lippincott Williams & Wilkins; 2008:203, Fig 12.7.)*

lesion such as a dimple, hair patch, dermal sinus tract, hemangioma, or lipoma, the presence of which should alert the clinician to possible underlying spinal column and/or cord anomalies (e.g., tethered cord).

Meningoceles are normally diagnosed prenatally by fetal ultrasonography or at birth by the presence of a dorsal spinal mass. By definition, only the meninges are affected without nerve tissue involvement. For this reason, these patients generally do not have neurologic deficits and are not at noticeable risk of developing long-term neurologic sequelae. Once the meningocele is discovered, expeditious surgical repair is needed to prevent sac injury, infection, and CSF leak. Although nerves are not involved, there can be nerve root entrapment by fibrous bands in the sac. Thus, nerve injury is a potential problem during surgical sac ligation.

Myelomeningocele, in which a portion of the spinal cord is extruded into the herniated meningeal sac, is the most common type of spina bifida. Often the spinal cord ends in the sac with the spinal canal exposed in a splayed-open fashion, a condition known as *neural placode.* Children born with a myelomeningocele have varying degrees of motor and sensory deficits as well as bowel and bladder dysfunction. Any damage to the cord and spinal nerves evident at birth is usually irreversible. In severe cases, children may be born paraplegic and are bound for a wheelchair-dependent life. Over 90% of children born with a myelomeningocele also have a Chiari II malformation (also known as *Arnold-Chiari malformation*) which consists of caudal displacement of the cerebellar vermis, fourth ventricle, and medulla down through the foramen magnum into the cervical spinal canal. Hydrocephalus and other developmental brain abnormalities are also common. In addition, myelomeningoceles are associated with a high incidence of cardiac, esophageal, intestinal, renal, urogenital, and orthopedic anomalies.

TREATMENT

Meticulous care at birth is needed to prevent sac rupture and damage to the spinal cord. If the spinal canal is exposed, the myelomeningocele also requires moistened sponge coverage to avoid drying of the neural tissues. Surgical closure usually takes place within 24 to 48 hours of birth. Hydrocephalus, if present, may also require surgical intervention. A recent study comparing prenatal with postnatal repair of myelomeningocele showed that prenatal repair was associated with a lower rate of need for shunt surgery as well as a lower rate of death at 12 months of postnatal age. It was also associated with improved long-term mental and motor function. Prenatal surgery, however, is offered only at a few centers, has many exclusion criteria, and is associated with preterm birth and maternal morbidity. The majority of children with myelomeningocele have lifelong motor and sensory neurologic impairment as well as fecal and urinary incontinence.

MANAGEMENT OF ANESTHESIA

Positioning is one of the most critical aspects in the perioperative care of the child with open spina bifida lesions (meningocele and myelomeningocele). Maintaining the patient in the prone or lateral decubitus position is essential to avoid sac and nerve injury, particularly for myelomeningoceles. In some cases, the patient may be elevated on soft rolls or a donut-shaped gel support to avoid compression of the defect, so that endotracheal intubation can be accomplished with the patient in the supine position. However, some defects may be too large to risk supine positioning, and the anesthesiologist must always be prepared for a difficult intubation with the patient in the lateral decubitus position. Regardless of positioning during induction, surgical repair is always performed with the patient in the prone position. Because of this, meticulous attention must be paid to avoid compression injury to the eyes, brachial plexus, and any ventral defects such as bladder exstrophy, as well as compression of the inferior vena cava with resultant impaired venous return.

A comprehensive preoperative assessment is needed to identify specific anesthetic risks, because myelomeningoceles are often associated with other congenital anomalies. Although an Arnold-Chiari malformation is present in almost all cases of myelomeningocele, a clinically significant increase in ICP is rare; nevertheless, this must always be a consideration in the management of anesthesia. Respiratory insufficiency and apnea are also important perioperative concerns because of potential brainstem compression. Thus, tracheal extubation must take place only after the patient has regained adequate spontaneous respiratory effort and ventilation.

Intraoperative neuromonitoring is usually carried out to guide surgical repair. For this reason, an anesthetic plan that minimizes signal interference is important. Latex precautions should be observed for all of these patients, because repeated exposure to latex products throughout their lifetime predisposes these children to the development of severe latex allergy. Finally, myelomeningocele repair can be associated with significant blood and evaporative fluid loss. This is especially true for large defects that require extensive skin undermining for closure. Adequate intravenous access must be established before the start of surgery.

Craniosynostosis

Craniosynostosis is defined as premature closure of one or more cranial sutures. At birth, the cranium consists of floating bone plates that allow for rapid postnatal brain growth require a proportionate increase in the intracranial space. Four major sutures separate these bone plates: (1) metopic suture separates the frontal bones, (2) sagittal suture separates the parietal bones, (3) coronal suture separates the frontal from the parietal bones, and (4) lambdoid suture separates the parietal bones from the occipital bone (Figure 27-3). The sagittal suture is affected in over half of all cases of premature closure. Craniosynostosis can involve one or more sutures. Single-suture craniosynostosis is usually an isolated finding. Multiple-suture closure is often associated with other skull base suture abnormalities as seen in Apert's and Crouzon's syndromes.

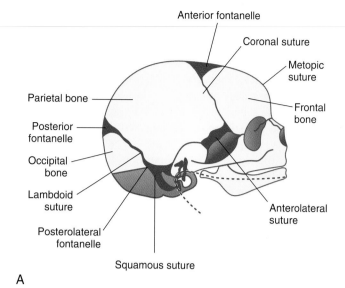

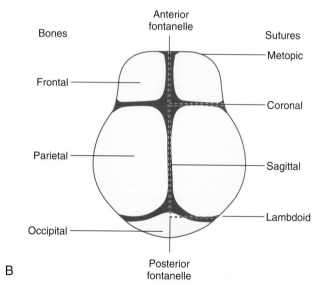

FIGURE 27-3 Cranial sutures and fontanelles. *(With permission from Holzman RS, Mancuso TJ, Polaner DM. A Practical Approach to Pediatric Anesthesia. 1st ed. Philadelphia, PA: Lippincott Williams & Wilkins; 2008:225, Fig 14.2.)*

PATHOGENESIS

Craniosynostosis can be a primary or a secondary event. In primary craniosynostosis, intrinsic bone ossification abnormalities cause premature closure of one or more sutures. In the secondary form, premature closure is due to slowed or arrested brain growth because bone plates are normally kept apart only by the outward force exerted by a growing brain. Brain growth failure causes premature closure of all sutures, resulting in a relatively normal-shaped but microcephalic head. On the other hand, closure of a single or an unbalanced combination of sutures results in various abnormal head shapes (Table 27-15). Because brain growth is restricted in one direction, brain growth can continue only along unrestricted suture lines, usually in a direction perpendicular to

the affected axis. For example, premature closure of the sagittal suture prevents normal lateral brain growth. Therefore, the brain can expand only in an anterior-posterior direction, which results in an elongated head shape or scaphocephaly. The exact mechanisms for primary craniosynostosis are unclear, but major theories include abnormal dural attachment that prevents bone plate separation and abnormal osteoblastic activity that causes accelerated bone fusion.

SIGNS AND SYMPTOMS

Craniosynostosis is usually evident at birth or during the first 2 years of life when rapid brain growth takes place (the brain achieves 75% of its adult size by 2 years of age; the rest occurs between 2 and 18 years of age). An increase in ICP occurs when brain growth continues against a nonexpanding calvaria. Thus, increased ICP is not usually seen in secondary craniosynostosis since there is little or no brain growth. Craniosynostosis involving one and even two sutures is also not associated with increased ICP because the brain can still expand in at least one other direction. Premature closure of multiple sutures frequently leads to increased ICP; children may present with lethargy, nausea and vomiting, and papilledema.

Head shape depends on the suture(s) involved. Scaphocephaly was discussed earlier. Other examples of abnormal head shapes are brachycephaly (flat, broad head resulting from coronal suture closure), plagiocephaly ("twisted head" resulting from unbalanced closure of the coronal or lambdoid suture), and trigonocephaly (triangular head shape with a peaked forehead resulting from metopic suture closure). The cloverleaf skull deformity, also known as *kleeblattschädel*, is the most severe type of craniosynostosis in which all sutures except the metopic and squamosal ones are fused.

In most cases of nonsyndromic craniosynostosis with only one or two sutures affected, the skull deformity poses only a cosmetic problem with no physiologic sequelae. However, the physical deformity can adversely impact the child's psychologic and social development if left untreated. Multiple-suture craniosynostosis is often associated with some degree of mental delay as well as hydrocephalus.

TREATMENT

Surgical repair may be done endoscopically (strip craniectomy) or may involve extensive calvarial reconstruction depending on the deformity. The latter usually requires a collaboration between specialists in neurosurgery and craniofacial plastic surgery and is associated with a much longer operative time and recovery period. Timing of the repair depends on the surgeon; some prefer to perform repair between 3 and 6 months of age and others between 8 and 12 months of age. Regardless, surgical correction is preferably performed before the age of 1 year to take advantage of the malleable skull, to optimize the potential for reossification, and to decrease the risk of neurologic damage, because this time period is associated with the greatest neural plasticity. Early intervention is also necessary to provide room for rapid brain growth during the first 2 years of life.

TABLE 27-15 ■ Classification of craniosynostosis based on involved cranial sutures

Affected suture	Morphology	Increased ICP	Mental retardation
Sagittal (40%)	Scaphocephaly (decreased biparietal and increased AP diameter)	Uncommon	Uncommon
Coronal			
Unilateral (15%)	Anterior plagiocephaly (marked craniofacial asymmetry, lopsided appearance)	Uncommon	Uncommon
Bilateral (20%)	Brachycephaly (short AP diameter and wide biparietal distance)	Common	Common
Metopic (4%)	Trigonocephaly (pointed forehead and narrow triangular skull)	Uncommon	Uncommon
Lambdoid (5%)			
Bilateral	Brachycephaly	Common	Common
Unilateral	Plagiocephaly	Uncommon	Uncommon
Multiple sutures			
Multisuture (most frequently the sagittal and coronal sutures)	Oxycephaly (high conical or pointed skull)	Common	Common
Kleeblattschädel (all sutures except the metopic and squamous)	Cloverleaf skull	Common	Common
All sutures10%)	Microcephaly	Common	Common

AP, Anteroposterior; *ICP,* intracranial pressure.

MANAGEMENT OF ANESTHESIA

A thorough preoperative evaluation is necessary, with particular attention to potential intracranial hypertension as well as co-existing morbidities. Associated anomalies of other organ systems (e.g., congenital heart disease) must be well delineated. In syndromic craniosynostosis other craniofacial abnormalities (midface and mandibular hypoplasia) are often present that can make airway management extremely challenging. For this reason, equipment for handling a potentially difficult airway must be prepared before the induction of anesthesia. When relevant, the anesthetic plan must also be tailored to avoid ICP increase.

Once the trachea is intubated, controlled ventilation should be set to maintain normocarbia unless hypocarbia is needed to minimize preexisting intracranial hypertension. Large-bore intravenous access is necessary, as is real-time blood pressure monitoring via an intraarterial catheter. The latter also allows for frequent blood sampling. Even in strip craniectomy procedures, excessive blood loss can still occur. Large-volume blood loss is usually the norm in open cranial vault reconstructive procedures (as high as one half to one blood volume in the majority of cases). Blood products must be available (preferably already in the operating room) before skin incision. Because most patients undergoing craniosynostosis repair are young infants, techniques to reduce blood loss (acute normovolemic hemodilution) and to minimize exposure to allogeneic blood (autodonation) are not feasible. Cell salvage can be done for small infants, because relevant cell saver reservoir sizes (as small as 25 mL) are now available. Use of antifibrinolytics such as aminocaproic acid and tranexamic acid have shown success in decreasing intraoperative blood loss and reducing the total transfusion volume.

However, large-scale studies involving the craniosynostosis population are lacking.

Other major intraoperative concerns are hypothermia, hypovolemia (large area of exposure for an extended period of time), and venous air embolism. Some practitioners elect to place a central venous catheter to evacuate air from the right atrium should a large air embolism occur. However, the small-sized catheter used in infants does not permit rapid air evacuation. Precordial Doppler imaging has a high sensitivity for detecting air embolism before hemodynamic changes are evident and is a valuable tool in all cases of open cranial vault reconstruction. Nitrous oxide should be avoided.

As much of the infant's body as possible should be covered with forced-hot-air blankets to minimize hypothermia because of the large area of exposure, lengthy surgical time, and large-volume fluid and blood resuscitation. Significant periorbital and facial edema can occur and may preclude immediate extubation. Unless there are concomitant craniofacial anomalies, most infants can be considered for extubation in the operating room if the edema is limited to the upper half of the face. Except for otherwise healthy infants who have undergone endoscopic repair, postoperative care in the ICU is required.

CRANIOFACIAL ANOMALIES

Cleft Lip and Palate

Orofacial clefts are a heterogeneous group of tissue approximation defects manifesting as cleft lip, cleft lip and palate, and cleft palate. These defects can occur in isolation or in association with a congenital syndrome.

PATHOGENESIS

Cleft lip is thought to result from failure of the fusion between the medial nasal and maxillary processes in early gestation. The defect usually occurs at the junction between the central and lateral portions of the upper lip on either side. Cleft lip may be limited to the upper lip or may extend into the alveolar ridge.

Cleft palate results from partial or complete failure in the apposition and fusion of the palatal shelves, which normally occurs between 8 and 12 weeks of gestation. *Complete cleft palate* denotes involvement of the uvula, soft palate, and hard palate. In some cases of cleft palate, the hard palate defect may be covered by a mucous membrane that may extend to partially cover the soft palate cleft as well; such defects are termed *submucous cleft palate.*

SIGNS AND SYMPTOMS

Newborns with orofacial clefts should have immediate evaluation and early referral to a craniofacial specialist. Depending on the defect, the child may be at risk for aspiration and airway obstruction, particularly if additional craniofacial anomalies are present. Feeding difficulty is universal, because the cleft defect prevents the generation of adequate negative pressure necessary for sucking. For this reason, failure to thrive is a common problem in children with cleft lip and cleft palate. Special feeding bottles and nipples are available that help to restore a more effective and energy-efficient feeding process. A multidisciplinary team of physicians, dentist, nutritionist, and speech therapist is recommended to address the physical and psychologic concerns that arise in different developmental stages of childhood.

Cleft palates are associated with a higher incidence of otitis media, because abnormal palatal muscle insertion impairs middle ear drainage. The threshold for performing myringotomy with ear tube placement is generally lower in these children.

TREATMENT

Cleft lip repair is typically performed between 6 and 12 weeks of age, whereas cleft palate repair is done at a later age, between 9 and 14 months. Timing and sequence of surgical repair (primary vs. staged repair) depend on surgeon preference in most cases. Timing of cleft palate repair is aimed at preventing further speech abnormalities and at minimizing distortion in facial growth (as can occur if repair is done too early).

Velopharyngeal insufficiency may persist even after complete cleft palate repair. The velopharyngeal sphincter or soft palate and the lateral and posterior pharyngeal walls normally appose to create velopharyngeal closure during speech, which prevents air from escaping out the nasal passage. Velopharyngeal insufficiency leads to a hypernasal voice, improper escape of air through the nose during speech, and improper pronunciation of certain consonants. Pharyngoplasty is performed to treat velopharyngeal insufficiency in older children.

MANAGEMENT OF ANESTHESIA

Children with cleft lip or palate generally undergo standard inhalation induction of anesthesia followed by endotracheal intubation via direct laryngoscopy uneventfully. Concurrent cleft lip and palate defects as well as syndromic orofacial clefts may portend difficult intubation, and appropriate preparations for a difficult airway must be made in advance. If a laryngeal mask airway is considered to aid intubation, the device must be placed carefully to prevent disruption of any previous cleft palate repairs.

Preformed oral RAE tracheal tubes are preferred for their low profile and better fit with the Dingman-Dott mouth retractor used during surgery. Meticulous attention must be paid to securing the endotracheal tube, because frequent surgical manipulations predispose to unintentional extubation. Cleft repair may also be done in positions that increase the risk of unplanned extubation (e.g., Rose's position, in which the patient's head is pulled over the edge of the operating table and placed in the surgeon's lap).

Significant edema of the tongue, palate, and pharyngeal tissues can occur from compression by the mouth retractor and may preclude immediate extubation. Placement of a nasopharyngeal airway by the surgeon in patients with known difficult airway or anticipated difficult extubation may be helpful in some cases.

Pain control must be balanced against the risk of respiratory depression. Intravenous or rectal acetaminophen as well as regional anesthesia (infraorbital blocks) should be considered.

Mandibular Hypoplasia

Hypoplasia of the mandible is a common congenital anomaly. Its presentation varies greatly depending on the cause and whether it is associated with other craniofacial skeletal and soft tissue abnormalities. It may arise as a result of extrinsic intrauterine constraint on development or intrinsic growth disturbance. The majority of cases occur as part of a co-existing syndrome; nonsyndromic isolated defects are rare. A universal feature in congenital mandibular hypoplasia is airway compromise resulting from the constricted mandibular space with resultant glossoptosis (posterior prolapse of the tongue). The following sections discuss several congenital disorders that share mandibular hypoplasia as a prominent feature.

PIERRE ROBIN SEQUENCE

Pierre Robin sequence, previously termed *Pierre Robin syndrome,* consists of three congenital orofacial abnormalities: micrognathia (small mandible) or retrognathia (posterior displacement of mandible), glossoptosis, and cleft palate (present in almost all cases). It is more appropriately termed *sequence* rather than *syndrome* because the latter is reserved to describe disorders of morphogenesis in which a single cause (e.g., chromosomal deletion) produces multiple defects simultaneously. In Pierre Robin sequence, the events occur in *sequence,* with one defect leading to the next. The most widely accepted theory for the cause of Pierre Robin sequence is one of mechanical constraint. Mandibular hypoplasia, either from physical intrauterine compression or intrinsic genetic growth deficiency, is thought to be the initial event. Mandibular crowding displaces the tongue posteriorly and superiorly, and thereby prevents closure of the palatal shelves with resultant cleft palate. Autosomal recessive and X-linked inheritance patterns are possible. Pierre Robin sequence can be syndromic or nonsyndromic. Some congenital disorders associated with Pierre Robin sequence are Stickler's syndrome, velocardiofacial syndrome, hemifacial microsomia, and fetal alcohol syndrome.

Affected newborns have varying degrees of airway obstruction, often in association with feeding difficulties and gastroesophageal reflux. Intervention is mostly aimed at restoring a patent airway. Additional anomalies that independently cause feeding problems are also addressed. Treatments for airway obstruction range from simple lateral or prone positioning to tongue-lip adhesion, mandibular distraction, and even tracheostomy. Particularly in nonsyndromic cases, airway obstruction decreases over time with mandibular growth, but most patients still require early surgical intervention to address glossoptosis.

HEMIFACIAL MICROSOMIA

Hemifacial microsomia is the one of the most common congenital facial anomalies (second only to cleft lip and palate). It is a facial asymmetry disorder that unilaterally affects bone, muscle, and soft tissue structures. Hemifacial microsomia typically affects the lower half of the face with prominent hypoplasia of the malar-maxillary-mandibular complex and variable involvement of the ear, temporomandibular joint, and orbit as well as the cervical spine. *Goldenhar's syndrome* (oculoauriculovertebral syndrome or OAV) can be considered the most severe form of syndromic hemifacial microsomia, characterized by colobomas and vertebral anomalies in addition to facial asymmetry. Beyond the obvious structural abnormality, osseous impingement on nerves can lead to neurologic deficits such as hearing loss. Some experts advocate the use of classification systems like OMENS (*o*cular/orbital anomaly, *m*andibular hypoplasia, *e*ar anomaly, *n*erve involvement, *s*oft tissue deficiency) to better categorize disease presentation, as this may allow for more targeted treatment plans. The exact cause of hemifacial microsomia is yet to be determined, but it is generally thought to be related to developmental abnormalities of the first and possibly second branchial arches.

TREACHER COLLINS SYNDROME

Treacher Collins syndrome, also known as *mandibulofacial dysostosis* (defective ossification or formation of bone), is a rare craniofacial anomaly with an autosomal dominant disorder mode of inheritance and variable expression. There is bilateral and symmetric underdevelopment of structures deriving from the first and second pharyngeal arch, groove, and pouch leading to hypoplasia of the supraorbital rims, zygoma, midfacial bones, and mandible as well as ear deformities and cleft palate (seen in 30%). The Treacher Collins syndrome facies features downward-sloping palpebral fissures, small or absent cheek bones, a normal-sized nose that may appear large against background hypoplasia, malformed pinnae, ear tags, abnormal external auditory canal, and receding chin. Occasionally,

choanal atresia may be present. Intelligence is usually not affected unless hearing loss is not promptly recognized and addressed. A small percentage of patients with Treacher Collins syndrome may have concomitant congenital heart disease.

Immediate concerns revolve around airway protection. Tracheostomy may be needed at birth to restore airway patency. Swallowing difficulties lead to failure to thrive, and early gastrostomy is frequently needed for feeding. Children with Treacher Collins syndrome typically require multiple craniofacial and dental corrective surgeries throughout their childhood and adolescence.

MANAGEMENT OF ANESTHESIA

Concerns central to the perioperative care of patients with mandibular hypoplasia relate mainly to airway management. A detailed preoperative assessment will reveal co-existing abnormalities, which occur in the majority of cases.

Patients with mandibular hypoplasia, especially in association with Treacher Collins syndrome and hemifacial microsomia, not only are difficult to intubate but may be nearly impossible to mask ventilate. Therefore, it is not always feasible to perform endotracheal intubation after the induction of general anesthesia. When anesthesia can be safely induced, maintenance of spontaneous ventilation is of utmost importance before the airway is secured. Maneuvers to pull the tongue forward are helpful, since glossoptosis is a major component of airway obstruction. A laryngeal mask airway may serve well to assist with ventilation and as a conduit for intubation. Intubating laryngeal mask airway devices such as the Air-Q now exist in pediatric sizes that accommodate most neonates and infants. Direct laryngoscopy is generally difficult regardless of blade type. Alternative means for visualizing the vocal cords such as traditional fiberscope, videolaryngoscope, and optical laryngoscope must be prepared and ready for use from the outset. Several surgical procedures specific to mandibular hypoplasia require nasotracheal intubation.

Drugs with respiratory-depressant effects should be used sparingly. Analgesic adjuncts including dexmedetomidine, ketamine, acetaminophen, and regional analgesia should be considered whenever possible. Timing of extubation is as important as, if not more important than, initial airway management, since significant postsurgical edema and in-situ distraction devices may be present that will make rescue mask ventilation and intubation extremely difficult or impossible. Some patients should be kept intubated for several days until better extubation conditions exist.

Midface Hypoplasia

Whereas syndromes with mandibular hypoplasia have underdevelopment of the lower half of the face, disorders with midface hypoplasia result in underdevelopment of the eye sockets, cheek bones, and upper jaw. Growth deficiency of the midface produces a characteristic concave appearance with wide-set eyes (hypertelorism) that are often proptotic, flattened nasal bridge, as well as a large underbite. Isolated mild forms of midface hypoplasia can occur and do not require treatment unless there is significant proptosis (predisposing to keratoconjunctivitis), severe malocclusion, and obstructive sleep apnea. Syndromic midface hypoplasia is frequently associated with multiple other congenital anomalies such as craniosynostosis, syndactyly, and congenital heart disease. Achondroplasia (dwarfism) is a well-recognized disorder featuring midface hypoplasia.

APERT'S SYNDROME

Apert's syndrome is a rare inherited disorder (autosomal dominant) characterized by acrocephalosyndactyly. The cranium, midface, and bones and soft tissues of the hands and feet are affected. The result is a combination of craniosynostosis, midface hypoplasia, and symmetric syndactyly of the extremities with cutaneous and bony fusion. Turribrachycephaly (towering of the skull), hypertelorism, and low-set ears are also prominent features. Occasionally, choanal atresia, tracheal stenosis, cervical spine fusion, congenital heart defects, and genitourinary anomalies are also present. Premature closure of the skull bones causing increased ICP may be an important cause of developmental delay.

Most patients with Apert's syndrome experience some degree of airway obstruction as a result of small nasopharyngeal and oropharyngeal dimensions, particularly if choanal atresia and/or tracheal stenosis are present. Obstructive sleep apnea is common and must be addressed early to avoid development of cor pulmonale. Eye complaints include proptosis and exophthalmos predisposing to corneal injury, amblyopia, strabismus, and optic nerve atrophy.

CROUZON'S SYNDROME

Crouzon's syndrome shares many clinical features with Apert's syndrome, but the viscera and extremities are spared. Also known as *craniofacial dysostosis* (malformation of the face and skull bones), it is a hereditary disorder (autosomal dominant) characterized by craniosynostosis, midface hypoplasia, mandibular prognathism, and shallow eye sockets with hypertelorism and proptosis. As a result of frequent premature fusion of the coronal sutures, brachycephaly (short and broad head) is usually seen. Mental delay is not an intrinsic part of Crouzon's syndrome but may occur due to increased ICP and hearing impairment. Conductive hearing loss is common due to ear canal abnormalities (atresia or stenosis). Airway obstructive problems are similar to those seen in Apert's syndrome. Of note, acanthosis nigricans is seen in approximately 5% of patients with Crouzon's syndrome.

MANAGEMENT OF ANESTHESIA

Patients with midface hypoplasia typically come to the operating room for midface advancement procedures, adenotonsillectomy, and cranial vault reconstruction if craniosynostosis is present. Some may require tracheostomy at an early age to establish airway patency. A thorough preoperative assessment is important to evaluate for degree of airway obstruction as well as presence of comorbid conditions.

As with mandibular hypoplasia, mask ventilation and tracheal intubation may be extremely difficult, especially if there are cervical spine abnormalities that limit neck extension. Preparations for a potentially difficult airway must be made, as would be done in any case with an anticipated challenging airway.

Given the characteristic proptosis, special attention must be paid to the eyes to avoid corneal and compression ophthalmic injury. A history of headache, vomiting, and somnolence should raise suspicion of increased ICP, and the anesthetic plan should be tailored accordingly. Finally, intravenous access may be extremely difficult in patients with Apert's syndrome depending on the severity of syndactyly.

UPPER AIRWAY DISORDERS

Acute Epiglottitis (Supraglottitis)

Acute epiglottitis, also termed *supraglottitis,* is a life-threatening infection of the epiglottis and adjacent supraglottic structures. Specifically, it is a cellulitis of the stratified squamous epithelium of these structures, including the lingular surface of the epiglottis, the aryepiglottic folds, and the arytenoids. Occasionally, the uvula is also affected. Subglottic structures, including the laryngeal surface of the epiglottis, are generally spared.

PATHOGENESIS

Acute epiglottitis results from direct bacterial invasion of the epithelial layer of the supraglottic structures, which leads to rapid and severe inflammation. The causative organism can be bacterial, viral, or fungal, and the posterior nasopharynx serves as the primary source of pathogens in many cases. A bacterial origin is most common in otherwise healthy children. Historically, *Haemophilus influenzae* type b (Hib) was the main pathogen and accounted for over 75% of cases. The institution of widespread immunization against Hib in the late 1980s has since dramatically decreased the overall incidence of epiglottitis. Today, immunization against Hib is recommended for all children younger than 5 years of age, with the first dose given at 2 months of age. Nonetheless, epiglottitis can still occur in fully Hib-immunized children, which may be due to the acellular composition of some Hib vaccines. In the postvaccination era, the primary pathogens include *Haemophilus parainfluenzae,* group A streptococci, pneumococci, and staphylococci. In immunocompromised patients, atypical pathogens such as *Candida* species, herpes simplex type 1, varicella-zoster virus, and parainfluenza virus must also be considered.

SIGNS AND SYMPTOMS

The highest incidence of epiglottitis has historically been seen in children aged 2 to 6 years, although this trend reflects mostly the pre–Hib vaccination era. Epiglottitis can also occur in infants, older children, and occasionally adults. The classic presentation of acute epiglottitis is that of a toxic-appearing, agitated child with a high fever and the so-called 4 Ds: dysphagia, dysphonia, dyspnea, and drooling. Parents typically report a history of the child's complaining of severe sore throat with muffled voice and sudden onset of high fever. Typical symptoms of upper respiratory tract infection such as rhinorrhea and cough are usually absent, although a croupy cough may be present in rare cases; the cough may confuse the clinical picture and make it more difficult to distinguish the condition from laryngotracheobronchitis, a different infectious entity (Table 27-16). The child often assumes a characteristic tripod posture with the trunk leaning forward supported by the arms and a hyperextended neck with the chin thrust forward in an effort to maximize airflow. Inspiratory stridor is a late feature and should alert the practitioner to impending complete upper airway obstruction. Indeed, the course of acute epiglottitis spirals downward rapidly, and the condition may be fatal within 6 to 12 hours of onset of initial symptoms. There is considerable variability among clinicians regarding the use of imaging in making the diagnosis. A lateral neck radiograph typically shows the thumb sign, representing the shadow created by a swollen epiglottis obstructing the airway. Because this is a rapidly fatal disease, the diagnosis is based principally on the clinical picture.

The most common and feared complication of acute epiglottitis is airway obstruction, thus the need for expeditious diagnosis and airway control. Other complications of epiglottitis include epiglottic abscess, secondary infection (e.g., pneumonia, cervical adenitis, meningitis, and bacteremia leading to distant infections such as septic arthritis), and necrotizing epiglottitis.

MANAGEMENT OF ANESTHESIA

The mainstay in the management of acute epiglottitis is airway control, and its achievement should always involve a team of a pediatric anesthesiologist, a pediatric intensivist, and an otolaryngologist. The child should be kept in the tripod posture. Any fear- or agitation-provoking maneuver or procedure such as establishment of intravenous access should be deferred until definitive airway protection is established. Expeditious transfer to the operating room should be undertaken with oxygen, pulse oximetry, and other resuscitative tools available, including medications and intubation equipment. The child should always be accompanied by a physician with expert airway management skills during transfer. Equipment for tracheal intubation and possible emergent tracheostomy–needle cricothyrotomy must be immediately available. Styletted endotracheal tubes in one to two sizes smaller than that predicted by the child's age must be prepared, because the airway caliber will invariably be reduced.

Anesthesia is induced via inhalation with the child in a sitting position. A calm induction with maintenance of spontaneous ventilation is paramount to safe practice. Application of moderate continuous positive pressure (10 to 15 cm H_2O) will help to minimize further reduction in airway caliber caused by collapse of the pharyngeal soft tissues with anesthesia induction. Once the child is adequately anesthetized, intravenous access can be established, followed by direct laryngoscopy and orotracheal intubation. An air leak around the endotracheal tube at or below 25 cm H_2O of pressure must be demonstrated to prevent additional tracheal damage.

Postoperative ICU care is mandatory. Timing of extubation depends on resolution of clinical signs and symptoms (abatement of fever, neutrophilia, and increasing air leak around the endotracheal tube) confirmed by repeat examination of the supraglottic structures by direct vision or flexible fibroscopy. In most cases, the child can be extubated in 24 to 48 hours after initiation of appropriate therapy (antibiotics with or without corticosteroids).

Croup (Laryngotracheitis and Laryngotracheobronchitis)

Croup is a common infectious disease of the subglottic airway structures, including but not limited to the larynx and trachea. Because of the variability in the level of involvement, the term *croup* has been used in the general literature to describe a variety of upper airway disorders, including laryngitis, laryngotracheitis, laryngotracheobronchitis, bacterial tracheitis, and spasmodic croup. For the purpose of this discussion, *croup* refers to laryngotracheitis and laryngotracheobronchitis (involvement of the bronchi in addition to the larynx and trachea) because the two are often clinically indistinguishable.

TABLE 27-16	Clinical features of acute epiglottitis and laryngotracheobronchitis	
Parameter	**Acute epiglottitis**	**Laryngotracheobronchitis**
Age group affected	2-6 yr	<2 yr
Incidence	Accounts for 5% of cases of stridor in children	Accounts for about 80% of cases of stridor in children
Etiologic agent	Bacterial	Viral
Onset	Rapid over 24 hr	Gradual over 24-72 hr
Signs and symptoms	4 Ds (dysphagia, dysphonia, dyspnea, drooling), high fever, tripod position	Inspiratory stridor, barking cough, rhinorrhea, mild fever (rarely >39° C)
Cell counts	Neutrophilia	Lymphocytosis
Lateral neck radiograph	Swollen epiglottis (thumb sign)	Subglottic narrowing (steeple sign)
Treatment	Oxygen, urgent tracheal intubation or tracheostomy under general anesthesia, fluids, antibiotics, corticosteroids (?)	Oxygen, aerosolized racemic epinephrine, humidification, fluids, corticosteroids, tracheal intubation for severe airway obstruction

PATHOGENESIS

Whereas acute epiglottitis is primarily a *bacterial* infection of the *supraglottic* structures, croup is primarily a *viral* infection of the *subglottic* structures. The inhaled pathogen initially infects the nasal and pharyngeal mucosal epithelium and then eventually spreads to the larynx and trachea. Cellular infiltration of the mucosal and submucosal layers of the subglottic structures leads to edema and inflammation, most pronounced at the cricoid ring because this is the narrowest part of the pediatric trachea. Since the inflammation is surrounded by a relatively firm and nonstretchable tube of cartilaginous ring structures, there is inward narrowing with early airflow obstruction. Fibrinous exudates and pseudomembranes may form, which further exacerbate airway narrowing.

The parainfluenza virus family (mostly type 1) accounts for the majority of cases. Other important viral pathogens are respiratory syncytial virus, influenza viruses type A and B, adenovirus, and less frequently human metapneumovirus, coronavirus, rhinovirus, and even measles during measles outbreaks. In the minority of cases attributable to a bacterial pathogen, *Mycoplasma pneumoniae* is the main culprit. Secondary bacterial infections leading to more severe laryngotracheobronchitis and even laryngotracheobronchopneumonitis are usually caused by *Staphylococcus aureus, Streptococcus pyogenes,* and *Streptococcus pneumoniae.*

SIGNS AND SYMPTOMS

In contrast to acute epiglottitis with its rapid progression, croup has a gradual onset starting with symptoms of an upper respiratory tract infection that progress to include upper airway obstructive symptoms over days to sometimes longer than a week. Croup occurs between 6 months and 3 years of age with a peak incidence around the second year of life. The child usually has a several-day history of rhinorrhea, cough, sore throat, and low-grade fever that progresses to the distinctive barking or seal-like cough along with hoarse voice and inspiratory stridor. Symptoms are worse in the supine position, and thus the child with croup prefers to sit or to be held upright.

Diagnosis is made clinically; radiologic and laboratory confirmatory tests are not needed. When radiographs are taken, one may see the classic steeple sign on an anteroposterior projection, which represents a long area of narrowing in the subglottic region. However, radiographic findings are not pathognomonic and generally do not correlate well with clinical severity. Inspiratory stridor is the key element in determining disease severity. Although determination of the causative agent is not needed to make the diagnosis of croup, such testing is useful in planning appropriate methods of patient isolation and potentially initiating antiviral therapy (particularly if influenza is suspected).

TREATMENT

Treatment is guided by disease severity based on a number of clinical parameters, including stridor, air entry, retractions, cyanosis, and level of consciousness. For much of the twentieth century, mist therapy (treatment with humidified air) was the cornerstone of the management of croup, but it has become largely obsolete with the introduction of steroid therapy. All experts now recommend routine administration of corticosteroid in the treatment of croup. The most cited regimens are (1) single-dose dexamethasone (0.6 mg/kg PO or IM) and (2) nebulized budesonide (2 mg in 4 mL of water). There is still some debate over the benefit of single versus multiple doses of corticosteroids as well as the exact dose of dexamethasone required (0.15 mg/kg vs. 0.6 mg/kg). Regardless, corticosteroid therapy has emerged as the single most important outpatient treatment of croup and has significantly reduced the rates of hospitalization. Children with severe croup should be treated with nebulized epinephrine (0.5 mL of 2.25% racemic epinephrine in 4.5 mL of normal saline or L-epinephrine diluted in 5 mL of normal saline at a ratio of 1:1000). Even if the plan is for potential discharge, children should be observed for at least 2 to 4 hours after the last nebulized epinephrine treatment for possible return of obstructive symptoms. Often nebulized epinephrine treatment needs to be repeated several times to minimize the need for endotracheal intubation.

Unless there is extensive distal spread to the lower airways, croup is generally a self-limited infection that lasts approximately 72 hours. However, life-threatening airway obstruction can occur in rare cases (<1%) and requires endotracheal intubation. As in the case of acute epiglottitis, children with croup should be intubated with a smaller endotracheal tube than that predicted for their age given the expected subglottic narrowing. Timing of extubation will depend on resolution of croup symptoms as well as treatment of any associated complications such as bacterial superinfection of the lower airways. Of note, children with recurrent croup should be evaluated for occult conditions such as subglottic stenosis, laryngeal clefts, and laryngomalacia.

MANAGEMENT OF ANESTHESIA

Endotracheal intubation in a child with croup, as in any child with airway disorders, should be carried out in a controlled setting such as the operating room with all necessary drugs and equipment available. The induction of anesthesia is carried out in a manner to similar that described for a child with acute epiglottitis.

Postintubation Laryngeal Edema

Postintubation laryngeal edema, also termed *postintubation croup* (not to be confused with infectious croup), is a potential complication of all tracheal intubations regardless of age. It is most commonly discussed in the context of pediatric patients, because infants and children have smaller absolute tracheal diameters and thus have the highest incidence of developing clinically significant postintubation laryngeal edema. Although there may be predisposing factors (Table 27-17), this is an iatrogenic disorder resulting directly from endotracheal intubation.

TABLE 27-17   ■   **Factors associated with postintubation laryngeal edema**

Age <4 yr
Tight-fitting endotracheal tube, no audible leak at or below
  25 cm H$_2$O pressure
Traumatic or repeated intubation
Prolonged intubation
Overinflation of endotracheal tube cuff
Inadequate anesthesia during intubation
Head repositioning while intubated
History of infectious or postintubation croup
Neck or airway surgery
Upper respiratory tract infection
Trisomy 21

PATHOGENESIS

The majority of cases of postintubation laryngeal edema are due to the use of an inappropriately large endotracheal tube. The tracheal mucosa requires perfusion just as do all other living tissues. Tracheal mucosal perfusion is impaired at pressures above 25 cm H$_2$O, and tracheal mucosal ischemia ensues once the pressure exceeds 30 cm H$_2$O. Severe consequences such as deep tracheal ulceration and tracheal rupture can also occur. Postintubation laryngeal edema has the highest incidence in children between the ages of 1 and 4 years. The pressure from a tightly fitting endotracheal tube causes tracheal mucosal ischemic damage, which leads to edema and narrowing of the subglottic airway. Occasionally, edema may also occur at the glottic level. Although a different entity from infectious croup, postintubation croup shares a similar pathophysiology with the same outcome of a reduction in the airway caliber.

SIGNS AND SYMPTOMS

Postintubation croup typically manifests within 30 to 60 minutes of extubation and is characterized by a barking or croupy cough, hoarseness, and stridor. As severity increases, nasal flaring, respiratory retractions, hypoxemia, cyanosis, and a decrease in the level of consciousness may also be observed. Treatment is aimed at reducing airway edema. Keeping the child calm is also important, because crying will further exacerbate symptoms. In mild cases of postintubation croup, mist therapy with cool, humidified air may be helpful. In general, repeated nebulized epinephrine treatments are needed to produce mucosal vasoconstriction to help shrink the swollen tissue. As in infectious croup, the recommended dose of nebulized racemic epinephrine is 0.5 mL of 2.25% solution diluted in 3 to 5 mL of normal saline. The patient must be observed for up to 4 hours after the last nebulized epinephrine treatment in case rebound obstructive symptoms occur. In severe cases, treatment with heliox (helium and oxygen mixture) may also be tried. The use of dexamethasone in both the treatment and prevention of postintubation laryngeal edema is widespread, but one must keep in mind the slower onset of action (4 to 6 hours to achieve maximum effect). Resolution of symptoms usually occurs within 24 hours; a child with persistent and recurrent respiratory distress should be admitted for further observation and management.

MANAGEMENT OF ANESTHESIA

The most important anesthetic consideration in postintubation laryngeal edema is its *prevention*. Although use of uncuffed endotracheal tubes is traditionally recommended in children younger than 8 years of age, repeat laryngoscopy may be needed to exchange for a larger-sized uncuffed tube in cases of large air leaks, and this may result in more laryngeal trauma. On the other hand, cuffed endotracheal tube use may be associated with overzealous cuff inflation, which also leads to tracheal mucosal injury. Although no consensus position or guidelines on endotracheal tube cuff pressure monitoring have been published, use of a manometer to directly and accurately determine cuff pressure, particularly in pediatric patients, should always be considered. Regardless of whether a cuffed or uncuffed endotracheal tube is used, one must be able to demonstrate an air leak around the tube at or below a pressure of 25 cm H$_2$O to prevent impaired perfusion to the tracheal mucosa.

Subglottic Stenosis

Subglottic stenosis is a congenital or acquired narrowing of the subglottic airway. It is the most common type of laryngeal stenosis; others are supraglottic and glottic stenosis. Specifically, *subglottic stenosis* refers to narrowing at the level of the cricoid ring. It is defined as a luminal diameter of less than 4 mm in the full-term neonate and less than 3 mm in those born prematurely. Most cases are acquired as a result of trauma.

PATHOGENESIS

In the congenital form, subglottic stenosis lies on a spectrum of diseases that result from recanalization abnormalities of the laryngeal lumen during embryogenesis. Recanalization defects can also lead to laryngeal atresia, laryngeal stenosis, and laryngeal webs. Congenital subglottic stenosis is divided into the membranous type and the cartilaginous type. The former consists of fibrous soft tissue thickening at the subglottic region and is generally a circumferential defect. The cartilaginous type is a consequence of thickening or deformity of the cricoid cartilage, the simplest form of which may be a mere change in the ring shape (e.g., unevenly large anterior or posterior lamina, elliptical shape) with little physical narrowing.

Acquired subglottic stenosis usually results from trauma associated with intubation, including pressure necrosis from use of an inappropriately large endotracheal tube and direct injury to the laryngeal structures during intubation. Additional factors suspected to play a role in causing subglottic stenosis include prematurity, duration of intubation, endotracheal tube movement, and concurrent conditions that increase local inflammatory response (gastroesophageal reflux disease, systemic infection, hypoxia).

SIGNS AND SYMPTOMS

Clinical presentation varies depending on the severity of the narrowing and can range from stridor to complete airway obstruction. Mild cases of congenital subglottic stenosis may not be clinically evident from the outset and may be diagnosed only after the child experiences recurrent croup. Subglottic stenosis should always be considered in neonates and infants in whom multiple attempts at successful extubation have failed.

Diagnosis of subglottic stenosis is made by endoscopic examination. The degree of stenosis correlates well with the ability to detect an air leak at pressures of less than 20 cm H_2O using endotracheal tubes of various sizes. Subglottic stenosis is graded on a severity scale from I to IV, with grade I indicating less than 50% luminal obstruction, grade II 50% to 70% obstruction, grade III 71% to 91% obstruction, and grade IV no discernible lumen. Congenital subglottic stenosis is a diagnosis of exclusion made only in the absence of trauma and other apparent postnatal causes.

TREATMENT

Grades I and II subglottic stenosis generally do not require surgical treatment and may be amenable to medical therapy alone using antiinflammatory and vasoconstrictive agents such as a corticosteroid and nebulized epinephrine. Grades III and IV subglottic stenosis need one or more forms of surgical treatment. Clinical symptoms ultimately dictate the need for surgical intervention regardless of grade. Concurrent gastroesophageal reflux disease must also be addressed.

Less severe subglottic stenosis may be treated endoscopically with steroid injection, serial dilations, and carbon dioxide laser ablation with or without topical mitomycin C. More severe subglottic stenosis may require an open surgical procedure. These procedures include anterior cricoid split, laryngotracheoplasty with cartilage graft (laryngotracheal reconstruction), and tracheotomy.

MANAGEMENT OF ANESTHESIA

Since most acquired cases of subglottic stenosis result from intubation-related trauma, extreme vigilance and caution must be used in every intubation, particularly intubation of infants and young children. One must always be able to demonstrate an air leak around the endotracheal tube at or below a pressure of 25 cm H_2O to minimize the risk of pressure ischemia and necrosis of the tracheal mucosa. With cuffed endotracheal tubes, inflated cuff pressure should also be kept below the predicted safe maximum of 25 cm H_2O, which can be easily and accurately achieved with commercially available manometers.

For patients coming for surgery to correct subglottic stenosis, standard anesthetic considerations pertaining to airway surgery are applicable. In particular, the risk of airway fire in the setting of laser use and electrocauterization must always be kept in mind. As with all airway surgeries, close communication between the anesthesiologist and surgeon is important.

In cases of open reconstruction, the postoperative management is as important as the actual surgery. Patients usually have in place an endotracheal tube (often larger than that predicted for age) that acts as a stent once the stenosis has been repaired and the lumen enlarged with a cartilage graft. Adequate sedation and frequently muscle relaxation are required to prevent patient movement, which may prove disastrous

should sutures lines be disrupted or accidental extubation occur with resultant complete airway obliteration.

Foreign Body Aspiration

Foreign body aspiration occurs when an object or substance nonnative to the laryngotracheobronchial pathway is inhaled and embedded anywhere from the level of the larynx down to the distal bronchus and beyond.

PATHOGENESIS

Commonly aspirated objects in the pediatric population include peanuts (up to 55% of all foreign body aspirations in Western societies), seeds, popcorn, other food particles, small toy parts, and metal objects. The size and shape of the aspirated object usually determine the level of entrapment. Although objects lodged at proximal locations can cause complete airway obstruction and lead to death from asphyxiation, smaller and more streamlined objects may travel down to the distal airways and cause milder and more subtle signs and symptoms. In addition to the physical airway obstruction posed by the aspirated foreign body, a secondary chemical or inflammatory reaction to the foreign body and postobstruction infection may occur. Over half of all aspirated foreign bodies are located in the right main bronchus, followed by the right lobar bronchi, left bronchi, trachea or carina, larynx, and bilateral locations.

SIGNS AND SYMPTOMS

Children between the ages of 1 and 3 years represent the overwhelming majority of patients with foreign body aspiration. This age period coincides with the intellectual and physical developmental stages of the typical inquisitive toddler, who explores the environment via the oral route and who has the locomotive ability to find objects and the fine motor skills to put such objects in the mouth. In older children and teenagers, neurologic disorders and substance abuse predispose to foreign body aspiration.

Signs and symptoms of bronchial aspiration include coughing, wheezing, dyspnea, and decreased air entry into the affected side. Laryngeal or tracheal foreign body aspiration presents with frank or impending respiratory failure with severe dyspnea, stridor, cyanosis, and altered mental status, and is associated with increased morbidity and mortality. Overall, the classic triad of cough, wheezing, and decreased breath sounds is present in fewer than 60% of all children with foreign body aspiration. A reported history of choking is highly suggestive of foreign body aspiration, but it may be missed because it is an early symptom typically lasting only seconds to minutes immediately after the incident. Chronically retained airway foreign bodies have a much more insidious presentation and are often misdiagnosed as upper respiratory tract infections, asthma, pneumonia, and undefined airway abnormalities. The diagnosis of foreign body aspiration can be easily established with plain radiographs when the object is radiopaque. However, most aspirated objects (nuts, other food items) are radiolucent and will not be obvious on radiographs unless there is evidence to suggest aspiration, such as postobstructive atelectasis, infiltrate or consolidation, or air trapping, in conjunction with the history and clinical findings.

TREATMENT

Rigid bronchoscopy is the procedure of choice for both the diagnosis and treatment of foreign body aspiration because it permits airway control, optimizes visualization, and allows removal of the foreign body with a variety of forceps. Dislodgment or fragmentation of the object into the contralateral bronchus is a potentially lethal complication if the initially affected side remains obstructed by the object and/or inflammation. When the foreign body cannot be removed, it is sometimes necessary to push it to a more distal location to restore ventilation to as large a portion of the lungs as possible. Rarely, aspirated foreign bodies require thoracotomy for retrieval.

MANAGEMENT OF ANESTHESIA

Flexibility in management and close communication between the anesthesiologist and surgeon are paramount to the safe care of children with foreign body aspiration. There is no gold standard anesthetic approach, and controversy still exists regarding whether to maintain spontaneous ventilation or to initiate controlled ventilation. It is best to remember that each child requires an individualized approach depending on the severity of symptoms and the location of the aspirated object. Therefore, a thorough history taking and physical examination as well as a review of radiographic films must be performed in planning anesthetic care. For example, the location of the object and associated findings such as air trapping may alert the anesthesiologist to avoid sudden changes in position (an object in the right main bronchus may dislodge proximally to cause complete obstruction) as well as the use of nitrous oxide (air trapping and areas of emphysema may expand rapidly). Urgent or emergent need for bronchoscopic examination takes precedence over NPO status.

Inhalation induction of anesthesia with maintenance of spontaneous ventilation is generally preferred, because positive pressure ventilation may force the foreign body into a potentially more precarious position. Intravenous induction may be acceptable in patients with relatively stable airways. Total intravenous anesthesia using propofol, remifentanil, and possibly dexmedetomidine, or a combination thereof, should be established as early as possible after induction to provide an uninterrupted source of anesthesia. Topical anesthesia of the larynx and trachea with up to 3 mg/kg of lidocaine (2% to 4%) is extremely useful in preventing laryngospasm and reaction to endoscopic manipulation. Anticholinergics such as atropine (10 to 20 mcg/kg IV) or glycopyrrolate (3 to 5 mcg/kg IV) should be readily available in case of pronounced vagal stimulation during bronchoscopy. Once the bronchoscope passes the glottis, the anesthesia circuit should immediately be connected to the side port to provide supplemental oxygen and to assist spontaneous ventilation or initiate gentle manual ventilation as needed. Close attention must be paid to the patient's respiratory excursions, and use of a precordial stethoscope can be invaluable in assessing respiratory effort and quality in these cases.

Spontaneous ventilation is desirable until the nature and location of the foreign body have been elucidated. Muscle relaxation is sometimes required to prevent movement during retrieval of the aspirated object. This may be particularly true when the foreign body is passing through the glottis along with the forceps and bronchoscope for removal as a unit. Any sudden movement from light anesthesia or lack of muscle relaxation may cause premature dislodgment of the object from the forceps. After completion of the bronchoscopic procedure, the child is usually intubated to allow for definitive airway control as well as tracheal and esophageal suctioning. In general, the child can be promptly extubated once appropriate criteria are met. Pneumothorax can be a complication, although it is rare, and should always be considered in case of rapid deterioration.

Dexamethasone (0.4 to 1.0 mg/kg, maximum of 20 mg) is given prophylactically to reduce subglottic edema. Nebulized epinephrine treatment may be needed to treat postoperative croup. Chest radiographs are sometimes obtained after bronchoscopy if dictated by clinical symptoms.

Laryngeal Papillomatosis

Laryngeal papillomatosis is one of the most common causes of hoarseness and airway obstruction in children. Also known as *recurrent respiratory papillomatosis* (warts), it is a benign neoplasm of the larynx and trachea caused by human papilloma virus (HPV) types 6 and 11.

PATHOGENESIS

Laryngeal papillomatosis is thought to occur as a result of ororespiratory exposure to HPV during vaginal birth. The etiology is not entirely clear, however, because adults who are exposed to HPV rarely develop warts of the larynx and trachea, and laryngeal papillomatosis is not generally considered a sexually transmitted disease. HPV infects the epithelial cell layer of the target site (cutaneous, anogenital, oral, or respiratory mucosa) producing benign, well-demarcated growths. In laryngeal papillomatosis, the larynx is the most commonly involved location, but distal spread to the trachea and lungs can also occur.

SIGNS AND SYMPTOMS

Children between the ages of 6 months and 10 years can have symptoms of an upper airway disorder at presentation. Dysphonia or change in voice quality (or altered cry in infants) is often the first and most prominent symptom. If lesions are left untreated, continued growth will lead to stridor, dyspnea, and airway obstruction. Although lesions in children and adults appear similar histologically and pathologically, the clinical course is quite different in the two patient populations. The main difference is the highly recurrent nature of the wart lesions in children, and often numerous surgical excisions are required over the course of childhood. Adults usually require only a few surgical procedures for complete eradication. Despite its being an aggressive "benign" disease, laryngeal papillomatosis in children tends to become quiescent in adolescence. Malignant degeneration is rare but can occur in older children (distal seeds may transform into squamous cell carcinoma of the airway).

TREATMENT

Surgical excision is the current standard of care in the treatment of laryngeal papillomatosis. Although not all warts seen during surgery may be removed, any symptomatic or clinically significant lesion must be excised. Adjuvant antiviral medical therapy (such as with cidofovir) has been tried but is still undergoing investigation. Carbon dioxide laser ablation in suspension microlaryngoscopy is the most common surgical modality. The procedure must be performed by experienced hands to minimize scarring, fibrosis, and potential laryngeal web formation. The laryngeal microdébrider, an adaptation of the endoscopic sinus instrument, has gained popularity in the treatment of many types of airway lesions including juvenile laryngeal papillomatosis. Some advocate its use over carbon dioxide laser ablation because of its more precise application and reported advantages such as better postsurgical voice quality, quicker recovery, and longer asymptomatic intervals between operations.

In rare cases of large obstructive lesions, tracheotomy may have to be performed to restore airflow. However, tracheotomy is strongly discouraged because of the risk of inducing distal spread of disease.

MANAGEMENT OF ANESTHESIA

Suspension microlaryngoscopic airway surgeries are some of the most challenging cases in pediatric anesthesia and require close cooperation between the otolaryngologist and anesthesiologist. Meticulous attention must be paid to the airway, because patients are usually turned 90 degrees away from the anesthesia station and are suspended in a hands-free laryngoscope setup that allows for microscopic binocular operative intervention. Traditionally, intubation with a smaller endotracheal tube during surgery has been the standard approach. However, the endotracheal tube may pose a problem in a number of ways. It can act as a fuel for combustion during laser surgery, and thus modified devices such as metal-, rubber-, or silicone-coated tubes wrapped in reflective foil may have to be used to minimize the risk of airway fire. In addition, the presence of the endotracheal tube may compromise the visualization and excision of the lesion. Tubeless techniques with or without spontaneous ventilation have become more popular to address these concerns.

Children generally undergo inhalation induction of general anesthesia with the aim of establishing intravenous access and a steady level of total intravenous anesthesia as early as possible. Topical anesthesia with weight-based doses of lidocaine, preferably delivered via an atomizer device for even distribution, should be instituted to further decrease reaction to surgical stimuli. Spontaneous ventilation should be maintained

at least until the nature and location of the lesion have been determined. Muscle relaxation for vocal cord paralysis is sometimes required for precise surgical excision of vocal cord lesions. Most children are intubated after completion of the surgery, even when tubeless techniques are used, and then allowed to awaken for extubation.

Laryngeal Clefts

Laryngeal clefts are a group of rare congenital abnormalities in the separation between the posterior laryngotracheal wall and the adjacent esophagus. As a result, varying degrees of communication exist between the larynx, trachea, and esophagus. Albeit rare, laryngeal clefts represent an important occult cause of chronic respiratory complaints in children. Laryngeal clefts have an incidence of 1 in 10,000 to 20,000 live births with a slight male predominance (male/female ratio of 5:3).

PATHOGENESIS

The trachea and esophagus share a common lumen embryologically until they are divided by the tracheoesophageal septum. Defects in the development of the septum or incomplete division of the lumen can lead to a variety of defects, including laryngeal cleft, tracheoesophageal fistula, and esophageal atresia. Laryngeal clefts are graded according the level of involvement, ranging from type I (interarytenoid defect superior to the true vocal folds) to type IV (defect extending into the posterior wall of the thoracic trachea with possible carinal involvement) (Figure 27-4).

SIGNS AND SYMPTOMS

The timing and nature of presentation depend on cleft severity. Stridor, choking, and regurgitation are typical manifestations. Some children may have recurrent croup or aspiration pneumonia and the cleft may remain undiagnosed for years. Diagnosis requires a high index of suspicion. The presence of a laryngeal cleft should be considered in any child with a history of feeding problems in association with respiratory complaints.

Microlaryngoscopic examination remains the gold standard in the diagnosis of laryngeal clefts. Symptoms and extent of the cleft defect will determine the timing and type of surgical repair. Minor clefts are usually amenable to minimally invasive surgery (suspension microlaryngoscopy, robotic surgery). Severe clefts such as those involving the thoracic trachea may require median sternotomy or lateral pharyngotomy with right thoracotomy to optimize exposure.

All patients with laryngeal clefts should undergo complete examination of the tracheobronchial tree and esophagus to rule out other associated abnormalities.

MANAGEMENT OF ANESTHESIA

Spontaneous ventilation under general anesthesia is optimal for endoscopic examination because spontaneous movement of the vocal cords and surrounding structures is maintained.

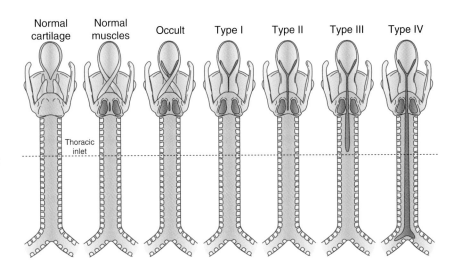

FIGURE 27-4 Laryngeal cleft: grading of the various lesions. *(With permission from Holzman RS, Mancuso TJ, Polaner DM. A Practical Approach to Pediatric Anesthesia. 1st ed. Philadelphia, PA: Lippincott Williams & Wilkins; 2008:264, Fig 14.28.)*

A tubeless procedure also allows for the best visualization of the area of concern, because some defects are subtle and may be easily masked by an in-situ endotracheal tube. Of course, the safety of the patient ultimately dictates the anesthetic technique. Anesthetic concerns discussed under laryngeal papillomatosis also apply here. After laryngeal cleft repair surgery, the child is usually transferred to the pediatric ICU for postoperative monitoring and management.

Macroglossia

Macroglossia is true enlargement of the tongue. This is to be differentiated from glossoptosis, in which a normal-sized tongue causes obstructive symptoms in an abnormally small oral cavity. Macroglossia can be focal or generalized.

SIGNS AND SYMPTOMS

The child's ability to swallow, breath, and speak may be impaired to varying degrees depending on the extent of macroglossia. Taste sensation may also be affected and cause feeding aversions. In addition, the impingement on surrounding structures may lead to facial and dental problems such as prognathism, bite deformities, malocclusion, and temporomandibular joint pain.

Drooling, speech impairment, failure to thrive, and stridor are all symptoms of macroglossia, with airway obstruction being the most feared consequence. In mild cases, speech therapy may be all that is needed. Surgical reduction is aimed at restoring normal functions such as mastication, deglutition, and articulation as well as restoring a patent airway.

MANAGEMENT OF ANESTHESIA

Preparations for a difficult airway must be made for any child with macroglossia coming for surgery. In some cases, induction of anesthesia may occur only after endotracheal intubation, because the tongue is both enlarged and relatively fixed in position, as is seen in advanced Hurler's syndrome. For children at an appropriate developmental stage, surgeries that can be performed under local anesthesia should be attempted with minimal sedation to avoid airway obstruction. Spontaneous ventilation is essential until a definitive airway is established.

Adenotonsillar Hypertrophy and Sleep-Disordered Breathing

Adenotonsillar hypertrophy is the most common cause of snoring in children. Snoring may or may not be associated with actual obstructive hypopnea and obstructive apnea. Sleep-disordered breathing represents a spectrum of nocturnal airflow-restrictive problems that may range in presentation from physiologically inconsequential snoring to complete obstructive sleep apnea.

PATHOGENESIS

The smallest cross-sectional area of the pediatric pharyngeal space is the retropalatal area where the tonsils and adenoids overlap. Hypertrophy of one or both groups of lymphoid tissue leads to expected decrease in airway caliber with resultant resistance and/or obstruction to airflow. However, the degree of hypertrophy does not necessarily predict or correlate with the severity of obstructive symptoms. Some children with large tonsils and adenoids display few or no symptoms of sleep-disordered breathing, whereas others with severe obstructive symptoms are found to have relatively normal-sized tonsils and adenoids. It is clear from these cases that obstruction to airflow also depends on the tone and volume of surrounding tissues. Thus, the presence of comorbid conditions such as obesity, craniofacial anomalies, and neuromuscular disorders must be considered in understanding the pathophysiology in each child. Whether the obstruction results from adenotonsillar hypertrophy alone or from additive collapse of surrounding tissues, the child must increase respiratory effort to maintain airflow. Increased intraluminal negative pressure against compliant pediatric airway structures leads to airway collapse and cessation of airflow via the Bernoulli effect. Abnormal peripheral and central neuromuscular regulation of respiratory function also contributes to the development of sleep-disordered breathing and obstructive symptoms.

Children and adolescents with adenotonsillar hypertrophy have a range of symptoms, including mouth breathing, snoring, and symptoms of obstructive sleep disorder. Whereas daytime sleepiness is frequently reported in adults with obstructive sleep apnea, children more often have nonspecific behavioral difficulties such as hyperactivity and learning disability. Parents may also report a history of chronic rhinorrhea, allergic rhinitis, and poor appetite. Examination of the child may reveal audible mouth breathing, dry lips, hyponasal speech, and the so-called adenoid face, an elongated or oblong face with the mouth open and an expression of being lost or apathetic.

Tonsillar hypertrophy is graded on a numeric scale from 0 to 4. The lowest grade denotes normally sized tonsils that fit within the tonsillar fauces and the highest indicates hypertrophic tonsils that obstruct at least 75% of the lateral oropharyngeal dimension. Flexible endoscopy and lateral radiography are helpful in diagnosing adenoid hypertrophy, although most cases are diagnosed clinically with examination of the adenoids performed at the time of surgery. Adenoids are located midline in the nasopharynx in close proximity to the opening of the eustachian tubes. For this reason, adenoid hypertrophy is frequently associated with chronic middle ear effusion, otitis media, and sinusitis.

History and physical examination alone are poor at differentiating simple snoring from obstructive sleep apnea. Snoring, as estimated from history, and adenotonsillar size on examination have relatively low positive and negative predictive values in the evaluation of children with sleep-disordered breathing. Polysomnography remains the gold standard for diagnosing obstructive sleep apnea. Breathing parameters that are usually monitored in pediatric patients include airflow, respiratory effort, and oxygen saturation via pulse oximetry. End-tidal carbon dioxide concentration, brain electrical potentials (via electroencephalography), chin muscle electrical potentials (vis electromyography), and leg movements may also be monitored.

Obstructive sleep apnea is usually defined as cessation of airflow with continued respiratory effort for at least two breaths or 10 seconds. Hypopnea is defined as at least 50% reduction in airflow with associated respiratory effort for at least two breaths or more than 3% decrease in oxygen saturation. Apnea and apnea-hypopnea indices (number of events divided by number of hours of sleep) are calculated for the entire duration of sleep. Ideally, all children suspected of having sleep apnea should undergo polysomnography, but young age is a limiting factor.

TREATMENT

Recognizing and treating sleep-disordered breathing is important, because untreated obstructive sleep apnea has neurocognitive, inflammatory, and cardiovascular sequelae. Adenotonsillectomy has been the treatment of choice, sometimes even in the absence of significant adenotonsillar hypertrophy when there are concomitant predisposing conditions to obstructive sleep apnea. In general, adenotonsillectomy is effective in relieving obstructive symptoms and can significantly improve quality of life. Despite being one of the most commonly performed surgeries in children (second only to myringotomy) with many advances in surgical technique, adenotonsillectomy is not without risk. Bleeding, laryngospasm, vomiting, pain, and dehydration are among the most common postoperative complications.

MANAGEMENT OF ANESTHESIA

Adenotonsillar hypertrophy in association with obstructive sleep disorder is not a contraindication to administering preoperative anxiolytic medication. As in all cases, the child should be closely monitored after pharmacologic intervention. Unless an intravenous catheter is already in place, induction of general anesthesia is usually accomplished with inhalation of sevoflurane and oxygen with or without nitrous oxide. Rapid airway obstruction can be expected, and oral airways of several sizes should always be readily available. Moderate continuous positive pressure is often needed to counteract the effects of a reduced upper airway muscle tone. Cuffed endotracheal tubes may be preferable to uncuffed tubes to minimize the chance of aspiration of blood. Air leak at or below a pressure of 25 cm H_2O should be confirmed and cuff pressure monitored. The choice of opioid is not as important as appropriate drug dosing; lower dosages are given to children who have symptoms or have obstructive sleep apnea documented by sleep study to minimize risks of prolonged emergence and postoperative upper airway obstruction. The use of nonsteroidal antiinflammatory drugs remains controversial and varies widely from center to center. The intravenous form of acetaminophen is becoming more available in U.S. centers and may become an important analgesic adjunct given its lack of bleeding risk and respiratory-depressant effect. High-dose intravenous dexamethasone (up to 1 mg/kg, maximum of 25 mg) has been shown to reduce postoperative swelling as well as nausea and vomiting. Most adenotonsillectomy procedures are not associated with excessive bleeding, but the amount of blood loss can be hard to estimate and is often larger than predicted. Fluid deficits must be replaced appropriately. Rarely, massive hemorrhage can occur when the carotid vessels are torn during the procedure.

Upper Respiratory Tract Infection

MANAGEMENT OF ANESTHESIA

The traditional approach of postponing elective surgery for 1 to 2 weeks in children with mild active or recent upper respiratory tract infections (URIs) and for 4 to 6 weeks in those with more severe symptoms (such as productive cough) may be too conservative and is often unrealistic. It may be difficult to find a block of completely "healthy" time lasting 4 to 6 weeks in peak URI seasons, because most children either have an active cold or are recovering from one.

The urgency and type of surgery must be considered. Emergent procedures must proceed regardless of the severity of the URI. Type of surgery is also an important consideration, because some procedures such as myringotomy and adenotonsillectomy may help to relieve chronic URI-like symptoms. In fact, many children coming for such procedures will have chronic symptoms that are difficult to distinguish from those of a URI. A detailed parental interview usually provides a helpful comparison of the child's current health status to baseline condition. In general, elective surgeries should be postponed if the child has high fever, croupy cough, general malaise, or evidence of lower respiratory tract infection.

General anesthesia via mask or laryngeal mask airway is preferable to endotracheal intubation and has been shown to be associated with a lower incidence of intraoperative and postoperative respiratory complications. Regional anesthesia should also be considered in appropriate cases. If intubation is required, the trachea should be instrumented only under a deep plane of anesthesia. A smaller than expected endotracheal tube should be considered, because children with active or recent URI have a higher incidence of postintubation laryngeal edema. Dexamethasone may also be given prophylactically to reduce postintubation croup.

GENITOURINARY DISORDERS

Vesicoureteral Reflux

Vesicoureteral reflux (VUR) is the abnormal reflux of urine from the bladder into the upper urinary tract, including the ureters and kidneys, and can be unilateral or bilateral. It is the most common urologic disorder in children. Prenatal hydroureter and hydronephrosis may suggest the presence of VUR.

SIGNS AND SYMPTOMS

Most children have a febrile urinary tract infection (UTI). Some are found to have VUR based on testing prompted by prenatal urologic abnormalities or a significant family history. Evaluation for VUR should be done in children with recurrent UTIs, any male child with a first UTI, any child younger than 5 years with a febrile UTI, and children with significant renal anomalies.

Diagnosis of VUR is most commonly based on the results of contrast voiding cystourethrography, which can be done with relative ease in most children. It does involve urethral catheterization for contrast injection, and some children may require sedation or even general anesthesia for catheter placement. VUR is diagnosed based on evidence of contrast reflux and is graded into one of five levels of severity (Table 27-18). Grades I and II are considered mild, grade III moderate, and grades IV and V severe. Treatment differs for primary and secondary VUR and is also dictated by reflux severity. A majority of children with mild VUR (80%) will experience spontaneous resolution by 5 years of age. Spontaneous resolution can also occur in moderate VUR but with variable rates; younger age at presentation and unilateral disease are favorable prognostic factors, whereas older age at presentation and bilateral disease

TABLE 27-18   ■   Grading of vesicoureteral reflux

Grade	Description
1	Urine refluxes into the ureter only.
2	Urine refluxes into the ureter, renal pelvis, and calyces.
3	Urine refluxes into the ureter and collecting system. There is mild dilation of the ureter and renal pelvis and calyces are mildly blunted.
4	Urine refluxes into the ureter and collecting system. There is moderate dilation of the ureter and renal pelvis. Calyces are moderately blunted.
5	Urine refluxes into the ureter and collecting system. The pelvis is severely dilated, ureters are tortuous, and the calyces are severely blunted.

Adapted from Holzman RS. Urogenital system. In: Holzman RS, Mancuso TJ, Polaner DM. *A Practical Approach to Pediatric Anesthesia.* 1st ed. Philadelphia, PA: Lippincott Williams & Wilkins; 2008:449.

predict a low chance of spontaneous resolution. The most severe cases of VUR (grade V) rarely resolve without surgical intervention.

TREATMENT

Treatment is aimed at preventing UTI with antibiotic prophylaxis and restoring ureterovesical junction competence or relieving downstream bladder obstruction. Untreated reflux increases the risks of pyelonephritis and renal scarring with subsequent reflux nephropathy. The most common surgical procedure for VUR is ureteral reimplantation or ureteroneocystostomy. The affected ureter is repositioned and retunneled into the bladder wall to create a new ureterovesical junction with the proper length/diameter ratio. Injection of a polysaccharide-based gel (Deflux) is a less invasive procedure that may be tried in less severe grades of VUR until spontaneous resolution occurs or until definitive surgical intervention is deemed necessary.

MANAGEMENT OF ANESTHESIA

Most children with VUR are otherwise healthy and undergo general anesthesia without problems. For those with severe VUR and/or co-existing renal anomaly, baseline renal indices should be checked to assess kidney function. Advanced VUR may be accompanied by symptoms of chronic renal disease, including hypertension.

Children with VUR may become frequent visitors to the operating room for repeat cystoscopic procedures and can exhibit overwhelming anxiety. A gentle approach in conjunction with appropriate preoperative anxiolysis is helpful in most cases.

Cystoscopic procedures are generally short, but a relatively deep plane of anesthesia must be established to minimize risk of laryngospasm during urethral stimulation. Care must also be taken to secure the airway device, since the child is usually moved to the far end of the operating table for cystoscopy.

Caudal or lumbar epidural analgesia is recommended for reimplantation procedures to treat both peri-incisional pain and postsurgical bladder spasm.

Posterior Urethral Valve

Posterior urethral valve is a common cause of bladder outlet obstruction in male children. Malformation of the posterior urethra in the form an obstructive membrane results in varying degrees of urethral obstruction. Urine outflow obstruction can cause bladder, ureteral, and renal damage.

SIGNS AND SYMPTOMS

Unless the obstruction is mild, posterior urethral valve is usually diagnosed prenatally via ultrasonography during evaluation for antenatal megaureter and hydronephrosis. Pulmonary insufficiency may be present. Symptoms of delayed presentation include dysuria, abnormal urinary stream, diurnal enuresis, UTI, and an abdominal mass representing a markedly distended bladder. Bladder hypertrophy causes abnormally high intravesicular pressure, which predisposes to VUR. Occasionally, the first presenting problem is renal failure with associated uremic symptoms. Approximately one third of patients with posterior urethral valve progress to end-stage renal disease, requiring lifelong renal replacement therapy or renal transplantation.

Bladder outlet obstruction is usually addressed immediately at birth by placement of a urethral catheter. The obstructive valves can be incised in the first few days of life. If the urethra is too small to accommodate the necessary surgical instruments, direct vesicocutaneous or ureterocutaneous urinary diversion procedures may be required.

MANAGEMENT OF ANESTHESIA

Children with posterior urethral valve come for a wide range of surgical procedures from simple valve incision to renal transplantation. Anesthetic care must be tailored to each individual with particular attention to fluid and electrolyte management, especially in the setting of advanced renal insufficiency.

Cryptorchidism

Cryptorchidism (hidden or obscure testis) is the congenital absence of one or both testes in the scrotum resulting from incomplete testicular descent. Undescended testes have an increased risk of malignant transformation compared with normally descended ones. In addition, there is usually a concurrent hernia with attendant risks of bowel incarceration and strangulation, as well as increased risk of infertility and testicular torsion.

SIGNS AND SYMPTOMS

Cryptorchidism is diagnosed by inability to palpate the testis or palpation of a malpositioned testis (e.g., inguinal canal location). Physical examination must be performed in a warm environment to prevent cold-induced testicular retraction, which may confound the clinical picture. Nonpalpable testes account for only one fifth of all cases of cryptorchidism; in 40% of cases the testis has an intraabdominal location, in another 40% a high inguinal location, and in the remainder shows atrophy or congenital absence. Most palpable undescended testes will spontaneously descend during infancy, but this rarely continues after 9 months of age.

TREATMENT

Orchiopexy is the treatment for all cases of cryptorchidism and involves identification, mobilization, and fixation of the malpositioned testis to the scrotum. Orchiopexy can be performed via an inguinal, suprainguinal, or laparoscopic approach. In cases in which the testis is in a high intraabdominal position and spermatic vessels are short, a two-stage procedure may be required to allow time for collateral vessel formation after initial vessel clipping, followed by mobilization and scrotal fixation of the testis.

MANAGEMENT OF ANESTHESIA

Unless the child has comorbid conditions, there are few special anesthetic considerations. An intense vagal response can be seen with surgical traction and manipulation of the spermatic cord and testicle; this may also occur with pneumoperitoneum as in all laparoscopic procedures. A high incidence of postoperative nausea and vomiting is observed, and thus prophylactic antiemetic treatment should be routinely given. Caudal analgesia is highly recommended in appropriate patients.

Hypospadias

Hypospadias is congenital malpositioning of the urethral meatus on the ventral aspect (underside) of the penis. The abnormal opening can occur anywhere from the glans penis to the penile shaft and even down to the scrotum and perineum. Hypospadias involving the glans penis, also known as *coronal hypospadias,* is the most common (50% of cases). Chordee, an abnormal ventral curvature of the penis, is commonly seen with hypospadias.

The defect is thought be an early gestational event, but the exact mechanism is still under investigation. A combination of genetic and environmental factors is likely. Distal and coronal hypospadias impose mostly cosmetic problems; more proximal lesions can affect urination and fertility. Treatment for hypospadias is surgical repair and in the majority of cases can be accomplished in a single stage. Multiple corrective surgeries are needed for proximal meatal locations (scrotum and perineum) and often preputial skin grafting is often required. Concurrent chordee deformity is also corrected. Most surgeons perform hypospadias repair between the ages of 4 and 18 months before the child has full genital awareness to minimize psychologic impact.

Hypospadias is generally an isolated finding, and most children do not have additional health problems that pose specific anesthetic concerns. General anesthesia supplemented with caudal analgesia is the preferred technique.

ORTHOPEDIC-MUSCULOSKELETAL DISORDERS

Clubfoot (Talipes Equinovarus)

Clubfoot is a common congenital foot deformity caused by malalignment of the calcaneotalar-navicular complex with a resultant combination of (1) excessive plantar flexion, (2) medially deviated forefoot, and (3) inward-facing sole. Bilateral involvement is seen in 30% to 50% of cases.

SIGNS AND SYMPTOMS

Clubfoot is evident at birth and can be diagnosed prenatally in some cases. All patients exhibit some degree of calf atrophy. Concomitant shortening of the tibia and fibula can also occur.

Nonoperative treatment includes taping and serial casting for positional clubfoot. Although normal alignment is maintained in some cases, there is a high rate of recurrence. For this reason, surgical Achilles tenotomy (clipping or release of the Achilles tendon) is often needed. Ponseti's method is the most popular treatment scheme for clubfoot and involves initial weekly stretching and casting (5 to 10 sessions), followed by percutaneous Achilles tenotomy, long leg casting with the foot in abduction and dorsiflexion, and finally a bracing program for 3 to 5 years. Rigid clubfoot deformities usually require more invasive surgical realignment such as anterior tibial tendon transfer. Prognosis depends on how severe the defect is and whether there are underlying structural and/or chromosomal abnormalities.

MANAGEMENT OF ANESTHESIA

Anesthetic considerations differ for cases of isolated clubfoot and those associated with genetic or congenital disorders. The most obvious concern is the potential anesthetic impact on patients whose neuromuscular integrity is compromised. Risks of pulmonary aspiration, prolonged muscle weakness, and delayed emergence must be considered. Some procedures are done with the patient in prone position, which requires special precautions to prevent the injuries commonly associated with prone positioning. The patient must be kept adequately anesthetized, sometimes with neuromuscular blockade, to allow adequate stretching and casting. Continuous epidural analgesia (in some cases with combined regional anesthesia) is highly recommended for invasive procedures, because there is often significant postoperative pain.

Slipped Capital Femoral Epiphysis

Slipped capital femoral epiphysis (SCFE) literally means a slippage of the femoral end cap (*epi,* "over"; *physis,* "growth plate") over the femoral neck as a result of a fracture in the growth plate. This is a disorder of adolescence, a period of rapid bone growth predisposing to increased growth plate instability. More and more cases are seen at an earlier age presumably because of early maturation and childhood obesity.

SIGNS AND SYMPTOMS

SCFE typically presents between the ages of 10 and 16 years and affects boys more than girls. Obesity is a risk factor. Medical disorders that are associated with a higher risk of SCFE, as well as an earlier age at onset, include Down's syndrome, endocrinopathies (hypothyroidism, precocious puberty, pituitary tumors), and renal osteodystrophy.

Patients have groin, thigh, and knee pain and often hold the affected hip in an externally rotated position. Gait pattern and weight-bearing ability may be affected. Twenty percent of patients have bilateral involvement even if only unilateral symptoms are present. Patients who are younger than 10 years, older than 16 years, or have short stature should undergo evaluation for an underlying medical cause. Diagnosis is made from findings of the physical examination and plain radiography. Treatment involves surgical pinning of the growth plate to prevent further displacement.

MANAGEMENT OF ANESTHESIA

Surgical treatment for SCFE is mostly done on an urgent basis to prevent further displacement with the attendant risk of vascular compromise. Full-stomach precautions must be observed when indicated, particularly for obese patients. There are few special anesthetic considerations unless comorbid conditions are present.

Blount's Disease

Blount's disease is a disorder of abnormal cartilage growth at the proximal tibial growth plate resulting in genu varum (bowleg) deformity that may lead to leg length discrepancy and joint instability. It is important to distinguish Blount's disease from other causes of genu varum (e.g., physiologic genu varum seen in children younger than 2 years of age, rickets) because treatment differs.

SIGNS AND SYMPTOMS

There are two forms of Blount's disease: infantile and adolescent. The infantile form typically presents before the age of 3 years and is usually bilateral (80% of cases). The adolescent form can be unilateral or bilateral. Risk factors include walking at an early age, African descent, and obesity. In addition to the obvious abnormal bowing, the physical examination often reveals a nontender prominence on the medial side of the proximal tibia. Radiography is the primary modality for diagnosis.

TREATMENT

The infantile form is often amenable to nonoperative treatment, namely, corrective bracing. If the condition is left untreated, surgical realignment may be needed. The adolescent form usually requires operative treatment. Hemiepiphysiodesis, better understood as a growth-guiding procedure, involves placement of screws into the growth plate on the side opposite the defect, to limit continued outward growth and bowing. Tibial osteotomy is a much more invasive procedure that may be needed to correct severe deformities and those that present after the growth spurt period. This procedure can have serious complications, including nonunion, neurovascular injury, and compartment syndrome.

MANAGEMENT OF ANESTHESIA

Significant postoperative pain is expected with osteotomy procedures. However, surgeons typically oppose the use of regional and neuraxial analgesia to avoid masking of symptoms related to potential nerve injury and compartment syndrome. A well-planned scheme of intraoperative and postoperative pain control should be implemented, often in consultation with the acute pain management team. As in the SCFE population, adolescents with Blount's disease are often obese, and appropriate anesthetic precautions (related to potential delayed gastric emptying and restrictive respiratory dysfunction) must be observed.

Developmental Dysplasia of the Hip

Developmental dysplasia of the hip (DDH) refers to abnormal growth of the hip caused by a combination of joint laxity and acetabular dysplasia (abnormal shape) resulting in joint instability and dislocation. It is also known as *hip dysplasia* and *congenital hip dislocation;* however, the latter term is inaccurate since DDH can occur at any point from the antenatal period to the time of skeletal maturity.

SIGNS AND SYMPTOMS

Otherwise healthy newborns can have DDH, which is usually due to ligamentous laxity and immature development of the acetabulum associated with young age. Thus, over half of cases will resolve by the first week of life and up to 90% will resolve by 2 months of age. DDH can be diagnosed and monitored using the Barlow (hip adduction with posterior pressure) and Ortolani (abduction and anterior pressure on the greater trochanter) maneuvers, which detect dislocation and reduction, respectively. Leg length discrepancy and gluteal fold asymmetry are also clues to possible DDH. Ultrasonography is the primary diagnostic modality until 5 months of age, at which time sufficient ossification permits adequate radiographic examination. Arthrograms are used infrequently in older children.

Untreated hip joint instability can lead to repetitive and chronic dislocations, contractures of adjoining muscles and tendon, as well as early hip osteoarthritis. DDH in association with connective tissue and neuromuscular disorders such as Ehlers-Danlos syndrome and cerebral palsy are particularly difficult to treat.

TREATMENT

DDH in otherwise healthy infants is treated with bracing (Pavlik's harness) and body casting (spica cast), both of which are abduction devices aimed at stabilizing the femoral head in the hip joint socket. Children in whom DDH presents after 2 years of age generally need open reduction. Residual DDH may even require pelvic and femoral osteotomy to remodel joint architecture. Unfortunately, chronic dislocations and DDH associated with neuromuscular disorders are generally not amenable to surgical intervention.

MANAGEMENT OF ANESTHESIA

During spica casting, infants are often elevated on a wood frame for cast application. Particular attention must be paid to securing any airway device and preventing accidental fall from the wood frame. In addition, any respiratory compromise caused by the spica cast must be communicated to the surgeon so the cast can be modified. There are few other specific anesthetic concerns for standard DDH-related surgeries.

Thoracic Insufficiency Syndrome

Thoracic insufficiency syndrome is the inability of the thorax to support postnatal lung growth and respiratory function. There are multiple causes but all belong to a spectrum of thoracospinal abnormalities. There can be isolated rib abnormalities (fused ribs, absence of ribs) and/or spinal deformities (shortened vertebrae, rotational deformities of the spine) that result in unilateral or bilateral defects. Regardless of cause, restrictive lung disease ensues. The most well-known causes of thoracic insufficiency syndrome are congenital and neuromuscular scoliosis; other important causes include syndromes associated with a shortened or narrowed thorax such as Jarcho-Levin syndrome and Jeune's syndrome, and congenital absence of ribs with flail chest.

PATHOGENESIS

Structural development of the thoracic cage (sternum, ribs, and spine) directly impacts lung growth because the two are intimately related processes. This is particularly true during the early childhood period since the most rapid lung growth takes place in the first 3 years of life. Thereafter, alveolar development continues until approximately 8 years of age and the lungs continue to grow, albeit at a much slower pace, until skeletal maturity is reached. Both the quantity and quality (shape) of the intrathoracic space are important for normal lung development. Studies have shown that thoracic spinal growth is greatest during the first 5 years of life (1.4 cm/yr from 0 to 5 years compared with 0.6 cm/yr from 5 to 10 years and 1.2 cm/yr from 10 to 18 years); thus, this is the most critical time period for overall lung and thoracospinal development. Restrictive lung dysfunction results from a combination of lung hypoplasia, perfusion defects, and impaired rib mechanics. Most patients with thoracic insufficiency syndrome are demonstrated to have consistently higher baseline levels of atelectasis than their healthy counterparts. In contrast to the high lung and chest wall compliance seen in healthy young children, low (stiff) lung and chest wall compliance are noted in children with thoracic insufficiency syndrome.

SIGNS AND SYMPTOMS

Progressive restrictive lung dysfunction associated with thoracic insufficiency syndrome leads to chronic respiratory failure, the earliest manifestations of which are intermittent nocturnal hypercarbia and hypoxemia. Recurrent lower respiratory tract infections may occur due to increased atelectasis and decreased airway clearance from inadequate forceful exhalation, particularly if there is concomitant neuromuscular weakness. Inefficient lung and rib cage mechanics also place higher metabolic demands on the child, which predisposes to poor nutritional status. Cardiovascular sequelae such as pulmonary hypertension and cor pulmonale may follow if thoracic insufficiency syndrome is left untreated.

Lung perfusion scan findings and measures of structural spinal deformity, such as the Cobb angle, correlate poorly with degree of lung dysfunction. However, young children cannot participate in voluntary lung function testing such as spirometry and plethysmography. Because of this, medical therapy must be initiated as early as possible based on clinical findings to mitigate chronic respiratory failure. This therapy includes noninvasive ventilation and chest percussion with postural drainage. Tracheostomy may be needed for progressive hypoventilation.

TREATMENT

Surgical therapy is aimed at correcting the skeletal deformities. The exact technique used depends on the age at presentation, the severity of the deformity, and the underlying cause. Spinal fusion is the definitive treatment for spinal abnormalities; fusion stunts spinal growth, however. Nonfusion techniques are designed to stabilize spinal deformities while preserving spinal growth in young children until fusion can be done at a later time.

The vertical expandable prosthetic titanium rib (VEPTR) procedure (Figure 27-5) is an example of nonfusion spine surgery and is indicated for thoracospinal deformities that also involve the rib cage. It is performed in skeletally immature children (ideally <5 years of age) to guide normal growth of the thoracic cage in hopes that normal lung growth and respiratory function will follow. The procedure starts with an open expansion thoracostomy in which separations are made between the ribs followed by rib cage expansion; congenitally fused ribs are also separated if needed. Vertical expandable titanium rods are then inserted onto healthy bony structures above and below the affected area (rib to distal rib, rib to spine, or rib to pelvis) to hold the expanded thorax. Children return at regular intervals during their growth period for rod lengthening. The immediate and long-term effects on pulmonary mechanics and function are still under investigation.

MANAGEMENT OF ANESTHESIA

Anesthetic considerations relevant for any patient with restrictive lung dysfunction undergoing extensive spinal fusion apply here as well; these are discussed extensively in Chapter 21. The patient's preoperative respiratory function must be thoroughly investigated. The child's cardiac function should be assessed with echocardiography whenever possible. Recognition of associated abnormalities is important, with particular attention paid to the baseline neurologic status. Surgery should be postponed if any acute respiratory illness is present, since most

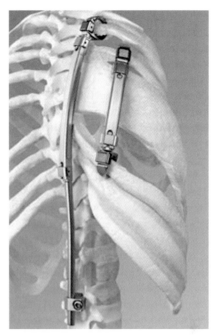

FIGURE 27-5 Vertical expandable prosthetic titanium rib device. *(With permission from Holzman RS, Mancuso TJ, Polaner DM. A Practical Approach to Pediatric Anesthesia. 1st ed. Philadelphia, PA: Lippincott Williams & Wilkins; 2008:488, Fig 23.16.)*

patients already have compromised respiratory functions. Like posterior spinal fusion, VEPTR procedures are done with the patient in the prone position, so standard precautions to prevent injuries related to this positioning must be observed. Blood transfusion is not usually required.

Patients who have undergone the initial VEPTR procedure require postoperative ICU care with or without mechanical ventilation. In general, there is minimal spinal manipulation during VEPTR placement. Early assessment of postoperative neurologic function is important, however. Subsequent VEPTR lengthening procedures are typically brief and do not require postoperative ICU management.

Juvenile Idiopathic Arthritis

Juvenile idiopathic arthritis refers to all types of juvenile arthritis, including what was formerly known as *juvenile rheumatoid arthritis* and other arthritides of unclear cause. *Juvenile idiopathic arthritis* is not synonymous with *juvenile rheumatoid arthritis* because the latter denotes a specific rheumatoid etiology and the former includes idiopathic conditions. Juvenile idiopathic arthritis is the most common autoimmune disease of childhood and is defined as joint pain, stiffness, and swelling that last longer than 6 weeks with the first occurrence before the age of 16 years.

SIGNS AND SYMPTOMS

Three categories of juvenile idiopathic arthritis are identified: systemic, polyarticular, and pauciarticular or oligoarticular. The latter two types affect girls more than boys.

Oligoarticular juvenile idiopathic arthritis accounts for approximately 50% of all cases with a peak incidence around 2 years of age. Four or fewer joints are affected after 6 months of illness with the knees commonly involved, and up to three quarters of patients test positive for antinuclear antibodies (ANAs). Clinical course is generally milder than in the other two variants and joint destruction is rare.

Polyarticular juvenile idiopathic arthritis refers to disease with involvement of more than four joints after 6 months of illness and represents 30% to 40% of cases. Peak incidence occurs at 3 years of age. Small joints of the hands are commonly involved. Fewer than half of these patients demonstrate ANAs and only 10% test positive for rheumatoid factor. Subcutaneous nodules and moderate systemic symptoms are occasionally seen.

Systemic juvenile idiopathic arthritis (formerly known as *Still's disease*) is the smallest subset (10% to 15% of cases) with clinical manifestations of symmetric polyarthritis, intermittent fever, macular rash, hematopoietic abnormalities (leukocytosis, thrombocytopenia, lymphadenopathy), and hepatosplenomegaly. Any joint can be involved, including those of the hands, hips, and shoulders. Cervical spine and temporomandibular joint involvement are not uncommon. Other systemic complications include uveitis, pleuritis, and pericarditis. The disorder can present after the age of 16 years, at which point it is termed *adult-onset Still's disease*. Progression of systemic and joint symptoms does not always occur in a congruent fashion. Some children can have years of persistent rash and spiking fevers with little progression of arthritis. Severe growth retardation, osteoporosis, and macrophage activation syndrome are the most important complications. The latter is characterized by unremitting fevers and a consumptive coagulopathy with resultant spontaneous bruising and bleeding that may lead to shock.

MANAGEMENT OF ANESTHESIA

A potentially difficult airway is one of the most important anesthetic concerns in the care of children with juvenile idiopathic arthritis. Temporomandibular joint arthritis typically limits mouth opening and can be compounded by a micrognathic mandible that results from the growth-stunting effect of the arthropathy. In addition, there may be concurrent cervical spine involvement that further complicates airway management because of limited neck range of motion. The patient must be evaluated for the presence of systemic complications such as pleuritis and pericarditis that affect perioperative cardiopulmonary function so that appropriate anesthetic adjustments can be made. Finally, the physiologic implications (e.g., immunosuppression) of medication used to treat juvenile idiopathic arthritis such as disease-modifying antirheumatic drugs and corticosteroids must be considered.

CHILDHOOD MALIGNANCIES

Wilms's Tumor

Wilms's tumor, or nephroblastoma, is the most common type of renal cancer in children as well as the most common pediatric abdominal malignancy. Overall, it is the fourth most prevalent childhood cancer. The overwhelming majority of patients have unilateral disease with only 6% showing bilateral renal involvement. Neonatal and adult presentations are rare.

PATHOGENESIS

Wilms's tumor can occur as part of a syndrome or as a sporadic lesion, or it can be familial. It is thought to arise from persistent primitive embryologic cells of the kidneys, known as *metanephric blastema cells* or *nephrogenic rests*. Nephrogenic rests that later undergo spontaneous regression are seen in 1% of normal newborn kidneys. In comparison, up to 35% of kidneys with unilateral Wilms's tumor and almost 100% of kidneys involved in bilateral disease have persistent nephrogenic rests. Loss of function of several tumor suppressor genes is thought to play a role, particularly in the familial form of the disease.

SIGNS AND SYMPTOMS

The peak incidence occurs between the ages of 1 and 3 years, and over 95% of cases are diagnosed before 10 years of age. The most common finding is an abdominal mass, which may or may not be painful. Additional signs and symptoms include fever, anemia, hypertension, and hematuria. Associated congenital syndromes include WAGR syndrome (*W*ilms's tumor, *a*niridia or agenesis of the iris and macular hypoplasia, *g*enitourinary anomalies, and *r*etardation or intellectual disabilities), Beckwith-Wiedemann syndrome, and Denys-Drash syndrome (triad of progressive renal disease, male pseudohermaphroditism, and Wilms's tumor). Additional congenital anomalies that predispose to the development of Wilms's tumor are Perlman's syndrome (fetal gigantism), Sotos's syndrome (cerebral gigantism), and isolated hemihypertrophy.

Wilms's tumor is typically surrounded by a pseudocapsule that may rupture with aggressive palpation, manifesting as a rapidly enlarging abdominal mass. Gross examination may reveal cystic, hemorrhagic, and necrotic areas. The lungs are the most common sites for metastasis, although associated respiratory complaints are rare. Local invasion is uncommon, and metastatic disease is usually spread via lymphatic and hematogenous channels. Up to 40% of cases show tumor extension into the renal vein; invasion into the inferior vena cava and right atrium is much less common. Coincidental acquired von Willebrand's disease is seen in 8% of patients. Prognosis depends on tumor stage (I to V) with higher stage and unfavorable histologic features (anaplasia) predicting a lower chance of survival. With current therapy, children with tumors with favorable histologic features have over 90% chance of survival at 5 years and 80% to 90% chance of cure. Tumors with less favorable histologic features are associated with an average lifetime survival rate of 50%. Diagnosis usually begins with imaging studies to evaluate the primary tumor and potential metastatic disease.

According to the protocol of the National Wilms Tumor Study Group, surgical staging should take place before adjuvant or neoadjuvant chemotherapy is begun to minimize the risk of treating a benign disease. Moreover, initiating chemotherapy before surgical staging may require changing what otherwise would have been the best treatment plan by necessitating the use of different modalities (surgical resection, alternative chemotherapy, and radiotherapy). When feasible (well-confined or relatively localized unilateral disease), radical nephrectomy is also performed at the time of staging. Extreme care to avoid tumor spillage during surgery is of utmost importance.

MANAGEMENT OF ANESTHESIA

Patients coming for Wilms's tumor staging and/or resection surgeries may be at higher risk of aspiration resulting from abdominal distention, and thus full-stomach precautions should be observed. Cardiopulmonary status must be determined for patients with known lung metastases and extensive caval involvement. The latter may be associated with sudden massive hemorrhage during dissection. For this reason at least one supradiaphragmatic large-bore intravenous line should be placed in case of inferior vena cava clamping. Specific tests to assess preoperative cardiac function should be performed in patients who have undergone chemotherapy, because the standard regimen includes doxorubicin. Even with bilateral disease, severe renal dysfunction is rare. Nonetheless, standard laboratory tests to evaluate renal function and electrolyte balance as well as cell counts should be performed.

Some surgeons use a laparoscopic approach, although most procedures are done with open incisions because of disease burden. Continuous epidural analgesia provides excellent postoperative pain control.

Hepatoblastoma

Hepatoblastoma is the most common pediatric hepatic malignancy, although liver cancer is an uncommon childhood cancer in general. It is a disease of infants and young children; adolescent and adult presentations are extremely rare.

PATHOGENESIS

Hepatoblastomas arise from immature liver precursor cells and display elements resembling normal hepatic structures (bile ducts, mature liver cells). Evidence of cirrhosis is uncommon. Specific genetic mutations such as chromosomal 11 abnormalities and loss of *APC* (adenomatous polyposis coli) tumor suppressor gene function have been observed in hepatoblastomas that occur in association with particular congenital disorders. Tumors are typically unifocal and affect the right lobe more often than the left lobe.

SIGNS AND SYMPTOMS

The median age at presentation is 1 year, and the overwhelming majority of hepatoblastomas occur in children younger than 3 years of age. There is a slight male predilection (male/female ratio of 1.7:1), and white children are affected five times more frequently than African American children. Children born prematurely with low birth weight (<2500 g) have a significantly increased risk of developing hepatoblastoma. A higher incidence is also observed in several congenital and genetic disorders, including Beckwith-Wiedemann syndrome, hemihypertrophy, and familial adenomatous polyposis.

Hepatoblastoma most commonly presents as an asymptomatic abdominal mass. Anorexia may occur in advanced disease. Some hepatoblastomas secrete β-human chorionic gonadotropin and may cause penile and testicular enlargement. Approximately 10% of children with hepatoblastomas have metastatic disease at presentation; the lungs are the most common sites.

The most important laboratory marker for hepatoblastoma is α-fetoprotein, although it is not specific to this disease. Regular monitoring of α-fetoprotein is important in assessing disease progression and response to treatment. Final diagnosis relies on tissue biopsy.

Prognosis is dependent on histologic features (anaplasia is unfavorable) and the ability to completely resect the tumor. Chemotherapy has emerged as an important part of a successful treatment plan. Cisplatin and doxorubicin are the most active agents against hepatoblastomas. Lesions that are amenable to complete resection at diagnosis are associated with a nearly 100% survival rate with adjuvant chemotherapy. Liver transplantation has become important in the treatment of unresectable lesions and disease that has failed to respond to initial surgical and medical therapy.

MANAGEMENT OF ANESTHESIA

Patients with hepatoblastomas can be in relatively robust health or can be acutely ill; specific anesthetic techniques will differ accordingly. In addition to the usual preoperative assessment, specific investigations to evaluate hepatic synthetic and metabolic functions should be carried out. In particular, coagulation status must be determined, and appropriate blood components reserved preoperatively, especially since hepatic resections are often associated with significant bleeding. Preoperative cardiac function should be assessed in patients being treated with an anthracycline-based chemotherapeutic regimen.

Extreme hemodynamic perturbations can be seen in hepatic surgeries. Invasive arterial blood pressure monitoring is highly recommended. In addition, large-bore intravenous access, preferably placed in the supradiaphragmatic venous circulation, should be established. Placement of a central venous catheter is helpful for monitoring central venous pressure, administering vasoactive drugs, and taking frequent blood samples. Hypothermia is an important concern given the large area of surgical exposure as well as the potentially large volume resuscitation with fluids and blood components. Unless preoperative coagulation abnormalities exist, continuous epidural analgesia should be considered.

Neuroblastoma

Neuroblastoma refers to a group of malignant neoplasms of the sympathetic nervous system (SNS). Neuroblastoma is the most common extracranial solid tumor in childhood and is the most common neoplasm seen in infants. Overall, it represents the third most common pediatric cancer, after leukemia and intracranial tumors. It is a disease of extreme heterogeneity in both presentation and clinical course.

PATHOGENESIS

As in the case of many cancer types, the exact mechanism and triggers for the development of neuroblastoma are not known. Neuroblastoma arises from primitive ganglion cells of the SNS. Since these primitive cells retain the potential for differentiation, neuroblastoma represents a spectrum of tumor cell types, ranging from undifferentiated small round cells (neuroblastoma) to mature ganglion (ganglioneuroblastoma). A combination of genetic and environmental factors likely cause a cascade of mutational events in the prenatal and perinatal period that ultimately lead to the formation of neuroblastic tumors.

SIGNS AND SYMPTOMS

A hallmark of neuroblastoma is the broad range of tumor location and clinical behavior. These tumors can occur anywhere throughout the SNS. The most common site is the adrenal glands (40% of cases), followed by abdominal, thoracic, cervical, and pelvic sympathetic ganglia. Clinical behavior can be relatively benign with some tumors undergoing spontaneous regression or can be aggressively malignant with disease that is widely metastatic and resistant to therapy. Common sites of metastases include the bone marrow, cortical bone, lymph nodes, orbits, dura, and liver. In contrast to Wilms's tumor and hepatoblastoma, metastasis to the lungs is uncommon. Fifty percent of patients have metastatic disease at presentation.

Two thirds of neuroblastomas have intraabdominal primary tumors and most commonly present with abdominal mass, pain, and fullness. Frequent metastatic involvement of cortical bone and bone marrow make bone pain another common symptom. Orbital involvement manifests as periorbital ecchymosis (raccoon eyes) and proptosis and may be the first detectable clinical signs in young infants who cannot verbalize specific complaints. Tumors arising from the paraspinal ganglion may impinge on nerve roots and cause spinal cord compression. Opsoclonus-myoclonus-ataxia is a paraneoplastic syndrome seen in 2% of neuroblastoma cases. These children exhibit involuntary random eye movements (opsoclonus) and myoclonic jerks that can persist even after curative treatment of the cancer. A subtype of neuroblastoma called *stage 4S* is seen in young infants (<6 months) and consists of a small primary tumor with metastatic disease limited to the liver and skin (subcutaneous nodules); this form of neuroblastoma carries a favorable prognosis. Finally, neuroblastoma cells actively synthesize catecholamines, the metabolites of which are accumulated and secreted. Urinary secretion of these substances (homovanillic acid and vanillylmandelic acid) can be measured to monitor disease activity.

Diagnostic evaluation begins with various forms of imaging, which may show calcified masses that help distinguish neuroblastoma from the noncalcifying lesions of Wilms's tumor. Tissue diagnosis is mandatory before treatment is initiated; this can be accomplished by biopsy of the obvious primary tumor or bone marrow aspiration if bone marrow metastases are present.

Risk stratification based on histologic features, age at presentation (younger age is better), and extent of disease helps in individualizing treatment plans, which consist of surgical resection, chemotherapy, and occasionally radiotherapy. A well-recognized prognostic factor in neuroblastoma regardless of age and stage is *MYCN* status: amplification of the N-Myc proto-oncogene predicts poor outcome. Localized neuroblastoma (stage I) can often be cured by surgical resection alone.

MANAGEMENT OF ANESTHESIA

Anesthetic considerations depend on clinical presentation and the planned surgical procedure, which can range from simple bone marrow biopsy to craniotomy for dural lesion biopsy. Location, size, and metabolic activity of the tumor will dictate the specific anesthetic management, including decisions to place arterial catheters, rapid-infusion intravenous catheters, and an epidural catheter for continuous neuraxial analgesia. In patients receiving anthracycline-based chemotherapy cardiac function should be evaluated preoperatively. Despite potential catecholamine release with tumor manipulation, intraoperative hypertension is infrequent.

Ewing's Sarcoma

Ewing's sarcoma is the most common primary bone malignancy in children and adolescents after osteosarcoma. It is part of the Ewing's sarcoma family of tumors that share a common neuroectodermal origin and include peripheral primitive neuroectodermal tumor, extraosseous Ewing's sarcoma, atypical Ewing's sarcoma, and Askin's tumor (malignant small round cell tumor of the chest wall). These are all small round cell neoplasms of varying differentiation. Ewing's sarcoma represents the least differentiated end of the spectrum.

PATHOGENESIS

The cause and histopathologic features of Ewing's sarcoma have been a source of controversy since it was first described in 1921 by James Ewing. Although tumors in the Ewing's sarcoma family share a common origin, the exact cell type giving rise to Ewing's sarcoma lesions is not known. What has been established is that nearly all tumors of the Ewing's sarcoma family have a reciprocal translocation of the *EWS* gene on chromosome 22, typically with chromosome 11, or t(22;11).

SIGNS AND SYMPTOMS

Ewing's sarcoma is primarily a disease of adolescence. However, approximately 30% of cases occur in children younger than 10 years of age and another 10% occur in the third decade of life. It preferentially affects whites and is uncommon in blacks (both in the United States and Africa) and Asians. Lesions typically develop in flat and long bones, mostly involving the long bones of the lower extremities followed by the pelvis and then the bones of the upper extremities. Soft tissues can also be involved. Localized pain, often in association with a palpable mass, is the most common presenting symptom. Pain may be initiated by minor trauma and is usually exacerbated by exercise and often worse at night. Pathologic fractures are seen in 15% of cases. Systemic symptoms such as fever and anorexia are uncommon (in contrast with osteosarcoma), but when they are present, metastatic disease is likely.

Between 20% and 25% of patients have clinically detectable metastatic disease at presentation. Most cases, however, are thought to have micrometastases from the outset. The most common sites are the lungs, bone, and bone marrow.

Definitive diagnosis is based on tissue biopsy. Experts recommend that bone marrow aspiration and biopsy, at least unilaterally, be a routine part of the initial workup given the predilection for bone marrow involvement. Plain radiography, CT, MRI, and positron emission tomography are all useful diagnostic modalities.

TREATMENT

Neoadjuvant chemotherapy has significantly increased overall survival. Even in nonmetastatic disease, intensive chemotherapy consisting of alternating courses of vincristine, cyclophosphamide, and doxorubicin with ifosfamide and etoposide is administered, followed by surgical resection. Radiotherapy is also used, especially in cases of unresectable disease and positive margins after tumor resection. Hematopoietic stem cell transplantation is being studied as an adjunctive treatment for metastatic disease involving bone and bone marrow.

The most important prognostic factor in Ewing's sarcoma is the presence or absence of metastasis. The 5-year survival rate for those with localized disease is approximately 70%, compared with 30% for those with clinically detectable metastatic disease.

MANAGEMENT OF ANESTHESIA

The most important consideration in the perioperative care of patients with Ewing's sarcoma is pain control. Patients typically have significant preoperative disease-related pain, which is compounded by peri-incisional pain after surgery. Regional and neuraxial analgesia should be strongly considered. Ewing's sarcomas are not associated with any particular congenital disorder, so few patients have significant comorbid conditions. The same principles described for any patient receiving anthracycline-based chemotherapy also apply here.

Tumors of the Central Nervous System

Primary malignancies of the CNS collectively represent the second most common cancer of childhood and adolescence (after leukemia). CNS malignancies have the highest morbidity of all childhood cancers, and the overall mortality approaches 50% despite advances in treatment modalities. The incidence is highest among infants and young children.

There are over 100 histologic subtypes of primary brain tumors, but only a few subtypes account for the majority of cases: astrocytomas, medulloblastomas (primitive neuroectodermal tumors), ependymomas, and craniopharyngiomas. Tumors can occur anywhere in the CNS, and the location is determined primarily by type and age at presentation. Children younger than 1 year of age most often have supratentorial tumors, which are

also the most common in adolescents. Among children between the ages of 1 and 10 years, infratentorial lesions predominate.

SIGNS AND SYMPTOMS

The clinical presentation depends on the location of the tumor, the effect of the tumor on ICP, and the age of the child. Tumors that obstruct the normal flow of CSF will result in increased ICP and hydrocephalus; the child may demonstrate changes in behavior or personality and may complain of headaches along with nausea and vomiting. An increasing head size can be seen in children whose cranial sutures have not closed. Midline infratentorial tumors are classic examples; these lesions can also cause visual disturbances such as nystagmus, diplopia, and blurry vision owing to their location. Supratentorial tumors generally cause widespread sensorimotor deficits as well as speech disorder (aphasia) and seizures. Tumors in the suprasellar and third ventricular regions often lead to neuroendocrine abnormalities caused by anterior and posterior pituitary dysfunctions. Brainstem tumors are associated with cranial nerve palsies and occasionally upper motor neuron deficits (hyperreflexia). Finally, tumors in the spinal cord, either primary lesions or metastatic seedings from leptomeningeal spread, can cause back pain, motor and/or sensory deficits, and possible bowel and bladder dysfunction.

Diagnosis must be made expeditiously given the high morbidity and mortality. Neuroimaging is important in both diagnosis and planning of surgical treatment. MRI remains the gold standard. Midline and suprasellar lesions also require additional laboratory testing to assess neuroendocrine disturbances.

Astrocytomas

Astrocytomas account for approximately 40% of CNS tumors and can occur throughout the CNS. As a group, astrocytomas are generally of low histologic grade and have an indolent clinical course. Juvenile pilocytic astrocytoma is the most common subtype and typically affects the cerebellum. Overall survival is 80% to 100% if complete surgical resection can be achieved. Aggressive subtypes such as anaplastic astrocytoma and glioblastoma multiforme are rare in children and are seen mostly in adults.

Medulloblastomas

Medulloblastomas belong to the family of primitive neuroectodermal tumors, not to be confused with peripheral primitive neuroectodermal tumor, which is part of the Ewing family of tumors as described previously. Primitive neuroectodermal tumors account for 25% of CNS tumors, with the majority being medulloblastomas. All primitive neuroectodermal tumors have a high histologic grade; clinically they demonstrate high metastatic activity within the neuraxis. Medulloblastomas are cerebellar tumors that affect boys more than girls with peak incidence between the ages of 5 and 7 years. Disseminated leptomeningeal disease is seen in approximately 30% of patients at presentation. Signs and symptoms related to increased ICP and cerebellar dysfunction (ataxia) are common. A multimodal treatment approach is standard.

Ependymomas

Ependymomas arise from the ependymal lining of the ventricular system. They account for 10% of CNS tumors in children, and the majority are located in the posterior fossa. Surgery is the primary treatment modality, although it is rarely curative without adjuvant radiotherapy and chemotherapy. Overall survival with a multimodal treatment approach is approximately 40%. Local recurrence is not uncommon.

Craniopharyngiomas

Craniopharyngiomas are the most common intracranial tumors of nonglial origin. They are tumors of epithelial origin deriving from the remnants of Rathke's pouch and occur in the suprasellar region in almost all cases. Craniopharyngiomas can be considered benign neoplasms, although malignant transformations have been reported. Nonetheless, these "benign" tumors are associated with significant morbidities because of their anatomic proximity to important structures such as the hypothalamus, pituitary gland, optic chiasm, ventricular system, and carotid arteries. Even when curative surgical resection can be accomplished, children are often left with serious neuroendocrine and visual complications. In the modern era treatment for craniopharyngiomas consists of surgery, radiotherapy, brachytherapy, and chemotherapy. Tumor recurrence is one of the most significant and commonly encountered complications.

Choroid Plexus Tumors

Choroid plexus tumors are the most common CNS tumors of infancy, although they are generally rare in children. Clinical symptoms are related to increased ICP caused by overproduction of CSF by the abnormal choroid plexus growths. Almost 100% of choroid plexus papillomas can be cured by surgical resection; choroid plexus carcinomas have a much worse prognosis (survival rate of 40%).

MANAGEMENT OF ANESTHESIA

Anesthetic concerns for children with CNS tumors fall into two general categories: those relating to increased ICP and those pertaining to neuroendocrine disturbances, particularly ones that impact perioperative fluid and electrolyte management. A thorough preoperative assessment must clearly establish the presence and severity of the aforementioned complications in addition to evaluating the general health and neurologic status of the patient.

Management of the patient with increased ICP has already been described, and the reader is referred to the previous discussion on hydrocephalus. In general, anesthetic management is aimed at limiting further increase in ICP and preserving cerebral perfusion. The head is often elevated above the level of the heart (even when the classic "sitting craniotomy" position is not used), so the risk of venous air embolism must be recognized. Precordial Doppler imaging is a sensitive means of detecting venous air embolism before hemodynamic changes are evident.

Of all the neuroendocrine disturbances that can result from CNS tumors, particularly from craniopharyngiomas, diabetes insipidus is the most important complication from a perioperative standpoint. Diabetes insipidus is diagnosed based on a rising serum sodium concentration (>145 mg/dL) in the setting of copious dilute urine production (specific gravity < 1.005). The patient may already have diabetes insipidus, and preoperative treatment (vasopressin infusion) must be continued intraoperatively along with isotonic fluid administration at two thirds of the maintenance rate. Blood and evaporative losses must also be replaced. Vasopressin is typically started at 0.5 milliunits/kg/hr and is increased in increments of 0.5 milliunits/kg/hr until urine osmolality is twice that of serum osmolality or is titrated to keep urine output to less than 2 mL/kg/hr. Desmopressin (DDAVP) can also be used; a single dose (0.5 to 4 mcg IV) lasts 8 to 12 hours, and thus it is less preferred than vasopressin because its effects are not easily titratable. Diabetes insipidus may also develop postoperatively, typically 4 to 6 hours after surgery. Intraoperative onset of diabetes insipidus is infrequent. An intraoperative need for mannitol complicates the management of diabetes insipidus. Urine output, urine and serum osmolality, and serum sodium must be strictly monitored throughout the perioperative period.

CNS tumor resections can be associated with excessive blood loss, especially if important vascular structures such as the sagittal sinus are compromised. Intraarterial blood pressure monitoring should be used in all cases of craniotomy for tumor resections. A sample for typing and cross matching should already have been processed and the necessary blood components reserved in case transfusion is necessary.

Modern procedures for CNS tumor resection at some centers include the use of perioperative MRI imaging to help guide the extent of resection. The patient undergoes MRI scanning in the operating room immediately after tumor resection while still under general anesthesia. Strict MRI precautions must be observed to prevent injury to the patient and operating room personnel. Meticulous attention must be paid to securing the endotracheal tube and the various intravenous and intraarterial catheters to avoid dislodgment.

ANTERIOR MEDIASTINAL MASS

There are many causes of anterior mediastinal mass in children, including both neoplastic and nonneoplastic diseases. In the neoplastic category, lymphomas (non-Hodgkin's and Hodgkin's disease) account for the majority of cases. Others include lymphangiomas (cystic hygroma), germ cell tumors (teratoma), and neurogenic tumors (neuroblastoma). Regardless of the cause, an anterior mediastinal mass can have serious cardiorespiratory consequences as a result of compression of adjacent structures.

Signs and Symptoms

The clinical presentation of an anterior mediastinal mass depends how large it is and, more importantly, on whether the mass is impinging on nearby important structures such as the trachea, the heart, and the great vessels. There is often discordance between the clinical presentation and radiologic findings. Some children with compressive cardiorespiratory symptoms have no radiologic evidence of compression, whereas others who have demonstrable mass compression on imaging studies remain asymptomatic.

Compression of the tracheobronchial tree leads to varying degrees of respiratory compromise. Patients can have tachypnea, wheezing, recurrent pneumonia, obstructive emphysema, and atelectasis. Some children are erroneously considered to have asthma until a mediastinal mass is found incidentally on a subsequent radiographic study. Asthmalike symptoms caused by a mediastinal mass do not respond to conventional bronchodilator treatment because the pathophysiology is different. Of all the respiratory complaints, orthopnea is most predictive of potential airway obstruction. Children often report worsening of their symptoms in the supine position. Chronic compression of the tracheobronchial tree can lead to weakened wall structures whose patency becomes dependent on the negative intrathoracic pressure created during spontaneous respiration.

Cardiovascular signs and symptoms can be caused by compression of the heart and/or the great vessels. Compression of the heart can cause symptoms of restrictive pericardial disease, either directly by tumor compression of the myocardium or indirectly by causing a reactive pericardial effusion. Signs and symptoms of cardiac tamponade may occur, including Beck's triad (increased jugular venous pressure, hypotension, and decreased heart sounds), tachycardia, tachypnea, and dyspnea. As with respiratory complaints, cardiovascular symptoms may become worse in the supine position. Compression of the superior vena cava impairs venous drainage from the upper body, which leads to upper body edema, a feature of the superior vena cava syndrome. Other features of superior vena cava syndrome include facial and periorbital edema, shortness of breath, engorged jugular veins, headaches, and visual disturbances.

Several imaging studies are useful in the evaluation of an anterior mediastinal mass, including plain radiography, CT, and MRI. Echocardiography can delineate the dynamic effects of the mass on the heart and the proximal great vessels. Flow volume loops obtained in the supine and upright positions provide the best estimation of the dynamic respiratory impact of the mass. Unfortunately, most young children cannot cooperate with such testing.

Definitive diagnosis is based on tissue biopsy, a procedure not easily accomplished without sedation or general anesthesia in young children. Since anterior mediastinal masses produce fixed and dynamic cardiorespiratory compressive symptoms, the potential loss of muscle tone and negative intrathoracic pressure associated with the administration of sedative and anesthetic drugs can lead to disastrous outcomes. Some patients with large lesions are pretreated with corticosteroids or radiation therapy to reduce mass size before tissue biopsy under sedation or anesthesia is performed. However, such prebiopsy treatments can affect the accuracy of future histologic evaluation and thus adversely impact the efficacy of future treatment plans.

Management of Anesthesia

The most important concern in the perioperative management of a child with an anterior mediastinal mass is the potential loss of airway. A detailed preoperative assessment of the child's respiratory status is mandatory. Specifically, details must be sought regarding the particular complaints, such as tachypnea and stridor, as well as maneuvers that improve or worsen those symptoms. Positional changes (e.g., upright to supine) that worsen symptoms should be avoided even if it interferes with optimal positioning for the operative procedure. Conversely, positions that minimize respiratory complaints should be maintained. Preoperative radiologic studies must be reviewed to delineate the location and extent of potential compression by the mass. A preoperative radiographic finding of a 50% reduction in the tracheal cross-sectional area portends respiratory complications with the induction of general anesthesia.

Tissue biopsy procedures that may be amenable to performance under local anesthesia with or without light sedation should be considered whenever possible (e.g., in an older child, biopsy of a peripheral lesion such as a cervical or supraclavicular node). If deep sedation or general anesthesia is required, spontaneous ventilation must be preserved, because airway patency may be entirely dependent on negative intrathoracic pressure. Carefully titrated inhaled volatile agents and intravenous ketamine and/or dexmedetomidine (1 to 3 mcg/kg/hr with or without a loading dose of 1 mcg/kg over 10 minutes) have been used successfully for maintenance in an anesthetized but spontaneously breathing child. Nitrous oxide should be avoided to maximize supplemental oxygen and to prevent rapid expansion of a potential pneumothorax that may occur during tissue biopsy. Titration of low doses of ketamine and/or dexmedetomidine, both of which lack significant respiratory-depressant effects, can produce a comfortably sedated child who may even tolerate deep tissue biopsy. Nonetheless, no one anesthetic technique can guarantee airway patency. For this reason, the ability to perform rigid bronchoscopy (availability of both equipment and an experienced bronchoscopist) must be ensured in case of airway collapse. Intubation alone may not reestablish airway patency, because the tracheobronchial tree beyond the end of the tracheal tube may be compressed by the mass.

Rapid cardiovascular deterioration may also occur with induction of general anesthesia, because the child may be barely maintaining stable hemodynamics in the awake and anxious state. Careless positional changes may also cause direct compression of cardiovascular structures by the mass, leading to impaired ventricular output and venous return. Because of its sympathomimetic effects, ketamine is a good choice to help maintain stable hemodynamic parameters. Its direct myocardial-depressant effects must be recognized, however. Adequate intravenous access in the lower extremities must be established, since compression of the superior great vessels can occur even in the absence of preexisting superior vena cava syndrome.

Should cardiorespiratory decompensation occur, the child should be turned to a lateral decubitus or prone position to help relieve the compression exerted by the mass. An extra bed or stretcher should be immediately available, especially for older children, to help facilitate quick prone positioning.

Children with hematologic malignancies may have coagulation abnormalities (thrombocytopenia). Therefore, available preoperative laboratory data should be reviewed.

Although children with an anterior mediastinal mass are at risk for significant perioperative morbidity and mortality, the actual incidence of perioperative complications is quite low due to the recognition of prognostic factors and the implementation of appropriate anesthetic techniques. In general, perioperative complications have occurred mostly in patients with preoperative compressive symptoms. In a recent study, the clinical and diagnostic imaging findings that were most predictive of anesthetic complications include orthopnea, upper body edema, great vessel compression, and main bronchus compression. The presence of pleural effusion and tracheal compression also appeared to be risk factors.

The potential for postanesthetic airway compromise is high given the propensity for tracheobronchomalacia. Vigilant monitoring in the postanesthesia care unit or ICU is required before the patient can be returned to a less acute care setting.

DOWN'S SYNDROME

Down's syndrome is the most common chromosomal abnormality, occurring in 1 in 700 to 1 in 800 live births. Advanced maternal age significantly increases the risk of this chromosomal aberration. Also known as *trisomy 21,* Down's syndrome can also occur with mosaicism and translocation of chromosome 21. Patients with Down's syndrome have characteristic dysmorphic features and have a higher incidence of many health problems than their healthy counterparts (Table 27-19). Some of these health issues are congenital and some occur later on in life. Although the overall life expectancy of patients with Down's syndrome has dramatically improved over the years, Down's syndrome still confers a shorter life span than would be expected for healthy individuals.

Signs and Symptoms

Down's syndrome is usually recognized at birth or soon thereafter by a constellation of characteristic dysmorphic features. These include upslanting palpebral fissures, epicanthal folds, flattened nasal bridge, flattened occiput and brachycephalic head shape, short broad hands with a palmar crease (simian crease), and hypotonia. Diagnosis is confirmed by karyotype analysis. Congenital anomalies of almost all organ systems are associated with Down's syndrome.

Down's syndrome is the most common cause of intellectual disability. Almost all affected children have some degree of mental retardation. Most are only mildly to moderately impaired, although severe mental retardation can occur. Individuals with Down's syndrome are also prone to developing early-onset

TABLE 27-19	Clinical findings associated with Down's syndrome

GENERAL
Low birth weight
Short stature

CENTRAL NERVOUS SYSTEM
Mental retardation
Seizure
Strabismus
Hypotonia

AIRWAY AND RESPIRATORY SYSTEM
High-arched narrow palate
Macroglossia
Micrognathia
Subglottic stenosis
Upper airway obstruction
Increased susceptibility to postintubation croup and respiratory infections
Obstructive sleep apnea

CARDIOVASCULAR SYSTEM
Congenital heart disease
Increased susceptibility to pulmonary hypertension
Atropine sensitivity
Bradycardia with sevoflurane induction

GASTROINTESTINAL SYSTEM
Duodenal obstruction
Gastroesophageal reflux
Hirschsprung's disease

MUSCULOSKELETAL SYSTEM
Atlantoaxial instability
Hyperextensibility/flexibility of joints
Dysplastic pelvis

IMMUNE AND HEMATOLOGIC FUNCTIONS
Immune deficiency
Leukemia (acute lymphocytic leukemia, acute myeloid leukemia)
Neonatal polycythemia

ENDOCRINE SYSTEM
Thyroid dysfunction
Low circulating levels of catecholamine

Adapted from Maxwell LG, Goodwin SR, Mancuso TJ, et al. Systemic disorders. In: Davis PJ, Cladis FP, Motoyama EK, eds. *Smith's Anesthesia for Infants and Children.* 8th ed. Philadelphia, PA: Mosby; 2011:1173.

dementia-like symptoms and Alzheimer's disease. Epilepsy occurs at a higher frequency than in the general population. Ocular disorders such as congenital and early-onset cataracts, strabismus, nystagmus, and refractive errors are common.

Children with Down's syndrome are at increased risk of developing obstructive sleep apnea resulting from soft tissue defects (low tone and redundancy) and skeletal abnormalities (midface hypoplasia, high arched palate, micrognathia). Moreover, poor tone and macroglossia further predispose to upper airway obstruction. Most children with Down's syndrome are observed to have a protruding tongue. Subglottic airway diameter is generally decreased; small insults can lead to clinically overt subglottic stenosis.

Approximately half of all patients with Down's syndrome have congenital heart disease. Endocardial cushion defects (atrioventricular septal defects) are the most common (40% to 50%), followed by ventral septal defects, secundum atrial septal defects, persistent patent ductus arteriosus, tetralogy of Fallot, and others (vascular rings). There can be single or multiple defects.

Gastrointestinal anomalies are also common, including gastroesophageal reflux, intestinal atresia, anorectal malformations, and Hirschsprung's disease. From a musculoskeletal standpoint, patients with Down's syndrome have hypotonia and their joints are hyperextensible. Dysplastic pelvis is also common. Atlantoaxial instability has potentially the gravest impact on neurologic function. Subluxation of the atlas (C1) and axis (C2) joint can cause spinal cord compression with resultant sensorimotor deficits as well as loss of bowel and bladder control. According to the current recommendations of the American Academy of Pediatrics on the management of patients with Down's syndrome, children should undergo radiographic screening for atlantoaxial instability between the ages of 3 and 5 years. Children may have asymptomatic atlantoaxial instability. Symptoms of cord compression include neck pain, torticollis, and gait abnormalities. Bowel and bladder dysfunction as well as paretic symptoms require immediate surgical stabilization of the atlantoaxial joint.

Thyroid hormonal disturbances are frequently seen; hypothyroidism is more common than hyperthyroidism. Endocrine abnormalities may play a role in the tendency toward obesity among patients with Down's syndrome; these patients have also been demonstrated to have a lower rate of metabolism. Finally, children with Down's syndrome have a high incidence of hematologic abnormalities such as neonatal polycythemia. They have a 10- to 20-fold increased risk of developing leukemia. Immune deficiencies are not uncommon.

Management of Anesthesia

Several clinical manifestations and associated congenital anomalies are of particular concern in the perioperative management of children with Down's syndrome. A thorough preoperative assessment must be done with specific focus on the cardiac, respiratory, and neurologic status. The presence of atlantoaxial instability may not be apparent, because most patients are asymptomatic. The parents should be questioned specifically about symptoms suggestive of atlantoaxial subluxation, such as neck pain, head tilt, and abnormal gait. Older infants and toddlers can be observed for poor head control, passive limited neck range of motion, and signs and symptoms of upper motor neuron dysfunction (spasticity, hyperreflexia,

clonus). Any existing neck radiographic studies should be reviewed. Elective surgery should be delayed if there is clinical or radiographic evidence of subluxation (posterior atlantodens interval of >4 to 5 mm), and a neurosurgeon should be consulted for further management. Even in the absence of overt atlantoaxial instability, neck manipulation should be kept to a minimum, especially during laryngoscopy.

Macroglossia compounded by potential micrognathia and midface hypoplasia predispose these children to rapid airway obstruction and hypoxemia with induction of anesthesia. Oral airways should always be available to help in reestablishing airway patency. These children are also at a higher risk for developing postintubation croup because they tend to have a smaller absolute subglottic airway diameter. Therefore, children with Down's syndrome should be intubated with a smaller endotracheal tube than predicted for age. As in all children, an air leak at or below a pressure of 25 cm H_2O must be demonstrated.

Significant bradycardia occurs with inhaled sevoflurane induction in up to 50% of children with Down's syndrome regardless of the presence or absence of co-existing congenital heart disease. It has been speculated that these children have ultrastructural myocardial defects that predispose them to conduction abnormalities. Anticholinergics (atropine, glycopyrrolate) should be immediately available in the appropriate weight-based doses. Increased sensitivity to atropine is occasionally seen, manifesting as mydriasis and profound tachycardia.

Co-existing congenital heart disease must be clearly delineated. Anesthetic management is guided by the in-situ pattern of blood flow and should be aimed at balancing the pulmonary and systemic circulations. In general, children with Down's syndrome undergoing cardiac surgery have a higher perioperative mortality than their counterparts without trisomy 21.

Patients must be closely observed for obstructive symptoms and hypoventilation in the postoperative period given the high incidence of obstructive sleep apnea and obesity.

MALIGNANT HYPERTHERMIA

Malignant hyperthermia (MH) is a potentially lethal genetic disorder of muscle hypermetabolism that occurs upon exposure to volatile anesthetic agents and succinylcholine. It has multiple inheritance patterns, including autosomal dominant, autosomal recessive, and unclassified. Both penetrance and expression are variable, and affected individuals demonstrate different sensitivity to triggering agents and manifest different levels of clinical severity. Overall incidence of MH is estimated to be anywhere between 1 in 3000 to 1 in 15,000 in children. The higher incidence represents cases in which both a volatile anesthetic agent and succinylcholine are used. Most cases occur in the first three decades of life, although cases of MH at the extremes of age have been reported.

The porcine model has provided much insight into the pathophysiology of MH. In addition to classic MH, pigs also demonstrate MH-like symptoms that occur in response to nonanesthetic stressors such as heat and human handling (porcine stress syndrome). All breeds of pigs that are susceptible to MH share a specific point mutation in the ryanodine receptor gene (*RYR1*). This same point mutation is seen in a minority of humans who are susceptible to MH. Mutations in multiple other loci of the RYR1 gene (located on chromosome 19) have been demonstrated in susceptible human families. In addition, abnormalities in other muscle membrane proteins such as the dihydropyridine receptor have been linked with MH. This explains the heterogeneous nature of MH in humans.

Pathogenesis

Normal muscle contraction depends on an increase in intracellular (sarcoplasmal) calcium (Ca^{2+}). Upon membrane depolarization, Ca^{2+} is released from the sarcoplasmic reticulum into the sarcoplasma via the dihydropyridine and ryanodine receptors, both of which are voltage-gated ion channels. Calcium interacts with troponin to allow cross-bridging between actin and myosin for muscle contraction to occur. MH-related mutations in the RYR1 gene decrease receptor threshold for Ca^{2+} release. In addition, affected RYR1 receptors are resistant to the negative feedback mechanisms (increased Ca^{2+} and magnesium levels) that normally decrease Ca^{2+} conductance. Exposure to triggers causes an exaggerated Ca^{2+} release at smaller levels of membrane depolarization.

Adenosine triphosphate (ATP) is consumed in all steps of intracellular Ca^{2+} handling. Decoupling of Ca^{2+} from troponin (muscle relaxation) requires ATP. Removal of intracellular Ca^{2+}, including return to the sarcoplasmic reticulum and mitochondria as well as extrusion into the extracellular milieu, also requires ATP. Because of this, the initial exaggerated release of Ca^{2+} via abnormal ryanodine receptors sets up a cascade of reactions that consumes an equally exaggerated amount of ATP, and hypermetabolism ensues.

Signs and Symptoms

MH in humans is a heterogeneous disorder, and thus clinical presentation varies greatly. Some susceptible individuals can receive multiple triggering anesthetics without apparent problems, whereas others demonstrate severe reactions to only traces of volatile agents. Time of onset is also variable; some have immediate reactions upon exposure to triggers and others do not manifest signs and symptoms of MH until well into the postoperative period.

Early clinical signs and symptoms of MH are nonspecific and reflect a hypermetabolic state such as would also be seen in conditions such as thyroid storm, fulminant sepsis, and pheochromocytoma (Table 27-20). Therefore, diagnosis requires a high index of suspicion along with consideration of the circumstances specific to each patient (trigger exposure, comorbid conditions, family history).

Early clinical signs of MH include sinus tachycardia, tachypnea (if there is spontaneous ventilation), hypercarbia (that

TABLE 27-20   Differential diagnosis of malignant hyperthermia (MH)

Diagnosis	Distinguishing features
Hyperthyroidism	Characteristic symptoms and physical findings often present, blood gas abnormalities increase gradually
Sepsis	Hypercarbia usually not seen, severe lactic acidosis may be present
Pheochromocytoma	Similar to MH except marked blood pressure swings
Metastatic carcinoid	Same as pheochromocytoma
Cocaine intoxication	Fever, rigidity, rhabdomyolysis similar to malignant neuroleptic syndrome
Heat stroke	Similar to MH except that patient is outside operating room
Masseter muscle rigidity	May progress to MH, with or without total body spasm
Malignant neuroleptic syndrome	Similar to MH, usually associated with the use of antidepressants
Serotonergic syndrome	Similar to MH and malignant neuroleptic syndrome, associated with the use of mood-elevating drug

Adapted from Bissonnette B, Ryan JF. Temperature regulation: normal and abnormal (malignant hyperthermia). In: Coté CJ, Todres ID, Goudsouzian NG, et al, eds. *A Practice of Anesthesia for Infants and Children*. 3rd ed. Philadelphia, PA: Saunders; 2001:621.

does not improve with compensatory increases in minute ventilation), and masseter muscle spasm (Table 27-21). Rapid exhaustion of the carbon dioxide absorber is usually evident along with obvious warming of the canister. Dysrhythmias and peaked T waves may also be seen on the electrocardiogram, reflecting progressive hyperkalemia. Increase in core temperature can occur within 15 minutes of exposure to culprit agents. However, overt hyperthermia may be a late sign. Laboratory analysis typically reveals a mixed respiratory and metabolic acidosis (lactic acidosis), arterial hypoxemia, and hyperkalemia. Because MH is a hypermetabolic disorder of skeletal muscles, later clinical manifestations are more specific to, but not pathognomonic of, an underlying muscle pathology. Masseter muscle spasm can progress to whole-body muscle rigidity with imminent rhabdomyolysis. At this stage, MH is considered to be fulminant; the patient will typically have cola-colored urine along with myoglobinuria and an elevated serum creatinine kinase (CK) level (characteristically in excess of 20,000 units/L) on laboratory testing. Ultimately, the body's capacity to support the exaggerated oxidative metabolism is exhausted, and cardiovascular collapse ensues. Severe hyperthermia is also associated with the development of disseminated intravascular coagulation.

A diagnosis of MH is made based on the clinical picture. Definitive diagnosis requires tissue biopsy to obtain a specimen for the caffeine-halothane contracture test. However, the caffeine-halothane contracture test has a specificity of only approximately 80%; thus, a negative result does not completely rule out MH. Because the clinical picture of MH is nonspecific

TABLE 27-21 ■ **Clinical feature of malignant hyperthermia**

Timing	Clinical signs	Changes in monitored variables	Biochemical changes
Early	Masseter spasm		
	Tachypnea	Increased minute ventilation	
	Rapid exhaustion of soda lime	Increasing end-tidal CO_2	Increased Pa_{CO_2}
	Warm soda lime canister		
	Tachycardia		Acidosis
	Irregular heart rate	Cardiac dysrhythmias Peaked T waves	Hyperkalemia
Intermediate	Patient warm to touch	Increasing core body temperature	
	Cyanosis	Decreasing oxygen saturation	
	Dark blood in surgical site		
	Irregular heart rate	Cardiac dysrhythmias Peaked T waves	Hyperkalemia
Late	Generalized skeletal muscle rigidity		Increased serum creatinine kinase level
	Prolonged bleeding		
	Cola-colored urine		Myoglobinuria
	Irregular heart rate	Cardiac dysrhythmias Peaked T waves Widened QRS Ventricular arrhythmias	Hyperkalemia

Adapted from Hopkins PM. Malignant hyperthermia: advances in clinical management and diagnosis. *Br J Anaesth.* 2000;85(1):118-128.

and most patients do not have a clear family history of susceptibility, constant vigilance is mandatory for early recognition and expeditious treatment. The introduction of dantrolene therapy has decreased overall mortality from 70% to less than 5%.

MASSETER SPASM

Masseter spasm is often the first clue to potential MH. However, transient jaw rigidity is a normal response to succinylcholine administration. There are several confusing terms describing masseter spasm, including *trismus* and *masseter muscle rigidity*. However, they are not synonymous but rather describe a spectrum of spasm intensity. Trismus is generally defined as masseter spasm that still permits enough mouth opening for intubation and *masseter muscle rigidity* is defined as masseter spasm that completely prevents mouth opening. Regardless, masseter spasm deserves immediate attention, because its presence in children is associated with a 50% chance of MH susceptibility and a 30% chance of an actual MH episode. Controversy still exists regarding whether or not to continue elective surgery and which anesthetic technique to choose once masseter spasm occurs. Worrisome signs include persistent or worsening masseter spasm and concurrent manifestations of hypermetabolism, in which case elective surgery should be aborted. If masseter spasm is mild and/or transient and is also an isolated finding, elective surgery may continue, but the child should receive ample intravenous hydration to maintain a urine output of at least 2 to 3 mL/kg/hr because myoglobinuria may occur. Significant serum CK elevations can be seen in isolated masseter spasm; thus, the patient must be monitored postoperatively for resolution. Experienced

anesthesiologists differ in their opinions on whether or not volatile agents should be immediately discontinued in these cases. However, it is difficult to justify continuing volatile drug–based anesthesia in these circumstances when currently available equipment and medications make it easy to transition to a nontriggering technique.

ANESTHESIA-INDUCED RHABDOMYOLYSIS

Dystrophinopathies (Duchenne's and Becker's muscular dystrophy) have long been linked with possible increased MH susceptibility. It has now become apparent that these patients do not have an increased susceptibility to MH. However, they can develop MH-like symptoms upon exposure to the same triggering agents. Specifically, these patients can develop anesthesia-induced rhabdomyolysis, which is frequently accompanied by the same hypermetabolic signs as those seen in MH. Instead of ryanodine receptor abnormalities, the absence of the dystrophin-glycoprotein complex in dystrophinopathies results in instability and increased permeability of the muscle cell membrane (sarcolemma) with resultant increased intracellular Ca^{2+} levels. Sarcolemma instability also predisposes to membrane breakdown leading to massive potassium release. For this reason, an acute onset of hyperkalemic cardiac arrest (without preceding hypermetabolic signs) can be the first manifestation of anesthesia-induced rhabdomyolysis, a presentation not typical of MH. The role of dantrolene in the treatment of anesthesia-induced rhabdomyolysis is unknown, but it likely has little efficacy because it does not possess membrane-stabilizing effects. Although only a small percentage of patients with dystrophinopathies may develop anesthesia-induced rhabdomyolysis, use of a nontriggering anesthetic technique is recommended given the potential life-threatening consequences.

Treatment

The only known antidote for MH is dantrolene; additional treatments consist of supportive and resuscitative measures (Table 27-22). Dantrolene is thought to inhibit Ca^{2+} conductance through ryanodine receptor channels. More recently, it has been shown that dantrolene blocks the external entry of Ca^{2+} into the sarcoplasma that normally occurs upon membrane depolarization. Regardless of the mechanism, dantrolene halts further rises in intracellular Ca^{2+} levels. The most common side effects of dantrolene are muscle weakness and vein irritation.

Once an acute episode of MH is suspected, all triggering agents must be stopped immediately and the anesthesia machine flushed with 100% oxygen at the highest possible flow rate. Dantrolene must be given expeditiously starting at 2.5 mg/kg, and occasionally a cumulative dose of more than 10 mg/kg is required to control the hypermetabolic signs and sequelae. Preparation of dantrolene solutions is a cumbersome task, and the need to call for additional help immediately cannot be overemphasized. Dantrolene powder must be diluted with sterile distilled water. Each vial contains 20 mg of dantrolene along with 3 g of mannitol, which must be mixed with 60 mL of sterile water. Newer formulations of dantrolene manufactured after 2008 solubilize more easily, but it is nonetheless a time-consuming process, especially in the face of a rapidly deteriorating clinical situation. The surgeon must be notified immediately to abort or to complete surgery as quickly as possible. Under no circumstance should volatile agents or succinylcholine be administered again.

Supportive and resuscitative measures are aimed at addressing the hypermetabolic consequences. Hyperventilation with 100% oxygen should be initiated to compensate for the increased carbon dioxide production and oxygen consumption. Aggressive hydration with room-temperature fluids and possible pharmacologic diuresis (furosemide, mannitol) should be started to maintain a urine output of at least 2 mL/kg/hr to minimize renal damage from myoglobinuria. One must be remember that dantrolene solutions contain mannitol in calculating the dose being administered. Active cooling can be done with surface cooling and intracavitary lavage of the stomach and bladder with cold saline solutions. An arterial catheter should be placed to continuously monitor the patient's hemodynamic parameters and to allow for repeat blood sampling. Metabolic disturbances such as metabolic acidosis and hyperkalemia should be treated with a combination of sodium bicarbonate, regular insulin with glucose (to drive potassium intracellularly), β-agonists, and calcium chloride, especially if there are electrocardiographic manifestations of hyperkalemia (peaked T waves, widened QRS complex), to prevent progression to hyperkalemic cardiac arrest. Calcium

TABLE 27-22 ■ Treatment of malignant hyperthermia

PRIMARY TREATMENT

Stop inhaled anesthetic immediately.
Call for help immediately.
Administer dantrolene (2.5 mg/kg IV) as initial bolus.
Repeat every 5-10 min until symptoms are controlled (may rarely exceed maximum of 10 mg/kg).
Prevent recrudescence (dantrolene 1 mg/kg IV every 6 hr for 72 hr).

SYMPTOMATIC TREATMENT

Abort or conclude surgery as soon as possible.
Hyperventilate the lungs with 100% oxygen at >10 L/min.
Initiate active cooling (iced saline 15 mL/kg IV every 10 min, gastric and bladder lavage with iced saline, surface cooling).
Correct metabolic acidosis (sodium bicarbonate 1-2 mEq/kg IV).
Treat hyperkalemia (calcium chloride 5-10 mg/kg IV or regular insulin 0.15 units/kg in 1 mL/kg of 50% dextrose).
Maintain urine output (hydration, mannitol* 0.25 g/kg IV, furosemide 1 mg/kg IV).
Treat cardiac dysrhythmias (procainamide 15 mg/kg IV, lidocaine 2 mg/kg IV, follow pediatric advanced life support guidelines).
Place peripheral arterial and central venous catheters.
Check blood gas concentrations every 15 min until abnormalities are corrected.
Monitor in an intensive care unit.

IV, Intravenous.
*Each 20-mg vial of dantrolene contains 3 g of mannitol.

channel blockers are contraindicated because they can worsen hyperkalemia.

After the acute episode of MH has been controlled, the patient must have continued care in an ICU setting. Recrudescence occurs in up to 25% of patients, with muscular body type, temperature increase, and increased latency between exposure and MH onset as risk factors. Recrudescence usually occurs within the first few hours after the initial episode, but late presentations (up to 36 hours after the initial episode) have been reported. Because of this, dantrolene therapy should continue (1 mg/kg every 6 hours) for 48 to 72 hours after the last observed sign of MH. Dantrolene may also be given as a continuous infusion (0.1 to 0.3 mg/kg/hr). Development of disseminated intravascular coagulation is an ominous sign and is a common finding in fatal MH. Laboratory coagulation test results should be followed throughout the course of MH management.

All patients with clinical MH or signs of anesthesia-induced hypermetabolism as well as those with significant masseter spasm should undergo the caffeine-halothane contracture test. At least 1 g of muscle must be harvested for satisfactory testing; this precludes some young children from undergoing the test because of their small size. The patient's immediate family members should be counseled and possibly referred for muscle and genetic testing as well (Table 27-23). All cases of suspected MH and significant masseter spasm should be reported to the North American Malignant Hyperthermia Registry (888-274-7899).

TABLE 27-23	Follow-up of patients with malignant hyperthermia (MH) or masseter muscle rigidity

1. Have patient wear a medical alert bracelet; patient and first-degree relatives must be assumed to have MH susceptibility.
2. Refer patient to Malignant Hyperthermia Association of the United States (MHAUS; http://www.mhaus.org). MHAUS can refer patient to an MH diagnostic center.
3. Review family history for adverse anesthetic events or suggestion of heritable myopathy.
4. Consider evaluation for temporomandibular joint disorder.
5. Consider neurologic consultation to evaluate for a potential myotonic disorder.
6. For severe rhabdomyolysis, consider evaluation for a dystrophinopathy (Duchenne's or Becker's muscular dystrophy) or heritable metabolic disorder (e.g., carnitine palmitoyltransferase II deficiency or McArdle's disease).

TABLE 27-24	Drugs that do not trigger malignant hyperthermia

Barbiturates
Propofol
Etomidate
Benzodiazepines
Opioids
Droperidol
Nitrous oxide
Nondepolarizing muscle relaxants
Anticholinesterases
Anticholinergics
Sympathomimetics
Local anesthetics (esters and amides)
α_2-Agonists (clonidine, dexmedetomidine)

Management of Anesthesia

Identification of susceptible patients is the most important first step. It would of course be ideal to be able to identify all MH-susceptible patients so that triggering agents can be avoided. This is neither possible nor feasible, especially in the pediatric populations in which the majority of patients are receiving their first anesthetic. Family history is unclear in many cases, particularly for adopted children. Preoperative serum CK levels are generally not predictive (some patients with elevated baseline CK levels are not MH susceptible, whereas others with a normal preoperative serum CK concentration go on to develop MH). There are currently only a few disorders that have been clearly linked with MH; these include central core disease, King-Denborough syndrome, and Evans's myopathy. They are all rare and well-defined clinical entities. Of note, a rare subset of MH-susceptible patients can develop MH in response to nonanesthetic triggers such as vigorous exercise, heat, and anxiety, as in pigs with porcine stress syndrome.

Preoperative dantrolene prophylaxis is not indicated. Some continue to administer prophylactic dantrolene (2 to 4 mg/kg IV 15 to 30 minutes before induction) when the patient has a documented history of severe MH. In addition to muscle weakness and vein irritation, other side effects of dantrolene include nausea, blurred vision, and diarrhea. For this reason, the drug must be given in a monitored setting, especially when the patient has underlying neuromuscular and/or respiratory dysfunctions.

Children should be given a liberal dose of oral anxiolytic(s) preoperatively. In addition to midazolam, ketamine (4 to 5 mg/kg if used with midazolam and 9 to 10 mg/kg if used alone) should be considered as an adjunct to maximize sedation while preserving respiratory efforts. Topical local anesthetics (lidocaine plus prilocaine [EMLA], 4% lidocaine [ELA-Max]) should be applied on anticipated intravenous catheter insertion sites to facilitate awake placement.

Once MH susceptibility is identified or suspected, a non-triggering anesthetic plan (Table 27-24) must be initiated that includes elimination of triggering agents and thorough preparation of the anesthesia machine to minimize even trace residues of volatile agents. If available, a dedicated MH-preventive anesthesia machine that was never exposed to volatile anesthetics should be used. Otherwise, the anesthesia station must be flushed with high-flow oxygen for the recommended length of time specific to each model (from 20 minutes to over 100 minutes). Most current models have an extensive internal flow circuitry that requires a much longer flush time to reduce residual volatile anesthetics to clinically insignificant levels. External parts such as the anesthesia circuit, ventilation bag, and carbon dioxide absorber should be changed and vaporizers removed. Dantrolene and other resuscitative drugs must be immediately available. The entire perioperative team should be made aware of the patient's condition and be educated on the recognition and treatment of MH. The presurgical time-out provides an ideal opportunity to voice anesthetic concerns and delineate a clear treatment plan should MH occur.

Use of nitrous oxide in oxygen can facilitate intravenous catheter placement in a child who is not adequately sedated with premedication. Intramuscular induction (e.g., ketamine 4 to 5 mg/kg) is an alternative for the unusually uncooperative and combative child. Maintenance of anesthesia relies mostly on intravenous hypnotics, with or without nitrous oxide; nondepolarizing muscle relaxants may be used if necessary. Dexmedetomidine is a useful adjunct for both its sedative and analgesic effects. Whenever possible, local anesthesia (both ester- and amide-based drugs are safe) or regional anesthesia should be used. Standard monitoring as prescribed by the American Society of Anesthesiologists (pulse oximetry, end-tidal carbon dioxide measurement, electrocardiography, noninvasive blood pressure monitoring, and temperature monitoring) usually suffices, and additional invasive monitoring such as peripheral arterial cannulation and central venous line placement are not necessary unless dictated for other reasons specific to the patient's condition or the surgical procedure.

If the patient does not show clinical signs of MH within the first hour after a nontriggering anesthetic technique is implemented, MH is unlikely to occur later. All patients must be monitored for at least 1 hour (preferably 4 hours) in the postoperative period. Discharge to home is acceptable if the usual discharge criteria are met.

These anesthetic considerations also apply to patients who come for muscle biopsy for the caffeine-halothane contracture test.

KEY POINTS

- Characteristics of the pediatric patient related to the airway include a relatively larger head and tongue, a more cephalad larynx, and a shorter cord-to-carina distance (4 mm in a term newborn). The cricoid cartilage is the narrowest part of the airway.
- Children have a resting oxygen consumption rate that is twice that of adults. Their functional residual capacity is similar to that in adults on a per-kilogram basis. Pulmonary and chest wall compliance is high. Not only does their larger tongue size predispose to upper airway obstruction, children are at risk for rapid onset of hypoxemia upon induction of general anesthesia.
- Pulmonary vascular resistance is high at birth and decreases to adult levels over days to months, but pulmonary vasculature remains reactive for a longer period of time. The ductus arteriosus and foramen ovale are only functionally closed at birth and may reopen under conditions of high pulmonary vascular resistance, hypercarbia, and hypoxemia with resultant reversion to fetal circulation patterns.
- The immature myocardium of neonates and infants have limited contractile and elastic reserves, which results in a relatively fixed stroke volume. Cardiac output and systemic blood pressure are dependent on heart rate.

- Physiologic anemia occurs between 2 and 3 months of age (nadir hematocrit of 29% to 31%). Obtaining a complete blood count preoperatively may be prudent in this age group if significant intraoperative blood loss is anticipated.
- Newborns generate heat via nonshivering brown fat metabolism. Hypothermic stress leads to increased oxygen consumption and thus increased risk of hypoxemia.
- Because of risks of apnea of prematurity and postanesthetic apnea, preterm infants younger than 60 weeks' postconceptual age should be observed overnight for apnea.
- Drug and fluid administration and ventilatory parameters should always be guided by the child's weight. Calculating doses on a per-kilogram basis and preparing drugs and fluids ahead of time is helpful, particularly in emergent and unexpected clinical situations. Estimates of blood volume and maximal allowable blood loss, also on a per-kilogram basis, are useful to guide transfusion therapy.
- The MAC for sevoflurane varies with age: for birth to 6 months of age it is 3.2%; for 6 months to 12 years of age, 2.5%. The MAC-awake (concentration required to block voluntary reflexes and control perceptive awareness) for sevoflurane in children is 0.2 to 0.3 of the MAC.
- Maintenance of spontaneous ventilation is usually key to successful airway management of children with airway disease and craniofacial abnormalities. Close communication between surgeon and anesthesiologist is also essential.
- An air leak around the endotracheal tube at or below a pressure of 25 cm H_2O must always be demonstrated to minimize risk of tracheal mucosal injury. When an appropriately sized cuffed endotracheal tube is used, cuff pressure should also be monitored and kept at 25 cm H_2O or less.

- Congenital anomalies can exist as isolated findings or as part of a syndrome. Additional congenital abnormalities such as congenital heart disease and renal defects are commonly seen. A brief but comprehensive preoperative assessment of all organ systems is usually in order.
- Antifibrinolytic therapy (aminocaproic acid, tranexamic acid) should be considered in children undergoing surgery with expected large-volume blood loss such as procedures to correct craniosynostosis and posterior spinal fusion. Children with syndromic conditions appear to have a higher risk of bleeding.
- CNS diseases may be accompanied by increased ICP, sensorimotor deficits, endocrine disturbance, and brainstem dysfunction. Appropriate anesthetic precautions must be taken. Monitoring for diabetes insipidus is especially important in patients with suprasellar lesions.
- Anterior mediastinal mass presents a formidable anesthetic challenge. Maintenance of spontaneous ventilation (negative intrathoracic pressure) is essential. Preparation must be made for rescue maneuvers (rigid bronchoscopy, prone positioning).
- Children with Down's syndrome may have atlantoaxial instability, so cervical manipulation should be kept to a minimum. Severe bradycardia is seen in up to 50% of children with Down's syndrome with sevoflurane inhalation induction.
- MH and anesthesia-induced rhabdomyolysis are distinct clinical entities that share similar clinical manifestations. Dantrolene is effective in the treatment of MH, but not of anesthesia-induced rhabdomyolysis. Only central core disease, King-Denborough syndrome, and Evans's myopathy have been clearly linked with MH susceptibility.

RESOURCES

Baraldi E, Filippone M. Chronic lung disease after premature birth. *N Engl J Med.* 2007;357:1946-1955.

Chen ML, Guo L, Smith L, et al. High or low oxygen saturation and severe retinopathy of prematurity: a meta-analysis. *Pediatrics.* 2010;125:e1483-e1492.

Cherry JD. Croup. *N Engl J Med.* 2011;358:384-391.

Feld LG, Mattoo TK. Urinary tract infections and vesicoureteral reflux in infants and children. *Pediatr Rev.* 2010;31:451-463.

Hartley JL, Davenport M, Kelly DA. Biliary atresia. *Lancet.* 2009;374:1704-1713.

Jenkins IA, Saunders M. Infections of the airway. *Paediatr Anaesth.* 2009;19(suppl 1):118-130.

Kim TW, Nemergut ME. Preparation of modern anesthesia workstations for malignant hyperthermia-susceptible patients: a review of past and present practice. *Anesthesiology.* 2010;114:205-212.

Kleinman ME, de Caen AR, Chameides L, et al. Part 10: pediatric basic and advanced life support: 2010 international consensus on cardiopulmonary resuscitation and emergency cardiovascular care science with treatment recommendations. *Circulation.* 2010;122:S466-S515.

Kraemer FW, Stricker PA, Gurnaney HG, et al. Bradycardia during induction of anesthesia with sevoflurane in children with Down syndrome. *Anesth Analg.* 2010;111:1259-1163.

Mayer OH. Management of thoracic insufficiency syndrome. *Curr Opin Pediatr.* 2009;21:333-343.

Neu JN, Walker WA. Necrotizing enterocolitis. *N Engl J Med.* 2011;364:255-264.

Stricker PA, Gurnaney HG, Litman RS. Anesthetic management of children with an anterior mediastinal mass. *J Clin Anesth.* 2010;22:159-163.

Vlastos IM. Hajiioannou. Diagnosis and treatment of childhood snoring. *Eur J Pediatr.* 2010;169:261-267.

CHAPTER 28

Geriatric Disorders

ZOLTAN G. HEVESI ■
LAURA L. HAMMEL ■

PUBLIC HEALTH AND AGING TRENDS

The median age of the world's population is increasing because of a decline in fertility and an increase in the average life span during the past century. Worldwide, the average life span is expected to extend another 10 years by 2050 (Table 28-1). The growing number of older adults increases demands on public health systems and on social services. In developed countries, the health care cost per capita for the elderly is three to five times greater than the cost for younger persons. Chronic diseases, which affect older adults disproportionately, contribute to disability and diminish quality of life. Increased

life expectancy reflects, in part, the success of public health interventions. Now public health programs must respond to the new challenges created by this achievement, including the growing concern about future health care costs of chronic illness, injuries, and disabilities.

In the United States, the elderly population—persons 65 years and older—numbered 47 million in 2010. This represented 17% of the total population. By 2030, there will be approximately 80 million elderly individuals. The number of persons older than 80 years is expected to increase from

TABLE 28-1 ■ Life expectancy at birth in the United States

Period	Both sexes combined	Males	Females
1950-1955	68.9	66.1	72.0
1955-1960	69.7	66.6	72.9
1960-1965	70.0	66.8	73.5
1965-1970	70.4	66.8	74.1
1970-1975	71.5	67.8	75.4
1975-1980	73.3	69.5	77.2
1980-1985	74.3	70.8	77.9
1985-1990	75.0	71.5	78.4
1990-1995	75.7	72.4	78.9
1995-2000	77.6	75.2	79.8
2000-2005	78.3	75.8	80.6
2005-2010	79.2	76.9	81.4
2010-2015	79.9	77.7	82.1
2015-2020	80.5	78.3	82.7
2020-2025	81.0	78.7	83.2
2025-2030	81.4	79.1	83.7
2030-2035	81.9	79.5	84.3
2035-2040	82.4	79.9	84.8
2040-2045	82.8	80.4	85.3
2045-2050	83.3	80.8	85.8

Data from United Nations. World population prospects: the 2008 revision. www.unpopulation.org. Accessed January 18, 2012.

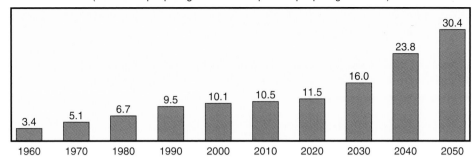

PARENT SUPPORT RATIOS: 1960 to 2050
(Number of people age 85 and over per 100 people age 50 to 64)

FIGURE 28-1 As more and more people live long enough to experience multiple chronic illnesses and/or disability, there will be more and more relatives in their 50s and 60s who will be facing the concern and expense of caring for them. *(Data from the U.S. Bureau of the Census.)*

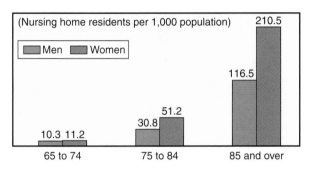

NURSING HOME RESIDENTS AMONG PEOPLE AGE 65 AND OVER BY AGE AND SEX: 1999

FIGURE 28-2 Care use increases with advanced age. The reference population for these data is nursing home residents, excluding residents in personal care or domiciliary care homes. *(Data from Centers for Disease Control and Prevention, National Center for Health Statistics.)*

9.3 million in 2000 to 19.5 million by 2030. The combined cost of Medicare and Social Security is predicted to grow from its current 8.4% to 11.2% of the gross domestic product as the number of elderly people grows to comprise 20% of the population by 2030 (Figure 28-1).

The overall health of older Americans is improving. Still, many are disabled and have chronic conditions. The proportion of older Americans with a disability has decreased significantly in recent decades, but still 14 million people aged 65 and older reported some level of disability in the census of 2000 (Figure 28-2). Currently individuals older than 65 years of age comprise only 17% of the population but undergo almost one third of the 25 million surgical procedures performed annually. In addition, they consume approximately one half of the $140 billion annual U.S. federal health care budget. The aging of the U.S. population will result in a significant growth in the demand for surgical services. Based on the assumption that age-specific per capita use of surgical services will remain constant, the amount of work in *all* surgical fields is predicted to increase. These increases will vary widely by specialty.

For anesthesiologists, it is a great responsibility to develop strategies to address this increased demand while maintaining quality of care for our senior patients. Elderly individuals can develop the same illnesses as the rest of the population, but their diminished physiologic reserve, the long-term persistence of disease, and the cumulative effect of comorbid conditions warrant separate and focused discussion of anesthetic management in this age group. This chapter describes age-related biologic alterations and discusses a few prevalent age-specific conditions affecting the elderly.

A sound understanding of age-related physiologic changes is an essential first step in providing high-quality care to elderly citizens. Emphasis should be placed on careful preanesthesia screening and evaluation, so that comorbid conditions are identified and thoughtfully considered in relation to the planned anesthetic management.

PHYSIOLOGY OF AGING

Nervous System Changes

There is a continual loss of neuronal substance with advancing age that is accompanied by a similarly reduced cerebral blood flow and diminished production of neurotransmitters such as norepinephrine and dopamine. However, this reduction in neuronal density is not directly proportional to the general level of mental functioning. This can be explained by the considerable redundancy of the neuronal network in younger individuals. Gray matter is more affected by atrophy than white matter, and there is a compensatory increase in cerebrospinal fluid volume. There is great individual variability in the degree to which these changes are manifested in the elderly. In general, nervous system function tends to decline with age, which leads to impairments in cognition and motor, sensory, and other behaviors. Much needs to be learned regarding the cellular and molecular mechanisms responsible for the selective vulnerability of brain cells and regions to age-dependent dysfunction and neurodegeneration, such as occur in parkinsonism and

Alzheimer's disease. Most pathologic processes involving the central nervous system are progressively more prevalent with increasing age. Examples are cerebral atherosclerosis, Parkinson's disease, depression, dementia, Alzheimer's disease, and delirium.

The autonomic nervous system is no exception in the overall decline of neural function. With advancing age, parasympathetic outflow diminishes, whereas sympathetic activity increases. However, most elderly patients manifest a reduced responsiveness to β-adrenergic stimulation. Changes in sympathetic and parasympathetic responsiveness are reflected in compromised thermoregulation, decreased baroreceptor sensitivity and dehydration. Hypothermia, heat stroke, orthostatic hypotension, and syncope are common problems in the elderly and can be worsened by co-existing diabetes-related autonomic dysfunction.

It is very important to note that most geriatric patients have a reduced requirement for anesthetic agents. Minimum alveolar concentration (MAC) is reduced. In addition, clearance of various pharmaceutical compounds can be compromised by reduced renal and hepatic function. The incidence of postoperative cognitive dysfunction is greatly increased in patients of advanced age, independent of the type of anesthetic technique employed.

Cardiovascular System Changes

"Seventy is the new fifty" is a common aphorism today. In fact, a large number of elderly individuals report strenuous and frequent athletic activity and look much younger than their stated age. As a result, there is a broad range of cardiovascular capacity in the older population, so individualized preoperative cardiac functional assessment cannot be overemphasized.

Whether aging is associated with a significant decrease in cardiac output and stroke volume at rest is controversial. However, exercise tolerance (maximal attainable heart rate, stroke volume, and cardiac output) is typically reduced in older adults. Progressive loss of vascular elasticity often leads to compensatory left ventricular hypertrophy and hypertension. Chronic elevation of blood pressure results in decreased baroreceptor sensitivity. The incidence of coronary arteriosclerosis and valvular heart disease is also higher with advancing age. In more severe cases of cardiac dysfunction, the presence of various forms of dysrhythmia and congestive heart failure may compound the problem of prescribing an appropriate anesthetic regimen. In the assessment of cardiac risk, patient self-report of daily physical activities and exercise tolerance may be the most valuable source of information for the clinician. Stress tests are frequently used to differentiate cardiac and noncardiac causes of limited exercise tolerance or atypical chest pain. When multiple risk factors are identified, stress echocardiography or cardiac catheterization may be indicated to provide a precise quantitative measurement of the degree of cardiac compromise.

Respiratory System Changes

Gradual tissue degeneration is the main cause of respiratory system aging. Protective reflexes, especially coughing and swallowing, are diminished with increasing age. The result can be chronic pulmonary inflammation and loss of alveolar surface area from repeated "microaspirations" and contamination of the lower respiratory tract with enteral organisms. In addition, exposure to environmental toxins may be a major contributing factor in smokers and various subgroups of agricultural and industrial workers.

In general, physiologic responsiveness to hypercapnia and hypoxemia is diminished in the elderly. Not only is the respiratory drive reduced, but the work of breathing is increased due to a reduction in chest wall elasticity and turbulent air flow that can be seen in narrowed air passages. Progressive mismatch between increasing respiratory work and weakened respiratory muscles results in an increased incidence of shortness of breath during regular daily activities and, in severe cases, at rest. As a result of these changes, forced vital capacity and forced expiratory volume in 1 second decline progressively in the elderly. Intraparenchymal elastic forces in some pulmonary segments may become insufficient to maintain patent distal airways. Consequently, air trapping can occur, and closing capacity and residual volume increase. Residual volume as a proportion of total lung capacity is 20% at 20 years of age and 40% at age 70.

Maldistribution of ventilation and, less often, perfusion leads to decreased efficiency of oxygenation and carbon dioxide removal. The two most frequently seen forms of ventilation/perfusion mismatch are dead space (regional excess of ventilation compared with perfusion) and pulmonary venous admixture (pulmonary perfusion in excess of ventilation). Dead space manifests primarily as reduced ventilatory efficiency, since increased minute ventilation is necessary to achieve the same alveolar ventilation and maintain the same arterial carbon dioxide level. Pulmonary venous admixture affects arterial oxygen tension. Deoxygenated blood from the pulmonary artery passes through inadequately ventilated areas of the lung, and this lowers pulmonary venous, and ultimately systemic, oxygen tension. Mean arterial oxygen tension on room air decreases from 95 mm Hg at age 20 to less than 70 mm Hg at age 80.

Hepatic, Gastrointestinal, and Renal Changes

Parenchymal atrophy, vascular sclerosis, and diminished function are often described when age-related changes in various viscera are discussed. Hepatic synthetic and metabolic capacity, renal blood flow and clearance, and gastrointestinal motility and sphincter function are frequently compromised in the elderly. These changes develop gradually and can persist at a subclinical level for long periods before the appearance of clinically observable signs such as abnormal laboratory test values and reduction in functional reserve. Hepatic tissue mass can be significantly reduced in old age, but baseline function

TABLE 28-2	Age differences in $T_{1/2}\beta$ (elimination half-life) for selected drugs	
Drug	**Young adults**	**Elderly adults**
Fentanyl	250 min	925 min
Midazolam	2.8 hr	4.3 hr
Vecuronium	16 min	45 min

is relatively well preserved. Renal tissue atrophy results in an approximately 50% reduction in the number of functioning nephrons by age 80, with a corresponding 1% to 1.5% decline per year in glomerular filtration rate compared with that of young adults. Creatinine clearance also declines with age, but the serum creatinine level frequently remains within normal limits because of the lesser skeletal muscle mass and lower creatinine production. Maintenance of adequate urine output (>0.5 mL/kg/hr) is crucial in preventing postoperative renal dysfunction, because postsurgical acute renal failure carries a very high mortality in the elderly. It can be a great challenge for the anesthesiologist to detect reduced organ function that may seem inconsequential preoperatively but will pose a significant risk during the stressful perioperative period.

Various pharmacodynamic and pharmacokinetic alterations, such as increased volume of distribution for lipid-soluble drugs, reduced plasma volume, reduced plasma protein binding, slower hepatic conjugation, and diminished renal elimination, will influence the anesthetic planning and decision-making process for elderly patients (Table 28-2).

Endocrine Function Changes

Like all other parenchymal organs, the endocrine glands tend to atrophy in the elderly, and reduced hormone production frequently leads to impaired endocrine function, such as impaired glucose homeostasis. Deficiencies of compounds like insulin, thyroxine, growth hormone, renin, aldosterone, and testosterone are often present. Diabetes, hypothyroidism, impotence, and osteoporosis are common, along with chronic electrolyte abnormalities. Of note, basal metabolic rate declines approximately 1% per year after age 30.

Hematologic, Oncologic, and Immune Function Changes

In the bone marrow and lymph nodes of elderly individuals, various cellular elements are produced at a lower rate than in healthy young adults. Anemia can be especially worrisome if this diminished oxygen-carrying capacity is present in combination with coronary artery disease.

Compromised cellular immunity (leukopenia, lymphopenia) results in increased vulnerability to a variety of infectious diseases, ranging from simple community-acquired infections to less common entities such as tuberculosis and herpes zoster. Age is the most significant risk factor for the development

Normal bone   Osteoporosis

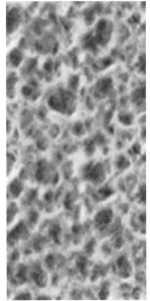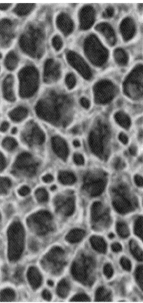

FIGURE 28-3 Comparison of normal (*left*) and osteoporotic (*right*) bone. With aging, bone becomes fragile because of loss of normal structure.

of cancer. The incidence of cancer is less than 2% before age 20 and more than 25% after age 65. The prevalence of auto-antibodies and autoimmune disorders is also higher with advanced age.

GERIATRIC SYNDROMES

Correlation between biologic and chronologic age is not always strong, but it is important to recognize that the unavoidable physiologic decline seen with advancing age always leads to similar pathologic conditions. In the geriatric population, the increased prevalence of these syndromes makes it essential for the anesthesiologist to be familiar with them.

Osteoporosis

Aging of the musculoskeletal system can be a change that is easily observable at the preoperative encounter with the patient. Loss of skeletal muscle (lean body mass) and increased percentage of body fat are typical changes associated with aging. Osteoporosis is characterized by microarchitectural deterioration of bone and decreased bone density, with consequent increased bone fragility and susceptibility to fracture. Osteoporosis is often asymptomatic until a fracture occurs. Some patients may note a loss of height or a gradually increasing kyphosis secondary to vertebral compression fractures. Prevention is a key aspect of management (Figure 28-3).

In the United States, approximately 10 million people have osteoporosis. Another 14 to 18 million have osteopenia. Approximately 1.5 million fractures per year are attributed to osteoporosis, and more than 37,000 people die of fracture-related complications. Among women who sustain a hip fracture, 50% spend time in a nursing home while recovering, and 14% of all patients with hip fractures are still in nursing homes 1 year later. Whites, especially of northern European descent, and Asians are at increased risk of osteoporosis. The peak incidence is in people aged 70 years and older. Besides demographic characteristics, estrogen deficiency, male hypogonadism, smoking, increased alcohol consumption, calcium deficiency, cancer, immobilization, and long-term corticosteroid therapy are well-documented risk factors for osteoporosis.

Plain radiography is not as accurate as bone mineral density testing in evaluating for the presence of osteoporosis, but in symptomatic patients, radiographs can be useful to identify osteopenia and fractures.

Regular weight-bearing exercise and adequate calcium and vitamin D intake are key elements of prevention. Hormone replacement therapy is considered an effective treatment for postmenopausal women. Parenteral or intranasal calcitonin is typically reserved for the treatment of cancer-related bone resorption.

Osteoarthritis

Osteoarthritis is the most common joint disease, affecting more than 20 million individuals in the United States alone. More than half of the population older than 65 years displays radiographic signs of osteoarthritis, although it is often asymptomatic. Prevalence increases with age. Middle-aged men and women are affected equally, but prevalence is greater in elderly women. Risk factors include obesity, joint trauma, infection, and metabolic and neuromuscular disorders.

Pathologic findings suggest that articular cartilage is the primary site of the abnormality, but reactive changes also affect periarticular tissues and surrounding bone. The weight-bearing joints such as the knees, hips, cervical and lumbosacral spine, and feet are most affected. Pain and dysfunction of the affected joints are major causes of long-term inactivity, disability and morbidity. No specific laboratory abnormalities are associated with osteoarthritis. The diagnosis is based on clinical assessment and positive radiographic findings for the affected joints (Figure 28-4).

Nonpharmacologic interventions are the cornerstones of therapy for osteoarthritis and include patient education, weight loss, physical therapy, occupational therapy, and a reduction in joint stress. Acetaminophen and nonsteroidal antiinflammatory drugs can be administered to improve mobility. Muscle relaxants are considered selectively for patients with evidence of muscle spasm. Intraarticular glucocorticoid injections, narcotics, and arthroplasty are reserved for patients with severe pain.

Decreased mobility and discomfort are concerns for all caregivers, but cervical spinal mobility and stability carry special implications for the anesthesiologist if laryngoscopy and tracheal intubation are planned. Cervical osteoarthritis may interfere with visualization of the glottic opening. Cervical flexion and extension radiographs may be helpful in deciding which technique offers the safest approach for endotracheal intubation without causing neck injury or compromising the spinal cord.

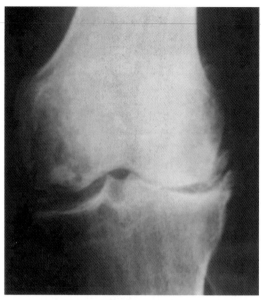

FIGURE 28-4 Classic osteoarthritis of the knee with associated changes in the articular cartilage.

Parkinson's Disease

Parkinson's disease deserves special mention because there are many perioperative concerns pertaining to the optimal management of affected patients. Parkinson's disease is a disorder of the extrapyramidal system and is one of the most common neurodegenerative diseases. Although the cause of Parkinson's disease is largely unknown, it has long been hypothesized that neurodegeneration is induced by genetic, environmental, or infectious factors. Age is the single most consistent risk factor, and it has been estimated that Parkinson's disease affects about 3% of the population older than 65 years of age. More than 50% of individuals older than 85 years of age have symptoms of Parkinson's disease.

Parkinson's disease is characterized by progressive depletion of selected neuronal populations, including dopaminergic neurons of the substantia nigra of the basal ganglia (Figure 28-5). Patients demonstrate clinical signs when approximately 80% of dopaminergic activity is lost. Imbalance between the inhibitory action of dopamine and the excitatory action of acetylcholine leads to the classic triad of rigidity, resting tremor, and bradykinesis. These clinical features are not exclusive to Parkinson's disease and may be exhibited by other syndromes.

There is no specific test to confirm the diagnosis of Parkinson's disease. The diagnosis is made on clinical grounds. The goal of treatment is to allow the patient to pursue normal daily activities. The mainstay of treatment is drug therapy using l-dopa or dopamine receptor agonists. Some promising developments have occurred in surgical treatment of Parkinson's disease in recent years, especially subthalamic deep brain stimulation and fetal mesencephalic tissue implantation. These modalities have been shown to improve outcome in certain patient populations.

When anesthesia care is needed, aspiration prophylaxis and monitoring of perioperative respiratory function are paramount. The usual drug or drugs used to treat the parkinsonian symptoms should be administered as close to the regular schedule as possible. Drugs that precipitate or exacerbate Parkinson's disease, including phenothiazines, butyrophenones (droperidol), and metoclopramide, should be avoided. If drug-induced extrapyramidal signs develop or sedation is required, diphenhydramine can be effective. Concomitant autonomic nervous system dysfunction is common in these patients, so monitoring of hemodynamic parameters is required.

Dementia

Intellectual decline is one of the early hallmarks of dementia. Major differences are seen in the elderly in their level of intellectual function compared with their own baseline in early adulthood. In any patient with a slowly progressive dementia,

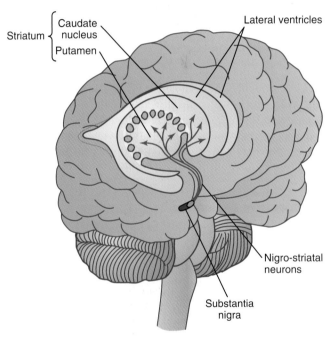

FIGURE 28-5 Dopaminergic neurons of the basal ganglia become depleted in Parkinson's disease.

sudden changes in cognitive, behavioral, or health status may occur. Mental status is often a barometer of health in these patients, and abrupt changes necessitate a search for any additional problem that may be occurring (Table 28-3). Numerous population-based studies report decreased longevity in elderly individuals who experience cognitive decline. Diminishing cognitive performance over any time interval is predictive of an early death. Perhaps the most important challenge in treating dementia is identifying cases of *reversible* dementia such as chronic drug intoxication, vitamin deficiencies, subdural hematoma, major depression, normal-pressure hydrocephalus, and hypothyroidism.

Unfortunately, most causes of dementia, including degenerative brain diseases such as Alzheimer's disease and other common multi-infarct states, are incurable. This does not mean, however, that symptoms cannot be treated and ameliorated. Pharmacotherapy for dementia is tailored to control the behavioral problems and sleep disorders that may be present and to prevent further intellectual decline and neurodegeneration. Those treatments include vitamin E, nonsteroidal antiinflammatory drugs, estrogen replacement therapy, and centrally acting acetylcholinesterase inhibitors.

For the anesthesiologist, the challenges in caring for elderly patients with declining mental capacity are many. Perioperative interactions with patient and family should take into account the patient's compromised ability to process general and medical information and capability to provide true informed consent. Establishment and documentation of baseline cognitive and neurologic function may become significant if postoperative alterations in mental function are encountered. If acute deterioration is suspected, a neurologic consultation is advised.

ANESTHETIC STRATEGIES FOR GERIATRIC PATIENTS

A hundred years ago, the age of 50 was considered a contraindication to many types of surgical procedures. With advances in health care, improved anesthetic and surgical techniques, and longer life expectancies, a greater number of geriatric patients are considered for and do undergo major or high-risk

TABLE 28-3 ■ **Comparison of different central nervous system disorders**

Diagnosis	Distinguishing features	Symptoms	Course
Dementia	Memory impairment	Disorientation, agitation	Slow onset, progressive, chronic
Delirium	Fluctuating level of consciousness, decreased attention	Disorientation, visual hallucinations, agitation, apathy, withdrawal, memory and attention impairment	Acute; most cases remit with correction of underlying medical condition
Psychotic disorders	Deficit in reality testing	Social withdrawal, apathy	Slow onset with prodromal syndrome; chronic with exacerbations
Depression	Sadness, loss of interest and pleasure in usual activities	Disturbances of sleep, appetite, concentration; low energy; feelings of hopelessness and worthlessness; suicidal ideation	Single episode or recurrent episodes; may be chronic

surgery at advanced ages. The decision to operate should not be based on age alone. The elderly are a nonhomogenous population and cannot be categorized as a single surgical group. There is often a disparity between chronologic and biologic age. Normal age-related changes do not increase the risk of perioperative complications and death. However, the elderly are often affected by a number of illnesses, and all have impairment in functional reserve that may become evident in times of stress. *Biologic age*—that is, the sum of physiologic aging processes, comorbid conditions, functional status, and genetic factors—is most important in determining an elderly patient's potential to undergo surgery and the perioperative risks associated with it. It is important that the anesthesiologist have knowledge of the physiology of aging and the ability to identify potential problems, develop a safe anesthetic strategy, and prevent complications that can arise during the perioperative period.

Surgical Mortality and Morbidity

It has been estimated that the elderly require surgery four times more often than the rest of the population. These patients will often have an American Society of Anesthesiologists (ASA) physical status score of 3 or higher. In fact, in several large prospective observational studies, including the Veterans Affairs National Surgical Quality Improvement Project, patients over the age of 70 had an ASA score of 3 or higher about two thirds of the time. Although the elderly do not have a monopoly on certain disease processes such as chronic obstructive lung disease, diabetes mellitus, coronary artery disease, hypertension, and renal failure, these diseases are present in geriatric patients at a much greater frequency than in younger age groups. In the previously mentioned studies, among patients older than age 70 the incidence of diabetes was 22%; of ischemic heart disease, 20%; of malnutrition, 17%; of renal impairment, 16%; of cerebrovascular disease, 14%; and of lung disease, 8%. The existence of these illnesses and others, such as cancer, increases the likelihood that this population will require major surgical interventions. As the elderly population increases, the practicing anesthesiologist will be required to care for an ever greater number of elderly patients, and it is likely that these patients will have at least one, and frequently two or more, significant disease process. This will clearly impact anesthetic management.

Functional reserve is the ability of an organism to maintain a steady state in the presence of physiologic stress. Age-related physiologic alterations negatively impact the elderly patient's ability to cope with stress such as surgery or injury. The elderly have a diminished functional reserve, and when facing a stressor, they lack the ability to preserve homeostasis. Lesser injuries can bring about greater degrees of shock, respiratory failure, thermoregulatory dysfunction, and so on, than are observed in younger patients. This reduction in functional reserve coupled with the existence of other diseases has negative consequences on perioperative outcome, both morbidity and mortality. Seemingly minor issues can create big problems when caring for someone with several compromised organ systems and diminished reserve. Attention to detail is rarely as important as when taking care of patients at the extremes of age.

The majority of complications occur in the postoperative period, rather than the intraoperative period, and can start even in the postanesthesia care unit. Perioperative complications, including myocardial infarction, dysrhythmias, cardiac arrest, reintubation, wound-related problems, acute renal impairment, stroke, prolonged mechanical ventilation, sepsis, and unplanned intensive care unit (ICU) admissions, increase linearly with each increasing decade of life. In patients 80 years of age or older, complications occur at rates at least two to three times those in patients younger than age 60. Thirty-day mortality rates increase exponentially for each decade over age 60. Nonsurvivors are more likely to be older than 80 years, to be male, to have a low albumin level, to exhibit impaired ability to accomplish the activities of daily living, to have an impaired functional status, to have an ASA score of 3 or higher, and to undergo emergency surgery. Indeed, the odds ratio for 30-day mortality triples with each increase in the ASA score above 2. In all studies, ASA scores of 3 or higher and emergency surgery are the most consistent predictors of perioperative morbidity and mortality.

Little evidence has been gathered about events during the first year after a major surgical intervention, but what has been noted is that independence and quality of life are often reduced. Mortality rates during that first year are higher in the elderly who have had surgery than in those who have not had surgery.

Preoperative Evaluation

In keeping with the ASA 2008 practice advisory on preanesthetic testing, it is important to remember that, for the elderly, performing undirected or routine testing results in no improvement in quality of care. Any testing performed should be directed by the type of surgical procedure, known co-existing conditions and symptoms, or findings on history taking and physical examination. For the elderly undergoing general anesthesia, it is prudent to obtain an electrocardiogram (ECG) if a relatively recent one is not available. Obtaining a baseline hemoglobin level and hematocrit value is also reasonable. The most important aspect of the preanesthetic evaluation is a thorough history taking and physical examination with close attention to functional status. The best predictor of postoperative functional status is preoperative functional status. Accurate assessment of functional status and overall health status in the elderly can be challenging and time consuming. Many elderly patients underreport potentially important symptoms, especially those that they consider to be a normal part of aging. The presence of mild dementia or cognitive deficits along with hearing or visual impairments can make precise history taking extremely difficult. Assessment of true functional capacity and health status may require the presence of a spouse, other family member, caregiver, or close friend. Determining the ability to perform activities of daily living and calculating the metabolic equivalents (METs) when assessing exercise capacity are usually adequate for evaluation of functional capacity.

In addition to assessing functional status, the preoperative evaluation should include organ-focused assessment with emphasis on the cardiac, pulmonary, renal, and hepatic systems and nutritional status, as well as assessment for the presence and therapeutic control of diabetes mellitus. The major clinical predictors of increased cardiovascular risk are an unstable coronary syndrome, decompensated congestive heart failure, significant or unstable dysrhythmias, and severe or critical valvular disease, especially aortic stenosis. In the presence of any of these indicators, consideration should be given to referral to a cardiologist. Cardiac testing should generally be reserved for those patients anticipating an intermediate- or high-risk surgery who cannot achieve 4 METs of activity and who have three or more additional risk factors for significant coronary artery disease. In general, the presence of adequate functional capacity, a normal or unchanged ECG, stable symptoms, and cardiac testing within the last 2 years or cardiac intervention within the last 5 years with stable symptoms suggests that no further testing is required.

Evaluation of the pulmonary system should include a thorough history taking and physical examination and perhaps chest radiography. In patients with known lung disease, consideration can be given to pulmonary function testing if it has not been performed recently. Referral to an internist or pulmonologist may be indicated if the patient has signs and symptoms of decompensated lung function or has severe disease that has not been previously evaluated or optimally treated. The most common complications following surgery are related to the respiratory system. The incidence of postoperative hypoxia is 20% to 60% in the elderly. Diminished laryngeal reflexes, declining respiratory drive, reduced respiratory muscle strength, increased ventilation/perfusion mismatch and drug-induced hypoventilation can all contribute to hypoxia. The risk of postoperative pneumonia is also significant, and when it occurs, postoperative pneumonia is associated with a 20% or higher 30-day mortality. Risk factors for postoperative pneumonia include inability to carry out activities of daily living at baseline, weight loss of 10% or more in the previous 6 months, history of stroke, impaired sensorium, ingestion of two or more alcoholic drinks daily, long-term steroid use, smoking, and underlying lung disease.

Acute renal failure contributes to one in five postoperative deaths. Considering the high rate of preexisting renal dysfunction in the elderly population, it is probably prudent to obtain serum electrolyte levels and creatinine concentration before surgical procedures that carry a risk of acute renal failure, such as those involving cardiopulmonary bypass or aortic aneurysm repair or surgeries in which large fluid shifts or significant blood losses are anticipated.

In the presence of known hepatic disease or before surgery that requires manipulation of the liver, it may be reasonable to perform baseline liver function tests. Prothrombin time or international normalized ratio and albumin level are better indicators of synthetic liver function than serum transaminase levels.

Diabetes mellitus is an independent predictor of a long-term decrease in quality of life following surgery. Poor glucose control (levels > 200 mg/dL) is associated with an increased risk of aspiration, poor wound healing, infection, cardiac and cerebrovascular events, and autonomic dysfunction causing hypotension and urinary retention. Whenever possible, time should be invested in ensuring adequate glucose control for several weeks before surgery. Serum glucose concentrations that range steadily between 120 and 180 mg/dL are probably adequate for surgery.

Malnutrition is an independent predictor of 30-day and 1-year postoperative mortality, as well as morbidity and loss of independence in the postoperative period. The elderly have rates of malnutrition of 15% to 26%. These rates may be even higher in certain subsets such as patients from lower socioeconomic classes, those with significant chronic disease, those with depression, and those who live alone without social support (shut-ins). Albumin concentration is a simple screening tool. A serum albumin level of less than 3 g/dL in conjunction with hypocholesterolemia and low body mass index is indicative of malnutrition and/or vitamin deficiency.

Pharmacokinetics and Pharmacodynamics in the Elderly

There is no evidence that that any specific inhaled or injected anesthetic agent is preferable for induction and/or maintenance of anesthesia in elderly patients. Some drugs may be better for use in the elderly, however, because of certain pharmacokinetic and pharmacodynamic properties. One result of the physiologic changes of aging is altered pharmacodynamics and pharmacokinetics. Changes in body composition can affect the distribution, metabolism, and clearance of drugs. In general, the plasma concentration and the volume of distribution (V_d) of a drug are inversely related. Compared with younger patients, the elderly tend to have decreased total body water, which results in a smaller V_d for hydrophilic drugs and, therefore, a higher plasma concentration for a given dose. Conversely, the elderly have a higher ratio of adipose tissue to lean muscle than the young and generally have increased body fat overall. The V_d of lipophilic drugs increases; this results in accumulation and prolongation of drug effects, which may become even more pronounced in the face of impaired hepatic metabolism or renal elimination. Circulating levels of important drug-binding proteins, such as albumin and α_1-acid glycoprotein, decrease with age. Qualitative changes in these proteins can occur and alter their ability to bind certain drugs, which results in an increased circulating free fraction of drug and therefore an increased drug effect. Propofol, for example, is extensively protein bound, and even modestly decreased albumin levels result in a higher free drug fraction and effect. The result is that smaller initial and subsequent doses of protein-bound drugs may be required.

Elderly patients with cardiac disease may have decreased cardiac output at baseline. This creates a prolonged circulation time to drug effect for anesthetics administered intravenously, but can result in a more rapid uptake of volatile anesthetics. Repeated intravenous dosing at short intervals or administration of high concentrations of volatile anesthetics can lead to cardiovascular collapse in a patient with an already tenuous cardiac status. Altered pharmacologic effects of muscle relaxants in geriatric patients are explained by altered pharmacokinetics in the elderly. There is a delayed onset of action caused by decreased muscle blood flow and cardiac output. Relaxants with hepatic and renal metabolism and elimination may have significantly prolonged effects, but relaxants eliminated by other means do not. Elderly patients are frequently taking several prescription medications, which increases the potential for undesirable drug interactions.

The effect of a drug depends not only on the concentration of the drug at its site of action, but also on the number and adequacy of function of receptors at the target tissue. The sensitivity to drugs in the geriatric population may be increased or decreased or the desired affect may be altered. The MAC of volatile anesthetics decreases with age, about 4% per decade for each decade after 40 years of age (Figure 28-6). Age-related changes occur in the number and subunit composition of γ-aminobutyric acid type A receptors, which may explain some of the increased sensitivity to both intravenous and inhaled anesthetics. The elderly can be very sensitive to the undesired cardiovascular and respiratory-depressant effects of benzodiazepines. Time for recovery of psychomotor function

is also slower for benzodiazepines than for shorter-acting drugs like propofol. Occasionally, geriatric patients may have an altered or paradoxical response to benzodiazepines that is characterized by restlessness, agitation, and hyperactivity. This can be reversed with a small dose of flumazenil without reversing the amnesic and anxiolytic effects of the benzodiazepine. The elderly show exaggerated respiratory and cardiovascular depression in response to most narcotics, and dose requirements decrease by approximately 50% between the ages of 20 and 80. In general it is wise to remember that the elderly will require smaller doses of anesthetic drugs and that the risk of undesirable effects is increased. It is smart to "start low and go slow" when administering medications, particularly drugs with the potential for adverse cardiovascular effects.

Anesthetic Plan

Choosing an anesthetic plan for an elderly patient requires consideration of many details. Several retrospective and prospective studies have failed to show a difference in outcome or a clear benefit for general anesthesia versus regional or neuraxial anesthesia. These studies failed to identify any meaningful difference in mortality and morbidity except for a clearly reduced incidence of deep vein thrombosis with regional anesthesia. There is some evidence that use of regional anesthesia may decrease intraoperative blood loss in certain subsets of

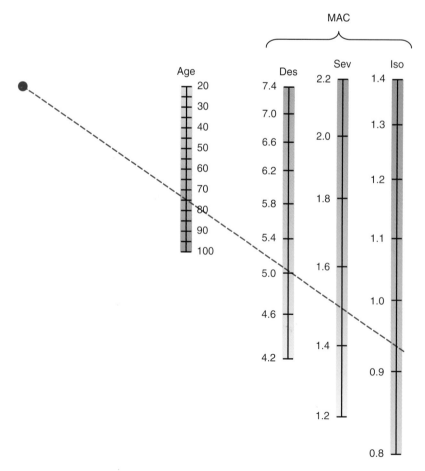

FIGURE 28-6 Nomogram for minimum alveolar concentration (MAC) as a function of age. The MACs for desflurane (Des), sevoflurane (Sev), and isoflurane (Iso) can be determined by placing a ruler on the dot at left and drawing a line through the age of the patient. The point at which this line crosses each MAC nomogram line yields the MAC value for the given drug for that age. As an example, the dotted line shows how to determine MAC for a 75-year-old patient. An approximation of the value for MAC-awake (the alveolar concentration of anesthetic at which a patient responds to verbal commands, e.g., "open your eyes") can be determined by dividing the MAC by 3. *(Adapted from Rivera R, Antognini J. Perioperative drug therapy in elderly patients. Anesthesiology. 2009;110[5]:1176-1181.)*

surgical patients. The choice of anesthetic technique must ultimately be based on patient preference, the anesthesiologist's experience or comfort with the technique, the patient's ASA physical status, and the planned surgery.

The standard ASA-recommended monitoring should be implemented. Age alone is not an indication for invasive monitoring such as transesophageal echocardiography or pulmonary artery catheterization. The decision to use these monitoring methods should be based, as always, on the potential benefits and risks, the potential for excessive blood loss or large fluid shifts, the patient's ASA physical status and concurrent illnesses, and the planned surgery.

The elderly have decreased skin elasticity and reduced skin and soft tissue perfusion, which increases the risk of skin breakdown or ulcerations. The presence of osteoarthritis and osteoporosis also poses a risk of injury. Bony prominences must be protected and padded.

Elderly patients are often dehydrated because of a diminished sensation of thirst, reduced renal capacity to conserve water and sodium, and frequent use of diuretics. Because of decreased left ventricular compliance and limited β-adrenergic receptor responsiveness, these patients are more prone to develop hypotension when hypovolemic and congestive heart failure when hypervolemic. A thorough assessment of intravascular volume status is essential before induction of anesthesia.

Measures to conserve body heat and decrease the risk of hypothermia should be implemented. Prolonged elimination of anesthetic agents and slower postoperative awakening can occur as a result of intraoperative heat loss. Elderly patients can respond to hypothermia by shivering during the early postoperative period. Shivering results in increased oxygen demand, which is a special concern in patients with coronary disease or in those with compromised cardiovascular reserve.

The same basic principles that guide acute pain management in the general population apply to the geriatric group. However, *optimal* analgesia for elderly individuals can be challenging to achieve. The elderly may experience the most potential harm as well as the greatest potential benefit from control of postoperative pain. Because of concomitant ischemic heart disease and diminished pulmonary capacity, elderly patients are more vulnerable to the physiologic consequences of inadequate analgesia and to the side effects of various analgesics. The belief that pain perception diminishes with age is a misconception. Cultural constraints and fear of addiction may prevent elderly patients from reporting pain. Dementia, delirium, or hearing and visual impairment can make it difficult to assess pain. Indeed, inadequate analgesia can contribute to postoperative delirium. Easy-to-understand pain scales and simple dosing schedules are most effective.

POSTOPERATIVE DELIRIUM AND COGNITIVE DYSFUNCTION

Postoperative delirium and postoperative cognitive dysfunction are not unique to the geriatric population, but there is a much greater incidence of these events in the elderly. Although

TABLE 28-4 ■ Components of delirium

For a diagnosis of delirium, each of the following criteria must be met:

- The patient shows a disturbance of consciousness (i.e., reduced clarity of awareness of the environment) with reduced ability to focus, sustain, or shift attention.
- The patient shows a change in cognition (e.g., memory deficit, disorientation, language disturbance) or a perceptual disturbance that is not better accounted for by a preexisting, established, or evolving dementia.
- The disturbance develops over a short period of time (usually hours to days) and tends to fluctuate during the course of a day.
- Evidence from the history, physical examination, or laboratory findings indicates that the disturbance is caused by direct physiologic consequences of a general medical condition.

TABLE 28-5 ■ Factors that can precipitate delirium

Drug use (especially when the drug is introduced or the dosage adjusted)
Electrolyte and physiologic abnormalities (e.g., hyponatremia, hypoxemia)
Lack of drugs (withdrawal)
Infection (especially urinary or respiratory infection)
Reduced sensory input (blindness, deafness, darkness, change in surroundings)
Intracranial problems (stroke, bleeding, meningitis, postictal state)
Urinary retention and fecal impaction
Myocardial problems (myocardial infarction, dysrhythmia, heart failure)

postoperative delirium and postoperative cognitive dysfunction are separate entities, they appear to have an association and are both linked to poor outcomes and higher mortality. The key characteristics of *delirium* include a decline in mental status; a reduced awareness of the environment; a disturbance in attention; cognitive dysfunction, which may include disorientation and memory impairment; mixed psychomotor impairments; and possibly hallucinations (Table 28-4). Postoperative delirium has a greater association with older age and occurs most commonly 1 to 3 days after surgery. Patients who experience postoperative delirium tend to be lucid initially after surgery but later begin to exhibit fluctuating mental status followed by the other characteristics of this disorder.

Almost any acute illness or exacerbation of a chronic illness can precipitate delirium in the geriatric population (Table 28-5). Delirium is estimated to affect 10% to 30% of elderly patients hospitalized for medical illness. Postoperative delirium has an incidence of 10% to 15% but can be much higher in certain high-risk groups. Risk factors for postoperative delirium include age older than 70 years, preexisting dementia, preoperative use of narcotics or benzodiazepines, alcohol abuse, previous episodes of postoperative delirium, visual impairment, severe illness, certain types of injuries (such as hip fractures), and elevated blood urea nitrogen level. Precipitating factors have been identified and include the use of physical restraints, malnutrition, introduction of three or more new medications within a 24- to 48-hour period, presence of an indwelling urinary catheter, and electrolyte or fluid derangements. Specific perioperative factors include greater intraoperative blood loss, transfusion of blood products, inadequate analgesia, and a postoperative hematocrit of less than 30%. Interestingly, the incidence of postoperative delirium is the same regardless of whether regional or general anesthesia is used.

The mechanism of postoperative delirium remains elusive, but it has been hypothesized that the stress of surgery and the associated inflammatory response resulting in leukocyte migration into the central nervous system may play an active role in the pathophysiology of postoperative delirium. Most patients with postoperative delirium experience complete recovery, but this disorder is far from benign. Hospitalized patients with delirium demonstrate up to a 10-fold higher risk of developing other medical complications and have longer hospital stays, increased medical costs, increased need for long-term care, and a higher 1-year mortality rate.

Postoperative delirium prevention focuses on interventions that consistently orient the patient, stimulate cognition, enhance nutritional and fluid intake, and promote exercise, as well as the use of nonpharmacologic sleep aids to prevent sleep disturbances and deprivation. Once postoperative delirium occurs, therapy should include identification and treatment of underlying medical disorders such as dehydration, infection, hypoxemia, and alcohol or drug withdrawal. Optimization of the environment and attempts at orientation as well as adequate analgesia are also important. Pharmacologic treatment may be necessary for extreme agitation that compromises the patient's safety or the ability of caregivers to perform necessary functions. Haloperidol is the preferred treatment and can be given orally, intravenously, or intramuscularly. Other drugs such as chlorpromazine and benzodiazepines have been used with mixed results. Quetiapine has been used successfully for both prevention and treatment of ICU delirium. Monitoring for oversedation is essential when using any of these drugs. In cases of severe agitation physical restraints should be considered only as a last resort when other strategies have failed.

Postoperative cognitive dysfunction is characterized by persistent deterioration of cognitive performance after surgery. Most cases of postoperative cognitive dysfunction are identified by conducting preoperative testing and comparing the results of this testing with the results of postoperative neuropsychologic testing at hospital discharge and 3 months later. Most cognitive impairment is mild and resolves during the first 3 months after surgery. However, at times postoperative cognitive dysfunction can be quite severe and negatively impact quality of life, overall functional capacity, and 1-year mortality. Some patients cannot return to employment or lose their independence.

Postoperative cognitive dysfunction has been associated with cardiac surgery and is well described in this setting, but little is known about the prevalence or scope of this problem in connection with noncardiac surgery. Even less is understood about the pathophysiology of this disorder and whether or not anesthesia can be implicated as a contributor to the problem The diagnosis of postoperative cognitive dysfunction requires neuropsychologic testing before and after surgery and anesthesia. Many issues contribute to the difficulties in defining and diagnosing postoperative cognitive dysfunction. Not the least are the lack of standardization in testing, including the timing of testing and patient exclusion or inclusion criteria, and agreement on the amount of change considered clinically significant. Frequently when postoperative cognitive dysfunction is studied, patients who may be at high risk, such as those with underlying cerebrovascular disease, are excluded. Subject attrition may also adversely affect follow-up testing. Patients are usually elderly with multiple co-existing illnesses and may die during the study period. Those with cognitive decline might fail to follow up, since they have less insight and may be less likely to seek care for problems. In fact, it is conceivable that the most severely affected may be the least likely to come for follow-up testing. Studies testing specifically for decline in memory and executive function found an equal distribution of impairment in memory, executive function, and combined memory–executive function at hospital discharge. In contrast, at 3 months more patients continued to exhibit mild memory impairment. In the majority of patients with either memory or executive decline the impairment was categorized as mild. Those with combined dysfunction seemed to be more severely affected. Interestingly, those with memory decline alone were much less likely to drop out of the study, whereas those with isolated executive function impairments were three times more likely to drop out before follow-up testing.

The only consistent risk factor that has been identified for postoperative cognitive dysfunction is advanced age. Rates of postoperative cognitive dysfunction are at least twice as high in the elderly (>60 years) than in middle-aged or younger age groups, both at hospital discharge and at 3 months. Other risk factors for postoperative cognitive dysfunction include lower educational level, history of cerebrovascular accident, and poorer ability to perform the activities of daily living at baseline. There is also evidence that longer time under anesthesia may be associated with a greater likelihood of development of postoperative cognitive dysfunction. Preexisting dementia, especially when mild, may be overlooked before surgery, but appears to be associated with higher rates of cognitive decline after surgery.

Whether general anesthesia causes postoperative cognitive dysfunction or simply unmasks a preexisting problem in unclear. Many hypotheses have been put forward to explain how general anesthesia might lead to postoperative cognitive dysfunction. These include direct neurotoxicity via altered calcium homeostasis, increased β-amyloid peptide production with enhancement of endogenous neurodegeneration, neuroinflammatory assault triggered by surgically induced systemic

TABLE 28-6 ■ Essential elements of informed consent
Sufficient information for patient
Competence of consenting individual
Voluntary decision making without pressure

TABLE 28-7 ■ Definition of palliative care by the World Health Organization
Affirms life and regards dying as a normal process
Neither hastens nor postpones death
Provides relief from pain and other distressing symptoms
Integrates the psychologic and spiritual aspects of patient care
Offers a support system to help the family cope during the patient's illness and deal with their own bereavement

inflammatory mediators, and suppression of stem cell proliferation and/or differentiation of central nervous system cells.

To date there are no data to support the hypothesis that volatile anesthetics administered at clinically relevant doses for clinically relevant durations cause neurotoxicity in humans. Further research is needed to ascertain the true incidence and severity of postoperative cognitive dysfunction and its association with anesthetic exposure if such an association exists. Until such research has been accomplished, there is no scientific basis for recommending changes in current anesthetic practices or avoidance of specific anesthetic agents. The goals of anesthesia are patient comfort and safety and the creation of optimal conditions for surgical procedures. The well-established benefits of general anesthesia should not be relinquished without substantial clinical evidence.

ETHICAL CHALLENGES IN GERIATRIC ANESTHESIA AND PALLIATIVE CARE

Ethical principles are identical for all adult patient populations. Common challenges include those involving patient autonomy, surrogate decision making, and do-not-resuscitate status in the hospital and in the operating room. The ultimate decision regarding which medical therapy is to be employed rests with the patient. The legal doctrine embodying this principle is *informed consent*. Essential criteria for informed consent include provision of sufficient information, patient competence, and voluntary decision making (Table 28-6). Patients with possible dementia should be referred for competency evaluations to assess mental function and decision-making capacity. If the patient is too compromised to give consent, a surrogate should be identified based on a living will or a durable power of attorney. Each state has a legal procedure for appointing a proxy decision maker if these documents are not available.

Cause and prognosis of cardiac arrest and the success rate of resuscitation are markedly different when the arrest occurs in the operating room than when it occurs outside it. However, informed consent for (or informed refusal of) medical intervention is guided by the same moral principles during end-of-life care, regardless of location. To ensure that institutional legal guidelines are followed, each anesthesiologist should refer to his or her institution's protocols and policies regarding do-not-resuscitate status in the operating room and postanesthesia care unit. For high-risk surgical procedures, detailed discussions of the patient's preferences are well advised.

It is established in the medical literature that a significant proportion of the elderly, cancer patients in particular, experience pain and discomfort of various origins during the last years of life. Palliative care is gaining more recognition, especially in the industrially developed aging societies. *Palliative medicine* is defined as the all-inclusive care of patients whose disease is not responsive to curative treatment (Table 28-7). This care requires a multidisciplinary approach to treat symptoms, control pain, and address the psychologic, social, and spiritual needs of the patient and his or her family. By training, anesthesiologists are invaluable experts on pharmacologic and procedural pain management. These modalities are key elements of successful palliative care.

SUMMARY

Aging is a multifactorial, all-encompassing process. It produces a gradual decline in the functional reserve of most of the major organ systems, which results in a decreased capacity for adaptation. Aging is not a disease but carries an increased potential for the development of various age-related pathologic conditions. Therefore, there is no one "ideal anesthetic" for the elderly patient. A sound understanding of aging-related physiologic changes and the altered pharmacokinetic and pharmacodynamic responses of these patients helps the anesthesiologist to design and implement an optimal anesthetic plan for each elderly patient. Since this patient subgroup is not only physiologically but also physically fragile, these patients require special attention throughout the perioperative period to prolong life and maintain good function and quality of living, including incorporation of their wishes regarding end-of-life issues.

KEY POINTS

■ As the age of the population increases, a thorough appreciation of age-related physiologic changes will allow for the provision of optimal perioperative care.

■ Aging is not a disease, but the incidence of various illnesses increases in the elderly.

■ The correlation between chronologic age and biologic age is variable, and calendar age and physiologic age can be significantly different in some individuals.

■ A thorough exploration of the patient's medical history, combined with a detailed physical examination and a sound understanding of age-related physiologic alterations, provides the foundation for delivery of optimal medical care in this patient population.

RESOURCES

Bekker A, Lee C, de Santi S, et al. Does mild cognitive impairment increase the risk of developing postoperative cognitive dysfunction? *Am J Surg.* 2010;199:782-788.

Bettelli G. Anaesthesia for the elderly outpatient: preoperative assessment and evaluation, anaesthetic technique and postoperative pain management. *Curr Opin Anesthesiol.* 2010;23:726-731.

Bittner EA, Zhongkong X. Brief review: anesthetic neurotoxicity in the elderly, cognitive dysfunction and Alzheimer's disease. *Can J Anaesth.* 2010;58:216-223.

Fabbri LM, Luppi F, Beghe B. Update in chronic obstructive pulmonary disease 2005. *Am J Respir Crit Care Med.* 2006;173:1056-1065.

Fleisher LA, et al. ACC/AHA 2007 guidelines on perioperative cardiovascular evaluation and care for noncardiac surgery: a report of the American College of Cardiology and the American Heart Association Task Force on Practice Guidelines (Writing Committee to Revise the 2002 Guidelines on Perioperative Cardiovascular Evaluation Guidelines for Noncardiac Surgery): developed in collaboration with the American Society of Echocardiography, American Society of Nuclear Cardiology, Heart Rhythm Society, Society of Cardiovascular Anesthesiologists, Society for Cardiovascular Angiography and Interventions, Society for Vascular Medicine and Biology, and Society for Vascular Surgery. *Circulation.* 2007;116:e418-e499.

Hamel MB, Henderson MG, Khuri SF, et al. Surgical outcomes for patients aged 80 and older: morbidity and mortality from major noncardiac surgery. *J Am Geriatr Soc.* 2005;53:424-429.

Monk TG, Weldon BC, Garvan CW, et al. Predictors of cognitive dysfunction after major noncardiac surgery. *Anesthesiology.* 2008;108:18-30.

Silverstein JH, Steinmetz J, Reichenberg A, et al. Postoperative cognitive dysfunction in patients with preoperative cognitive impairment. Which domains are most vulnerable?. *Anesthesiology.* 2007;106:431-435.

Story DA, Leslie K, Myles PS, et al. Complications and mortality in older surgical patients in Australia and New Zealand (the REASON study): a multicentre, prospective, observational study. *Anaesthesia.* 2010;65:1022-1030.

Tang J, Eckenhoff MF, Eckenhoff RG. Anesthesia and the old brain. *Anesth Analg.* 2010;110:421-426.

INDEX

Page numbers followed by "b" indicate boxes; "f" figures; "t" tables